Chapter Codes

The Physicians' Drug Manual

Prescription and Nonprescription Drugs

Editors

Rubin Bressler, M.D.

Professor and Head
Departments of Medicine and Pharmacology
University of Arizona Health Sciences Center

Morton D. Bogdonoff, M.D.

Professor of Medicine
Cornell University College of Medicine

Genell J. Subak-Sharpe, M.S.

A Biomedical Information Corporation Book

DOUBLEDAY & COMPANY INC.
Garden City, N.Y. 1981

Library of Congress Cataloging in Publication Data

Main entry under title: Physicians' Drug Manual.

"Originally published as The Physician's Compendium of Drug Therapy."

Includes index.

1. Drugs—Handbooks, manuals, etc.

2. Chemotherapy—Handbooks, manuals, etc.

I. Biomedical Information Corporation.

DNLM: 1. Drugs—Standards—Periodicals.

W1 PH787G

RM300.P53 1981 615'.1'0202

ISBN 0-385-17477-2

Library of Congress Catalogue Card Number: 80-2846 AACR2

Printed in the United States of America
First Edition

The Physicians' Drug Manual

Prescription and Nonprescription Drugs

Preface

The Physicians' Drug Manual should be one of the most frequently consulted books in any home health library. It has evolved over the last two years with painstaking care and research and is a direct outgrowth of *The Physician's Compendium of Drug Therapy*—a comprehensive reference designed to provide doctors with important information about the most frequently used drugs.

Shortly after *The Compendium* was introduced to physicians, we began receiving letters from doctors throughout the United States pointing out that the book contained information invaluable to patients, too. Why is it important for patients to know about drugs? More and more, patients from all walks of life are assuming a greater role in their own health care, including participation in important decisions regarding treatment. Obviously, an informed and educated patient is better equipped for such participation than one with little understanding of what is involved.

In part, the need for a book like this reflects the tremendous advances that have taken place in medicine in recent years. A few decades ago, the number of effective drugs was rather limited and their use fairly simple. There were few medical specialists, and the average family doctor had more time to get to know each patient, even though his ability to treat or cure was often limited. Today, quite the opposite is true. Hundreds of new drugs have been introduced in recent years and they have revolutionized the practice of medicine. Three out of four Americans now use at least one drug on a fairly regular basis.

The family doctor who had ample time to spend with each patient is also a thing of the past; instead, there are specialists for virtually every type of disorder. Few have the time or means to establish an ongoing rapport with their patients. Instead, patients are bombarded by health advice from dozens of sources. Much of this information is conflicting, misleading, or confusing. Who and what to believe is a major problem faced by any consumer who wants to assume a more informed approach to his or her own health care.

After pondering the problem at length, and consulting with numerous physicians and nonphysicians alike, we decided to adapt *The Physician's Compendium of Drug Therapy* into a reference that would be useful to doctors and also understandable to patients. *The Physicians' Drug Manual* is the result of those efforts. Presented in this book are the actual drug information tables that physicians use in their daily practice of medicine as well as extensive material written especially to help the lay reader understand the more technical information. Drugs often come in colorful and benign-looking forms, an appearance that belies their true properties. Drugs can be highly, even miraculously beneficial, but they can also be dangerous and even lethal if used carelessly. It is essential that you always know what drug you are taking and why. The well-informed patient knows and understands what is involved in using any drug, whether it is a nonprescription painkiller or vitamin, or a more potent medication to treat a serious disease.

Of course, the prescribing physician should still be the major source of specific drug information. He or she should tell you exactly how and when to take the drug, in what quantity, and what to expect. If any questions or doubts persist, you should not hesitate to raise them with your doctor. The pharmacist is still another health professional who can answer questions about drugs and their effects.

This book is intended to *reinforce* the information provided by your doctor and pharmacist, and to give additional information in a concise, understandable format. **In no instance should you use this book to alter your physician's instructions without his or her clear agreement.** Very often, dosages and therapeutic regimens are individualized to meet the needs of a particular patient. If you find information in this book that seems to contradict your doctor's advice, or raises questions about medication, do not hesitate to discuss your questions with your doctor or pharmacist. Much of the information in this book is derived from the government-approved prescribing information that is developed for each drug, and although every effort has been made to ensure maximum accuracy, the publisher has not independently tested or verified the information. Therefore, your prescribing physician should be the final authority.

This manual covers more than 95 percent of all medications prescribed by primary care physicians, plus the most frequently used nonprescription drugs as of January 1981. **The drugs listed were chosen in collaboration with the Medical Consultants based upon clinical usage and classification. The publisher does not advocate the use of, and takes no responsibility for, any of the products described here.**

Before looking up a specific drug, it is important that you read the introductory chapter *How to Use This Book*, as well as the general discussion that introduces each section. This will give you the background information needed to understand the individual drug charts. We hope that *The Physicians' Drug Manual* will remove the mystique and confusion surrounding drugs and their use, and will help you become a more informed participant in your own health care decisions.

—The Editors

Acknowledgments

Editors

Rubin Bressler, M.D.
Professor and Head
Departments of Medicine and Clinical Pharmacology
University of Arizona Health Sciences Center
Tucson

Morton D. Bogdonoff, M.D.
Professor of Medicine
Cornell University College of Medicine
New York

Genell J. Subak-Sharpe, M.S.
Vice President
Biomedical Information Corporation
New York

Leo E. Hollister, M.D.
Professor of Medicine, Psychiatry, and Pharmacology
Stanford University School of Medicine and Veterans Administration Medical Center
Palo Alto, Calif.

Medical Consultants

E. Everett Anderson, M.D.
Professor of Urologic Surgery
Duke University Medical Center
Durham, N.C.

Alan D. Barreuther, Pharm.D.
Assistant Professor of Pharmacy Practice
Arizona Health Sciences Center
Tucson

Gary S. Berger, M.D.
Clinical Assistant Professor of Obstetrics and Gynecology
University of North Carolina School of Medicine
Chapel Hill, N.C.

David R. Bickers, M.D.
Professor and Chairman
Department of Dermatology
University Hospitals of Cleveland
Cleveland, Ohio

Thomas Boyden, M.D.
Assistant Professor of Endocrinology
Veterans Administration Hospital
Tucson, Ariz.

Noble J. David, M.D.
Professor of Neurology
University of Miami School of Medicine
Miami, Fla.

David N. Fairbanks, M.D.
Clinical Professor of Otolaryngology
School of Medicine and Health Sciences
George Washington University
Washington, D.C.

Mark A. Goodman, M.D.
Director, Coronary Care Unit
Nassau Hospital
Mineola, N.Y.

Robert E. Hermann, M.D.
Chairman
Department of General Surgery
Cleveland Clinic Foundation
Cleveland, Ohio

Bernard Jacobs, M.D.
Clinical Professor of Orthopedics
Cornell University College of Medicine
New York

Ronald C. Hansen, M.D.
Assistant Professor of Dermatology
University of Arizona Health Sciences Center
Tucson

Edward Jackson, M.D.
Clinical Pharmacology Fellow
University of Arizona Health Sciences Center
Tucson

William N. Jones, M.S.
Clinical Pharmacy Coordinator
Tucson Veterans Administration Hospital
Tucson

Michael D. Katz, Pharm. D.
Assistant Professor of Pharmacy Practice
University of Arizona Health Sciences Center
Tucson

Louis G. Keith, M.D.
Professor of Obstetrics and Gynecology
Northwestern University Medical School
Chicago

Norman Levine, M.D.
Assistant Professor of Dermatology
University of Arizona Health Sciences Center
Tucson

Keith E. Likes, M.S.
Assistant Professor of Pharmacy Practice
University of Arizona Health Sciences Center
Tucson

Robert E. Mancini, Ph.D., D.O.
Chairman, Department of Pharmacology and Toxicology
New York College of Osteopathic Medicine
Old Westbury, N.Y.

Joseph A. Markenson, M.D.
Assistant Professor of Medicine
Cornell University College of Medicine
New York

Robert S. Martin, M.S.
Assistant Professor of Pharmacy Practice
University of Arizona Health Sciences Center
Tucson

Marvin Moser, M.D.
Clinical Professor of Medicine
New York Medical College
Valhalla, N.Y.

Robert H. Moser, M.D.
Executive Vice President
American College of Physicians
Philadelphia

Lawrence C. Parish, M.D.
Clinical Associate Professor of Dermatology
Thomas Jefferson Medical College
Philadelphia

Robert Powell, Pharm. D.
Associate Professor of Clinical Pharmacy
University of North Carolina
Chapel Hill, N.C.

Robert H. Seller, M.D.
Professor and Chairman
Department of Family Medicine
Professor of Medicine
State University of New York School of Medicine
Buffalo

James P. Shinnick, D.O.
Assistant Professor of Medicine
Director, Respiratory Intensive Care Unit
The Hahnemann Medical College and Hospital
Philadelphia

Gilbert I. Simon, D.Sc.
Director
Department of Pharmacy
Lenox Hill Hospital
New York

J. Kelly Smith, M.D.
Professor and Associate Chairman
Department of Medicine
Chief, Infectious Diseases, Allergy and Immunology
East Tennessee Quillen-Dishner College of Medicine
Johnson City, Tenn.

Harold C. Strauss, M.D.
Associate Professor of Medicine
Duke University Medical Center
Durham, N.C.

Donald P. Swartz, M.D.
Professor of Obstetrics and Gynecology
Albany Medical College
Albany, N.Y.

Louis Tuft, M.D.
Clinical Professor of Medicine (Emeritus)
Temple University Health Sciences Center
Philadelphia

William Thomas Vaughn Jr.
Pharmacist-Physician Assistant
Duke University Medical Center
Durham, N.C.

Ray A. Wolf, Pharm. D.
Assistant Professor of Pharmacy Practice
Arizona Health Sciences Center
Tucson

Sumner J. Yaffe, M.D.
Professor of Pediatrics and Pharmacology
University of Pennsylvania Children's Hospital
Philadelphia

Special Tributes

Over the last two years, scores of people have been involved in the creation of *The Physicians' Drug Manual.* While it is impossible to cite all of the many dedicated writers, researchers, and others who have worked so diligently on this book, there are some whose contributions cannot be overlooked. These include May Annexton, William Check, Ph.D., Audrey Dawson, Dr. Arthur S. Freese, Leonard Gross, Marcia Holly, Ph.D., Dr. M. Philip S. Kasofsky, Helene MacLean, Jane Clark Shannon, Seymour Shubin, and Constance Young. Special recognition is also due Ellen H. Datloff and Edwin S. Geffner of the Biomedical Information Corporation Staff, as well as Joan Simpson, Executive Art Director of this book, and Nancy Lou Gahan, illustrator. Finally, our thanks to Barry Lippman, our untiring editor at Doubleday.

Table of Contents

Special Updates

To keep your *Physicians' Drug Manual* current, a special newsletter, THE PDM DRUG UPDATE, has been created. Each month, it will bring subscribers information about new drugs as well as different approaches to using old ones. Details on how to subscribe to this newsletter and an order form may be found on the last page of this book.

How To Use This Book

The Physicians' Drug Manual is a unique home health reference book with many uses. It is, first and foremost, a comprehensive manual of drugs. It is also an illustrated medical encyclopedia, covering more than one hundred different diseases and their treatments. The glossary doubles as a medical dictionary for laymen, designed to make the often incomprehensible language of medical doctors more understandable to the nonphysician. The full-color section on drug identification makes it easy to confirm whether the correct drug is being taken or to identify an unknown one. And the manual is a guide to important health care resources, such as Comprehensive Cancer Centers.

The various chapters are arranged according to disease states, with each section introduced by a general discussion of the disease, followed by charts outlining the most pertinent information about the drugs used to treat the various disorders covered in the introductory text. These charts are designed to enable both the physician and patient to determine quickly what should be known about a drug before it is prescribed or administered.

GENERAL OVERVIEW

Before examining each feature of this manual in detail, we feel it is important to discuss the rationale of drug therapy and the steps an individual can take to help ensure safe and effective drug use. In the last few decades, increased understanding of body chemistry and many disease processes has led to the development of hundreds of drugs that can cure or at least control many formerly fatal or disabling diseases. At the outset, it should be emphasized that the majority of drugs, *when used as directed by people who are not allergic to them*, are safe. Contrary to popular belief, serious adverse drug reactions are rare and, for the most part, confined to potent medications used to treat serious diseases, such as cancer. Still, all drugs have multiple effects, including *potentially* desirable and undesirable ones. In simple terms, drugs are nothing more than chemical compounds that, by a variety of mechanisms, alter the body's natural chemical processes to aid in overcoming or controlling a disease process. In some instances, a drug's effects are clearly defined and reasonably predictable; in others, the wanted and unwanted effects may reflect varying degrees of the drug's usual actions. Other adverse effects can occur due unpredictably to individual sensitivity or dose difference. The effectiveness of penicillin, for example, against certain types of bacterial infections is well documented and fairly predictable, depending upon the site and nature of the infection. Some people, however, have unpredictable adverse reactions, ranging from rashes and gastrointestinal upsets to life-threatening allergic responses (anaphylaxis). With other drugs, whether an effect is desirable or not depends upon the situation. For example, many of the drugs used to treat depression can cause drowsiness, an undesirable side effect for people who drive or operate machinery, but one that is welcome to those also suffering from insomnia.

In any case, one should always be aware of the various possible effects—both wanted and unwanted—before taking a drug. Clearly, a medication should not be used if the potential harm outweighs the anticipated benefits. This is particularly true during pregnancy.

Another potential problem area involves the use of more than one drug. In many instances, such as the treatment of high blood pressure, cancer, heart failure, and some types of mental illness and arthritis, a multiple drug regimen may be required to control the disease. In others, however, multiple drug use may be unintentional—people who use antacids like Tums or Rolaids or nonprescription cold or allergy remedies often do not realize that these preparations also are drugs that may interact with another medication to produce an adverse reaction. In general, the potential for adverse reactions increases with the number of drugs being used. One drug may negate or reduce the beneficial effect of another, as in the case of antacids taken with tetracyclines, digitalis, and a number of other drugs. In others, the second drug may increase the effect of a medication, as when aspirin, taken with a drug that reduces the blood's ability to clot, leads to a danger of serious bleeding. To minimize the danger of drug interactions, a patient should always tell a prescribing physician all the other medications, including antacids, megadose vitamins, and other nonprescription drugs, that are being used. In addition, some foods, which, after all, also contain chemical compounds, may interact with certain drugs to produce undesired effects. Patients should always ask a doctor if there are any foods or beverages, particularly alcohol, that should be avoided while taking a medication.

Sensitivity or allergic reactions account for still another kind of adverse drug reaction. These are unpredictable—a person may use a drug for years without problems, and then experience an allergic response. A family history of allergies or an allergy to substances chemically similar to a drug often points to potential problems. This is why a physician usually asks for any background of allergies before prescribing a drug. It should be remembered, however, that many nonprescription drugs can also provoke an allergic response and should be used with caution by those with allergies.

The presence of other diseases is still another important consideration in determining whether a drug should be used. This is particularly true for patients with kidney or liver disorders, since most drugs are inactivated and/or cleared from the body through one or both of these vital organs. The presence of heart disease, asthma, high blood pressure, or blood disorders, among others, dictates special caution in using drugs that may affect the function of diseased vital organs.

Age may affect the metabolism, body clearance, and actions of many drugs. A drug given to an infant or child may produce responses quite different from those in adults. This is especially true of drugs given to elderly persons.

PREVENTING DRUG-RELATED PROBLEMS

These are but a few of the many factors that should be examined before taking any medication, either prescription or nonprescription. All medications should be taken only as directed, either according to a physician's instructions or those printed on the label. Prescription drugs should never be shared with family members or others without specific instructions from a physician. It is important to know the proper names of all drugs in use at any given time and to keep a record of all drugs or vaccines that have provoked an adverse or allergic reaction in the past.

Many adverse drug reactions can be attributed to carelessness. Medicines should be kept in their original containers and stored, out of the reach of children, according to directions. Drugs should never be taken in the dark; always know what you are taking by checking the label first. The chemical nature of many drugs changes with time; therefore, old drugs should be discarded, especially after the expiration date printed on the label. The recommended dosage should never be exceeded or altered without checking first with the prescribing physician. Any untoward symptom or adverse reaction should be reported promptly to the prescribing physician. Some drugs should not be discontinued abruptly; therefore, it is important to follow a doctor's instructions for both starting and stopping a medication.

ORGANIZATION OF THIS BOOK

The Physicians' Drug Manual is organized primarily according to disease state or problem area; for example, the various forms of heart and circulatory disorders are grouped in the *Cardiovascular Diseases* chapter, the various mental and emotional disorders are covered in the chapter on *Psychological Problems*, etc. The chapters are further divided into sections covering specific diseases, such as asthma, hypertension, diabetes, and so forth.

Each section is introduced by a comprehensive discussion of the various disorders, followed by the information on individual drugs. It is important to read the introductory sections before turning to the drug charts, which are the ones used by physicians to answer a multitude of questions that arise in prescribing a drug: What is the correct dosage? What are the potential side effects? Are there any contraindications (instances in which the drug should not be used) or specific precautions? Should it be given to a pregnant or nursing woman? What about use in children? Doctors have the education to fully understand the information in these charts. It is also important, however, that the consumer know about the drugs. The introductory sections provide the essential background information that a nonphysician needs to understand the information in the drug charts. Where appropriate, illustrations have been included to make the text even clearer and more comprehensible.

Even so, the words that appear in the text and particularly in the drug charts may be unfamiliar to many nonphysicians. These words are clearly defined in laymen's terms in the *Glossary*, which also includes the abbreviations used throughout the charts; to further facilitate use of the drug charts, a complete list of abbreviations is also included at the end of this introduction.

HOW TO READ A DRUG CHART

After carefully reading the introduction to the section, turn to the individual drug chart. The charts are arranged alphabetically, with an overall chart on common nonprescription products (where applicable) following the prescription drugs. This manual covers the most used drugs in each category; while every effort has been made to include as many drugs as possible, it would require several volumes this size to include them all. In some instances, a single listing may contain useful information about identical or very similar drugs available under other brand names. The brand covered in the chart should not be considered to be better or more commonly used than those listed in the notes at the end of the chart; this is simply a space-saving device that enables us to include as many different drugs as possible. A good example is aspirin; while only one brand name appears at the top of the chart, the information can be applied to other analgesics in which aspirin is the major ingredient. This does not necessarily mean that all brands of aspirin are identical—there are individual differences, and the selection of a particular brand depends upon patient preference and needs. On the other hand, the same general precautions, indications for use, etc. can be applied to most aspirin products.

As noted earlier, many drugs have multiple uses. Propranolol (Inderal), for example, is used to treat high blood pressure, chest pains, cardiac arrhythmias, and migraine headaches. In these instances, an abbreviated form of the drug chart will appear in one section, with a reference to the full chart in another section. If a drug cannot be found readily, consult the index; all drugs in the manual are listed in the index under both their trade and generic names. The drug charts have been designed to present the most important information about each medication in a consistent, easy-to-use format. At the top of each chart appears the drug brand or trade name in bold type, followed by the generic name in parentheses, and the name of the manufacturer. Drugs requiring a prescription are marked with the Rx symbol. (Prescription laws vary from state to state, however, and what is a prescription drug in some states may be nonprescription in others.)

Directly under the drug name is the form and strength in which the drug is marketed; for example, an entry reading "Tabs: 100, 300 mg" means that the drug is available in tablets of 100- and 300-milligram strength.

Any legal restrictions on a drug are signified by the letter C (for control), followed by a Roman numeral. Caution should be exercised in long-term use of these drugs, since they have a high potential for addiction and abuse. (See list of abbreviations for specific definitions of these categories.)

Next comes the listing of indications and dosages. These are based on the manufacturer's prescribing information, which must be approved by the Food and Drug Administration. In addition, important information on use by pregnant or nursing women, effects on laboratory tests, and other factors that should be considered in taking a particular drug are included in the charts. In some cases, a physician may prescribe a drug in a dosage or for an indication that varies from the official recommendations. In these instances, the physician's instructions should be followed; *in no instance should a person use this book to alter a prescribed regimen without first consulting the prescribing physician.*

The columns on administration and dosage adjustments, contraindications, warnings and precautions, adverse reactions, overdosage, drug interactions, and altered laboratory values are self-explanatory. In the last two, the arrows pointing upwards signify an increase, while those pointing down signify a decrease. (For example, "⇧ CNS depression" means the drug increases depression of the central nervous system.) Italicized entries in the adverse reactions section signify those that are most common. A • symbol is used to separate unrelated entries in the contraindications section.

Particular attention should be paid to the special entries on use of the drug in children or pregnant or nursing women. Many drugs affect growth and development and should be used with caution, if at all, in children. As a rule, all drugs should be avoided during pregnancy unless they are absolutely necessary for the health of the mother or the fetus. Obviously a diabetic woman should be particularly careful to take the correct amount of insulin to avoid complications for both herself and her baby. On the other hand, the indiscriminate use of painkillers to relieve minor discomfort may be detrimental to both mother and infant.

In most chapters, nonprescription drugs are covered in an overall chart after the prescription drugs. (Exceptions include nonprescription drugs that have important systemic effects or are often treated like prescription medications—for example, aspirin or drugs to treat diarrhea.) These charts for nonprescription medications list the drug's major ingredients, the action of these ingredients, and a brief description of dosage or how the drug is used.

THE GLOSSARY

As noted earlier, the drug charts contain many words that may be unfamiliar to the nonphysician. These words are clearly defined in the glossary, which should be used like any other dictionary.

DRUG IDENTIFICATION SECTION

The full-color Drug Identification Section shows the various drugs arranged and pictured according to actual size, shape, and color, making it easier to identify an unknown drug by matching its physical characteristics with the corresponding photograph. Many drugs also have identifying code numbers, which are also visible in these photographs.

DIRECTORY OF MANUFACTURERS

Most pharmaceutical manufacturers will provide additional information about their products. This directory lists the names, addresses, and telephone numbers of manufacturers whose products are included in this manual. Most queries can be handled by mail, but in an emergency situation, such as an accidental overdosage, the manufacturers can be telephoned for instructions or information.

INDEX

All products included in this manual are listed alphabetically in the index under both their brand and generic names. In instances where a drug has multiple uses, the various disease categories will be listed under the drug's brand name. For example, the entry for Inderal will indicate page numbers for use in angina pectoris, cardiac arrhythmias, hypertension, and migraine. The index also includes the major diseases covered in the introductory section.

A FEW DO'S AND DON'TS

The Physicians' Drug Manual, although originally created to give doctors comprehensive and accurate drug information in a single reference book, is also an important information source for the nonphysician. To gain the most value from this manual, however, it should be properly used. Following are suggestions for how to best use *The Physicians' Drug Manual*:

- Read the introductory section before consulting the individual drug charts.
- Read through the warnings, contraindications, and other precautions and raise any questions or misgivings with your physician.
- Read through the lists of ingredients of nonprescription drugs, paying particular attention to intended action. This will enable you to select the drug that will be most appropriate for your needs.
- Do not use this book to alter your physician's instructions or as a do-it-yourself manual.

IN CONCLUSION

This manual is designed to give the consumer the same information about drugs that physicians have. In addition, each section contains important explanatory material to give the nonphysician reader the necessary background to use *The Physicians' Drug Manual* properly. By following the instructions in this introduction, the nonphysician reader also will benefit from this reference book. This may well become the most important and most frequently used book in your home medical reference/health care library. Achieving better health and medical care is everyone's goal.

Abbreviations and Terms Used in Drug Charts

Following is a listing of abbreviations that appear in the drug information charts. Definitions for the various terms are included in the *Glossary*.

ACTH	adrenocorticotropic hormone
ADH	antidiuretic hormone
amps	ampuls
ANA	antinuclear antibody
ASA	acetylsalicylic acid (aspirin)
ATP	adenosine triphosphate
ATPase	adenosine triphosphatase
AV	atrioventricular
bid	*bis in die*, twice a day
BSP	sulfobromophthalein
BUN	blood urea nitrogen
C	Celsius, centigrade
cap	capsule
CBC	complete blood count
CCr	creatinine clearance rate
CNS	central nervous system
conc	concentrate
CSF	cerebrospinal fluid
CVP	cardiovascular pressure
div	in equally divided doses
dl	deciliters
ECG	electrocardiogram
ECT	electroconvulsive therapy
EEG	electroencephalogram
F	Fahrenheit
FBS	fasting blood sugar level
fl oz	fluid ounces
FSH	follicle-stimulating hormone
g	grams
gal	gallons
GI	gastrointestinal
gr	grains
h	hours
HCG	human chorionic gonadotropins
IA	intra-arterial
IM	intramuscular
IV	intravenous
IU	international units
kg	kilograms
l	liters
lb	pounds
LDH	lactate dehydrogenase
LE	lupus erythematosus
LH	luteinizing hormone
liq	liquid
M	molar
m	meters
MAO	monoamine oxidase
mEq	milliequivalents
mg	milligrams
min	minutes *or* minims
ml	milliliters
mm	millimeters
mo	months
msec	milliseconds
mU	milliunits
ng	nanograms
OTC	over the counter; sold without a prescription
oz	ounces
PBI	protein-bound iodine
ped	pediatric
pH	hydrogen ion concentration
PO	*per os*, by mouth
pt	pints
q	*quaque*, every (as in q4h, every four hours)
qd	every day
qid	*quater in die*, four times a day
qs	*quantum sufficit*, as much as is needed
RBC	red blood cell *or* red blood count
RDA	recommended daily allowance
REM	rapid eye movement
s	seconds
SC	subcutaneous
SGOT	serum glutamic oxaloacetic transaminase
SGPT	serum glutamic pyruvic transaminase
sol	solution
supp	suppository
susp	suspension
sust rel	sustained release
tab	tablet
tbsp	tablespoon
tid	*ter in die*, three times a day
tsp	teaspoons
VMA	vanillylmandelic acid
WBC	white blood cell *or* white blood count
wk	weeks
w/v	weight per volume
yr	years
μg	micrograms

Probably effective **Possibly effective** **Lacks substantial evidence of effectiveness as a fixed combination**	Indications considered less than effective by the FDA based on a review of the drug by the National Academy of Sciences—National Research Council and/or other information; final classification of such indications requires further investigation
Safe use not established during pregnancy	Insufficient information exists to establish whether human fetal development will be adversely affected; the potential hazard to the fetus must be carefully weighed against the expected benefits of therapy to the mother
Adult dosage	The manufacturer's recommended dosage for adult patients with normal renal and hepatic function and, except where noted, children over twelve years of age
Altered laboratory values	Changes in blood/serum or urine chemistry values at therapeutic dosages resulting from either a direct physiologic effect of the drug or, where noted, interference with the test method
General guidelines not established	Indicates that physicians should contact manufacturers or consult other medical authorities regarding use in specific individuals
Controlled substances	Ranking of drugs under Comprehensive Drug Abuse Prevention and Control Act[1] is signified by letter C and Roman numerals following dosage form (e.g., C-I, C-II, etc.) Categories and their definitions are as follows:

Category	**Definition**	**Criteria for use**	**Examples**
C-I	High abuse potential No currently accepted medical use For research, instructional use, or chemical analysis only	Approved protocol necessary	Marijuana, levomoramide, dihydromorphine, morphine methylsulfonate, nicocodeine, and others[2]
C-II	High abuse potential Currently accepted for medical use May lead to severe psychological and/or physical dependence	Written prescription only 34-day supply limit No refills Emergency dispensing without written prescription permitted Container must carry warning label[3]	Morphine, codeine, meperidine (Demerol), methadone (Dolophine), straight amphetamines, methaqualone (Parest, Mequin, Somnafac, Sopor), pentobarbital (Nembutal), and others[2]
C-III	Less abuse potential than drugs in C-I or II Currently accepted for medical use May lead to moderate or low physical dependence or high psychological dependence	Written or oral prescription required Prescription expires in six months No more than five prescription refills Container must carry warning label[3]	Any compound, mixture, or preparation containing limited quantities of codeine, hydrocodone, dihydrocodeine, ethylmorphine, opium, or morphine and some nonnarcotic drugs
C-IV	Low abuse potential relative to C-III substances Currently accepted for medical use May lead to limited physical or psychological dependence	Written or oral prescription required Prescription expires in six months No more than five prescription refills Container must carry warning label[3]	Most of the drugs prescribed to treat anxiety[2]
C-V	Low abuse potential relative to C-IV substances Currently accepted for medical use May lead to limited physical or psychological dependence	May require written prescription or be sold without prescription Check state law	With the exception of paregoric, these substances consist of those preparations formerly known as "exempt" narcotics (preparations containing nonnarcotic ingredients with narcotic-like actions)

[1]These specifications also apply to the State Uniform Controlled Substances Act. Check state law for variations.

[2]For complete list of controlled substances, write to: Superintendent of Documents, U.S. Government Printing Office, Washington, D.C. 20402

[3]The label of any controlled substance in Schedules II, III, or IV, when dispensed to, or for, a patient pursuant to a prescription order, must contain the following warning:
Caution: Federal law prohibits the transfer of this drug to any person other than the patient for whom it was prescribed.

Cardiovascular Diseases

1

Coronary Artery Disease

Despite the recent ten-year decline in cardiovascular mortality, heart attacks remain the leading cause of death in the United States, claiming more than 600,000 lives a year. About five million Americans have coronary artery disease—the major cause of heart attacks—which is characterized by a narrowing of the blood vessels that nourish the heart muscle. Of these five million, about 20 percent will experience myocardial infarction (heart attack).

Many persons with coronary artery disease have no obvious symptoms: The narrowing of their vital coronary vessels may progress for many years before any adverse effects are evident. Indeed, in many instances a heart attack is the first overt sign of the disease. Half or more of the victims of coronary artery disease will, however, experience a warning, usually in the form of angina pectoris—chest pains caused by a temporary shortage of oxygen to the heart muscle. This section will be devoted to a discussion of the major causes and modes of treatment of angina pectoris, heart attacks, rhythm disturbances, and cardiac failure.

ANGINA PECTORIS

Angina pectoris—commonly referred to simply as "angina"—may be present for years, even decades, without significant complications, or it may progress quickly to disabling heart disease, most often a heart attack. Prognosis is determined largely by the site and degree of narrowing of the coronary arteries and what long-term effect this has had on the myocardium (heart muscle). Coexisting factors such as hypertension, high levels of cholesterol and other lipids (particularly low-density lipoproteins), cigarette smoking, chronic anxiety, and diabetes mellitus may accelerate the process. Other risk factors include a family history of heart attacks, advancing age, and sex (men are more susceptible than women).

Atherosclerosis, the build-up of fatty deposits in the inner lining of the blood vessels, is responsible for about 90 percent of all coronary artery disease. Numerous studies have shown that at least one of the three major coronary arteries must be narrowed by 80 percent or more before angina develops; in many patients, two—or even all three—of the major coronary vessels are involved.

Another type of chest pain, variant or Prinzmetal's angina, is caused by a spasm in a coronary artery. Unlike angina pectoris, variant angina occurs during rest and is not precipitated by exercise. Although variant angina is receiving increased attention as a cause of cardiac-derived chest pain—and even heart attacks—important details concerning frequency and cause have not yet been established.

Site and Character of Angina

Angina is manifested mainly by varying degrees of discomfort in the chest. The term discomfort is appropriate since the sensation can vary from mild pressure ("a weight on the chest") to agonizing pain. Many physicians use the SAVES criteria to define angina: *S*udden pain in the *A*nterior chest wall that is *V*aguely localized, brought on by *E*xcitement, *E*xertion, *E*motion, or *E*xercise, and is of *S*hort duration.

Patients often deny that the sensation in the chest is pain; instead they may describe it as oppression, heaviness, breathlessness, tightness, or a band-like feeling. The pain of angina pectoris is seldom knife-like or stabbing. A person experiencing an attack of angina may be aware of rapid beating of the heart (tachycardia), and there is often a concomitant asymptomatic rise in the blood pressure.

Precipitating Factors

A number of factors may precipitate an attack of angina. They include, among others, physical exertion (especially sudden or vigorous effort, such as chopping wood or shoveling snow); emotional stress; cold weather; a heavy meal; vigorous arm movements (such as rubbing oneself down briskly after a shower); and sexual activity. When an attack is precipitated by physical exertion, rest often relieves the symptoms in a short time. Respite from emotional stress will also bring relief. Most often, however, one of the fast-acting antianginal drugs is needed to effect relief.

Diagnosis of Angina Pectoris

Angina can often be diagnosed by a careful review of symptoms. Physical examination—listening to the heart, feeling the pulses, measuring blood pressure and heart rate, etc.—may not be particularly helpful, even during an attack. And an electrocardiogram, unless made during an actual anginal episode, may be perfectly normal. Among other diagnostic procedures, the exercise tolerance or stress test is now widely used in establishing the diagnosis of coronary artery disease. In approximately 70 percent of patients with angina pectoris or other symptoms of coronary heart disease, a properly performed treadmill exercise test, in which the heart rate is raised to 90 percent of its maximum capacity as predicted for age and sex, will show an abnormality. The only test capable of pinpointing the precise area and degree of narrowing (stenosis) of the coronary arteries, however, is coronary angiography. This procedure involves inserting a catheter into a vein in the arm and threading it along the vein into and through the heart, injecting an opaque dye or other radioactive contrast material, and following its flow through cardiac chambers and the coronary arteries with motion pictures.

Other Causes of Chest Pain

Not all chest pain is caused by angina pectoris. Musculoskeletal chest pains can be experienced by individuals with perfectly normal hearts. Anxiety may produce chest pains and other symptoms suggestive of heart disease. Other heart disorders, such as inflammation of the pericardium (covering of the heart) or damaged or deformed heart valves may produce angina-like discomfort. Pleurisy, manifestations of hiatus hernia, and even simple indigestion (heartburn) are sometimes mistaken for angina. Even so, whenever chest pain occurs, the possibility of a heart attack must be considered. The pain of myocardial infarction is usually much more prolonged and severe than that of angina, and the onset of a heart attack is seldom related to exercise or exertional effort. But the difference may be subtle (e.g., the pain of a myocardial infarction may fail to respond to nitroglycerin in the usual time or may spread differently and may be accompanied by light-headedness, sweating, or a feeling of impending disaster).

TREATMENT OF ANGINA

Treatment of angina is aimed at: (1) relieving symptoms, (2) identifying factors that may be modified (i.e., adopting a less stressful life-style), and (3) preventing a heart attack.

General Health Measures

The long-range outlook for many angina patients may be enhanced by reducing or eliminating certain

ANATOMY OF ATHEROSCLEROTIC CORONARY DISEASE

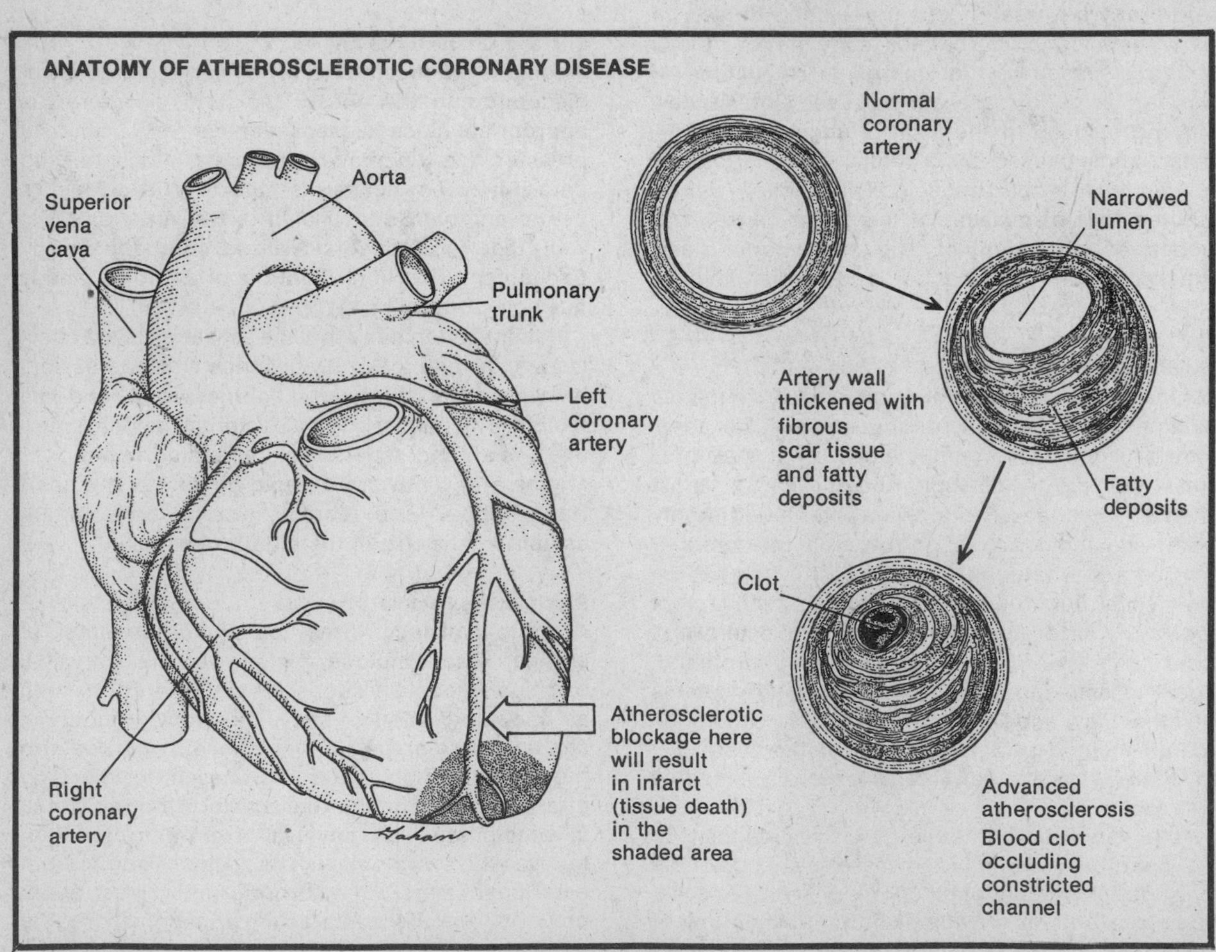

risk factors. These include sustained weight reduction, cessation of cigarette smoking, programmed physical activity, lowering of high blood cholesterol (particularly low-density lipoproteins), and control of high blood pressure and diabetes. Although there is disagreement over whether these measures will actually prevent a heart attack, most experts agree that they will improve general health and well-being, and thus, at the least, will add to the patient's quality of life.

Nitroglycerin

Nitroglycerin, which has been used for almost 100 years to relieve angina pectoris, remains the most widely prescribed drug for this condition. The exact mechanism of action of nitroglycerin and the other organic nitrates is unknown, but it is assumed that the pain is relieved through dilation of both the coronary and systemic blood vessels, which increases the delivery of oxygen to the heart muscle. Nitroglycerin taken sublingually (under the tongue) relieves pain in about two minutes, with the effect lasting about forty-five minutes. Nitroglycerin is also available as an oral tablet, to be chewed or swallowed, for persons who cannot tolerate or use the sublingual route. Since absorption is through the intestinal tract, these oral tablets take longer to become effective. In addition, nitroglycerin is available as an ointment, which is absorbed through the skin. Both the ointment and oral tablets are used for long-term preventive effects. It is particularly important for the patient to learn to use nitroglycerin properly, both to relieve pain that has been identified as angina pectoris and to prevent an attack by taking the drug in anticipation of physical effort or emotional stress.

Nitroglycerin is available as Nitrostat, which is administered only sublingually, and Nitro-Bid, which is available as an oral capsule as well as an ointment to be applied to the site of pain.

Nitroglycerin should not be used by persons during a myocardial infarction or by persons with severe anemia, glaucoma, or a known sensitivity to nitroglycerin. Patients on nitroglycerin should carry the medication with them at all times. Nitroglycerin sublingual tablets should be kept in the tightly stoppered, dark container in which they are dispensed. Since heat reduces the potency of nitroglycerin, the container should not be carried next to the body or stored in a warm, damp place, such as a bathroom medicine chest. The cotton in the top of the container should be removed to prevent absorption. Failure of the nitroglycerin to cause a slight burning or bitterness under the tongue means that it has lost its potency and that a new supply should be obtained.

Long-Acting Nitrates

Long-acting nitrate preparations are less consistent in therapeutic effectiveness than nitroglycerin, having a duration of action of forty-five minutes to two or more hours. Drugs in this group include Cardilate, Isordil, Sorbitrate, Peritrate, and Persantine. The first three drugs may be administered sublingually and take effect in about five minutes. These agents are also available in tablet form for oral ingestion for those who cannot tolerate a tablet under the tongue. (Oral tablets that are intended to be chewed or swallowed must not be used sublingually.) Peritrate and Persantine, however, come only in oral form.

Adverse reactions to the long-acting nitrate preparations include headache, dizziness, weakness, nausea, vomiting, skin rash, and flushing; such reactions or any untoward symptoms should be reported immediately to the physician. All of the nitrates, including nitroglycerin, interact when taken with alcohol and can produce symptoms of decreasing blood supply to the brain, including light-headedness and fainting.

Beta-Adrenergic Blocking Drugs

Introduction of the so-called beta blockers represented a major advance in the management of angina pectoris. Until recently, propranolol (Inderal) was the only drug of this type indicated for treatment of angina in the United States. At the end of 1979, however, a second beta blocker, nadolol (Corgard), also became available in this country for the treatment of angina. Beta-adrenergic blocking agents reduce the oxygen demand of the heart muscle, slow the heart rate, reduce blood pressure, and diminish cardiac contraction velocity, thus helping prevent attacks of angina. They may be used in conjunction with nitroglycerin and similar agents. Many beta blockers also have an antihypertensive action, making them doubly useful for those anginal patients who also have hypertension. The major contraindications of these drugs are bronchial asthma, which they may exacerbate, and peripheral vascular disease, because of the vasoconstrictive properties of these agents. Consequently, beta blockers should be used with caution in patients with diabetes mellitus, who are likely to have impaired circulation. Beta blockers also should not be used in patients with variant angina.

When the physician determines that a beta blocker is no longer needed, it should be withdrawn slowly over a period of time. Abrupt withdrawal may lead to sudden worsening of the angina; it may also precipitate myocardial infarction. *Under no circumstances should the patient stop the drug on his own initiative.*

MYOCARDIAL INFARCTION

Myocardial infarction—defined literally as death of heart muscle—is caused by a sudden and catastrophic reduction in the blood supply to the heart that may be precipitated by a number of poorly understood factors. Nearly all patients who suffer a heart attack have atherosclerosis of one or more of the major coronary arteries. The infarction may be precipitated by a complete blockage of one or more of these vessels caused by rupture of a fatty plaque deposit in the inner wall. The extent of tissue damage depends on the site of occlusion and the state of the other coronary vessels and is of prime importance in morbidity (illness) and mortality.

Pain, which may come on suddenly or develop gradually over a period of minutes or hours, is the major initial symptom. It usually lasts for thirty minutes to several hours, but sometimes is felt for only a few minutes. The pain usually occurs in the middle or upper sternal area, although it may be felt lower in the chest. It may radiate to one or both sides of the chest, move to the neck or lower jaw, and to one or both arms. In addition, persons having a heart attack commonly experience sweating, light-headedness, nausea, vomiting, and very often, an unfamiliar sense of foreboding. The diagnosis of a heart attack is established by characteristic abnormalities in the electrocardiogram as well as by enzyme changes in the blood. Although the chances of surviving a heart attack have increased markedly in the last decade, the mortality rate is still high. About 20 to 25 percent of heart attack victims will die in the first four weeks, with half of these deaths occurring within two hours of the onset of the heart attack, generally before the patient reaches a hospital. Most of those who survive the initial period make a satisfactory recovery.

TREATMENT OF MYOCARDIAL INFARCTION

The primary goals of treatment are to (1) restore heart action and breathing when these have ceased; (2) relieve pain and discomfort; (3) reduce the oxygen demands of the heart muscle to minimize the extent of tissue death, and (4) prevent or correct complications. In many instances, heart beat and breathing can be restored with cardiopulmonary resuscitation or administration of a drug or electrical shock to start the heart beating again. Pain relief is usually achieved by administering morphine sulfate either intravenously or intramuscularly.

By the time a patient enters a hospital coronary care unit, the most dangerous stage of the attack has passed. Bed rest is mandatory but rarely extends beyond a few days to a week or two.

Most patients receive oxygen to counteract any hypoxemia (too little oxygen in the blood). Administration of lidocaine (Xylocaine) may help prevent dangerous tachyarrhythmias (rapid irregular heartbeats). Smoking is, of course, prohibited.

Drug Therapy

The types of drugs administered to heart attack patients are dictated by individual circumstances. In the past, anticoagulant drugs were often given to prevent thromboembolism and similar complications stemming from prolonged bed rest. Most physicians today no longer use anticoagulants routinely in myocardial infarction; instead, these drugs are reserved for those patients with severe cardiac failure, shock, persistent arrhythmia (especially fibrillation), or those with a history of deep vein thrombosis or pulmonary embolism.

Irregular heartbeats that may be precursors of ventricular fibrillation (very rapid uncoordinated heartbeats that may lead to death) require prompt detection and treatment. As noted earlier, injection of lidocaine is considered the most effective drug in this situation and is often used prophylactically to prevent disturbances in heart rhythm. Other drugs include procainamide (Procan SR and Pronestyl), which is an alternative to lidocaine, or bretylium tosylate (Bretylol), a drug that suppresses ventricular fibrillation.

Another common cardiac arrhythmia is bradycardia, which is defined as a heart rate of less than sixty beats per minute in an adult (or less than 120 beats per minute in an infant). Bradycardia is not considered detrimental in myocardial infarction unless there is evidence of inadequate pumping of blood (hemodynamic failure) or ventricular extra beats from the slow rhythm. Although atropine, an anticholinergic agent, is useful in some patients, persistent symptomatic bradycardia may call for implantation of a cardiac pacemaker—a device that helps both to control the electrical activity of the heart and maintain a regular heartbeat.

In contrast, there are also a number of cardiac arrhythmias characterized by rapid (tachycardia) or irregular heartbeats such as premature ventricular contractions. These arrhythmias also may impede the normal pumping action of the heart and prove life-threatening. Aside from lidocaine and procainamide, drugs that are derivatives of quinidine (Quinaglute, Quinidex, and Quinidine Sulfate), as well as disopyramide (Norpace), which has properties similar to quinidine, are commonly prescribed in these circumstances because they help control the tachycardia by suppressing heart action. They must be monitored very carefully, however, since even a small overdose may have serious consequences. Other agents prescribed to control tachycardia and similar arrhythmias are the beta-blocking drugs such as propranolol (Inderal). Some patients experience a combination of arrhythmias, characterized by alternating periods of rapid and slow heartbeats. Since the drugs that are normally given for tachycardia alone may exacerbate the bradycardia, an electrical pacemaker often is the treatment of choice in this condition.

Cardiogenic Shock

Shock, which is the result of a severe reduction in circulatory blood volume due to the heart's failure to pump the blood adequately, is another potential complication of a myocardial infarction. Since it has a mortality of about 50 percent, its prevention is of critical importance. Drugs used to prevent or manage shock syndrome include those that stimulate the sympathetic nervous system. These drugs act by increasing the heart rate, strengthening myocardial contraction, or altering vascular resistance (afterload reduction). The use of vasopressor drugs, such as norepinephrine and isoproterenol, is controversial because these drugs may increase the size of the infarction by stimulating the heart to work harder. Dopamine (Intropin) or vasodilator agents such as nitroprusside (Nipride), prazosin (Minipress), and hydralazine are alternatives that, in some circumstances, will increase cardiac output without putting undue strain on the heart. Using a catheter with an intra-aortic balloon to help the heart's pumping action, followed by coronary bypass surgery, has been lifesaving in some instances.

CARDIAC FAILURE

Cardiac failure, also referred to as congestive heart failure, is a chronic inadequacy of the heart to pump sufficient blood. It is often a complication of myocardial infarction or advanced heart disease from another cause such as hypertension. It is characterized by dyspnea (difficult breathing) and pulmonary edema (the build-up of fluid in the lungs). Treatment of acute cardiac failure consists of reducing the build-up of body fluids, usually by administering a potent diuretic such as furosemide (Lasix), and improving the contractile strength of the heart. Long-term treatment of congestive heart disease often entails using the thiazide diuretics, which are also used in the treatment of hypertension. (For detailed information on these drugs, see *Hypertension*, page 54.) Digitalis glycosides, such as digoxin (Lanoxin), in combination with a diuretic, are often used to combat congestive heart failure. There are instances, however, in which vasodilators, such as nitroprusside (Nipride) or hydralazine (Apresoline), may be used either alone or in conjunction with digitalis.

ELEVATED LIPID LEVELS

As noted earlier, elevated levels of cholesterol, particularly low-density lipoproteins, is considered by many authorities to be a major risk factor in the development of atherosclerosis. Although there is some disagreement on what constitutes elevated lipid levels, a fasting cholesterol measurement of 220 mg per deciliter and a triglyceride measurement of 140 mg per deciliter are considered high.

There is ongoing controversy about the contribution of diet to atherosclerosis, but most authorities recommend reduction in caloric intake and lower consumption of saturated fats (i.e., animal fats) as a prudent course. In some rare instances, a genetic defect can produce a group of conditions known as familial hyperlipidemia. One of these conditions, familial hypercholesterolemia, often manifests itself as advanced coronary artery disease at a very early age. Its victims often suffer a heart attack in their teens or twenties. Xanthomas—yellowish, fatty growths that often appear on the eyelids and just under the skin, particularly on the elbows, knees, and along the spine—are a common hallmark of the disease.

Treatment

Diet remains the mainstay of treatment to reduce cholesterol and other blood lipids. Weight reduction, especially if it is accompanied by increased exercise, usually produces a reduction in cholesterol and triglycerides. In addition, reduced consumption of cholesterol and other saturated fats (in general, animal fats or fats that are solid rather than liquid at room temperature) is also recommended as a strategy in lowering blood lipids.

For persons with familial hyperlipidemia as well as those with very high cholesterol and/or triglyceride levels, lipid-lowering drugs may be prescribed. These include clofibrate (Atromid-S), dextrothyroxine sodium (Choloxin), probucol (Lorelco), and cholestyramine (Questran). Some (e.g., cholestyramine and probucol) act by increasing the excretion of fats from the intestinal tract, while the others are systemic drugs and have a variety of mechanisms of action.

IN CONCLUSION

The improved outlook in the treatment of coronary artery disease and its complications in recent years may be attributed to a variety of factors, including improved therapies, the introduction of new drugs and increased understanding in the use of older agents, new surgical procedures, and increased emphasis on prevention. The following tables cover the major drugs used to treat angina pectoris; cardiac arrhythmias, including emergency situations; and hyperlipidemia. The diuretics that are used to treat congestive heart failure are generally the same ones used to treat hypertension, and are included in that section. (See page 54.) Drugs used to treat other cardiovascular disorders may be found in the sections on *Clotting Disorders* (page 130) and *Peripheral Circulatory Disorders* (page 143).

CARDILATE (Erythrityl tetranitrate) Burroughs Wellcome

Tabs (oral, sublingual): 5, 10, 15 mg **Tabs (chewable):** 10 mg

INDICATIONS	SUBLINGUAL DOSAGE	ORAL DOSAGE
Prophylaxis and long-term management of **angina pectoris**	**Adult:** 10 mg to start prior to stressful situations and at bedime for patients subject to nocturnal attacks, followed by larger or smaller doses, as needed, up to 100 mg/day	**Adult:** 10 mg to start before each meal, as well as midmorning, midafternoon, and at bedtime for patients subject to nocturnal attacks, followed by larger or smaller doses, as needed, up to 100 mg/day; chewable tabs: same as sublingual dosage

ADMINISTRATION/DOSAGE ADJUSTMENTS

Management of headache during dosage adjustment period — If headache occurs, reduce dosage for a few days and, if necessary, give an analgesic

CONTRAINDICATIONS

Idiosyncratic reaction to erythrityl tetranitrate

WARNINGS/PRECAUTIONS

Early, acute myocardial infarction — Safe use not established

Increased intraocular pressure — Use with caution in patients with glaucoma

Tolerance — May develop, as well as cross-tolerance to other nitrites and nitrates

ADVERSE REACTIONS

Frequent reactions are italicized

Central nervous system — *Headache* (sometimes severe and persistent); transient dizziness, weakness, and other signs of cerebral ischemia associated with postural hypotension; restlessness

Cardiovascular — Cutaneous vasodilation with flushing, pallor

Gastrointestinal — Nausea, vomiting

Dermatological — Rash, exfoliative dermatitis

Other — Sweating , collapse

OVERDOSAGE

Signs and symptoms — See ADVERSE REACTIONS

Treatment — Discontinue use of drug; treat symptomatically

DRUG INTERACTIONS

Alcohol — ⇧ Cerebral ischemic symptoms (dizziness, weakness, palpitations, syncope) due to nitrate-induced vasodilation

Norepinephrine — ⇩ Pressor effect

Acetylcholine — ⇩ Cholinergic-receptor stimulation

Histamine — ⇩ Histamine effect

ALTERED LABORATORY VALUES

No clinically significant alterations in blood/serum or urinary values occur at therapeutic dosages

Use in children

General guidelines not established

Use in pregnancy or nursing mothers

General guidelines not established

CORGARD (Nadolol) Squibb

Tabs: 40, 80, 120, 160 mg

INDICATIONS	ORAL DOSAGE
Angina pectoris	**Adult:** 40 mg qd to start, followed by increments of 40–80 mg/day every 3–7 days until optimal response is achieved or pronounced slowing of heart rate occurs; usual maintenance dosage: 80–240 mg qd
Hypertension	**Adult:** 40 mg qd (alone or with a diuretic) to start, followed by increments of 40–80 mg/day, as needed, up to 640 mg/day; usual maintenance dosage: 80–320 mg qd

ADMINISTRATION/DOSAGE ADJUSTMENTS

Patients with renal impairment	Increase interval between doses as follows: administer q24h when creatinine clearance rate (CCr)>50 ml/min; q24–36h when CCr = 31–50 ml/min; q24–48h when CCr = 10–30 ml/min; q40–60h when CCr <10 ml/min
Combination therapy	May be used at full dosage in combination with other antihypertensive agents, especially thiazide-type diuretics
Discontinuation of therapy	Reduce dosage gradually over 1–2 wk, if possible, and monitor patient closely. Caution patients with angina or hyperthyroidism against interruption or abrupt cessation of therapy (see WARNINGS/PRECAUTIONS).

CONTRAINDICATIONS

Bronchial asthma ●	Conduction block greater than first degree ●	Overt cardiac failure (see WARNINGS/PRECAUTIONS) ●
Sinus bradycardia ●	Cardiogenic shock ●	

WARNINGS/PRECAUTIONS

Cardiac failure	May be precipitated by further or continued depression of myocardial contractility; discontinue use (gradually, if possible) if cardiac failure occurs or persists despite adequate digitalization and diuretic therapy. In cases of well-compensated congestive heart failure, use with caution.
Abrupt discontinuation	May exacerbate angina pectoris and, in some cases, lead to myocardial infarction in patients with ischemic heart disease
Impaired response to reflex adrenergic stimuli	May augment the risks of general anesthesia and surgery, resulting in protracted hypotension or low cardiac output, and, occasionally, difficulty in restarting and maintaining heart beat. If possible, discontinue use well before surgery takes place. Excessive beta blockade occurring during emergency surgery can be reversed by IV administration of a beta-receptor agonist (eg, isoproterenol, dopamine, dobutamine, or levarterenol).
Diabetes mellitus	Beta blockade may mask symptoms of hypoglycemia and potentiate insulin-induced hypoglycemia; use with caution, especially in patients with labile diabetes
Thyrotoxicosis	Clinical signs of hyperthyroidism may be masked; abrupt withdrawal may precipitate thyroid storm
Nonallergic bronchospasm	Use with caution in patients with bronchospastic diseases, since bronchodilation produced by beta stimulation may be blocked
Hepatic or renal impairment	Use with caution and monitor for signs of excessive drug accumulation (see OVERDOSAGE)

Table continued on following page

CORGARD continued

ADVERSE REACTIONS[1]

Frequent reactions are italicized

Cardiovascular	*Heart rate <40 beats/min and/or symptomatic bradycardia (2%), peripheral vascular insufficiency (2%), cardiac failure (1%), hypotension (1%), rhythm and/or conduction disturbances (1%),* first- and third-degree heart block, intensified AV block[1]
Central nervous system	*Dizziness (2%), fatigue (2%),* paresthesias, sedation, changed behavior, headache, slurred speech, reversible mental depression progressing to catatonia,[1] visual disturbances,[1] hallucinations,[1] an acute reversible syndrome characterized by disorientation, short-term memory loss, emotional lability, clouded sensorium, and decreased neuropsychometric performance[1]
Respiratory	Bronchospasm, cough, nasal stuffiness
Gastrointestinal	Nausea, diarrhea, abdominal discomfort, constipation, vomiting, indigestion, anorexia, bloating, flatulence, dry mouth, mesenteric arterial thrombosis,[1] ischemic colitis[1]
Dermatological	Rash, pruritus, dry skin, facial swelling, diaphoresis, erythematous rash[1]
Ophthalmic	Dry eyes, blurred vision
Genitourinary	Impotence or decreased libido
Hematological	Agranulocytosis,[1] thrombocytopenic or nonthrombocytopenic purpura[1]
Allergic	Fever,[1] aching,[1] sore throat,[1] laryngospasm,[1] respiratory distress[1]
Other	Weight gain, tinnitus, reversible alopecia,[1] Peyronie's disease[1]

OVERDOSAGE

Signs and symptoms	Excessive bradycardia, cardiac failure, hypotension, bronchospasm
Treatment	Empty stomach by gastric lavage. Hemodialysis may be useful. For excessive bradycardia, administer 0.25-1.0 mg atropine; if there is no response to vagal blockade, administer isoproterenol cautiously. For cardiac failure, administer digitalis and a diuretic; IV glucagon may be helpful. For hypotension, administer a vasopressor, such as levarterenol or (preferably) epinephrine. Treat bronchospasm with a beta$_2$-stimulating agent (eg, isoproterenol) and/or a theophylline derivative.

DRUG INTERACTIONS

Digitalis	⇩ AV conduction
Reserpine, *Rauwolfia* alkaloids	⇧ Risk of vertigo, syncope, or orthostatic hypotension

ALTERED LABORATORY VALUES

No clinically significant alterations in blood/serum or urinary values have yet been reported at therapeutic dosages

Use in children

Safety and effectiveness in children have not been established

Use in pregnancy or nursing mothers

Safe use during pregnancy not established. Embryo- and fetotoxicity have been observed in rabbits, but not in rats or hamsters. Excretion in human breast milk unknown; use with caution in nursing mothers.

[1]Adverse reactions associated with other beta blockers which, although they have not been reported in patients treated with nadolol, should be considered as potential adverse effects of nadolol

INDERAL (Propranolol hydrochloride) Ayerst

Tabs: 10, 20, 40, 80 mg **Amps:** 1 mg/ml (1 ml)

INDICATIONS	ORAL DOSAGE	PARENTERAL DOSAGE
Prophylaxis of moderate to severe **angina pectoris**	**Adult:** 10–20 mg/day tid or qid, before meals and at bedtime, to start, followed by gradual increments every 3–7 days until optimal response is achieved, up to 320 mg/day; usual maintenance dosage: 160 mg/day	—
Hypertension	**Adult:** 40 mg bid (alone or with a diuretic) to start, followed by gradual increases until optimal response is achieved, up to 640 mg/day; usual maintenance dosage: 160–480 mg/day	—
Cardiac arrhythmias, including supraventricular arrhythmias, ventricular tachycardias, digitalis-induced tachyarrhythmias, and resistant tachyarrhythmias due to excessive catecholamine activity during anesthesia	**Adult:** 10–30 mg tid or qid, before meals and at bedtime	**Adult:** 1–3 mg IV, slowly (see ADMINISTRATION/DOSAGE ADJUSTMENTS)
Hypertrophic subaortic stenosis	**Adult:** 20–40 mg tid or qid, before meals and at bedtime	—
As an adjunct to alpha-adrenergic blocking agents in the management of **pheochromocytoma**	**Adult:** 60 mg/day div for 3 days prior to surgery, concomitantly with an alpha-adrenergic blocking agent, or 30 mg/day div for inoperable tumors	—
Migraine prophylaxis	**Adult:** 80 mg/day div to start, followed by gradual increments until optimal response is achieved; usual maintenance dosage: 160–240 mg/day	—

ADMINISTRATION/DOSAGE ADJUSTMENTS

Intravenous use — Limited to life-threatening arrhythmias or those occurring under anesthesia. To minimize risk of hypotension and possibility of cardiac standstill, administer slowly (≤1 mg/min) and monitor ECG and CVP continuously. Initial dose may be repeated after 2 min; thereafter, wait at least 4 h before administering additional propranolol.

Selection of patients with angina — Reserve for patients with moderate to severe angina pectoris unresponsive to conventional therapy, including weight control, rest, cessation of smoking, use of sublingual nitroglycerin, and avoidance of precipitating circumstances. Monitor patient closely and re-evaluate therapy periodically.

Inadequate control of hypertension — Twice daily dosing is usually effective. Some patients, however, experience a modest rise in blood pressure toward the end of the 12-h dosing interval, especially when lower dosages are used. If control is inadequate, a larger dose or tid therapy may be indicated.

Discontinuation of therapy — Reduce dosage gradually over several weeks, if possible, and monitor patient closely. Caution patients with angina or hyperthyroidism against interruption or abrupt cessation of therapy (see WARNINGS/PRECAUTIONS).

CONTRAINDICATIONS

Sinus bradycardia ●

Greater than first-degree heart block ●

Cardiogenic shock ●

Right ventricular failure secondary to pulmonary hypertension ●

Congestive heart failure not resulting from propranolol-treatable tachyarrhythmias ●

Bronchial asthma ●

Allergic rhinitis during the pollen season ●

Concomitant therapy with adrenergic-augmenting psychotropic agents, including MAO inhibitors (both during therapy and for 2 wk after such drugs are withdrawn) ●

WARNINGS/PRECAUTIONS

Cardiac failure — May be precipitated by further or continued depression of myocardial contractility; discontinue use if cardiac failure persists despite adequate digitalization and diuretic therapy, except when managing tachyarrhythmias

Abrupt discontinuation of therapy — May exacerbate angina pectoris, lead to myocardial infarction in patients with coronary artery disease, or precipitate thyrotoxicosis in hyperthyroid patients

Thyrotoxicosis — Clinical signs of hyperthyroidism may be masked

Wolff-Parkinson-White syndrome — Tachycardia may be replaced by severe bradycardia requiring a demand pacemaker

Table continued on following page

WARNINGS/PRECAUTIONS continued

Impaired response to reflex stimuli	Withdraw drug 48 h prior to surgery unless surgery is for pheochromocytoma. Patients undergoing emergency surgery may experience protracted severe hypotension and, occasionally, difficulty in restarting and maintaining heart beat. Excessive beta blockade may be reversed during surgery by IV administration of a beta-receptor agonist (eg, isoproterenol or levarterenol).
Myocardial depression during anesthesia	May occur with inhalation anesthetics that depend on endogenous catecholamine release to maintain adequate cardiac function; when treating arrhythmias occurring during anesthesia, titrate dosage carefully (see ADMINISTRATION/DOSAGE ADJUSTMENTS)
Nonallergic bronchospasm	Use with caution, since bronchodilation produced by beta stimulation may be blocked
Diabetes, hypoglycemia	Beta blockade may prevent appearance of premonitory signs and symptoms of acute hypoglycemia, especially in patients with labile diabetes
Renal or hepatic impairment	Use with caution and monitor for signs of excessive drug accumulation (see OVERDOSAGE)

ADVERSE REACTIONS

Cardiovascular	Bradycardia, congestive heart failure, AV-block intensification, hypotension, paresthesia of the hands, Raynaud-type arterial insufficiency, thrombocytopenic purpura
Central nervous system	Lightheadedness, depression, insomnia, weakness, fatigue, lassitude, catatonia, visual disturbances, hallucinations, disorientation, short-term memory loss, emotional lability, slightly clouded sensorium, decreased neuropsychometric performance
Gastrointestinal	Nausea, vomiting, epigastric distress, abdominal cramps, diarrhea, constipation, mesenteric arterial thrombosis, ischemic colitis
Respiratory	Bronchospasm
Allergic	Pharyngitis, agranulocytosis, erythematous rash, fever with aching and sore throat, laryngospasm and respiratory distress
Other	Reversible alopecia

OVERDOSAGE

Signs and symptoms	Severe bradycardia, congestive heart failure, hypotension, bronchospasm
Treatment	For excessive bradycardia, administer 0.25–1.0 mg atropine IV; if there is no response to vagal blockade, administer isoproterenol cautiously. For cardiac failure, administer digitalis and a diuretic. For hypotension, use levarterenol or (preferably) epinephrine. Treat bronchospasm with isoproterenol and aminophylline.

DRUG INTERACTIONS

Digitalis	⇩ AV conduction
Ephedrine, isoproterenol, and other beta-adrenergic bronchodilating agents	⇩ Bronchodilation
Reserpine, *Rauwolfia* alkaloids	⇧ Risk of vertigo, syncope, or orthostatic hypotension

ALTERED LABORATORY VALUES

Blood/serum values	⇧ BUN ⇧ SGOT ⇧ SGPT ⇧ Alkaline phosphatase ⇧ Lactate dehydrogenase

No clinically significant alterations in urinary values occur at therapeutic dosages

Use in children

Safe use not established

Use in pregnancy or nursing mothers

Safe use during pregnancy not established. In animal studies, propranolol has demonstrated embryotoxicity at doses ~ 10 times greater than the maximum recommended human dose. General guidelines not established for use in nursing mothers.

ISORDIL (Isosorbide dinitrate) Ives

Tabs (sublingual): 2.5, 5, 10 mg **Tabs (chewable):** 10 mg **Tabs (oral):** 5, 10, 20, 30 mg **Tabs, caps (sust rel):** 40 mg

INDICATIONS	SUBLINGUAL DOSAGE	ORAL DOSAGE
Acute angina pectoris[1]	**Adult:** 2.5–10 mg, as needed	—
Prophylaxis in situations likely to provoke **angina**[1]	**Adult:** 2.5–10 mg q2-3h	—
Prophylaxis and long-term management of **angina pectoris**[2]	—	**Adult:** 5–30 mg qid (usual dosage: 10–20 mg qid); sust-rel tabs or caps: 40 mg q6–12h, as needed (*do not chew*)

ADMINISTRATION/DOSAGE ADJUSTMENTS

Chewable tablets — See SUBLINGUAL DOSAGE, but do not initiate therapy with more than 5 mg to avoid severe hypotension

Supplemental therapy — Stressful conditions may provoke anginal attacks despite prophylactic treatment; supplement sust-rel therapy with sublingual isosorbide dinitrate or nitroglycerin

CONTRAINDICATIONS

Idiosyncracy to isosorbide dinitrate

WARNINGS/PRECAUTIONS

Early, acute myocardial infarction — Safe use not established

Tolerance — May develop, as well as cross-tolerance to other nitrites and nitrates

Functional or organic GI hypermotility, malabsorption syndrome — Sustained-release tablets are not recommended for use in patients with these conditions

ADVERSE REACTIONS Frequent reactions are italicized

Central nervous system — *Headache* (sometimes severe and persistent); transient dizziness, weakness, and other signs of cerebral ischemia associated with postural hypotension; restlessness

Cardiovascular — Cutaneous vasodilation with flushing, pallor,

Gastrointestinal — Nausea, vomiting

Dermatological — Rash, exfoliative dermatitis

Other — Sweating, collapse

OVERDOSAGE

Signs and symptoms — See ADVERSE REACTIONS

Treatment — Discontinue use of drug; treat symptomatically

DRUG INTERACTIONS

Alcohol — ⇧ Cerebral ischemic symptoms (dizziness, weakness, palpitations, syncope)

Norepinephrine, acetylcholine, histamine — ⇩ Physiologic effect

ALTERED LABORATORY VALUES

No clinically significant alterations in blood/serum or urinary values occur at therapeutic dosages

Use in children

General guidelines not established

Use in pregnancy or nursing mothers

General guidelines not established

[1]Probably effective
[2]Possibly effective

NITRO-BID (Nitroglycerin) Marion

Ointment: 2% (20, 60 g) **Caps (sust rel):** 2.5, 6.5, 9 mg

INDICATIONS	TOPICAL DOSAGE	ORAL DOSAGE
Prevention and treatment of **angina pectoris attacks,** especially at night[1]	**Adult:** apply 1–2 inches of ointment q3–4h, if necessary (some patients may require up to 4–5 inches); one application at bedtime frequently suffices for the entire night (consult package insert for details of administration)	—
Management, prophylaxis, and treatment of **anginal attacks**[1]	—	**Adult:** 1 cap q12h or, if needed, 1 cap q8h *(do not chew)*

ADMINISTRATION/DOSAGE ADJUSTMENTS

Discontinuation of topical therapy —— To prevent sudden withdrawal reactions, reduce the dosage and frequency gradually over 4–6 wk

CONTRAINDICATIONS

For both topical and oral use	For topical use only	For oral use only
Marked or severe anemia●	Increased intraocular pressure●	Acute or recent myocardial infarction●
Increased intracranial pressure●		Closed-angle glaucoma●
Idiosyncracy to nitrites or nitroglycerin●		Postural hypotension●

WARNINGS/PRECAUTIONS

Glaucoma —— Intraocular pressure may increase; use medication with caution, if at all

Postural hypotension and fainting —— May occur with ointment in elderly patients upon suddenly arising

Blurred vision, dry mouth —— May occur with oral dosage form; discontinue medication

Tolerance —— May develop, as well as cross-tolerance to other nitrites and nitrates

ADVERSE REACTIONS

Central nervous system —— Headache (transient with topical use, severe and persistent with oral use), dizziness, weakness (with oral use)

Cardiovascular —— Cutaneous flushing, postural hypotension and tachycardia (with topical use)

Gastrointestinal —— Nausea and vomiting (with oral use)

Dermatological —— Rash and exfoliative dermatitis (with oral use)

OVERDOSAGE

Signs and symptoms —— Severe headache, flushing, tachycardia, dizziness, blurred vision, dry mouth

Treatment —— Discontinue use of drug; treat symptomatically

DRUG INTERACTIONS

Alcohol —— ⇧ Cerebral ischemic symptoms (dizziness, weakness, palpitations, syncope) due to nitrate-induced vasodilation

ALTERED LABORATORY VALUES

No clinically significant alterations in blood/serum or urinary values occur at therapeutic dosages

Use in children

General guidelines not established

Use in pregnancy or nursing mothers

General guidelines not established

[1]Possibly effective

NITROSTAT (Nitroglycerin) Parke-Davis

Tabs (sublingual): 0.15, 0.3, 0.4, 0.6 mg

INDICATIONS	SUBLINGUAL DOSAGE
Acute angina pectoris Management of **angina pectoris** due to coronary insufficiency, coronary-artery disease, coronary occlusion, or subacute myocardial infarction	**Adult:** 1 tab (smallest effective dose) dissolved under tongue or in the buccal pouch immediately upon indication of attack; repeat, as needed, until relief is obtained

CONTRAINDICATIONS

Early myocardial infarction●

Increased intracranial pressure●

Hypersensitivity to nitroglycerin●

Severe anemia●

WARNINGS/PRECAUTIONS

Blurred vision, dry mouth — May occur; discontinue medication

Tolerance — May develop, especially with excessive use

ADVERSE REACTIONS

Central nervous system — Transient headache; vertigo, weakness, and other signs of cerebral ischemia associated with postural hypotension

Cardiovascular — Palpitations, syncope

OVERDOSAGE

Signs and symptoms — Violent headache, blurred vision, dry mouth

Treatment — Discontinue use of drug; treat symptomatically

DRUG INTERACTIONS

Alcohol — ⇧ Cerebral ischemic symptoms (dizziness, weakness, palpitations, syncope) due to nitrate-induced vasodilation

ALTERED LABORATORY VALUES

No clinically significant alterations in blood/serum or urinary values occur at therapeutic dosages

Use in children

General guidelines not established

Use in pregnancy or nursing mothers

General guidelines not established

PERITRATE/PERITRATE SA (Pentaerythritol tetranitrate) Parke-Davis

Tabs: 10, 20, 40 mg **Tabs (sust rel):** 80 mg

INDICATIONS	ORAL DOSAGE
Prophylaxis and long-term management of **angina pectoris**[1]	**Adult:** 10–20 mg qid to start, followed by up to 40 mg qid, taken ½ h before or 1 h after meals and at bedtime; sust-rel tabs: 80 mg bid

CONTRAINDICATIONS

Hypersensitivity to pentaerythritol tetranitrate

WARNINGS/PRECAUTIONS

Early, acute myocardial infarction	Safe use not established
Increased intraocular pressure	Administer with caution in patients with glaucoma
Tolerance	May develop, as well as cross-tolerance to other nitrites and nitrates

ADVERSE REACTIONS Frequent reactions are italicized

Central nervous system	*Headache* (sometimes severe and persistent), dizziness, weakness, and other signs of cerebral ischemia associated with postural hypotension; restlessness
Cardiovascular	Cutaneous vasodilation with flushing, pallor
Gastrointestinal	*Distress*, nausea, vomiting
Dermatological	*Rash*
Other	Sweating, collapse

OVERDOSAGE

Signs and symptoms	See ADVERSE REACTIONS
Treatment	Discontinue use of drug; treat symptomatically

DRUG INTERACTIONS

Alcohol	⇧ Cerebral ischemic symptoms (dizziness, weakness, palpitations, syncope) due to vasodilation
Norepinephrine	⇩ Pressor effect
Acetylcholine	⇩ Cholinergic-receptor stimulation
Histamine	⇩ Histamine effect

ALTERED LABORATORY VALUES

No clinically significant alterations in blood/serum or urinary values occur at therapeutic dosages

Use in children

General guidelines not established

Use in pregnancy or nursing mothers

General guidelines not established

[1]Possibly effective

PERSANTINE (Dipyridamole) **Boehringer Ingelheim**

Tabs: 25, 50, 75 mg

INDICATIONS	ORAL DOSAGE
Chronic angina pectoris[1]	**Adult:** 50 mg tid, at least 1 h before meals

ADMINISTRATION/DOSAGE ADJUSTMENTS

Therapeutic response	Reduction in frequency of anginal attacks and need for nitroglycerin, as well as improvement in exercise tolerance, may not be evident before 2nd or 3rd mo of continuous therapy. Higher doses, while sometimes necessary, significantly increase risk of side effects.

CONTRAINDICATIONS

None

WARNINGS/PRECAUTIONS

Peripheral vasodilation	Use with caution in patients with hypotension
Tartrazine sensitivity	May cause allergic-type reactions, including bronchial asthma, in susceptible individuals

ADVERSE REACTIONS

Central nervous system	Headache, dizziness, weakness
Gastrointestinal	Nausea, mild distress
Cardiovascular	Flushing, syncope, aggravated angina pectoris (rare)
Dermatological	Rash

OVERDOSAGE

Signs and symptoms	See ADVERSE REACTIONS
Treatment	Discontinue use of drug; treat symptomatically

DRUG INTERACTIONS

No clinically significant drug interactions have been observed

ALTERED LABORATORY VALUES

No clinically significant alterations in blood/serum or urinary values occur at therapeutic dosages

Use in children	**Use in pregnancy or nursing mothers**
General guidelines not established	General guidelines not established

[1]Possibly effective

SORBITRATE (Isosorbide dinitrate) Stuart

Tabs (sublingual): 2.5, 5 mg **Tabs (chewable):** 5, 10 mg **Tabs (oral):** 5, 10, 20 mg **Tabs (sust rel):** 40 mg

INDICATIONS	SUBLINGUAL DOSAGE	ORAL DOSAGE
Acute angina pectoris[1]	**Adult:** 2.5–10 mg, as needed	—
Prophylaxis in situations likely to provoke **angina**[1]	**Adult:** 2.5–10 mg (or up to 30 mg, if needed) q4–6h	—
Prophylaxis and long-term management of **angina pectoris**[2]	—	**Adult:** 2.5–10 mg (or up to 30 mg, if needed) tid or qid; sust-rel tabs: 40 mg q12h, as needed

ADMINISTRATION/DOSAGE ADJUSTMENTS

Chewable tablets — See SUBLINGUAL DOSAGE; severe hypotension may occur occasionally with this dosage form, even with doses as low as 5 mg

Oral doses — Should be taken on an empty stomach

Vascular headache — May be minimized by taking drug with meals if uncontrollable by decreasing dosage or use of analgesics

CONTRAINDICATIONS

Hypersensitivity to isosorbide dinitrate

WARNINGS/PRECAUTIONS

Early, acute myocardial infarction — Safe use not established

Tartrazine sensitivity — Presence of FD&C Yellow No. 5 (tartrazine) in both chewable and sust-rel tabs and 5- and 10-mg oral tabs may cause allergic-type reactions, including bronchial asthma, in susceptible individuals

Tolerance — May develop, as well as cross-tolerance to other nitrites and nitrates

ADVERSE REACTIONS

Frequent reactions are italicized

Central nervous system — *Headache* (sometimes severe and persistent); transient dizziness, weakness, and other signs of cerebral ischemia associated with postural hypotension; restlessness

Cardiovascular — Cutaneous vasodilation with flushing, pallor

Gastrointestinal — Nausea, vomiting

Dermatological — Rash, exfoliative dermatitis

Other — Sweating, collapse

OVERDOSAGE

Signs and symptoms — See ADVERSE REACTIONS

Treatment — Discontinue use of drug; treat symptomatically

DRUG INTERACTIONS

Alcohol — ⇧ Cerebral ischemic symptoms (dizziness, weakness, palpitations, syncope) due to nitrate-induced vasodilation

Norepinephrine — ⇩ Pressor effect

Acetylcholine — ⇩ Cholinergic-receptor stimulation

Histamine — ⇩ Histamine effect

ALTERED LABORATORY VALUES

No clinically significant alterations in blood/serum or urinary values occur at therapeutic dosages

Use in children

General guidelines not established

Use in pregnancy or nursing mothers

General guidelines not established

[1]Possibly effective
[2]Occurs more frequently in children

BRETYLOL (Bretylium tosylate) American Critical Care

Amps: 50 mg/ml (10 ml)

INDICATIONS	PARENTERAL DOSAGE
Immediately life-threatening ventricular arrhythmias, such as ventricular fibrillation, that have failed to respond to adequate doses of a first-line antiarrhythmic agent (such as lidocaine or procainamide)	**Adult:** 5 mg/kg IV (rapidly) to start, followed by 10 mg/kg every 15–30 min, if needed, up to a total dose of 30 mg/kg
Other life-threatening ventricular arrhythmias that have failed to respond to adequate doses of a first-line antiarrhythmic agent (such as lidocaine or procainamide)	**Adult:** 5–10 mg/kg IM or by IV infusion over a period >8 min; repeat in 1–2 h if arrhythmia persists

ADMINISTRATION/DOSAGE ADJUSTMENTS

Maintenance regimen	Give 5–10 mg/kg IM q6–8h or intermittently by IV infusion over a period >8 min q6h or give 1–2 mg/min by constant IV infusion. Reduce dosage and discontinue treatment in 3–5 days; if indicated, substitute appropriate antiarrhythmic agents.
Intramuscular administration	Do not inject more than 5 ml into any one site; vary injection site if drug is used repeatedly, to avoid atrophy and necrosis of muscle tissue, fibrosis, vascular degeneration and inflammation
Preparation of solution for intravenous infusion	Dilute contents of one ampul (10 ml containing 500 mg bretylium) with at least 40 ml of Dextrose Injection USP or Sodium Chloride Injection USP. For immediately life-threatening arrhythmias or IM use, bretylium should be injected undiluted.
Patients with renal impairment	Reduce dosage to avoid excessive accumulation, since drug is eliminated mainly by the kidney

CONTRAINDICATIONS

None

WARNINGS/PRECAUTIONS

Orthostatic hypotension	Occurs frequently, characterized by dizziness, lightheadedness, vertigo, or faintness; keep patient supine until tolerance develops
Transient hypertension and increased frequency of arrhythmias	May occur early in treatment due to release of norepinephrine from adrenergic postganglionic nerve terminals
Severe aortic stenosis or pulmonary hypertension	Severe hypotension may result from a fall in peripheral resistance without a compensatory increase in cardiac output; combat with vasoconstrictive catecholamines
Digitalis toxicity	May be enhanced; avoid concomitant administration of digitalis glycosides and bretylium
Nausea, vomiting	May occur in about 3% of patients, generally because of overly rapid IV administration

ADVERSE REACTIONS

Frequent reactions are italicized

Cardiovascular	*Hypotension, postural hypotension,* bradycardia, increased frequency of premature ventricular contractions, transitory hypertension, initial increase in arrhythmias, anginal attacks, substernal pressure
Gastrointestinal	*Nausea, vomiting,* diarrhea, abdominal pain, hiccoughs
Central nervous system	Vertigo, dizziness, lightheadedness, syncope, hyperthermia, confusion, paranoid psychosis, emotional lability, lethargy, anxiety
Genitourinary	Renal dysfunction
Dermatological	Erythematous macular rash
Other	Flushing, generalized tenderness, shortness of breath, diaphoresis, nasal stuffiness, mild conjunctivitis

Table continued on following page

OVERDOSAGE

Signs and symptoms	Hypotension (supine systolic blood pressure < 75 mm Hg)
Treatment	To raise blood pressure, administer a diluted solution of dopamine or norepinephrine and monitor pressure closely. If indicated, administer blood or plasma to expand blood volume and IV fluids to correct dehydration.

DRUG INTERACTIONS

Digitalis glycosides	⇧ Risk of digitalis toxicity
Catecholamines	⇧ Pressor effect
Procainamide, quinidine	⇧ Hypotension
Tricyclic antidepressants	⇩ Hypotension

ALTERED LABORATORY VALUES

No clinically significant alterations in blood/serum or urinary values occur at therapeutic dosages

Use in children

Safety and effectiveness have not been established

Use in pregnancy or nursing mothers

Safe use not established during pregnancy. General guidelines not established for use in nursing mothers

INDERAL (Propranolol hydrochloride) Ayerst

Tabs: 10, 20, 40, 80 mg **Amps:** 1 mg/ml (1 ml)

INDICATIONS	ORAL DOSAGE	PARENTERAL DOSAGE
Cardiac arrhythmias, including supraventricular arrhythmias, ventricular tachycardias, digitalis-induced tachyarrhythmias, and resistant tachyarrhythmias due to excessive catecholamine activity during anesthesia	**Adult:** 10–30 mg tid or qid, before meals and at bedtime	**Adult:** 1–3 mg IV, slowly (see ADMINISTRATION/DOSAGE ADJUSTMENTS)
Prophylaxis of moderate to severe **angina pectoris**	**Adult:** 10–20 mg/day tid or qid, before meals and at bedtime, to start, followed by gradual increments every 3–7 days until optimal response is achieved, up to 320 mg/day; usual maintenance dosage: 160 mg/day	—
Hypertension	**Adult:** 40 mg bid (alone or with a diuretic) to start, followed by gradual increases until optimal response is achieved, up to 640 mg/day; usual maintenance dosage: 160–480 mg/day	—
Hypertrophic subaortic stenosis	**Adult:** 20–40 mg tid or qid, before meals and at bedtime	—
As an adjunct to alpha-adrenergic blocking agents in the management of **pheochromocytoma**	**Adult:** 60 mg/day div for 3 days prior to surgery, concomitantly with an alpha-adrenergic blocking agent, or 30 mg/day div for inoperable tumors	—
Migraine prophylaxis	**Adult:** 80 mg/day div to start, followed by gradual increments until optimal response is achieved; usual maintenance dosage: 160–240 mg/day	—

ADMINISTRATION/DOSAGE ADJUSTMENTS

Intravenous use	Limited to life-threatening arrhythmias or those occurring under anesthesia. To minimize risk of hypotension and possibility of cardiac standstill, administer slowly (≤1 mg/min) and monitor ECG and CVP continuously. Initial dose may be repeated after 2 min; thereafter, wait at least 4 h before administering additional propranolol.

Note: Full chart appears on page 15.

NORPACE (Disopyrámide phosphate) Searle

Caps: 100, 150 mg

INDICATIONS	ORAL DOSAGE
Premature ventricular contractions, ventricular tachycardia	**Adult:** 400–800 mg/day in 4 divided doses, preceded, if rapid control is essential, by a loading dose of 300 mg; usual therapeutic dosage: 150 mg q6h

ADMINISTRATION/DOSAGE ADJUSTMENTS	
Small patients (weight <110 lb)	Give 100 mg q6h, preceded, if rapid control is essential, by a loading dose of 200 mg
Patients with cardiomyopathy or possible cardiac decompensation	Limit initial dosage to 100 mg q6h and omit loading dose
Hepatic or renal insufficiency	For patients with hepatic insufficiency or *moderate* renal impairment (creatinine clearance rate [CCr] >40 ml/min), limit dosage to 100 mg q6h, with or without a loading dose of 200 mg. For patients with *severe* renal impairment, reduce loading dose to 150 mg and lengthen interval between maintenance doses, as follows: Give 100 mg q8h if CCr=30–40 ml/min; give 100 mg q12h if CCr=15–30 ml/min; or give 100 mg q24h if CCr<15 ml/min.
Transferring patients with normal renal function from procainamide or quinidine to disopyramide	Use normal maintenance dosage, without a loading dose, 3–6 h after last dose of procainamide or 6–12 h after last dose of quinidine
Concomitant antiarrhythmic therapy	Reserve for patients with life-threatening arrhythmias who are unresponsive to single-agent antiarrhythmic therapy
Refractory patients	If patient neither responds nor shows signs of toxicity within 6 h of loading dose, increase maintenance dosage to 200 mg q6h; if there is still no response within 48 h of starting this maintenance regimen, either discontinue use of the drug or consider hospitalizing the patient for careful monitoring while subsequent doses of 250–300 mg q6h are given

CONTRAINDICATIONS		
Second- or third-degree AV block ● (if no pacemaker is present)	Cardiogenic shock ●	Hypersensitivity to disopyramide ●

WARNINGS/PRECAUTIONS	
Congestive heart failure	May be precipitated or worsen; do not use in patients with uncompensated or marginally compensated heart failure, unless failure is due to an arrhythmia. May be used in patients with a history of heart failure, provided that cardiac function is being adequately maintained. If congestive heart failure worsens, discontinue disopyramide therapy and reinstitute at a lower dosage only after cardiac failure has been adequately compensated.
Severe hypotension	May occur, particularly in patients with primary cardiomyopathy or inadequately compensated congestive heart failure; do not use in patients with hypotension, unless hypotension is secondary to cardiac arrhythmia. If hypotension occurs during disopyramide therapy, discontinue use of the drug and, if necessary, reinstitute therapy at a lower dosage.
Heart block	If first-degree heart block develops, reduce dosage; if the block persists despite dosage reduction, the benefits of continuing therapy should be weighed against the risk of higher degrees of heart block. If second- or third-degree AV block or unifascicular, bifascicular, or trifascicular block develops, discontinue use of disopyramide, unless ventricular rate is controlled with an artificial pacemaker.
Atrial tachyarrhythmias	Patients with atrial flutter or fibrillation should be digitalized prior to initiating disopyramide therapy to prevent an excessive increase in ventricular rate
Conduction abnormalities	Use with caution in patients with sick sinus syndrome, Wolff-Parkinson-White syndrome, or bundle branch block
Anticholinergic activity	Unless adequate overriding measures have been taken, do not use in patients with glaucoma, myasthenia gravis, or urinary retention. Urinary retention may occur during disopyramide administration, particularly in males with benign prostatic hypertrophy. Before initiating therapy in patients with a family history of glaucoma, measure intraocular pressure to rule out glaucoma. Use with particular caution in patients with myasthenia gravis due to increased risk of myasthenic crisis.
Hypoglycemia	May occur in rare instances; follow blood glucose levels closely in patients with congestive heart failure, chronic malnutrition, hepatic, renal, or other diseases, or who are taking drugs that could compromise normal glucoregulation in the absence of food, such as beta blockers or alcohol.
Renal or hepatic impairment	May lead to excessive drug accumulation; reduce dosage (see ADMINISTRATION/DOSAGE ADJUSTMENTS) and monitor ECG for signs of toxicity
Hypokalemia	Correct any existing potassium deficit before instituting disopyramide therapy to ensure an adequate antiarrhythmic effect

Table continued on following page

NORPACE continued

ADVERSE REACTIONS	Frequent reactions are italicized
Autonomic nervous system	*Dry mouth (32 %), urinary hesitancy (14%), constipation (11%), blurred vision (3-9%), dry nose, eyes, and throat (3-9%), urinary retention (1-3%)*
Genitourinary	*Urinary frequency and urgency (3-9%),* impotence, dysuria
Gastrointestinal	*Nausea (3-9%), pain, bloating, and flatulence (3-9%), anorexia (1-3%), diarrhea (1-3%), vomiting (1-3%)*
Central nervous system	*Dizziness (3-9%), fatigue and muscle weakness (3-9%), headache (3-9%), malaise (3-9%), aches and pains (3-9%), nervousness (1-3%),* depression, insomnia, numbness and tingling, acute psychoses (rare)
Cardiovascular	*Hypotension (1-3%), congestive heart failure (1-3%), cardiac conduction disturbances (1-3%), edema and weight gain (1-3%), shortness of breath (1-3%), syncope (1-3%), chest pain (1-3%),* AV block
Dermatological	*Rash (1-3%), dermatoses (1-3%), itching (1-3%)*
Hepatic	Cholestatic jaundice (rare)
Other	Hypoglycemia, reversible agranulocytosis (rare)

OVERDOSAGE

Signs and symptoms	Hypotension, worsening of heart failure, widening of QRS complex (>0.04 s) or prolongation of the Q-T interval (>25%), conduction disturbances, bradycardia, asystole, anticholinergic effects (eg, dry mouth, nose, and throat; blurred vision; urinary hesitancy or retention)
Treatment	Withhold disopyramide and other antiarrhythmic agents, especially quinidine and procainamide. Insert pacemaker, if necessary. Institute supportive measures to treat hypotension; if indicated, isoproterenol and/or dopamine may be used. Use other supportive measures, as needed, including digitalization, diuretic therapy, hemoperfusion with charcoal, hemodialysis, intra-aortic balloon counterpulsation, and mechanically assisted ventilation.

DRUG INTERACTIONS

Other antiarrhythmic agents	⇧ Conduction time ⇩ Myocardial contractility

ALTERED LABORATORY VALUES

Blood/serum values	⇧ SGOT ⇧ SGPT ⇧ BUN ⇧ Creatinine ⇧ Cholesterol ⇧ Triglycerides ⇩ Potassium ⇩ Glucose ⇩ Hemoglobin ⇩ Hematocrit

No clinically significant alterations in urinary values occur at therapeutic dosages

Use in children

Safety and effectiveness not established

Use in pregnancy or nursing mothers

Safe use not established during pregnancy or during labor and delivery; may stimulate uterine contractions. Patient should stop nursing if drug is prescribed.

PROCAN SR (Procainamide hydrochloride) **Parke-Davis**

Tabs (sust rel): 250, 500 mg

INDICATIONS	ORAL DOSAGE
Premature ventricular contractions and ventricular tachycardia	**Adult:** initiate therapy with regular procainamide hydrochloride; for maintenance, give 50 mg/kg/day of Procan SR div q3h for premature ventricular contractions or q6h for ventricular tachycardia (see ADMINISTRATION/DOSAGE ADJUSTMENTS)
Atrial fibrillation and paroxysmal atrial tachycardia	**Adult:** initiate therapy with regular procainamide hydrochloride; for maintenance, give 1 g of Procan SR q6h

ADMINISTRATION/DOSAGE ADJUSTMENTS

Oral administration	Treat with regular procainamide hydrochloride until tachycardia or arrhythmia is interrupted or the tolerance limit is reached
Oral dosage schedule	To provide 50 mg/kg/day, give patients weighing <120 lb 500 mg q6h; for patients weighing between 120 and 200 lb, give 750 mg q6h; and for patients weighing >200 lb, give 1g q6h
Chronic therapy	Evaluate antinuclear antibody (ANA) titer periodically and watch for signs of lupus erythematosus syndrome (eg, polyarthralgia, arthritis, pleuritic pain, fever, myalgia, skin lesions; see WARNINGS/PRECAUTIONS)

CONTRAINDICATIONS

Myasthenia gravis	
Hypersensivity to procainamide	Cross-sensitivity to procaine and related drugs may exist
Second- and third-degree AV block	Unless pacemaker is present
Complete AV heart block	

WARNINGS/PRECAUTIONS

Sudden increase in ventricular rate	May result from slowing of atrial rate in atrial fibrillation or flutter; adequate digitalization reduces but does not abolish this danger. If myocardial damage exists, ventricular tachysystole is particularly hazardous.
Embolization	May result from dislodgment of mural thrombi caused by forceful contractions of the atrium with conversion to sinus rhythm; if the patient is already discharging emboli however, procainamide is more likely to stop rather than to aggravate the process
Ventricular tachycardia during occlusive coronary episode	Adjust heart rate with extreme caution
Marked AV conduction disturbances	Use with caution in patients with AV block, bundle-branch block, or severe digitalis intoxication, to avoid additional depression of conduction and ventricular asystole or fibrillation
Asystole	May result if ventricular rate is slowed without attaining regular AV conduction, especially in patients with severe organic heart disease and ventricular tachycardia who may also have undiagnosed complete heart block
Hepatic and renal impairment	May cause drug accumulation, leading to signs and symptoms of overdosage (principally, ventricular tachycardia and severe hypotension)
Positive ANA test	May develop, with or without symptoms of lupus erythematosus, and necessitate alternative antiarrhythmic therapy. If discontinuation of the drug does not induce remission of lupus erythematosus symptoms, steroid therapy may be effective. Concomitant steroid therapy may be used if the syndrome develops in a patient with recurrent life-threatening arrhythmias uncontrollable by other antiarrhythmics.
Potassium balance	Hypokalemia may reduce antiarrhythmic effectiveness, while hyperkalemia may aggravate toxicity[1]

[1]Hoffman BF et al: Electrophysiology and pharmacology of cardiac arrhythmas. VII. Cardiac effects of quinidine and procaine amide. B., in DeGraff A, Frieden J (eds): Appraisal and reappraisal of cardiac therapy. *Am Heart J* 90:117–122, 1975

Table continued on following page

PROCAN SR continued

ADVERSE REACTIONS

Cardiovascular	Hypotension (rare)
Gastrointestinal	Anorexia, nausea, bitter taste, diarrhea
Dermatological	Urticaria, pruritus
Central nervous system	Weakness, mental depression, giddiness, psychosis, hallucinations
Hematological	Agranulocytosis (occasionally fatal)
Hypersensitivity reactions	Angioneurotic edema, maculopapular rash
Systemic	Fever and chills; lupus erythematosus-like syndrome characterized by polyarthralgia, arthritis, pleuritic pain, myalgia, skin lesions, pleural effusion, pericarditis, thrombocytopenia (rare); Coomb's positive hemolytic anemia (rare)

OVERDOSAGE

Signs and symptoms	Hypotension, heart failure, ventricular arrhythmias, widening of QRS complex (>0.04 s), prolongation of Q-T interval (>25%), bradycardia, heart block
Treatment	Withhold procainamide and other antiarrhythmic agents, especially quinidine and disopyramide. Insert pacemaker, if necessary. Institute supportive therapy. Counteract severe hypotension with phenylephrine or levarterenol.

DRUG INTERACTIONS

Other antiarrhythmic agents	⇧ Depression of excitabilty and/or conduction ⇩ Myocardial contractility

ALTERED LABORATORY VALUES

Blood/serum values	⇧ Alkaline phosphatase ⇩ Bilirubin ⇧ Lactate dehydrogenase ⇧ SGOT ⇧ ANA titer

No clinically significant alterations in urinary values occur at therapeutic dosages

Use in children

General guidelines not established

Use in pregnancy or nursing mothers

General guidelines not established

PRONESTYL (Procainamide hydrochloride) Squibb

Caps: 250, 375, 500 mg **Tabs:** 250, 375, 500 mg **Vials:** 100 mg/ml (10 ml), 500 mg/ml (2 ml)

INDICATIONS	ORAL DOSAGE	PARENTERAL DOSAGE
Premature ventricular contractions	**Adult:** 50 mg/kg/day div q3h (see ADMINISTRATION/DOSAGE ADJUSTMENTS)	—
Ventricular tachycardia	**Adult:** 1 g to start, followed by 50 mg/kg/day div q3h (see ADMINISTRATION/DOSAGE ADJUSTMENTS)	—
Atrial fibrillation and paroxysmal atrial tachycardia	**Adult:** 1.25 g to start, followed 1 h later by 0.75 g and then 0.5–1.0 g q2h until arrhythmia is interrupted or tolerance is reached; usual maintenance dosage: 0.5–1.0 g q4–6h	—
Ventricular extrasystoles and tachycardia, atrial fibrillation, and paroxysmal atrial tachycardia	—	**Adult:** 0.5–1.0 g IM q4–8h until oral therapy is possible, or 100 mg IV (25–50 mg/min) until arrhythmia is suppressed or a total dose of 1 g is given, followed by 2–6 mg/min by IV infusion, depending on patient's body weight, circulatory condition, and adrenal function; alternative regimen: 500–600 mg by IV infusion at a constant rate for 25–30 min to start, followed by 2–6 mg/min by IV infusion
Cardiac arrhythmias associated with anesthesia and surgery	—	**Adult:** 0.1–0.5 g IM (preferably) or IV (slowly)

ADMINISTRATION/DOSAGE ADJUSTMENTS

Oral administration	Preferred for treatment of arrhythmias that do not require immediate suppression or for continuation of treatment after control of serious arrhythmias with parenteral form or other antiarrhythmic therapy
Oral dosage schedule	To provide 50 mg/kg/day, give patients weighing <120 lb 250 mg q3h; for patients weighing between 120 and 200 lb, give 375 mg q3h; and for patients weighing >200 lb, give 500 mg q3h
Intramuscular administration	May be preferable to oral route in patients who are vomiting, or who should receive nothing by mouth before surgery, or when there is reason to believe that absorption may be unreliable
Intravenous administration	Blood pressure and ECG must be monitored before each dose is given. Terminate parenteral therapy as soon as basic cardiac rhythm stabilizes. Wait 3–4 h after giving last IV dose before instituting oral antiarrhythmic therapy, if indicated.
Chronic therapy	Evaluate antinuclear antibody (ANA) titer periodically and watch for signs of lupus erythematosus syndrome (eg, polyarthralgia, arthritis, pleuritic pain, fever, myalgia, skin lesions; see WARNINGS/PRECAUTIONS)

CONTRAINDICATIONS

Myasthenia gravis	
Hypersensivity to procainamide	Cross-sensitivity to procaine and related drugs may exist
Second- and third-degree AV block	Unless pacemaker is present
Complete AV heart block	

WARNINGS/PRECAUTIONS

Sudden increase in ventricular rate	May result from slowing of atrial rate in atrial fibrillation or flutter; adequate digitalization reduces but does not abolish this danger. If myocardial damage exists, ventricular tachysystole is particularly hazardous.
Embolization	May result from dislodgment of mural thrombi caused by forceful contractions of the atrium with conversion to sinus rhythm; if the patient is already discharging emboli, however, procainamide is more likely to stop rather than to aggravate the process

Table continued on following page

PRONESTYL continued

WARNINGS/PRECAUTIONS continued

Ventricular tachycardia during occlusive coronary episode	Adjust heart rate with extreme caution
Marked AV conduction disturbances	Use with caution in patients with second- or third-degree AV block, bundle-branch block, or severe digitalis intoxication, to avoid additional depression of conduction and ventricular asystole or fibrillation
Asystole	May result if ventricular rate is slowed without attaining regular AV conduction, especially in patients with severe organic heart disease and ventricular tachycardia who may also have undiagnosed complete heart block
Hepatic and renal impairment	May cause drug accumulation, leading to signs and symptoms of overdosage (principally, ventricular tachycardia and severe hypotension)
Positive ANA test	May develop, with or without symptoms of lupus erythematosus, and necessitate alternative antiarrhythmic therapy. If discontinuation of the drug does not induce remission of lupus erythematosus symptoms, steroid therapy may be effective. Concomitant steroid therapy may be used if the syndrome develops in a patient with recurrent life-threatening arrhythmias uncontrollable by other antiarrhythmic agents.
Potassium balance	Hypokalemia may reduce antiarrhythmic effectiveness, while hyperkalemia may aggravate toxicity[1]

ADVERSE REACTIONS

Cardiovascular	Hypotension (most common with IV use); ventricular arrhythmias, including asystole, tachycardia, and fibrillation (most common with IV use)
Gastrointestinal	Anorexia (with oral use), nausea (with oral use), bitter taste, diarrhea
Dermatological	Urticaria and pruritus (with oral use)
Central nervous system	Weakness, mental depression, giddiness, psychosis, hallucinations
Hematological	Agranulocytosis (occasionally fatal)
Hypersensitivity reactions	Angioneurotic edema, maculopapular rash
Systemic	Fever and chills; lupus erythematosus-like syndrome characterized by polyarthralgia, arthritis, pleuritic pain, myalgia, skin lesions, pleural effusion, pericarditis, and thrombocytopenia (rare); Coombs' positive hemolytic anemia (rare)

OVERDOSAGE

Signs and symptoms	Hypotension, heart failure, ventricular arrhythmias, widening of QRS complex (>0.04 s), prolongation of Q-T interval (>25%), prolongation of P-R interval, bradycardia, heart block
Treatment	Withhold procainamide and other antiarrhythmic agents, especially quinidine and disopyramide. Insert pacemaker, if necessary. Institute supportive therapy. Counteract severe hypotension with phenylephrine or levarterenol.

DRUG INTERACTIONS

Other antiarrhythmic agents	⇧ Depression of excitability and/or conduction ⇩ Myocardial contractility

ALTERED LABORATORY VALUES

Blood/serum values	⇧ Alkaline phosphatase ⇩ Bilirubin ⇧ Lactate dehydrogenase ⇧ SGOT ⇧ ANA titer

No clinically significant alterations in urinary values occur at therapeutic dosages

Use in children	Use in pregnancy or nursing mothers
General guidelines not established	General guidelines not established

[1]Hoffman BF et al: Electrophysiology and pharmacology of cardiac arrhythmas. VII. Cardiac effects of quinidine and procaine amide. B., in DeGraff A, Frieden J (eds): Appraisal and reappraisal of cardiac therapy. *Am Heart J* 90:117-122, 1975

QUINAGLUTE (Quinidine gluconate) Berlex

Tabs (sust rel): 324 mg

INDICATIONS	ORAL DOSAGE
Prevention of premature atrial, nodal, or ventricular contractions	**Adult:** 324–648 mg (1–2 tabs) q8–12h
Maintenance of normal sinus rhythm following conversion of atrial fibrillation, tachycardia, or flutter	**Adult:** 648 mg (2 tabs) q12h or 486–648 mg (1½–2 tabs) q8h

ADMINISTRATION/DOSAGE ADJUSTMENTS	
Dosage range for individual patients	Normal sinus rhythm may be maintained in some patients with 324 mg (1 tab) q8–12h, while other patients may require larger doses or more frequent administration (eg, q6h)
Gastrointestinal disturbances	May be minimized by administering drug with food

CONTRAINDICATIONS	
Aberrant impulses and abnormal rhythms	Due to escape mechanisms
Partial AV or complete heart block, or intraventricular conduction defects	Especially those exhibiting marked widening of QRS complex
Renal disease	Resulting in significant azotemia or in the development of cardiotoxic effects, including conduction defects
Premature ventricular beats, ventricular tachycardia, or flutter	While patient is receiving quinidine
Marked cardiac enlargement	Particularly when accompanied by congestive heart failure, poor renal function, and especially, renal tubular acidosis
Idiosyncratic reaction or hypersensitivity	To quinidine

WARNINGS/PRECAUTIONS	
Extremely rapid ventricular rate	May result during the treatment of atrial flutter, from progressive reduction in the degree of AV block to a 1:1 ratio preceding reversion to sinus rhythm
Hypersensitivity to quinidine	Although rare, should be considered constantly, especially during first weeks of therapy; symptons of cinchonism (ringing in ears, headache, nausea, and/or visual disturbances) may appear in sensitive patients after a single dose
Idiosyncratic reaction to quinidine	May be determined by administering a preliminary test dose of 1 tab
Special-risk patients, high dosages	Use with extreme caution in senile patients and in those with severe heart disease, hypotension, or digitalis intoxication; hospitalization for close clinical observation, ECG monitoring, and, possibly, determination of plasma quinidine levels may be required

Table continued on following page

QUINAGLUTE continued

ADVERSE REACTIONS

Central nervous system	Headache, fever, vertigo, apprehension, excitement, confusion, delirium, syncope
Auditory	Tinnitus, decreased acuity
Ophthalmic	Mydriasis, blurred vision, disturbed color perception, reduced visual field, photophobia, diplopia, night blindness, scotomata, optic neuritis
Cardiovascular	Widening of QRS complex, cardiac asystole, ectopic ventricular beats, idioventricular rhythms (including ventricular tachycardia and fibrillation) paradoxical tachycardia, arterial embolism, hypotension
Gastrointestinal	Nausea, vomiting, abdominal pain, diarrhea
Dermatological	Cutaneous flushing with intense pruritus
Hematological	Acute hemolytic anemia, hypoprothrombinemia, thrombocytopenic purpura, agranulocytosis
Hypersensitivity	Angioedema, acute asthmatic episodes, vascular collapse, respiratory arrest

OVERDOSAGE

Signs and symptoms	Hypotension, heart failure, ventricular arrhythmias, widening of QRS complex (>0.04 s), prolongation of Q-T interval (>25%), bradycardia, heart blockage, symptoms of cinchonism (see ADVERSE REACTIONS)
Treatment	Withhold quinidine and other antiarrythmic agents, especially procainamide and disopyramide. Insert pacemaker, if necessary. Institute supportive therapy. Correct acidosis or hyperkalemia, if present.

DRUG INTERACTIONS

Other antiarrhythmic agents	⇧ Depression of excitability ⇩ Myocardial contractility
Oral anticoagulants	⇧ Hypoprothrombinemia, possibly resulting in hemorrhage
Neuromuscular blocking agents	⇧ Neuromuscular blockade
Phenobarbital, phenytoin	⇩ Serum half-life of quinidine
Digoxin	⇧ Digoxin serum level, possibly resulting in toxicity

ALTERED LABORATORY VALUES

No clinically significant alterations in blood/serum or urinary values occur at therapeutic dosages

Use in children

General guidelines not established

Use in pregnancy or nursing mothers

General guidelines not established

QUINIDEX (Quinidine sulfate) Robins

Tabs (sust rel): 300 mg

INDICATIONS	ORAL DOSAGE
Premature atrial and ventricular contractions; paroxysmal atrial tachycardia; paroxysmal atrioventricular junctional rhythm; atrial flutter; paroxysmal atrial fibrillation; established atrial fibrillation when therapy is appropriate; **paroxysmal ventricular tachycardia** when not associated with complete heart block; **maintenance therapy** after electrical conversion of atrial fibrillation and/or flutter	**Adult:** 600 mg q8–12h

ADMINISTRATION/DOSAGE ADJUSTMENTS

Gastrointestinal disturbances	May be minimized by administering drug with food

CONTRAINDICATIONS

Intraventricular conduction defects	
Atrioventricular block	
Hypersensitivity or idiosyncratic reaction	To quinidine sulfate
Aberrant impulses and abnormal rhythms	Resulting from escape mechanisms

WARNINGS/PRECAUTIONS

Extremely rapid ventricular rate	May result during the treatment of atrial flutter from progressive reduction in degree of AV block preceding reversion to sinus rhythm
Cardiotoxicity	Discontinue therapy immediately if QRS complex widens by 50%, or if frequent ectopic ventricular beats appear. Monitor ECG closely; if necessary, administer 1 M sodium lactate.
Vagal stimulation	May fail to terminate paroxysmal supraventricular tachycardia
Asystole, complete heart block	May occur in patients with incomplete AV block; use with extreme caution
Other antiarrhythmic agents	Use with extreme caution in quinidine-treated patients
Concomitant treatment with digitalis	Unpredictable rhythm abnormalities may occur; use with particular caution in the presence of digitalis intoxication
Potassium serum levels	Hypokalemia may reduce antiarrhythmic effect, while hyperkalemia may enhance toxicity
Congestive heart failure, hypotension	Cardiac contractility and arterial blood pressure are depressed; use only if heart failure or hypotension are due to, or aggravated by, the arrhythmia
Hepatic and/or renal insufficiency	May delay excretion, increase serum levels, and lead to systemic accumulation (see OVERDOSAGE); use with caution
Special-risk patients	Use with extreme caution in patients with bronchial asthma or other respiratory disorders, myasthenia gravis, muscle weakness, acute infection, or hyperthyroidism
Long-term therapy	Perform periodic blood counts and liver- and kidney-function tests; discontinue use if blood dyscrasias or signs of hepatic or renal impairment occur

Table continued on following page

QUINIDEX continued

ADVERSE REACTIONS	
Allergic and idiosyncratic	Fever, skin eruptions, thrombocytopenia (extremely rare)
Central nervous system	Tinnitus, blurred vision, dizziness, lightheadedness, tremor
Gastrointestinal	Nausea, vomiting, diarrhea, colic
Cardiovascular	Ventricular extrasystoles, widening of QRS complex, complete AV block, ventricular tachycardia

OVERDOSAGE	
Signs and symptoms	See ADVERSE REACTIONS
Treatment	Withhold quinidine and other antiarrhythmic agents, especially procainamide and disopyramide. Insert pacemaker, if necessary, and institute supportive therapy. For hypotension, use a vasoconstrictor and/or catecholamine. Correct acidosis or hyperkalemia, if present. Cardiotoxic signs may be reversed by administering 1 M sodium lactate.

DRUG INTERACTIONS	
Other antiarrhythmic agents	⇧ Depression of excitability ⇩ Myocardial contractility
Oral anticoagulants	⇧ Hypoprothrombinemia, possibly resulting in hemorrhage
Neuromuscular blocking agents	⇧ Neuromuscular blockade
Phenobarbital, phenytoin	⇩ Serum half-life of quinidine
Digoxin	⇧ Digoxin serum level, possibly resulting in toxicity

ALTERED LABORATORY VALUES

No clinically significant alterations in blood/serum or urinary values occur at therapeutic dosages

Use in children

General guidelines not established

Use in pregnancy or nursing mothers

General guidelines not established

QUINIDINE SULFATE Parke-Davis

Tabs: 200 mg

INDICATIONS	ORAL DOSAGE
Premature atrial and ventricular contractions	**Adult:** 200–300 mg tid or qid **Child:** 30 mg/kg/24 h, or 900 mg/m²/24 h, in 5 divided doses
Paroxysmal supraventricular tachycardias	**Adult:** 400–600 mg q2–3h until paroxysm is terminated **Child:** same as above
Conversion of atrial fibrillation	**Adult:** 200 mg q2–3h for 5–8 doses, followed by daily increases, up to 3–4 g/day, until sinus rhythm is restored or toxicity occurs **Child:** same as above
Maintenance therapy following electrical conversion of atrial fibrillation and/or flutter	**Adult:** 200–300 mg tid or qid **Child:** same as above

ADMINISTRATION/DOSAGE ADJUSTMENTS

Preliminary test dose	Often administered to determine presence of hypersensitivity or idiosyncratic reaction. Adults may be given 200 mg as a test dose; for children, use 2 mg/kg, or 60 mg/m².
Atrial flutter	Patient should be started on digitalis before quinidine therapy is instituted; dosage must be individualized
Atrial fibrillation	Ventricular rate and congestive heart failure, if present, must be brought under control by digitalization before quinidine therapy is instituted
High-dosage therapy	Monitor ECG continuously and determine plasma quinidine levels when large doses (>2 g/day) are used

CONTRAINDICATIONS

Hypersensitivity or idiosyncratic reaction	To quinidine sulfate
Thrombocytopenic purpura	Associated with previous use of quinidine
Digitalis intoxication	Manifested by AV conduction disturbances
Complete atrioventricular block	With AV nodal or idioventricular pacemaker
Ectopic impulses and rhythms	Resulting from escape mechanisms

WARNINGS/PRECAUTIONS

Extremely rapid ventricular rate	May result in the treatment of atrial flutter from progressive reduction in degree of AV block preceding reversion to sinus rhythm; potential risk may be lessened by digitalization prior to treatment with quinidine
Cardiotoxicity	Discontinue therapy immediately if QRS complex widens by 50%, or if frequent ectopic ventricular beats appear. Monitor ECG closely; if necessary, administer 1 M sodium lactate.
Vagal stimulation	May fail to terminate paroxysmal supraventricular tachycardia
Asystole, complete heart block	May occur in patients with incomplete AV block; use with extreme caution
Other cardiac agents	Use with extreme caution in quinidine-treated patients
Concomitant treatment with digitalis	Unpredictable rhythm abnormalities may occur; use with particular caution in the presence of digitalis intoxication
Potassium serum levels	Hypokalemia may reduce antiarrhythmic effect, while hyperkalemia may enhance toxicity
Congestive heart failure, hypotension	Cardiac contractility and arterial blood pressure are depressed; use only if heart failure or hypotension are due to, or aggravated by, the arrhythmia

Table continued on following page

Hepatic and/or renal insufficiency	May delay excretion, increase serum levels, and lead to systemic accumulation (see OVERDOSAGE); use with caution
Special-risk patients	Use with extreme caution in patients with bronchial asthma or other respiratory disorders, myasthenia gravis, muscle weakness, acute infection, or hyperthyroidism
Long-term therapy	Perform periodic blood counts and liver- and kidney-function tests; discontinue use if blood dyscrasias or signs of hepatic or renal impairment occur

ADVERSE REACTIONS

Central nervous system	Headache, vertigo, apprehension, excitement, confusion, delirium, syncope
Otic	Tinnitus, decreased acuity
Ophthalmic	Mydriasis, blurred vision, disturbed color perception, photophobia, diplopia, night blindness, scotomata, optic neuritis
Cardiovascular	Widening of QRS complex, cardiac asystole, ectopic ventricular beats, idioventricular rhythms (including ventricular tachycardia and fibrillation), paradoxical tachycardia, arterial embolism
Gastrointestinal	Diarrhea, nausea, vomiting, abdominal pain
Hematological	Acute hemolytic anemia, hypoprothrombinemia, thrombocytopenic purpura, agranulocytosis
Dermatological	Cutaneous flushing with intense pruritus
Hypersensitivity	Angioedema, acute asthmatic episodes, vascular collapse, respiratory arrest
Other	Fever

OVERDOSAGE

Signs and symptoms	Tinnitus, headache, visual disturbances, hypotension, heart failure, widening of QRS complex (>50%), prolongation of Q-T interval (>25%), frequent ectopic ventricular beats, bradycardia, heart block
Treatment	Withhold quinidine and other antiarrhythmic agents, especially procainamide and disopyramide. Insert pacemaker, if necessary, and institute supportive therapy. For hypotension, use a vasoconstrictor and/or catecholamine. Correct acidosis or hyperkalemia, if present. Cardiotoxic signs may be reversed by administering 1 M sodium lactate.

DRUG INTERACTIONS

Other antiarrhythmic agents	⇧ Depression of excitability ⇩ Myocardial contractility
Oral anticoagulants	⇧ Hypoprothrombinemia, possibly resulting in hemorrhage
Neuromuscular blocking agents	⇧ Neuromuscular blockade
Phenobarbital, phenytoin	⇩ Serum half-life of quinidine
Digoxin	⇧ Digoxin serum level, possibly resulting in toxicity

ALTERED LABORATORY VALUES

No clinically significant alterations in blood/serum or urinary values occur at therapeutic dosages

Use in children

See INDICATIONS

Use in pregnancy or nursing mothers

Reserve use during pregnancy only for cases in which benefits outweigh potential hazards to patient and fetus. Quinidine is excreted in breast milk; use with extreme caution in nursing mothers.

XYLOCAINE (Lidocaine hydrocloride) Astra

Amps: 20 mg/ml (5 ml) for direct IV injection; 100 mg/ml (5 ml) for IM use **Vial:** 40 mg/ml (25, 50 ml) for IV infusion
Syringe: 20 mg/ml (5 ml) for direct IV injection **Additive syringes:** 200 mg/ml (5, 10 ml) for IV infusion

INDICATIONS	PARENTERAL DOSAGE
Ventricular arrhythmias occurring during cardiac manipulation, such as cardiac surgery **Life-threatening arrhythmias,** particularly ventricular arrhythmias, such as those occurring during acute myocardial infarction	**Adult:** 50–100 mg IV (20–50 mg/min), repeated in 5 min, if necessary; no more than 200–300 mg should be given over 1 h

ADMINISTRATION/DOSAGE ADJUSTMENTS

Patients with recurrent arrhythmias	Following a single 100-mg IV dose, begin IV infusion at a rate of 1–4 mg/min (20–50 μg/min in the average 70-kg man) under constant ECG monitoring. Terminate IV infusion as soon as basic cardiac rhythm stabilizes or signs of toxicity appear; if indicated, switch to maintenance oral antiarrhythmic regimen at earliest opportunity.
Intramuscular administration	Use 100 mg/ml concentration. Inject 4.3 mg/kg (~2 mg/lb), preferably into the deltoid muscle, when (1) ECG equipment is unavailable to verify the diagnosis, but potential benefits outweigh possible risks, or (2) facilities for IV administration are unavailable. Paramedical personnel in a mobile coronary-care unit may administer drug at the direction of the physician viewing the transmitted ECG. If necessary, repeat IM dose 60–90 min after initial injection. Change to IV or oral therapy as soon as possible, if indicated.

CONTRAINDICATIONS

Hypersensitivity to amide-type local anesthetics●

Wolff-Parkinson-White syndrome (for IV use)●

Stokes-Adams syndrome●

Severe sinoatrial, atrioventricular, or intraventricular block●

WARNINGS/PRECAUTIONS

ECG monitoring	Constant monitoring is essential for proper IV administration and recommended during IM administration
Accelerated ventricular rate	May occur during IV administration in patients with atrial fibrillation
Inadvertent intravascular administration	Aspirate frequently during IM administration
Hepatic or renal impairment	May cause accumulation of drug and/or its metabolites with repeated use, resulting in toxicity (see OVERDOSAGE)
Sinus bradycardia, incomplete heart block	More frequent and serious ventricular arrhythmias or complete heart block may occur following either IV administration or failure to accelerate heart rate (eg, by isoproterenol or electric pacing)
Special-risk patients	Use with caution in patients with hypovolemia, shock, and all forms of heart block

ADVERSE REACTIONS

Central nervous system	Lightheadedness, drowsiness, dizziness, apprehension, euphoria, tinnitus, blurred or double vision; sensation of heat, cold, or numbness; twitching, tremors, convulsions, unconsciousness, respiratory depression and arrest
Gastrointestinal	Vomiting
Cardiovascular	Hypotension, collapse, and bradycardia, leading to cardiac arrest
Hypersensitivity	Allergic reactions (infrequent)
Other	Soreness at IM injection site (occasional)

Table continued on following page

XYLOCAINE continued

OVERDOSAGE

Signs and symptoms	Drowsiness, confusion, dyspnea, prolongation of P-R interval, widening of QRS complex, increase in arrhythmias, severe convulsions, respiratory depression and arrest, circulatory collapse
Treatment	Discontinue use and institute emergency resuscitative procedures. Maintain patent airway and adequate ventilation. For severe convulsions, administer small doses of diazepam or an ultra-short-acting barbiturate (eg, thiopental or thiamylal), or if these are unavailable, a short-acting barbiturate (eg, pentobarbital or secobarbital); if patient is under anesthesia, a short-acting muscle relaxant (eg, succinylcholine) may be given IV. For circulatory depression, a vasopressor, such as ephedrine or metaraminol, may be used.

DRUG INTERACTIONS

Phenobarbital, phenytoin (chronic administration)	⇩ Antiarrhythmic effect
Isoniazid, chloramphenicol	⇧ Antiarrhythmic effect and toxicity
Propranolol	⇧ Antiarrhythmic effect

ALTERED LABORATORY VALUES

Blood/serum values	⇧ Creatine phosphokinase (with IM use)

No clinically significant alterations in urinary values occur at therapeutic dosages

Use in children

General guidelines not established

Use in pregnancy or nursing mothers

Safe use not established

CRYSTODIGIN (Digitoxin) Lilly

Tabs: 0.05, 0.1, 0.15, 0.2 mg **Amps:** 0.2 mg/ml (1 ml)

INDICATIONS	ORAL DOSAGE	PARENTERAL DOSAGE
Congestive heart failure **Atrial fibrillation and flutter** **Paroxysmal atrial tachycardia**	**Adult:** 0.2 mg bid for 4 days to start, or 0.6 mg initially, then 0.4 and 0.2 mg 4–6 h apart, followed by 0.05–0.3 mg/day for maintenance **Premature infants, newborns under 2 wk of age, and infants with reduced renal function or myocarditis:** 0.022 mg/kg in 3 or more divided doses at least 6 h apart; maintenance dosage: 1/10 digitalizing dosage **Infant (2 wk–1 yr):** 0.045 mg/kg in 3 or more divided doses at least 6 h apart; maintenance dosage: 1/10 digitalizing dosage **Child (1–2 yr):** 0.04 mg/kg in 3 or more divided doses at least 6 h apart; maintenance dosage: 1/10 digitalizing dosage **Child (>2 yr):** 0.03 mg/kg in 3 or more divided doses at least 6 h apart; maintenance dosage: 1/10 digitalizing dosage	**Adult:** 1.2–1.6 mg IV (slowly) div to start, or 0.6 mg initially, then 0.4 and 0.2 mg q4–6h until full therapeutic effect is evident, followed by 0.05–0.3 mg/day **Premature infants, newborns under 2 wk of age, and infants with reduced renal function or myocarditis:** 0.022 mg/kg IV (slowly) in 3 or more divided doses at least 6 h apart; maintenance dosage: 1/10 digitalizing dosage **Infant (2 wk to 1 yr):** 0.045 mg/kg IV (slowly) in 3 or more divided doses at least 6h apart; maintenance dosage: 1/10 digitalizing dosage **Child (1–2 yr):** 0.04 mg/kg IV (slowly) in 3 or more divided doses at least 6 h apart; maintenance dosage: 1/10 digitalizing dosage **Child (>2 yr):** 0.03 mg/kg IV (slowly) in 3 or more divided doses at least 6 h apart; maintenance dosage: 1/10 digitalizing dosage

CONTRAINDICATIONS

Ventricular tachycardia ● Beriberi heart disease ● Digitalis toxicity or hypersensitivity ●

Carotid sinus hypersensitivity ●

WARNINGS/PRECAUTIONS

Arrhythmias	May reflect digitalis toxicity or may be caused by underlying heart disease; to ascertain which, withhold drug temporarily if clinical situation permits
Nausea and vomiting	May reflect digitalis toxicity or may be caused by underlying heart disease; determine cause before continuing use of drug
Idiopathic hypertrophic subaortic stenosis	Outflow obstruction may worsen; digitalis therapy probably should not be employed unless cardiac failure is severe
Acute glomerulonephritis accompanying congestive heart failure	Use with extreme care; total dose for digitalization should be relatively low and given in divided doses with concomitant use of reserpine or other antihypertensive therapy and continual ECG monitoring. Discontinue use of digitoxin as soon as possible.
Rheumatic carditis	Rhythm disturbances may occur; if heart failure develops, use relatively low doses and cautiously increase dosage until benefit is obtained. If no improvement is obtained, discontinue use of digitoxin.
Potassium depletion, hypokalemia	Toxicity is likely to occur even with usual dosage; positive inotropic effect of digitoxin may be reduced. Use with caution in malnourished or elderly patients, patients with long-standing congestive heart failure, and those receiving hemodialysis or diuretic or corticosteroid therapy.
Calcium	May produce serious arrhythmias; calcium salts should not be given intravenously
Myxedema	Decreases rate of excretion of digitoxin, raising blood level; reduce dosage accordingly
Incomplete AV heart block	May worsen, especially in patients with Stokes-Adams attacks; alternative therapy for heart failure should be considered
Chronic constrictive pericarditis	Response is likely to be unfavorable
Renal insufficiency	Delays excretion of digitoxin, raising blood level; reduce dosage accordingly
Cardioversion	Dose may need to be decreased before electrical conversion of arrhythmias
Special-risk patients	Use with caution in patients with hypercalcemia or multiple ventricular extrasystoles and in patients with acute myocardial infarction or acute myocarditis, severe pulmonary disease, or far-advanced heart failure to minimize risk of rhythm disturbances

Table continued on following page

WARNINGS/PRECAUTIONS continued

Patients already taking digitalis	Should not receive rapid digitalizing dose
Impaired liver function	May necessitate dosage reduction

ADVERSE REACTIONS

Gastrointestinal	Anorexia, nausea, vomiting, diarrhea, abdominal pain or discomfort
Central nervous system	Headache, weakness, apathy, visual disturbances (blurred or yellow vision), depression, confusion, disorientation, delirium
Endocrinological	Gynecomastia
Cardiovascular	Arrhythmias, including ventricular premature beats (except in infants and young children), paroxysmal and nonparoxysmal nodal rhythms, AV dissociation, and paroxysmal atrial tachycardia with block, ventricular tachycardia, ventricular fibrillation, atrial fibrillation

OVERDOSAGE

Signs and symptoms	See ADVERSE REACTIONS
Treatment	Discontinue use of digitoxin. To control arrhythmias in patients with adequate renal function, administer potassium in divided oral doses of 4–6 g/day for adults and 1–2 g/day for children. If correction of the arrhythmia is urgent, potassium may be given IV in 5% dextrose-in-water, provided that the serum potassium level is normal or low and that severe or complete heart block due to digitalis and unrelated to any tachyarrhythmia is absent. Adults may be given 40–100 mEq (in a concentration of 40 mEq/500 ml) at a rate of 40 mEq/h, or more slowly if pain occurs at the injection site; children may be given 5–10 mEq/h at a concentration of 5–10 mEq/100 ml. Additional amounts may be given if the arrhythmia is uncontrolled and the potassium is well tolerated. If potassium fails or is contraindicated, arrhythmias may be controlled with disodium EDTA or, if necessary, an appropriate antiarrhythmic agent (eg, quinidine, procainamide, propranolol).

DRUG INTERACTIONS

Potassium-depleting diuretics	⇧ Digitoxin toxicity
Corticosteroids	⇧ Digitoxin toxicity may occur secondary to resulting hypokalemia
Antacids	⇩ Digitoxin absorption
Kaolin-pectin	⇩ Digitoxin absorption
Neomycin	⇩ Digitoxin absorption
Cholestyramine	⇩ Digitoxin absorption
Quinidine	⇧ Serum digitoxin level
Propranolol	⇧ Risk of AV block; combination often used advantageously for control of atrial fibrillation
Sympathomimetic agents, calcium, succinylcholine	May precipitate or exacerbate digitalis-induced arrhythmias
Antihistamines	⇧ Digitoxin metabolism
Anticonvulsants	⇧ Digitoxin metabolism
Barbiturates	⇧ Digitoxin metabolism
Oral hypoglycemics	⇧ Digitoxin metabolism

ALTERED LABORATORY VALUES

No clinically significant alterations in blood/serum or urinary values occur at therapeutic dosages; hyperkalemia occurs with massive overdosage

Use in children

See INDICATIONS; dosage must be carefully titrated with continuous ECG monitoring to avoid toxicity

Use in pregnancy or nursing mothers

Safe use in pregnancy not established; give only when clearly indicated. Use with caution in nursing mothers.

DYRENIUM (Triamterene) Smith Kline & French

Caps: 50, 100 mg

INDICATIONS	ORAL DOSAGE
Edema associated with congestive heart failure, hepatic cirrhosis, the nephrotic syndrome, steroid therapy, idiopathic causes, and secondary hyperaldosteronism	**Adult:** 100 mg bid after meals, or up to 300 mg/day in resistant cases

ADMINISTRATION/DOSAGE ADJUSTMENTS	
Combination therapy	Reduce daily dosage of each agent initially, then adjust to patient's needs; discontinue potassium supplementation

CONTRAINDICATIONS	
Anuria	
Severe or progressive kidney disease	With possible exception of nephrosis
Severe hepatic disease	
Hypersensitivity	To triamterene
Pre-existing hyperkalemia	In patients with azotemia or impaired renal function or developing during therapy
Concurrent potassium supplementation	As medication or in the form of a potassium-rich diet

WARNINGS/PRECAUTIONS	
Blood dyscrasias, liver damage, and other idiosyncratic reactions	May occur; monitor patients regularly
Kidney function	Monitor BUN and serum potassium periodically, especially in the elderly and in patients with suspected or confirmed renal insufficiency or diabetes
Hyperkalemia	May occur, especially with prolonged therapy at high dosage; rarely causes cardiac irregularities. If hyperkalemia develops, discontinue use; to avoid rebound kaliuresis, withdraw drug gradually.
Concomitant spironolactone therapy	May cause hyperkalemia; use with caution, if at all, and determine serum potassium levels frequently
Electrolyte imbalances	May occur or worsen, especially in patients with congestive heart failure, renal disease, or cirrhosis; measure serum electrolytes periodically
Megaloblastosis	May occur in cirrhotic patients with splenomegaly; periodic blood studies are advisable
Low-salt syndrome	May occur with full dosage in salt-restricted patients
Metabolic acidosis	May occur due to drug-induced decrease in alkali reserve
Nitrogen retention	May be minimized by alternate-day therapy
Hyperuricemia	May occur, especially in patients predisposed to gouty arthritis
Lithium therapy	Renal clearance is reduced, increasing risk of lithium toxicity; coadministration generally should be avoided unless adequate precautions are taken

ADVERSE REACTIONS[1]	
Central nervous system	Weakness, headache
Gastrointestinal	Nausea,[2] vomiting,[2] dry mouth, other GI disturbances
Hypersensitivity	Anaphylaxis, photosensitivity, rash
Other	Renal stones[3]

[1]Rarely necessitate discontinuation of therapy
[2]May also indicate electrolyte imbalance
[3]Triamterene has been found in renal stones in association with other usual calculus components

Table continued on following page

DYRENIUM continued

OVERDOSAGE

Signs and symptoms	Electrolyte imbalance; hyperkalemia; nausea, vomiting, and other GI disturbances; weakness; hypotension
Treatment	Empty stomach by inducing emesis, followed by gastric lavage and activated charcoal. Monitor electrolyte levels and fluid balance. Treat hypotension by elevating feet and by volume expansion alone, if possible. Treat GI effects symptomatically.

DRUG INTERACTIONS

Antihypertensive agents	⇩ Blood pressure
Spironolactone	⇧ Risk of hyperkalemia
Potassium salts	⇧ Risk of hyperkalemia
Lithium	⇩ Lithium clearance

ALTERED LABORATORY VALUES

Blood/serum values	⇧ Uric acid[4] ⇧ Lactate dehydrogenase ⇩ Sodium ⇧ Potassium ⇩ Chloride ⇧ or ⇩ Glucose ⇧ BUN ⇧ Creatinine
Urinary values	⇧ Sodium ⇩ Potassium ⇧ Chloride ⇧ Uric acid[4]

Use in children

General guidelines not established

Use in pregnancy or nursing mothers

Safe use has not been established during pregnancy. Triamterene crosses the placental barrier of ewes and appears in cord blood, which may also occur in humans. In general, diuretics should not be given to pregnant women except for pathologic edema; however, a short course of diuretic therapy may be appropriate for hypervolemia-dependent edema that is causing extreme discomfort unrelieved by rest. Triamterene also appears in cow's milk and may be excreted in human breast milk. Patient should stop nursing if drug is prescribed.

[4]Especially in patients predisposed to gouty arthritis

LANOXIN (Digoxin) Burroughs Wellcome

Tabs: 0.125, 0.25, 0.5 mg **Elixir (ped):** 0.05 mg/ml **Amps:** 0.25 mg/ml (2 ml) **Amps (ped inj):** 0.1 mg/ml (1 ml)

INDICATIONS	ORAL DOSAGE	PARENTERAL DOSAGE
Congestive heart failure **Atrial fibrillation and flutter** **Re-entrant supraventricular arrhythmias,** such as paroxysmal atrial tachycardia **Cardiogenic shock**	**Adult:** 0.5–0.75 mg to start, then 0.25–0.50 mg q6–8h to achieve full digitalization (average total loading dose, 1.0–1.5 mg/24 h), followed by 0.125–0.5 mg qd for maintenance; loading dose may be omitted, if desired **Newborn (≤ 1 mo):** 40–60 μg/kg; maintenance dosage: 20–30% digitalizing dose **Infant (1 mo to 2 yr):** ~60–80 μg/kg; maintenance dosage: 20–30% digitalizing dose **Child (2–10 yr):** 40–60 μg/kg; maintenance dosage: 20–30% digitalizing dose	**Adult and child (≥10 yr):** 0.25–0.5 mg IV (slowly) to start, then 0.25 mg q4–6h to achieve full digitalization (average total loading dose, 0.5–1.0 mg/24 h), followed by 0.125–0.5 mg qd for maintenance **Premature and newborns < 2 wk:** 25–40 μg/day; ¼ to ½ total digitalizing dose to start, then ¼ total dose q6h until patient is completely digitalized; total daily maintenance dosage: 20–30% digitalizing dose in one or divided doses **Infant (2 wk to 2 yr):** 35–50 μg/kg; ¼ to ½ total digitalizing dose to start, then ¼ total dose q6h until patient is completely digitalized; total daily maintenance dosage: 20–30% digitalizing dose in one or divided doses **Child (2–10 yr):** 25–40 μg/kg; ¼ to ½ total digitalizing dose to start, then ¼ total dose q6h until patient is completely digitalized; total daily maintenance dosage: 20–30% digitalizing dose in one or divided doses

ADMINISTRATION/DOSAGE ADJUSTMENTS

Serum concentration	Usual therapeutic range, 0.8–2.0 ng/ml; levels >3 ng/ml are often associated with toxicity
Atrial arrhythmias	May require higher dosages than treatment of congestive heart failure
Intramuscular doses	Approximately equal oral doses; however, IM route is extremely painful and offers no advantage unless other routes are contraindicated

CONTRAINDICATIONS

Ventricular fibrillation ●	Hypersensitivity to digoxin (rare) ●

WARNINGS/PRECAUTIONS

Arrhythmias	May reflect digitalis toxicity or may be caused by underlying heart disease; to ascertain which, withhold drug temporarily if clinical situation permits
Anorexia, nausea, and vomiting	May reflect digitalis toxicity or may be caused by underlying heart disease; determine cause before continuing use of drug
Electrolyte disturbances	Hypokalemia, hypomagnesemia, or hypercalcemia may predispose to or enhance toxicity
Idiopathic hypertrophic subaortic stenosis	Outflow obstruction may worsen; digoxin therapy probably should not be employed unless cardiac failure is severe
Incomplete AV heart block	May worsen, especially in patients with Stokes-Adams attacks; alternative therapy for heart failure should be considered
Wolff-Parkinson-White syndrome and atrial fibrillation	Ventricular response rate may increase
Sick-sinus syndrome	May be aggravated
Cardioversion	Dose may need to be decreased before electrical conversion of arrhythmias
Hyperthyroidism	Usually requires higher doses, increasing the risk of toxicity
Special-risk patients	Use with caution in premature and immature infants and patients with severe rheumatic carditis, renal failure, severe pulmonary disease, acute myocardial infarction, or far-advanced heart failure
Unwarranted uses	Constrictive pericarditis, obesity
Acute glomerulonephritis accompanying congestive heart failure	Use with extreme care; total dose for digitalization should be relatively low and given in divided doses with concomitant use of antihypertensive therapy and continual ECG monitoring. Discontinue use of digoxin as soon as possible.
Calcium	May produce serious arrhythmias
Myxedema	Decreases excretion of digoxin, raising blood level; reduce dosage accordingly
Renal insufficiency	Delays excretion and prolongs serum half-life of digoxin; reduce dosage accordingly

Table continued on following page

LANOXIN continued

ADVERSE REACTIONS	Frequent reactions are italicized
In adults	
Gastrointestinal	*Anorexia, nausea, vomiting, diarrhea*
Central nervous system	Visual disturbances (blurred or yellow vision), headache, weakness, apathy
Cardiovascular	*Ventricular premature beats, paroxysmal and nonparoxysmal nodal rhythms, AV dissociation, paroxysmal atrial tachycardia with block,* AV block of increasing degree
Other	Gynecomastia
In infants and children	
Gastrointestinal	Vomiting, diarrhea (rare)
Central nervous system	Neurologic and visual disturbances (rare)
Cardiovascular	*Atrial arrhythmias, atrial ectopic rhythms, paroxysmal atrial tachycardia with block,* nodal and atrial systoles; premature ventricular systoles, ventricular arrhythmias (rare)
Other	Gynecomastia

OVERDOSAGE	
Signs and symptoms	See ADVERSE REACTIONS; undue slowing of the sinus rate, sinoatrial arrest, and prolongation of P-R interval are premonitory signs of toxicity in newborn
Treatment	Discontinue use of digitoxin. To control arrhythmias in patients with adequate renal function, administer potassium in divided oral doses of 50–80 mEq/day for adults and 1–1.5 mEq/kg/day for children. If correction of the arrhythmia is urgent, potassium may be given IV in 5% dextrose-in-water, provided that the serum potassium level is normal or low and that severe or complete heart block due to digitalis and unrelated to any tachyarrhythmia is absent. Adults may be given 40–100 mEq (in a concentration of 30 mEq/500 ml) at a rate of 40 mEq/h, or more slowly if pain occurs at the injection site; children may be given up to 2 mEq/kg (in a concentration of not greater than 20 mEq/500 ml) at a rate of 0.5 mEq/kg/h. Additional amounts may be given if the arrhythmia is uncontrolled and the potassium is well tolerated. If potassium fails or is contraindicated, administer lidocaine, quinidine, phenytoin (experimental), propranolol, or procainamide. Correct hypercalcemia or hypomagnesemia, if present. Advanced heart block may require a temporary pacemaker. For massive overdose, digoxin-specific antibody fragments may be used (experimental).

DRUG INTERACTIONS	
Potassium-depleting diuretics	⇧ Digoxin toxicity
Corticosteroids	⇧ Digoxin toxicity may occur secondary to resulting hypokalemia
Antacids	⇩ Digoxin absorption
Kaolin-pectin	⇩ Digoxin absorption
Neomycin	⇩ Digoxin absorption
Cholestyramine	⇩ Digoxin absorption
Quinidine	⇧ Serum digoxin level
Propranolol	⇧ Risk of AV block; combination often used advantageously for control of atrial fibrillation
Sympathomimetic agents, calcium, succinylcholine	May precipitate or exacerbate digitalis-induced arrhythmias

ALTERED LABORATORY VALUES

No clinically significant alterations in blood/serum or urinary values occur at therapeutic dosages; hyperkalemia occurs with massive overdosage

Use in children

See INDICATIONS

Use in pregnancy or nursing mothers

General guidelines not established

ATROMID-S (Clofibrate) Ayerst

Caps: 500 mg

INDICATIONS	ORAL DOSAGE
Primary hyperlipidemia (adjunctive therapy) **Significant hyperlipidemia with high risk of coronary artery disease** (adjunctive therapy) **Primary dysbetalipoproteinemia** (type III hyperlipidemia) **Recognized disorders of fat metabolism** predisposing to increased risk of heart disease	**Adult:** 2 g/day div, or less in some patients

ADMINISTRATION/DOSAGE ADJUSTMENTS

Selection of patients	Reserve for patients with significant hyperlipidemia and at a high risk of coronary artery disease (eg, strong family history of coronary heart disease, low serum levels of high-density lipoprotein, marked obesity, continued smoking, use of oral contraceptives, unsatisfactorily controlled hypertension) who do not respond adequately to diet and weight loss. Young patients and patients with a history of pancreatitis or abdominal pain associated with marked hypertriglyceridemia are particularly good candidates for clofibrate therapy; however, in view of the serious adverse effects of this drug, consideration should also be given to other hypolipidemic agents.

CONTRAINDICATIONS

Significant hepatic or renal dysfunction ●	Primary biliary cirrhosis ●

WARNINGS/PRECAUTIONS

Cardiovascular morbidity and mortality	There is no substantial evidence that clofibrate exerts a beneficial effect on cardiovascular mortality or reduces the incidence of fatal myocardial infarction; an increased incidence of cardiac arrhythmias, intermittent claudication, definite or suspected thromboembolism, and angina has been reported in patients treated with clofibrate
Risk of malignancy	May be increased, contributing to the increased incidence of noncardiovascular deaths among clofibrate users reported in one large clinical trial; hepatic tumorigenicity has been demonstrated in rodents receiving high doses for prolonged periods
Biliary disease	Risk of cholelithiasis and cholecystitis requiring surgery is increased twofold; perform appropriate diagnostic tests if signs and symptoms of biliary disease occur
Adjunctive therapy	Attempt to control serum lipids by appropriate dietary measures, weight reduction, control of diabetes mellitus, etc, before instituting clofibrate therapy
Serum lipid values	Determine that the patient has significantly elevated serum lipid levels before initiating therapy. Obtain frequent determinations of serum lipids during the first few months of therapy and periodic determinations thereafter. Discontinue medication after 3 mo if lipid response is inadequate, unless patient has xanthoma tuberosum and is responding to therapy. Perform subsequent determinations to detect a paradoxical rise in serum cholesterol or triglyceride levels. Clofibrate does not alter seasonal variations in serum cholesterol levels. Elevated serum triglycerides are generally reduced to a greater extent than elevated serum cholesterol, although both may be lowered substantially in type III hyperlipidemia.
Hepatic impairment	May occur; obtain frequent serum transaminase determinations and perform other liver-function tests and hepatic biopsy, if necessary. Discontinue medication if tests reveal excessive abnormality. Use with caution in patients with past jaundice or hepatic disease.
Flu-like symptoms	May occur, including muscle ache, soreness, and cramping; distinguish this from actual viral and/or bacterial disease
Peptic ulcer	Reactivation may occur; use with caution
Leukopenia, anemia	May occur; obtain complete blood counts periodically
Concomitant anticoagulant therapy	May lead to bleeding complications; reduce anticoagulant dosage by about 50%; obtain frequent prothrombin determinations until prothrombin level has been definitely stabilized
Discontinuation of therapy	Continue the patient on an appropriate hypolipidemic diet; monitor serum lipids until stabilized

Table continued on following page

ATROMID-S continued

ADVERSE REACTIONS

Gastrointestinal	Nausea, vomiting, loose stools, dyspepsia, flatulence, bloating, abdominal distress, hepatomegaly, gallstones, stomatitis, gastritis; peptic ulcer and GI bleeding (causal relationship not established)
Dermatological	Rash, alopecia, urticaria, dry skin, brittle hair, pruritus
Musculoskeletal	Muscle cramping, aching, and weakness; arthralgia "flu-like" symptoms; rheumatoid arthritis (causal relationship not established)
Central nervous system	Headache, dizziness, fatigue, drowsiness, weakness; tremors and blurred vision (causal relationship not established)
Hematological	Leukopenia, anemia, eosinophilia; thrombocytopenic purpura (causal relationship not established)
Cardiovascular	Increased or decreased angina, arrhythmias, swelling and phlebitis at site of xanthomas
Genitourinary	Impotence, decreased libido, dysuria, hematuria, proteinuria, decreased urine output
Other	Weight gain, polyphagia; systemic lupus erythematosus and gynecomastia (causal relationship not established)

OVERDOSAGE

Signs and symptoms	See ADVERSE REACTIONS
Treatment	Discontinue medication; treat symptomatically and institute supportive measures, as required

DRUG INTERACTIONS

Oral anticoagulants	⇧ Prothrombin time
Furosemide	Muscular pain, stiffness, and diuresis

ALTERED LABORATORY VALUES

Blood/serum values	⇧ SGOT ⇧ SGPT ⇧ Sulfobromophthalein retention ⇧ Thymol turbidity ⇧ Creatine phosphokinase ⇧ Beta-lipoprotein ⇩ Fibrinogen
Urinary values	⇧ Protein

Use in children

Safety and effectiveness have not been established

Use in pregnancy or nursing mothers

Contraindicated during pregnancy and nursing period; withdraw medication several months before conception. Strict birth control must be exercised by women of childbearing potential.

CHOLOXIN (Dextrothyroxine sodium) Flint

Tabs: 1, 2, 4, 6 mg

INDICATIONS	ORAL DOSAGE
Hypercholesterolemia, as an adjunct to diet and other measures in euthyroid patients with no known evidence of organic heart disease	**Adult:** 1–2 mg/day to start, followed by increases of 1–2 mg at intervals of 1 mo or more, up to 4–8 mg/day **Child:** 0.05 mg/kg to start, followed by increases of up to 0.05 mg/kg at intervals of 1 mo, up to 4 mg/day, if needed
Hypothyroidism in patients with cardiac disease who cannot tolerate other types of thyroid medication	**Adult:** 1 mg/day to start, followed by increases of 1 mg at intervals of 1 mo or more, up to 4–8 mg/day

CONTRAINDICATIONS	
Known organic heart disease	Including angina pectoris, history of myocardial infarction, cardiac arrhythmias or tachycardia, rheumatic heart disease, history of congestive heart failure, decompensated or borderline compensated cardiac status
Hypertensive states	Other than mild, labile systolic hypertension
Advanced liver or kidney disease	
History of iodism	

WARNINGS/PRECAUTIONS	
Cardiovascular morbidity and mortality	It has not been established whether drug-induced lowering of serum cholesterol or lipid levels has a beneficial or detrimental effect (or no effect) on morbidity or mortality due to atherosclerosis or coronary heart disease
Concomitant digitalis therapy	May stimulate the myocardium excessively in patients with significant myocardial impairment; do not administer more than 4 mg/day of dextrothyroxine to patients on digitalis therapy; carefully monitor the total effect of both drugs
Obesity	Doses within the range of daily hormonal requirements are ineffective for weight reduction in euthyroid patients, but larger doses may produce serious or life-threatening toxicity, particularly when given in combination with sympathomimetic amines
Anticoagulant effect	May be potentiated by concomitant therapy; reduce anticoagulant dosage by 1/3 when initiating dextrothyroxine therapy; readjust dosage on the basis of prothrombin time and observe at least weekly during the first few weeks of treatment; consider withdrawal of dextrothyroxine 2 wk prior to surgery if the use of anticoagulants during surgery is contemplated
Coronary-artery disease or other cardiac disease	Myocardial oxygen requirements may increase, especially at high dosage levels, in hypothyroid patients; use with caution, especially in patients with a history of angina pectoris or myocardial infarction; reduce dosage or discontinue use if aggravation of angina or increased myocardial ischemia, cardiac failure, or clinically significant arrhythmia develops
Concomitant thyroid therapy	Hypothyroid patients are more sensitive to thyroactive drugs than euthyroid patients; adjust dosage accordingly
Coronary insufficiency	May be precipitated by injection of epinephrine and enhanced by dextrothyroxine in patients with coronary-artery disease; use with caution
Cardiac arrhythmias	May occur during surgery in patients taking thyroid hormones; discontinue use 2 wk before elective surgery; when impossible or inadvisable, careful observation is required
Diabetes	May increase blood sugar levels, with a resultant increase in insulin or oral hypoglycemic requirements
Renal or hepatic impairment	Use with caution
Increased serum PBI values (10–25 μg/dl)	Indicate absorption and transport of dextrothyroxine; do not interpret these values as hypermetabolism or use them for dosage titration
Iodism	Discontinue use if manifestations appear
Tartrazine sensitivity	Presence of FD&C Yellow No. 5 (tartrazine) in 2- and 6-mg tablets may cause allergic-type reactions, including bronchial asthma, in susceptible individuals

Table continued on following page

CHOLOXIN continued

ADVERSE REACTIONS

Gastrointestinal	Dyspepsia, nausea, vomiting, constipation, diarrhea, anorexia, jaundice, gallstones
Cardiovascular	Angina pectoris, palpitations, extrasystoles, ectopic beats, supraventricular tachycardia, ECG evidence of myocardial ischemia, cardiac enlargement, peripheral edema, worsened peripheral vascular disease; myocardial infarction (causal relationship not established)
Central nervous system and neuromuscular	Insomnia, nervousness, tremor, headache, tinnitus, dizziness, malaise, fatigue, psychic changes, paresthesia, muscle pain, altered sensorium
Ophthalmic	Visual disturbances, exophthalmos, retinopathy
Dermatological	Alopecia, rash, itching
Genitourinary	Diuresis, menstrual irregularities, increased or decreased libido
Other	Increased metabolism, weight loss, lid lag, sweating, flushing, hyperthermia, hoarseness

OVERDOSAGE

Signs and symptoms	See ADVERSE REACTIONS
Treatment	Discontinue medication; institute supportive measures, as required

DRUG INTERACTIONS

Digitalis	⇧ Risk of excessive myocardial stimulation
Oral anticoagulants	⇧ Prothrombin time
Catecholamines	⇧ Risk of coronary insufficiency

ALTERED LABORATORY VALUES

Blood/serum values	⇧ PBI

No clinically significant alterations in urinary values occur at therapeutic dosages

Use in children

General guidelines not established for use in pediatric hypothyroid patients. In children with familial hypercholesterolemia, continued therapy (over 1 yr) is recommended only if a significant serum cholesterol-lowering effect is observed.

Use in pregnancy or nursing mothers

Contraindicated for use during pregnancy and in nursing mothers; may be given to women of childbearing age who exercise strict birth-control procedures

LORELCO (Probucol) **Dow**

Tabs: 250 mg

INDICATIONS	ORAL DOSAGE
Primary hypercholesterolemia (adjunctive therapy) **Combined hypercholesterolemia and hypertriglyceridemia** (adjunctive therapy)	**Adult:** 500 mg bid with morning and evening meals

CONTRAINDICATIONS

Hypersensitivity to probucol

WARNINGS/PRECAUTIONS

Cardiovascular morbidity and mortality	It has not been established whether drug-induced lowering of serum cholesterol or triglyceride levels has a beneficial or detrimental effect (or no effect) on morbidity or mortality due to atherosclerosis, including coronary heart disease
Adjunctive therapy	Attempt to control serum cholesterol by dietary regimens, weight reduction, and treatment of any underlying disorder which might be the cause of hypercholesterolemia before instituting probucol therapy
Serum cholesterol levels	Should be determined during the first few months of treatment and periodically thereafter; a decision should be made by the 6th mo whether adequate reduction is being attained. Discontinue use if serum cholesterol level has not been lowered satisfactorily.
Serum triglyceride levels	Should be determined periodically; discontinue use if hypertriglyceridemia persists despite improved diet compliance, alcohol abstinence, and further caloric restriction or adjustment of carbohydrate intake

ADVERSE REACTIONS	Frequent reactions are italicized
Gastrointestinal	*Diarrhea (10%), flatulence, abdominal pain, nausea, vomiting,* anorexia, heartburn, indigestion, bleeding
Idiosyncratic	Dizziness, palpitations, syncope, nausea, vomiting, chest pain
Central nervous system	*Headache (2%), dizziness (2%), paresthesias (2%),* insomnia, tinnitus, diminished senses of taste and smell
Ophthalmic	Conjunctivitis, lacrimation, blurred vision
Dermatological	Hyperhidrosis, fetid sweat, rash, pruritus, ecchymoses, petechiae
Hematological	*Eosinophilia (2%), consistently low hemoglobin and/or hematocrit (1%),* thrombocytopenia
Genitourinary	Impotence, nocturia
Other	Enlarged multinodular goiter, angioneurotic edema, peripheral neuritis

DRUG INTERACTIONS

No clinically significant drug interactions have been observed

ALTERED LABORATORY VALUES

Blood/serum values	⇧ SGOT ⇧ SGPT ⇧ Alkaline phosphatase ⇧ Bilirubin ⇧ Creatine phosphokinase ⇧ Uric acid ⇧ BUN ⇧ Glucose

No clinically significant alterations in urinary values occur at therapeutic dosages

Use in children

Safety and effectiveness have not been established

Use in pregnancy or nursing mothers

Not recommended during pregnancy and nursing period; if patient wishes to become pregnant, withdraw medication and advise patient to use birth control measures for at least 6 mo

NICOTINIC ACID various manufacturers

Tabs: 25, 50, 100, 500 mg **Tabs (sust-rel):** 150 mg **Caps:** 500 mg **Caps (sust-rel):** 125, 200, 250, 300, 400, 500 mg
Elixir: 50 mg/5 ml **Amps:** 50 mg/ml (2 ml) **Vials:** 100 mg/ml (30 ml)

INDICATIONS	ORAL DOSAGE	PARENTERAL DOSAGE
Hypercholesterolemia and hyperbetalipoproteinemia (adjunctive therapy)	**Adult:** 1.5–6 g/day divided into 2–4 doses; sust-rel caps: 400 mg bid to start, followed by a gradual increase to 800 mg tid	——

WARNINGS/PRECAUTIONS

Initiating hypolipidemic therapy	Attempt to control serum cholesterol by appropriate dietary measures, weight reduction, and treatment of any underlying disorder that might be the cause of the hypercholesterolemia before initiating nicotinic acid therapy
Cardiovascular morbidity and mortality	It has not been established whether drug-induced lowering of serum cholesterol or triglyceride levels has a beneficial or detrimental effect (or no effect) on morbidity and mortality due to atherosclerosis, including coronary artery disease
Serum cholesterol and triglyceride levels	Should be determined prior to nicotinic acid therapy and regularly thereafter; serum cholesterol and triglyceride levels usually decrease within the first 2 wk of therapy. Continue treatment as long as serum lipid levels remain below baseline values. If no appreciable effect occurs after 1–2 mo of therapy, discontinue use of drug.

Note: For complete chart, see page 147

QUESTRAN (Cholestyramine) Mead Johnson

Powder: 4 g/packet or level scoopful (9-g packets, 378-g cans)

INDICATIONS	ORAL DOSAGE
Primary hypercholesterolemia (adjunctive therapy) **Combined hypercholesterolemia and hypertriglyceridemia** (adjunctive therapy) **Pruritus** associated with partial biliary obstruction	**Adult:** 1 packet or level scoopful tid or qid

ADMINISTRATION/DOSAGE ADJUSTMENTS

Preparation	Must not be taken in dry form; advise patient to mix powder with 2–6 fl oz of water, milk, fruit juice, or other noncarbonated beverage before ingestion; may also be mixed with highly fluid soups or pulpy fruits with high moisture content (eg, applesauce, crushed pineapple)

CONTRAINDICATIONS

Hypersensitivity to any component ●	Complete biliary obstruction ●

WARNINGS/PRECAUTIONS

Cardiovascular morbidity and mortality	It has not been established whether drug-induced lowering of serum cholesterol or triglyceride levels has a beneficial or detrimental effect (or no effect) on morbidity or mortality due to atherosclerosis, including coronary heart disease
Adjunctive therapy	Attempt to control serum cholesterol by dietary measures, weight reduction, and treatment of any underlying disorder which might be the cause of hypercholesterolemia before instituting cholestyramine therapy
Serum cholesterol levels	Should be measured frequently during the first few months of therapy and periodically thereafter; a favorable trend in cholesterol reduction should be evident during the first month of treatment
Triglyceride levels	Should be measured periodically to detect any significant change
Vitamin deficiency	May result from altered absorption of fat-soluble vitamins (such as A, D, and K) with long-term therapy; provide daily vitamin A and D supplements in water-miscible or parenteral form. For increased bleeding due to hypoprothrombinemia, administer vitamin K_1 parenterally; prevent recurrences by administering the oral form.
Folic acid absorption	May be reduced; consider folic acid supplementation for these patients
Concurrent medication	Absorption may be impeded; patient should take other medications at least 1 h before or 4–6 h after cholestyramine
Hyperchloremic acidosis	May occur after prolonged use, especially in smaller and younger patients
Constipation	May occur or worsen, especially with high doses and in patients over 60 yr of age; reduce dosage to prevent fecal impaction and aggravated hemorrhoids
Gastrointestinal dysfunction	Should be evaluated prior to therapy; avert severe constipation, especially in patients with clinically symptomatic coronary-artery disease
Tartrazine sensitivity	Presence of FD&C Yellow No. 5 (tartrazine) may cause allergic-type reactions, including bronchial asthma, in susceptible individuals

ADVERSE REACTIONS

Gastrointestinal	Constipation, fecal impaction, hemorrhoids (with or without bleeding), abdominal discomfort, flatulence, nausea, vomiting, diarrhea, heartburn, anorexia, indigestion, steatorrhea, biliary colic (one case); gallbladder calcification, rectal bleeding, black stools, bleeding from known duodenal ulcer, dysphagia, hiccoughs, ulcer attack, sour taste, pancreatitis, rectal pain, and diverticulitis (causal relationship not established)
Dermatological	Rash; irritation of skin, tongue, and perianal area and ecchymoses (causal relationship not established)
Hematological	Bleeding tendencies (due to hypoprothrombinemia); decreased prothrombin time, and anemia (causal relationship not established)
Metabolic	Hyperchloremic acidosis in children, osteoporosis
Cardiovascular	Claudication, xanthomata of hands and fingers, angina, arteritis, thrombophlebitis, myocardial infarction, myocardial ischemia, increased postprandial angina, and chest pains (causal relationship not established)

Table continued on following page

QUESTRAN continued

ADVERSE REACTIONS continued

Musculoskeletal	Backache, muscle and joint pains, and arthritis (causal relationship not established)
Central nervous system	Headache, anxiety, vertigo, dizziness, fatigue, tinnitus, syncope, drowsiness, femoral nerve pain, and paresthesias (causal relationship not established)
Hypersensitivity	Urticaria, asthma, wheezing, and shortness of breath (causal relationship not established)
Ophthalmic	Night blindness due to vitamin A deficiency (one case), arcus juvenilis, and uveitus (causal relationship not established)
Genitourinary	Hematuria, dysuria, burnt odor to urine, and diuresis (causal relationship not established)
Other	Weight loss or gain; increased libido, swollen glands, edema, and dental bleeding (causal relationship not established)

OVERDOSAGE

Signs and symptoms	Gastrointestinal obstruction
Treatment	Discontinue medication; treat according to location and degree of obstruction and status of gut motility

DRUG INTERACTIONS

Phenylbutazone, warfarin, chlorothiazide, tetracycline, phenobarbital, thyroid preparations, digitalis, other medications	⇩ Rate and/or extent of absorption

ALTERED LABORATORY VALUES

Blood/serum values	⇧ Triglycerides ⇩ Bile acids ⇩ Beta-lipoprotein/low-density lipoprotein ⇩ Cholesterol ⇩ Vitamins A, D, and K

No clinically significant alterations in urinary values occur at therapeutic dosages

Use in children

A practical dosage schedule has not been established; long-term effects in children are unknown

Use in pregnancy or nursing mothers

Safe use not established during pregnancy or in women of childbearing age. General guidelines not established for use in nursing mothers

Hypertension

Hypertension—the medical term for high blood pressure—is one of the most common serious health problems in the United States. An estimated thirty-five million Americans have high blood pressure, and although significant gains have been made in its detection and treatment, about a third or more of these people still are not receiving adequate treatment.

Hypertension itself usually does not have any symptoms, but since it places undue strain on the heart, arteries, and kidneys, it contributes to degenerative changes in these organs and increases the risk of heart attack, stroke, or kidney disease.

DEFINITION OF HYPERTENSION

Blood pressure is the force of the blood against the arterial walls. It is usually measured by a sphygmomanometer (pronounced SFIG-mo-ma-nom-e-tur), a simple instrument containing a cuff and a column of mercury. The cuff is placed on the upper arm and inflated to a pressure slightly more than the pressure of blood coursing through the arteries. As the cuff is slowly deflated, the mercury column falls, first indicating the systolic pressure—the higher of the two numbers in a blood pressure reading—which is the maximum pressure exerted against the arterial walls as the heart contracts. The diastolic pressure—the lower number in a reading—is the minimum pressure exerted between heart contractions or beats.

Blood pressure is regulated by arterioles (the smallest arteries), which supply blood to the capillaries—the minute vessels that deliver blood and its nutrients to body tissues. The more difficult it is for blood to pass through the arterioles, the higher the blood pressure.

Blood pressure normally varies with mood and activity, rising during periods of strenuous activity, stress, or anxiety. The first blood pressure reading taken in a physician's office often coincides with a feeling of anxiety or stress, and therefore may be

EFFECTS OF HYPERTENSION ON HEART AND KIDNEY

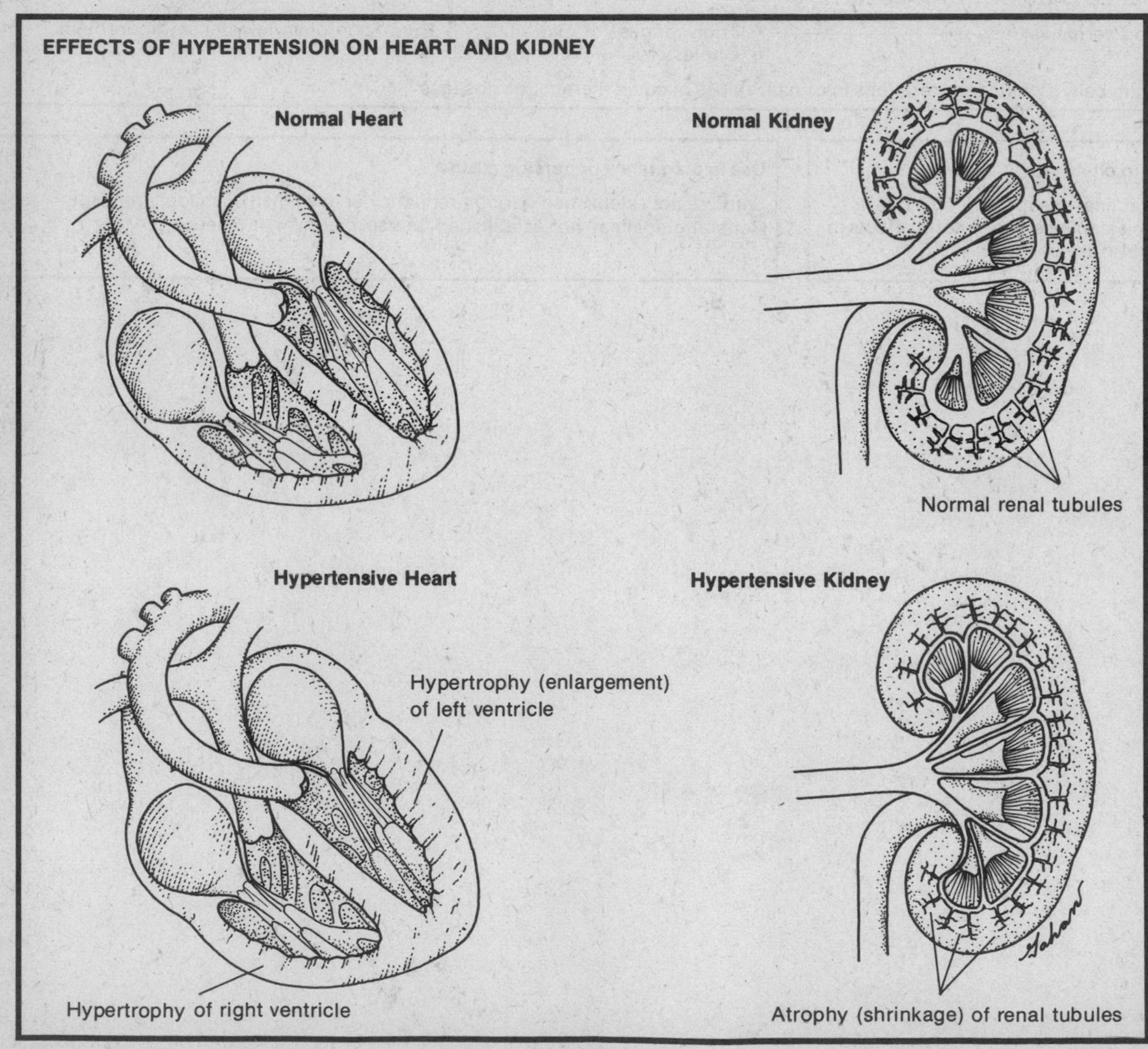

higher than usual. This is why several measurements taken at different times and in different positions or settings may be required to establish a diagnosis of hypertension.

There is some disagreement as to what constitutes hypertension. A reading of 120/80 millimeters of mercury (mm Hg) is considered normal. A diastolic pressure of 90 to 104 mm Hg is generally considered mild or borderline hypertension, especially in persons under the age of fifty, but there is disagreement as to whether persons in this range should undergo treatment. If the systolic pressure is also elevated—over 140 mm Hg—and the patient exhibits other cardiovascular risk factors, such as high blood cholesterol and other lipids, cigarette smoking, and overweight, a physician may recommend a dietary and exercise regimen to lower the blood pressure. At any rate, the blood pressure should be measured every few months. If this approach is unsuccessful and the blood pressure remains elevated or even continues to rise, drug therapy may be recommended. Most authorities agree that diastolic blood pressures of 100 to 105 mm Hg or higher constitute moderate hypertension and should be treated, usually by drugs and hygienic preventive measures, such as stopping smoking, weight loss, and reduced salt intake.

CAUSES OF HYPERTENSION

In the vast majority of hypertensive patients, there is no discernible physical cause for the elevated blood pressure. The disease in these persons is referred to as primary (or essential) hypertension. In rare instances, the hypertension is secondary to an organic cause, such as kidney disease.

Heredity is thought to be a factor since high blood pressure tends to "run in families." Blood pressure tends to rise with age; women have slightly lower pressures than men in the third and fourth decades of life, and slightly higher levels thereafter. Recent studies have found that children whose blood pressures are at the upper range for their age groups remain in the upper ranges into adulthood and are more likely to develop hypertension than those in the middle or lower ranges. Blacks tend to have a higher incidence of hypertension than whites. Epidemiological studies have found that populations with high salt intake tend to have higher blood pressures than those seen in groups with low salt consumption, but there is no conclusive evidence that salt actually causes high blood pressure. Salt does tend to increase fluid retention and, until the introduction of antihypertensive drugs, a salt-restricted diet, such as one consisting of rice and fruit, was the only effective treatment of high blood pressure.

Of the controllable risk factors, obesity seems to be the only one that can be altered to achieve a preventive effect. Body weight is correlated with both systolic and diastolic blood pressures, particularly in young and middle-aged adults. Weight gain is associated with a rise in blood pressure and, among those who are obese, weight loss appears to lessen the risk of developing hypertension. Although weight loss tends to be associated with a lowering of blood pressure, it is not known whether this is due to the weight reduction or to a combination of factors, including dietary changes, reduced salt intake, and increased physical activity.

Hypertension in Pregnancy

Since blood pressure generally decreases somewhat during pregnancy, a reading of even 130/80 mm Hg would be considered high in a pregnant woman. Hypertension during pregnancy often leads to impaired placental function and a low-birth-weight baby. It increases the risk of both fetal and newborn death, as well as of complications for the mother.

Hypertension provoked by pregnancy is characterized by excessive fluid retention and the presence of proteins in the urine. In the past, pregnant women with hypertension often were hospitalized and had to spend many weeks in bed. Now treatment is usually similar to that for other hypertensive patients, although the safety of some antihypertensive drugs has not been established for pregnant women.

Drug-Induced Hypertension

Several types of drugs tend to increase blood pressure. These include oral contraceptives, corticosteroids, certain anti-inflammatory agents, and vasoconstrictors (often used for migraine). The high blood pressure in these instances generally is not severe.

TREATMENT OF HYPERTENSION

Although there is no cure for hypertension, the disease can now be controlled in most patients. In persons who have mild to moderate hypertension, reduction in weight and salt consumption, increased physical activity, and, where applicable, stopping smoking, may be sufficient. For most persons who are diagnosed as having hypertension, however, drug therapy is necessary to control the blood pressure. It is important to recognize that the treatment is lifelong; once it is stopped, the blood pressure returns to pretreatment levels (or higher).

ANTIHYPERTENSIVE DRUGS

A number of drugs and combinations of drugs are commonly used to lower blood pressure. Although some of these drugs may produce unpleasant side effects in certain individuals, the availability of a wide variety of drugs usually permits the physician to select a drug or combination of drugs that will achieve the desired results with a minimum of side effects. Therefore, if the first one or two regimens that are recommended are unsatisfactory, it is important to keep trying until a combination suitable to individual needs is found.

The major categories of antihypertensive drugs are (1) diuretics, (2) beta-adrenergic blockers,

(3) centrally acting drugs, (4) vasodilators, (5) alpha-adrenergic blocking agents, and (6) combination agents.

Diuretics

Diuretics act by reducing the body's sodium chloride (salt) and water volume, thereby lowering blood pressure. The most commonly used antihypertensive diuretics are the thiazides and thiazide-type agents, which include Esidrix, Diuril, and HydroDIURIL. Treatment of mild to moderate hypertension usually begins with a thiazide diuretic, and, in many patients, this alone is sufficient to control the blood pressure. If additional reduction is required, a second drug may be added.

The main adverse effects of long-term thiazide diuretic use are potassium depletion, an increased risk of gout, and impaired glucose metabolism. Potassium balance can usually be maintained by reducing the intake of salt. Eating potassium-rich foods, such as oranges, bananas, or tomatoes, or taking a potassium supplement may be recommended for some patients. There are also potassium-sparing diuretics, such as spironolactone (Aldactone).

The so-called loop diuretics have a different mechanism of action than that of the thiazides, although they also reduce blood pressure by promoting the excretion of sodium chloride from the body. The major loop diuretic—furosemide (Lasix)—is a potent blood-pressure-lowering drug; therefore, it is often used during a hypertensive crisis. Loop diuretics also may be prescribed for patients with impaired kidney function. Still other types of diuretics lower blood pressure by unknown mechanisms of action. An example is chlorthalidone (Hygroton).

Beta-Adrenergic Blocking Agents

Beta-adrenergic blocking agents are among the newest drugs used to treat hypertension. So far, three beta-blocking drugs—propranolol (Inderal), metoprolol (Lopressor), and nadolol (Corgard)—have been introduced in the United States. Although the mechanism by which these drugs lower blood pressure is not fully understood, their usefulness in treating hypertension has been firmly established. They are frequently prescribed in conjunction with a diuretic when a diuretic alone does not sufficiently lower blood pressure. A beta blocker may be prescribed alone for patients who cannot tolerate a diuretic (i.e., hypertensive patients who also have gout). Since beta blockers also are effective in treating angina and arrhythmias, they are often prescribed for hypertensive patients who have symptoms of coronary artery disease as well.

Centrally Acting Drugs

These drugs lower blood pressure by working through the sympathetic nervous system, which controls involuntary muscle action, such as the heartbeat. They usually are given in conjunction with a thiazide diuretic.

Centrally acting antihypertensive drugs include clonidine (Catapres), reserpine (Serpasil), and methyldopa (Aldomet). (The latter two also have peripheral actions.) All tend to decrease the heart rate and output of blood from the heart.

Vasodilators

As their name implies, vasodilators act by dilating or expanding the blood vessels, thereby enabling the blood to flow through them with less resistance. These drugs are often used in combination with other antihypertensive agents, particularly the thiazide diuretics or the beta blockers. Drugs in this category include hydralazine (Apresoline), diazoxide (Hyperstat I.V.), minoxidil (Loniten), and nitroprusside (Nipride). These agents act very quickly to lower blood pressure—often within minutes, especially when administered intravenously. Minoxidil and nitroprusside are particularly useful in treating hypertensive emergencies.

Alpha-Adrenergic Blocking Agents

Alpha receptors are instrumental in the constriction of blood vessels; by blocking some of these receptors, peripheral vascular resistance is reduced, the blood vessels are dilated or slightly expanded, and consequently blood pressure is lowered. The major antihypertensive agent with this mechanism of action is prazosin (Minipress). This drug is often administered along with a diuretic.

Combination Antihypertensive Agents

As noted earlier, antihypertensive agents often are used in combination, both to increase effectiveness and to minimize the possibility of side effects. Once the most effective dosage of each individual drug has been established, a physician often will prescribe a drug that contains the desired combination in a single tablet or capsule.

IN CONCLUSION

High blood pressure almost always can be controlled, either by a single antihypertensive drug or a combination of two or more agents. A major problem in treating hypertension is long-term patient adherence to the prescribed regimen. In most cases, the hypertension itself does not cause any symptoms. Indeed, since many patients find that they actually feel worse after beginning therapy than they did before, they simply stop taking their medication. Discontinuing treatment is potentially life-threatening because untreated high blood pressure frequently leads to premature death from heart attack, stroke, or kidney failure. Side effects can usually be eliminated or minimized by trying different drugs or combinations of drugs, but only under the supervision of a physician. In addition, good health practices such as weight control, not smoking, reduced salt intake, and regular physical activity also may be important.

The following charts are divided into two overall categories: antihypertensive agents, both single and in combination, and diuretics, which also may be prescribed for edema and congestive heart failure.

ALDOMET (Methyldopa) Merck Sharp & Dohme

Tabs: 125, 250, 500 mg methyldopa **Vial:** 250 mg methyldopate hydrochloride/5 ml (5 ml)

INDICATIONS	ORAL DOSAGE	PARENTERAL DOSAGE
Hypertension	**Adult:** 250 mg bid or tid to start, followed by up to 3 g/day in 2-4 divided doses; usual maintenance dosage: 500 mg to 2 g/day **Child:** 10 mg/kg/day in 2-4 divided doses to start, followed by divided doses totaling up to 65 mg/kg/day or 3 g/day, whichever is less	**Adult:** 250-500 mg IV q6h, as needed, up to 1 g q6h **Child:** 20-40 mg/kg/day IV div q6h, as needed, up to 65 mg/kg/day or 3 g/day, whichever is less
Hypertensive crisis	—	**Adult:** same as above **Child:** same as above

ADMINISTRATION/DOSAGE ADJUSTMENTS

Initiating therapy	Allow at least 48 h between dosage adjustments. Increase or decrease dosage until optimal blood-pressure response is obtained; to minimize sedation, increase dosage in evenings.
Intravenous administration	Add the desired dose to 100 ml of 5% dextrose-in-water and give by slow IV infusion over a period of 30-60 min; decline in blood pressure generally begins in 4-6 h and may last 10-16 h after injection
Combination therapy	Thiazide dosages do not need to be altered; when adding methyldopa to other antihypertensive regimens, limit initial dosage to 500 mg/day
Tolerance	May develop occasionally, usually between 2nd and 3rd mo of therapy; to restore control, add a diuretic or increase dosage of methyldopa
Refractory patients	Add a thiazide diuretic if therapy has not been started with a diuretic or if blood pressure cannot be controlled with 2 g/day of methyldopa

CONTRAINDICATIONS

Hypersensitivity	To methyldopa
Active hepatic disease	Including acute hepatitis and active cirrhosis
Liver disorders	Associated with prior methyldopa therapy

WARNINGS/PRECAUTIONS

Coombs'-positive hemolytic anemia	May occur in less than 4% of patients, with potentially fatal complications. Obtain a blood count and Coombs' test before initiating therapy and at 6 and 12 mo after inception. With prolonged use of methyldopa, 10-20% of patients develop a positive direct Coombs' test; while this is not a contraindication to further use of the drug, therapy should be discontinued immediately if hemolytic anemia also develops in such patients. Usually, the anemia remits promptly. If it is related to methyldopa use,however, do not reinstitute the drug.
Drug-induced hepatitis	May occur at any time during therapy. Obtain liver-function studies (eg, SGOT, bilirubin) periodically, especially during first 2-3 mo of therapy or if unexplained fever or rash occurs. If drug-related, abnormalities will revert to normal after drug is stopped; do not reinstitute therapy.
Orthostatic hypotension	May occur; reduce dosage
Edema and weight gain	May occur and can usually be relieved with a diuretic; discontinue therapy if edema progresses or signs of heart failure appear
Reversible leukopenia	May occur rarely, manifested primarily by a reduction in granulocytes; discontinue therapy

Table continued on following page

ALDOMET continued

WARNINGS/PRECAUTIONS continued

Circulatory instability during anesthesia	May occur; if necessary, reduce anesthetic dosage. If hypotension does occur, use a vasopressor.
Paradoxical pressor response	May occur with parenteral administration
Involuntary choreoathetotic movements	**May occur rarely in patients with severe bilateral cerebrovascular disease; discontinue therapy**
Special-risk patients	Use with caution in patients with previous liver disease or dysfunction or in those with severe renal impairment; the latter may respond adequately to lower doses
Suspected pheochromocytoma	**Urinary catecholamine level may appear to be elevated due to fluorescence of methyldopa; measurement of vanillylmandelic acid (VMA) by methods that convert VMA to vanillin is not affected**
Dialysis patients	May be difficult to control, since drug is removed by dialysis

ADVERSE REACTIONS

Central nervous system and neuromuscular	Sedation, headache, asthenia, weakness, dizziness, lightheadedness, symptoms of cerebrovascular insufficiency, paresthesias, parkinsonism, Bell's palsy, decreased mental acuity, involuntary choreoathetotic movements, psychic disturbances (including nightmares and reversible mild psychoses or depression)
Cardiovascular	Bradycardia, aggravation of angina pectoris, orthostatic hypotension, edema (and weight gain)
Gastrointestinal	Nausea, vomiting, distention, constipation, flatus, diarrhea, mild dryness of the mouth, sore or black tongue, pancreatitis, sialadenitis
Hepatic	Abnormal liver-function tests, jaundice, liver disorders
Metabolic and endocrinological	Breast enlargement, gynecomastia, lactation, impotence, decreased libido
Hematological	Hemolytic anemia, leukopenia, granulocytopenia, thrombocytopenia
Hypersensitivity	Drug-related fever, lupus-like syndrome, myocarditis
Other	Nasal stuffiness, dermatological reactions (including eczema and lichenoid eruptions), mild arthralgia, myalgia

OVERDOSAGE

Signs and symptoms	Sedation, hypotension
Treatment	Institute supportive measures, as indicated. Treat hypotension by elevating feet and by volume expansion, if possible.

DRUG INTERACTIONS

Other antihypertensive agents	⇧ Antihypertensive effect

ALTERED LABORATORY VALUES

Blood/serum values	⇧ Alkaline phosphatase ⇧ SGOT ⇧ SGPT ⇧ Bilirubin ⇧ Creatinine (with alkaline picrate method) ⇩ Plasma renin activity + Coombs' test + LE cell reaction + Rheumatoid factor + ANA
Urinary values	⇧ Uric acid (with phosphotungstate method) ⇧ Catecholamines (with fluorescence methods)

Use in children

See INDICATIONS

Use in pregnancy or nursing mothers

Use with caution if drug is essential. Methyldopa crosses the placental barrier and appears in cord blood and breast milk. No unusual adverse effects have been reported during pregnancy, nor is there any evidence of teratogenicity. However, the possibility of injury to the fetus or nursing infant cannot be excluded.

APRESOLINE (Hydralazine hydrochloride) Ciba

Tabs: 10, 25, 50, 100 mg **Amps:** 20 mg/ml (1 ml)

INDICATIONS	ORAL DOSAGE	PARENTERAL DOSAGE
Essential hypertension	**Adult:** 10 mg qid for the first 2-4 days, followed by 25 mg qid for the balance of the 1st wk and 50 mg qid thereafter	—
Severe essential hypertension when oral administration is impossible or when the need to lower blood pressure is urgent	—	**Adult:** 20-40 mg IM or IV (very slowly), repeated as needed

CONTRAINDICATIONS

Hypersensitivity	To hydralazine
Coronary artery disease	Anginal attacks may be precipitated or may worsen
Rheumatic mitral-valve disease	Congestive heart failure may be precipitated

WARNINGS/PRECAUTIONS

Lupus erythematosus-like syndrome	May occur; obtain CBC, LE cell preparation, and antinuclear antibody (ANA) titer before and periodically during prolonged therapy or if arthralgia, fever, chest pain, continued malaise, or other unexplained symptoms develop. In general, unless hydralazine is essential, discontinue therapy if clinical symptoms occur, ANA titer rises, or LE cell reaction is positive.
Profound hypotension	May occur with concomitant use of other potent parenteral antihypertensive agents, such as diazoxide; patient should be observed for several hours
Peripheral neuritis	May occur, evidenced by paresthesias, numbness, and tingling; combat with pyridoxine
Blood dyscrasias	May occur (see ADVERSE REACTIONS); obtain periodic blood counts during prolonged therapy and withdraw if abnormalities develop
Special-risk patients	Use with caution in patients with suspected coronary-artery disease, specific cardiovascular inadequacies (eg, mitral valvular disease), cerebrovascular accidents, or advanced renal disease, or those on MAO inhibitor therapy
Tartrazine sensitivity	Presence of FD&C Yellow No. 5 (tartrazine) in 10- and 100-mg tablets may cause allergic-type reactions, including bronchial asthma, in susceptible individuals

ADVERSE REACTIONS

Frequent reactions are italicized

Central nervous system and neuromuscular	*Headache, anorexia,* peripheral neuritis (paresthesias, numbness, tingling), dizziness, tremors, muscle cramps, psychotic reactions (eg, depression, disorientation, anxiety)
Cardiovascular	*Palpitations, tachycardia, angina pectoris,* hypotension, paradoxical pressor response
Gastrointestinal	*Nausea, vomiting, diarrhea,* constipation, paralytic ileus
Hematological	Reduction in hemoglobin level and erythrocyte count, leukopenia, agranulocytosis, purpura
Ophthalmic	Lacrimation, conjunctivitis
Hypersensitivity	Rash, urticaria, pruritus, fever, chills, arthralgia, eosinophilia, hepatitis (rare)
Other	Nasal congestion, flushing, difficult micturition, dyspnea, lymphadenopathy, splenomegaly

Table continued on following page

OVERDOSAGE

Signs and symptoms — Hypotension, tachycardia, headache, generalized skin flushing, myocardial ischemia, cardiac arrhythmia, profound shock (in severe overdosage)

Treatment — Empty stomach, taking care to prevent pulmonary aspiration; if conditions permit, instill activated charcoal to remove any remaining drug from the stomach. Cardiovascular support is primary. Use volume expansion without resorting to vasopressors, if possible. If a vasopressor is required, use one that is least likely to precipitate or aggravate cardiac arrhythmias. Digitalization may be necessary. Monitor renal function and institute supportive measures, as required.

DRUG INTERACTIONS

Beta blockers — ⇧ Antihypertensive effect of hydralazine

Other antihypertensive agents — ⇧ Antihypertensive effect of both drugs

ALTERED LABORATORY VALUES

Blood/serum values — + ANA titer + LE-cell reaction + Direct Coombs' test
⇧ Plasma renin activity

No clinically significant alterations in urinary values occur at therapeutic dosages

Use in children

General guidelines not established

Use in pregnancy or nursing mothers

Safe use not established during pregnancy; hydralazine is teratogenic in mice and possibly rabbits, but not in rats. General guidelines not established for use in nursing mothers.

CATAPRES (Clonidine hydrochloride) Boehringer Ingelheim

Tabs: 0.1, 0.2, 0.3 mg

INDICATIONS	ORAL DOSAGE
Hypertension	**Adult:** 0.1 mg bid to start, followed by increments of 0.1 or 0.2 mg/day, up to 2.4 mg/day, until desired response is achieved; usual maintenance dosage: 0.2–0.8 mg/day div

ADMINISTRATION/DOSAGE ADJUSTMENTS

Discontinuation of therapy	Reduce dosage gradually over 2–4 days, whenever possible, to avoid severe increase in blood pressure (usually observed in patients receiving more than 0.6–0.8 mg/day). If blood pressure rises excessively, resume clonidine therapy or administer IV phentolamine and propranolol, as in treating pheochromocytoma. Caution patients against interrupting or abruptly discontinuing therapy.

CONTRAINDICATIONS

None

WARNINGS/PRECAUTIONS

Tolerance	May develop; re-evaluate therapy
Hypertensive encephalopathy, death	May occur, in rare instances, after abrupt cessation of therapy (see ADMINISTRATION/DOSAGE ADJUSTMENTS)
Visual impairment	Periodic eye examinations (every 6–12 mo) are recommended during prolonged therapy, based on observation of retinal degeneration in rats
Drowsiness, sedation	Performance of potentially hazardous activities may be impaired; caution patients accordingly
Special-risk patients	Use with caution in patients with severe coronary insufficiency, recent myocardial infarction, cerebrovascular disease, or chronic renal failure

ADVERSE REACTIONS
Frequent reactions are italicized

Gastrointestinal	*Dry mouth (~40%),* constipation, anorexia, malaise, nausea, vomiting, parotid pain, mild transient abnormalities in liver-function tests, drug-induced hepatitis without icterus or hyperbilirubinemia (one case)
Metabolic and endocrinological	Weight gain, gynecomastia
Cardiovascular	Congestive heart failure, Raynaud's phenomenon, ECG abnormalities manifested as Wenckebach's period or ventricular trigeminy
Central nervous system	*Drowsiness (~35%), sedation (~8%),* dizziness, headache, fatigue, vivid dreams or nightmares, insomnia, other behavioral changes, nervousness, restlessness, anxiety, mental depression
Dermatological	Rash, angioneurotic edema, hives, urticaria, thinning of hair, pruritus not associated with rash
Genitourinary	Impotence, urinary retention
Other	Increased sensitivity to alcohol; dryness, itching, or burning of the eyes; dryness of the nasal mucosa; pallor; weakly positive Coombs' test

OVERDOSAGE

Signs and symptoms	Profound hypotension, weakness, somnolence, diminished or absent reflexes, vomiting
Treatment	Use gastric lavage to empty stomach. Administer an analeptic and a vasopressor or, alternatively, 10 mg tolazoline IV every 30 min. Institute supportive measures, as needed.

Table continued on following page

CATAPRES continued

DRUG INTERACTIONS

Alcohol, tranquilizers, sedative-hypnotics, and other CNS depressants	⇧ CNS depression
Diuretics	⇧ Antihypertensive effect of clonidine
Tricyclic antidepressants	⇩ Antihypertensive effect

ALTERED LABORATORY VALUES

Blood/serum values	⇧ Glucose (transient) ⇧ Creatine phosphokinase ⇩ Plasma renin activity
Urinary values	⇧ Aldosterone ⇧ Catecholamines

Use in children

Safety and effectiveness have not been established

Use in pregnancy or nursing mothers

Not recommneded for use in women who are or who may become pregnant, unless potential benefit outweighs risk. General guidelines not established for use in nursing mothers.

CORGARD (Nadolol) Squibb

Tabs: 40, 80, 120, 160 mg

INDICATIONS	ORAL DOSAGE
Hypertension	**Adult:** 40 mg qd (alone or with a diuretic) to start, followed by increments of 40–80 mg/day, as needed, up to 640 mg/day; usual maintenance dosage: 80–320 mg qd
Angina pectoris	**Adult:** 40 mg qd to start, followed by increments of 40–80 mg/day every 3–7 days until optimal response is achieved or pronounced slowing of heart rate occurs; usual maintenance dosage: 80–240 mg qd

ADMINISTRATION/DOSAGE ADJUSTMENTS

Patients with renal impairment	Increase interval between doses as follows: administer q24h when creatinine clearance rate (CCr)>50 ml/min; q24–36h when CCr = 31–50 ml/min; q24–48h when CCr = 10–30 ml/min; q40–60h when CCr <10 ml/min
Combination therapy	May be used at full dosage in combination with other antihypertensive agents, especially thiazide-type diuretics
Discontinuation of therapy	Reduce dosage gradually over 1–2 wk, if possible, and monitor patient closely. Caution patients with angina or hyperthyroidism against interruption or abrupt cessation of therapy (see WARNINGS/PRECAUTIONS).

Note: Full chart appears on page 13.

INDERAL (Propranolol hydrochloride) **Ayerst**

Tabs: 10, 20, 40, 80 mg **Amps:** 1 mg/ml (1 ml)

INDICATIONS	ORAL DOSAGE	PARENTERAL DOSAGE
Hypertension	**Adult:** 40 mg bid (alone or with a diuretic) to start, followed by gradual increases until optimal response is achieved, up to 640 mg/day; usual maintenance dosage: 160–480 mg/day	—
Cardiac arrhythmias, including supraventricular arrhythmias, ventricular tachycardias, digitalis-induced tachyarrhythmias, and resistant tachyarrhythmias due to excessive catecholamine activity during anesthesia	**Adult:** 10–30 mg tid or qid, before meals and at bedtime	**Adult:** 1–3 mg IV, slowly (see ADMINISTRATION/DOSAGE ADJUSTMENTS)
Prophylaxis of moderate to severe **angina pectoris**	**Adult:** 10–20 mg/day tid or qid, before meals and at bedtime, to start, followed by gradual increments every 3–7 days until optimal response is achieved, up to 320 mg/day; usual maintenance dosage: 160 mg/day	—
Hypertrophic subaortic stenosis	**Adult:** 20–40 mg tid or qid, before meals and at bedtime	—
As an adjunct to alpha-adrenergic blocking agents in the management of **pheochromocytoma**	**Adult:** 60 mg/day div for 3 days prior to surgery, concomitantly with an alpha-adrenergic blocking agent, or 30 mg/day div for inoperable tumors	—
Migraine prophylaxis	**Adult:** 80 mg/day div to start, followed by gradual increments until optimal response is achieved; usual maintenance dosage: 160–240 mg/day	—

Note: Full chart appears on page 15.

ISMELIN (Guanethidine sulfate) Ciba

Tabs: 10, 25 mg

INDICATIONS	ORAL DOSAGE
Moderate to severe essential hypertension **Renal hypertension,** including hypertension secondary to pyelonephritis, renal amyloidosis, and renal artery stenosis	**Adult (ambulatory):** 10 mg qd to start; blood pressure must be taken at 5–7-day intervals to determine if there is a need for an increase in dosage (see ADMINISTRATION/DOSAGE ADJUSTMENTS); if needed on 2nd visit, increase dosage to 20 mg qd; if needed on 3rd visit, increase dosage to 30 or 37.5 mg qd; if needed on 4th visit, increase dosage to 50 mg qd; if needed on 5th or subsequent visits, increase dosage by 12.5 or 25 mg/day; usual maintenance dosage: 25–50 mg qd **Adult (hospitalized):** 25–50 mg to start, followed by increases of 25 or 50 mg/day or every other day, as needed

ADMINISTRATION/DOSAGE ADJUSTMENTS

Initial titration of dosage	Take blood pressure, with patient in supine position, after he has been standing for 10 min, and immediately after exercise, if feasible. Increase dosage only if there is *no* decrease in standing blood pressure from previous levels. Reduce dosage if pressure is normal in the supine position or if patient evidences either an excessive orthostatic fall in pressure or severe diarrhea.
Combination therapy	Add gradually to thiazides or hydralazine. When thiazide diuretics are added, it is usually necessary to reduce guanethidine dosage.
Patients with fever	Dosage requirements may be reduced
Transferring patients from ganglionic blockers	Withdraw blocker gradually to prevent a spiking blood-pressure response during period of transition

CONTRAINDICATIONS

Hypersensitivity	To guanethidine
Pheochromocytoma	Either known or suspected
Frank congestive heart failure	Not due to hypertension
Use of MAO inhibitors	Wait 1 wk after discontinuing MAO-inhibitor therapy before initiating guanethidine

WARNINGS/PRECAUTIONS

Orthostatic hypotension	Occurs frequently; caution ambulatory patients to sit or lie down at the first sign of dizziness or weakness and to avoid sudden or prolonged standing or exercise. Hospitalized patients should be warned not to get out of bed without assistance during initial dosage adjustment period.
Cardiovascular instability during surgery	If possible, withdraw therapy 2 wk prior to elective surgery to minimize risk of vascular collapse and cardiac arrest. For emergency surgery, reduce dosage of preanesthetic and anesthetic agents. Use vasopressors with extreme caution if vascular collapse occurs.
Bronchial asthma	May be exacerbated due to hypersensitivity to catecholamine depletion; use with particular care in patients with a history of bronchial asthma
Long-term therapy	Effects of guanethidine are cumulative; increase dosage slowly (see ORAL DOSAGE)
Special-risk patients	Use very cautiously in patients with severe renal disease and nitrogen retention or rising BUN levels; or coronary disease with insufficiency or recent myocardial infarction; or cerebral vascular disease, especially with encephalopathy
Peptic ulcer	May be exacerbated by relative increase in parasympathetic tone; use with caution in patients with a history of peptic ulcer
Severe cardiac failure	May interfere with compensatory role of adrenergic system in producing circulatory adjustments; use with extreme caution
Incipient cardiac decompensation	Observe patient for possible weight gain or edema; can be averted by concomitant administration of a thiazide diuretic
Severe diarrhea	May occur, necessitating discontinuation of therapy
Tartrazine sensitivity	Presence of FD&C Yellow No. 5 (tartrazine) in 10-mg tablets may cause allergic-type reactions, including bronchial asthma, in susceptible individuals

Table continued on following page

ISMELIN continued

ADVERSE REACTIONS

Frequent reactions are italicized

Central nervous system and neuromuscular	***Dizziness, weakness, lassitude, and syncope due to postural or exertional hypotension,*** fatigue, myalgia, muscle tremor, mental depression
Cardiovascular	***Orthostatic hypotension, bradycardia, fluid retention and edema, with occasional development of congestive heart failure,*** dyspnea, chest pains (angina), chest paresthesias
Gastrointestinal	*Increased bowel movements, diarrhea,* nausea, vomiting, dry mouth
Genitourinary	*Inhibition of ejaculation,* nocturia, urinary incontinence, priapism (causal relationship not established)
Hematological	Anemia, thrombocytopenia, and leukopenia (causal relationship not established)
Other	Dermatitis, scalp-hair loss, ptosis of eyelids, blurred vision, parotid tenderness, nasal congestion, weight gain, asthma (in susceptible individuals)

OVERDOSAGE

Signs and symptoms	Postural hypotension (with dizziness, blurring of vision, and like symptoms, progressing to syncope when standing), bradycardia, diarrhea (possibly severe), unconsciousness
Treatment	Evacuate stomach contents, taking care to prevent aspiration. Begin monitoring of serum electrolytes and renal function. Support vital functions and control cardiac irregularities, as needed. Keep patient in supine position. Use vasopressors only with extreme caution because of heightened sensitivity (see DRUG INTERACTIONS). Treat diarrhea symptomatically to reduce intestinal hypermotility; maintain hydration and electrolyte balance.

DRUG INTERACTIONS

MAO inhibitors	⇧ Hypertension to crisis proportions
Digitalis	⇩ Heart rate
Amphetamine-like compounds, ephedrine, methylphenidate, and other stimulants; tricyclic antidepressants; phenothiazines; other psychotropic agents	⇩ Antihypertensive effect
Oral contraceptives	⇩ Antihypertensive effect
Rauwolfia derivatives	Excessive postural hypotension, bradycardia, mental depression
Norepinephrine and other vasopressors	⇧ Pressor effect and risk of cardiac arrhythmias

ALTERED LABORATORY VALUES

Blood/serum values	⇧ BUN ⇧ Creatinine ⇧ Plasma renin activity
Urinary values	⇧ Catecholamines (initially) ⇩ Catecholamines (subsequently) ⇩ VMA

Use in children

General guidelines not available

Use in pregnancy or nursing mothers

Safe use not established during pregnancy. General guidelines not established for use in nursing mothers.

LONITEN (Minoxidil) Upjohn

Tabs: 2.5, 10 mg

INDICATIONS	ORAL DOSAGE
Severe hypertension that is symptomatic or associated with target-organ damage and that is not manageable with maximum therapeutic doses of a diuretic plus two other antihypertensive agents	**Adult:** 5 mg qd to start, followed by increases to 10, 20, and then 40 mg/day, in single or divided doses, as needed for optimal control, up to 100 mg/day; usual maintenance dosage: 10–40 mg/day **Child (<12 yr):** 0.2 mg/kg/day to start, followed by increases in 50–100% increments, as needed for optimal control, up to 50 mg/day; usual maintenance dosage: 0.25–1.0 mg/kg/day

ADMINISTRATION/DOSAGE ADJUSTMENTS

Dose frequency	If supine diastolic pressure has been reduced <30 mm Hg, administer only once daily; if reduced >30 mm Hg, divide the daily dose into 2 equal parts
Frequency of dosage adjustments	Titrate dosage according to patient response. Allow at least 3 days between dosage adjustments. When rapid control of hypertension is required, dose adjustments can be made every 6 h, with careful monitoring.
Mandatory concomitant therapy	At least 24 h before starting minoxidil, administer (1) the equivalent of 80–160 mg/day of propranolol div or, if beta blockers are contraindicated, 250–750 mg methyldopa bid or possibly 0.1–0.2 mg clonidine bid and (2) the equivalent of 50 mg hydrochlorothiazide bid, 50–100 mg chlorthalidone qd, or 40 mg furosemide bid

CONTRAINDICATIONS

Pheochromocytoma	Catecholamine secretion from tumor may be stimulated

WARNINGS/PRECAUTIONS

Salt and water retention, congestive heart failure	Must be prevented by concomitant diuretic therapy; a high-ceiling (loop) diuretic is almost always required. If excessive salt and water retention results in a weight gain >5 lb on a thiazide-type diuretic, switch to furosemide. If the patient is already taking furosemide and is experiencing edema, increase the dosage. Rarely, refractory fluid retention may require discontinuing minoxidil therapy. Refractory salt retention may resolve by discontinuing minoxidil for 1 or 2 days and then reinstituting treatment in conjunction with vigorous diuretic therapy.
Tachycardia, anginal symptoms	Can be partly or entirely prevented by concomitant administration of a beta-adrenergic-blocking drug or other sympathetic-nervous-system suppressant, such as methyldopa
Pericardial effusion with or without tamponade	May occur in ~3% of patients not on dialysis; more vigorous diuretic therapy, dialysis, pericardiocentesis, or surgery may be required. If the effusion persists, consider withdrawal of minoxidil.
Rapid blood-pressure control	Can precipitate cerebrovascular accidents and myocardial infarction
Use within 1 mo of myocardial infarction	Might further limit blood flow to the myocardium
Hypersensitivity	May be manifested as a skin rash in <1% of patients
Patients with renal failure or on dialysis	May require smaller doses and should be closely supervised medically to prevent exacerbation of renal failure or precipitation of cardiac failure
Hypertrichosis	Elongation, thickening, and increased pigmentation of fine body hair may occur in ~80% of patients 3–6 wk after starting therapy; after therapy is discontinued, new hair growth stops, but 1–6 mo may elapse before normal appearance is restored

Table continued on following page

LONITEN continued

ADVERSE REACTIONS

Frequent reactions are italicized

Cardiovascular	*T-wave changes (~60%)*, tachycardia, angina, pericardial effusion and tamponade
Hematological	Transient decrease in hematocrit, hemoglobin, and RBC count
Hypersensitivity	Rash (<1%)
Other	*Hypertrichosis (~80%), transient edema (7%)*, breast tenderness (<1%)

OVERDOSAGE

Signs and symptoms	Exaggerated hypotension
Treatment	To help maintain blood pressure and promote urine formation, administer normal saline IV. Avoid sympathomimetic drugs, such as norepinephrine or epinephrine. If underperfusion of a vital organ is present, administer phenylephrine, angiotensin II (investigational), vasopressin (investigational), or dopamine.

DRUG INTERACTIONS

Guanethidine	Profound orthostatic hypotension

ALTERED LABORATORY VALUES

Blood/serum values	⇧ Alkaline phosphatase ⇧ Creatinine ⇧ BUN

No clinically significant alterations in urinary values occur at therapeutic dosages

Use in children

See INDICATIONS. Dosage recommendations should be considered only as a rough guide; careful titration is essential, particularly in infants.

Use in pregnancy or nursing mothers

Safe use has not been established during pregnancy. A reduction in fertility and fetal survival has been observed in animal reproductive studies, but, so far, no teratogenic effects have been reported. Excretion into breast milk unknown; in general, patient should stop nursing if drug is prescribed.

LOPRESSOR (Metoprolol tartrate) **Geigy**

Tabs: 50, 100 mg

INDICATIONS	**ORAL DOSAGE**
Hypertension	**Adult:** 50 mg bid (alone or with a diuretic) to start, followed by weekly (or less frequent) increases until optimal response is achieved, up to 450 mg/day; usual maintenance dosage: 100 mg bid

ADMINISTRATION/DOSAGE ADJUSTMENTS

Inadequate control	Twice daily dosing is usually effective. Some patients, however, experience a modest rise in blood pressure toward the end of the 12-h dosing interval, especially when lower dosages are used. If control is inadequate, a larger dose or tid therapy may be indicated.
$Beta_1$ (cardiac) selectivity	Decreases as dosage of metoprolol is increased
Combination therapy	May be used in combination with other antihypertensive agents, especially thiazide-type diuretics
Discontinuation of therapy	Reduce dosage gradually and monitor patient closely. Caution patients with angina or hyperthyroidism against interruption or abrupt cessation of therapy (see WARNINGS/PRECAUTIONS).

CONTRAINDICATIONS

Sinus bradycardia ●	Cardiogenic shock ●
Heart block greater than first degree ●	Overt cardiac failure (see WARNINGS/PRECAUTIONS) ●

WARNINGS/PRECAUTIONS

Cardiac failure	May be precipitated by further or continued depression of myocardial contractility; discontinue use if cardiac failure persists despite adequate digitalization and diuretic therapy. In cases of well-compensated congestive heart failure, use with caution.
Abrupt discontinuation of therapy	May exacerbate angina pectoris and, in some cases, lead to myocardial infarction in patients with ischemic heart disease
Bronchospastic disease	Administer with caution, using the lowest possible dose; since $beta_1$ selectivity is not absolute, a $beta_2$-stimulating agent should be given concomitantly
Impaired response to reflex adrenergic stimuli	May augment the risks of general anesthesia and surgery. Patients undergoing emergency surgery may experience protracted severe hypotension and, occasionally, difficulty in restarting and maintaining heart beat. Excessive beta blockade may be reversed during surgery by IV administration of a beta-receptor agonist (eg, dobutamine or isoproterenol).
Protracted severe hypotension	May develop after administration of beta-receptor agonists, such as dobutamine or isoproterenol
Diabetes mellitus	Beta blockade may mask symptoms of hypoglycemia and potentiate insulin-induced hypoglycemia; use with caution, especially in patients with labile diabetes
Thyrotoxicosis	Clinical signs of hyperthyroidism may be masked; abrupt withdrawal may precipitate thyroid storm
Hepatic or renal impairment	Use with caution and monitor for signs of excessive drug accumulation (see ADVERSE REACTIONS)

Table continued on following page

LOPRESSOR continued

ADVERSE REACTIONS

Frequent reactions are italicized

Central nervous system	*Tiredness (10%), dizziness (10%), depression (5%),* headache, nightmares, insomnia, reversible mental depression progressing to catatonia,[1] visual disturbances,[1] an acute, reversible syndrome characterized by disorientation, short-term memory loss, emotional lability, clouded sensorium, and decreased neuropsychometric performance[1]
Cardiovascular	*Shortness of breath (3%), bradycardia (3%),* cold extremities, arterial insufficiency, palpitations, congestive heart failure, intensified AV block[1]
Respiratory	Bronchospasm
Gastrointestinal	*Diarrhea (5%), nausea (1%), gastric pain (1%), constipation (1%), flatulence (1%), heartburn (1%)*
Hematological	Agranulocytosis,[1] nonthrombocytopenic purpura,[1] thrombocytopenic purpura[1]
Allergic	Pruritus, erythematous rash,[1] fever,[1] aching,[1] sore throat,[1] laryngospasm,[1] respiratory distress[1]
Other	Peyronie's disease, reversible alopecia[1]

OVERDOSAGE

Signs and symptoms	Severe bradycardia, hypotension, cardiac failure, bronchospasm
Treatment	Empty stomach by gastric lavage. For excessive bradycardia, administer 0.25–1.0 mg atropine IV. If there is no response to vagal blockade, administer isoproterenol cautiously. For hypotension, use a vasopressor, such as levarterenol or (preferably) epinephrine. For cardiac failure, administer a digitalis glycoside and a diuretic; dobutamine may be helpful if shock results from inadequate cardiac contractility. A $beta_2$ stimulant (eg, isoproterenol) and/or theophylline derivative may be given for bronchospasm.

DRUG INTERACTIONS

Digitalis	⇩ AV conduction
Reserpine, *Rauwolfia* alkaloids	⇧ Risk of vertigo, syncope, or orthostatic hypotension

ALTERED LABORATORY VALUES

Blood/serum values	⇧ BUN ⇧ SGOT ⇧ SGPT ⇧ Alkaline phosphatase ⇧ Lactate dehydrogenase

No clinically significant alterations in urinary values occur at therapeutic dosages

Use in children

Safety and effectiveness in children have not been established

Use in pregnancy or nursing mothers

Use in pregnant women only when clearly needed. Increased postimplantation loss and decreased neonatal survival have been noted in rats. Excretion into breast milk is unknown; patient should stop nursing if drug is prescribed.

[1]Adverse reactions associated with other beta blockers which should be considered as potential adverse effects of metoprolol

MINIPRESS (Prazosin hydrochloride) Pfizer

Caps: 1, 2, 5 mg

INDICATIONS	ORAL DOSAGE
Hypertension	**Adult:** 1 mg bid or tid, followed by up to 20 mg/day div; usual maintenance dosage: 6–15 mg/day div

ADMINISTRATION/DOSAGE ADJUSTMENTS

Dosage schedule	After initial titration, some patients can be maintained adequately on a bid dosage regimen
Combination therapy	When adding a diuretic or other antihypertensive agent, reduce prazosin dosage to 1 or 2 mg tid, then retitrate
Refractory patients	May benefit from additional increases in dosage up to 40 mg/day div

CONTRAINDICATIONS

None

WARNINGS/PRECAUTIONS

Syncope, accompanied by dizziness, lightheadedness, or sudden loss of consciousness	May occur, usually within 30–90 min of initial dose and occasionally in association with rapid dose increases or when other antihypertensive agents are added. Severe tachycardia (heart rate, 120–160 beats/min) may precede syncopal episode. May be minimized by limiting initial dose to 1 mg, by increasing dosage slowly, and by using caution when other antihypertensive agents are introduced (see ADMINISTRATION/ DOSAGE ADJUSTMENTS).

ADVERSE REACTIONS

Frequent reactions are italicized

Gastrointestinal	*Nausea (4.9%)*, vomiting, diarrhea, constipation, abdominal discomfort and/or pain, dry mouth
Cardiovascular	*Palpitations (5.3%)*, edema, dyspnea, syncope, tachycardia
Central nervous system	*Dizziness (10.3%), headache (7.8%), drowsiness (7.6%), lack of energy (6.9%), weakness (6.5%)*, nervousness, vertigo, depression, paresthesias
Ophthalmic	Blurred vision, reddened sclera, pigmentary mottling, serious retinopathy, cataracts (causal relationship not established)
Dermatological	Rash, pruritis
Genitourinary	Urinary frequency, incontinence, impotence
Other	Diaphoresis, epistaxis, tinnitus, nasal congestion

OVERDOSAGE

Signs and symptoms	Drowsiness, depressed reflexes, hypotension, shock
Treatment	Support cardiovascular system if hypotension occurs. Keep patient in supine position to restore blood pressure and normalize heart rate. Volume expanders should be used first to treat shock; then, if necessary, use a vasopressor. Monitor renal function, and institute supportive measures, as needed. Dialysis is not beneficial, since drug is protein-bound.

DRUG INTERACTIONS

Beta blockers	⇧ Risk of hypotension
Other antihypertensive agents	⇧ Antihypertensive effect and risk of syncope

ALTERED LABORATORY VALUES

No clinically significant alterations in blood/serum or urinary values occur at therapeutic dosages

Use in children

Safety and effectiveness not established

Use in pregnancy or nursing mothers

Safe use not established during pregnancy. General guidelines not established for use in nursing mothers.

SERPASIL (Reserpine) Ciba

Tabs: 0.1, 0.25, 1 mg **Elixir:** 0.2 mg/4 ml **Amps:** 2.5 mg/2 ml (2 ml)

INDICATIONS	ORAL DOSAGE	PARENTERAL DOSAGE
Mild essential hypertension and adjunctively in more severe forms of hypertension	**Adult:** 0.5 mg/day for 1–2 wk, followed by 0.1–0.25 mg/day	——
Hypertensive emergencies (eg, acute hypertensive encephalopathy)	——	**Adult:** 0.5–1 mg IM, followed by 2–4 mg q3h, as needed
Psychiatric disorders (eg, schizophrenia)	**Adult:** 0.1–1 mg/day to start (usual initial dosage, 0.5 mg); readjust dosage upward or downward according to patient response	——
Psychiatric emergencies	——	**Adult:** 2.5–5 mg IM

ADMINISTRATION/DOSAGE ADJUSTMENTS

Combination therapy	Titrate dosage carefully when used concomitantly with other antihypertensive agents
Utility in hypertensive crisis	Because of the slow, unpredictable onset of action, usefulness is limited in hypertensive emergencies; if 4 mg is ineffective, use another antihypertensive agent
Selection of psychiatric patients	Use oral form primarily in patients in agitated psychotic states, such as schizophrenia, who are unable to tolerate phenothiazines or who require antihypertensive medication. Use parenteral form only to initiate treatment in patients unable to accept oral therapy or unable to control extreme agitation; always give a small initial dose to test responsiveness.

CONTRAINDICATIONS

Hypersensitivity to *Rauwolfia* alkaloids ●

Mental depression, especially with suicidal tendencies ●

Active peptic ulcer ●

Ulcerative colitis ●

Electroconvulsive therapy ●

WARNINGS/PRECAUTIONS

History of mental depression	Use with extreme caution; discontinue therapy at first sign of despondency, early morning insomnia, loss of appetite, impotence,or self-deprecation. Mental depression may be increased by higher doses; increase dosage cautiously.
Persistence of symptoms following withdrawal	Drug-induced depression may persist for several months after drug withdrawal and may be severe enough to result in suicide; cardiovascular effects may also persist
Increased GI motility and secretion	Use with caution in patients with a history of peptic ulcer, which may be reactivated by high dosages, or in those with ulcerative colitis
Biliary colic	May be precipitated in patients with a history of gallstones
Renal insufficiency	May make it difficult for patients to adjust easily to lowered blood-pressure levels; concomitant use of diuretic is usually necessary
Circulatory instability and hypotension	May occur during surgery, even if drug is withdrawn preoperatively; combat with anticholinergic and/or adrenergic agents (eg, metaraminol or norepinephrine)
MAO inhibitors	Avoid, if possible, or use with extreme caution
Severe hypotension	May be precipitated, especially in patients with cerebral hemorrhage, by initial parenteral doses greater than 0.5 mg

Table continued on following page

SERPASIL continued

ADVERSE REACTIONS

Gastrointestinal	Hypersecretion, nausea, vomiting, anorexia, diarrhea, dry mouth
Central nervous system and neuromuscular	Drowsiness, depression, nervousness, paradoxical anxiety, nightmares, dulled sensorium, deafness, dizziness, headache, muscle aches, parkinsonism and other extrapyramidal symptoms (rare)
Ophthalmic	Glaucoma, uveitis, optic atrophy, conjunctival injection
Cardiovascular	Angina-like symptoms, arrhythmias, bradycardia, dyspnea, syncope, water retention and edema (rare)
Dermatological	Pruritus, rash
Hematological	Purpura, epistaxis, other hematological reactions
Endocrinological	Impotence or decreased libido, breast engorgement, pseudolactation, gynecomastia
Other	Nasal congestion, dysuria, weight gain

OVERDOSAGE

Signs and symptoms	Impairment of consciousness, ranging from drowsiness to coma; flushing, conjunctival injection, pupillary constriction; *severe overdosage:* hypotension, hypothermia, respiratory depression, bradycardia, diarrhea
Treatment	Induce emesis or use gastric lavage, followed by activated charcoal, to empty stomach if drug is taken orally. Institute supportive measures, as required. Treat hypotension by elevating feet and by volume expansion, if possible. If a vasopressor is needed, use phenylephrine, levarterenol, or metaraminol. Treat significant bradycardia with vagal blocking agents, along with other appropriate measures. Observe patient for at least 72 h.

DRUG INTERACTIONS

Digitalis	⇧ Risk of cardiac arrhythmias, bradycardia, heart block
Quinidine	⇧ Risk of cardiac arrhythmias
MAO inhibitors	Severe hypertension

ALTERED LABORATORY VALUES

Blood/serum values	Carbohydrate intolerance ⇩ Thyroxine (T_4) ⇩ Plasma renin activity
Urinary values	⇧ 5-HIAA ⇩ 17-Ketosteroids

Use in children

General guidelines not established

Use in pregnancy or nursing mothers

Safe use not established. Reserpine crosses the placental barrier, appears in cord blood, and may cause increased respiratory-tract secretions, nasal congestion, cyanosis, and anorexia in newborns. Reserpine also appears in breast milk; patient should stop nursing if drug is prescribed.

ALDOCLOR (Methyldopa and chlorothiazide) Merck Sharp & Dohme

Tabs: 250 mg methyldopa and 150 mg chlorothiazide (Aldoclor-150); 250 mg methyldopa and 250 mg chlorothiazide (Aldoclor-250)

INDICATIONS	ORAL DOSAGE
Hypertension	**Adult:** 1 tab bid or tid to start, followed by up to 3 g/day of methyldopa and 1-2 g/day of chlorothiazide (see WARNINGS/PRECAUTIONS)

ADMINISTRATION/DOSAGE ADJUSTMENTS

Initiating therapy	Allow at least 48 h between dosage adjustments. Increase or decrease dosage until optimal blood-pressure response is obtained; to minimize sedation, increase dosage in evenings.
Combination therapy	Dosage of other antihypertensive agents may need to be adjusted to effect a smooth transition when initiating therapy; limit initial methyldopa dosage to 500 mg/day when adding combination to antihypertensives other than thiazides
Tolerance	May develop occasionally, usually between 2nd and 3rd mo of therapy; to restore control, increase dosage of methyldopa and/or chlorothiazide
Refractory patients	If blood pressure is not adequately controlled with maximal doses of Aldoclor, give additional methyldopa separately

CONTRAINDICATIONS

Anuria	
Hypersensitivity	To chlorothiazide, other sulfonamide derivatives, or methyldopa
Active hepatic disease	Including acute hepatitis and active cirrhosis
Liver disorders	Associated with prior methyldopa therapy

WARNINGS/PRECAUTIONS

Fixed combination	Not indicated for initial therapy of hypertension; dosages of component drugs must be individually titrated and then periodically reviewed, as conditions warrant
Coombs'-positive hemolytic anemia	May occur in less than 4% of patients, with potentially fatal complications. Obtain a blood count and Coombs' test before initiating therapy and at 6 and 12 mo after starting. With prolonged use of methyldopa, 10-20% of patients develop a positive direct Coombs' test; while this is not a contraindication to further use of the drug, therapy should be discontinued immediately if hemolytic anemia also develops in such patients. Usually, the anemia remits promptly. If it is related to methyldopa, do not reinstitute the drug.
Drug-induced hepatitis	May occur at any time during therapy. Obtain liver-function studies (eg, SGOT, bilirubin) periodically, especially during first 2-3 mo of therapy, or if unexplained fever or rash occurs. If drug-related, abnormalities will revert to normal after methyldopa is stopped; do not reinstitute therapy.
Hepatic coma	May be precipitated by minor changes in fluid and electrolyte balance in patients with hepatic impairment or progressive liver disease
Special-risk patients	Use with caution in patients with previous liver disease or dysfunction or in those with severe renal impairment; the latter may respond adequately to lower doses
Azotemia	May be precipitated in patients with renal disease
Lithium therapy	Renal clearance is reduced, increasing risk of lithium toxicity; coadministration generally should be avoided unless adequate precautions are taken
Circulatory instability during anesthesia	May occur; if necessary, reduce anesthetic dosage. If hypotension does occur, use a vasopressor.
Orthostatic hypotension	May occur; reduce dosage
Edema and weight gain	May occur; discontinue use of methyldopa if edema progresses or signs of heart failure appear
Suspected pheochromocytoma	Urinary catecholamine level may appear to be elevated due to fluorescence of methyldopa; measurement of vanillylmandelic acid (VMA) by methods that convert VMA to vanillin is not affected
Reversible leukopenia	May occur rarely, manifested primarily by a reduction in granulocytes; discontinue therapy
Involuntary choreoathetotic movements	May occur rarely in patients with severe bilateral cerebrovascular disease; discontinue therapy
Sensitivity reactions	May occur in patients with or without a history of allergy or bronchial asthma
Systemic lupus erythematosus	May be activated or exacerbated

Table continued on following page

WARNINGS/PRECAUTIONS continued

Electrolyte imbalances	Measure serum and urine electrolytes periodically, especially when patient is vomiting excessively or receiving parenteral fluids. Observe patient for such symptoms as dry mouth, thirst, weakness, lethargy, drowsiness, restlessness, muscle pains or cramps, muscular fatigue, hypotension, oliguria, tachycardia, and GI disturbances.
Hypokalemia	May develop, especially with brisk diuresis, concomitant corticosteroid or ACTH therapy, interference with adequate oral intake of electrolytes, or in the presence of severe cirrhosis; may be minimized by including potassium-rich foods in diet or, if necessary, with potassium supplements
Dilutional hyponatremia	May occur in edematous patients when weather is hot; restrict water and use salt replacement only for life-threatening hyponatremia
Hyperuricemia or frank gout	May occur or be precipitated in certain patients
Insulin requirements	May increase, decrease, or remain unchanged; latent diabetes may become active
Dialysis patients	May be difficult to control, since methyldopa is removed by dialysis
Postsympathectomy patients	Antihypertensive effect may be enhanced
Parathyroid function tests	Discontinue drug before testing

ADVERSE REACTIONS

Central nervous system and neuromuscular	Sedation, headache, asthenia, weakness, dizziness, lightheadedness, symptoms of cerebrovascular insufficiency, paresthesias, parkinsonism, Bell's palsy, decreased mental acuity, involuntary choreoathetotic movements, psychic disturbances (including nightmares and reversible mild psychoses or depression), vertigo, restlessness, muscle spasm
Ophthalmic	Transient blurred vision, xanthopsia
Cardiovascular	Bradycardia, aggravation of angina pectoris, orthostatic hypotension, edema (and weight gain)
Gastrointestinal	Nausea, vomiting, distention, constipation, flatus, diarrhea, mild dryness of the mouth, sore or "black" tongue, anorexia, gastric irritation, cramping, pancreatitis, sialadenitis
Hepatic	Abnormal liver-function tests, jaundice, liver disorders, intrahepatic cholestatic jaundice
Metabolic and endocrinological	Breast enlargement, gynecomastia, lactation, impotence, decreased libido
Hematological	Leukopenia, agranulocytosis, thrombocytopenia, aplastic anemia, hemolytic anemia
Hypersensitivity	Fever, lupus-like syndrome, myocarditis, purpura, photosensitivity, rash, urticaria, necrotizing angiitis, respiratory distress (including pneumonitis), anaphylactic reactions
Other	Nasal stuffiness, dermatological reactions (including eczema and lichenoid eruptions), mild arthralgia, myalgia

OVERDOSAGE

Signs and symptoms	*Methyldopa-related effects:* sedation, hypotension; *chlorothiazide-related effects:* diuresis, lethargy progressing to coma with minimal cardiorespiratory depression, GI irritation, hypermotility, elevated BUN, serum electrolyte changes
Treatment	Monitor serum electrolyte levels and renal function, and institute supportive measures, as required. Treat hypotension by elevating feet and by volume expansion alone, if possible. Treat GI effects symptomatically.

DRUG INTERACTIONS

Beta-adrenergic blockers	⇩ Antihypertensive effect (rare)
Other antihypertensive agents	⇧ Antihypertensive effect
Tubocurarine	⇧ Skeletal-muscle relaxation
Norepinephrine	⇩ Vasopressor effect
Steroids, ACTH	⇧ Risk of hypokalemia
Lithium	⇩ Lithium clearance
Alcohol, barbiturates, narcotic analgesics	⇧ Risk of orthostatic hypotension

Table continued on following page

ALDOCLOR continued

ALTERED LABORATORY VALUES

Blood/serum values	⇧ Alkaline phosphatase ⇧ SGOT ⇧ SGPT ⇧ Bilirubin ⇧ Creatinine (with alkaline picrate method) ⇧ Uric acid ⇧ Calcium ⇩ Sodium ⇩ Potassium ⇩ Chloride ⇩ Bicarbonate ⇩ Phosphate ⇩ PBI ⇧ or ⇩ Glucose ⇩ Plasma renin activity + Coombs' test + LE-cell reaction + Rheumatoid factor + ANA titer
Urinary values	⇧ Sodium ⇧ Potassium ⇧ Chloride ⇧ Bicarbonate ⇧ Uric acid ⇧ Catecholamines (with fluorescence methods) ⇩ Calcium

Use in children

General guidelines not established

Use in pregnancy or nursing mothers

Safe use not established during pregnancy. Both methyldopa and thiazides cross the placental barrier and appear in cord blood and breast milk. No unusual adverse effects of methyldopa have been reported during pregnancy, nor is there any evidence of teratogenicity. The possibility of fetal injury cannot be excluded, however. Thiazides may cause fetal or neonatal jaundice, thrombocytopenia, and other possible reactions. Patient should stop nursing if drug is prescribed.

ALDORIL (Methyldopa and hydrochlorothiazide) Merck Sharp & Dohme

Tabs: 250 mg methyldopa and 15 mg hydrochlorothiazide (Aldoril-15); 250 mg methyldopa and 25 mg hydrochlorothiazide (Aldoril-25); 500 mg methyldopa and 30 mg hydrochlorothiazide (Aldoril-D30); 500 mg methyldopa and 50 mg hydrochlorothiazide (Aldoril-D50)

INDICATIONS	ORAL DOSAGE
Hypertension	**Adult:** 1 tab bid or tid to start, followed by up to 3 g/day of methyldopa and 100–200 mg/day of hydrochlorothiazide (see WARNINGS/PRECAUTIONS)

ADMINISTRATION/DOSAGE ADJUSTMENTS

Initiating therapy	Allow at least 48 h between dosage adjustments. Increase or decrease dosage until optimal blood-pressure response is obtained; to minimize sedation, increase dosage in evenings.
Combination therapy	Dosage of other antihypertensive agents may need to be adjusted to effect a smooth transition when initiating therapy; limit initial methyldopa dosage to 500 mg/day when adding combination to antihypertensives other than thiazides
Tolerance	May develop occasionally, usually between 2nd and 3rd mo of therapy; to restore control, increase dosage of methyldopa and/or hydrochlorothiazide
Refractory patients	If blood pressure is not adequately controlled with maximal doses of Aldoril, give additional methyldopa separately

CONTRAINDICATIONS

Anuria	
Hypersensitivity	To hydrochlorothiazide, other sulfonamide derivatives, or methyldopa
Active hepatic disease	Including acute hepatitis and active cirrhosis
Liver disorders	Associated with prior methyldopa therapy

WARNINGS/PRECAUTIONS

Fixed combination	Not indicated for initial therapy of hypertension; dosages of component drugs must be individually titrated and then periodically reviewed, as conditions warrant
Coombs'-positive hemolytic anemia	May occur in less than 4% of patients, with potentially fatal complications. Obtain a blood count and Coombs' test before initiating therapy and at 6 and 12 mo after starting. With prolonged use of methyldopa, 10–20% of patients develop a positive direct Coombs' test; while this is not a contraindication to further use of the drug, therapy should be discontinued immediately if hemolytic anemia also develops in such patients. Usually, the anemia remits promptly. If it is related to methyldopa, do not reinstitute the drug.
Drug-induced hepatitis	May occur at any time during therapy. Obtain liver-function studies (eg, SGOT, bilirubin) periodically, especially during first 2–3 mo of therapy, or if unexplained fever or rash occurs. If drug-related, abnormalities will revert to normal after methyldopa is stopped; do not reinstitute therapy.
Hepatic coma	May be precipitated by minor changes in fluid and electrolyte balance in patients with hepatic impairment or progressive liver disease
Special-risk patients	Use with caution in patients with previous liver disease or dysfunction or in those with severe renal impairment; the latter may respond adequately to lower doses
Azotemia	May be precipitated in patients with renal disease
Lithium therapy	Renal clearance is reduced, increasing risk of lithium toxicity; coadministration generally should be avoided unless adequate precautions are taken
Circulatory instability during anesthesia	May occur; if necessary, reduce anesthetic dosage. If hypotension does occur, use a vasopressor.
Orthostatic hypotension	May occur; reduce dosage
Edema and weight gain	May occur; discontinue use of methyldopa if edema progresses or signs of heart failure appear
Suspected pheochromocytoma	Urinary catecholamine level may appear to be elevated due to fluorescence of methyldopa; measurement of vanillylmandelic acid (VMA) by methods that convert VMA to vanillin is not affected
Reversible leukopenia	May occur rarely, manifested primarily by a reduction in granulocytes; discontinue therapy
Involuntary choreoathetotic movements	May occur rarely in patients with severe bilateral cerebrovascular disease; discontinue therapy
Sensitivity reactions	May occur in patients with or without a history of allergy or bronchial asthma
Systemic lupus erythematosus	May be activated or exacerbated

Table continued on following page

ALDORIL continued

WARNINGS/PRECAUTIONS continued	
Electrolyte imbalances	Measure serum and urine electrolytes periodically, especially when patient is vomiting excessively or receiving parenteral fluids. Observe patient for such symptoms as dry mouth, thirst, weakness, lethargy, drowsiness, restlessness, muscle pains or cramps, muscular fatigue, hypotension, oliguria, tachycardia, and GI disturbances.
Hypokalemia	May develop, especially with brisk diuresis, concomitant corticosteroid or ACTH therapy, interference with adequate oral intake of electrolytes, or in the presence of severe cirrhosis; may be minimized by including potassium-rich foods in diet or, if necessary, with potassium supplements
Dilutional hyponatremia	May occur in edematous patients when weather is hot; restrict water and use salt replacement only for life-threatening hyponatremia
Hyperuricemia or frank gout	May occur or be precipitated in certain patients
Insulin requirements	May increase, decrease, or remain unchanged; latent diabetes may become active
Dialysis patients	May be difficult to control, since methyldopa is removed by dialysis
Postsympathectomy patients	Antihypertensive effect may be enhanced
Parathyroid function tests	Discontinue drug before testing
ADVERSE REACTIONS	
Central nervous system and neuromuscular	Sedation, headache, asthenia, weakness, dizziness, lightheadedness, symptoms of cerebrovascular insufficiency, paresthesias, parkinsonism, Bell's palsy, decreased mental acuity, involuntary choreoathetotic movements, psychic disturbances (including nightmares and reversible mild psychoses or depression), vertigo, restlessness, muscle spasm
Ophthalmic	Transient blurred vision, xanthopsia
Cardiovascular	Bradycardia, aggravation of angina pectoris, orthostatic hypotension, edema (and weight gain)
Gastrointestinal	Nausea, vomiting, distention, constipation, flatus, diarrhea, mild dryness of the mouth, sore or "black" tongue, anorexia, gastric irritation, cramping, pancreatitis, sialadenitis
Hepatic	Abnormal liver-function tests, jaundice, liver disorders, intrahepatic cholestatic jaundice,
Metabolic and endocrinological	Breast enlargement, gynecomastia, lactation, impotence, decreased libido
Hematological	Leukopenia, agranulocytosis, thrombocytopenia, aplastic anemia, hemolytic anemia
Hypersensitivity	Fever, lupus-like syndrome, myocarditis, purpura, photosensitivity, rash, urticaria, necrotizing angiitis, respiratory distress (including pneumonitis), anaphylactic reactions
Other	Nasal stuffiness, dermatological reactions (including eczema and lichenoid eruptions), mild arthralgia, myalgia
OVERDOSAGE	
Signs and symptoms	*Methyldopa-related effects:* sedation, hypotension; *hydrochlorothiazide-related effects:* diuresis, lethargy progressing to coma with minimal cardiorespiratory depression, GI irritation, hypermotility, elevated BUN, serum electrolyte changes
Treatment	Monitor serum electrolyte levels and renal function, and institute supportive measures, as required. Treat hypotension by elevating feet and by volume expansion alone, if possible. Treat GI effects symptomatically.
DRUG INTERACTIONS	
Beta-adrenergic blockers	⇩ Antihypertensive effect (rare)
Other antihypertensive agents	⇧ Antihypertensive effect
Tubocurarine	⇧ Skeletal-muscle relaxation
Norepinephrine	⇩ Vasopressor effect
Steroids, ACTH	⇧ Risk of hypokalemia
Lithium	⇩ Lithium clearance
Alcohol, barbiturates, narcotic analgesics	⇧ Risk of orthostatic hypotension

Table continued on following page

ALDORIL continued

ALTERED LABORATORY VALUES

Blood/serum values	⇧ Alkaline phosphatase ⇧ SGOT ⇧ SGPT ⇧ Bilirubin ⇧ Creatinine (with alkaline picrate method) ⇧ Uric acid ⇧ Calcium ⇩ Sodium ⇩ Potassium ⇩ Chloride ⇩ Bicarbonate ⇩ Phosphate ⇩ PBI ⇧ or ⇩ Glucose ⇩ Plasma renin activity + Coombs' test + LE - cell reaction + Rheumatoid factor + ANA titer
Urinary values	⇧ Sodium ⇧ Potassium ⇧ Chloride ⇧ Bicarbonate ⇧ Uric acid ⇧ Catecholamines (with fluorescence methods) ⇩ Calcium

Use in children

General guidelines not established

Use in pregnancy or nursing mothers

Safe use not established during pregnancy. Both methyldopa and thiazides cross the placental barrier and appear in cord blood and breast milk. No unusual adverse effects of methyldopa have been reported during pregnancy, nor is there any evidence of teratogenicity. However, the possibility of fetal injury cannot be excluded. Thiazides may cause fetal or neonatal jaundice, thrombocytopenia, and other possible reactions. Patient should stop nursing if drug is prescribed.

APRESAZIDE (Hydralazine hydrochloride and hydrochlorothiazide) Ciba

Caps: 25 mg hydralazine hydrochloride and 25 mg hydrochlorothiazide (Apresazide 25/25); 50 mg hydralazine hydrochloride and 50 mg hydrochlorothiazide (Apresazide 50/50); 100 mg hydralazine hydrochloride and 50 mg hydrochlorothiazide (Apresazide 100/50)

INDICATIONS	ORAL DOSAGE
Hypertension	**Adult:** 1 cap bid (see WARNINGS/PRECAUTIONS); adjust dosage to lowest effective level for maintenance

ADMINISTRATION/DOSAGE ADJUSTMENTS

Combination therapy	Other antihypertensive agents, such as sympathetic inhibitors, may be added gradually in reduced dosages; monitor patient closely

CONTRAINDICATIONS

Anuria	
Hypersensitivity	To hydrochlorothiazide, other sulfonamide derivatives, or hydralazine
Coronary-artery disease	Anginal attacks may be precipitated or may worsen
Rheumatic mitral-valve disease	Congestive heart failure may be precipitated

WARNINGS/PRECAUTIONS

Fixed combination	Not indicated for initial therapy of hypertension; dosages of component drugs must be individually titrated and then periodically reviewed, as conditions warrant
Lupus erythematosus-like syndrome	May occur; obtain CBC, LE cell preparation, and antinuclear antibody (ANA) titer before and periodically during prolonged therapy or if arthralgia, fever, chest pain, continued malaise, or other unexplained symptoms develop. In general, unless hydralazine component is essential, discontinue therapy if clinical symptoms occur, ANA titer rises, or LE cell reaction is positive.
Profound hypotension	May occur with concomitant use of potent parenteral antihypertensive agents, such as diazoxide; patient should be observed for several hours
Peripheral neuritis	May occur (see ADVERSE REACTIONS); combat with pyridoxine
Blood dyscrasias	May occur (see ADVERSE REACTIONS); obtain periodic blood counts during prolonged therapy and withdraw drug if abnormalities develop
Renal impairment	Use with caution and monitor for signs of excessive drug accumulation
Azotemia	May be precipitated in patients with renal disease
Hepatic coma	May be precipitated by minor changes in fluid and electrolyte balance in patients with hepatic impairment or progressive liver disease
Sensitivity reactions	May occur in patients with a history of allergy or bronchial asthma
Electrolyte imbalances	Measure serum electrolytes periodically, especially when patient is vomiting excessively or receiving parenteral fluids. Watch for dry mouth, thirst, weakness, lethargy, drowsiness, restlessness, muscle pains or cramps, muscular fatigue, hypotension, oliguria, tachycardia, and GI disturbances.
Hypokalemia	May develop, especially with brisk diuresis, concomitant corticosteroid or ACTH therapy, interference with adequate oral intake of electrolytes, or in the presence of severe cirrhosis; may be minimized by including potassium-rich foods in diet or, if necessary, with potassium supplements
Dilutional hyponatremia	May occur in edematous patients when weather is hot; restrict water and use salt replacement only for life-threatening hyponatremia

Table continued on following page

APRESAZIDE continued

WARNINGS/PRECAUTIONS continued	
Special-risk patients	Use with caution following sympathectomy or in patients with suspected coronary-artery disease, specific cardiovascular inadequacies (eg, mitral valvular disease), cerebrovascular accidents, or advanced renal disease, or those on MAO inhibitor therapy
Insulin requirements	May increase, decrease, or remain unchanged; latent diabetes may become active
Hyperuricemia or frank gout	May occur or be precipitated in certain patients
Parathyroid function tests	Discontinue drug before testing
Tartrazine sensitivity	Presence of FD&C Yellow No. 5 (tartrazine) in Apresazide 100/50 capsules may cause allergic-type reactions, including bronchial asthma, in susceptible individuals
ADVERSE REACTIONS Frequent reactions are italicized	
Central nervous system and neuromuscular	*Headache,* dizziness, vertigo, peripheral neuritis (paresthesias, numbness, tingling), tremors, muscle cramps, psychotic reactions (depression, disorientation, anxiety), muscle spasm, weakness, restlessness
Cardiovascular	*Palpitations, tachycardia, angina pectoris,* orthostatic hypotension, paradoxical pressor response, edema
Gastrointestinal	*Nausea, vomiting, diarrhea, anorexia,* gastric irritation, cramping, constipation, paralytic ileus, intrahepatic cholestatic jaundice, pancreatitis, sialadenitis
Hematological	Reduction in hemoglobin level and erythrocyte count, leukopenia, thrombocytopenia, agranulocytosis, purpura, aplastic anemia
Ophthalmic	Lacrimation, conjunctivitis, xanthopsia
Hypersensitivity	Rash, urticaria, pruritus, fever, chills, arthralgia, eosinophilia, purpura, photosensitivity, necrotizing angiitis, Stevens-Johnson syndrome, hepatitis (rare)
Other	Nasal congestion, flushing, difficult micturition, dyspnea, lymphadenopathy, splenomegaly
OVERDOSAGE	
Signs and symptoms	*Hydralazine-related effects:* hypotension, tachycardia, headache, generalized skin flushing, myocardial ischemia, cardiac arrhythmia, profound shock (in severe overdosage); *hydrochlorothiazide-related effects:* diuresis, lethargy progressing to coma with minimal cardiorespiratory depression, GI irritation, hypermotility, elevated BUN, serum electrolyte changes
Treatment	Empty stomach, taking care to prevent pulmonary aspiration; if conditions permit, instill activated charcoal to remove any remaining drug from the stomach. Cardiovascular support is primary. Use volume expanders without resorting to vasopressors, if possible. If a vasopressor is required, use one that is least likely to precipitate or aggravate cardiac arrhythmias. Digitalization may be necessary. Monitor serum electrolyte levels and renal function and institute supportive measures, as required. Treat GI effects symptomatically.
DRUG INTERACTIONS	
Beta blockers	⇧ Antihypertensive effect of hydralazine component
Other antihypertensive agents	⇧ Antihypertensive effect of both drugs
Tubocurarine	⇧ Skeletal-muscle relaxation
Norepinephrine	⇩ Vasopressor effect
Steroids, ACTH	⇧ Risk of hypokalemia
Lithium	⇩ Lithium clearance
Alcohol, barbiturates, narcotic analgesics	⇧ Risk of orthostatic hypotension

Table continued on following page

APRESAZIDE continued

ALTERED LABORATORY VALUES

Blood/serum values	⇧ Uric acid ⇧ Calcium ⇧ Plasma renin activity ⇩ Sodium ⇩ Potassium ⇩ Chloride ⇩ Bicarbonate ⇩ Phosphate ⇩ PBI + ANA titer + LE-cell reaction + Direct Coombs' test ⇧ or ⇩ Glucose
Urinary values	⇧ Sodium ⇧ Potassium ⇧ Chloride ⇧ Bicarbonate ⇧ Uric acid ⇩ Calcium

Use in children

General guidelines not established

Use in pregnancy or nursing mothers

Safe use not established during pregnancy. Hydralazine is teratogenic in mice and possibly rabbits, but not in rats. Thiazides cross the placental barrier, appear in cord blood, and may cause fetal or neonatal jaundice, thrombocytopenia, and other possible reactions. Thiazides also appear in breast milk; patient should stop nursing if drug is prescribed.

COMBIPRES (Clonidine hydrochloride and chlorthalidone) Boehringer Ingelheim

Tabs: 0.1 mg clonidine hydrochloride and 15 mg chlorthalidone (Combipres 0.1); 0.2 mg clonidine hydrochloride and 15 mg chlorthalidone (Combipres 0.2)

INDICATIONS	ORAL DOSAGE
Hypertension	**Adult:** determine patient dose by individual titration of separate components (see Catapres and Hygroton)

ADMINISTRATION/DOSAGE ADJUSTMENTS

Discontinuation of therapy	Reduce dosage gradually over 2–4 days, whenever possible, to avoid severe increases in blood pressure (usually observed in patients receiving more than 0.6–0.8 mg/day of clonidine). If blood pressure rises excessively, resume Combipres therapy or administer IV phentolamine and propranolol, as in treating pheochromocytoma. Caution patients against interrupting or abruptly discontinuing therapy.

CONTRAINDICATIONS

Hypersensitivity to chlorthalidone●	Severe renal or hepatic disease●

WARNINGS/PRECAUTIONS

Fixed combination	Not indicated for initial therapy of hypertension; dosages of component drugs must be individually titrated and then periodically reviewed, as conditions warrant
Tolerance	May develop; re-evaluate therapy
Hypertensive encephalopathy, death	May occur, in rare instances, after abrupt cessation of therapy (see ADMINISTRATION/DOSAGE ADJUSTMENTS)
Drowsiness, sedation	Performance of potentially hazardous activities may be impaired; caution patients accordingly
Special-risk patients	Use with caution in patients with severe coronary insufficiency, recent myocardial infarction, cerebrovascular disease, or chronic renal failure
Visual impairment	Periodic eye examinations are recommended during prolonged therapy, based on observation of retinal degeneration in rats
Decreased glucose tolerance	May occur; periodically test patients predisposed toward or affected by diabetes
Renal failure	Determine BUN periodically; if rise in BUN is significant, stop therapy
Sodium and/or potassium depletion	May occur, resulting in muscular weakness, muscle cramps, anorexia, nausea, vomiting, constipation, lethargy, or mental confusion; severe dietary salt restriction is not recommended
Potassium deficiency, hypokalemia	May develop, often preceded by hypochloremic acidosis. Patients taking corticosteroids, ACTH, or digitalis concomitantly must be closely monitored. Risk of potassium deficiency may be minimized by including potassium-rich foods in diet or, if necessary, with oral potassium supplements supplying 3.0–4.5 g/day of KCl.
Hyperuricemia or acute gout	May occur or be precipitated by chlorthalidone; for significant or prolonged hyperuricemia, administer a uricosuric agent while continuing Combipres therapy

ADVERSE REACTIONS
Frequent reactions are italicized

Gastrointestinal	*Dry mouth (~40%)*, anorexia, malaise, nausea, vomiting, parotid pain, mild transient abnormalities in liver-function tests, gastric irritation, constipation, cramping, pancreatitis, jaundice, drug-induced hepatitis without icterus or hyperbilirubinemia (one case)
Metabolic and endocrinological	Weight gain, gynecomastia, hyperglycemia, glycosuria, hypokalemia, gout, hyperuricemia
Cardiovascular	Congestive heart failure, Raynaud's phenomenon, ECG abnormalities manifested as Wenckebach's period or ventricular trigeminy, orthostatic hypotension
Central nervous system and neuromuscular	*Drowsiness (~35%), sedation (~8%)*, dizziness, headache, vivid dreams or nightmares, insomnia, other behavioral changes, nervousness, restlessness, anxiety, mental depression, paresthesias, fatigue, weakness

Table continued on following page

COMBIPRES continued

ADVERSE REACTIONS continued

Ophthalmic	Dry, itching, or burning eyes, xanthopsia
Dermatological	Rash, angioneurotic edema, hives, urticaria, thinning of hair, pruritus not associated with a rash, purpura, photosensitization
Genitourinary	Impotence, urinary retention, dysuria
Hematological (idiosyncratic)	Aplastic anemia, thrombocytopenia, leukopenia, agranulocytosis, necrotizing angiitis
Other	Increased sensitivity to alcohol, dryness of the nasal mucosa, pallor, weakly positive Coombs' test

OVERDOSAGE

Signs and symptoms	*Clonidine-related effects:* profound hypotension, weakness, somnolence, diminished or absent reflexes, vomiting; *chlorthalidone-related effects:* nausea, weakness, dizziness, electrolyte balance disturbances
Treatment	Use gastric lavage to empty stomach. Administer an analeptic and vasopressor or, alternatively, 10 mg tolazoline every 30 min. Treat chlorthalidone-related effects supportively, including, when necessary, IV dextrose and saline with potassium, administered with caution.

DRUG INTERACTIONS

Alcohol, barbiturates, narcotic analgesics	⇧ CNS depression ⇧ Risk of orthostatic hypotension
Tricyclic antidepressants	⇩ Antihypertensive effect
Tubocurarine	⇧ Skeletal-muscle relaxation
Norepinephrine	⇩ Vasopressor effect
Steroids, ACTH	⇧ Risk of hypokalemia
Lithium	⇩ Lithium clearance

ALTERED LABORATORY VALUES

Blood/serum values	⇧ Glucose (transient) ⇧ Creatine phosphokinase ⇧ Uric acid ⇩ Sodium ⇩ Potassium ⇩ Chloride ⇩ Plasma renin activity
Urinary values	⇧ Aldosterone ⇧ Catecholamines ⇧ Sodium ⇧ Potassium ⇧ Chloride ⇧ Uric acid

Use in children

Safety and effectiveness have not been established

Use in pregnancy or nursing mothers

Not recommended for use in women who are or who may become pregnant unless potential benefit outweighs risk. General guidelines not established for use in nursing mothers.

DIUPRES (Chlorothiazide and reserpine) Merck Sharp & Dohme

Tabs: 250 mg chlorothiazide and 0.125 mg reserpine (Diupres-250); 500 mg chlorothiazide and 0.125 mg reserpine (Diupres-500)

INDICATIONS	ORAL DOSAGE
Hypertension	**Adult:** 1–2 Diupres-250 tabs or 1 Diupres-500 tab qd or bid (see WARNINGS/PRECAUTIONS)

CONTRAINDICATIONS

Hypersensitivity to chlorothiazide, other sulfonamide derivatives, or reserpine●

Mental depression, especially in patients with suicidal tendencies●

Active peptic ulcer●

Ulcerative colitis●

Anuria●

Electroconvulsive therapy●

WARNINGS/PRECAUTIONS

Fixed combination	Not indicated for initial therapy of hypertension; dosages of component drugs must be individually titrated and then periodically reviewed, as conditions warrant
Renal impairment	Use with caution and monitor for signs of excessive drug accumulation (see OVERDOSAGE); patient may adjust poorly to lowered blood pressure
Azotemia	May be precipitated in patients with renal disease
Hepatic coma	May be precipitated by minor changes in fluid and electrolyte balance in patients with hepatic impairment or progressive liver disease
Sensitivity reactions	May occur in patients with or without a history of allergy or bronchial asthma
Postsympathectomy patients	Antihypertensive effect may be enhanced
Systemic lupus erythematosus	May be activated or exacerbated
Electrolyte imbalances	Measure serum and urine electrolytes periodically, especially when patient is vomiting excessively or receiving parenteral fluids. Observe patient for such symptoms as dry mouth, thirst, weakness, lethargy, drowsiness, restlessness, muscle pains or cramps, muscular fatigue, hypotension, oliguria, tachycardia, and GI disturbances.
Hypokalemia	May develop, especially with brisk diuresis, concomitant corticosteroid or ACTH therapy, interference with adequate oral intake of electrolytes, or in the presence of severe cirrhosis; may be minimized by including potassium-rich foods in diet or, if necessary, with potassium supplements
Dilutional hyponatremia	May occur in edematous patients when weather is hot; restrict water and use salt replacement only for life-threatening hyponatremia
Hyperuricemia or frank gout	May occur or be precipitated in certain patients
Insulin requirements	May increase, decrease, or remain unchanged; latent diabetes may become active
History of mental depression	Use with extreme caution; discontinue therapy at first sign of despondency, early morning insomnia, loss of appetite, impotence, or self-deprecation. Mental depression is unusual with reserpine doses of 0.25 mg/day or less.
Patients undergoing electroconvulsive therapy	Discontinue drug at least 7 days before giving electroshock treatments; severe and even fatal reactions have occurred
Increased gastric secretion and motility	Use with caution in patients with history of peptic ulcer, ulcerative colitis, or other GI disorders
Biliary colic	May be precipitated in patients with gallstones
Bronchial asthma	May be precipitated in susceptible patients
Lithium therapy	Renal clearance is reduced, increasing risk of lithium toxicity; coadministration generally should be avoided unless adequate precautions are taken
Circulatory disturbances	May develop during surgical anesthesia; vagal blocking agents may be needed to prevent or reverse hypotension and/or bradycardia
Parathyroid function tests	Discontinue drug before testing

ADVERSE REACTIONS

Gastrointestinal	Anorexia, gastric irritation, hypersecretion and increased motility, nausea, vomiting, cramps, diarrhea, constipation, dry mouth, increased salivation, intrahepatic cholestatic jaundice, pancreatitis, sialadenitis
Central nervous system and neuromuscular	Dizziness, syncope, nervousness, vertigo, paresthesias, headache, excessive sedation, mental depression, nightmares, paradoxical anxiety, dulled sensorium, deafness, muscle spasm, weakness, restlessness, muscle aches, parkinsonism (usually reversible)
Ophthalmic	Transient blurred vision, glaucoma, uveitis, optic atrophy, conjunctival injection, xanthopsia

Table continued on following page

ADVERSE REACTIONS continued

Cardiovascular	Orthostatic hypotension, bradycardia, angina pectoris, arrhythmia, premature ventricular contractions, fluid retention, congestive heart failure
Hematological	Leukopenia, agranulocytosis, thrombocytopenia, aplastic anemia, hemolytic anemia, excessive bleeding following prostatic surgery, thrombocytopenic purpura, epistaxis
Genitourinary	Dysuria, impotence, decreased libido
Hypersensitivity	Purpura, photosensitivity, pruritus, rash, urticaria, flushing, necrotizing angiitis, fever, respiratory distress (including pneumonitis), anaphylactic reactions
Other	Nasal congestion, dyspnea, increased susceptibility to colds, weight gain, nonpuerperal lactation

OVERDOSAGE

Signs and symptoms	*Chlorothiazide-related effects:* diuresis, lethargy progressing to coma with minimal cardiorespiratory depression, GI irritation, hypermotility, elevated BUN, serum electrolyte changes; *reserpine-related effects:* impairment of consciousness ranging from drowsiness to coma, flushing, conjunctival injection, miosis, hypotension, hypothermia, respiratory depression, bradycardia, diarrhea
Treatment	Induce emesis or use gastric lavage, followed by activated charcoal, to empty stomach. Treat hypotension by elevating feet and by volume expansion, if possible. If a vasopressor is neeeded, use phenylephrine, levarterenol, or metaraminol. Treat significant bradycardia with vagal blocking agents, along with other appropriate measures. Monitor serum electrolytes and renal function, and institute supportive measures, as required. Treat GI effects symptomatically. Observe patient for at least 72 h.

DRUG INTERACTIONS

Other antihypertensive agents	⇧ Antihypertensive effect
Digitalis	⇧ Risk of cardiac arrhythmias, bradycardia, heart block
Quinidine	⇧ Risk of cardiac arrhythmias
MAO inhibitors	Severe hypertension
Tubocurarine	⇧ Skeletal-muscle relaxation
Norepinephrine	⇩ Vasopressor effect
Steroids, ACTH	⇧ Risk of hypokalemia
Lithium	⇩ Lithium clearance
Alcohol, barbiturates, narcotic analgesics	⇧ Risk of orthostatic hypotension

ALTERED LABORATORY VALUES

Blood/serum values	Carbohydrate intolerance ⇧ Uric acid ⇧ Calcium ⇩ Sodium ⇩ Potassium ⇩ Chloride ⇩ Bicarbonate ⇩ Phosphate ⇩ PBI ⇩ Thyroxine (T_4) ⇩ Plasma renin activity
Urinary values	⇧ Sodium ⇧ Potassium ⇧ Chloride ⇧ Bicarbonate ⇧ Uric acid ⇧ 5-HIAA ⇩ Calcium ⇩ 17-Ketosteroids

Use in children

General guidelines not established

Use in pregnancy or nursing mothers

Safe use not established during pregnancy. Thiazides cross the placental barrier, appear in cord blood, and may cause fetal or neonatal jaundice, thrombocytopenia, and other possible reactions. Reserpine crosses the placental barrier, appears in cord blood, and may cause nasal congestion, lethargy, depressed Moro reflex, and bradycardia in newborns. Both drugs also appear in breast milk; patient should stop nursing if drug is prescribed.

ENDURONYL/ENDURONYL FORTE (Methyclothiazide and deserpidine) Abbott

Tabs: 5 mg methyclothiazide and 0.25 mg deserpidine (Enduronyl); 5 mg methyclothiazide and 0.5 mg deserpidine (Enduronyl Forte)

INDICATIONS	ORAL DOSAGE
Mild to moderately severe hypertension	**Adult:** ½–2 tabs/day (see WARNINGS/PRECAUTIONS)

ADMINISTRATION/DOSAGE ADJUSTMENTS

Frequency of dosage adjustments	Titrate dosage to individual needs; allow at least 10 days to 2 wk between dosage adjustments for full drug effects to become evident
Combination therapy	Addition of other antihypertensive drugs should be gradual; ganglionic blocking agents should be given at only ½ the usual dose since their effect is potentiated

CONTRAINDICATIONS

Hypersensitivity to methyclothiazide, other sulfonamide derivatives, or deserpidine●	Active peptic ulcer●	Renal decompensation●
	Ulcerative colitis●	
Mental depression, especially in patients with suicidal tendencies●	Electroconvulsive therapy●	

WARNINGS/PRECAUTIONS

Fixed combination	Not indicated for initial therapy of hypertension; dosages of component drugs must be individually titrated and then periodically reviewed, as conditions warrant
Renal impairment	Use with caution and monitor for signs of excessive drug accumulation (see OVERDOSAGE); patient may adjust poorly to lowered blood pressure
Azotemia	May be precipitated in patients with renal disease
Hepatic coma	May be precipitated by minor changes in fluid and electrolyte balance in patients with hepatic impairment or progressive liver disease
Sensitivity reactions	May occur in patients with a history of allergy or bronchial asthma
Systemic lupus erythematosus	May be activated or exacerbated
Electrolyte imbalances	Measure serum and urine electrolytes periodically, especially when patient is vomiting excessively or receiving parenteral fluids. Observe patient for such symptoms as dry mouth, thirst, weakness, lethargy, drowsiness, restlessness, muscle pains or cramps, muscular fatigue, hypotension, oliguria, tachycardia, and GI disturbances.
Hypokalemia	May develop, especially with brisk diuresis, concomitant corticosteroid or ACTH therapy, interference with adequate oral intake of electrolytes, or in the presence of severe cirrhosis; may be minimized by including potassium-rich foods in diet or, if necessary, with potassium supplements
Dilutional hyponatremia	May occur in edematous patients when weather is hot; restrict water and use salt replacement only for life-threatening hyponatremia
Hyperuricemia or frank gout	May occur or be precipitated in certain patients
Insulin requirements	May increase, decrease, or remain unchanged; latent diabetes may become active
Postsympathectomy patients	Antihypertensive effect may be enhanced
History of mental depression	Use with extreme caution; discontinue treatment at first sign of despondency, early morning insomnia, loss of appetite, impotence, or self-deprecation
Persistence of drug effects	Drug-induced depression may persist for several months after withdrawal and may be severe enough to result in suicide; cardiac effects may also persist
Increased GI motility and secretion	Use with caution in patients with a history of peptic ulcer or ulcerative colitis
Biliary colic	May be precipitated in patients with gallstones
Circulatory instability and hypotension	May occur during anesthesia; anticholinergic and/or adrenergic agents (metaraminol, norepinephrine) may be needed to correct adverse vagocirculatory effects

Table continued on following page

ENDURONYL/ENDURONYL FORTE continued

ADVERSE EFFECTS

Gastrointestinal	Anorexia, gastric irritation, nausea, vomiting, cramping, diarrhea, constipation, intrahepatic cholestatic jaundice, pancreatitis, hypersecretion
Central nervous system and neuromuscular	Dizziness, vertigo, paresthesias, headache, drowsiness, depression, nervousness, paradoxical anxiety, nightmares, extrapyramidal tract symptoms, dulled sensorium, deafness, muscle spasm, muscular aches, weakness, restlessness
Ophthalmic	Glaucoma, uveitis, optic atrophy, conjunctival injection, xanthopsia
Cardiovascular	Orthostatic hypotension, angina-like symptoms, arrhythmias, bradycardia
Hematological	Leukopenia, agranulocytosis, thrombocytopenia, aplastic anemia, thrombocytopenic purpura
Hypersensitivity	Purpura, photosensitivity, rash, urticaria, necrotizing angiitis, pruritus, and asthma (in asthmatic patients)
Other	Nasal congestion, weight gain, impotence or decreased libido, dysuria, dyspnea

OVERDOSAGE

Signs and symptoms	*Methyclothiazide-related effects:* electrolyte imbalance, confusion, dizziness, muscular weakness, GI disturbances; *deserpidine-related effects:* flushing, conjunctival injection, pupillary constriction, sedation ranging from drowsiness to coma; in severe cases: hypotension, hypothermia, central respiratory depression, bradycardia
Treatment	Carefully evacuate stomach contents. Treat CNS depression symptomatically. For severe hypotension, use a direct-acting vasopressor, such as levarterenol. Monitor serum electrolytes and renal function, and replace fluids and electrolytes, as needed.

DRUG INTERACTIONS

Other antihypertensive agents	⇧ Antihypertensive effect
Tubocurarine	⇧ Skeletal-muscle relaxation
Norepinephrine	⇩ Vasopressor effect
Steroids, ACTH	⇧ Risk of hypokalemia
Lithium	⇩ Lithium clearance
Digitalis	⇧ Risk of cardiac arrhythmias ⇧ Risk of heart block
Quinidine	⇧ Risk of cardiac arrhythmias
Alcohol, barbiturates, narcotic analgesics	⇧ Risk of orthostatic hypotension

ALTERED LABORATORY VALUES

Blood/serum values	⇧ Uric acid ⇧ Calcium ⇩ Sodium ⇩ Potassium ⇩ Chloride ⇩ Bicarbonate ⇩ Phosphate ⇩ PBI ⇧ or ⇩ Glucose
Urinary values	⇧ Sodium ⇧ Potassium ⇧ Chloride ⇧ Bicarbonate ⇧ Uric acid ⇩ Calcium

Use in children

General guidelines not established

Use in pregnancy or nursing mothers

Safe use has not been established during pregnancy. Thiazides cross the placental barrier, appear in cord blood, and may cause fetal or neonatal jaundice, thrombocytopenia, and other possible reactions. *Rauwolfia* alkaloids such as deserpidine also cross the placental barrier, appear in cord blood, and have caused increased respiratory secretions, nasal congestion, cyanosis, and anorexia in neonates. Both drugs appear in breast milk; patient should stop nursing if drug is prescribed.

ESIMIL (Guanethidine monosulfate and hydrochlorothiazide) Ciba

Tabs: 10 mg guanethidine monosulfate and 25 mg hydrochlorothiazide

INDICATIONS	ORAL DOSAGE
Hypertension	**Adult:** 1 tab/day to start, followed by increases of 1 tab/day at weekly intervals, up to 4 tabs/day, as needed; usual maintenance dosage: 2 tabs/day (see WARNINGS/PRECAUTIONS)

ADMINISTRATION/DOSAGE ADJUSTMENTS

Initial titration of dosage	Take blood pressure with patient in supine position and again after patient has been standing for 10 min. Increase dosage only if there is *no* decrease in standing blood pressure from previous levels.
Transferring from other antihypertensive agents	Begin with 1 tab/day of Esimil and ½ the usual dose of the antihypertensive agent to be substituted. One week later, increase Esimil dosage to 2 tabs/day and give ¼ the usual dose of the previous agent. The following week, discontinue the previous drug and begin titrating Esimil dosage at weekly intervals.
Refractory patients	If blood pressure is not adequately controlled at maximum dosage (4 tabs/day), add guanethidine alone
Patients with fever	Dosage requirements may be reduced

CONTRAINDICATIONS

Anuria	
Hypersensitivity	To hydrochlorothiazide, other sulfonamide derivatives, or guanethidine
Pheochromocytoma	Either known or suspected
Frank congestive heart failure	Not due to hypertension
Use of MAO inhibitors	Wait 1 wk after discontinuing MAO inhibitor therapy before starting Esimil

WARNINGS/PRECAUTIONS

Fixed combination	Not indicated for initial therapy of hypertension; dosages of component drugs must be individually titrated and then periodically reviewed, as conditions warrant
Orthostatic hypotension	Occurs frequently; caution patient to sit or lie down at the first sign of dizziness or weakness and to avoid sudden or prolonged standing or exercise
Cardiovascular instability during surgery	If possible, withdraw therapy 2 wk prior to elective surgery to minimize risk of vascular collapse and cardiac arrest. For emergency surgery, reduce dosage of pre-anesthetic and anesthetic agents. Use vasopressors with extreme caution if vascular collapse occurs.
Bronchial asthma	May be exacerbated due to hypersensitivity to catecholamine depletion; thiazide sensitivity reactions are also more apt to occur. Exercise special care when treating patients with a history of bronchial asthma.
Long-term therapy	Since effects of guanethidine are cumulative, increase dosage slowly (see ORAL DOSAGE)
Special-risk patients	Use very cautiously in patients with severe renal disease and nitrogen retention or rising BUN levels; coronary disease with insufficiency or recent myocardial infarction; or cerebral vascular disease, especially with encephalopathy
Peptic ulcer	May be exacerbated by relative increase in parasympathetic tone; use with caution in patients with a history of peptic ulcer
Severe cardiac failure	May interfere with compensatory role of adrenergic system in producing circulatory adjustment; use with extreme caution
Incipient cardiac decompensation	Observe patient for possible weight gain or edema
Severe diarrhea	May occur, necessitating discontinuation of therapy
Azotemia	May be precipitated in patients with renal disease
Excessive drug accumulation	May occur in patients with impaired renal function (see OVERDOSAGE)

Table continued on following page

ESIMIL continued

WARNINGS/PRECAUTIONS continued

Hepatic coma	May be precipitated by minor changes in fluid and electrolyte balance in patients with hepatic impairment or progressive liver disease
Sensitivity reactions	May occur with increased frequency in patients with a history of allergy
Systemic lupus erythematosus	May be activated or exacerbated
Electrolyte imbalances	Measure serum and urine electrolytes periodically, especially when patient is vomiting excessively or receiving parenteral fluids. Observe patient for such symptoms as dry mouth, thirst, weakness, lethargy, drowsiness, restlessness, muscle pains or cramps, muscular fatigue, hypotension, oliguria, tachycardia, and GI disturbances.
Hypokalemia	May develop, especially with brisk diuresis, concomitant corticosteroid or ACTH therapy, interference with adequate oral intake of electrolytes, or in the presence of severe cirrhosis; may be minimized by including potassium-rich foods in diet or, if necessary, with potassium supplements
Dilutional hyponatremia	May occur in edematous patients when weather is hot; restrict water and use salt replacement only for life-threatening hyponatremia
Hyperuricemia or frank gout	May occur or be precipitated in certain patients
Insulin requirements	May increase, decrease, or remain unchanged; latent diabetes may become active
Postsympathectomy patients	Antihypertensive effect may be enhanced
Parathyroid function tests	Discontinue drug before testing

ADVERSE REACTIONS
Frequent reactions are italicized

Central nervous system and neuromuscular	*Dizziness, weakness, lassitude, and syncope due to postural or exertional hypotension,* fatigue, myalgia, muscle tremor, mental depression, vertigo, paresthesias, headache, restlessness, muscle spasm
Ophthalmic	Ptosis, blurred vision, xanthopsia
Cardiovascular	*Orthostatic hypotension, bradycardia, fluid retention and edema, with occasional development of congestive heart failure,* dyspnea, chest pains (angina), chest paresthesias
Gastrointestinal	*Increased bowel movements, diarrhea,* nausea, vomiting, anorexia, gastric irritation, cramping, constipation, dry mouth, intrahepatic cholestatic jaundice, pancreatitis, sialadenitis
Genitourinary	*Inhibition of ejaculation,* nocturia, urinary incontinence, priapism (causal relationship not established)
Hematological	Anemia, thrombocytopenia, leukopenia, agranulocytosis, aplastic anemia (first three conditions have been linked to guanethidine, but not conclusively)
Hypersensitivity	Purpura, photosensitivity, rash, urticaria, necrotizing angiitis, Stevens-Johnson syndrome
Other	Dermatitis, scalp-hair loss, parotid tenderness, nasal congestion, weight gain, asthma (in susceptible individuals)

OVERDOSAGE

Signs and symptoms	*Guanethidine-related effects:* postural hypotension (with dizziness, blurring of vision, and like symptoms, progressing to syncope when standing), bradycardia, diarrhea (possibly severe), unconsciousness; *hydrochlorothiazide-related effects:* diuresis, lethargy progressing to coma with minimal cardiorespiratory depression, GI irritation and hypermotility, temporarily elevated BUN, serum electrolyte changes
Treatment	Evacuate stomach contents, taking care to prevent aspiration. Begin monitoring serum electrolytes and renal function. Support vital functions and control cardiac irregularities, as needed. Keep patient in supine position. Use vasopressors only with extreme caution because of heightened sensitivity (see DRUG INTERACTIONS). Treat diarrhea and other GI effects symptomatically and maintain hydration and electrolyte balance.

Table continued on following page

ESIMIL continued

DRUG INTERACTIONS

MAO inhibitors	⇧ Hypertension to crisis proportions
Digitalis	⇩ Heart rate
Amphetamine-like compounds, ephedrine, methylphenidate, and other stimulants; tricyclic antidepressants, phenothiazines, and other psychotropic agents	⇩ Antihypertensive effect
Oral contraceptives	⇩ Antihypertensive effect
Rauwolfia derivatives	Excessive postural hypotension, bradycardia, mental depression
Norepinephrine and other vasopressors	⇧ Pressor effect ⇧ Risk of cardiac arrhythmias
Tubocurarine	⇧ Skeletal-muscle relaxation
Steroids, ACTH	⇧ Risk of hypokalemia
Lithium	⇩ Lithium clearance
Alcohol, barbiturates, narcotic analgesics	⇧ Risk of orthostatic hypotension

ALTERED LABORATORY VALUES

Values	Alteration
Blood/serum values	⇧ BUN ⇧ Creatinine ⇧ Uric acid ⇧ Calcium ⇧ Plasma renin activity ⇩ Sodium ⇩ Potassium ⇩ Chloride ⇩ Bicarbonate ⇩ Phosphate ⇩ PBI ⇧ or ⇩ Glucose
Urinary values	⇧ Sodium ⇧ Potassium ⇧ Chloride ⇧ Bicarbonate ⇧ Uric acid ⇧ Catecholamines (initially) ⇩ Catecholamines (subsequently) ⇩ VMA ⇩ Calcium

Use in children

General guidelines not established

Use in pregnancy or nursing mothers

Safety of guanethidine during pregnancy not established. Thiazides cross the placental barrier, appear in cord blood, and may cause fetal or neonatal jaundice, thrombocytopenia, and possibly other reactions. Thiazides also appear in breast milk; patient should stop nursing if drug is prescribed.

HYDROPRES (Hydrochlorothiazide and reserpine) **Merck Sharp & Dohme**

Tabs: 25 mg hydrochlorothiazide and 0.125 mg reserpine (Hydropres-25); 50 mg hydrochlorothiazide and 0.125 mg reserpine (Hydropres-50)

INDICATIONS	ORAL DOSAGE
Hypertension	**Adult:** 1–2 Hydropres-25 tabs or 1 Hydropres-50 tab qd or bid, as needed (see WARNINGS/PRECAUTIONS)

CONTRAINDICATIONS

Hypersensitivity to hydrochlorothiazide, other sulfonamide derivatives, or reserpine●

Mental depression, especially in patients with suicidal tendencies●

Active peptic ulcer●

Ulcerative colitis●

Anuria●

Electroconvulsive therapy●

WARNINGS/PRECAUTIONS

Fixed combination	Not indicated for initial therapy of hypertension; dosages of component drugs must be individually titrated and then periodically reviewed, as conditions warrant
Renal impairment	Use with caution and monitor for signs of excessive drug accumulation (see OVERDOSAGE); patient may adjust poorly to lowered blood pressure
Azotemia	May be precipitated in patients with renal disease
Hepatic coma	May be precipitated by minor changes in fluid and electrolyte balance in patients with hepatic impairment or progressive liver disease; use with caution
Sensitivity reactions	May occur in patients with or without a history of allergy or bronchial asthma
Postsympathectomy patients	Antihypertensive effect may be enhanced
Systemic lupus erythematosus	May be activated or exacerbated
Electrolyte imbalances	Measure serum and urine electrolytes periodically, especially when patient is vomiting excessively or receiving parenteral fluids. Observe patient for such symptoms as dry mouth, thirst, weakness, lethargy, drowsiness, restlessness, muscle pains or cramps, muscular fatigue, hypotension, oliguria, tachycardia, and GI disturbances.
Hypokalemia	May develop, especially with brisk diuresis, concomitant corticosteroid or ACTH therapy, interference with adequate oral intake of electrolytes, or in the presence of severe cirrhosis; may be minimized by including potassium-rich foods in diet or, if necessary, with potassium supplements
Dilutional hyponatremia	May occur in edematous patients when weather is hot; restrict water and use salt replacement only for life-threatening hyponatremia
Hyperuricemia or frank gout	May occur or be precipitated in certain patients
Insulin requirements	May increase, decrease, or remain unchanged; latent diabetes may become active
History of mental depression	Use with extreme caution; discontinue therapy at first sign of despondency, early morning insomnia, loss of appetite, impotence, or self-deprecation. Mental depression is unusual with reserpine doses of 0.25 mg/day or less.
Patients undergoing electroconvulsive therapy	Discontinue drug at least 7 days before giving electroshock treatments; severe and even fatal reactions have occurred
Increased gastric secretion and motility	Use with caution in patients with a history of peptic ulcer, ulcerative colitis, or other GI disorders
Biliary colic	May be precipitated in patients with gallstones
Bronchial asthma	May be precipitated in susceptible patients
Lithium therapy	Renal clearance is reduced, increasing risk of lithium toxicity; coadministration generally should be avoided unless adequate precautions are taken
Circulatory disturbances	May develop during surgical anesthesia; vagal blocking agents may be needed to prevent or reverse hypotension and/or bradycardia
Parathyroid function tests	Discontinue drug before testing

ADVERSE REACTIONS

Gastrointestinal	Anorexia, gastric irritation, hypersecretion and increased motility, nausea, vomiting, cramps, diarrhea, constipation, dry mouth, increased salivation, intrahepatic cholestatic jaundice, pancreatitis, sialadenitis
Central nervous system and neuromuscular	Dizziness, syncope, nervousness, vertigo, paresthesias, headache, excessive sedation, mental depression, nightmares, paradoxical anxiety, dulled sensorium, deafness, muscle spasm, weakness, restlessness, muscle aches, parkinsonism (usually reversible)

Table continued on following page

HYDROPRES continued

ADVERSE REACTIONS continued

Ophthalmic	Transient blurred vision, glaucoma, uveitis, optic atrophy, conjunctival injection, xanthopsia
Cardiovascular	Orthostatic hypotension, bradycardia, angina pectoris, arrhythmia, premature ventricular contractions, fluid retention, congestive heart failure
Hematological	Leukopenia, agranulocytosis, thrombocytopenia, aplastic anemia, hemolytic anemia, excessive bleeding following prostatic surgery, thrombocytopenic purpura, epistaxis
Genitourinary	Dysuria, impotence, decreased libido
Hypersensitivity	Purpura, photosensitivity, pruritus, rash, urticaria, flushing, necrotizing angiitis, fever, respiratory distress (including pneumonitis), anaphylactic reactions
Other	Nasal congestion, dyspnea, increased susceptibility to colds, weight gain, nonpuerperal lactation

OVERDOSAGE

Signs and symptoms	*Hydrochlorothiazide-related effects:* diuresis, lethargy progressing to coma with minimal cardiorespiratory depression, GI irritation, hypermotility, elevated BUN, serum electrolyte changes; *reserpine-related effects:* impairment of consciousness ranging from drowsiness to coma, flushing, conjunctival injection, miosis, hypothermia, respiratory depression, bradycardia, diarrhea
Treatment	Induce emesis or use gastric lavage, followed by activated charcoal, to empty stomach. Treat hypotension by elevating feet and by volume expansion, if possible. If a vasopressor is needed, use phenylephrine, levarterenol, or metaraminol. Treat significant bradycardia with vagal blocking agents, along with other appropriate measures. Monitor serum electrolytes and renal function, and institute supportive measures, as required. Treat GI effects symptomatically. Observe patient for at least 72 h.

DRUG INTERACTIONS

Other antihypertensive agents	⇧ Antihypertensive effect
Digitalis	⇧ Risk of cardiac arrhythmias, bradycardia, heart block
Quinidine	⇧ Risk of cardiac arrhythmias
MAO inhibitors	Severe hypertension
Tubocurarine	⇧ Skeletal-muscle relaxation
Norepinephrine	⇩ Vasopressor effect
Steroids, ACTH	⇧ Risk of hypokalemia
Lithium	⇩ Lithium clearance
Alcohol, barbiturates, narcotic analgesics	⇧ Risk of orthostatic hypotension

ALTERED LABORATORY VALUES

Blood/serum values	Carbohydrate intolerance ⇧ Uric acid ⇧ Calcium ⇩ Sodium ⇩ Potassium ⇩ Chloride ⇩ Bicarbonate ⇩ Phosphate ⇩ PBI ⇩ Thyroxine (T_4) ⇩ Plasma renin activity
Urinary values	⇧ Sodium ⇧ Potassium ⇧ Chloride ⇧ Bicarbonate ⇧ Uric acid ⇧ 5-HIAA ⇩ Calcium ⇩ 17-Ketosteroids

Use in children

General guidelines not established

Use in pregnancy or nursing mothers

Safe use not established during pregnancy. Thiazides cross the placental barrier, appear in cord blood, and may cause fetal or neonatal jaundice, thrombocytopenia, and other possible reactions. Reserpine crosses the placental barrier, appears in cord blood, and may cause nasal congestion, lethargy, depressed Moro reflex, and bradycardia in newborns. Both drugs also appear in breast milk; patient should stop nursing if drug is prescribed.

INDERIDE (Propranolol hydrochloride and hydrochlorothiazide) Ayerst

Tabs: 40 mg propranolol hydrochloride and 25 mg hydrochlorothiazide (Inderide-40/25); 80 mg propranolol hydrochloride and 25 mg hydrochlorothiazide (Inderide-80/25)

INDICATIONS	ORAL DOSAGE
Hypertension	**Adult:** 1–2 tabs bid (see WARNINGS/PRECAUTIONS)

ADMINISTRATION/DOSAGE ADJUSTMENTS

Combination therapy	Reduce usual recommended starting dosage of other antihypertensive agents by ½ to avoid an excessive fall in blood pressure
Discontinuation of therapy	Reduce dosage gradually and monitor patient closely. Caution patients with angina or hyperthyroidism against interruption or abrupt cessation of therapy (see WARNINGS/PRECAUTIONS).

CONTRAINDICATIONS

Sinus bradycardia ●

Greater than first-degree heart block ●

Cardiogenic shock ●

Right ventricular failure secondary to pulmonary hypertension ●

Congestive heart failure not resulting from propranolol-treatable tachyarrhythmias ●

Hypersensitivity to hydrochlorothiazide or other sulfonamide derivatives ●

Concomitant therapy with adrenergic-augmenting psychotropic agents, including MAO inhibitors (both during therapy and for 2 wk after such drugs are withdrawn) ●

Anuria ●

Bronchial asthma ●

Allergic rhinitis during the pollen season ●

WARNINGS/PRECAUTIONS

Fixed combination	Not indicated for initial therapy of hypertension; dosages of component drugs must be individually titrated and then periodically reviewed, as conditions warrant
Cardiac failure	May be precipitated by further or continued depression of myocardial contractility; discontinue use if cardiac failure persists despite adequate digitalization and diuretic therapy
Abrupt discontinuation of therapy	May exacerbate angina pectoris, lead to myocardial infarction in patients with coronary artery disease, or precipitate thyrotoxicosis in hyperthyroid patients
Thyrotoxicosis	Clinical signs of hyperthyroidism may be masked
Wolff-Parkinson-White syndrome	Tachycardia may be replaced by severe bradycardia requiring a demand pacemaker
Impaired response to reflex adrenergic stimuli	Withdraw drug 48 h prior to surgery, unless surgery is for pheochromocytoma. Patients undergoing emergency surgery may experience protracted severe hypotension and, occasionally, difficulty in restarting and maintaining heartbeat. Excessive beta blockade may be reversed during surgery by IV administration of a beta-receptor agonist (eg, isoproterenol or levarterenol).
Nonallergic bronchospasm	Use with caution, since bronchodilation produced by beta stimulation may be blocked
Diabetes, hypoglycemia	Beta blockade may prevent appearance of premonitory signs and symptoms of acute hypoglycemia, especially in patients with labile diabetes
Renal or hepatic impairment	Use with caution and monitor for signs of excessive drug accumulation (see OVERDOSAGE)
Azotemia	May be precipitated in patients with renal disease
Hepatic coma	May be precipitated by minor changes in fluid and electrolyte balance in patients with hepatic impairment or progressive liver disease
Sensitivity reactions	May occur in patients with a history of allergy or bronchial asthma
Systemic lupus erythematosus	May be activated or exacerbated
Electrolyte imbalances	Measure serum and urine electrolytes periodically, especially when patient is vomiting excessively or receiving parenteral fluids. Watch for dry mouth, thirst, weakness, lethargy, drowsiness, restlessness, muscle pains or cramps, muscular fatigue, hypotension, oliguria, tachycardia, and GI disturbances.
Hypokalemia	May develop, especially with brisk diuresis, concomitant corticosteroid or ACTH therapy, interference with adequate oral intake of electrolytes, or in the presence of severe cirrhosis; may be minimized by including potassium-rich foods in diet or, if necessary, with potassium supplements
Dilutional hyponatremia	May occur in edematous patients when weather is hot; restrict water and use salt replacement only for life-threatening hyponatremia
Hyperuricemia or frank gout	May occur or be precipitated in certain patients
Insulin requirements	May increase, decrease, or remain unchanged; latent diabetes may become active
Postsympathectomy patients	Antihypertensive effect may be enhanced
Parathyroid function tests	Discontinue drug before testing

Table continued on following page

INDERIDE continued

ADVERSE REACTIONS

Cardiovascular	Bradycardia, congestive heart failure, intensified AV block, hypotension, Raynaud-type arterial insufficiency, orthostatic hypotension
Central nervous system and neuromuscular	Lightheadedness, insomnia, lassitude, weakness, fatigue, reversible mental depression progressing to catatonia, visual disturbances, hallucinations, acute reversible syndrome of disorientation, short-term memory loss, emotional lability, clouded sensorium, decreased neuropsychometric performance, dizziness, vertigo, paresthesias, headache, restlessness, muscle spasm
Ophthalmic	Transient blurred vision, xanthopsia
Gastrointestinal	Nausea, vomiting, epigastric distress, abdominal cramping, diarrhea, constipation, mesenteric arterial thrombosis, ischemic colitis, anorexia, gastric irritation, intrahepatic cholestatic jaundice, pancreatitis, sialadenitis
Allergic or hypersensitivity	Pharyngitis, agranulocytosis, erythematous rash, purpura, photosensitivity, urticaria, necrotizing angiitis, fever, aching, sore throat, laryngospasm, respiratory distress (including pneumonitis), anaphylactic reactions
Respiratory	Bronchospasm
Hematological	Agranulocytosis, nonthrombocytopenic purpura, thrombocytopenic purpura, leukopenia, thrombocytopenia, aplastic anemia
Other	Reversible alopecia

OVERDOSAGE

Signs and symptoms	*Propranolol-related effects:* severe bradycardia, congestive heart failure, hypotension, bronchospasm; *hydrochlorothiazide-related effects:* diuresis, lethargy progressing to coma with minimal cardiorespiratory depression, GI irritation, hypermotility, temporarily elevated BUN, serum electrolyte changes
Treatment	Empty stomach, taking care to prevent pulmonary aspiration. For bradycardia, administer 0.25–1.0 mg atropine IV; if there is no response to vagal blockade, administer isoproterenol cautiously. For cardiac failure, administer digitalis and a diuretic. For hypotension, use levarterenol or (preferably) epinephrine. Treat bronchospasm with isoproterenol and aminophylline. For stupor or coma, employ supportive measures. Treat GI effects symptomatically. Monitor serum electrolyte levels and renal function, and institute supportive measures, as required.

DRUG INTERACTIONS

Other antihypertensive agents	⇧ Antihypertensive effect
MAO inhibitors	Severe hypertension
Alcohol, barbiturates, narcotic analgesics	⇧ Risk of orthostatic hypotension
Digitalis	⇩ AV conduction
Ephedrine, isoproterenol, and other beta-adrenergic bronchodilating agents	⇩ Bronchodilation
Reserpine, *Rauwolfia* alkaloids	⇧ Risk of vertigo, syncope, or orthostatic hypotension
Tubocurarine	⇧ Skeletal-muscle relaxation
Norepinephrine	⇩ Vasopressor effect
Steroids, ACTH	⇧ Risk of hypokalemia
Lithium	⇩ Lithium clearance

ALTERED LABORATORY VALUES

Blood/serum values	⇧ BUN ⇧ Alkaline phosphatase ⇧ Lactate dehydrogenase ⇧ SGOT ⇧ SGPT ⇧ Uric acid ⇧ Calcium ⇩ Sodium ⇩ Potassium ⇩ Chloride ⇩ Bicarbonate ⇩ Phosphate ⇩ PBI ⇧ or ⇩ Glucose
Urinary values	⇧ Sodium ⇧ Potassium ⇧ Chloride ⇧ Bicarbonate ⇧ Uric acid ⇩ Calcium

Use in children

General guidelines not established

Use in pregnancy or nursing mothers

Safe use not established during pregnancy. In animal studies, propranolol has demonstrated embryotoxicity at doses ~10 times greater than the maximum recommended human dose. Thiazides cross the placental barrier, appear in cord blood, and may cause fetal or neonatal jaundice, thrombocytopenia, and other possible reactions. Thiazides also appear in breast milk; patient should stop nursing if drug is prescribed.

MINIZIDE (Prazosin hydrochloride and polythiazide) Pfizer

Caps: 1 mg prazosin hydrochloride and 0.5 mg polythiazide (Minizide 1); 2 mg prazosin hydrochloride and 0.5 mg polythiazide (Minizide 2); 5 mg prazosin hydrochloride and 0.5 mg polythiazide (Minizide 5)

INDICATIONS	ORAL DOSAGE
Hypertension	**Adult:** determine patient dose by individual titration of separate components; usual dosage: 1 cap bid or tid (see WARNINGS/PRECAUTIONS)

CONTRAINDICATIONS	
Anuria●	Hypersensitivity to thiazides or other sulfonamide derivatives●

WARNINGS/PRECAUTIONS	
Fixed combination	Not indicated for initial therapy of hypertension; dosages of component drugs must be individually titrated and then periodically reviewed, as conditions warrant
Syncope, accompanied by dizziness, lightheadedness, or sudden loss of consciousness	May occur due to prazosin component, usually within 30–90 min of initial administration and occasionally in association with rapid dose increases or when other antihypertensive agents are added to prazosin. Severe tachycardia (heart rate, 120–160 beats/min) may precede a syncopal episode. May be minimized by limiting initial dose to 1 mg of prazosin, by increasing dosage slowly, and by using caution when other antihypertensive agents are introduced.
Renal impairment	May result in excessive drug accumulation (see OVERDOSAGE); use with caution in patients with severe renal disease. If renal impairment progresses, consider withholding or discontinuing diuretic therapy.
Azotemia	May be precipitated in patients with renal disease
Hepatic coma	May be precipitated by minor changes in fluid and electrolyte balance in patients with hepatic impairment or progressive liver disease; use with caution
Postsympathectomy patients	Antihypertensive effect may be enhanced
Systemic lupus erythematosus	May be activated or exacerbated
Insulin requirements	May increase, decrease, or remain unchanged; latent diabetes may become active
Electrolyte imbalances	Measure serum and urine electrolytes periodically, especially when patient is vomiting excessively or receiving parenteral fluids or digitalis. Observe patient for such symptoms as dry mouth, thirst, weakness, lethargy, drowsiness, restlessness, muscle pains or cramps, muscular fatigue, hypotension, oliguria, tachycardia, and GI disturbances (nausea, vomiting, diarrhea).
Hypokalemia	May develop, especially with brisk diuresis, concomitant corticosteroid or ACTH therapy, interference with adequate oral intake of electrolytes, or in the presence of severe cirrhosis; hypokalemia may result in digitalis cardiotoxicity
Dilutional hyponatremia	May occur in edematous patients in hot weather; replace salt only for actual salt depletion or when hyponatremia is life-threatening
Sensitivity reactions	May occur in patients with a history of bronchial asthma or allergy
Hyperuricemia or frank gout	May occur or be precipitated in certain patients due to thiazide component

ADVERSE REACTIONS	Frequent reactions are italicized
Central nervous system	*Dizziness (10.3%), headache (7.8%), drowsiness (7.6%), lack of energy (6.9%), weakness (6.5%),* nervousness, vertigo, depression, paresthesia, restlessness
Gastrointestinal	*Nausea (4.9%),* vomiting, diarrhea, constipation, abdominal discomfort and/or pain, dry mouth, anorexia, gastric irritation, cramping, intrahepatic cholestatic jaundice, pancreatitis
Cardiovascular	*Palpitations (5.3%),* edema, dyspnea, syncope, tachycardia, orthostatic hypotension
Dermatological	Rash, pruritus, purpura, photosensitivity, urticaria, necrotizing angiitis
Genitourinary	Urinary frequency, incontinence, impotence
Ophthalmic	Blurred vision, reddened sclera, xanthopsia, pigmentary mottling and serous retinopathy (rare)
Hematological	Leukopenia, agranulocytosis, thrombocytopenia, aplastic anemia
Other	Epistaxis, tinnitus, nasal congestion, diaphoresis, muscle spasm

Table continued on following page

MINIZIDE continued

OVERDOSAGE

Signs and symptoms	*Prazosin-related effects:* profound drowsiness, depressed reflexes, hypotension, shock; *polythiazide-related effects:* electrolyte imbalance; lethargy progressing to coma, with minimal cardiorespiratory depression and with or without significant serum electrolyte changes or dehydration; GI irritation; hypermotility; transient elevation in BUN level
Treatment	Empty stomach by gastric lavage. Support cardiovascular system if hypotension occurs. Keep patient supine to restore blood pressure and normalize heart rate. Treat shock with volume expanders and, if necessary, vasopressors. Institute supportive measures, as needed, to maintain hydration, electrolyte balance, respiration, and cardiovascular and renal function. Treat GI effects symptomatically. Dialysis is not beneficial for the removal of prazosin, since it is protein-bound.

DRUG INTERACTIONS

Beta blockers	⇧ Risk of hypotension
Other antihypertensive agents	⇧ Antihypertensive effect and risk of syncope
Steroids, ACTH	⇧ Risk of hypokalemia
Digitalis	⇧ Risk of digitalis toxicity associated with hypokalemia
Tubocurarine	⇧ Skeletal-muscle relaxation
Norepinephrine	⇩ Vasopressor effect; however, interaction does not preclude therapeutic use of norepinephrine
Alcohol, barbiturates, narcotic analgesics	⇧ Risk of orthostatic hypotension
Lithium	⇧ Risk of lithium toxicity due to reduced renal clearance

ALTERED LABORATORY VALUES

Blood/serum values	⇧ Glucose ⇧ Uric acid ⇩ Sodium ⇩ Potassium ⇩ Chloride ⇧ Calcium ⇩ Bicarbonate ⇩ Phosphate ⇩ PBI
Urinary values	⇧ Glucose ⇧ Sodium ⇧ Potassium ⇧ Chloride ⇧ Bicarbonate ⇧ Uric acid ⇩ Calcium

Use in children

Safety and effectiveness not established

Use in pregnancy or nursing mothers

In rats, the combination of polythiazide at 40 times the usual maximum human dose and prazosin at 8 times the usual maximum human dose increased the number of stillbirths, prolonged gestation, and decreased survival before weaning. No teratogenic effects have been observed in rats or rabbits at oral doses more than 100 times the usual maximum human dose. Studies in humans are inadequate. Thiazides appear in breast milk; patient should stop nursing if drug is prescribed.

RAUZIDE (*Rauwolfia serpentina* and bendroflumethiazide) Squibb

Tabs: 50 mg *Rauwolfia serpentina* and 4 mg bendroflumethiazide

INDICATIONS	ORAL DOSAGE
Hypertension	**Adult:** 1-4 tabs/day (see WARNINGS/PRECAUTIONS)

ADMINISTRATION/DOSAGE ADJUSTMENTS

Combination therapy	May potentiate actions of ganglionic or peripheral adrenergic-blocking agents; titrate dosage carefully

CONTRAINDICATIONS

Hypersensitivity to thiazides, other sulfonamide derivatives, or *Rauwolfia* ●

Mental depression, especially in patients with suicidal tendencies ●

Active peptic ulcer ●

Ulcerative colitis ●

Electroconvulsive therapy ●

Anuria ●

WARNINGS/PRECAUTIONS

Fixed combination	Not indicated for initial therapy of hypertension; dosages of component drugs must be individually titrated and then periodically reviewed, as conditions warrant
History of mental depression	Use with extreme caution; discontinue therapy at first sign of despondency, early morning insomnia, loss of appetite, impotence, or self-deprecation
Persistence of symptoms following withdrawal	Drug-induced depression may persist for several months after drug withdrawal and may be severe enough to result in suicide; cardiovascular effects may also persist
Circulatory instability and hypotension	May occur during surgery, even if drug is withdrawn preoperatively; combat with anticholinergic and/or adrenergic agents (eg, metaraminol or norepinephrine)
Increased GI motility and secretion	Use with caution in patients with a history of peptic ulcer (which may be reactivated by high dosages) or ulcerative colitis
Biliary colic	May be precipitated in patients with a history of gallstones
Renal impairment	Use with caution and monitor for signs of excessive drug accumulation (see OVERDOSAGE); patient may adjust poorly to lowered blood pressure
Azotemia	May be precipitated in patients with renal disease
Hepatic coma	May be precipitated by minor changes in fluid and electrolyte balance in patients with hepatic impairment or progressive liver disease; use with caution
Sensitivity reactions	May occur in patients with a history of allergy or bronchial asthma
Systemic lupus erythematosus	May be activated or exacerbated
Electrolyte imbalances	Measure serum and urine electrolytes periodically, especially when patient is vomiting excessively or receiving parenteral fluids. Observe patient for such symptoms as dry mouth, thirst, weakness, lethargy, drowsiness, restlessness, muscle pains or cramps, muscular fatigue, hypotension, oliguria, tachycardia, and GI disturbances.
Hypokalemia	May develop, especially with brisk diuresis, concomitant corticosteroid or ACTH therapy, interference with adequate oral intake of electrolytes, or in the presence of severe cirrhosis; may be minimized by including potassium-rich foods in diet or, if necessary, with potassium supplements
Dilutional hyponatremia	May occur in edematous patients when weather is hot; restrict water and use salt replacement only for life-threatening hyponatremia
Hyperuricemia or frank gout	May occur or be precipitated in certain patients
Insulin requirements	May increase, decrease, or remain unchanged; latent diabetes may become active
Postsympathectomy patients	Antihypertensive effect may be enhanced
Tartrazine sensitivity	Presence of FD&C Yellow No. 5 (tartrazine) in tablets may cause allergic-type reactions, including bronchial asthma, in susceptible individuals

ADVERSE REACTIONS

Gastrointestinal	Hypersecretion, anorexia, gastric irritation, nausea, vomiting, cramping, diarrhea, constipation, dry mouth, intrahepatic cholestatic jaundice, pancreatitis
Central nervous system and neuromuscular	Drowsiness, depression, dizziness, vertigo, paresthesias, nervousness, paradoxical anxiety, nightmares, dulled sensorium, deafness, dizziness, headache, extrapyramidal symptoms (rare), muscle spasm, muscle aches, weakness, restlessness
Ophthalmic	Glaucoma, uveitis, optic atrophy, xanthopsia, conjunctival injection
Cardiovascular	Angina-like symptoms, arrhythmias, bradycardia, orthostatic hypotension

Table continued on following page

RAUZIDE continued

ADVERSE REACTIONS continued

Hematological	Leukopenia, agranulocytosis, thrombocytopenia, aplastic anemia
Hypersensitivity	Purpura, photosensitivity, pruritus, rash, urticaria, necrotizing angiitis, allergic glomerulonephritis
Genitourinary	Impotence or decreased libido, dysuria
Other	Nasal congestion, dyspnea, metabolic acidosis (in diabetics), weight gain

OVERDOSAGE

Signs and symptoms	*Rauwolfia-related effects:* impairment of consciousness ranging from drowsiness to coma, flushing, conjunctival injection, pupillary constriction; severe overdosage: hypotension, hypothermia, respiratory depression, bradycardia, diarrhea; *bendroflumethiazide-related effects:* diuresis, lethargy progressing to coma with minimal cardiorespiratory depression, GI irritation, hypermotility, elevated BUN, serum electrolyte changes
Treatment	Induce emesis or use gastric lavage, followed by activated charcoal, to empty stomach. Treat hypotension by elevating feet and by volume expansion, if possible. If a vasopressor is needed, use phenylephrine, levarterenol, or metaraminol. Treat significant bradycardia with vagal blocking agents, along with other appropriate measures. Monitor serum electrolytes and renal function, and institute supportive measures, as required. Treat GI effects symptomatically.

DRUG INTERACTIONS

Other antihypertensive agents	⇧ Antihypertensive effect
Digitalis	⇧ Risk of cardiac arrhythmias, bradycardia, heart block
Quinidine	⇧ Risk of cardiac arrhythmias
MAO inhibitors	Severe hypertension
Tubocurarine	⇧ Skeletal-muscle relaxation
Norepinephrine	⇩ Vasopressor effect
Steroids, ACTH	⇧ Risk of hypokalemia
Lithium	⇩ Lithium clearance
Alcohol, barbiturates, narcotic analgesics	⇧ Risk of orthostatic hypotension

ALTERED LABORATORY VALUES

Blood/serum values	Carbohydrate intolerance ⇧ Uric acid ⇧ Calcium ⇩ Sodium ⇩ Potassium ⇩ Chloride ⇩ Bicarbonate ⇩ Phosphate ⇩ PBI ⇩ Thyroxine (T_4) ⇩ Plasma renin activity
Urinary values	⇧ Sodium ⇧ Potassium ⇧ Chloride ⇧ Bicarbonate ⇧ Uric acid ⇧ 5-HIAA ⇩ Calcium ⇩ 17-Ketosteroids

Use in children

General guidelines not established

Use in pregnancy or nursing mothers

Safe use not established during pregnancy. *Rauwolfia* preparations cross the placental barrier, appear in cord blood, and have caused increased respiratory secretions, nasal congestion, cyanosis, and anorexia in newborns. Thiazides also cross the placental barrier, appear in cord blood, and may cause fetal or neonatal jaundice, thrombocytopenia, and other possible reactions. Both drugs also appear in breast milk; patient should stop nursing if drug is prescribed.

REGROTON (Chlorthalidone and reserpine) USV

Tabs: 50 mg chlorthalidone and 0.25 mg reserpine

DEMI-REGROTON (Chlorthalidone and reserpine) USV

Tabs: 25 mg chlorthalidone and 0.125 mg reserpine

INDICATIONS	ORAL DOSAGE
Hypertension	**Adult:** 1–2 tabs qd, in AM with food (see WARNINGS/PRECAUTIONS)

ADMINISTRATION/DOSAGE ADJUSTMENTS

Initial titration of dosage	Optimal effect on blood pressure may require 2 wk or more to appear, because of slow onset of action of reserpine component; wait at least this long before adjusting dosage
Combination therapy	In more severe cases, other antihypertensive agents may be added gradually at dosages at least 50% lower than customary; monitor patient closely. When used concomitantly, reduce dosage of ganglionic blocking agents, other potent antihypertensive agents, and curare by at least 50% and provide close supervision.

CONTRAINDICATIONS

Hypersensitivity to chlorthalidone or reserpine●	Most cases of severe renal or hepatic disease●	Electroconvulsive therapy●
Mental depression or history of depression●		

WARNINGS/PRECAUTIONS

Fixed combination	Not indicated for initial therapy of hypertension; dosages of component drugs must be individually titrated and then periodically reviewed, as conditions warrant
Renal impairment	Use with caution in patients with severe renal disease; monitor for signs of excessive drug accumulation
Azotemia	May be precipitated in patients with severe renal disease
Hepatic coma	May be precipitated by minor changes in fluid and electrolyte balance in patients with hepatic impairment or progressive liver disease; discontinue therapy if liver-function abnormalities increase
Sensitivity reactions	May occur in patients with a history of allergy or bronchial asthma
Mental depression	May occur; discontinue therapy at first sign of despondency, early morning insomnia, loss of appetite, impotence, self-deprecation, or other symptoms of depression
Patients undergoing electroconvulsive therapy	Discontinue drug at least 7 days before giving electroshock treatments; severe and even fatal reactions have occurred
Peptic ulcer	May be precipitated or aggravated in susceptible patients; discontinue therapy
Postsympathectomy patients	Antihypertensive effect may be enhanced; use with caution
Electrolyte imbalances	Measure serum and urine electrolytes periodically, especially when patient is vomiting excessively or receiving parenteral fluids. Observe patient for such symptoms as dry mouth, thirst, weakness, lethargy, drowsiness, restlessness, muscle pains or cramps, muscular fatigue, hypotension, oliguria, tachycardia, and GI disturbances.
Hypokalemia	May develop, especially with brisk diuresis, concomitant corticosteroid or ACTH therapy, interference with adequate oral intake of electrolytes, or in the presence of severe cirrhosis; may be minimized by including potassium-rich foods in diet or, if necessary, with potassium supplements
Dilutional hyponatremia	May occur in edematous patients when weather is hot; restrict water and use salt replacement only for life-threatening hyponatremia
Hyperuricemia or frank gout	May occur or be precipitated in certain patients; combat with a uricosuric agent if serious
Insulin requirements	May increase, decrease, or remain unchanged; latent diabetes may become active
Decreased glucose tolerance	May occur, evidenced by hyperglycemia and glycosuria; discontinue therapy. Monitor diabetics and other susceptible patients closely.
Increased GI motility and secretion	Use with caution in patients with ulcerative colitis
Biliary colic	May be precipitated in patients with gallstones
Hypotension during surgery	May occur; discontinue therapy at least 2 wk before elective surgery. For emergency surgery, use anticholinergic and/or adrenergic agents (eg, metaraminol or norepinephrine) to prevent vagocirculatory responses; other supportive measures may also be indicated.
Progressive renal damage	May occur; perform kidney-function tests periodically. Discontinue therapy if BUN rises.
Bronchial asthma	May occur in susceptible patients

Table continued on following page

REGROTON/DEMI-REGROTON continued

ADVERSE REACTIONS	Frequent reactions are italicized
Gastrointestinal	*Anorexia, gastric irritation, nausea, vomiting, diarrhea, constipation,* dry mouth, pancreatitis (rare)
Central nervous system and neuromuscular	*Muscle cramps, dizziness, weakness, headache, drowsiness, mental depression* (rare at recommended dosages), restlessness, lassitude, paradoxical anxiety, nightmares, dulled sensorium, muscle aches, paralysis agitans-like syndrome (reversible), deafness
Ophthalmic	Transient myopia, blurred vision, conjunctival injection, uveitis, optic atrophy, glaucoma
Dermatological	Skin rash, urticaria, pruritis, eruptions, flushing, ecchymosis (one case)
Cardiovascular	Orthostatic hypotension, bradycardia, ectopic cardiac rhythms, angina pectoris
Genitourinary	Decreased libido, impotence, dysuria
Idiosyncratic	Aplastic anemia, purpura, thrombocytopenia, leukopenia, agranulocytosis, necrotizing angiitis, Lyell's syndrome (toxic epidermal necrolysis)
Other	*Nasal congestion,* increased susceptibility to colds, dyspnea, weight gain

OVERDOSAGE	
Signs and symptoms	Nausea, weakness, dizziness, syncope, electrolyte-balance disturbances, marked hypotension
Treatment	Use gastric lavage, followed by activated charcoal, to empty stomach. Institute supportive measures, as required. Intravenous dextrose-saline with potassium chloride may be given. Vasopressors may be used for marked hypotension.

DRUG INTERACTIONS	
Other antihypertensive agents	⇧ Antihypertensive effect
Digitalis	⇧ Risk of cardiac arrhythmias, bradycardia, heart block
Quinidine	⇧ Risk of cardiac arrhythmias
MAO inhibitors	Severe hypertension
Tubocurarine	⇧ Skeletal-muscle relaxation
Norepinephrine	⇩ Vasopressor effect
Steroids, ACTH	⇧ Risk of hypokalemia
Lithium	⇩ Lithium clearance
Alcohol, barbiturates, narcotic analgesics	⇧ Risk of orthostatic hypotension

ALTERED LABORATORY VALUES	
Blood/serum values	Carbohydrate intolerance ⇧ Uric acid ⇧ Calcium ⇩ Sodium ⇩ Potassium ⇩ Chloride ⇩ Bicarbonate ⇩ Phosphate ⇩ PBI ⇩ Thyroxine (T_4) ⇩ Plasma renin activity
Urinary values	⇧ Sodium ⇧ Potassium ⇧ Chloride ⇧ Bicarbonate ⇧ Uric acid ⇧ 5-HIAA ⇩ Calcium ⇩ 17-Ketosteroids

Use in children

General guidelines not established

Use in pregnancy or nursing mothers

Safe use not established during pregnancy. Reserpine crosses the placental barrier, appears in cord blood, and has caused increased respiratory secretions, nasal congestion, cyanosis, and anorexia in newborns. Although chlorthalidone has not demonstrated teratogenicity in animal reproduction studies, thiazides—to which it is related—do cross the placental barrier and appear in cord blood. Both thiazides and reserpine also appear in breast milk; patient should stop nursing if drug is prescribed.

SALUTENSIN (Hydroflumethiazide and reserpine) **Bristol**

Tabs: 50 mg hydroflumethiazide and 0.125 mg reserpine

SALUTENSIN-Demi (Hydroflumethiazide and reserpine) **Bristol**

Tabs: 25 mg hydroflumethiazide and 0.125 mg reserpine

INDICATIONS	**ORAL DOSAGE**
Hypertension	**Adult:** 1 tab qd or bid (see WARNINGS/PRECAUTIONS)

ADMINISTRATION/DOSAGE ADJUSTMENTS

Refractory patients	Up to 3 or 4 tabs/day div may be given. Follow closely serum uric acid, fasting blood sugar, BUN/NPN, and serum electrolytes. Reduce dosage to minimum effective level after desired blood pressure reduction is attained.
Combination therapy	Reduce dosage of other antihypertensives, especially ganglionic blockers, by at least 50%, to avoid excessive drop in blood pressure. Further dosage reduction or discontinuance may be necessary.

CONTRAINDICATIONS

Hypersensitivity to hydroflumethiazide or reserpine●	Active peptic ulcer●	Severe depression●
Anuria or oliguria●	Ulcerative colitis●	Electroconvulsive therapy●

WARNINGS/PRECAUTIONS

Fixed combination	Not indicated for initial therapy of hypertension; dosages of component drugs must be individually titrated and then periodically reviewed, as conditions warrant
Renal impairment	Use with caution and monitor for signs of excessive drug accumulation (see OVERDOSAGE); patient may adjust poorly to lowered blood pressure
Azotemia	May be precipitated in patients with renal disease
Hepatic coma	May be precipitated by minor changes in fluid and electrolyte balance in patients with hepatic cirrhosis
Sensitivity reactions	May occur in patients with a history of allergy or bronchial asthma
Postsympathectomy patients	Antihypertensive effect may be enhanced
Systemic lupus erythematosus	May be activated or exacerbated
Electrolyte imbalances	Measure serum and urine electrolytes periodically, especially when patient is vomiting excessively or receiving parenteral fluids. Observe patient for such symptoms as dry mouth, thirst, weakness, lethargy, drowsiness, restlessness, muscle pains or cramps, muscular fatigue, hypotension, oliguria, tachycardia, and GI disturbances.
Hypokalemia	May develop, especially with brisk diuresis, concomitant corticosteroid or ACTH therapy, interference with adequate oral intake of electrolytes, or in the presence of severe cirrhosis; may be minimized by including potassium-rich foods in diet or, if necessary, with potassium supplements. Use enteric-coated potassium tablets only when adequate dietary supplementation is impractical; discontinue immediately if abdominal pain, distention, nausea, vomiting, or GI bleeding occurs.
Dilutional hyponatremia	May occur in edematous patients when weather is hot; restrict water and use salt replacement only for life-threatening hyponatremia
Hyperuricemia or frank gout	May occur or be precipitated in certain patients
Insulin requirements	May increase, decrease, or remain unchanged; latent diabetes may become active
History of mental depression	Use with extreme caution; discontinue therapy at first sign of despondency, early morning insomnia, loss of appetite, impotence, or self-deprecation. Mental depression is unusual with reserpine doses of 0.25 mg/day or less.
Increased gastric secretion and motility	Use with caution in patients with history of peptic ulcer, ulcerative colitis, or other GI disorders
Biliary colic	May be precipitated in patients with gallstones
Circulatory disturbances	May develop during surgical anesthesia; discontinue therapy 2 wk before elective surgery. For emergency procedures, vagal blocking agents may be needed to prevent or reverse hypotension and/or bradycardia.
Parathyroid function tests	Discontinue drug before testing

Table continued on following page

SALUTENSIN/SALUTENSIN-Demi continued

ADVERSE REACTIONS

Gastrointestinal	Anorexia, gastric irritation, nausea, vomiting, cramps, increased intestinal motility, diarrhea, constipation, dry mouth, increased salivation, intrahepatic cholestatic jaundice, pancreatitis
Central nervous system and neuromuscular	Dizziness, vertigo, paresthesias, headache, excessive sedation, mental depression, nightmares, nervousness, paradoxical anxiety, dulled sensorium, deafness, muscle spasm, weakness, restlessness, muscle aches, parkinsonism (usually reversible)
Ophthalmic	Blurred vision, glaucoma, uveitis, optic atrophy, conjunctival injection, xanthopsia
Cardiovascular	Orthostatic hypotension, angina pectoris, premature ventricular contractions, fluid retention, congestive heart failure, syncope
Hematological	Leukopenia, agranulocytosis, thrombocytopenia, aplastic anemia, thrombocytopenic purpura, epistaxis
Genitourinary	Dysuria, impotence, decreased libido
Hypersensitivity	Purpura, photosensitivity, rash, urticaria, flushing, pruritis, necrotizing angiitis
Other	Nasal congestion, dyspnea, increased susceptibility to colds, weight gain, non-puerperal lactation

OVERDOSAGE

Signs and symptoms	*Hydroflumethiazide-related effects:* diuresis, lethargy progressing to coma with minimal cardiorespiratory depression, GI irritation, hypermotility, elevated BUN, serum electrolyte changes; *reserpine-related effects:* impairment of consciousness ranging from drowsiness to coma, flushing, conjunctival injection, miosis, hypotension, hypothermia, respiratory depression, bradycardia, diarrhea
Treatment	Induce emesis or use gastric lavage, followed by activated charcoal, to empty stomach. Treat hypotension by volume expansion, if possible. If a vasopressor is needed, use phenylephrine, levarterenol, or metaraminol. Treat significant bradycardia with vagal blocking agents, along with other appropriate measures. Monitor serum electrolytes and renal function, and institute supportive measures, as required. Treat GI effects symptomatically. Observe patient for at least 72 h.

DRUG INTERACTIONS

Other antihypertensive agents	⇧ Antihypertensive effect
Digitalis	⇧ Risk of cardiac arrhythmias, bradycardia, heart block
Quinidine	⇧ Risk of cardiac arrhythmias
MAO inhibitors	Severe hypertension
Tubocurarine	⇧ Skeletal-muscle relaxation
Norepinephrine	⇩ Vasopressor effect
Steroids, ACTH	⇧ Risk of hypokalemia
Lithium	⇩ Lithium clearance
Alcohol, barbiturates, narcotic analgesics	⇧ Risk of orthostatic hypotension

ALTERED LABORATORY VALUES

Blood/serum values	Carbohydrate intolerance ⇧ Uric acid ⇧ Calcium ⇩ Sodium ⇩ Potassium ⇩ Chloride ⇩ Bicarbonate ⇩ Phosphate ⇩ PBI ⇩ Thyroxine (T_4) ⇩ Plasma renin activity
Urinary values	⇧ Sodium ⇧ Potassium ⇧ Chloride ⇧ Bicarbonate ⇧ Uric acid ⇧ 5-HIAA ⇩ Calcium ⇩ 17-Ketosteroids

Use in children

General guidelines not established

Use in pregnancy or nursing mothers

Safe use not established during pregnancy. Thiazides cross the placental barrier, appear in cord blood, and may cause fetal or neonatal jaundice, thrombocytopenia, and other possible reactions. Reserpine crosses the placental barrier, appears in cord blood, and may cause nasal congestion, lethargy, depressed Moro reflex, and bradycardia in newborns. Both drugs also appear in breast milk; patient should stop nursing if drug is prescribed.

SER-AP-ES (Reserpine, hydralazine hydrochloride, and hydrochlorothiazide)

Tabs: 0,1 mg reserpine, 25 mg hydralazine hydrochloride, and 15 mg hydrochlorothiazide

INDICATIONS	ORAL DOSAGE
Hypertension	**Adult:** 1-2 tabs tid (see WARNINGS/PRECAUTIONS); for maintenance, adjust dosage to lowest effective level

ADMINISTRATION/DOSAGE ADJUSTMENTS

Initial titration of dosage	Optimal effect on blood pressure may require up to 2 wk to appear, because of slow onset of action of reserpine; wait at least this long before adjusting dosage
Combination therapy	In resistant cases, more potent antihypertensive agents may be added gradually at dosages at least 50% lower than customary; monitor patient closely

CONTRAINDICATIONS

Anuria	
Hypersensitivity	To hydrochlorothiazide, other sulfonamide derivatives, reserpine, or hydralazine
Mental depression	Especially in patients with suicidal tendencies
Active peptic ulcer, ulcerative colitis	May be exacerbated
Electroconvulsive therapy	
Coronary artery disease	Anginal attacks may be precipitated or may worsen
Rheumatic mitral valve disease	Congestive heart failure may be precipitated

WARNINGS/PRECAUTIONS

Fixed combination	Not indicated for initial therapy of hypertension; dosages of component drugs must be individually titrated and then periodically reviewed, as conditions warrant
History of mental depression	Use with extreme caution; discontinue therapy at first sign of despondency, early morning insomnia, loss of appetite, impotence, or self-deprecation. Mental depression may be increased by higher doses of reserpine; increase dosage cautiously.
Persistence of symptoms following withdrawal	Drug-induced depression may persist for several months after drug withdrawal and may be severe enough to result in suicide; cardiovascular effects may also persist
Circulatory instability and hypotension	May occur during surgery, even if drug is withdrawn preoperatively; combat with anticholinergic and/or adrenergic agents (eg, metaraminol or norepinephrine)
Increased GI motility and secretion	Use with caution in patients with a history of peptic ulcer (which may be reactivated by high dosages) or ulcerative colitis
Biliary colic	May be precipitated in patients with a history of gallstones
MAO inhibitors	Avoid, if possible, or use with extreme caution
Lupus erythematosus-like syndrome	May occur; obtain CBC, LE-cell preparation, and antinuclear antibody (ANA) titer before and periodically during prolonged therapy or if arthralgia, fever, chest pain, continued malaise, or other unexplained symptoms develop. In general, unless hydralazine component is essential, discontinue therapy if clinical symptoms occur, ANA titer rises, or LE-cell preparation is positive.
Profound hypotension	May occur with concomitant use of potent parenteral antihypertensive agent, such as diazoxide; patient should be observed for several hours
Peripheral neuritis	May occur, evidenced by paresthesias, numbness, and tingling; combat with pyridoxine
Blood dyscrasias	May occur (see ADVERSE REACTIONS); obtain periodic blood counts during prolonged therapy and withdraw drug if abnormalities develop
Renal impairment	Use with caution and monitor for signs of excessive drug accumulation (see OVERDOSAGE)
Azotemia	May be precipitated in patients with renal disease

Table continued on following page

WARNINGS/PRECAUTIONS continued	
Hepatic coma	May be precipitated by minor changes in fluid and electrolyte balance in patients with hepatic impairment or progressive liver disease
Sensitivity reactions	May occur in patients with a history of allergy or bronchial asthma
Systemic lupus erythematosus	May be activated or exacerbated
Electrolyte imbalances	Measure serum and urine electrolytes periodically, especially when patient is vomiting excessively or receiving parenteral fluids. Observe patient for such symptoms as dry mouth, thirst, weakness, lethargy, drowsiness, restlessness, muscle pains or cramps, muscular fatigue, hypotension, oliguria, tachycardia, and GI disturbances.
Hypokalemia	May develop, especially with brisk diuresis, concomitant corticosteroid or ACTH therapy, interference with adequate oral intake of electrolytes, or in the presence of severe cirrhosis; may be minimized by including potassium-rich foods in diet or, if necessary, with potassium supplements
Dilutional hyponatremia	May occur in edematous patients when weather is hot; restrict water and use salt replacement only for life-threatening hyponatremia
Hyperuricemia or frank gout	May occur or be precipitated in certain patients
Special-risk patients	Use with caution following sympathectomy or in patients with suspected coronary artery disease, specific cardiovascular inadequacies (eg, mitral valvular disease), cerebral vascular accidents, or advanced renal disease
Insulin requirements	May increase, decrease, or remain unchanged; latent diabetes may become active
Parathyroid function tests	Discontinue drug before testing

ADVERSE REACTIONS	
Gastrointestinal	Hypersecretion, nausea, vomiting, anorexia, diarrhea, constipation, paralytic ileus, gastric irritation, cramping, dry mouth, intrahepatic cholestatic jaundice, pancreatitis, sialadenitis
Cardiovascular	Angina-like symptoms, arrhythmias, bradycardia, tachycardia, orthostatic hypotension, syncope, palpitations, water retention with edema, paradoxical pressor response
Central nervous system and neuromuscular	Drowsiness, depression, nervousness, paradoxical anxiety, nightmares, dulled sensorium, deafness, dizziness, headache, vertigo, paresthesias, numbness, tingling, tremors, muscle cramps and aches, muscle spasm, weakness, restlessness, psychotic reactions, parkinsonism and other extrapyramidal symptoms (rare)
Ophthalmic	Glaucoma, uveitis, optic atrophy, xanthopsia, lacrimation, conjunctivitis, conjunctival injection
Hematological	Purpura, epistaxis, reduction in hemoglobin level and erythrocyte count, leukopenia, agranulocytosis, thrombocytopenia, aplastic anemia
Genitourinary	Difficult micturition, impotence, decreased libido, dysuria
Metabolic and endocrinological	Weight gain, breast engorgement, pseudolactation, gynecomastia
Hypersensitivity	Pruritus, rash, urticaria, fever, chills, arthralgia, eosinophilia, photosensitivity, necrotizing angiitis, Stevens-Johnson syndrome, hepatitis (rare)
Other	Nasal congestion, flushing, dyspnea, lymphadenopathy, splenomegaly

Table continued on following page

SER-AP-ES continued

OVERDOSAGE

Signs and symptoms	*Reserpine-related effects:* impaired consciousness ranging from drowsiness to coma, flushing, conjunctival injection, pupillary constriction; severe overdosage: hypotension, hypothermia, respiratory depression, bradycardia, diarrhea; *hydralazine-related effects:* hypotension, tachycardia, headache, flushing, myocardial ischemia, cardiac arrhythmia, shock; *hydrochlorothiazide-related effects:* diuresis, lethargy progressing to coma, GI irritation, hypermotility, temporarily elevated BUN, serum electrolyte changes
Treatment	Induce emesis or use gastric lavage, followed by activated charcoal, to empty stomach, taking care to prevent aspiration. Treat hypotension and shock by elevation of feet and volume expansion, not with vasopressors, when possible. If a vasopressor must be used, administer phenylephrine, levarterenol, or metaraminol. Digitalization may be necessary. Treat GI effects symptomatically. Employ supportive measures, as indicated, to maintain adequate hydration, electrolyte balance, respiration, and cardiovascular and renal function. Observe patient for at least 72 h.

DRUG INTERACTIONS

Beta blockers	⇧ Antihypertensive effect of hydralazine component
Other antihypertensive agents	⇧ Antihypertensive effect of both drugs
MAO inhibitors	Severe hypertension
Digitalis	⇧ Risk of cardiac arrhythmias, bradycardia, heart block
Quinidine	⇧ Risk of cardiac arrhythmias
Tubocurarine	⇧ Skeletal-muscle relaxation
Norepinephrine	⇩ Vasopressor effect
Steroids, ACTH	⇧ Risk of hypokalemia
Epinephrine	⇩ Pressor response
Lithium	⇩ Lithium clearance
Alcohol, barbiturates, narcotic analgesics	⇧ Risk of orthostatic hypotension

ALTERED LABORATORY VALUES

Blood/serum values	⇧ Uric acid ⇧ Calcium ⇧ Plasma renin activity ⇩ Sodium ⇩ Potassium ⇩ Chloride ⇩ Bicarbonate ⇩ Phosphate ⇩ PBI + ANA + LE-cell reaction + Direct Coombs' test ⇧ or ⇩ Glucose
Urinary values	⇧ Sodium ⇧ Potassium ⇧ Chloride ⇧ Bicarbonate ⇧ Uric acid ⇩ Calcium

Use in children

General guidelines not established

Use in pregnancy or nursing mothers

Safe use not established during pregnancy. Reserpine and thiazides cross the placental barrier and appear in cord blood. Hydralazine is teratogenic in mice and possibly rabbits, but not in rats. Reserpine and thiazides also appear in breast milk; patient should stop nursing if drug is prescribed.

ALDACTAZIDE (Spironolactone and hydrochlorothiazide) Searle

Tabs: 25 mg spironolactone and 25 mg hydrochlorothiazide

INDICATIONS	ORAL DOSAGE
Essential hypertension	**Adult:** 2–4 tabs/day (see WARNINGS/PRECAUTIONS)
Edema associated with congestive heart failure, hepatic cirrhosis, or the nephrotic syndrome (adjunctive therapy) **Diuretic-induced hypokalemia**	**Adult:** 1–8 tabs/day (see WARNINGS/PRECAUTIONS); usual maintenance dosage: 1 tab qid; additional spironolactone or hydrochlorothiazide may be administered, if necessary **Child:** 0.75–1.5 mg spironolactone/lb/day (1.65–3.3 mg/kg/day) (see WARNINGS/PRECAUTIONS)

CONTRAINDICATIONS

Anuria ●	Hyperkalemia ●	Hypersensitivity to hydrochlorothiazide or other sulfonamide derivatives ●
Acute renal insufficiency ●	Acute or severe hepatic failure (relative) ●	
Significant renal impairment ●		

WARNINGS/PRECAUTIONS

Fixed combination	Not indicated for initial therapy of edema or hypertension; dosages of component drugs must be individually titrated and then periodically reviewed, as conditions warrant
Tumorigenicity	Has been shown in chronic toxicity studies in rats, with proliferative changes occurring in endocrine organs and the liver
Hyperkalemia	May occur in patients with impaired renal function or excessive potassium intake; avoid potassium supplements and potassium-rich food. Potentially fatal cardiac irregularities may occur. Significant hyperkalemia can be promptly corrected by rapid IV infusion of 20–50% glucose with regular insulin (0.25–0.50 units/g glucose); repeat, as needed.
Electrolyte imbalances	Measure serum and urine electrolytes periodically, especially when patient is vomiting excessively or receiving parenteral fluids. Observe patient for such symptoms as dry mouth, thirst, weakness, lethargy, drowsiness, restlessness, muscle pain or cramps, muscular fatigue, hypotension, oliguria, tachycardia, and GI disturbances.
Hypokalemia	May develop, especially with brisk diuresis, concomitant loop diuretic, corticosteroid, or ACTH therapy, or interference with adequate oral intake of electrolytes; hypokalemia may result in digitalis cardiotoxicity at previously tolerated dosage levels
Dilutional hyponatremia	May be precipitated, especially if other diuretics are given simultaneously. Observe patient for tell-tale signs (dry mouth, thirst, lethargy, drowsiness); a low serum sodium level confirms diagnosis. Rarely, a true low-salt syndrome may develop, signaled by progressive mental confusion resembling that of hepatic coma; discontinue drug and administer sodium.
Gynecomastia	May develop, especially with high dosages or prolonged therapy; usually reverses when drug is withdrawn. Rarely, some breast enlargement may persist.
Hyperuricemia, gout, decreased glucose tolerance	May develop, due to thiazide-induced changes in metabolism of uric acid and carbohydrates; abnormal glucose metabolism may develop in latent diabetics or may worsen in diabetics
Postsympathectomy patients	Antihypertensive effect may be enhanced
Transient elevation of BUN	May occur; progressive rise in BUN suggests pre-existing renal impairment
Parathyroid changes with hypercalcemia and hypophosphatemia	May occur with prolonged therapy
Systemic lupus erythematosus	May be activated or exacerbated

Table continued on following page

ADVERSE REACTIONS

Gastrointestinal	Cramping, diarrhea, anorexia, nausea, vomiting, acute pancreatitis, jaundice
Central nervous system and neuromuscular	Drowsiness, lethargy, headache, mental confusion, dizziness, vertigo, paresthesias, ataxia, muscle spasm, weakness, restlessness
Ophthalmic	Xanthopsia, photosensitivity
Endocrine, genitourinary	Gynecomastia, impotence, irregular menses, amenorrhea, postmenopausal bleeding, deepening of voice, breast carcinoma (causal relationship not established)
Hematological	Purpura, thrombocytopenia, leukopenia, agranulocytosis, aplastic anemia
Cardiovascular	Orthostatic hypotension
Dermatological and hypersensitivity	Maculopapular or erythematous eruptions, pruritus, purpura, photosensitivity, urticaria, necrotizing angiitis, drug fever, erythema multiforme, hirsutism

OVERDOSAGE

Signs and symptoms	Hyperkalemia, cardiac irregularities
Treatment	Discontinue drug; hyperkalemia can be promptly corrected by rapid IV infusion of 20–50% glucose with regular insulin (0.25–0.5 units/g glucose); repeat, as needed

DRUG INTERACTIONS

Other antihypertensive agents	⇧ Antihypertensive effect
Tubocurarine	⇧ Skeletal-muscle relaxation
Norepinephrine	⇩ Vasopressor effect
Steroids, ACTH	⇧ Risk of hypokalemia
Potassium supplements, other potassium-sparing diuretics	⇧ Risk of hyperkalemia

ALTERED LABORATORY VALUES

Blood/serum values	⇧ Uric acid ⇧ Calcium ⇩ Sodium ⇧ Potassium ⇩ Chloride ⇧ BUN ⇩ Bicarbonate ⇩ Phosphate ⇩ PBI ⇧ or ⇩ Glucose
Urinary values	⇧ Sodium ⇩ Potassium ⇧ Chloride ⇧ Bicarbonate ⇧ Uric acid ⇩ Calcium

Use in children

General guidelines not established

Use in pregnancy or nursing mothers

Safe use has not been established during pregnancy. Thiazides cross the placental barrier and appear in cord blood, and spironolactone may do so as well. In general, diuretics should not be given to pregnant women except for pathologic edema; however, a short course of diuretic therapy may be appropriate for hypervolemia-dependent edema that is causing extreme discomfort unrelieved by rest. Canrenone, a metabolite of spironolactone, and hydrochlorothiazide also appear in breast milk; use of this drug may cause fetal or neonatal jaundice, thrombocytopenia, and other possible reactions. Patient should stop nursing if drug is prescribed.

ALDACTONE (Spironolactone) Searle

Tabs: 25 mg

INDICATIONS	ORAL DOSAGE
Essential hypertension	**Adult:** 50–100 mg/day div to start, followed by larger or smaller doses until optimal response is achieved
Edema associated with congestive heart failure, hepatic cirrhosis, or the nephrotic syndrome (adjunctive therapy)	**Adult:** 25–200 mg/day div to start; recommended initial dosage: 100 mg/day div **Child:** 3.3 mg/kg/day (1.5 mg/lb/day) div to start
Hypokalemia when oral potassium supplementation or other potassium-sparing regimens are deemed inappropriate or inadequate	**Adult:** 25–100 mg/day
Short-term treatment of **primary hyperaldosteronism** prior to surgery	**Adult:** 100–400 mg/day
Long-term maintenance of patients with discrete **inoperable aldosterone-producing adrenal adenomas** or bilateral micro- or macronodular **adrenal hyperplasia** (idiopathic hyperaldosteronism)	**Adult:** use lowest effective dosage

ADMINISTRATION/DOSAGE ADJUSTMENTS

Initiating therapy	For hypertension, continue initial dosage for at least 2 wk; for edema, continue 5 days. If response is inadequate, second diuretic may be added.
Combination therapy	Effects of other diuretics or antihypertensive agents, especially ganglionic-blocking agents, are potentiated; reduce dosage of such agents by at least 50% when spironolactone is added to regimen
Diagnosis of hyperaldosteronism	*Long test:* Administer 400 mg/day for 3–4 wk; correction of hypokalemia and hypertension provides presumptive evidence of primary hyperaldosteronism. *Short test:* Administer 400 mg/day for 4 days; if serum potassium increases during spironolactone administration but drops when drug is discontinued, a presumptive diagnosis of primary hyperaldosteronism should be considered.
Small children	Tablets may be pulverized and administered as a suspension in cherry syrup; refrigerated suspension is stable for 1 mo

CONTRAINDICATIONS

Anuria●	Significant renal impairment●	Hyperkalemia●
Acute renal insufficiency●		

WARNINGS/PRECAUTIONS

Tumorigenicity	Has been shown in chronic toxicity studies in rats, with proliferative changes occurring in endocrine organs and the liver
Hyperkalemia	May occur in patients with impaired renal function or excessive potassium intake; avoid potassium supplements and potassium-rich food. Potentially fatal cardiac irregularities may occur. Significant hyperkalemia can be promptly corrected by rapid IV infusion of 20–50% glucose with regular insulin (0.25–0.50 units/g glucose); repeat, as needed; discontinue spironolactone and restrict potassium intake.
Hyponatremia	May be precipitated or may worsen, especially if other diuretics are given simultaneously. Observe patient for such symptoms as dry mouth, thirst, lethargy, and drowsiness; a low serum sodium level confirms the diagnosis.
Gynecomastia	May develop, especially with high dosages or prolonged therapy; usually reverses when drug is withdrawn. Rarely, some breast enlargement may persist.
Fluid and electrolyte imbalance	May develop; carefully evaluate patients

Table continued on following page

WARNINGS/PRECAUTIONS continued

Transient elevation of BUN	May occur, especially in patients with pre-existing renal impairment
Mild acidosis	May occur

ADVERSE REACTIONS

Gastrointestinal	Cramping, diarrhea
Central nervous system	Drowsiness, lethargy, headache, mental confusion, ataxia, drug fever
Dermatological	Maculopapular or erythematous eruptions, urticaria, hirsutism
Endocrinological and genitourinary	Gynecomastia, irregular menses, amenorrhea, postmenopausal bleeding, impotence, deepening of voice, breast carcinoma (causal relationship not established)

OVERDOSAGE

Signs and symptoms	See ADVERSE REACTIONS
Treatment	Discontinue medication; treat symptomatically and institute supportive measures, as required

DRUG INTERACTIONS

Other antihypertensive agents	⇧ Antihypertensive effect
Norepinephrine	⇩ Vasopressor effect
Potassium supplements, other potassium-sparing diuretics	⇧ Risk of hyperkalemia
Digitoxin	⇩ Digitoxin effect (possible)

ALTERED LABORATORY VALUES

Blood/serum values	⇩ Sodium ⇧ Potassium ⇩ Chloride ⇧ BUN
Urinary values	⇧ Sodium ⇩ Potassium ⇧ Chloride

Use in children

See INDICATIONS and ADMINISTRATION/ DOSAGE ADJUSTMENTS

Use in pregnancy or nursing mothers

Safe use has not been established during pregnancy. Spironolactone or its metabolites may cross the placental barrier. In general, diuretics should not be given to pregnant women except for pathological edema; however, a short course of spironolactone therapy may be appropriate for hypervolemia-dependent edema causing extreme discomfort unrelieved by rest. Canrenone, a metabolite of spironolactone, appears in breast milk; patient should stop nursing if drug is prescribed.

DIULO (Metolazone) Searle

Tabs: 2.5, 5, 10 mg

INDICATIONS	ORAL DOSAGE
Mild to moderate hypertension	**Adult:** 2.5–5 mg qd
Edema associated with congestive heart failure	**Adult:** 5–10 mg qd
Edema associated with renal disease and dysfunction (including the nephrotic syndrome)	**Adult:** 5–20 mg qd

ADMINISTRATION/DOSAGE ADJUSTMENTS

Paroxysmal nocturnal dyspnea	May occur in patients with congestive heart failure; dosage near upper end of range may help ensure 24-h duration of diuretic and saluretic effects
Combination therapy	Dosage of other antihypertensive agents or diuretics and metolazone should be carefully adjusted, particularly during initial therapy; dosage of other agents, especially ganglionic blockers, should be reduced. Concurrent administration of metolazone and furosemide should be initiated under hospital conditions (see WARNINGS/PRECAUTIONS).
Optimal dosage	Initial dose should be reduced to lowest maintenance level as soon as desired effect is obtained; the time interval may range from days for edematous states to 3–4 wk for hypertension. Dosage adjustment is usually necessary during course of therapy, based on clinical and laboratory evaluations.
Side effects	Reduce dosage or discontinue therapy if side effects are moderate or severe (see ADVERSE REACTIONS)

CONTRAINDICATIONS

Anuria●	Hepatic coma or pre-coma●	Hypersensitivity to metolazone●

WARNINGS/PRECAUTIONS

Azotemia	May be precipitated in patients with renal disease; if azotemia and oliguria worsen during treatment, discontinue drug
Hyperuricemia, gouty attacks	May occur in patients with a history of gout; use with caution
Electrolyte imbalances	May occur; measure serum and urine electrolytes periodically, especially when patient is vomiting excessively or receiving parenteral fluids. Monitor BUN, uric acid, and glucose levels. Observe patient for such symptoms as dry mouth, thirst, weakness, lethargy, drowsiness, restlessness, muscle pain or cramps, muscular fatigue, hypotension, oliguria, tachycardia, and GI disturbances.
Concurrent use of furosemide	May result in unusually large or prolonged effects on volume and electrolytes; if necessary, administer in hospital setting to provide for adequate monitoring
Hypokalemia	May develp, especially with intensive or prolonged diuresis, concomitant corticosteroid or ACTH therapy, or inadequate electrolyte intake; may require potassium supplementation. Hypokalemia may result in dangerous or fatal arrhythmias in digitalized patients.
Potassium-sparing diuretics	Concurrent use may potentiate diuresis; dosages of both diuretics should be reduced and potassium supplements discontinued
Chloride deficit and hypochloremic alkalosis	May occur
Orthostatic hypotension	May occur; may be potentiated by alcohol, barbiturates, narcotics, or concurrent antihypertensive therapy
Insulin requirements	May increase, decrease, or remain unchanged; latent diabetes may become active
Elective surgery	Discontinue metolazone 3 days before elective surgery; related diuretics (but not metolazone) have increased responsiveness to tubocurarine and decreased arterial responsiveness to norepinephrine

Table continued on following page

WARNINGS/PRECAUTIONS continued

Cross-allergy[1]	Theoretically may occur in patients allergic to sulfonamide derivatives, thiazides, or quinethazone
Parathyroid changes with hypercalcemia and hypophosphatemia[1]	May occur rarely with diuretics

ADVERSE REACTIONS

Gastrointestinal	Constipation, nausea, vomiting, anorexia, diarrhea, abdominal bloating, epigastric distress, intrahepatic cholestatic jaundice, hepatitis
Central nervous system	Syncope, dizziness, drowsiness, vertigo, headache
Hematological	Leukopenia
Cardiovascular	Orthostatic hypotension, excess volume depletion, hemoconcentration, venous thrombosis, palpitations, chest pain
Hypersensitivity	Urticaria, other skin rashes
Other	Dry mouth, hypokalemia (symptomatic and asymptomatic), hyponatremia, hypochloremia, hypochloremic alkalosis, hyperuricemia, hyperglycemia, glycosuria, fatigue, muscle cramps or spasms, weakness, restlessness, chills, acute gouty attacks

OVERDOSAGE

Signs and symptoms	Diuresis; lethargy progressing to coma, with minimal cardiorespiratory depression and with or without significant serum electrolyte changes or dehydration; GI irritation; hypermotility; transient elevation in BUN level
Treatment	Empty stomach by gastric lavage, taking care to avoid aspiration. Monitor serum electrolyte levels and renal function, and institute supportive measures, as required, to maintain hydration, electrolyte balance, respiration, and cardiovascular and renal function. Treat GI effects symptomatically.

DRUG INTERACTIONS

Other antihypertensive agents	⇧ Antihypertensive effect
Steroids, ACTH	⇧ Risk of hypokalemia
Lithium	⇩ Lithium clearance
Alcohol, barbiturates, narcotic analgesics	⇧ Risk of orthostatic hypotension

ALTERED LABORATORY VALUES

Blood/serum values	⇧ Uric acid ⇧ Calcium ⇩ Sodium ⇩ Potassium ⇩ Chloride ⇩ Bicarbonate ⇩ Phosphate ⇩ PBI ⇧ or ⇩ Glucose ⇧ BUN ⇧ Creatinine
Urinary values	⇧ Sodium ⇧ Potassium ⇧ Chloride ⇧ Bicarbonate ⇧ Uric acid ⇧ Phosphate ⇧ Magnesium

Use in children

Not recommended

Use in pregnancy or nursing mothers

Safe use has not been established during pregnancy. Metolazone crosses the placental barrier and appears in cord blood. In general, diuretics should not be given to pregnant women except for pathologic edema; however, a short course of metolazone therapy may be appropriate for hypervolemia-dependent edema that is causing extreme discomfort unrelieved by rest. Metolazone also appears in breast milk and may cause fetal or neonatal jaundice, thrombocytopenia, and other possible reactions. Patient should stop nursing if drug is prescribed.

[1]Not reported to date for metolazone

DIURIL (Chlorothiazide) **Merck Sharp & Dohme**

Tabs: 250, 500 mg **Susp:** 250 mg/5 ml

DIURIL Intravenous Sodium (Chlorothiazide sodium) **Merck Sharp & Dohme**

Vial: 0.5 g

INDICATIONS	ORAL DOSAGE	PARENTERAL DOSAGE
Hypertension	**Adult:** 0.5–1.0 qd or div to start; increase or decrease dosage according to blood-pressure response	—
Edema associated with congestive heart failure, hepatic cirrhosis, corticosteroid and estrogen therapy, and renal dysfunction (adjunctive therapy)	**Adult:** 0.5–1.0 g qd or bid **Infant (<2 yr):** 125–375 mg/day in 2 divided doses, according to weight (<6 mo, up to 15 mg/lb/day; older infants, 10 mg/lb/day) **Child (2–12 yr):** 375 mg to 1.0 g/day in 2 divided doses, according to weight (10 mg/lb/day)	**Adult:** 0.5–1.0 g IV qd or bid

ADMINISTRATION/DOSAGE ADJUSTMENTS

Refractory hypertension (rare)	Increase oral dosage to 2.0 g/day div
Combination therapy	Dosage of other antihypertensive agents must be reduced when chlorothiazide is added to the regimen to prevent excessive blood-pressure drop; further reductions or even discontinuation of other agents may be necessary as blood pressure continues to fall
Intermittent treatment of edema	Administer normal daily oral or IV dose on alternate days or 3–5 days each week to reduce risk of excessive response and resultant electrolyte imbalance
Side effects	Reduce dosage or discontinue diuretic therapy if side effects are moderate or severe (see ADVERSE REACTIONS)
Intravenous use	Reserve for patients unable to take drug orally or for emergencies. Extravasation must be avoided; do not give SC or IM or simultaneously with whole blood or derivatives. Dilute contents of vial with 18 ml of Sterile Water for Injection.

CONTRAINDICATIONS

Anuria ●	Hypersensitivity to chlorothiazide or other sulfonamide derivatives ●

WARNINGS/PRECAUTIONS

Renal impairment	May result in excessive drug accumulation (see OVERDOSAGE); if renal impairment progresses, consider withholding or discontinuing diuretic therapy
Azotemia	May be precipitated in patients with renal disease
Electrolyte imbalances	Measure serum and urine electrolytes periodically, especially when patient is vomiting excessively or receiving parenteral fluids. Observe patient for such symptoms as dry mouth, thirst, weakness, lethargy, drowsiness, restlessness, muscle pain or cramps, muscular fatigue, hypotension, oliguria, tachycardia, and GI disturbances.
Hypokalemia	May develop, especially with brisk diuresis, concomitant corticosteroid or ACTH therapy, interference with adequate oral intake of electrolytes, or in the presence of severe cirrhosis; may be minimized by including potassium-rich foods in diet or, if necessary, with potassium supplements. Hypokalemia may result in digitalis toxicity.
Dilutional hyponatremia	May occur in edematous patients when weather is hot; restrict intake of water. Replace salt only for actual salt depletion or when hyponatremia is life-threatening.
Hepatic coma	May be precipitated by minor changes in fluid and electrolyte balance in patients with hepatic impairment or progressive liver disease; use with caution
Sensitivity reactions	May occur in patients with or without a history of allergy or bronchial asthma
Insulin requirements	May increase, decrease, or remain unchanged; latent diabetes may become active
Hyperuricemia or frank gout	May occur in certain patients

Table continued on following page

DIURIL continued

WARNINGS/PRECAUTIONS continued	
Lithium therapy	Renal clearance is reduced, increasing risk of lithium toxicity; coadministration generally should be avoided unless adequate precautions are taken
Systemic lupus erythematosus	May be activated or exacerbated
Postsympathectomy patients	Antihypertensive effect may be enhanced
Parathyroid-function tests	Discontinue drug before testing; parathyroid changes with hypercalcemia and hypophosphatemia may occur with prolonged therapy

ADVERSE REACTIONS	
Gastrointestinal	Anorexia, gastric irritation, nausea, vomiting, cramping, diarrhea, constipation, intrahepatic cholestatic jaundice, pancreatitis, sialadenitis
Central nervous system	Dizziness, vertigo, paresthesias, headache, weakness, restlessness
Ophthalmic	Xanthopsia, transient blurred vision
Hematological	Leukopenia, agranulocytosis, thrombocytopenia, aplastic anemia, hemolytic anemia
Cardiovascular	Orthostatic hypotension
Hypersensitivity	Purpura, photosensitivity, rash, urticaria, necrotizing angiitis, fever, respiratory distress (including pneumonitis), anaphylactic reactions
Other	Hyperglycemia, glycosuria, hyperuricemia, muscle spasm, hematuria[1]

OVERDOSAGE	
Signs and symptoms	Diuresis; lethargy progressing to coma, with minimal cardiorespiratory depression and with or without significant serum electrolyte changes or dehydration; GI irritation; hypermotility; transient elevation in BUN level
Treatment	Empty stomach by gastric lavage, taking care to avoid aspiration. Monitor serum electrolyte levels and renal function, and institute supportive measures, as required, to maintain hydration, electrolyte balance, respiration, and cardiovascular and renal function. Treat GI effects symptomatically.

DRUG INTERACTIONS	
Other antihypertensive agents	⇧ Antihypertensive effect
Tubocurarine	⇧ Skeletal-muscle relaxation
Norepinephrine	⇩ Vasopressor effect
Steroids, ACTH	⇧ Risk of hypokalemia
Lithium	⇩ Lithium clearance
Alcohol, barbiturates, narcotic analgesics	⇧ Risk of orthostatic hypotension

ALTERED LABORATORY VALUES	
Blood/serum values	⇧ Uric acid ⇧ Calcium ⇩ Sodium ⇩ Potassium ⇩ Chloride ⇩ Bicarbonate ⇩ Phosphate ⇩ PBI ⇧ or ⇩ Glucose
Urinary values	⇧ Sodium ⇧ Potassium ⇧ Chloride ⇧ Bicarbonate ⇧ Uric acid ⇩ Calcium

Use in children

See INDICATIONS for use of oral form: IV use in infants and children has been limited and is not recommended

Use in pregnancy or nursing mothers

Safe use has not been established during pregnancy. Thiazides cross the placental barrier and appear in cord blood. In general, thiazides should not be given to pregnant women except for pathologic edema; however, a short course of diuretic therapy may be appropriate for hypervolemia-dependent edema that is causing extreme discomfort unrelieved by rest. Thiazides also appear in breast milk and may cause fetal or neonatal jaundice, thrombocytopenia, and other possible reactions. Patient should stop nursing if drug is prescribed.

[1]One case following IV use

DYAZIDE (Triamterene and hydrochlorothiazide) Smith Kline & French

Caps: 50 mg triamterene and 25 mg hydrochlorothiazide

INDICATIONS	ORAL DOSAGE
Hypertension **Edema** associated with congestive heart failure, hepatic cirrhosis, the nephrotic syndrome, corticosteroid and estrogen therapy, and idiopathic edema (adjunctive therapy)	**Adult:** 1–2 caps bid after meals, or up to 4 caps/day, if needed (see WARNINGS/PRECAUTIONS); some patients may be maintained on 1 cap/day or every other day

ADMINISTRATION/DOSAGE ADJUSTMENTS

Combination therapy	If indicated, other antihypertensive agents may be added cautiously to regimen. Additions should be gradual; reduce starting dosage by at least 50%, particularly of ganglionic blockers, to prevent excessive blood-pressure drop. Potassium supplementation should be discontinued unless triamterene component fails to compensate for potassium loss.

CONTRAINDICATIONS

Anuria, progressive renal dysfunction	Including increasing oliguria and azotemia
Hyperkalemia	Developing during therapy
Hypersensitivity	To triamterene, hydrochlorothiazide, or other sulfonamide derivatives
Pre-existing hyperkalemia	
Progressive hepatic dysfunction	

WARNINGS/PRECAUTIONS

Fixed combination	Not indicated for initial therapy of edema or hypertension; dosages of component drugs must be individually titrated and then periodically reviewed, as conditions warrant
Hyperkalemia	May occur, especially in the severely ill, in those with small urine volumes (<1 liter/day), or in elderly or diabetic patients with known or suspected renal insufficiency; acute transient hyperkalemia has occurred during IV glucose-tolerance testing of triamterene-treated diabetics
Potassium supplementation	Should not be used concurrently unless hypokalemia develops or potassium intake is markedly impaired. If supplementation is needed, avoid potassium in tablet form: small-bowel lesions may occur with potassium tablets. With spironolactone, frequent serum potassium determinations are necessary; two deaths have been reported.
Electrolyte imbalances	Measure serum electrolytes and urine periodically, especially when patient is vomiting excessively or receiving parenteral fluids. Observe patient for such symptoms as dry mouth, thirst, weakness, lethargy, drowsiness, restlessness, muscle pain or cramps, muscular fatigue, hypotension, oliguria, tachycardia, and GI disturbances.
Hypokalemia (rare)	May develop and result in digitalis cardiotoxicity at previously tolerated dosages
Prerenal azotemia	May develop, but rarely occurs with alternate-day therapy. Periodic BUN and creatinine determinations are advisable, especially in the elderly or in those with suspected or confirmed renal insufficiency. If azotemia increases, discontinue therapy.
Transient elevation of BUN and/or serum creatinine level	May occur; levels return to normal after drug is discontinued
Hepatic coma	May be precipitated by minor changes in fluid and electrolyte balance in patients with hepatic impairment or progressive liver disease; use with caution. Observe patient for signs of impending coma (eg, confusion, drowsiness, tremor); if mental confusion persists, withhold drug for a few days.
Hyperuricemia or frank gout	May occur or be precipitated in certain patients
Blood dyscrasias, liver damage, other idiosyncratic reactions	May occur; monitor patients regularly
Insulin requirements	May increase, decrease, or remain unchanged
Apparent megaloblastosis	Cirrhotic patients with splenomegaly have marked hematological variations. Periodic blood studies should be performed; apparent megaloblastosis may be due to depletion of folic acid stores by folic acid antagonistic effect of drug.
Postsympathectomy patients	Antihypertensive effect may be enhanced
Metabolic acidosis	May occur due to depletion of alkali reserve
Quinidine serum-level determinations	Fluorescent measurement may be disturbed, owing to similarity of spectra of triamterene and quinidine; discontinue use of triamterene before measuring quinidine serum level
Lithium therapy	Renal clearance is reduced, increasing risk of lithium toxicity; coadministration generally should be avoided unless adequate precautions are taken

Table continued on following page

ADVERSE REACTIONS

Central nervous system	Weakness, dizziness, headache, paresthesias
Ophthalmic	Xanthopsia
Gastrointestinal	Dry mouth, nausea and vomiting,[1] diarrhea, jaundice, pancreatitis, constipation, other GI disturbances
Dermatological and hypersensitivity	Anaphylaxis, rash, urticaria, photosensitivity, purpura, necrotizing vasculitis, other skin conditions
Other	Muscle cramps, allergic pneumonitis (rare), renal stones[2]

OVERDOSAGE

Signs and symptoms	Polyuria, nausea, vomiting, weakness, lassitude, fever, flushed face, hyperactive deep-tendon reflexes
Treatment	Discontinue medication; immediately empty stomach by emesis or gastric lavage. Maintain fluid and electrolyte balance; treat hypotension with pressor agents, such as levarterenol. If hyperkalemia develops, discontinue drug and any potassium supplementation; substitute a thiazide alone, and obtain an ECG. Absence of arrhythmia or of widening of QRS complex indicates steps taken are sufficient; *widened QRS or arrhythmia in presence of hyperkalemia necessitates prompt additional therapy.* For tachyarrhythmia: give 44 mEq sodium bicarbonate or 10 ml of 10% calcium gluconate or calcium chloride IV over several minutes; for asystole, bradycardia, or AV block: also institute transvenous pacing, and repeat, as needed. Dialysis or oral or rectal administration of sodium polystyrene sulfonate may be used to help remove excess potassium; infusion of glucose and insulin also may be used to treat hyperkalemia.

DRUG INTERACTIONS

Other antihypertensive agents	⇧ Antihypertensive effect
Spironolactone, potassium salts	⇧ Risk of hyperkalemia
Tubocurarine	⇧ Skeletal-muscle relaxation
Norepinephrine	⇩ Vasopressor effect
Lithium	⇩ Lithium clearance
Alcohol, barbiturates, narcotic analgesics	⇧ Risk of orthostatic hypotension

ALTERED LABORATORY VALUES

Blood/serum values	⇧ Uric acid ⇧ Calcium ⇩ Sodium ⇧ Potassium ⇩ Chloride ⇧ Creatinine ⇧ BUN ⇧ or ⇩ Glucose ⇩ Folic acid
Urinary values	⇧ Sodium ⇩ Potassium ⇧ Chloride ⇧ Bicarbonate ⇧ Uric acid ⇩ Calcium ⇧ Folic acid ⇧ Glucose

Use in children

Safe use not established; no adequate information available

Use in pregnancy or nursing mothers

Safe use has not been established during pregnancy. Thiazides cross the placental barrier and appear in cord blood. In rare instances, newborns whose mothers received thiazides during pregnancy developed thrombocytopenia, jaundice, or pancreatitis. In general, thiazides should not be given to pregnant women except for pathologic edema; however, a short course of diuretic therapy may be appropriate for hypervolemia-dependent edema that is causing extreme discomfort unrelieved by rest. Thiazides appear, and triamterene may appear, in breast milk. Patient should stop nursing if drug is prescribed.

[1]May indicate electrolyte imbalance; other nausea preventable by giving drug with meals

[2]Triamterene has been found in renal stones in association with other usual calculus components

ENDURON (Methyclothiazide) Abbott

Tabs: 2.5, 5 mg

INDICATIONS	ORAL DOSAGE
Hypertension	**Adult:** 2.5–5.0 mg qd, or up to 10 mg qd in resistant cases
Edema associated with congestive heart failure, hepatic cirrhosis, corticosteroid and estrogen therapy, and renal dysfunction (adjunctive therapy)	**Adult:** 2.5–10 mg qd

ADMINISTRATION/DOSAGE ADJUSTMENTS

Combination therapy	Other antihypertensive agents should be added gradually; dosage of ganglionic blockers must be reduced by at least 50% to prevent excessive blood-pressure drop
Side effects	Discontinue diuretic therapy if side effects are severe (see

CONTRAINDICATIONS

Renal decompensation	Hypersensitivity to methyclothiazide or other sulfonamide derivatives

WARNINGS/PRECAUTIONS

Renal impairment	May result in excessive drug accumulation (see OVERDOSAGE); if renal impairment progresses, consider withholding or discontinuing diuretic therapy
Azotemia	May be precipitated in patients with renal disease
Electrolyte imbalances	Measure serum and urine electrolytes periodically, especially when patient is vomiting excessively or receiving parenteral fluids. Observe patient for such symptoms as dry mouth, thirst, weakness, lethargy, drowsiness, restlessness, muscle pain or cramps, muscular fatigue, hypotension, oliguria, tachycardia, and GI disturbances.
Hypokalemia	May develop, especially with brisk diuresis, concomitant corticosteroid or ACTH therapy, interference with adequate oral intake of electrolytes, or in the presence of severe cirrhosis; may be minimized by including potassium-rich foods in diet or, if necessary, with potassium supplements. Hypokalemia may result in digitalis toxicity.
Dilutional hyponatremia	May occur in edematous patients when weather is hot; restrict intake of water. Replace salt only for actual salt depletion or when hyponatremia is life-threatening.
Hepatic coma	May be precipitated by minor changes in fluid and electrolyte balance in patients with hepatic impairment or progressive liver disease; use with caution
Hyperuricemia or frank gout	May occur in certain patients
Sensitivity reactions	May occur in patients with a history of allergy or bronchial asthma
Insulin requirements	May increase, decrease, or remain unchanged; latent diabetes may become active
Systemic lupus erythematosus	May be activated or exacerbated
Postsympathectomy patients	Antihypertensive effect may be enhanced

ADVERSE REACTIONS

Gastrointestinal	Anorexia, gastric irritation, nausea, vomiting, cramping, diarrhea, constipation, intrahepatic cholestatic jaundice, pancreatitis
Central nervous system	Dizziness, vertigo, paresthesias, headache, weakness, restlessness
Ophthalmic	Xanthopsia
Hematological	Leukopenia, agranulocytosis, thrombocytopenia, aplastic anemia
Cardiovascular	Orthostatic hypotension

Table continued on following page

ENDURON continued

OVERDOSAGE

Signs and symptoms	Electrolyte imbalance, signs of potassium deficiency, confusion, dizziness, muscular weakness, and GI disturbances
Treatment	Institute general supportive measures, as indicated, including fluid and electrolyte replacement

DRUG INTERACTIONS

Other antihypertensive agents	⇧ Antihypertensive effect
Tubocurarine	⇧ Skeletal-muscle relaxation
Norepinephrine	⇩ Vasopressor effect
Steroids, ACTH	⇧ Risk of hypokalemia
Lithium	⇩ Lithium clearance
Alcohol, barbiturates, narcotic analgesics	⇧ Risk of orthostatic hypotension

ALTERED LABORATORY VALUES

Blood/serum values	⇧ Uric acid ⇧ Calcium ⇩ Sodium ⇩ Potassium ⇩ Chloride ⇩ Bicarbonate ⇩ Phosphate ⇩ PBI ⇧ Glucose
Urinary values	⇧ Sodium ⇧ Potassium ⇧ Chloride ⇧ Bicarbonate ⇧ Uric acid ⇩ Calcium

Use in children

General guidelines not established

Use in pregnancy or nursing mothers

Safe use has not been established during pregnancy. Thiazides cross the placental barrier and appear in cord blood. In general, thiazides should not be given to pregnant women except for pathologic edema; however, a short course of diuretic therapy may be appropriate for hypervolemia-dependent edema that is causing extreme discomfort unrelieved by rest. Thiazides also appear in breast milk and may cause fetal or neonatal jaundice, thrombocytopenia, and other possible reactions. Patient should stop nursing if drug is prescribed.

ESIDRIX (Hydrochlorothiazide) Ciba

Tabs: 25, 50, 100 mg

INDICATIONS	ORAL DOSAGE
Hypertension	**Adult:** 75 mg/day to start; adjust dosage after 1 wk to 25–100 mg/day, depending on clinical response
Edema associated with congestive heart failure, hepatic cirrhosis, corticosteroid and estrogen therapy, and renal dysfunction (adjunctive therapy)	**Adult:** 25–200 mg/day for several days or until dry weight is attained, followed by 25–100 mg daily or intermittently, depending on clinical response **Infant (< 2 yr):** 12.5–37.5 mg/day in 2 divided doses, according to weight (<6 mo, up to 1.5 mg/lb/day; older infants, 1 mg/lb/day) **Child (2–12 yr):** 37.5–100 mg/day in 2 divided doses, according to weight (1 mg/lb/day)

ADMINISTRATION/DOSAGE ADJUSTMENTS

Refractory edema (rare)	Increase dosage to 200 mg/day (adults)
Combination therapy	If indicated, other antihypertensive agents may be added cautiously to regimen. Additions should be gradual; reduce starting dosage of ganglionic blockers, in particular, by 50% to prevent excessive blood-pressure drop
Side effects	Reduce dosage or discontinue diuretic therapy if side effects (see ADVERSE REACTIONS) are moderate or severe

CONTRAINDICATIONS

Anuria ●	Hypersensitivity to hydrochlorothiazide or other sulfonamide derivatives ●

WARNINGS/PRECAUTIONS

Renal impairment	May result in excessive drug accumulation (see OVERDOSAGE); if renal impairment progresses, consider withholding or discontinuing diuretic therapy
Azotemia	May be precipitated in patients with renal disease
Electrolyte imbalances	Measure serum and urine electrolytes periodically, especially when patient is vomiting excessively or receiving parenteral fluids. Observe patient for such symptoms as dry mouth, thirst, weakness, lethargy, drowsiness, restlessness, muscle pain or cramps, muscular fatigue, hypotension, oliguria, tachycardia, and GI disturbances.
Hypokalemia	May develop, especially with brisk diuresis, concomitant corticosteroid or ACTH therapy, interference with adequate oral intake of electrolytes, or in the presence of severe cirrhosis; hypokalemia may result in digitalis cardiotoxicity
Dilutional hyponatremia	May occur in edematous patients when weather is hot; restrict intake of water. Replace salt only for actual salt depletion or when hyponatremia is life-threatening.
Hepatic coma	May be precipitated by minor changes in fluid and electrolyte balance in patients with hepatic impairment or progressive liver disease; use with caution
Hyperuricemia or frank gout	May occur in certain patients
Sensitivity reactions	Are more likely to occur in patients with a history of allergy or bronchial asthma
Insulin requirements	May increase, decrease, or remain unchanged; latent diabetes may become active
Systemic lupus erythematosus	May be activated or exacerbated
Postsympathectomy patients	Antihypertensive effect may be enhanced
Parathyroid-function tests	Discontinue drug before testing; parathyroid changes with hypercalcemia and hypophosphatemia may occur with prolonged therapy

Table continued on following page

ESIDRIX continued

ADVERSE REACTIONS

Gastrointestinal	Anorexia, gastric irritation, nausea, vomiting, cramping, diarrhea, constipation, intrahepatic cholestatic jaundice, pancreatitis, sialadenitis
Central nervous system	Dizziness, vertigo, paresthesias, headache
Ophthalmic	Xanthopsia
Hematological	Leukopenia, agranulocytosis, thrombocytopenia, aplastic anemia
Cardiovascular	Orthostatic hypotension
Hypersensitivity	Purpura, photosensitivity, rash, urticaria, necrotizing angiitis, Stevens-Johnson syndrome
Other	Hyperglycemia, glycosuria, hyperuricemia, muscle spasm, weakness, restlessness

OVERDOSAGE

Signs and symptoms	Diuresis; lethargy progressing to coma, with minimal cardiorespiratory depression and with or without significant serum electrolyte changes or dehydration; GI irritation; hypermotility; transient elevation in BUN level
Treatment	Empty stomach by gastric lavage, taking care to avoid aspiration. Monitor serum electrolyte levels and renal function, and institute supportive measures, as required, to maintain hydration, electrolyte balance, respiration, and cardiovascular and renal function. Treat GI effects symptomatically.

DRUG INTERACTIONS

Other antihypertensive agents	⇧ Antihypertensive effect
Tubocurarine	⇧ Skeletal-muscle relaxation
Norepinephrine	⇩ Vasopressor effect
Steroids, ACTH	⇧ Risk of hypokalemia
Lithium	⇩ Lithium clearance
Alcohol, barbiturates, narcotic analgesics	⇧ Risk of orthostatic hypotension

ALTERED LABORATORY VALUES

Blood/serum values	⇧ Uric acid ⇧ Calcium ⇩ Sodium ⇩ Potassium ⇩ Chloride ⇩ Bicarbonate ⇩ Phosphate ⇩ PBI ⇧ or ⇩ Glucose
Urinary values	⇧ Sodium ⇧ Potassium ⇧ Chloride ⇧ Bicarbonate ⇧ Uric acid ⇩ Calcium

Use in children

See INDICATIONS

Use in pregnancy or nursing mothers

Safe use not established during pregnancy; thiazides cross the placental barrier and appear in cord blood. In general, thiazides should not be given to pregnant women except for pathologic edema; however, a short course of diuretic therapy may be appropriate for hypervolemia-dependent edema that is causing extreme discomfort unrelieved by rest. Thiazides also appear in breast milk and may cause fetal or neonatal jaundice, thrombocytopenia, and other possible reactions. Patient should stop nursing if drug is prescribed.

HydroDIURIL (Hydrochlorothiazide) **Merck Sharp & Dohme**

Tabs: 25, 50, 100 mg

INDICATIONS	ORAL DOSAGE
Hypertension	**Adult:** 50–100 mg/day, as a single dose or div, or up to 200 mg/day div, if needed
Edema associated with congestive heart failure, hepatic cirrhosis, corticosteroid and estrogen therapy, and renal dysfunction (adjunctive therapy)	**Adult:** 50–100 mg qd or bid **Infant (< 2 yr):** 12.5–37.5 mg/day in 2 divided doses, according to weight (<6 mo, up to 1.5 mg/lb/day; older infants, 1.0 mg/lb/day) **Child (2–12 yr):** 37.5–100 mg/day in 2 divided doses, according to weight (1.0 mg/lb/day)

ADMINISTRATION/DOSAGE ADJUSTMENTS

Combination therapy	Dosage of other antihypertensive agents must be reduced when hydrochlorothiazide is added to the regimen to prevent excessive blood-pressure drop
Intermittent treatment of edema	Administer normal daily dose on alternate days or 3–5 days each week to reduce risk of excessive response and resultant electrolyte imbalance
Side effects	Reduce dosage or discontinue diuretic therapy if side effects (see ADVERSE REACTIONS) are moderate or severe

CONTRAINDICATIONS

Anuria ●	Hypersensitivity to hydrochlorothiazide or other sulfonamide derivatives ●

WARNINGS/PRECAUTIONS

Renal impairment	May result in excessive drug accumulation (see OVERDOSAGE); if renal impairment progresses, consider withholding or discontinuing diuretic therapy
Azotemia	May be precipitated in patients with renal disease
Electrolyte imbalances	Measure serum and urine electrolytes periodically, especially when patient is vomiting excessively or receiving parenteral fluids. Observe patient for such symptoms as dry mouth, thirst, weakness, lethargy, drowsiness, restlessness, muscle pain or cramps, muscular fatigue, hypotension, oliguria, tachycardia, and GI disturbances.
Hypokalemia	May develop, especially with brisk diuresis, concomitant corticosteroid or ACTH therapy, interference with adequate oral intake of electrolytes, or in the presence of severe cirrhosis; may be minimized by including potassium-rich foods in diet or, if necessary, with potassium supplements. Hypokalemia may result in digitalis toxicity.
Dilutional hyponatremia	May occur in edematous patients when weather is hot; restrict intake of water. Replace salt only for actual salt depletion or when hyponatremia is life-threatening.
Hepatic coma	May be precipitated by minor changes in fluid and electrolyte balance in patients with hepatic impairment or progressive liver disease; use with caution
Hyperuricemia or frank gout	May occur in certain patients
Sensitivity reactions	May occur in patients with or without a history of allergy or bronchial asthma
Insulin requirements	May increase, decrease, or remain unchanged; latent diabetes may become active
Lithium therapy	Renal clearance is reduced, increasing risk of lithium toxicity; coadministration generally should be avoided unless adequate precautions are taken
Systemic lupus erythematosus	May be activated or exacerbated
Postsympathectomy patients	Antihypertensive effect may be enhanced
Parathyroid-function tests	Discontinue drug before testing; parathyroid changes with hypercalcemia and hypophosphatemia may occur with prolonged therapy

Table continued on following page

ADVERSE REACTIONS

Gastrointestinal	Anorexia, gastric irritation, nausea, vomiting, cramping, diarrhea, constipation, intrahepatic cholestatic jaundice, pancreatitis, sialadenitis
Central nervous system	Dizziness, vertigo, paresthesias, headache, weakness, restlessness
Ophthalmic	Xanthopsia, transient blurred vision
Hematological	Leukopenia, agranulocytosis, thrombocytopenia, aplastic anemia, hemolytic anemia
Cardiovascular	Orthostatic hypotension
Hypersensitivity	Purpura, photosensitivity, rash, urticaria, necrotizing angiitis, fever, respiratory distress (including pneumonitis), anaphylactic reactions
Other	Hyperglycemia, glycosuria, hyperuricemia, muscle spasm

OVERDOSAGE

Signs and symptoms	Diuresis; lethargy progressing to coma, with minimal cardiorespiratory depression and with or without significant serum electrolyte changes or dehydration; GI irritation; hypermotility; transient elevation in BUN level
Treatment	Empty stomach by gastric lavage, taking care to avoid aspiration. Monitor serum electrolyte levels and renal function, and institute supportive measures, as required, to maintain hydration, electrolyte balance, respiration, and cardiovascular and renal function. Treat GI effects symptomatically.

DRUG INTERACTIONS

Other antihypertensive agents	⇧ Antihypertensive effect
Tubocurarine	⇧ Skeletal-muscle relaxation
Norepinephrine	⇩ Vasopressor effect
Steroids, ACTH	⇧ Risk of hypokalemia
Lithium	⇩ Lithium clearance
Alcohol, barbiturates, narcotic analgesics	⇧ Risk of orthostatic hypotension

ALTERED LABORATORY VALUES

Blood/serum values	⇧ Uric acid ⇧ Calcium ⇩ Sodium ⇩ Potassium ⇩ Chloride ⇩ Bicarbonate ⇩ Phosphate ⇩ PBI ⇧ or ⇩ Glucose
Urinary values	⇧ Sodium ⇧ Potassium ⇧ Chloride ⇧ Bicarbonate ⇧ Uric acid ⇩ Calcium

Use in children

See INDICATIONS

Use in pregnancy or nursing mothers

Safe use not established during pregnancy; thiazides cross the placental barrier and appear in cord blood. In general, thiazides should not be given to pregnant women except for pathologic edema; however, a short course of diuretic therapy may be appropriate for hypervolemia-dependent edema that is causing extreme discomfort unrelieved by rest. Thiazides also appear in breast milk and may cause fetal or neonatal jaundice, thrombocytopenia, and other possible reactions. Patient should stop nursing if drug is prescribed.

HYGROTON (Chlorthalidone) USV

Tabs: 25, 50, 100 mg

INDICATIONS	ORAL DOSAGE
Hypertension	**Adult:** 25 or 50 mg qd with breakfast to start, then adjust dosage to clinical response
Edema associated with congestive heart failure, hepatic cirrhosis, corticosteroid and estrogen therapy, and renal dysfunction (adjunctive therapy)	**Adult:** 50–100 mg qd with breakfast or 100 mg on alternate days to start, then adjust dosage to clinical response

ADMINISTRATION/DOSAGE ADJUSTMENTS	
Resistant cases	Increase initial dosage to 150-200 mg on alternate days or up to 200 mg/day (for edema) or 100 mg/day (for hypertension)
Side effects	Reduce dosage or discontinue diuretic therapy if side effects are moderate or severe (see ADVERSE REACTIONS)

CONTRAINDICATIONS	
Anuria ●	Hypersensitivity to chlorthalidone or other sulfonamide derivatives ●

WARNINGS/PRECAUTIONS	
Renal impairment	May result in excessive drug accumulation (see OVERDOSAGE); if renal impairment progresses, consider withholding or discontinuing diuretic therapy
Azotemia	May be precipitated in patients with renal disease
Electrolyte imbalances	Measure serum and urine electrolytes periodically, especially when patient is vomiting excessively or receiving parenteral fluids. Observe patient for such symptoms as dry mouth, thirst, weakness, lethargy, drowsiness, restlessness, muscle pain or cramps, muscular fatigue, hypotension, oliguria, tachycardia, and GI disturbances.
Hypokalemia	May develop, especially with brisk diuresis, concomitant corticosteroid or ACTH therapy, interference with adequate oral intake of electrolytes, or in the presence of severe cirrhosis; may be minimized by including potassium-rich foods in diet or, if necessary, with potassium supplements. Hypokalemia may result in digitalis toxicity.
Dilutional hyponatremia	May occur in edematous patients when weather is hot; restrict intake of water. Replace salt only for actual salt depletion or when hyponatremia is life-threatening.
Hepatic coma	May be precipitated by minor changes in fluid and electrolyte balance in patients with hepatic impairment or progressive liver disease; use with caution
Hyperuricemia or frank gout	May occur in certain patients
Sensitivity reactions	May occur in patients with a history of allergy or bronchial asthma
Insulin requirements	May increase, decrease, or remain unchanged; latent diabetes may become active
Postsympathectomy patients	Antihypertensive effect may be enhanced

ADVERSE REACTIONS	
Gastrointestinal	Anorexia, gastric irritation, nausea, vomiting, cramping, diarrhea, constipation, intrahepatic cholestatic jaundice, pancreatitis
Central nervous system	Dizziness, vertigo, paresthesias, headache, weakness, restlessness
Ophthalmic	Xanthopsia
Hematological	Leukopenia, agranulocytosis, thrombocytopenia, aplastic anemia
Cardiovascular	Orthostatic hypotension
Hypersensitivity	Purpura, photosensitivity, rash, urticaria, necrotizing angiitis, Lyell's syndrome (toxic epidermal necrolysis)
Other	Hyperglycemia, glycosuria, hyperuricemia, muscle spasm, impotence

Table continued on following page

OVERDOSAGE

Signs and symptoms	Nausea, weakness, dizziness, and disturbance of electrolyte balance
Treatment	Empty stomach by gastric lavage, taking care to avoid aspiration. Monitor serum electrolyte levels and renal function, and institute supportive measures, as required, to maintain hydration, electrolyte balance, respiration, and cardiovascular and renal function. Treat GI effects symptomatically. If necessary, IV dextrose-saline with potassium may be administered with caution.

DRUG INTERACTIONS

Other antihypertensive agents	⇧ Antihypertensive effect
Tubocurarine	⇧ Skeletal-muscle relaxation
Norepinephrine	⇩ Vasopressor effect
Steroids, ACTH	⇧ Risk of hypokalemia
Lithium	⇩ Lithium clearance
Alcohol, barbiturates, narcotic analgesics	⇧ Risk of orthostatic hypotension

ALTERED LABORATORY VALUES

Blood/serum values	⇧ Uric acid ⇧ Calcium ⇩ Sodium ⇩ Potassium ⇩ Chloride ⇩ Bicarbonate ⇩ Phosphate ⇩ PBI ⇧ or ⇩ Glucose
Urinary values	⇧ Sodium ⇧ Potassium ⇧ Chloride ⇧ Bicarbonate ⇧ Uric acid ⇩ Calcium

Use in children

General guidelines not established

Use in pregnancy or nursing mothers

Safe use has not been established during pregnancy. Thiazides cross the placental barrier and appear in cord blood. In general, thiazides should not be given to pregnant women except for pathologic edema; however, a short course of diuretic therapy may be appropriate for hypervolemia-dependent edema that is causing extreme discomfort unrelieved by rest. Thiazides also appear in breast milk and may cause fetal or neonatal jaundice, thrombocytopenia, and other possible reactions. Patient should stop nursing if drug is prescribed.

LASIX (Furosemide) Hoechst-Roussel

Tabs: 20, 40, 80 mg **Oral sol:** 10 mg/ml (60, 120 ml) **Amps:** 10 mg/ml (2, 4, 10 ml) **Syringe:** 10 mg/ml (2, 4 ml)

INDICATIONS	ORAL DOSAGE	PARENTERAL DOSAGE
Hypertension	**Adult:** 40 mg bid; adjust dosage according to patient response	—
Edema associated with congestive heart failure, hepatic cirrhosis, and renal disease (including the nephrotic syndrome)	**Adult:** 20–80 mg to start; larger doses, up to 600 mg/day, may be given in increments of 20–40 mg 6–8 h after previous dose until adequate diuresis ensues, followed by same dose qd or bid **Child:** 2 mg/kg to start; larger doses, up to 6 mg/kg, may be given in increments of 1–2 mg/kg 6–8 h after previous dose until adequate diuresis ensues; reduce to minimum effective level for maintenance	**Adult:** 20–40 mg IM or IV (slowly) to start; larger doses may be given in increments of 20 mg 2 h after previous dose until adequate diuresis ensues, followed by same dose qd or bid **Child:** 1 mg/kg IM or IV (slowly) to start; larger doses, up to 6 mg/kg, may be given in increments of 1 mg/kg 2 h after previous dose until adequate diuresis ensues
Acute pulmonary edema (adjunctive therapy)	—	**Adult:** 40 mg IV (slowly) to start, followed by 80 mg IV (slowly) 1 h later, if needed

ADMINISTRATION/DOSAGE ADJUSTMENTS

Intermittent use	For edema, drug may be given 2–4 consecutive days per week
High-dose parenteral therapy	Administer controlled infusion at a rate not exceeding 4 mg/min; titrate dosage by therapeutic response and closely monitor patient
Combination antihypertensive therapy	Reduce dosage of other antihypertensive agents by at least 50% as soon as furosemide is added to the regimen to prevent an excessive fall in blood pressure; as blood pressure falls under furosemide's potentiating effect, a further reduction in dosage or discontinuation of other antihypertensive drugs may be required

CONTRAINDICATIONS

Anuria ●	Hypersensitivity to furosemide ●	Concomitant cephaloridine therapy ●

WARNINGS/PRECAUTIONS

Electrolyte depletion	May occur, especially with high dosages and salt restriction; monitor patients for hyponatremia, hypochloremic alkalosis, and hypokalemia; obtain serum and urine electrolyte determinations regularly, especially when patient is vomiting excessively or receiving parenteral fluids. Observe patient for such symptoms as dry mouth, thirst, weakness, lethargy, drowsiness, restlessness, muscle pain or cramps, muscular fatigue, hypotension, oliguria, tachycardia, and GI disturbances.
Hypokalemia	May develop, especially with brisk diuresis, concomitant corticosteroid or ACTH therapy, interference with adequate oral intake of electrolytes, or in the presence of severe cirrhosis; effects may be exaggerated by digitalis; may be prevented with supplemental potassium chloride and, if necessary, an aldosterone antagonist
Hyperuricemia or frank gout	May occur
Active or latent diabetes	Blood glucose may be increased and glucose tolerance tests may be altered; check urine and blood glucose periodically
Serum calcium	May be reduced and (rarely) lead to tetany; obtain periodic serum calcium determinations
Dehydration	May occur with reduction in blood volume, circulatory collapse, and possible vascular thrombosis, particularly in elderly patients; monitor patients, especially those with renal insufficiency, for associated reversible elevations in BUN
Prolonged high-dose therapy	Careful clinical and laboratory observation is advisable with prolonged administration of doses exceeding 80 mg/day

Table continued on following page

LASIX continued

WARNINGS/PRECAUTIONS continued	
Concomitant lithium therapy	Generally should be avoided because of the high risk of lithium toxicity
Concomitant indomethacin therapy	Diuretic and antihypertensive effects may be reduced; plasma renin levels and aldosterone excretion may be affected
Severe, progressive renal disease	If increasing azotemia and oliguria occur during treatment, discontinue therapy
Blood dyscrasias, liver damage, other idiosyncratic reactions	May occur; monitor patients regularly
Allergic reactions	May occur in patients with sulfonamide sensitivity
Systemic lupus erythematosus	May be activated or exacerbated
Concomitant use of aminoglycosides	Should be avoided, especially in patients with renal impairment, except in life-threatening situations
Tartrazine sensitivity	Presence of FD&C Yellow No. 5 (tartrazine) in oral solution may cause allergic-type reactions, including bronchial asthma, in susceptible individuals
ADVERSE REACTIONS	
Gastrointestinal	Anorexia, oral and gastric irritation, nausea, vomiting, cramping, diarrhea, constipation, cholestatic jaundice, pancreatitis
Central nervous system	Dizziness, vertigo, paresthesias, headache, blurred vision, tinnitus, xanthopsia, hearing loss,[1] muscle spasm, weakness, restlessness
Hematological	Anemia, leukopenia, agranulocytosis (rare), thrombocytopenia, aplastic anemia (rare)
Hypersensitivity	Purpura, photosensitivity, rash, urticaria, necrotizing angiitis, exfoliative dermatitis, erythema multiforme, pruritus
Cardiovascular	Orthostatic hypotension
Other	Hyperglycemia, glycosuria, hyperuricemia, urinary bladder spasm, thrombophlebitis, transient pain at IM injection site
OVERDOSAGE	
Signs and symptoms	See ADVERSE REACTIONS
Treatment	Discontinue medication; treat symptomatically and institute supportive measures, as required
DRUG INTERACTIONS	
Other antihypertensive agents	⇧ Antihypertensive effect
Digitalis glycosides	⇧ Digitalis toxicity
Steroids, ACTH	⇧ Risk of hypokalemia
Lithium	⇩ Lithium excretion
Aminoglycosides	⇧ Aminoglycoside ototoxicity
Salicylates	⇧ Salicylate toxicity
Cephaloridine	⇧ Nephrotoxicity of cephaloridine
Muscle relaxants	⇧ Muscle relaxation
Norepinephrine	⇩ Arterial responsiveness
Indomethacin	⇩ Diuretic and/or antihypertensive effect of furosemide
Oral hypoglycemics	⇩ Hypoglycemic effect
Alcohol, barbiturates, narcotics	⇧ Risk of orthostatic hypotension

Table continued on following page

ALTERED LABORATORY VALUES

Blood/serum values — ⇧ Glucose ⇧ BUN ⇧ Uric acid ⇩ Sodium ⇩ Potassium ⇩ Chloride ⇩ Calcium ⇩ Magnesium

Urinary values — ⇧ Glucose ⇧ Sodium ⇧ Potassium ⇧ Chloride

Use in children

See INDICATIONS

Use in pregnancy or nursing mothers

Animal reproductive studies show that furosemide may cause fetal abnormalities. Use in women of childbearing potential is contraindicated, except in life-threatening situations where parenteral use is paramount over use of alternative drugs. Furosemide appears in breast milk. If use is deemed essential, patient should stop nursing.

[1]Usually following high-dose parenteral therapy in patients with severe renal impairment receiving other ototoxic drugs

ZAROXOLYN (Metolazone) Pennwalt

Tabs: 2.5, 5, 10 mg

INDICATIONS	ORAL DOSAGE
Hypertension	**Adult:** 2.5–5 mg qd
Edema associated with congestive heart failure	**Adult:** 5–10 mg qd
Edema associated with renal disease and dysfunction (including the nephrotic syndrome)	**Adult:** 5–20 mg qd

ADMINISTRATION/DOSAGE ADJUSTMENTS

Paroxysmal nocturnal dyspnea	May occur in patients with congestive heart failure; dosage near upper end of range may help ensure 24-h duration of diuretic and saluretic effects
Combination therapy	Dosage of other antihypertensive agents or diuretics and metolazone should be carefully adjusted, particularly during initial therapy; dosage of other agents, especially ganglionic blockers, should be reduced. Concurrent administration of metolazone and furosemide should be initiated under hospital conditions (see WARNINGS/PRECAUTIONS).
Optimal dosage	Initial dose should be reduced to lowest maintenance level as soon as desired effect is obtained; the time interval may range from days for edematous states to 3–4 wk for hypertension. Dosage adjustment is usually necessary during course of therapy, based on clinical and laboratory evaluations.
Side effects	Reduce dosage or discontinue therapy if side effects are moderate or severe (see ADVERSE REACTIONS)

CONTRAINDICATIONS

Anuria ●	Hepatic coma or pre-coma ●	Hypersensitivity to metolazone ●

WARNINGS/PRECAUTIONS

Severe renal impairment	May result in excessive drug accumulation (see OVERDOSAGE); if renal impairment progresses, consider withholding or discontinuing diuretic therapy
Azotemia	May be precipitated in patients with renal disease; if azotemia and oliguria worsen during treatment, discontinue drug
Hyperuricemia, gouty attacks	May occur in patients with history of gout; use with caution
Electrolyte imbalances	May occur; measure serum and urine electrolytes periodically, especially when patient is vomiting excessively or receiving parenteral fluids. Monitor BUN, uric acid, and glucose levels. Observe patient for such symptoms as dry mouth, thirst, weakness, lethargy, drowsiness, restlessness, muscle pain or cramps, muscular fatigue, hypotension, oliguria, tachycardia, and GI disturbances.
Concurrent use of furosemide	May result in unusually large or prolonged effects on volume and electrolytes; if necessary, administer in hospital setting to provide for adequate monitoring
Hypokalemia	May develop, especially with intensive or prolonged diuresis, concomitant corticosteroid or ACTH therapy, or inadequate electrolyte intake; may require potassium supplementation. Hypokalemia may result in dangerous or fatal arrhythmias in digitalized patients.
Potassium-sparing diuretics	Concurrent use may potentiate diuresis; dosages of both diuretics should be reduced and potassium supplements discontinued
Dilutional hyponatremia	May occur in patients with severe edema accompanying cardiac failure or renal disease, especially in hot weather, or in those with a low salt intake
Chloride deficit and hypochloremic alkalosis	May occur
Orthostatic hypotension	May occur; may be potentiated by alcohol, barbiturates, narcotics, or concurrent antihypertensive therapy
Insulin requirements	May increase, decrease, or remain unchanged; latent diabetes may become active

Table continued on following page

WARNINGS/PRECAUTIONS continued

Elective surgery	Discontinue metolazone 3 days before elective surgery; related diuretics (but not metolazone) have increased responsiveness to tubocurarine and decreased arterial responsiveness to norepinephrine
Parathyroid changes with hypercalcemia and hypophosphatemia[1]	May occur rarely with diuretics

ADVERSE REACTIONS

Gastrointestinal	Constipation, nausea, vomiting, anorexia, diarrhea, abdominal bloating, epigastric distress, intrahepatic cholestatic jaundice, hepatitis
Central nervous system	Syncope, dizziness, drowsiness, vertigo, headache
Hematological	Leukopenia
Cardiovascular	Orthostatic hypotension, excess volume depletion, hemoconcentration, venous thrombosis, palpitations, chest pain
Hypersensitivity	Urticaria, other skin rashes
Other	Dry mouth, hypokalemia (symptomatic and asymptomatic), hyponatremia, hypochloremia, hypochloremic alkalosis, hyperuricemia, hyperglycemia, glycosuria, fatigue, muscle cramps or spasm, weakness, restlessness, chills, acute gouty attacks

OVERDOSAGE

Signs and symptoms	Diuresis; lethargy progressing to coma, with minimal cardiorespiratory depression and with or without significant serum electrolyte changes or dehydration; GI irritation; hypermotility; transient elevation in BUN level
Treatment	Empty stomach by gastric lavage, taking care to avoid aspiration. Monitor serum electrolyte levels and renal function, and institute supportive measures, as required, to maintain hydration, electrolyte balance, respiration, and cardiovascular and renal function. Treat GI effects symptomatically.

DRUG INTERACTIONS

Other antihypertensive agents	⇧ Antihypertensive effect
Steroids, ACTH	⇧ Risk of hypokalemia
Lithium	⇩ Lithium clearance
Alcohol, barbiturates, narcotic analgesics	⇧ Risk of orthostatic hypotension

ALTERED LABORATORY VALUES

Blood/serum values	⇧ Uric acid ⇧ Calcium ⇩ Sodium ⇩ Potassium ⇩ Chloride ⇩ Bicarbonate ⇩ Phosphate ⇩ PBI ⇧ or ⇩ Glucose ⇧ BUN ⇧ Creatinine
Urinary values	⇧ Sodium ⇧ Potassium ⇧ Chloride ⇧ Bicarbonate ⇧ Glucose ⇧ Uric acid ⇧ Phosphate ⇧ Magnesium

Use in children

Not recommended

Use in pregnancy or nursing mothers

Safe use has not been established during pregnancy. Metolazone crosses the placental barrier and appears in cord blood. In general, diuretics should not be given to pregnant women except for pathologic edema; however, a short course of metolazone therapy may be appropriate for hypervolemia-dependent edema that is causing discomfort unrelieved by rest. Metolazone also appears in breast milk and may cause fetal or neonatal jaundice, thrombocytopenia, and other possible reactions. Patient should stop nursing if drug is prescribed.

[1]Not reported to date for metolazone

Clotting Disorders

Blood is a substance that can change from a fluid to a solid and back to a fluid. Thus it regulates a delicate balance between the formation of clots to seal off cuts and other breaks in the circulatory system, and dissolution of those clots when further coagulation (clotting) would impede essential blood flow.

To achieve this balance, at least thirteen known factors or processes are involved. With this number of variables, it is not surprising that the process sometimes goes awry. This section will review the major clotting disorders and the drugs used to treat them.

FACTORS AFFECTING COAGULATION

Coagulation may be disrupted by disease or by exposure to drugs or other chemicals that impair or destroy a blood component essential for clotting. In some rare cases, the blood cannot coagulate because of a genetic defect, such as in hemophilia. If the clotting mechanism fails and effective measures are not taken to prevent hemorrhage, the consequence can be fatal.

Equally life-threatening is spontaneous clot formation that may eventually block blood vessels. When these blockages occur in vital organs—e.g., the heart, lungs, or brain—heart attack, pulmonary failure, or stroke may result. A number of factors may trigger abnormal clot formation, including a transfusion of an incompatible blood type and prolonged bed rest following surgery or childbirth. Certain drugs, such as oral contraceptives, also may increase the risk of clotting disorders.

THROMBOEMBOLIC DISEASES

Clotting disorders that interfere with normal circulation are referred to as thromboembolic disease. The most insidious clots form where there is a change in the shape or inner surface of a blood vessel wall. Such changes are usually associated with atherosclerosis, in which arterial walls are gradually hardened, roughened, and narrowed by an accumulation of fatty deposits.

Inflammation, infection, a burn, or a deep wound also may roughen or change the texture of the vessel wall, causing some constituents of the blood to adhere to it and eventually form a clot. Certain disorders of the blood vessels, such as varicose veins, are still other causes of clotting abnormalities.

A clot formed within a blood vessel, whether in a vein or an artery, is called a thrombus, while the process resulting in the clot is known as thrombosis. A thrombus that detaches itself from its place of origin is an embolus; when it is carried by the bloodstream and lodges in some other part of the circulatory system, impeding blood flow, the

MECHANISM OF PULMONARY THROMBOEMBOLISM

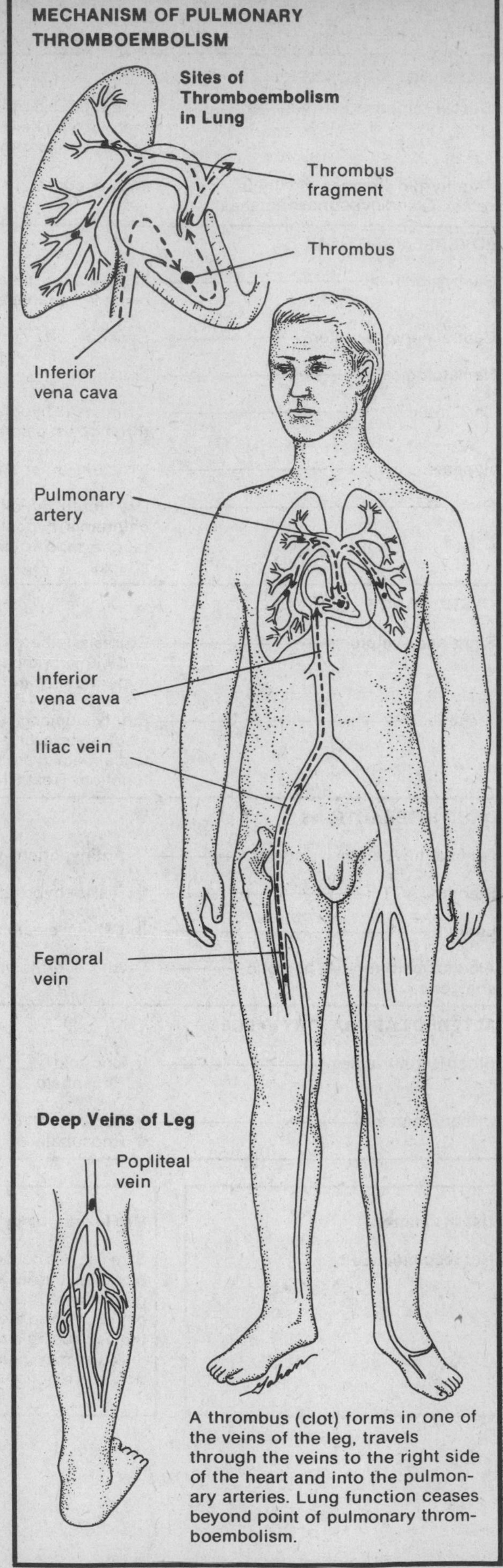

A thrombus (clot) forms in one of the veins of the leg, travels through the veins to the right side of the heart and into the pulmonary arteries. Lung function ceases beyond point of pulmonary thromboembolism.

3

condition is known as an embolism.

Thrombosis is more common in veins than in arteries because venous blood flows more slowly. It is more common still in the superficial vessels of the leg, especially if they are varicose. (Varicose veins are discussed in the section on *Peripheral Circulatory Disorders.*) Inflammation of a vein with subsequent clot formation is called thrombophlebitis, a condition that causes the affected part of the leg to become red, swollen, and sore. Suspected thrombophlebitis should be evaluated by a physician. Analgesics are usually recommended to relieve the pain, and if they contain aspirin, they will also contribute to the dissolution of the clot. Support hosiery or a properly applied elastic bandage also may be recommended.

At one time, thrombosis in the deep veins posed a serious threat to women following childbirth or to persons recuperating from surgery. Such cases have decreased significantly since the routine use of anticoagulant drugs and the practice of having these patients get out of bed—or at least exercise their legs—to prevent venous blood from pooling in the vessels of the lower leg.

While embolization is an ever present danger where venous thrombosis exists, arterial thrombosis is a more frequent cause of medical emergency. The most serious types of arterial thrombosis are usually a result of atherosclerosis, although in some instances they may follow infection or injury. In coronary thrombosis, a blood clot in a coronary artery blocks off a significant amount of the blood supply to the heart muscle, resulting in a heart attack (myocardial infarction). (For a more complete discussion of heart attacks, see the section on *Coronary Artery Disease.*)

A similarly dangerous situation prevails when a clot blocks the blood supply to the brain, as occurs in cerebral thrombosis, commonly referred to as stroke. Strokes are usually caused by hardening of the arteries of the brain and nearby areas, although a stroke may also be directly related to hypertension or may result from an acute injury to a diseased blood vessel, leading to a hemorrhage.

If the stroke is caused by the total blocking of an artery by an embolism, unconsciousness occurs swiftly and suddenly. In contrast, clotting in a smaller vessel that spreads into the internal carotid artery—the major artery that runs up the neck to the brain—produces early warning signs such as distorted speech, weakness, and confusion. Severe headache may be another warning of an impending stroke. Transient ischemic attacks—commonly referred to as TIAs—are also important warning signs of stroke. TIAs are characterized by temporary loss of sight, numbness, temporary paralysis on one side of the face or in a limb, difficulty in speaking or finding the right words, inability to recognize a familiar object or face, and fainting or dizziness.

Drug therapy for both stroke and TIAs—including the use of anticoagulants—is determined by the cause of the circulatory disruption, particularly whether the symptoms are caused by occluded vessels or hemorrhage.

A clotting disorder common in the elderly and in diabetics is peripheral thrombosis, which most frequently affects the arteries of the legs. In some cases, a clot may block the remaining passageway in a diseased or narrowed vessel, depriving the area of circulation. This deprivation can lead to tissue death or gangrene. Its onset, which may be sudden, is signaled by a tingling sensation, or the affected part may become cold and numb. In some instances, surgery to remove the thrombus is essential and is usually followed by anticoagulant therapy.

OTHER USES OF ANTICOAGULANT DRUGS

Surgical removal of severely occluded or diseased blood vessels and replacement with grafts—particularly coronary bypass surgery to treat heart disease—has become a common approach to treating or preventing thromboembolic disease. When surgery is the treatment of choice, however, anticoagulant drugs are often used concomitantly to prevent clots in the grafts.

Anticoagulant drugs also are used in patients with diseased heart valves, particularly those who have had artificial valves implanted. These drugs help prevent the formation of clots associated with the valve replacements, although this danger has been reduced somewhat by the development of heart valves made from natural substances, such as pig heart valves.

DRUGS USED TO TREAT CLOTTING DISORDERS

As noted earlier, at least thirteen factors or processes are involved in normal coagulation. Drugs to prevent clotting or promote clot dissolution fall into three general categories.

Anticoagulants

Anticoagulants are drugs that interfere with the conversion of fibrinogen, a blood protein, into an insoluble substance called fibrin. When a blood vessel is cut, for example, an enzyme called thrombin is released, which stimulates fibrinogen to produce fibrin. The fibrin creates a web that enmeshes red blood cells, forming the clot, and stops the bleeding through the cut. An enzyme called plasmin (also fibrinolysin), is capable of dissolving the fibrin. Plasmin is produced by the same injury that sets the clotting process in motion, thus giving the body an automatic reversal system.

The body manufactures another substance, heparin, that is capable of retarding or preventing clotting. Heparin is concentrated in the mucous membranes of the intestines and in the muscles, and is especially abundant in the liver and lungs. Heparin effectively aborts the clotting process by interfering with the action of thrombin on fibrinogen, thus preventing the formation of fibrin. Injections of heparin sodium are used to treat or prevent a variety of thromboembolic disorders, including stroke, pulmonary embolism, and venous thrombosis, and in the prevention of thrombosis and pulmonary embolism in surgery patients.

Other anticoagulants that are based on chemicals that interfere with or block production of prothrombin, the inactive form of thrombin, include warfarin (Coumadin, Panwarfin, and other brands). These drugs may be administered in either oral or injection form; therefore, patients on long-term anticoagulant therapy usually use one of the oral forms of these drugs, as opposed to heparin, which is given by intravenous injection.

Fibrinolytic Agents

Although anticoagulant drugs may be useful in preventing the formation of clots, they are of little value in dissolving established clots. To dissolve clots, drugs known as fibrinolytic agents are used. These drugs act by stimulating the production of plasmin to dissolve the clot. The two most commonly used fibrinolytic agents are streptokinase (Streptase), an enzymatic protein, and urokinase (Abbokinase), a protein found in kidney cells. Both drugs are digested when given orally, and therefore must be administered intravenously, virtually always in a hospital setting. They are relatively new drugs, and since bleeding problems occur more frequently and are harder to manage with fibrinolytic agents than those occurring with anticoagulant therapy, these drugs should be used by physicians experienced in treating thromboembolic disorders.

Antiplatelet Drugs

Platelets are still another blood constituent that plays a vital role in the formation of clots. In recent years, increased attention has been paid to the role of platelets in thrombotic disease, particularly stroke and heart attacks. A number of drugs interfere with platelet function, including aspirin, sulfinpyrazone (Anturane), and dipyridamole (Persantine). The use of these drugs to prevent clot formation is still, for the most part, considered experimental. One exception is the recent Food and Drug Administration approval of the use of aspirin to treat TIAs in certain male patients to prevent stroke.

USE OF ANTICOAGULANTS

Since the balance between clotting and hemorrhage is so critical, blood tests should always be given before administering anticoagulant drugs. Frequent laboratory checks of the changes in the blood should continue during anticoagulant therapy so that dosages can be adjusted for optimum results.

IN CONCLUSION

Outpatients using anticoagulants should make a special point of asking the prescribing physician which side effects are essentially harmless and within a normal range and which ones must be promptly reported. Since many drugs interfere with the action of anticoagulants (and vice versa), it is particularly important that the physician be aware of any other drugs—including nonprescription medications—that are being used. For example, when an anticoagulant is taken with antidepressants such as Elavil or Triavil, anti-inflammatory agents such as Indocin, and any analgesic containing aspirin, a hemorrage may result. Diabetics (especially those on oral medications), epileptics on anticonvulsants, and children of any age require particularly vigilant supervision during anticoagulant therapy. Eating habits and the use of alcohol also should be reviewed in detail with a physician to determine whether they may have any impact on therapy.

In the following drug tables, only the major anticoagulants are included. Fibrinolytic agents are used only under close supervision in a hospital setting and are not as widely used as the anticoagulants. As noted earlier, the effect of antiplatelet drugs on thrombotic disorders is still under investigation. However, the two most commonly used antiplatelet agents are aspirin and sulfinpyrazone (Anturane).

ABBOKINASE (Urokinase) Abbott

Vial: 250,000 IU

INDICATIONS	PARENTERAL DOSAGE
Pulmonary embolism	**Adult:** 2,000 IU/lb by IV infusion over 10 min to start, followed by 2,000 IU/lb/h for 12 h

ADMINISTRATION/DOSAGE ADJUSTMENTS	
Reconstruction and dilution	Add 5.2 ml of sterile water without preservatives to vial immediately before using; discard any unused portion of the reconstituted material. Dilute reconstituted urokinase with 0.9% normal saline prior to intravenous infusion to a total volume of 195 ml. Total fluid volume administered should not exceed 200 ml.
Posttreatment anticoagulation	To prevent recurrent thrombosis, administer heparin by continuous IV infusion when thrombin time has decreased to less than twice the normal control value

CONTRAINDICATIONS[1]	
Surgery (within 10 days)	Including liver or kidney biopsy, lumbar puncture, thoracentesis or paracentesis, extensive or multiple cutdowns
Intra-arterial diagnostic procedure (within 10 days)	
Ulcerative wound	
Recent trauma	With possibility of internal injuries
Visceral or intracranial malignancy	
Ulcerative colitis, diverticulitis	Or actively bleeding lesion (or one with a significant potential for bleeding) of the gastrointestinal or genitourinary tract
Severe hypertension	
Renal insufficiency	Acute or chronic
Hepatic insufficiency	Acute or chronic
Uncontrolled hypocoagulable state	Including one that may be caused by a coagulation factor deficiency, thrombocytopenia, spontaneous fibrinolysis, or another purpuric or hemorrhagic disorder
Chronic lung disease	With cavitation (eg, tuberculosis)
Subacute bacterial endocarditis or rheumatic valvular disease	
Recent cerebral embolism, thrombosis, or hemorrhage	Wait at least 2 mo before using urokinase
Other conditions	In which bleeding might constitute a significant hazard or be particularly difficult to manage because of its location

WARNINGS/PRECAUTIONS	
Bleeding, hematoma formation	May occur, particularly at injection sites; avoid IM injections and nonessential handling of the patient. If arterial puncture is absolutely necessary, avoid femoral artery and use radial or brachial artery instead; apply pressure for at least 15 min, then a pressure dressing. Frequently check puncture site for evidence of bleeding. Perform venipunctures carefully and as infrequently as possible.
Spontaneous internal bleeding	May occur, especially in patients with preexisting hemostatic defects; discontinue use if serious spontaneous bleeding occurs and institute appropriate measures (see OVERDOSAGE)
Special-risk patients	Use with caution in patients with atrial fibrillation or other conditions in which there is possible risk of cerebral embolism
Concomitant use of anticoagulants	Not recommended (see ADMINISTRATION/DOSAGE ADJUSTMENTS)

ADVERSE REACTIONS	
Hematological	Minor bleeding, severe bleeding, cerebral hemorrhage (sometimes fatal), oozing of blood from sites of percutaneous trauma
Allergic	Bronchospasm, skin rash (rare)
Other	Febrile episodes (causal relationship not established)

[1]Contraindications are not absolute; the risk of hemorrhage must be weighed against the anticipated benefits of urokinase, and the risks and benefits of urokinase therapy should be compared to those associated with other forms of treatment

Table continued on following page

ABBOKINASE continued

OVERDOSAGE

Signs and symptoms	See ADVERSE REACTIONS
Treatment	For uncontrollable bleeding, discontinue urokinase and administer large, packed red cells. Replace blood volume deficit with plasma volume expanders other than Dextran. Whole blood may be used. If hemorrhage is unresponsive to blood replacement, consider using aminocaproic acid. Treat fever symptomatically, using acetaminophen rather than aspirin.

DRUG INTERACTIONS

Aspirin, indomethacin, phenylbutazone	⇧ Risk of bleeding
Anticoagulants	⇧ Risk of bleeding

ALTERED LABORATORY VALUES

Blood/serum values	⇧ Thrombin time ⇧ Activated partial thromboplastin time ⇧ Prothrombin time ⇧ FDP ⇩ Hematocrit

No clinically significant alterations in urinary values occur at therapeutic dosages

Use in children

Safety and effectiveness not established

Use in pregnancy or nursing mothers

Contraindicated during pregnancy and first 10 days of postpartum period; general guidelines not established for use in nursing mothers

COUMADIN (Warfarin sodium) Endo

Tabs: 2, 2.5, 5, 7.5, 10 mg **Vial:** 50 mg/2 ml after reconstitution

INDICATIONS	ORAL DOSAGE	PARENTERAL DOSAGE
Venous thrombosis **Atrial fibrillation with embolization** **Pulmonary embolism** **Coronary occlusion** (adjunctive therapy) **Transient cerebral ischemic attacks** (adjunctive therapy)[1]	**Adult:** 40–60 mg in a single dose to start, or 10–15 mg/day for 2–3 days, followed in each case by 2–10 mg/day, as determined by the prothrombin-time response, for maintenance	**Adult:** 40–60 mg in a single IM or IV dose to start, or 10–15 mg/day IM or IV for 2–3 days, followed in each case by 2–10 mg/day orally, as determined by the prothrombin-time response, for maintenance

ADMINISTRATION/DOSAGE ADJUSTMENTS

Coagulation tests	Determine prothrombin time daily after initiating therapy until the results stabilize in the therapeutic range (1½–2½ times the normal value); subsequent determinations may be made at intervals of 1–4 wk
Elderly and/or debilitated patients	Reduce starting dose to 20–30 mg
Concomitant use of heparin	Draw blood for prothrombin-time determinations just prior to next heparin dose (at least 5 h after last IV injection or 24 h after last SC injection). In emergency situations, heparin and injectable warfarin may be coadministered to initiate anticoagulant therapy; the two drugs may be given together in the same syringe.
Withdrawal of therapy	Taper dosage gradually over 3–4 wk

CONTRAINDICATIONS

Hemorrhagic tendencies or blood dyscrasias	
Recent or contemplated surgery	CNS surgery, eye surgery, traumatic surgery resulting in large open surfaces
Bleeding tendencies associated with active ulceration or overt bleeding	Gastrointestinal, genitourinary, or respiratory-tract bleeding or ulceration, cerebrovascular hemorrhage, cerebral or dissecting aortic aneurysm, pericarditis and pericardial effusions, subacute bacterial endocarditis
Obstetric complications	Threatened abortion, eclampsia, pre-eclampsia
Major regional or lumbar block anesthesia	
Malignant hypertension	
Lack of supervision	Of senile, alcoholic, or psychotic patients
Lack of patient cooperation	
Inadequate laboratory facilities	
Diagnostic or therapeutic procedures	With potential for uncontrolled bleeding, such as spinal puncture

WARNINGS/PRECAUTIONS

Laboratory monitoring	Control dosage by periodic determinations of prothrombin time or by use of other suitable coagulation tests (see ADMINISTRATION/DOSAGE ADJUSTMENTS); additional determinations should be made in the period immediately after discharge from the hospital and whenever other medications are initiated, discontinued, or taken haphazardly
Congestive-heart-failure patients	May become more sensitive to warfarin; monitor prothrombin response more frequently and reduce dosage, if necessary
Increased risk of bleeding and/or hemorrhage	Use with caution in patients with moderate to severe hepatic or renal insufficiency, prolonged dietary deficiencies (cachexia, vitamin K deficiency), infectious diseases, disturbances of intestinal flora (sprue, antibiotic therapy), indwelling catheters, moderate to severe hypertension, polycythemia vera, vasculitis, severe diabetes, severe allergic and anaphylactic disorders, trauma which may result in internal bleeding, or in surgery or trauma resulting in large exposed raw surfaces
Increased prothrombin-time response	May result from carcinoma, collagen disease, congestive heart failure, diarrhea, elevated temperature, infectious hepatitis, jaundice, poor nutritional states, vitamin K deficiency (steatorrhea), prolonged hot weather, warfarin overdosage, unreliable prothrombin-time determinations, and a variety of drugs (see DRUG INTERACTIONS)

[1]Possibly effective

Table continued on following page

COUMADIN continued

WARNINGS/PRECAUTIONS continued

Decreased prothrombin-time response	May result from diabetes mellitus, edema, hereditary resistance to warfarin therapy, hyperlipemia, hypothyroidism, warfarin underdosage, a diet high in vitamin K (leafy green vegetables, fish, fish oil, onions), and a variety of drugs (see DRUG INTERACTIONS)
Dental and surgical procedures	May be performed without undue risk of hemorrhage by limiting the operative site to permit effective use of local procedures for hemostasis, including absorbable hemostatic agents, sutures, and pressure dressings; the prothrombin time should be 1½–2½ times the normal (control) value

ADVERSE REACTIONS

Hematological	Bleeding, hemorrhage, "purple toes" syndrome
Dermatological	Alopecia, urticaria, dermatitis, hemorrhagic infarction and skin necrosis
Gastrointestinal	Nausea, diarrhea, abdominal cramping
Hypersensitivity	Fever, other reactions
Other	Priapism (causal relationship not established)

OVERDOSAGE

Signs and symptoms	Excessive prothrombinopenia with or without bleeding, as manifested by microscopic hematuria, excessive menstrual bleeding, melena, petechiae, and/or oozing from shaving nicks
Treatment	For mild or no bleeding, omit 1 or more doses; if necessary, administer 2.5–10 mg vitamin K_1 orally. For persistent minor bleeding or frank bleeding, administer 5–25 mg vitamin K_1 IV (slowly). For severe bleeding or bleeding unresponsive to vitamin K_1, transfuse fresh whole blood.

DRUG INTERACTIONS

Allopurinol, aminosalicylic acid, anabolic steroids, antibiotics, bromelains, chloramphenicol, chymotrypsin, cimetidine, cinchophen, clofibrate, dextran, dextrothyroxine, diazoxide, disulfiram, drugs affecting blood elements, ethacrynic acid, glucagon, hepatotoxic drugs, indomethacin, inhalation anesthetics, MAO inhibitors, mefenamic acid, methyldopa, methylphenidate, methylthiouracil, metronidazole, nalidixic acid, narcotics (with prolonged use), nortriptyline, oxolinic acid, oxyphenbutazone, phenylbutazone, phenyramidol, phenytoin, propylthiouracil, quinidine, quinine, salicylates, sulfinpyrazone, sulfonamides (long-acting), sulindac, thyroid drugs, tolbutamide, triclofos sodium, trimethoprim-sulfamethoxazole	⇧ Prothrombin-time response
Adrenocorticosteroids, antacids, antihistamines, barbiturates, carbamazepine, chlordiazepoxide, cholestyramine, ethchlorvynol, estrogens, glutethimide, griseofulvin, haloperidol, meprobamate, oral contraceptives, paraldehyde, phenytoin, primidone, rifampin, vitamin C, vitamin K	⇩ Prothrombin-time response
Alcohol, chloral hydrate, diuretics	⇧ or ⇩ Prothrombin-time response
Alkylating agents, antimetabolites, corticosteroids, dipyridamole, indomethacin, oxyphenbutazone, phenylbutazone, quinidine, salicylates, streptokinase, sulfinpyrazone, urokinase	⇧ Risk of bleeding

Table continued on following page

COUMADIN continued

DRUG INTERACTIONS continued

Chlorpropamide, tolbutamide	⇧ Hypoglycemic effect
Phenobarbital, phenytoin	⇧ Anticonvulsant blood level and/or toxicity

ALTERED LABORATORY VALUES

Blood/serum values	⇧ Prothrombin time

No clinically significant alterations in urinary values occur at therapeutic dosages

Use in children

General guidelines not established

Use in pregnancy or nursing mothers

Contraindicated during pregnancy, as use may cause congenital malformations or fatal fetal hemorrhage; patients who become pregnant while taking warfarin should be apprised of the potential risks to the fetus, and the possibility of terminating the pregnancy should be discussed. Use in nursing mothers may cause a prothrombinopenic state in the nursing infant.

Note: Warfarin sodium also marketed as **PANWARFIN** (Abbott); warfarin potassium marketed as **ARTHROMBIN-K** (Purdue Frederick)

HEPARIN SODIUM various manufacturers

Amps: 1,000 units/ml (1, 5 ml), 5,000 units/ml (1 ml), 10,000 units/ml (1 ml) **Vials:** 1,000 units/ml (1, 2, 10, 30 ml), 5,000 units/ml (1, 5, 10 ml), 10,000 units/ml (1, 4, 5, 10 ml), 20,000 units/ml (1, 2, 5, 10 ml), 40,000 units/ml (1, 2, 4, 5 ml) **Syringes:** 1,000 units/ml (1 ml), 5,000 units/ml (1 ml), 7,500 units/ml (1 ml), 10,000 units/ml (1 ml), 20,000 units/ml (1 ml) **Cartridge-needle units:** 1,000 units/ml (1 ml), 2,500 units/ml (1 ml), 5,000 units/ml (1 ml), 7,500 units/ml (1 ml), 10,000 units/ml (1 ml), 15,000 units/ml (1 ml), 20,000 units/ml (1 ml)

INDICATIONS	PARENTERAL DOSAGE
Venous thrombosis **Atrial fibrillation with embolism** **Pulmonary embolism** Acute and chronic **consumption coagulopathies** (disseminated intravascular coagulation) Prevention of **cerebral thrombosis** in evolving stroke **Coronary occlusion with acute myocardial infarction** (adjunctive therapy) **Peripheral arterial embolism** (adjunctive therapy)	**Adult:** 5,000 units (undiluted) IV followed by 10,000–20,000 units of concentrated solution SC (deeply) to start, followed by 8,000–10,000 units of concentrated solution SC (deeply) q8h or 15,000–20,000 units q12h; for intermittent IV injection, 10,000 units (undiluted or in 50–100 ml of isotonic NaCl) IV to start, followed by 5,000–10,000 units (undiluted or in 50–100 ml of isotonic NaCl) IV q4–6h; for continuous IV infusion, 5,000 units (undiluted) IV to start, followed by 20,000–40,000 units (in 1 liter of isotonic NaCl)/24 h
Prevention of postoperative deep venous thrombosis and pulmonary embolism	**Adult:** 5,000 units (undiluted) by deep SC injection 2 h before surgery, followed by 5,000 units q8–12h for 7 days or until patient is fully ambulatory, whichever is longer
Prevention of clotting in arterial and heart surgery	**Adult:** not less than 150 units/kg to start; for procedures lasting <60 min, 300 units/kg; for procedures lasting >60 min, 400 units/kg

ADMINISTRATION/DOSAGE ADJUSTMENTS

As an anticoagulant in extracorporeal dialysis	Follow equipment manufacturer's operating directions carefully
As an anticoagulant in blood transfusions	Add 400–600 units to each 100 ml of whole blood; usually, 7,500 units of heparin is first added to 100 ml of Sterile Sodium Chloride Injection, and then 6–8 ml of this solution is added to 100 ml of whole blood
As an anticoagulant in blood samples for laboratory purposes	Add 70–150 units to 10–20 ml of whole blood; WBC counts should be performed within 2 h of adding heparin. Heparinized blood should not be used for isoagglutinin, complement, or erythrocyte fragility tests or for platelet counts.
Selection of patients for low-dose prophylaxis of postoperative thromboembolism	Reserve for patients over 40 yr of age undergoing major surgery. Exclude patients with bleeding disorders, those having neurosurgery, spinal anesthesia, eye surgery, or potentially sanguinous operations, as well as patients receiving oral anticoagulants or drugs that interfere with platelet aggregation (see WARNINGS/PRECAUTIONS and DRUG INTERACTIONS).
Blood coagulation tests	Regulate dosage by frequent testing. During 1st day of treatment, determine clotting time just prior to each injection. Dosage is considered adequate when clotting time is 2½–3 times the control value. When using continuous IV infusion, perform coagulation tests q4h during early stages of therapy. When using intermittent IV or SC injections, perform coagulation tests before each injection during the early stages of therapy and daily thereafter. In patients with normal coagulation parameters, there is usually no need for daily monitoring of *low-dose* heparin therapy.
Concomitant use of coumarin anticoagulants	Since heparin may prolong the one-stage prothrombin time, wait at least 5 h after the last IV dose or 24 h after the last SC dose before drawing blood, in order to obtain valid prothrombin times

CONTRAINDICATIONS

When suitable blood coagulation tests cannot be performed at required intervals●

Hypersensitivity to heparin●

Uncontrollable bleeding●

Table continued on following page

HEPARIN SODIUM continued

WARNINGS/PRECAUTIONS	
Increased risk of bleeding and hemorrhage	Use with caution in patients with subacute bacterial endocarditis, arterial sclerosis, increased capillary permeability, hemophilia, some purpuras, thrombocytopenia, or inaccessible ulcerative lesions of the GI tract; during continuous tube drainage of the stomach or small intestine; and during and immediately after a spinal tap, spinal anesthesia, or major surgery (especially involving the brain, spinal cord, or eye)
Unduly prolonged coagulation tests or hemorrhage	Discontinue anticoagulation therapy promptly (see OVERDOSAGE); significant GI- or urinary-tract bleeding may indicate the presence of an underlying occult lesion
Antiplatelet therapy	Bleeding may occur with concomitant use of drugs, such as acetylsalicylic acid, that interfere with platelet-aggregation reactions (see DRUG INTERACTIONS); use with caution in patients receiving heparin
Febrile state	Increased doses of heparin may be required
Special-risk patients	Use with caution in patients with mild hepatic or renal disease, hypertension, or indwelling catheters, as well as during menstruation and in women over 60 yr of age
Hypersensitive patients	If feasible, administer a trial dose of 1,000 units before giving a therapeutic dose to a patient with a history of allergy
Acute adrenal hemorrhage or insufficiency	Discontinue anticoagulant therapy; measure plasma cortisol levels immediately and promptly institute vigorous IV corticosteroid therapy. Do not delay treatment for laboratory confirmation of diagnosis, as death may result.
Vasospastic reactions	May develop 6–10 days after initiating therapy, causing pain, ischemia, and cyanosis in the affected limb which may last 4–6 h. After repeated injection, the reaction may become generalized, with cyanosis, tachypnea, a feeling of oppression, and headache. Chest pain, increased blood pressure, arthralgias, and/or headache may also occur in the absence of definite peripheral vasospasm. Protamine has no effect on the reaction.
ADVERSE REACTIONS	
Hematological	Bleeding, overly prolonged bleeding time, hemorrhage, acute reversible thrombocytopenia (with IV use), vasospasm
Hypersensitivity	Chills, fever, urticaria, asthma, rhinitis, lacrimation, anaphylactoid reactions, anaphylactic shock (following IV injection; rare)
Metabolic	Osteoporosis (with long-term, high-dose therapy), rebound hyperlipemia upon discontinuation of heparin therapy
Genitourinary	Suppression of renal function (with long-term, high-dose therapy), priapism
Other	Local irritation, mild pain, or hematoma at injection site (frequently with IM injection, less often with deep SC administration), histamine-like reactions at injection site, suppression of aldosterone secretion, delayed transient alopecia
OVERDOSAGE	
Signs and symptoms	See ADVERSE REACTIONS
Treatment	Administer 1.0–1.5 mg of 1% protamine sulfate by slow infusion for every 100 units of heparin to be neutralized (30 min after a dose of heparin, ~0.5 mg of protamine is usually sufficient to neutralize 100 units of heparin). No more than 50 mg should be given very slowly in any 10-min period. Blood or plasma transfusions may be necessary; such transfusions dilute but do not neutralize heparin.
DRUG INTERACTIONS	
Acetylsalicylic acid (aspirin), coumarin anticoagulants, dextran, dipyramidole, hydroxychloroquine, ibuprofen, indomethacin, oxyphenbutazone, phenylbutazone, streptokinase, sulfinpyrazone, urokinase	⇧ Risk of bleeding and hemorrhage
Corticotropin, ethacrynic acid, glucocorticoids, mefenamic acid, nonsteroidal anti-inflammatory agents	⇧ Risk of GI bleeding and hemorrhage
Antihistamines, digitalis, nicotine, tetracyclines	⇩ Anticoagulant effect

Table continued on following page

HEPARIN SODIUM continued

ALTERED LABORATORY VALUES

Blood/serum values — ⇧ Whole-blood clotting time ⇧ Activated partial thromboplastin time ⇧ Prothrombin time ⇧ Thyroxine (T_4) ⇧ Triiodothyronine (T_3) uptake False-positive BSP tests ⇩ Cholesterol (with doses of 15,000–20,000 units)

No clinically significant alterations in urinary values occur at therapeutic dosages

Use in children

General guidelines not established

Use in pregnancy or nursing mothers

Increases the risk of maternal hemorrhage; use with caution during pregnancy, especially during the last trimester and immediately postpartum. Heparin sodium does not cross the placental barrier. It is not excreted in human breast milk.

STREPTASE (Streptokinase) Hoechst-Roussel

Vial: 250,000, 750,000 IU

INDICATIONS	PARENTERAL DOSAGE
Pulmonary embolism	**Adult:** 250,000 IU by IV infusion over 30 min to start, followed by 100,000 IU/h for 24 h (up to 72 h if concurrent deep vein thrombosis is suspected)
Deep vein thrombosis	**Adult:** 250,000 IU by IV infusion over 30 min to start, followed by 100,000 IU/h for 72 h
Arterial thrombosis or embolism	**Adult:** 250,000 IU by IV infusion over 30 min to start, followed by 100,000 IU/h for 24–72 h
Arteriovenous cannula occlusion	**Adult:** 250,000 IU by slow instillation in 2 ml IV solution into each occluded limb of cannula; after clamping off cannula limb(s) for 2 h, aspirate contents, flush with saline, and reconnect cannula

ADMINISTRATION/DOSAGE ADJUSTMENTS

Reconstitution and dilution	To minimize flocculation, slowly add 5 ml sodium chloride to vial; gently roll and tilt vial to reconstitute. Avoid shaking. Dilute contents to a total volume of 45 ml. If necessary, total volume may be increased, in increments of 45 ml, to a maximum of 180 ml, with pump infusion setting increased accordingly.
Pretreatment monitoring	Obtain thrombin time (TT), activated partial thromboplastin time (APTT), prothrombin time (PT), hematocrit, and platelet count; if heparin has been given, it should be discontinued and the TT or APTT should be less than twice the normal control value before starting streptokinase
Excessive resistance to streptokinase	If after 4 h of therapy, thrombin time or other parameter of lysis is $< 1\frac{1}{2}$ times normal control value, discontinue therapy
Posttreatment anticoagulation	To prevent recurrent thrombosis, administer heparin by continuous IV infusion when thrombin time has decreased to less than twice the normal control value; follow with oral anticoagulation
Pretreatment of arteriovenous cannula occlusion	Attempt to clear the cannula by careful syringe technique, using heparinized saline solution; if adequate flow is not re-established, streptokinase may be employed. Allow the effect of pretreatment anticoagulants to diminish.

CONTRAINDICATIONS

Active internal bleeding●

Intracranial neoplasm●

Recent (within 2 mo) cerebrovascular accident, or intracranial or intraspinal surgery●

WARNINGS/PRECAUTIONS

Minor bleeding	May occur, particularly at injection sites; avoid IM injections and nonessential handling of patient. Perform venipunctures carefully and as infrequently as possible. If arterial puncture is necessary, upper extremity vessels are preferable; apply pressure for at least 30 min, then a pressure dressing. Frequently check puncture site for evidence of bleeding.
Special-risk patients	Use with extreme caution in patients with severe uncontrolled arterial hypertension, high likelihood of left heart thrombosis (eg, mitral stenosis with atrial fibrillation), subacute bacterial endocarditis, hemostatic defects including those secondary to severe hepatic or renal disease, cerebrovascular disease, diabetic hemorrhagic retinopathy, prior severe allergic reaction to streptokinase, septic thrombophlebitis or occluded AV cannula at seriously infected site, or any condition in which bleeding constitutes a significant hazard or would be difficult to manage because of its location; and in those who have recently had major surgery (within 10 days), obstetrical delivery, organ biopsy, previous puncture of noncompressible vessels, serious GI bleeding (within 10 days), or trauma, including cardiopulmonary resuscitation
Serious uncontrollable bleeding	May occur; discontinue use and institute appropriate measures (see OVERDOSAGE)
Concomitant use of anticoagulants	Not recommended (see ADMINISTRATION/DOSAGE ADJUSTMENTS)

Table continued on following page

STREPTASE continued

ADVERSE REACTIONS

Hematological	Minor bleeding; severe gastrointestinal, genitourinary, retroperitoneal, cerebral, or other internal hemorrhage (sometimes fatal)
Allergic	Minor breathing difficulty, bronchospasm, periorbital swelling, angioneurotic edema, urticaria, itching, flushing, nausea, headache, musculoskeletal pain

OVERDOSAGE

Signs and symptoms	See ADVERSE REACTIONS
Treatment	For uncontrollable bleeding, discontinue streptokinase and administer whole blood (preferably fresh), packed red blood cells, and cryoprecipitate or fresh frozen plasma; consider use of aminocaproic acid in emergency situations. For mild to moderate allergic reactions, administer concomitant antihistamine and/or corticosteriod therapy. For severe allergic reactions, discontinue streptokinase and administer adrenergics, antihistamines, or corticosteroids IV, as required.

DRUG INTERACTIONS

Aspirin, indomethacin, phenylbutazone	⇧ Risk of bleeding
Anticoagulants	⇧ Risk of bleeding

ALTERED LABORATORY VALUES

Blood/serum values	⇧ Thrombin time ⇧ Activated partial thromboplastin time ⇧ Prothrombin time ⇧ FDP

No clinically significant alterations in urinary values occur at therapeutic dosages

Use in children	**Use in pregnancy or nursing mothers**
Safety and effectiveness not established	Safety and effectiveness not established during pregnancy; general guidelines not established for use in nursing mothers

Peripheral Circulatory Disorders

In less than a minute, the nearly six quarts of blood in the human body make a complete circuit through a vascular network of more than 60,000 miles. In times of good health, most people are rarely aware of this vital process in which the blood carries oxygen and nutrients to all the body's cells and transports waste products away from them. However, the circulatory system is vulnerable to various disorders involving the heart, blood pressure, clotting abnormalities, the deterioration of the blood vessels themselves, injury, and other factors.

In this section, the causes and treatment of peripheral vascular disease—particularly disorders affecting the blood vessels of the extremities—will be discussed. Other vascular disorders, such as transient ischemic attack and thromboembolism, are discussed in the section on *Clotting Disorders*.

TYPES OF PERIPHERAL VASCULAR DISEASES

In general, peripheral vascular disorders are characterized—depending upon the site of circulatory disturbance—by sensitivity to cold, especially in the hands and feet; leg cramps, usually in the calf muscles during sleep; unusual fatigue from standing or walking; and occasional pain and spasms severe enough to interfere with walking. While rest usually relieves this latter symptom, which is known as intermittent claudication (after the Latin verb *claudicare*, to limp), it should not be ignored—without proper diagnosis and treatment, it is likely to become more severe and limiting.

Arteriosclerosis Obliterans

This condition, also called peripheral arteriosclerosis, is caused by the hardening and narrowing of the arterial walls (arteriosclerosis) in the leg so that the resulting diminished blood supply leads to muscular stiffness, shooting pain, and varying degrees of impaired function.

As arterial channels become progressively narrowed, even moderate use may bring on muscle fatigue. Many persons experience night leg cramps severe enough to disrupt sleep. In this disorder, the feet and toes are especially sensitive to cold, and their appearance may alternate between abnormal pallor and purplish discoloration. Because the skin of the affected parts is deprived of essential nourishment, it becomes shiny and thin, and, in more severe cases, it may ulcerate. Hemorrhages of the diseased arteries are not uncommon.

Diabetics are especially vulnerable to this form of arteriosclerosis. It is also associated with obesity, sedentary life-style, and high blood cholesterol.

Treatment is directed towards relief of symptoms and includes a regimen of exercise and suitable diet, plus vasodilator medications. These drugs dilate the blood vessels, thus increasing the supply of oxygen and other essential nutrients to the affected areas. In some cases, such as the possibility of gangrene, surgery may be considered necessary. The operation consists of resectioning (grafting) portions of the arterial system to channel the blood through healthier vessels.

The choice of clothing is also important in controlling arteriosclerosis obliterans. Constricting girdles or garters that interfere with circulation to the lower legs should be avoided. The same applies to elasticized knee socks or anklets. Tight shoes that cramp the toes should be discarded in favor of footwear wide enough to permit unimpeded circulation.

Buerger's Disease

Thromboangiitis obliterans, more commonly called Buerger's disease, is an inflammation of the blood vessels resulting in a thrombosis, or clotting that impairs or blocks circulation. It typically affects the smaller arteries and veins of the lower leg, and if not arrested promptly, presents the threat of gangrene.

Buerger's disease is directly related to nicotine sensitivity—it occurs most commonly in heavy smokers, especially men under thirty-five, and discontinuation of the smoking results in abatement of symptoms. It is rarely seen in women or nonsmokers.

In a typical case, the first manifestations occur soon after walking or other physical activity involving the legs. A tingling sensation, followed by coldness and numbness in the affected area, may precede the onset of acute pain. If the thrombosis continues to obstruct the arterial channels, ulceration occurs, followed by tissue death (gangrene). In severe cases, amputation of the gangrenous area may be necessary.

Therapy in the early stages of Buerger's disease—in addition to cessation of smoking—involves taking medications, such as nylidrin hydrochloride (Arlidin) or isoxsuprine hydrochloride (Vasodilan), which act as vasodilators. Nicotinic acid in the form of niacin tablets may also be prescribed for its vasodilating effect. Anticoagulant drugs may be used to halt the progress of thrombosis. As always, careful supervision of drug combinations must be observed when using these medications.

Raynaud's Disease
Another relatively common vascular disorder is Raynaud's disease, which is characterized by arterial spasm in the fingers and toes. The affected parts become cyanotic (bluish), cold, and then numb and white as a result of deprivation of oxygenated blood.

Raynaud's disease is more common in women than men, especially those past the age of forty. It may be triggered by exposure to extreme cold, emotional stress, or, in some cases, it may be an inherited tendency. Nicotine sensitivity also may be a factor, and in some persons, the phenomenon is a complication of a neurological or endocrine disease, rheumatoid arthritis, scleroderma, general circulatory deterioration, or constant jarring or trauma to the fingertips.

Occasionally the arterial spasms are chronic, lasting a half hour or more, and lead to thrombosis or superficial ulceration and severe pain of the affected area. Attacks often can be averted by avoiding exposure to cold or other precipitating circumstances, such as stressful situations. Patients with Raynaud's disease also are advised not to smoke. Treatment with vasodilator medications is usually effective. In the rare cases of severe, frequent, and long-lasting spasms that are unresponsive to drug therapy, surgery may be considered. The operation involves removal of the nervous system ganglia that serve the affected blood vessels.

Varicose Veins
Varicose veins are vessels that become swollen, ropy, and distended. The veins of the leg are the most commonly afflicted, and because they are likely to bulge out, they are vulnerable to bleeding, ulceration, and infection.

Varicose veins are caused by a failure of the valves within the veins to prevent the back flow of blood, leading to sluggish flow or pooling of blood in the veins. The legs are particularly vulnerable because the veins must overcome the pull of gravity in returning the blood to the heart. Early symptoms are leg cramps, fatigue, and in some cases, swollen ankles. The tendency may be inherited, and it is especially prevalent among people who sit or stand in one position for extended periods—for example, barbers, dentists, salespersons, typists, etc. Pregnancy and obesity are also contributing factors.

Mild cases can be arrested through a regimen of rest with the legs elevated, exercise, frequent changes in position and posture, and the use of lightly elasticized stockings or elastic bandages. In more troublesome cases, injections of a solution of sodium tetradecyl into the diseased vessels may be recommended. This causes a "withering away" of the treated veins so that circulation can be rechanneled into healthier ones. Surgical removal of the varicose veins is another approach, but this is usually reserved for the more severe or disabling cases. If ulcers develop, bed rest with the legs elevated may be necessary to promote healing. Saline dressing may be helpful.

Chilblains
As their name implies, chilblains are associated with exposure to cold and are characterized by congestion and swelling, accompanied by severe itching and/or burning sensations. The ears, face, hands, and feet are usually affected. In severe cases, blisters may develop that turn into painful sores.

Chilblains may be a recurrent problem, especially among the aged. They are most likely to occur in persons with impaired circulation. Treatment consists of avoiding exposure to the cold, exercise to improve circulation, and, in some instances, the prescribing of vasodilator medications.

USE OF VASODILATORS IN PERIPHERAL VASCULAR DISEASE

As noted earlier, vasodilators act by dilating the blood vessels, thus increasing blood flow. In addition to the disorders described in this section, vasodilating agents also are prescribed to treat the circulatory disturbances of the inner ear that cause tinnitus, vertigo, or the combination of symptoms called Meniere's syndrome.

One of the major effects of vasodilating drugs is a lowering of blood pressure that may lead to postural or orthostatic hypotension. This results in dizziness or, more rarely, fainting when getting up suddenly from a sitting position, or when getting out of bed immediately after waking up. The simplest countermeasure is to change postures slowly, or to sit on the edge of the bed for a few moments before standing upright and walking. If these corrective measures are ineffective, a doctor should be consulted about whether a change in dosage or medication may be indicated.

Vasodilators should be used with caution, if at all, in patients with glaucoma, diabetes, heart disease, and bleeding disorders. Some persons experience dermatological sensitivity to these drugs, and gastrointestinal effects also may occur. An added caution: the routine use of alcoholic beverages to "warm up" or increase circulatory flow to the extremities is not recommended, especially if the patient is taking drugs for any other condition. It has been estimated that alcohol interacts with at least one ingredient in about half of all drugs.

IN CONCLUSION
The following drug charts cover the drugs most commonly prescribed to treat peripheral vascular disorders affecting the extremities. Some are also prescribed to treat circulatory disturbances of the inner ear, and others such as dihydrogenated ergot alkaloids (Hydergine) are sometimes recommended to treat early symptoms of senile dementia. It should be noted that no cure for true senility has as yet been developed, and any beneficial effect of these drugs is limited to ameliorating symptoms in some patients in the early stages of mental deterioration. It also should be noted that most senile dementia is not caused by reduced blood flow to the brain.

ARLIDIN (Nylidrin hydrochloride) USV

Tabs: 6, 12 mg

INDICATIONS	ORAL DOSAGE
Peripheral vascular disease, including arteriosclerosis obliterans, thromboangiitis obliterans, diabetic vascular disease, nocturnal leg cramps, Raynaud's phenomenon and disease, ischemic ulcer, frostbite, acrocyanosis, acroparesthesia, thrombophlebitis, and cold feet, legs, and hands[1] **Circulatory disturbances of the inner ear,** including primary cochlear cell ischemia, cochlear stria vascular ischemia, macular or ampullar ischemia, other disturbances due to labyrinthine-artery spasm or obstruction[1]	**Adult:** 3-12 mg tid or qid

CONTRAINDICATIONS

Acute myocardial infarction●	Progressive angina pectoris●
Paroxysmal tachycardia●	Thyrotoxicosis●

WARNINGS/PRECAUTIONS

Cardiac disease	Use with caution in patients with tachyarrhythmias and uncompensated congestive heart failure

ADVERSE REACTIONS

Central nervous system	Trembling, nervousness, weakness, dizziness (not associated with labyrinthine-artery insufficiency)
Cardiovascular	Palpitations, postural hypotension
Gastrointestinal	Nausea, vomiting

OVERDOSAGE

Toxicity of nylidrin in humans has not been characterized

DRUG INTERACTIONS

No clinically significant drug interactions have been observed

ALTERED LABORATORY VALUES

No clinically significant alterations in blood/serum or urinary values occur at therapeutic dosages

Use in children	Use in pregnancy or nursing mothers
General guidelines not established	General guidelines not established

[1]Possibly effective

CYCLOSPASMOL (Cyclandelate) Ives

Tabs: 100 mg **Caps:** 200, 400 mg

INDICATIONS	ORAL DOSAGE
Intermittent claudication (adjunctive therapy)[1] **Arteriosclerosis obliterans**[1] **Thrombophlebitis**[1] **Nocturnal leg cramps**[1] **Raynaud's phenomenon**[1] **Ischemic cerebral vascular disease** (selected cases)[1]	**Adult:** 1200–1600 mg/day div before meals and at bedtime to start, followed by 400–800 mg/day in 2–4 divided doses

ADMINISTRATION/DOSAGE ADJUSTMENTS

Maintenance therapy — Improvement may be gradual, taking several weeks at initial dose level. When clinical response is noted, reduce dosage in 200-mg decrements until maintenance dosage is reached (see ORAL DOSAGE).

CONTRAINDICATIONS

Hypersensitivity to cyclandelate

WARNINGS/PRECAUTIONS

Severe, obliterative coronary-artery or cerebrovascular disease — Diseased areas may be compromised by vasodilation elsewhere in the body

Active bleeding or bleeding tendency — Prolongation of bleeding time has been demonstrated in animals at very large doses

Glaucoma — Use with caution

ADVERSE REACTIONS

Gastrointestinal — Distress (pyrosis, pain, eructation)[2]

Cardiovascular — Tachycardia

Central nervous system — Weakness, headache

Dermatological — Mild flushing

OVERDOSAGE

Toxicity of cyclandelate in humans has not been characterized

DRUG INTERACTIONS

No clinically significant drug interactions have been observed

ALTERED LABORATORY VALUES

No clinically significant alterations in blood/serum or urinary values occur at therapeutic dosages

Use in children

General guidelines not established

Use in pregnancy or nursing mothers

Safe use not established in pregnancy or nursing mothers; use only if essential

[1]Possibly effective
[2]May be relieved by taking drug with meals or by concomitant use of antacids

HYDERGINE (Dihydrogenated ergot alkaloids) Sandoz

Tabs (oral): 1 mg, containing 0.333 mg dihydroergocornine mesylate, 0.333 mg dihydroergocristine mesylate, and 0.333 mg dihydroergocryptine mesylate **Tabs (sublingual):** 0.5 mg, containing 0.167 mg dihydroergocornine mesylate, 0.167 mg dihydroergocristine mesylate, and 0.167 mg dihydroergocryptine mesylate; or 1 mg, containing 0.333 mg dihydroergocornine mesylate, 0.333 mg dihydroergocristine mesylate, and 0.333 mg dihydroergocryptine mesylate

INDICATIONS	ORAL AND SUBLINGUAL DOSAGE
Poor self care, mood depression, unsociability, dizziness, and confusion in the elderly	**Adult:** 1 mg tid

ADMINISTRATION/DOSAGE ADJUSTMENTS

Therapeutic response — Alleviation of symptoms is gradual and may not be observed for 3–4 wk

CONTRAINDICATIONS

Hypersensitivity to components

WARNINGS/PRECAUTIONS

Symptoms of unknown etiology — Before initiating therapy, careful diagnosis must be made to rule out underlying organic disease

ADVERSE REACTIONS

Gastrointestinal — Transient nausea, gastric disturbances

Other — Sublingual irritation

OVERDOSAGE

Toxicity of dihydrogenated ergot alkaloids in humans has not been characterized

DRUG INTERACTIONS

No clinically significant drug interactions have been observed

ALTERED LABORATORY VALUES

No clinically significant alterations in blood/serum or urinary values occur at therapeutic dosages

Use in children	**Use in pregnancy or nursing mothers**
General guidelines not established	**General guidelines not established**

NICOTINIC ACID various manufacturers

Tabs: 25, 50, 100, 500 mg **Tabs (sust-rel):** 150 mg **Caps:** 500 mg **Caps (sust-rel):** 125, 200, 250, 300, 400, 500 mg
Elixir: 50 mg/5 ml **Amps:** 50 mg/ml (2 ml) **Vials:** 100 mg/ml (30 ml)

INDICATIONS	ORAL DOSAGE	PARENTERAL DOSAGE
Peripheral vascular insufficiency, including vascular spasm, peripheral arteriosclerosis, and Raynaud's disease **Prevention and treatment of pellagra** **Circulatory inner ear disturbances**	**Adult:** 150–500 mg/day divided into 3–10 doses; sust-rel caps: 400–800 mg bid or tid, or up to 6 g/day, if needed	**Adult:** 150–500 mg/day IM or IV (slowly) divided into 3–10 doses
Hypercholesterolemia and hyperbetalipoproteinemia (adjunctive therapy)	**Adult:** 1.5–6 g/day divided into 2–4 doses; sust-rel caps: 400 mg bid to start, followed by a gradual increase to 800 mg tid	—

CONTRAINDICATIONS

Severe hypotension● Arterial hemorrhage● Active peptic ulcer● Hepatic dysfunction●

WARNINGS/PRECAUTIONS

Orthostatic hypotension	May occur in hypertensive patients being treated with ganglionic blocking agents
Decreased glucose tolerance	Use with caution in diabetic patients
Hyperuricemia	Use with caution in patients predisposed to gout
Special-risk patients	Use with caution in patients with gallbladder disease or a past history of jaundice, liver disease, or peptic ulcer
Initiating hypolipidemic therapy	Attempt to control serum cholesterol by appropriate dietary measures, weight reduction, and treatment of any underlying disorder before initiating nicotinic acid therapy
Serum cholesterol and triglyceride levels	Should be determined prior to nicotinic acid therapy and regularly thereafter If no appreciable effect occurs after 1–2 mo of therapy, discontinue use of drug.
Gastrointestinal upset	Occurs frequently during initial phase of therapy; may be minimized by dividing and/or reducing daily dose or by giving the drug on a full stomach or with of antacids

ADVERSE REACTIONS

Frequent reactions are italicized

Gastrointestinal	*Nausea, bloating, flatulence, hunger pains, heartburn, cramps, diarrhea,* vomiting, xerostomia, activation of peptic ulcer
Hepatic	Abnormal liver-function tests, jaundice
Central nervous system	Transient headache; sensation of burning, stinging, or tingling of the skin
Ophthalmic	Blurred vision, toxic amblyopia, proptosis, loss of central vision cystoid macular edema
Cardiovascular	Hypotension, tachycardia, syncope, vasovagal attacks
Dermatological	*Warmth, severe generalized flushing, pruritus,* increased sebaceous gland activity, dry skin, rash, keratosis nigricans
Other	Brief activation of fibrinolysis, metallic taste, and anaphylaxis (with IV administration)

OVERDOSAGE

Signs and symptoms	See ADVERSE REACTIONS
Treatment	Discontinue use and provide symptomatic and supportive treatment, as needed

DRUG INTERACTIONS

Antihypertensive ganglionic blocking agents	⇧ Risk of orthostatic hypotension

ALTERED LABORATORY VALUES

Blood/serum values	⇧ Alkaline phosphatase ⇧ SGOT ⇧ SGPT ⇧ Lactate dehydrogenase ⇧ Uric acid ⇧ Bilirubin ⇧ Sulfobromophthalein (BSP) retention ⇧ Glucose ⇩ Albumin
Urinary values	⇧ Glucose ⇧ Catecholamines (with fluorometric methods)

Use in children

Safety and effectiveness of large doses of nicotinic acid in children have not been established

Use in pregnancy or nursing mothers

Safe use not established during pregnancy or in nursing mothers; administration of supplemental amounts of nicotinic acid during pregnancy and lactation has had no adverse effects

[1]Possibly effective

PAVABID (Papaverine hydrochloride) **Marion**

Caps (sust rel): 150 mg

PAVABID HP (Papaverine hydrochloride) **Marion**

Caps (sust rel): 300 mg

INDICATIONS

Cerebral and peripheral ischemia associated with arterial spasm
Myocardial ischemia complicated by arrhythmias

ORAL DOSAGE

Adult: 150 mg q12h

ADMINISTRATION/DOSAGE ADJUSTMENTS

Difficult cases	Increase dosage to 150–300 mg q8h or 300 mg q12h

CONTRAINDICATIONS

None

WARNINGS/PRECAUTIONS

Glaucoma	Use with caution
Hepatic hypersensitivity	Discontinue use if GI symptoms, jaundice, or eosinophilia occur, or if liver-function tests are altered

ADVERSE REACTIONS

Gastrointestinal	Nausea, abdominal distress, anorexia, constipation, diarrhea
Central nervous system	Drowsiness, vertigo, headache, malaise
Dermatological	Rash
Other	Diaphoresis

OVERDOSAGE

Toxicity of papaverine in humans has not been characterized

DRUG INTERACTIONS

No clinically significant drug interactions have been observed

ALTERED LABORATORY VALUES

No clinically significant alterations in blood/serum or urinary values occur at therapeutic dosages

Use in children

General guidelines not established

Use in pregnancy or nursing mothers

General guidelines not established

VASODILAN (Isoxsuprine hydrochloride) Mead Johnson

Tabs: 10, 20 mg **Amps:** 5 mg/ml (2 ml) for IM use only

INDICATIONS	ORAL DOSAGE	PARENTERAL DOSAGE
Cerebral vascular insufficiency[1] **Arteriosclerosis obliterans**[1] **Thromboangiitis obliterans** (Buerger's disease)[1] **Raynaud's disease**[1]	**Adult:** 10–20 mg tid or qid	**Adult:** 5–10 mg IM bid or tid

CONTRAINDICATIONS

Arterial bleeding ● Hypotension (parenteral use only) ● Tachycardia (parenteral use only) ●

WARNINGS/PRECAUTIONS

Intravenous administration — Increases risk of side effects and is not recommended

Hypotension, tachycardia — May be produced by 10-mg doses IM; do not exceed recommended dosages

ADVERSE REACTIONS

Cardiovascular — **Hypotension, tachycardia (with IM use)**

Gastrointestinal — Nausea, vomiting, abdominal distress

Central nervous system — Dizziness

Dermatological — Severe rash[2]

OVERDOSAGE

Toxicity of isoxsuprine in humans has not been characterized

DRUG INTERACTIONS

No clinically significant drug interactions have been observed

ALTERED LABORATORY VALUES

No clinically significant alterations in blood/serum or urinary values occur at therapeutic dosages

Use in children

General guidelines not established

Use in pregnancy or nursing mothers

General guidelines not established for use during pregnancy or in nursing mothers; contraindicated during immediate postpartum period

[1]Possibly effective
[2]Discontinue therapy

Eye, Ear, and Mouth Disorders

Eye Diseases

The eye, although generally thought of as a distinct organ in itself, is actually in part an external extension of the brain. As the fetal brain develops, the eyes are formed from an elongated prominence known as the optic vesicle. The stalk-like portion of this vesicle eventually becomes the optic nerve, which is a tract of the brain rather than an actual nerve, while the ball-like ends become the eye globes.

The eye is a compact, extremely complex structure that has three layers and three fluid-filled compartments (see illustration). The outer layer is composed of the cornea, the clear "window of the eye," and the sclera, the white portion. The center layer is made up of the choroid, which contains blood vessels; the iris, which gives the eye its color; and the pupil, the opening that admits the light. The inner layer contains the retina, the thin sheet of tissue that is analogous to the film in a camera. The light rays fall upon the retina, and are projected into an image transmitted to the nerve endings in the retina. This image is relayed to the back of the brain, where it is interpreted.

Each eye is held in place by six muscles, which must work in concert if the eyes are to perceive a single image rather than seeing double.

THE EYE AS A DIAGNOSTIC TOOL

Examination of the eye is an important part of any routine checkup, not only to detect disorders of the eye itself, but also to look for symptoms of other diseases. Since the eye is an extension of the brain, and also the only place where a physician can view exposed blood vessels, it is often the first place where signs of disease are readily apparent. For example, diabetes, high blood pressure, leukemia, glaucoma, and certain types of tumors all produce characteristic changes in the blood vessels of the fundus (the back of the eyeball). Obviously, further tests and examinations are needed to confirm the presence of any of these diseases, but this is one reason why physicians carefully examine the eye with a bright light and magnifying mirrors during a routine checkup.

The eye itself is also vulnerable to a number of diseases, ranging from simple irritation to sight-threatening glaucoma and infections. This discussion will concentrate on the various types of glaucoma and their treatment and some of the more common eye infections.

GLAUCOMA

Glaucoma is a disease in which increased pressure within the eyeball causes blindness by gradually destroying the optic nerve. Ten to 20 percent of all blindness in the United States is caused by glaucoma. The disease occurs most frequently in persons over the age of fifty. Since glaucoma is asymptomatic in its early stages, it is important that everyone over the age of forty undergo periodic testing for glaucoma with a tonometer, a simple instrument that measures pressure within the eye (intraocular pressure). The rise in intraocular pressure is due to a buildup of the fluid known as aqueous humor, a normal component of the posterior chamber of the eye. There are two main ways in which a buildup of aqueous humor can occur, both involving obstruction of the angles or drainage channels for the aqueous humor.

Open-Angle Glaucoma

In open-angle glaucoma, also called chronic simple or noncongestive glaucoma, the obstruction is thought to be due to a primary abnormality of the outflow system.

Open-angle glaucoma is the more common form of the disease. It progresses gradually, and although early symptoms include blurred vision and the presence of colored haloes around lights, a person may not notice any visual impairment until a major part of the field of vision is lost.

The use of one or more drugs is the usual treatment of open-angle glaucoma, with surgery contemplated only if pressure in the eye remains high despite drug therapy. The following drugs or classes of drugs are those used most often in treating open-angle glaucoma:

Miotics The miotics cause the pupil to constrict and the ciliary muscle to contract, which is thought

THE EYE

Anterior chamber (containing aqueous fluid)
Lens
Iris
Cornea
Posterior chamber
Ciliary body
Suspensory ligament
Conjunctiva
Ciliary process
Lateral rectus muscle
Sclera
Medial rectus muscle
Lateral rectus muscle
Choroid
Vitreous
Retina
Optic nerve
Central retinal artery and veins

PATHOGENESIS OF CATARACTS

The normal lens of the eye is transparent. As a cataract starts to develop, the lens or its capsule (or both) begin to lose their transparency, eventually becoming opaque, with resultant loss of vision. As long as the iris shadow is visible through the lens, the cataract is considered immature. When it is no longer visible, the cataract is "ripe" and operable.

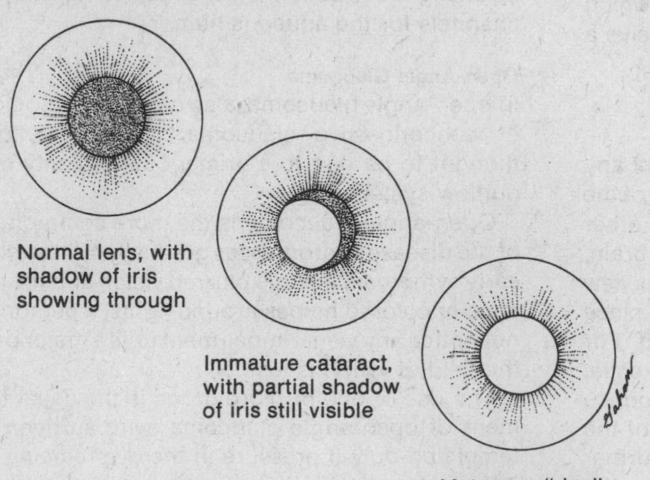

Normal lens, with shadow of iris showing through

Immature cataract, with partial shadow of iris still visible

Mature or "ripe" cataract, now in operable stage

GLAUCOMA

The normal round shape of the eye is maintained by steady pressure within its chambers, due to an equal inflow and outflow of aqueous fluid. If this balance is disrupted, aqueous fluid may be retained in one of the chambers, most commonly the anterior (open-angle glaucoma), but sometimes in the posterior chamber (closed-angle glaucoma).

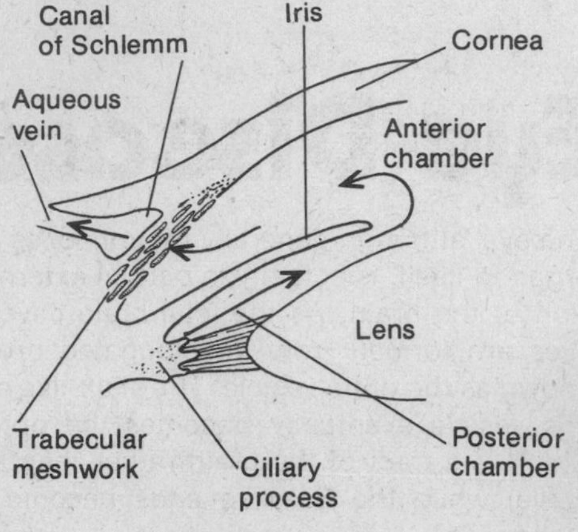

Open-Angle Glaucoma

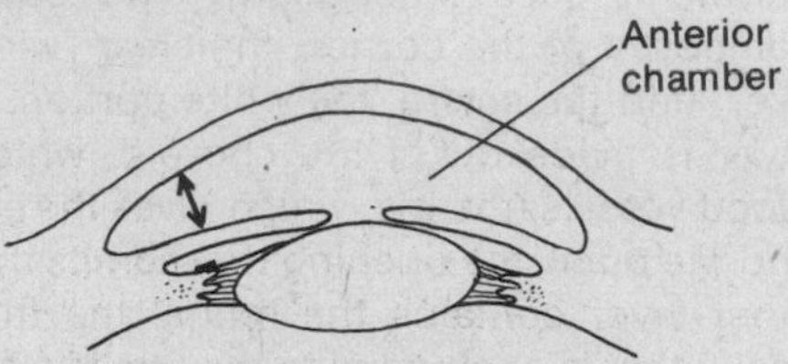

Fluid is retained in the anterior chamber, exerting pressure on the iris and flattening it. The cornea is also pressed outward.

Closed-Angle Glaucoma

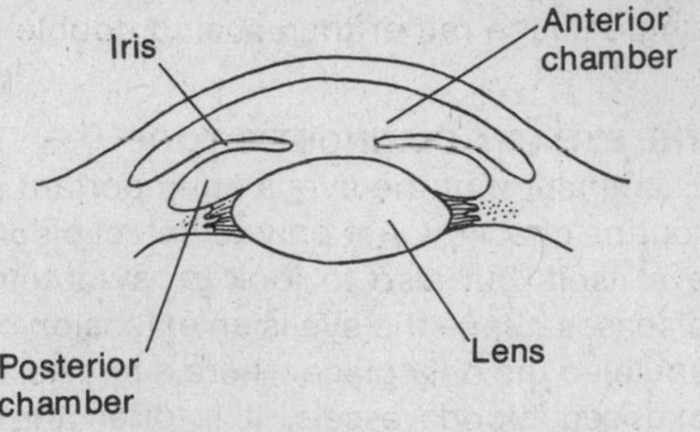

The anterior chamber is narrowed due to retention of aqueous fluid in posterior chamber, pushing iris forward.

If unchecked, blood vessel destruction will occur, leading to damage of the optic nerve and eventual blindness.

to decrease the intraocular pressure by facilitating the outflow of the aqueous humor.

Since the pupil is made to constrict by the nerve transmitter acetylcholine, there are two types of miotic agents. One reinforces the action of acetylcholine and the other inhibits the breakdown of this chemical, thereby prolonging its action. Drugs that reinforce the acetylcholine transmitter include pilocarpine (Isopto-Carpine, Pilocar, and other brands) and carbachol (Carbacel or Isopto Carbachol).

Drugs that inhibit the breakdown of acetylcholine include physostigmine (Isopto Eserine) and other, longer-acting compounds. These drugs are not often used because of the frequency of allergic-like reactions and the potential for causing cataracts.

Epinephrine Epinephrine, an adrenergic drug, acts by decreasing resistance to outflow of the aqueous humor, as well as reducing secretion of this fluid. It is sometimes used in conjunction with a miotic agent to gain an additive effect in reducing intraocular pressure, because epinephrine stimulates a different set of nerves. Drugs in this category include Epitrate, Epifrin, and Eppy.

Timolol maleate In 1978, the Food and Drug Administration approved the introduction of timolol maleate (Timoptic), the first new drug for use against glaucoma to be developed in twenty-five years. This drug, a beta-adrenergic blocking agent, represents a new approach to glaucoma therapy. It acts primarily to decrease the production of aqueous humor by a mechanism different from that of epinephrine. In addition, timolol is longer-acting than most other anti-glaucoma agents. It causes few side effects, and many physicians now prescribe it as the initial drug in treating uncomplicated glaucoma. Since it is absorbed into the bloodstream, however, timolol should be used with caution in patients with heart disease or asthma, as well as those who are already taking a beta-blocking agent, such as propranolol (Inderal).

Carbonic anhydrase inhibitors These drugs are usually used for long-term therapy. A major drug in this category is acetazolamide (Diamox). The carbonic anhydrase inhibitors were originally used as diuretics, but were found to lower intraocular pressure, probably by reducing aqueous fluid production.

Narrow-Angle Glaucoma

This type of glaucoma, also known as angle-closure, acute, or congestive glaucoma, is a very different condition. It results from a lens that is unusually far forward in the eye and raises pressure in the posterior chamber. This increased pressure pushes the iris toward the trabecular meshwork, which is essential in draining fluid from the eye interior. Emotional stress, drugs, or darkness may provoke dilation of the pupil, which then causes an acute blockage of the outflow tract. Such an acute attack is characterized by pain, very red eyes, headache, and loss of vision. This form of glaucoma is treated surgically, with drugs used temporarily before the operation.

EYE INFECTIONS

The eye frequently becomes infected with bacteria, fungi, or viruses. Conjunctivitis, bacterial infection of the lid or conjunctiva (the membrane lining the underside of the eyelid and the surface of the cornea) is common, but is usually not dangerous to sight. *Staphylococcus aureus,* for example, often causes sties, which are infections of the eyelid. Most of these infections clear up on their own, but topical antibiotics can hasten the healing process.

When bacteria such as *Staphylococcus* or *Pseudomonas* cause an ulcer on the cornea or grow within the eye, sight may be damaged. In these cases, antibiotics are necessary and are sometimes injected directly into the eye.

Fungal infections are found mostly in persons whose immune defenses are weakened from illness, drug therapy, or surgery, or who become more vulnerable because of another disease, such as diabetes. Long-term administration of corticosteroids can also make the eye more vulnerable to fungi. Many topical antifungal agents are available to treat these infections.

The most serious viral infection of the eye is herpes keratitis, an infection of the cornea by the herpes virus. If unchecked, this infection can damage the cornea and cause blindness. Two drugs, idoxuridine (Dendrid, Herplex, and Stoxil) and vidarabine (Vira-A) can control most cases of herpes keratitis.

MISCELLANEOUS EYE PREPARATIONS

The eye is vulnerable to strain, noninfectious conjunctivitis, and itching and redness due to allergy, and a number of nonprescription eyewashes and other preparations are available to relieve these minor irritations. Common ingredients in these preparations include zinc sulfate, boric acid, and antihistamines.

As noted earlier, a number of diseases, such as diabetes or high blood pressure, also affect the eye as well as other organs. Diabetes is particulary detrimental to the eye, and is a leading cause of blindness in the United States. Treatment of the underlying disease is the only known way to prevent serious ocular complications.

Still other eye disorders are not treated by drugs. Cataracts, a clouding of the crystalline lens or its capsule, is one of the most common disorders in this category. Surgery to remove the clouded lens is the major treatment of cataracts, and this approach is usually successful in restoring sight.

IN CONCLUSION

Many serious eye diseases, including glaucoma and most sight-threatening infections, can be effectively treated with drugs. The following charts cover the major agents used to treat these disorders. A representative selection of nonprescription eyewashes and other nonprescription preparations is also included.

DARANIDE (Dichlorphenamide) Merck Sharp & Dohme

Tabs: 50 mg

INDICATIONS

Chronic open-angle glaucoma (adjunctive therapy)
Secondary glaucoma (adjunctive therapy)
Preoperatively for **acute narrow-angle glaucoma** (adjunctive therapy)

ORAL DOSAGE

Adult: 100–200 mg to start, followed by 100 mg q12h until response is obtained; for maintenance, 25–50 mg qd, bid, or tid

ADMINISTRATIVE/DOSAGE ADJUSTMENTS

Combination therapy — Dichlorphenamide may be given with miotics such as isoflurophate, demecarium bromide, pilocarpine, physostigmine, or carbachol. For acute narrow-angle glaucoma, dichlorphenamide may be given concomitantly with miotics and osmotic agents.

CONTRAINDICATIONS

Hypersensitivity to dichlorphenamide●
Hyperchloremic acidosis●
Severe pulmonary obstruction with impaired alveolar ventilation●
Hyponatremia●
Renal failure●
Hepatic insufficiency●
Hypokalemia●
Adrenocortical insufficiency●

WARNINGS/PRECAUTIONS

Hypokalemia — May develop with brisk diuresis, concomitant corticosteroid or ACTH therapy, or interference with adequate oral electrolyte intake, or in presence of severe cirrhosis; avoid or treat with dietary potassium supplements. Hypokalemia can sensitize or exaggerate the response of the heart to the cardiotoxic effects of digitalis.

Special-risk patients — Use with caution in patients with severe respiratory acidosis

ADVERSE REACTIONS

Gastrointestinal — Anorexia, nausea, vomiting, constipation

Genitourinary — Renal colic, urinary frequency, renal calculi

Dermatological — Mild skin eruptions, pruritus

Hematological — Leukopenia, agranulocytosis, thrombocytopenia

Central nervous system and neuromuscular — Headache, weakness, nervousness, globus hystericus, sedation, lassitude, depression, confusion, disorientation, dizziness, ataxia, tremor, tinnitus, paresthesias of the hands, feet, and tongue

Other — Weight loss

OVERDOSAGE

Toxicity of dichlorphenamide in humans has not been characterized

DRUG INTERACTIONS

No clinically significant drug interactions have been reported

ALTERED LABORATORY VALUES

Blood/serum values — ⇩ Potassium ⇧ Uric acid

No clinically significant alterations in urinary values occur at therapeutic dosages

Use in children

General guidelines not established

Use in pregnancy or nursing mothers

Do not administer during pregnancy, especially during first trimester, unless essential. Teratogenic effects have been reported in rats given high doses, but have not been confirmed in man. General guidelines not established for use in nursing mothers.

DIAMOX (Acetazolamide) Lederle

Tabs: 125, 250 mg **Caps (sust rel):** 500 mg **Vial:** 500 mg

INDICATIONS	ORAL DOSAGE	PARENTERAL DOSAGE
Chronic open-angle glaucoma (adjunctive therapy)	**Adult:** 250 mg to 1 g/24 h (divide doses over 250 mg); sust-rel caps: 1 cap bid in AM and PM	—
Secondary glaucoma (adjunctive therapy)	**Adult:** 250 mg q4h; for short-term therapy, 250 mg bid may suffice; sust-rel caps: 1 cap bid in AM and PM	—
Preoperatively for **acute narrow-angle glaucoma**	**Adult:** 250 mg q4h, or 500 mg to start, followed by 125 or 250 mg q4h; sust-rel caps: 1 cap bid in AM and PM	**Adult:** for rapid relief, 250 mg q4h IV, or 500 mg IV to start, followed by 125 or 250 mg IV q4h
Centrencephalic epilepsy	**Adult:** 8–30 mg/kg/day div, up to 1 g/day; optimum range: 375–1,000 mg/day div **Child:** same as for adult	—
Edema associated with congestive heart failure (adjunctive therapy)	**Adult:** 250–375 mg (5 mg/kg) qd in AM to start, followed by 250–375 mg/day on alternate days or for 2 days on and 1 day off	—
Drug-induced edema	**Adult:** 250–375 mg qd on alternate days or for 2 days on and 1 day off	—

ADMINISTRATION/DOSAGE ADJUSTMENTS

Refractory congestive heart failure — Very high doses of acetazolamide may be given concomitantly with other diuretics to secure diuresis

Combination therapy for acute narrow-angle glaucoma — May be given with miotics or mydriatics, as needed

Combination anticonvulsant therapy — Give 250 mg qd in addition to existing medications to start, followed by gradual increases to dosage recommended above

CONTRAINDICATIONS

Hyponatremia●

Chronic, noncongestive narrow-angle glaucoma (prolonged therapy only)●

Hypokalemia●

Suprarenal gland failure●

Hypochloremic acidosis●

Marked kidney disease or dysfunction●

Marked liver disease or dysfunction●

WARNINGS/PRECAUTIONS

Excessive dosage — May decrease diuresis or cause drowsiness or paresthesias; do not exceed recommended dosage

Acidosis — May be precipitated or exacerbated in patients with impaired alveolar ventilation due to pulmonary obstruction or emphysema

Side effects — Discontinue drug and institute appropriate therapy if blood dyscrasias, renal complications, or hypersensitivity reactions occur (See ADVERSE REACTIONS)

ADVERSE REACTIONS[1]

Hematological — Bone marrow depression, thrombocytopenic purpura, hemolytic anemia, leukopenia, pancytopenia, agranulocytosis

Central nervous system and neuromuscular — Paresthesias, "tingling" sensation in extremities, drowsiness, confusion, flaccid paralysis, convulsions

Renal — Crystalluria, renal calculi, polyuria, hematuria, glycosuria

Dermatological — Rash, urticaria

Other — Fever, decreased appetite, acidosis (with long-term therapy), transient myopia, hepatic insufficiency, melena

OVERDOSAGE

Signs and symptoms — See ADVERSE REACTIONS

Treatment — Discontinue medication; treat symptomatically and institute general supportive measures, as indicated

[1]Includes reactions common to sulfonamides in general

DIAMOX continued

DRUG INTERACTIONS

Other diuretics	⇧ Diuretic effect and risk of hypokalemia
Lithium, phenobarbital, salicylates	⇧ Excretion, resulting in diminished pharmacologic activity
Amphetamines, procainamide, quinidine, tricyclic antidepressants	⇩ Excretion, resulting in enhanced pharmacologic activity and/or prolonged duration of action
Methenamine	Inactivation of antimicrobial effect
Nitrofurantoin	⇩ Antimicrobial effect
Insulin, oral hypoglycemics	⇩ Hypoglycemic effect
Digitalis	⇧ Risk of cardiotoxicity due to hypokalemia
Amphotericin B, corticosteroids	⇧ Risk of severe hypokalemia
Phenytoin, primidone	Possible osteomalacia

ALTERED LABORATORY VALUES

Blood/serum values	⇩ Bicarbonate ⇧ Chloride ⇩ Sodium ⇧ Ammonia ⇧ Bilirubin ⇧ Uric acid ⇩ Potassium (rare) ⇧ ^{131}I thyroid uptake (in euthyroid and hyperthyroid patients only) ⇧ Glucose (in prediabetic and diabetic patients)
Urinary values	⇧ Bicarbonate ⇧ Sodium ⇧ Potassium ⇩ Chloride ⇧ Phosphate ⇩ Citrate ⇩ Uric acid ⇩ Ammonia ⇧ Urobilinogen ⇧ Glucose (in prediabetic and diabetic patients) ⇧ Protein (with bromophenol blue reagent, sulfosalicylic acid, heat and acetic acid, or nitric acid ring test methods)

Use in children

See INDICATIONS

Use in pregnancy or nursing mothers

Contraindicated during pregnancy, especially during first trimester, unless expected benefits outweigh potential risk to fetus. Embryocidal and teratogenic effects have been reported in rats and mice, but have not been confirmed in man. General guidelines not established for use in nursing mothers.

E-CARPINE (Epinephrine bitartrate and pilocarpine hydrochloride) Alcon

Sol: 1% epinephrine bitartrate and 1%, 2%, 3%, 4%, or 6% pilocarpine hydrochloride (15 ml) for topical use only; do not apply to soft contact lenses

INDICATIONS	TOPICAL DOSAGE
Open-angle glaucoma	**Adult:** 1-2 drops in affected eye(s) up to 4 times/day

ADMINISTRATION/DOSAGE ADJUSTMENTS

Combination therapy	May be used with other miotics, beta blockers, carbonic anhydrase inhibitors, or hyperosmotic agents, as indicated

CONTRAINDICATIONS

Acute iritis or any condition in which pupillary construction is undesirable●	Hypersensitivity to any component●	Narrow-angle glaucoma●

WARNINGS/PRECAUTIONS

Impaired adaptation in poor light	Advise patient to exercise caution while driving at night and while performing other hazardous activities under conditions of poor illumination
Narrow-angle glaucoma	May be induced; estimate depth of angle of anterior chamber prior to use
Maculopathy with decreased visual acuity	May occur in the aphakic eye; discontinue medication promptly
Retinal detachment	May occur in predisposed individuals
General anesthesia	If used, consult anesthesiologist
Special-risk patients	Use with caution in patients with a history of hyperthyroidism, hypertension, organic cardiac disease, or long-standing bronchial asthma

ADVERSE REACTIONS

Ophthalmic	Slight ciliary spasm,[1] conjunctival vascular congestion,[1] induced myopia,[1] reduced visual acuity in poor light[2]; conjunctival or corneal pigmentation and lens opacity (with prolonged use)
Hypersensitivity	Ocular irritation (with prolonged use)
Cardiovascular	Palpitation, faintness, tachycardia, extrasystoles, hypertension, arrhythmias
Other	Temporal headache[1]

OVERDOSAGE

Signs and symptoms	Toxic effects primarily attributable to pilocarpine: nausea, vomiting, diarrhea, abdominal pain, intestinal cramps, frequent urination, excessive salivation, lacrimation, sweating, pallor, cyanosis, bronchoconstruction, nasal congestion, rhinorrhea; *in severe cases:* vertigo, tremors, muscle weakness, paresthesia, bradycardia, arrhythmias, hypotension, syncope, increased systemic vascular resistance, and CNS excitation, progressing to depression, confusion, ataxia, convulsions, coma, and respiratory or, more rarely, cardiovascular collapse
Treatment	Primary attention should be given to maintaining a patent airway and adequate respiratory exchange; if necessary, provide mechanically assisted ventilation and oxygen. To reverse the parasympathomimetic effects of the miotic, administer atropine sulfate, 1-4 mg SC, IM, or IV (in children, 40-80 μg/kg, up to 4 mg IM or IV). Repeat every 3-60 min, as needed, to control muscarinic symptoms. (Administer atropine with caution if patient is cyanotic.) If the drug has been accidentally ingested, perform gastric lavage, using a 0.02% solution of potassium permanganate.

DRUG INTERACTIONS

Other miotics; timolol; acetazolamide and other systemic carbonic anhydrase inhibitors	⇩ Intraocular pressure
Ophthalmic anticholinesterases	⇩ Miotic effect due to competitive inhibition

[1]Especially in younger patients during initial stages of therapy
[2]Especially in the elderly or in those with lens opacity

Table continued on following page

E-CARPINE continued

DRUG INTERACTIONS continued

Atropine	⇩ Mydriatic effect of atropine
Cyclopropane, chloroform, halothane, trichlorethylene, mercurial diuretics, digitalis glycosides	Cardiac arrhythmias
Tricyclic antidepressants	⇧ Cardiac effects of epinephrine

ALTERED LABORATORY VALUES

Blood/serum levels	⇧ Glucose

No clinically significant alterations in urinary values occur at therapeutic dosages

Use in children

General guidelines not established

Use in pregnancy or nursing mothers

General guidelines not established

Note: Other solutions containing epinephrine bitartrate and pilocarpine hydrochloride as major ingredients are marked as **E-PILO** (SMP); **P1E1, P2E1, P3E1,** and **P6E1** (Alcon)

[1]Especially in younger patients during initial stages of therapy
[2]Especially in the elderly or in those with lens opacity

EPIFRIN (Epinephrine hydrochloride) **Allergan**
Sol: 0.25% (15 ml), 0.50% (5, 15 ml), 1% (5, 15 ml), 2% (5, 15 ml)

INDICATIONS	**TOPICAL DOSAGE**
Chronic open-angle glaucoma	**Adult:** 1 drop in affected eye(s) qd or bid

CONTRAINDICATIONS	
History of acute narrow-angle glaucoma	Dilation of the pupil may trigger an attack

WARNINGS/PRECAUTIONS	
Patients with a narrow angle	Use with caution; pupil dilation may trigger an acute attack of narrow-angle glaucoma
Special-risk patients	Use with caution in patients with hypertension or coronary artery disease
Reversible macular edema	May occur; use with caution in aphakic patients
Local discomfort	May occur during instillation, especially with higher concentrations
Unwarranted use	Do not administer parenterally
Carcinogenesis, mutagenesis, and impairment of fertility	No studies have been conducted to evaluate the potential of these effects

ADVERSE REACTIONS	
Local	Eye pain or ache, conjunctival hyperemia, allergic lid reactions; adenochrome deposits in conjunctiva and cornea (with prolonged use)
Other	Browache, headache

OVERDOSAGE	
Signs and symptoms	For ophthalmic overdosage, see ADVERSE REACTIONS; accidental oral ingestion is inconsequential
Treatment	For ophthalmic overdosage, flush eyes with water or normal saline

DRUG INTERACTIONS	
Beta and alpha blocking agents	⇩ Antiglaucoma effect of ephinephrine
Cyclopropane, chloroform, halothane, trichlorethylene, mercurial diuretics, digitalis glycosides	Cardiac arrhythmias
Tricyclic antidepressants	⇧ Cardiac effects of epinephrine

ALTERED LABORATORY VALUES

No clinically significant alterations in blood/serum or urinary values occur at therapeutic dosages

Use in children

Safety and efficacy not established

Use in pregnancy or nursing mothers

Safe use during pregnancy is not established; use only if essential. General guidelines not established for use in nursing mothers.

ISOPTO-CARBACHOL (Carbachol) Alcon

Sol: 0.75%, 1.5%, 2.25%, 3.0% (15, 30 ml)

INDICATIONS	TOPICAL DOSAGE
Glaucoma	**Adult:** instill 2 drops in the eye(s) 1–4 times/day

CONTRAINDICATIONS

Acute iritis or other conditions in which constriction is undesirable	Hypersensitivity to any component

WARNINGS/PRECAUTIONS

Systemic toxicity	May occur with excessive penetration; use with caution in patients with corneal abrasion
Special-risk patients	Use with caution in patients with acute cardiac failure, bronchial asthma, active peptic ulcer, hyperthyroidism, gastrointestinal spasm, urinary tract obstruction, and Parkinson's disease
Retinal detachment	Has been reported when miotics are used in certain susceptible individuals (causal relationship not established)

ADVERSE REACTIONS

Local	Transient ciliary and conjunctival injection, headache, ciliary spasm with temporary decrease of visual acuity
Systemic	Salivation, syncope, cardiac arrhythmia, gastrointestinal cramping, vomiting, asthma, diarrhea

OVERDOSAGE

Signs and symptoms	See ADVERSE REACTIONS
Treatment	Discontinue use. Maintain adequate respiration. Administer 1–4 mg atropine parenterally; give additional doses every 3–60 min, as needed, for 24–48 h.

DRUG INTERACTIONS

Topical epinephrine, topical timolol, and/or systemic carbonic anhydrase inhibitors	⇧ Lowering of intraocular pressure
Corticosteroids, anticholinergics, antihistamines, meperidine, sympathomimetics, tricyclic antidepressants	Antagonism of miotic and/or ocular hypotensive effects

ALTERED LABORATORY VALUES

No clinically significant alterations in blood/serum or urinary values occur at therapeutic dosages

Use in children	Use in pregnancy or nursing mothers
General guidelines not established	General guidelines not established

Note: Carbachol also marketed as **CARBACEL** (Professional Pharmacal).

ISOPTO CARPINE (Pilocarpine hydrochloride) Alcon

Sol: 0.25% (15 ml), 0.5% (15, 30 ml), 1% (15, 30 ml), 1.5% (15 ml), 2% (15, 30 ml), 3% (15, 30 ml), 4% (15, 30 ml), 5% (15 ml), 6% (15, 30 ml), 8% (15 ml), 10% (15 ml) for topical use only

INDICATIONS	TOPICAL DOSAGE
Increased intraocular pressure	**Adult:** 2 drops in affected eye(s) up to 3–4 times/day

ADMINISTRATION/DOSAGE ADJUSTMENTS

Combination therapy — May be used with other miotics, beta blockers, carbonic anhydrase inhibitors, or hyperosmotic agents, as indicated

CONTRAINDICATIONS

Hypersensitivity to any component — Acute iritis or any condition in which pupillary constriction is undesirable

WARNINGS/PRECAUTIONS

Impaired adaptation in poor light — Advise patient to exercise caution while driving at night and while performing other hazardous activities under conditions of poor illumination

Retinal detachment — May occur in predisposed individuals (causal relationship not established)

ADVERSE REACTIONS

Ophthalmic — Slight ciliary spasm,[1] conjunctival vascular congestion,[1] induced myopia,[1] reduced visual acuity in poor light[2]; lens opacity (with prolonged use)

Other — Temporal or supraorbital headache[1]

OVERDOSAGE

Signs and symptoms — Nausea, vomiting, diarrhea, abdominal pain, intestinal cramps, frequent urination, excessive salivation, lacrimation, sweating, pallor, cyanosis, bronchoconstriction, nasal congestion, rhinorrhea; *in severe cases:* vertigo, tremors, muscle weakness, paresthesia, bradycardia, arrhythmias, hypotension, syncope, increased systemic vascular resistance, and CNS excitation, progressing to depression, confusion, ataxia, convulsions, coma, and respiratory or, more rarely, cardiovascular collapse

Treatment — Primary attention should be given to maintaining a patent airway and adequate respiratory exchange; if necessary, provide mechanically assisted ventilation and oxygen. To reverse the parasympathomimetic effects of the miotic, administer atropine sulfate, 1–4 mg SC, IM, or IV (in children, 40–80 µg/kg, up to 4 mg IM or IV). Repeat every 3–60 min, as needed, to control muscarinic symptoms. (Administer atropine with caution if patient is cyanotic.) If the drug has been accidentally ingested, perform gastric lavage, using a 0.02% solution of potassium permanganate

DRUG INTERACTIONS

Other miotics; timolol; topical epinephrine; acetazolamide and other systemic carbonic anhydrase inhibitors — ⇩ Intraocular pressure

Ophthalmic anticholinesterases — ⇩ Miotic effect due to competitive inhibition

Atropine — ⇩ Mydriatic effect of atropine

ALTERED LABORATORY VALUES

No clinically significant alterations in blood/serum or urinary values occur at therapeutic dosages

Use in children	**Use in pregnancy or nursing mothers**
General guidelines not established	General guidelines not established

NOTE: Pilocarpine hydrochloride also marketed as **ABSORBOCARPINE** (Burton, Parson); **PILOCAR** (Smith, Miller & Patch); and **PILOCEL** (Professional Pharmacal)

[1]Especially in younger patients during initial stages of therapy
[2]Especially in the elderly or in those with lens opacity

P.V. CARPINE (Pilocarpine nitrate) Allergan

Sol: 0.5%, 1%, 2%, 3%, 4%, 6% (15 ml) for topical use only

INDICATIONS	TOPICAL DOSAGE
Increased intraocular pressure associated with glaucoma	**Adult:** 1-2 drops 2-4 times/day
Mydriasis in acute glaucomatous emergencies	**Adult:** 1-2 drops of high concentration solution
Mydriasis associated with cycloplegic therapy	**Adult:** varies depending on cycloplegic used

CONTRAINDICATIONS

None

WARNINGS/PRECAUTIONS

Mucosal sensitization — May occur with prolonged therapy

ADVERSE REACTIONS

See WARNINGS/PRECAUTIONS

OVERDOSAGE

Signs and symptoms — Nausea, vomiting, diarrhea, abdominal pain, intestinal cramps, frequent urination, excessive salivation, lacrimation, sweating, pallor, cyanosis, bronchoconstriction, nasal congestion, rhinorrhea; *in severe cases:* vertigo, tremors, muscle weakness, paresthesia, bradycardia, arrhythmias, hypotension, syncope, increased systemic vascular resistance, and CNS excitation, progressing to depression, confusion, ataxia, convulsions, coma, and respiratory or, more rarely, cardiovascular collapse

Treatment — Primary attention should be given to maintaining a patient airway and adequate respiratory exchange; if necessary, provide mechanically assisted ventilation and oxygen. To reverse the parasympathomimetic effects of the miotic, administer atropine sulfate, 1-4 mg SC, IM, or IV (in children, 40-80 μg/kg, up to 4 mg IM or IV). Repeat every 3-60 min, as needed, to control muscarinic symptoms. (Administer atropine with caution if patient is cyanotic.) If the drug has been accidentally ingested, perform gastric lavage, using a 0.02% solution of potassium permanganate.

DRUG INTERACTIONS

Other miotics; timolol; topical epinephrine; acetazolamide and other systemic carbonic anhydrase inhibitors — ⇩ Intraocular pressure

Ophthalmic anticholinesterases — ⇩ Miotic effect due to competitive inhibition

Atropine — ⇩ Mydriatic effect of atropine

ALTERED LABORATORY VALUES

No clinically significant alterations in blood/serum or urinary values occur at therapeutic dosages

Use in children

General guidelines not established

Use in pregnancy and nursing mothers

General guidelines not established

TIMOPTIC (Timolol maleate) Merck Sharp & Dohme

Sol: 0.25%, 0.5% (5, 10 ml)

INDICATIONS	TOPICAL DOSAGE
Elevated intraocular pressure associated with **chronic open-angle glaucoma, aphakic glaucoma,** selected cases of **secondary glaucoma,** and **ocular hypertension**	**Adult:** 1 drop of 0.25% solution in each eye bid to start, followed by 1 drop of 0.5% solution in each eye bid, if needed; for maintenance, 1 drop (0.25% or 0.5%) in each eye qd

ADMINISTRATIVE/DOSAGE ADJUSTMENTS

Combination therapy	If response is not satisfactory with 1 drop of 0.5% solution bid, pilocarpine and other miotics, and/or epinephrine, and/or systemic carbonic anhydrase inhibitors may be given concomitantly
Transferring patients from other anti-glaucoma agents	On day 1, continue other agent and add 1 drop of 0.25% timolol solution in each eye bid; on day 2, discontinue previously used agent and adjust timolol dosage, as needed, up to 1 drop of 0.5% solution in each eye bid. To transfer patients from several agents, discontinue one agent at a time, as above, at intervals of usually not less than 1 wk.

CONTRAINDICATIONS

Hypersensitivity to any component

WARNINGS/PRECAUTIONS

Concurrent use of oral beta blockers	Monitor patient for additive effects on intraocular pressure or systemic effects of beta blockade
Narrow-angle glaucoma	Safety and efficacy not established
Acute bronchospasm	May occur in patients with bronchospastic disease
Special-risk patients	Use with caution in patients with bronchial asthma, sinus bradycardia, heart block greater than first degree, cardiogenic shock, right ventricular failure secondary to pulmonary hypertension, congestive heart failure, or in those receiving adrenergic-augmenting psychotropic agents; check pulse rates in patients with a history of severe cardiac disease

ADVERSE REACTIONS

Ophthalmologic	Mild ocular irritation
Hypersensitivity	Localized and generalized rash (rare)
Cardiovascular	Slight reduction in resting heart rate (average reduction, 2.9 ± 10.2 beats/min)

OVERDOSAGE

Toxicity has not been reported in clinical use

DRUG INTERACTIONS

Propranolol and other beta blockers	⇧ Systemic effect of beta blockage ⇩ Intraocular pressure
Pilocarpine and other topical miotics; topical epinephrine; acetazolamide and other systemic carbonic anhydrase inhibitors	⇩ Intraocular pressure

ALTERED LABORATORY VALUES

No clinically significant alterations in blood/serum or urinary values occur at therapeutic dosages

Use in children

Not recommended

Use in children or nursing mothers

Safe use not established during pregnancy; general guidelines not established for use in nursing mothers

BLEPH-10 (Sulfacetamide sodium) Allergan

Sol: 10% (5, 15 ml)

INDICATIONS

Conjunctivitis, corneal ulcer, and other **superficial ocular infections** caused by susceptible microorganisms

TOPICAL DOSAGE

Adult: instill 1-2 drops into lower conjunctival sac q2-3h during the day and less often at night

CONTRAINDICATIONS

Hypersensitivity to sulfonamides

WARNINGS/PRECAUTIONS

Silver preparations	Incompatible with this preparation
Nonsusceptible organisms, including fungi	May proliferate
Purulent exudates	Contain aminobenzoic acid, which will inactivate sulfonamides
Discoloration	Do not use if discolored; protect from light and excessive heat

ADVERSE REACTIONS

Sensitivity	Discontinue use immediately

Use in children

General guidelines not established

Use in pregnancy or nursing mothers

General guidelines not established

CHLOROMYCETIN Ophthalmic (Chloramphenicol) Parke-Davis

Ointment: 1% (3.5 g) **Sol:** 25 mg/15 ml after reconstitution (15 ml)

INDICATIONS

Superficial ocular infections involving the conjunctiva and/or cornea caused by susceptible organisms

TOPICAL DOSAGE

Adult: apply a small amount of ointment to the lower conjunctival sac or instill 2 drops of solution in the affected eye q3h for 48 h, or more often, if necessary; thereafter, lengthen intervals between applications

ADMINISTRATION/DOSAGE ADJUSTMENTS

Duration of therapy	Continue treatment for at least 48 h after the eye appears normal
Preparation of solution	Dilute contents of 15-ml vial with sterile distilled water supplied; solutions ranging in strength from 0.16% to 0.5% may be prepared by varying the quantity of diluent used
Supplementary systemic therapy	Administer appropriate systemic agents in all but very superficial infections

CONTRAINDICATIONS

Sensitivity to any component

WARNINGS/PRECAUTIONS

Hypersensitivity reactions	Including bone-marrow hypoplasia, may occur; avoid prolonged or frequent intermittent use
Overgrowth of nonsusceptible organisms, including fungi	May occur with prolonged use; discontinue and institute appropriate measures
Bacteriological studies	Should be performed to determine the causative organisms and their sensitivity to chloramphenicol

ADVERSE REACTIONS

Hematological	Blood dyscrasias (associated with systemic use)
Hypersensitivity	Bone-marrow hypoplasia, other reactions

Use in children

General guidelines not established

Use in pregnancy or nursing mothers

General guidelines not established

CHLOROPTIC (Chloramphenicol) Allergan

Sol: 0.5% (7.5 ml)

INDICATIONS	TOPICAL DOSAGE
Superficial ocular infections involving the conjunctiva and/or cornea, caused by susceptible organisms	**Adult:** instill 1-2 drops 4-6 times daily for 72 h; thereafter, lengthen the intervals between applications

ADMINISTRATION/DOSAGE ADJUSTMENTS

Duration of therapy	Continue for at least 48 h after condition appears to be cured

CONTRAINDICATIONS

Hypersensitivity to chloramphenicol

WARNINGS/PRECAUTIONS

Overgrowth of nonsusceptible organisms	May occur with prolonged use; if superinfection occurs or if clinical improvement is not noted within a reasonable period, discontinue use and institute appropriate therapy
Bone-marrow hypoplasia, depression of erythropoiesis, aplastic anemia, visual disturbances	Have occurred with systemic chloramphenicol; one case of bone-marrow hypoplasia has been reported after prolonged use (23 mo) of the ophthalmic solution

ADVERSE REACTIONS

Sensitivity	Stinging, itching, angioneurotic edema, urticaria, vesicular and maculopapular dermatitis

Use in children

General guidelines not established

Use in pregnancy or nursing mothers

General guidelines not established

ECONOCHLOR (Chloramphenicol) Alcon

Ointment: 1% (3.5 g) **Sol:** 0.5% (2.5, 15 ml)

INDICATIONS	TOPICAL DOSAGE
Superficial ocular infections involving the conjunctiva and/or cornea caused by susceptible organisms	**Adult:** for severe cases, instill 2 drops into the eye(s) qh; for mild cases, instill 2 drops into the eye(s) qid; when condition improves, reduce dosage gradually and eventually withdraw

ADMINISTRATION/DOSAGE ADJUSTMENTS

Supplementary therapy	Apply a small amount of chloramphenicol ointment to the lower conjunctival sac(s) at bedtime; administer appropriate systemic medication in all but very superficial infections

CONTRAINDICATIONS

Hypersensitivity to any component

WARNINGS/PRECAUTIONS

Overgrowth of nonsusceptible organisms, including fungi	May occur with use of ophthlamic ointment
Bacteriological studies	Should be performed to determine the causative organisms and their sensitivity to chloramphenicol
Hypersensitivity	Including bone-marrow hypoplasia, possible leading to aplastic anemia, may occur; avoid prolonged use or frequent intermittent use
Retardation of corneal wound healing	May occur with use of ophthalmic ointment

ADVERSE REACTIONS

Hematological	Blood dyscrasias (associated with systemic use)
Hypersensitivity	Bone-marrow hypoplasia (1 case)

Use in children

General guidelines not established

Use in pregnancy or nursing mothers

General guidelines not established

GANTRISIN Ophthalmic (Sulfisoxazole diolamine) Roche

Ointment: 4% (⅛ oz) **Sol:** 4% (½ oz)

INDICATIONS	TOPICAL DOSAGE
Conjunctivitis, corneal ulcer, and other **superficial ocular infections** caused by susceptible organisms **Trachoma** (adjunctive therapy)	**Adult:** apply a small amount of ointment to lower conjunctival sac qd, bid, or tid and at bedtime, or instill 2–3 drops in the eye at least tid

CONTRAINDICATIONS

Hypersensitivity to sulfonamides

WARNINGS/PRECAUTIONS

Silver preparations	Incompatible with these preparations
Retarded corneal healing	May occur with use of ophthalmic ointment
Overgrowth of nonsusceptible organisms, including fungi	May occur
Purulent exudates	Contain para-aminobenzoic acid, which will inactivate sulfonamides
Undesirable reactions	May occur; discontinue use immediately
Contamination of solution	May occur; do not touch dropper tip to any surface

ADVERSE REACTIONS

Sensitivity	Discontinue use immediately

Use in children	Use in pregnancy or nursing mothers
General guidelines not established	General guidelines not established

GARAMYCIN Ophthalmic (Gentamicin sulfate) Schering

Ointment: equivalent to 3.0 mg gentamicin per gram (⅛ oz) **Sol:** equivalent to 3.0 mg gentamicin per gram (5 ml)

INDICATIONS	TOPICAL DOSAGE
Infections of the external eye and its adnexa, including **conjuctivitis, keratitis and keratoconjunctivitis, corneal ulcers, blepharitis and blepharoconjunctivitis, acute meibomianitis,** and **dacryocystitis,** when caused by susceptible bacteria	**Adult:** instill 1–2 drops into affected eye q4h or apply a small amount of ointment to the affected eye bid or tid; for severe infections, instill as much as 2 drops qh

CONTRAINDICATIONS

Hypersensitivity to any component

WARNINGS/PRECAUTIONS

Unwarranted uses	Never inject solution subconjunctivally or introduce directly into the anterior chamber of the eye
Overgrowth of nonsusceptible organisms, including fungi	May occur with prolonged use; discontinue use and institute appropriate therapy
Irritation or hypersensitivity	May occur; discontinue use and institute appropriate therapy
Retardation of corneal healing	May occur with use of ophthalmic ointment

ADVERSE REACTIONS

Local	Transient irritation (with use of solution), occasional burning or stinging (with use of ointment)

Use in children	Use in pregnancy or nursing mothers
General guidelines not established	General guidelines not established

ILOTYCIN Ophthalmic (Erythromycin) Dista

Ointment: 5 mg/g (⅛ oz)

INDICATIONS	TOPICAL DOSAGE
Superficial ocular infections involving the conjunctiva and/or cornea caused by susceptible organisms	**Adult:** apply directly to the infected structure qd or more often, depending on the severity of the infection

CONTRAINDICATIONS

Hypersensitivity to erythromycin

WARNINGS/PRECAUTIONS

Sensitivity reactions	May occur in certain individuals

ADVERSE REACTIONS

Sensitivity	Discontinue use immediately

Use in children

General guidelines not established

Use in pregnancy or nursing mothers

General guidelines not established

ISOPTO CETAMIDE (Sulfacetamide sodium) Alcon

Sol: 15% (5, 15 ml)

INDICATIONS	TOPICAL DOSAGE
Conjunctivitis, corneal ulcer, and other **superficial ocular infections** due to susceptible microorganisms **Trachoma and other chlamydial infections** (adjunctive therapy)	**Adult:** instill 1-2 drops into the conjunctival sac q1-2h to start, increasing the time interval as condition responds

CONTRAINDICATIONS

Hypersensitivity to sulfonamides

WARNINGS/PRECAUTIONS

Severe sensitivity reactions (eg, Stevens-Johnson syndrome)	Have been identified in patients with no prior history of sulfonamide hypersensitivity
Silver preparations	Incompatible with this preparation
Overgrowth of nonsusceptible organisms, including fungi	May occur
Purulent exudates	May contain aminobenzoic acid, which will inactivate sulfonamides

ADVERSE REACTIONS

Hypersensitivity	Erythema multiforme (Stevens-Johnson syndrome), other reactions

Use in children

General guidelines not established

Use in pregnancy or nursing mothers

General guidelines not established

NEOSPORIN Ophthalmic Ointment (Polymyxin B sulfate, bacitracin zinc, and neomycin sulfate)

Burroughs Wellcome

Ointment: 5,000 units polymyxin B sulfate, 400 units bacitracin zinc, equivalent to 3.5 mg neomycin base per gram (⅛ oz)

INDICATIONS	TOPICAL DOSAGE
Short-term treatment of **superficial ocular infections** caused by susceptible organisms	**Adult:** apply q3–4h, depending on severity of the infection

CONTRAINDICATIONS

Sensitivity to any component

WARNINGS/PRECAUTIONS

Overgrowth of nonsusceptible organisms	May occur with prolonged use
Retardation of corneal healing	May occur
Culture and susceptibility tests	Should be performed during treatment
Allergic cross-reactions	May occur and could prevent the future use of any or all of the following antibiotics: kanamycin, paromomycin, streptomycin, and possibly gentamicin
Cutaneous sensitivity	May occur due to neomycin component; literature indicates an increase in the prevalence of persons allergic to neomycin

ADVERSE REACTIONS

Sensitivity	Discontinue use immediately

Use in children

General guidelines not established

Use in pregnancy or nursing mothers

General guidelines not established

NEOSPORIN Ophthalmic Solution (Polymyxin B sulfate, neomycin sulfate, and gramicidin)

Burroughs Wellcome

Sol: 5,000 units polymyxin B sulfate, equivalent to 1.75 mg neomycin base, and 0.025 mg gramicidin per ml (10 ml)

INDICATIONS	TOPICAL DOSAGE
Short-term treatment of **superficial ocular infections** caused by susceptible organisms	**Adult:** instill 1–2 drops into affected eye bid, tid, qid, or more often, as required; for acute infections, instill 1–2 drops every 15–30 min, reducing the frequency of instillation as infection is controlled

CONTRAINDICATIONS

Sensitivity to any component

WARNINGS/PRECAUTIONS

Overgrowth of nonsusceptible organisms	May occur with prolonged use
Culture and susceptibility tests	Should be performed during treatment
Allergic cross-reactions	May occur and could prevent the future use of any or all of the following antibiotics: kanamycin, paromomycin, streptomycin, and possibly gentamicin
Cutaneous sensitivity	May occur due to neomycin component; literature indicates an increase in the prevalence of persons allergic to neomycin

ADVERSE REACTIONS

Sensitivity	Discontinue use immediately

Use in children

General guidelines not established

Use in pregnancy or nursing mothers

General guidelines not established

POLYSPORIN Ophthalmic (Polymyxin B sulfate and bacitracin zinc) Burroughs Wellcome

Ointment: 10,000 units polymyxin B sulfate and 500 units bacitracin zinc per gram (⅛ oz)

INDICATIONS	TOPICAL DOSAGE
Superficial ocular infections involving the conjunctiva and/or cornea caused by susceptible organisms	**Adult:** apply q3–4h, depending on severity of the infection

CONTRAINDICATIONS

Hypersensitivity to any component

WARNINGS/PRECAUTIONS

Retardation of corneal healing	May occur
Overgrowth of nonsusceptible organisms, including fungi	May occur with prolonged use; institute appropriate measures

ADVERSE REACTIONS

Sensitivity	Discontinue use immediately

Use in children

General guidelines not established

Use in pregnancy or nursing mothers

General guidelines not established

SODIUM SULAMYD (Sulfacetamide sodium) **Schering**

Ointment: 10% (3.5 g) **Sol:** 10% (5 ml), 30% (15 ml)

INDICATIONS	TOPICAL DOSAGE
Conjunctivitis, corneal ulcer	**Adult:** 1–2 drops of 10% solution q2–3h during the day and less often at night, or 1 drop of 30% solution q2h or less often, instilled into the lower conjunctival sac, or small amount of ointment qid and at bedtime
Other **superficial ocular infections** due to susceptible microorganisms	**Adult:** variable, according to severity of the infection (see above dosages)
Trachoma (adjunctive therapy)	**Adult:** 2 drops of 30% solution q2h

ADMINISTRATION/DOSAGE ADJUSTMENTS

Supplemental therapy	For conjunctivitis or corneal ulcer, apply a small amount of ophthalmic ointment qid and at bedtime. For trachoma, concomitant systemic sulfonamide therapy is indicated.

CONTRAINDICATIONS

Hypersensitivity to any component

WARNINGS/PRECAUTIONS

Silver preparations	Incompatible with these preparations
Retardation of corneal healing	May occur with use of ophthalmic ointment
Overgrowth of nonsusceptible organisms, including fungi	May occur
Purulent exudates	Contain para-aminobenzoic acid, which will inactivate sulfonamides
Sensitization	May recur with readministration of sulfonamide, regardless of the route; discontinue use
Cross-sensitivity	May occur between different sulfonamides; discontinue use
Adverse reactions	Discontinue use if untoward reactions occur

ADVERSE REACTIONS

Local	Irritation; transient stinging or burning (with 30% solution)
Sensitivity	Erythema multiforme (Stevens-Johnson syndrome) (1 case), local hypersensitivity progressing to a fatal syndrome resembling systemic lupus erythematosus (1 case)

Use in children

General guidelines not established

Use in pregnancy or nursing mothers

General guidelines not established

STOXIL (Idoxuridine) Smith Kline & French

Ointment: 0.5% (4 g) **Sol:** 0.1% (15 ml)

INDICATIONS	TOPICAL DOSAGE
Herpes simplex keratitis[1]	**Adult:** instill 1 drop in each affected eye qh during day and q2h at night until definite improvement is noted; thereafter, reduce dosage to 1 drop q2h during day and q4h at night; or apply ointment to lower conjunctival sac 5 times/day at 4-h intervals

ADMINISTRATION/DOSAGE ADJUSTMENTS

Duration of therapy	Continue therapy for 3–5 days after healing appears complete, to minimize recurrences; monitor patient frequently
Epithelial infections	If improvement is noted after 7–8 days, continue therapy for up to 21 days longer
Herpes simplex with stromal lesions, corneal edema, or iritis	If topical corticosteroids are used concomitantly, continue idoxuridine therapy for several days after the steroid has been withdrawn (see WARNINGS/PRECAUTIONS)
Concomitant use of atropine	Atropine preparations may be employed adjunctively, as indicated

CONTRAINDICATIONS

Hypersensitivity to any component

WARNINGS/PRECAUTIONS

Resistant strains	May emerge; consider other forms of therapy for epithelial infections that fail to respond after 7–8 days
Unwarranted use	Not effective in corneal inflammations following herpes simplex keratitis in which the virus is not present
Concomitant use of corticosteroids	May accelerate the spread of viral infection and are usually contraindicated in herpes simplex keratitis (see ADMINISTRATION/DOSAGE ADJUSTMENTS)
Concomitant use of boric acid	May cause irritation; do not administer during idoxuridine therapy
Mutagenic potential	Chromosome aberrations in mice and mutations in mammalian cells in culture and in a host-mediated assay system have been reported
Oncogenic potential	Regard idoxuridine as potentially carcinogenic; idoxuridine can inhibit DNA synthesis or function and is incorporated into the DNA of mammalian cells as well as into the genome of DNA viruses
Accidental ingestion	No untoward effects should occur even from ingestion of entire contents; no treatment is indicated
Secondary infections	May be controlled with concomitant use of antibiotics
Corneal defects	May occur with overly frequent application; discontinue use, either temporarily or permanently, as indicated, after close observation of the progress of the infection

ADVERSE REACTIONS

Local	Irritation, pain, pruritis, inflammation, edema, corneal clouding and stippling; small punctate defects in the corneal epithelium (causal relationship not established)
Allergic	Photophobia, other reactions (rare)

Use in children

General guidelines not established

Use in pregnancy or nursing mothers

Administer with caution in pregnancy or in women of childbearing potential; idoxuridine has been reported to cross the placental barrier and to produce fetal malformations in some animal studies. Whether idoxuridine appears in breast milk is unknown; as a general rule, nursing should not be undertaken during therapy.

[1] Epithelial infections, especially initial attacks, have responded better than stromal infections; recurrences are common. Idoxuridine will often control the infection, but will have no effect on accumulated scarring and vascularization or on the resultant progressive loss of vision.

VIRA-A Ophthalmic Ointment (Vidarabine monohydrate) Parke-Davis

Ointment: 3% vidarabine monohydrate equivalent to 28.11 mg vidarabine per gram (3.5 g)

INDICATIONS	TOPICAL DOSAGE
Acute keratoconjunctivitis and **recurrent epithelial keratitis** due to herpes simplex virus types 1 and 2 **Superficial herpes simplex keratitis** when resistant to idoxuridine or when toxic or hypersensitivity reactions to idoxuridine have occurred	**Adult:** apply approximately ½ inch of ointment to the lower conjunctival sac 5 times/day at 3-h intervals; to prevent recurrence after re-epithelialization has occurred, continue treatment at a reduced dosage (eg, bid) for 7 days

ADMINISTRATION/DOSAGE ADJUSTMENTS

Duration of therapy	If there are no signs of improvement after 7 days, or if complete re-epithelialization has not occured by 21 days, other forms of therapy should be considered; severe cases may require longer treatment
Concomitant topical antibiotic therapy	Gentamicin, erythromycin, and chloramphenicol have been administered concurrently with this preparation without an increase in adverse reactions
Concomitant topical steroid therapy	Prednisolone and dexamethasone have been administered concurrently with this preparation without an increase in adverse reactions; however, steroid-induced ocular side effects, including glaucoma, cataract formation, and progression of bacterial or viral infection, must be considered when steroids are given concurrently with this preparation
Prior to therapy	The diagnosis of keratoconjunctivitis due to herpes simplex virus should be established clinically

CONTRAINDICATIONS

Hypersensitivity to vidarabine

WARNINGS/PRECAUTIONS

Mutagenic potential	Vidarabine may produce mutagenic effects in male germ cells; in vitro studies suggest that the drug can be incorporated into mammalian DNA and can induce mutations in mammalian cells. Vidarabine may cause chromosome breaks and gaps when added to human leukocytes in vitro; such effects correlate well with ability to produce heritable genetic damage.
Oncogenic potential	Liver tumors; kidney, intestinal, testicular, and thyroid neoplasia; and hepatic megalocytosis have been found in vidarabine-treated rodents
Temporary visual haze	May occur; patients should be forewarned
Viral resistance	Has not been observed but may exist
Accidental ingestion	Should produce no untoward effects
Overly frequent administration	Should be avoided

ADVERSE REACTIONS

Local	Lacrimation, foreign body sensation, conjunctival injection, burning, irritation, superficial punctate keratitis, pain, photophobia, punctal occlusion, sensitivity; uveitis, stromal edema, secondary glaucoma, trophic defects, corneal vascularization, and hyphema (casual relationship not established)

Use in children

General guidelines not established

Use in pregnancy or nursing mothers

Use during pregnancy only when clearly indicated. A 10% preparation of this ointment induced fetal abnormalities in rabbits, and the parenteral form is teratogenic in rats and rabbits. It is not known whether vidarabine is excreted in human milk. Nursing should not be undertaken during treatment.

NONPRESCRIPTION EYE DROPS

Product (Manufacturer)	Ingredients	Actions
Clear Eye (Abbott) **Dosage** 1 or 2 drops into each eye 2 to 3 times daily	Methylcellulose	Aids in wetting eye by increasing fluid's tendency to spread
	0.012% Naphazoline hydrochloride	Whitens reddened eyes by limiting local vascular response (constricts blood vessels)
	0.1% Edetate disodium	Preservative
	0.01% Benzalkonium chloride	Preservative
	Boric acid	Buffer
	Sodium borate	Buffer
Murine (Abbott) **Dosage** 1 or 2 drops into each eye several times daily or as directed by physician	Methylcellulose	Aids in wetting eye by increasing fluid's tendency to spread
	0.1% Benzalkonium chloride	Preservative
	0.05% Edetate sodium	Preservative
	Mono- and dibasic sodium phosphate	Buffer
	Glycerin	Emollient and demulcent
Murine Plus (Abbott) **Dosage** 1 or 2 drops into each eye several times daily or as directed by physician	Methylcellulose	Aids in wetting eye by increasing fluid's tendency to spread
	0.05% Tetrahydrozoline hydrochloride	Whitens reddened eyes by limiting local vascular response (constricts blood vessels)
	0.01% Benzalkonium chloride	Preservative
	0.1% Edetate sodium	Preservative
	Boric acid	Buffer
	Sodium borate	Buffer
Naphcon (Alcon) **Dosage** 2 drops into each eye 2 or 3 times daily or as needed	0.012% Naphazoline hydrochloride	Whitens reddened eyes by limiting local vascular response (constricts blood vessels)
	0.01% Benzalkonium chloride	Preservative
Visine (Leeming) **Dosage** 1 or 2 drops into each eye 2 to 3 times daily or as directed by physician	0.05% Tetrahydrozoline	Whitens reddened eyes by limiting local vascular response (constricts blood vessels)
	0.1% Edetate disodium	Preservative
	0.01% Benzalkonium chloride	Preservative
	Boric acid	Buffer
	Sodium borate	Buffer

Product (Manufacturer)	Ingredients	Actions
Collyrium (Wyeth) **Dosage** Fill enclosed eye cup and flush eyes 3 to 4 times daily as needed	Boric acid	Buffer
	Sodium borate	Buffer
	0.002% Thimerosal	Preservative
	0.4% Antipyrine	Whitens reddened eyes by limiting local vascular response (constricts blood vessels)
	0.056% Sodium salicylate	Buffer
Enuclene (Alcon) **Dosage** Put 1 or 2 drops into each eye 3 to 4 times daily	0.2% Benzalkonium chloride	Preservative
	0.25% Tyloxapol	Aids in wetting eye by increasing fluid's tendency to spread.
Eye-Stream (Alcon) **Dosage** Flush eyes as needed	Sodium citrate	Buffer
	Sodium acetate	Buffer
	Benzalkonium chloride	Preservative
	Sodium chloride Potassium chloride Calcium chloride Magnesium chloride	Forms a balanced salt solution (similar to eye fluid)
Murine Plus (Abbott) **Dosage** Squeeze 1 or 2 drops into each eye several times daily or as directed by physician	Methylcellulose	Aids in wetting eye by increasing fluid's tendency to spread
	0.05% Tetrahydrozoline hydrochloride	Whitens reddened eyes by limiting local vascular response (constricts blood vessels)
	0.01% Benzalkonium chloride	Preservative
	0.1% Edetate sodium	Preservative
	Boric acid	Buffer
	Sodium borate	Buffer
Op-thal-zin (Alcon) **Dosage** 2 drops into each eye 3 times daily	0.01% Benzalkonium chloride	Preservative
	Zinc sulfate	Astringent

Product (Manufacturer)	Ingredients	Actions
Isopto Alkaline (Alcon) **Dosage** 2 drops into each eye 3 times daily	Hydroxypropyl methylcellulose	Aids in wetting eye by increasing fluid's tendency to spread
	0.01% Benzalkonium chloride	Preservative
Isopto Plain (Alcon) **Dosage** 1 or 2 drops into each eye 3 times daily or as needed	0.5% Hydroxypropyl methylcellulose	Aids in wetting eye by increasing fluid's tendency to spread
	0.01% Benzalkonium chloride	Preservative
Lacril (Allergan) **Dosage** 1 or 2 drops into each eye or as directed by physician	Hydroxypropyl methylcellulose-gelatin	Aids in wetting eye by increasing fluid's tendency to spread
	0.5% Chlorobutanol	Preservative
	Polysorbate 80	Wetting agent (vehicle)
	Gelatin	Aids in wetting eye by increasing fluid's tendency to spread
	Sodium chloride Potassium chloride Calcium chloride Magnesium chloride	Tonicity agents (form an isotonic solution similar to eye fluid)
	Sodium acetate	Buffer
	Sodium citrate	Buffer
	Acetic acid	Buffer
	Sodium borate	Buffer
	Dextrose	Aids in wetting eye by increasing fluid's tendency to spread
Liquifilm Forte (Allergan) **Dosage** 1 drop in each eye as needed or as directed by physician	3.0% Polyvinyl alcohol	Aids in wetting eye by increasing fluid's tendency to spread
	0.002% Thimerosal	Preservative
	Edetate disodium	Preservative
		Isotonic solution
Liquifilm Tears (Allergan) **Dosage** 1 drop in each eye as needed	1.4% Polyvinyl alcohol	Aids in wetting eye by increasing fluid's tendency to spread
	0.5% Chlorobutanol	Preservative
	Sodium chloride	Induces solution osmolality the equal to that of tears

Table continued on following page

Product (Manufacturer)	Ingredients	Actions
Tears Naturale (Alcon) **Dosage** 1 or 2 drops into each eye as required to relieve eye irritation symptoms or as directed by physician	Water-soluble polymeric system	Aids in wetting eye by increasing fluid's tendency to spread
	0.01% Benzalkonium chloride	Preservative
	0.05% Edetate disodium	Preservative
Ultra Tears (Alcon) **Dosage** 1 or 2 drops into each eye 2 to 3 times daily or as needed	1% Hydroxypropyl methylcellulose	Aids in wetting eye by increasing fluid's tendency to spread
	0.01% Benzalkonium chloride	Preservative

Ear Disorders

As the organ of hearing and balance, the ear contains sensory receptors that send information for both functions to the brain. When this information is correctly transmitted and processed, a normal person in good health can literally hear a pin drop (on an uncarpeted floor) and can maintain bodily equilibrium in relation to the environment.

When the ear does not function properly, either because of injury or disease, the consequences are likely to be some degree of deafness, impairment of balance, or both. Also, because of the delicacy, minuteness, and interrelations of many structures within the ear, any malfunction or inflammation is likely to be accompanied by acute discomfort: earache, itching, formation of pus, ringing or buzzing sensations, and dizziness (vertigo) with or without nausea, in addition to hearing impairment.

EAR STRUCTURE

The visible part of the ear, called the outer ear or auricle, consists of a flap of cartilage and flesh that collects and condenses sounds, and the external auditory canal through which the sounds travel to the eardrum or tympanic membrane. The outer part of the canal is made up primarily of cartilage; the inner part passes through bone and is lined with skin containing glands that secrete wax.

The middle ear is not visible since it lies beyond the eardrum. It is the cavity in the temporal bone that contains the ossicles, the three bones of hearing. The movements of these bones convey the vibrations of the eardrum to the organs of hearing in the inner ear. The eustachian tube, which forms a tunnel between the middle ear and the mouth, equalizes the pressure on both sides of the eardrum.

It is the eustachian tube through which infectious bacteria travel from the upper throat and tonsils or adenoids to the middle ear. Infection can also travel from the middle ear to the mastoid bone that protrudes just behind the outer ear.

The inner ear, which is separated from the middle ear by a delicate membrane known as the oval window, is composed of a group of fluid-filled chambers within the hardest portion of the temporal bone. These chambers, called the cochlea, are coiled like the snail shell from which their name derives. Within the heart of this tiny spiral is the most important single structure in the hearing process: the organ of Corti. This structure contains many thousands of hairlike nerve endings that project from the lining of the cochlea and respond to the infinitely delicate and varied stimuli created by the movements of the fluid within the inner ear. The nature of these movements is determined by the forces exerted on the oval window by the bones of hearing as they respond to sound waves.

The nerve endings group themselves into a bundle at the base of the cochlea, forming the auditory nerve, which in turn sends its information to the brain for processing.

ANATOMY OF THE EAR AND SITES OF COMMON PROBLEMS

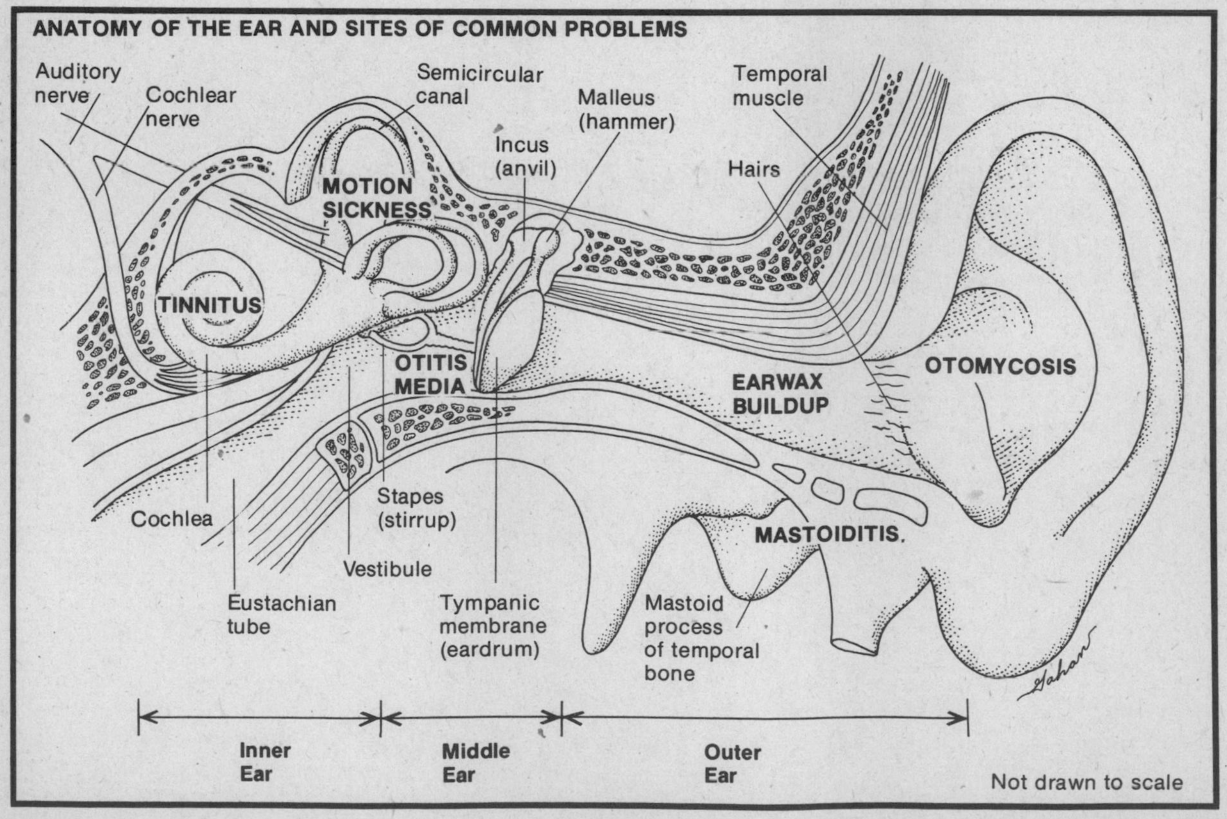

The inner ear also contains the organ of balance. This consists of three semicircular canals originating in the central portion of the labyrinth system known as the vestibule. The semicircular canals, which lie in different spatial planes at right angles to each other, are U-shaped tubes containing a fluid called endolymph. The behavior of this fluid in relation to the hairlike nerve cells at one end of each tube conveys information similar to that of a gyroscope, so that the brain can send appropriate messages to the muscles for the maintenance of bodily balance. This aspect of equilibrium is the kinetic sense, or sense of movement. The static sense, which senses the position of the head, originates in another set of hair cells to which are attached deposits of calcium carbonate. These crystals, called otoliths, respond to gravitational forces in a manner that provides information to the brain about whether the head is erect, tilted, or upside down. Thus, if the labyrinth of the inner ear is inflamed or impaired, the brain is likely to receive the kind of faulty information that results in vertigo.

DISORDERS OF THE OUTER EAR AND EAR CANAL

Itching

Itching in the ear may be the result of an allergy, or it may be a symptom of otomycosis, the technical term for a fungus infection of the ear. Neurodermatitis, inflamed patches of thickened, leathery skin, is another source of itching.

Fungal ear infections are commonly associated with swimming in polluted waters, hence the term "swimmer's ear." Fungi are microscopic organisms that multiply rapidly in the dark and damp, and when they settle in the outer ear, they cause the skin to become swollen and inflamed. The affected area itches and is usually covered by a flaky crust, from which there is a seepage of clear fluid.

Under no circumstances should anything be poked into the ear as a way of reducing the discomfort or itching. The condition should be called to a doctor's attention so that the cause can be determined, and if appropriate, the proper eardrops or ointment can be prescribed. Such medications are likely to contain antibiotics as well as corticosteroids, and they should be used *exactly* as instructed.

Even though swimming in and of itself rarely causes ear problems, breathing correctly—that is, breathing in through the mouth and out through the nose—is the best way to keep infection from spreading to the ears. On leaving the water, the ears should be dried thoroughly, and if water remaining in the ear canal does not run out of its own accord, lying down on one's side with the ear tilted downward will drain it.

Earwax Buildup

Earwax, technically called cerumen, may accumulate over the years and harden to the point that it blocks sound waves from passing through the auditory canal. Fortunately, this form of conduction deafness is simple to correct. When the impacted wax is softened by a few drops of 3 percent hydrogen peroxide, mixed with an equal amount of warm water, it can usually be removed by rotating a pointed wad of cotton against it. Special earwax softeners (e.g., Debrox or Cerumenex) may also be used. In cases resistant to this approach, a physician should be consulted so that the obstructive wax can be flushed out with a syringe. In any event, the wax should not be removed with a toothpick, hairpin, or other sharp instrument.

Aerotitis

Aerotitis, also called barotitis, is caused by a rapid change in barometric pressure. The resulting discomfort may range from a feeling of fullness with symptoms of deafness to sharp pain. Such a change typically occurs during the descent of a plane, and is caused by a failure of the eustachian tube to equalize the pressure on both sides of the eardrum. When the pressure in the middle ear is lower than the air pressure outside, the pain may be acute, sometimes lasting for several days, especially if there is a prior swelling caused by an upper respiratory infection or allergy. In extreme cases, the eardrum may rupture, and hemorrhage may occur in the middle ear. If possible, air travel should be avoided when one has a cold or nasal or sinus congestion.

Travelers in normal health can help mimimize discomfort by yawning, chewing gum, or swallowing. Since alcohol intensifies the problem, avoid drinking before takeoff or during the flight. The use of a nasal decongestant spray or decongestant (e.g., Sudafed) about an hour before landing time may also ease the problem.

DISORDERS OF THE MIDDLE EAR

Otitis is the term for any infection or inflammation of the ear. When the outer ear and the canal are affected, it is called otitis externa, while otitis media refers to middle ear infections. These are very common, especially among children, and until the development of penicillin and other antibiotics, such infections were the greatest single cause of hearing loss.

The large number of otitis media cases is attributable to the structural connection between the ear and the throat by way of the eustachian tube. In some instances, the infection begins in the upper respiratory tract—for example, a simple cold or a sore throat—and moves into the middle ear. More seriously, the ear infection may be a consequence of influenza, or in children, measles, mumps, or diseased tonsils or adenoids.

The onset of acute otitis media is signaled by pain in one or both ears, sometimes accompanied by a ringing in the affected ear, hearing loss, and fever. Prompt treatment with antibiotics is mandatory, usually with one of the penicillins or, where sensitivity to these drugs is a factor, erythromycin. It is of the utmost importance that the entire course of medication be completed to help prevent reinfection. To ease the earache, aspirin or acetaminophen may be taken, while a decongestant may help diminish the discomfort of stuffiness in the ear canal. There are also otic analgesics, such as a combination of benzocaine and antipyrine (Auralgan).

The importance of prompt drug therapy in dealing with middle ear infections cannot be overemphasized, especially in the case of children. Where treatment is unduly postponed, or where the condition is altogether neglected, the consequence may be some loss of hearing. An untreated ear infection also may lead to inflammation of the mastoid bone, a condition known as mastoiditis. Immediate surgery—inevitably resulting in a loss of hearing—is usually required to prevent spread of the infection to the brain.

DISORDERS OF THE INNER EAR

Motion Sickness

Motion sickness is a disorder that may be experienced by passengers in any moving vehicle—plane, train, car, boat, or amusement park ride such as a Ferris wheel. The discomfort is a result of a disturbance of the three semicircular canals in the inner ear that control equilibrium. Symptoms may range from a mild queasiness to acute nausea and vomiting. Pallor, a cold sweat, and a dull headache accompanied by dizziness are other typical manifestations.

Seasickness is likely to produce the most unpleasant reactions because of the vessel's combined motions of pitching from front to back, and rolling from side to side. Alcohol and a number of drugs may produce sensations that resemble motion sickness. Those prone to car sickness should sit in the front seat, if possible, and refrain from reading. A window should be kept open, and with the onset of queasiness, the most effective treatment is to get out of the car and take a brief walk. Advice regarding seasickness varies. Some persons find relief by lying down with the head lowered, while others fare better on deck, facing into the the wind and either sitting or standing, with eyes fixed on a stable object, such as the horizon. The discomfort of airsickness may be reduced by sitting as far down in the seat as possible and keeping one's eyes closed.

For those who chronically suffer from motion sickness, drugs may be prescribed. These include antinauseants that are largely antihistamines, such as hydroxyzine (Antivert) or dimenhydrinate (Dramamine), or in some instances, a mild tranquilizer such as Valium.

Tinnitus

Tinnitus, commonly referred to as a ringing or buzzing in the ears, is the perception of noises that do not originate in the environment. It should not be confused with the auditory hallucinations (hearing voices) that characterize certain psychotic episodes or that may be induced by drugs such as LSD.

In many cases, the disorder can be traced to specific underlying causes, such as irreversible damage to the delicate hair cells within the cochlea resulting from long-term exposure to destructive noise levels (e.g., loud rock music or the noise of factory machinery); tumors of the auditory nerve; cardiovascular disease affecting the blood vessels of the inner ear; and otosclerosis, a condition characterized by spongy bone formation in the labyrinth of the inner ear. Tinnitus may also result from food allergies, accumulated earwax, and in a significant number of cases, as a side effect of some drugs, especially aspirin, quinine, or certain antihypertensives. When tinnitus cannot be attributed to an underlying cause that can be corrected or removed, unorthodox alternative treatments, such as biofeedback or masking the tinnitus by playing recordings of "white noise," may be tried.

Meniere's Disease

Meniere's disease or syndrome is a poorly understood disorder of the labyrinth of the inner ear characterized by a triad of tinnitus, deafness, and vertigo. It usually affects one ear, although in about 20 percent of all cases, both ears are involved. The cause of Meniere's disease is unknown. Most patients experience alternating remission and intensification of symptoms; it is not unusual for symptom-free periods to last for months or even years, followed by flare-ups of the disease for no apparent reason.

Therapy includes a restriction of salt intake, combined with the prescription of diuretics, to reduce distention of the affected tissues by fluid, and sedatives, to reduce the effect of vertigo. In some cases resistant to drug therapy, vestibular surgery may be recommended, especially if the symptoms are so frequent and intense as to disrupt normal functioning.

IN CONCLUSION

Although most of it lies protected within the head, the ear is subject to a number of disorders, ranging from infections to little-understood syndromes such as Meniere's disease, that affect both hearing and balance. The following drug charts cover antibiotic agents used specifically for ear infections (other anti-infectives that may be prescribed for otitis are in the *Bacterial Infections* section, page 339). Also included are earwax softeners and otic analgesics.

AEROSPORIN Otic Solution (Polymyxin B sulfate) Burroughs Wellcome

Otic drops: 10,000 units/ml (10 ml)

INDICATIONS	TOPICAL DOSAGE
Acute and chronic **otitis externa,** including swimmer's ear, **otitis media** (if the tympanic membrane is perforated), **postoperative aural cavities,** and **otomycosis**[1]	**Adult:** instill 3–4 drops tid or qid **Child:** instill 2–3 drops tid or qid

ADMINISTRATION/DOSAGE ADJUSTMENTS

Instillation of drops	Thoroughly cleanse and dry affected ear with sterile cotton applicator; drops should be instilled with affected ear turned upward; this position should be maintained for a few minutes
Perforated eardrum	To induce flow into the middle ear, apply gentle intermittent pressure on the tragus
Saturation technique	Saturate gauze or cotton wick with solution and leave in canal for 24–48 h, keeping the wick moist by adding a few drops of solution, as required

CONTRAINDICATIONS

Hypersensitivity to polymyxin B

WARNINGS/PRECAUTIONS

Loss of antibiotic potency	Caution patients who prefer to warm the medication before use to avoid heating it above body temperature
Superinfection	Overgrowth of nonsusceptible organisms may occur with prolonged use; take appropriate measures
Middle-ear infections	Sterilize dropper or other applicator before each use; take measures to prevent contamination of dropper or solution

ADVERSE REACTIONS

Hypersensitivity	May occur; discontinue use

Use in children

See INDICATIONS

Use in pregnancy or nursing mothers

General guidelines not established

[1]Possibly effective

CHLOROMYCETIN OTIC (Chloramphenicol) Parke-Davis

Otic drops: 5 mg/ml (15 ml)

INDICATIONS	TOPICAL DOSAGE
Superficial infections of the external auditory canal caused by susceptible strains of *Staphylococcus aureus, Escherichia coli, Hemophilus influenzae, Pseudomonas aeruginosa, Aerobacter aerogenes, Klebsiella pneumoniae*, and *Proteus*	**Adult:** instill 2–3 drops into the ear bid or tid **Child:** same as adult

CONTRAINDICATIONS

Hypersensitivity to chloramphenicol

WARNINGS/PRECAUTIONS

Hypersensitivity reactions	Including bone-marrow hypoplasia, may occur with prolonged or frequent intermittent use; discontinue medication
Superinfection	Overgrowth of nonsusceptible organisms, including fungi, may occur; discontinue use and institute appropriate therapeutic measures
Appropriate systemic therapy	Should supplement topical therapy in all except very superficial infections

ADVERSE REACTIONS

Hypersensitivity	Local irritation with itching, burning, angioneurotic edema, urticaria, vesicular and maculopapular dermatitis

Use in children	Use in pregnancy or nursing mothers
See INDICATIONS	General guidelines not established

COLY-MYCIN S OTIC (Colistin sulfate, neomycin sulfate, thonzonium bromide, and hydrocortisone acetate) Parke-Davis

Otic drops: 3 mg colistin sulfate, 3.3 mg neomycin sulfate, 0.5 mg thonzonium bromide, and 10 mg (1%) hydrocortisone acetate per ml (5, 10 ml)

INDICATIONS	TOPICAL DOSAGE
Superficial bacterial infections of the external auditory canal caused by susceptible organisms, notably *Pseudomonas aeruginosa, Escherichia coli, Klebsiella-Aerobacter, Staphylococcus aureus,* and *Proteus*	**Adult:** instill 4 drops into the affected ear tid or qid for no more than 10 days **Child:** instill 3 drops into the affected ear tid or qid for no more than 10 days

ADMINISTRATION/DOSAGE ADJUSTMENTS

Instillation of drops	Drops should be instilled with patient lying down with affected ear turned upward; this position should be maintained for 5 min after instillation. Repeat, if necessary, for opposite ear.
Alternative technique using a cotton wick	Insert a cotton wick saturated with medication into the ear canal; add more solution q4h to keep wick moist. Replace wick at least once every 24 h.

CONTRAINDICATIONS

Hypersensitivity to any component● | Herpes simplex infection● | Vaccinia or varicella●

WARNINGS/PRECAUTIONS

Loss of antibiotic potency	Caution patients who prefer to warm the medication before use to avoid heating it above body temperature
Superinfection	Overgrowth of nonsusceptible organisms, including fungi, may occur; if infection does not improve after 1 wk, repeat culture and susceptibility tests to determine whether therapy should be changed
Sensitization or irritation	May occur; discontinue medication promptly
Ototoxicity	May occur; use with caution in patients with perforated eardrum or long-standing chronic otitis media
Allergic cross-reactions	May occur; thus precluding future use of kanamycin, paromomycin, streptomycin, and possibly gentamicin

ADVERSE REACTIONS

Dermatological	Cutaneous sensitization

Use in children	Use in pregnancy or nursing mothers
See INDICATIONS	General guidelines not established

CORTISPORIN OTIC Solution (Polymyxin B sulfate, neomycin sulfate, and hydrocortisone)

Burroughs Wellcome

Sol: 10,000 units polymyxin B sulfate, 5 mg neomycin sulfate, and 10 mg hydrocortisone per ml (10 ml)

INDICATIONS	TOPICAL DOSAGE
Superficial bacterial infections of the external auditory canal caused by susceptible organisms	**Adult:** instill 4 drops into affected ear(s) tid or qid **Child, infant:** instill 3 drops into affected ear(s) tid or qid

CORTISPORIN OTIC Suspension (Polymyxin B sulfate, neomycin sulfate, and hydrocortisone)

Burroughs Wellcome

Susp: 10,000 units polymyxin B sulfate, 5 mg neomycin sulfate, and 10 mg hydrocortisone per ml (10 ml)

INDICATIONS	TOPICAL DOSAGE
Superficial bacterial infections of the external auditory canal caused by susceptible organisms **Infections of mastoidectomy and fenestration cavities** caused by susceptible organisms	**Adult:** instill 4 drops into affected ear(s) tid or qid **Child, infant:** instill 3 drops into affected ear(s) tid or qid

ADMINISTRATION/DOSAGE ADJUSTMENTS

Instillation	Thoroughly clean auditory canal; patient should lie with affected ear upward and maintain position for 5 minutes after drops are instilled. Caution patient to avoid contaminating dropper. If preferred, a saturated cotton wick may be used. Moisten wick every 4 h and replace after 24 h.
Warm medication	If preferred, do not heat above body temperature to avoid loss of potency
Duration of treatment	Do not administer for longer than 10 days

CONTRAINDICATIONS

Hypersensitivity to any component● Herpes simplex● Vaccinia●

Varicella●

WARNINGS/PRECAUTIONS

Superinfection	Overgrowth of nonsusceptible organisms, including fungi, may occur with prolonged use. Institute appropriate anti-infective therapy and repeat cultures and susceptibility tests if superinfection does not improve after 1 wk.
Neomycin sensitization	May occur with prolonged use, especially during treatment of chronic dermatoses; discontinue medication if low-grade reddening with swelling, dry scaling, or itching occurs, and do not use neomycin-containing products thereafter
Allergic cross-reactions	May occur and may preclude future administration of kanamycin, paromomycin, streptomycin, and possibly gentamicin
Ototoxicity	May occur; use solution with caution when integrity of tympanic membrane is in question. Use suspension with caution in cases of perforated eardrum and in long-standing cases of chronic otitis media.

ADVERSE REACTIONS

Local	Stinging and burning if drug reaches middle ear (with use of solution); cutaneous sensitization (due to neomycin component)

Use in children

See INDICATIONS

Use in pregnancy or nursing mothers

General guidelines not established

LIDOSPORIN Otic Solution (Polymyxin B sulfate and lidocaine hydrochloride) Burroughs Wellcome

Otic drops: 10,000 units polymyxin B sulfate, and 50 mg lidocaine hydrochloride per ml (10 ml)

INDICATIONS	TOPICAL DOSAGE
Infection, pain, and itching associated with **otitis** and **furunculosis**[1]	**Adult:** instill 3–4 drops into infected ear tid or qid **Child:** instill 2–3 drops into infected ear tid or qid

ADMINISTRATION/DOSAGE ADJUSTMENTS

Instillation of drops	Drops should be instilled with affected ear turned upward; this position should be maintained for a few minutes
Perforated eardrum	To induce flow into the middle ear, apply gentle intermittent pressure on the tragus
Saturation technique	Saturate gauze or cotton wick with solution and leave in ear canal for 24–48 h, keeping the wick moist by adding a few drops of solution, as required

CONTRAINDICATIONS

Hypersensitivity to polymyxin B or lidocaine

WARNINGS/PRECAUTIONS

Loss of antibiotic potency	Caution patients who prefer to warm the medication before use to avoid heating it above body temperature
Long-term safety	Has been established for repeated or prolonged uninterrupted use
Superinfection	Overgrowth of nonsusceptible organisms may occur with prolonged use; take appropriate measures
Middle-ear infections	Sterilize dropper or other applicator before each use; take measures to prevent contamination of dropper or solution

ADVERSE REACTIONS

Hypersensitivity	May occur; discontinue use

Use in children	Use in pregnancy or nursing mothers
See INDICATIONS	General guidelines not established

[1]Possibly effective

OTOBIONE Otic Suspension (Neomycin sulfate, polymyxin B sulfate, and hydrocortisone) **Schering**

Otic drops: 5 mg neomycin sulfate (equivalent to 3.5 mg neomycin), 10,000 units polymyxin B sulfate, and 10 mg hydrocortisone per ml (5 ml)

INDICATIONS	TOPICAL DOSAGE
Superficial bacterial infections of the external auditory canal caused by susceptible organisms **Infections of mastoidectomy and fenestration cavities** caused by susceptible organisms	**Adult:** instill 4 drops into affected ear tid or qid for no more than 10 days **Child:** instill 3 drops into affected ear tid or qid for no more than 10 days

ADMINISTRATION/DOSAGE ADJUSTMENTS

Instillation of drops	Thoroughly cleanse and dry the affected ear; drops should be instilled with affected ear turned upward; this position should be maintained for 5 min after instillation. Repeat, if necessary, for the opposite ear. To preserve sterility of solution, do not allow dropper to touch affected area, fingers, or any other surface.
Alternative technique using a cotton wick	Insert a cotton wick saturated with medication into the ear canal; add more solution q4h to keep wick moist. Replace wick at least once every 24 h.

CONTRAINDICATIONS

Hypersensitivity to neomycin, polymyxin B, or hydrocortisone ●	Herpes simplex infection ●	Vaccinia or varicella ●

WARNINGS/PRECAUTIONS

Loss of antibiotic potency	Caution patients who prefer to warm the medication before use to avoid heating it above body temperature
Superinfection	Overgrowth of nonsusceptible organisms, including fungi, may occur; if infection does not improve after 1 wk, repeat culture and susceptibility tests to determine whether therapy should be changed
Sensitization or irritation	May occur; discontinue use promptly
Ototoxicity	May occur; use with caution in patients with perforated eardrum or long-standing chronic otitis media
Allergic cross-reactions	May occur, thus precluding future use of kanamycin, paromomycin, streptomycin, and possibly gentamicin

ADVERSE REACTIONS

Dermatological	Cutaneous sensitization

Use in children

See INDICATIONS

Use in pregnancy or nursing mothers

General guidelines not established

VōSoL HC Otic Solution (Hydrocortisone and acetic acid) **Wallace**

Otic drops: 1% hydrocortisone and 2% acetic acid (10 ml)

INDICATIONS	TOPICAL DOSAGE
Superficial infections, complicated by inflammation, of the external auditory canal caused by susceptible organisms	**Adult:** saturate a cotton wick and place in ear; keep wick moist for 24 h by occasionally adding a few drops; thereafter, remove wick and instill 5 drops tid or qid **Child:** same as adult

ADMINISTRATION/DOSAGE ADJUSTMENTS

Prevention of infection in unaffected ear	During treatment, instill acetic acid into unaffected ear tid

CONTRAINDICATIONS

Hypersensitivity to hydrocortisone or acetic acid ●	Perforated tympanic membrane ●	Vaccinia or varicella ●

WARNINGS/PRECAUTIONS

Sensitization or irritation	May occur; discontinue medication promptly
Systemic side effects	May occur with extensive use

ADVERSE REACTIONS

Hypersensitivity	May occur; discontinue use

Use in children

General guidelines not established

Use in pregnancy or nursing mothers

Safe use of topical steroids in pregnant women has not been established; do not use for extended period during pregnancy. General guidelines not established for use in nursing mothers.

VōSoL Otic Solution (Acetic acid) **Wallace**

Otic drops: 2% (15, 30 ml)

INDICATIONS	TOPICAL DOSAGE
Superficial infections of the external auditory canal caused by susceptible organisms	**Adult:** saturate a cotton wick and place in ear; keep wick moist for 24 h by occasionally adding a few drops; thereafter, remove wick and instill 5 drops tid or qid **Child:** same as adult
Prevention of otitis externa in swimmers and other susceptible individuals[1]	**Adult:** instill 2 drops bid, in AM and PM **Child:** same as adult

ADMINISTRATION/DOSAGE ADJUSTMENTS

Prevention of infection in unaffected ear	During treatment, instill acetic acid into unaffected ear tid

CONTRAINDICATIONS

Hypersensitivity to acetic acid ●	Perforated tympanic membrane ●

WARNINGS/PRECAUTIONS

Sensitization or irritation	May occur; discontinue medication promptly

ADVERSE REACTIONS

Hypersensitivity	May occur; discontinue use

Use in children

General guidelines not established

Use in pregnancy or nursing mothers

General guidelines not established

[1]Possibly effective

AMERICAINE-OTIC (Benzocaine) **American Critical Care**

Drops: 20% benzocaine

INDICATIONS	TOPICAL DOSAGE
Pain and pruritus of acute congestive and serous otitis media, acute swimmer's ear, and otitis externa	**Adult:** after ear has been cleaned with solution-saturated swab, instill 4–5 drops warm solution along side of ear canal (to prevent air pocket) and insert cotton pledget in meatus; patient should be laid on side with affected ear up and should remain in this position for several minutes after instillation of drops **Child (1–12 yr):** same as adult

CONTRAINDICATIONS

None

WARNINGS/PRECAUTIONS

Sensitivity	May occur; discontinue use
Fulminating middle-ear infection	Symptoms may be masked by indiscriminate use of anesthetic ear drops

ADVERSE REACTIONS

Hypersensitivity	May occur; discontinue use

Use in children	Use in pregnancy or nursing mothers
See INDICATIONS; contraindicated for use in infants under 1 yr of age	General guidelines not established

AURALGAN Otic Solution (Antipyrine and benzocaine) **Ayerst**

Drops: 54 mg antipyrine and 14 mg benzocaine per ml

INDICATIONS	TOPICAL DOSAGE
Pain and inflammation of acute congestive and serous otitis media **As an adjunct to systemic antibiotics for resolution of acute otitis media**	**Adult:** instill solution, permitting it to run along wall of ear canal until filled, and insert cotton pledget moistened with solution into meatus; repeat q1–2h until pain and congestion are relieved **Child:** same as adult
Removal of cerumen	**Adult:** instill solution and insert cotton pledget moistened with solution into meatus tid for 2–3 days **Child:** same as adult

CONTRAINDICATIONS

Spontaneous perforation or discharge ●	Hypersensitivity to components or related substances ●

WARNINGS/PRECAUTIONS

See CONTRAINDICATIONS

ADVERSE REACTIONS

Hypersensitivity	May occur; discontinue use

Use in children	Use in pregnancy or nursing mothers
See INDICATIONS	General guidelines not established

TYMPAGESIC (Phenylephrine hydrochloride, antipyrine, and benzocaine) Warren-Teed

Drops: 0.25% phenylephrine hydrochloride, 5% antipyrine, and 5% benzocaine

INDICATIONS	TOPICAL DOSAGE
Pain and inflammation of acute nonsuppurative otitis media and/or otitis externa	**Adult:** fill ear canal with solution and plug with cotton; may be repeated q4h, as needed **Child:** same as adult

CONTRAINDICATIONS

Hypersensitivity to benzocaine

WARNINGS/PRECAUTIONS

(see CONTRAINDICATIONS)

ADVERSE REACTIONS

Dermatological——— Dermatitis (rare)

Use in children

See INDICATIONS

Use in pregnancy or nursing mothers

General guidelines not established

CERUMENEX Drops (Triethanolamine polypeptide oleate-condensate) **Purdue Frederick**

Drops: 10% triethanolamine polypeptide oleate-condensate (8, 15 ml)

INDICATIONS	TOPICAL DOSAGE
Removal of cerumen **Removal of impacted cerumen** prior to ear examination, otologic therapy, or audiometry	**Adult:** fill ear canal with solution with patient's head tilted at a 45° angle and insert cotton plug for 30 min; *gently* flush ear with lukewarm water, using a soft rubber syringe; for unusually hard impactions, procedure may be repeated **Child:** same as above

CONTRAINDICATIONS

Previous untoward reaction to triethanolamine polypeptide oleate-condensate●	Positive patch test (see WARNINGS/PRECAUTIONS)●	Perforated ear drum or otitis media (relative contraindication)●

WARNINGS/PRECAUTIONS

Dermatological idiosyncrasies or history of allergic reactions	Use with extreme caution in known cases of idiosyncratic or allergic skin reactions. In doubtful cases, perform patch test by placing a drop of solution on flexor surface of arm or forearm and covering it with a small bandage strip; positive reaction 24 h later indicates probability of an allergic reaction following instillation in ear (see CONTRAINDICATIONS)
Duration of exposure	Ear canal should not be exposed to solution for more than 15–30 min
Contact with periaural skin	Should be avoided; if such undue exposure occurs, wash area with soap and water
External otitis	Use with caution
Local reactions	Occur in 1% of patients; reaction generally lasts for 2–10 days and clears with no residual complications. Treatment in mild cases is symptomatic and may include anti-inflammatory agents, when indicated.
Patient instructions	Advise patients not to exceed time of exposure, not to use drops more frequently than directed, and to discontinue use and consult physician if adverse reaction occurs

ADVERSE REACTIONS	Frequent reactions are italicized
Dermatological	*Local dermatitis, ranging from mild erythema and pruritis of external canal to a severe eczematoid reaction involving external ear and periauricular tissue (1%)*

Use in children	**Use in pregnancy or nursing mothers**
See INDICATIONS	General guidelines not established

DEBROX Drops (Carbamide peroxide) **Marion**

Drops: 6.5% carbamide peroxide

INDICATIONS	TOPICAL DOSAGE
Removal of cerumen	**Adult:** instill 5–10 drops into ear canal, with patient's head tilted to the side, and allow drops to remain in ear for several minutes; repeat bid for at least 3–4 days; any remaining wax may be removed by flushing with warm water, using a soft rubber bulb syringe

CONTRAINDICATIONS

None

WARNINGS/PRECAUTIONS

Eye irritant	Use with caution to avoid contact of solution with eyes
Persistent ear symptoms	Patient is advised to seek medical attention if redness, irritation, swelling, or pain persists or increases

ADVERSE REACTIONS

Hypersensitivity	May occur; discontinue use

Use in children	**Use in pregnancy or nursing mothers**
See INDICATIONS	General guidelines not established

Dental and Oral Problems

Dental problems are hardly new—mankind has been plagued by dental caries (tooth decay) since at least the Stone Age. The Babylonians recorded their toothache remedies some 7,000 years ago, and the early Egyptian physicians prescribed special mouthwashes for gums with what is now called periodontal disease. This section will discuss modern approaches to dental disease and other common oral problems.

DENTAL PLAQUE

Dental plaque, a sticky, colorless film of bacteria that forms on all teeth, especially around the gum line, can lead to both caries and periodontal disease. All of us develop plaque, but if it is allowed to accumulate and seep (infiltrate) under the gums, it hardens to form dental tartar. This substance is rough and porous, forming a protected environment in which the bacteria grow and multiply.

The bacteria in plaque thrive on sugar, which they convert to enamel-dissolving acids. As plaque and tartar increase, so do the bacteria, forming even more acid, which is retained in intimate contact with tooth surface. The tartar can be removed only by cleaning and scaling by a dentist or dental hygienist.

PREVENTIVE DENTISTRY

Modern preventive dentistry emphasizes the daily removal of plaque through proper flossing and brushing techniques (see illustration). A number of dental aids, such as various types of brushes, disclosing dyes and lights to make the plaque visible, picks, and water jets are available to promote effective plaque control, but a dentist or dental hygienist is generally the best guide as to what is best for individual oral problems.

In addition to regular home care and dental checkups, fluoridation of water is a powerful weapon against tooth decay. Studies have found that fluoridation can prevent up to 60 percent of caries. A recent study of elementary schoolchildren in a fluoride-deficient area found that a daily fluoride tablet, weekly use of a fluoride solution as a mouthrinse, and daily brushing with a toothpaste containing fluoride reduced decay between the teeth (the worst kind) by 85 percent. Even in areas where water is fluoridated, however, fluoride toothpaste can add further protection against caries.

Another useful measure is the application of a plastic sealant to the pits and cracks of the chewing surfaces of the back teeth. This sealant, which is

THE CORRECT WAY TO FLOSS AND BRUSH THE TEETH

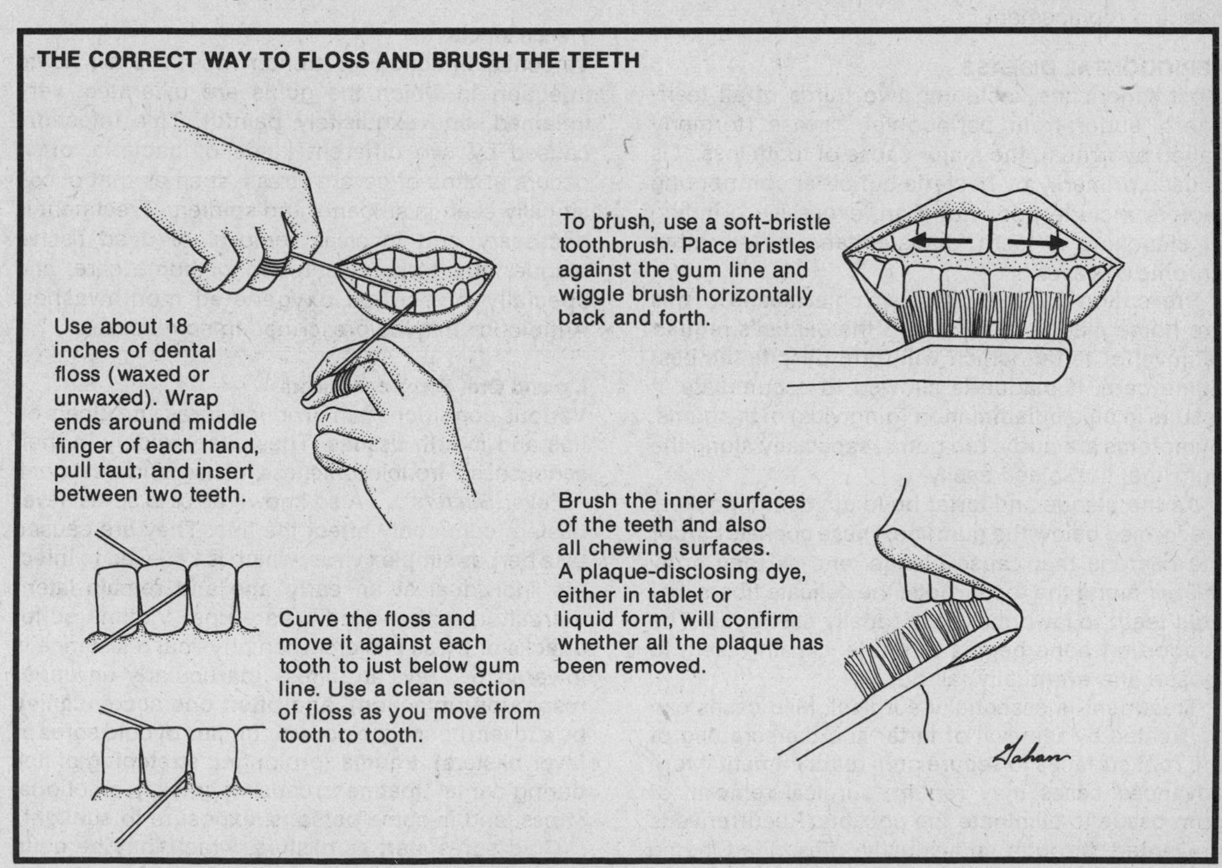

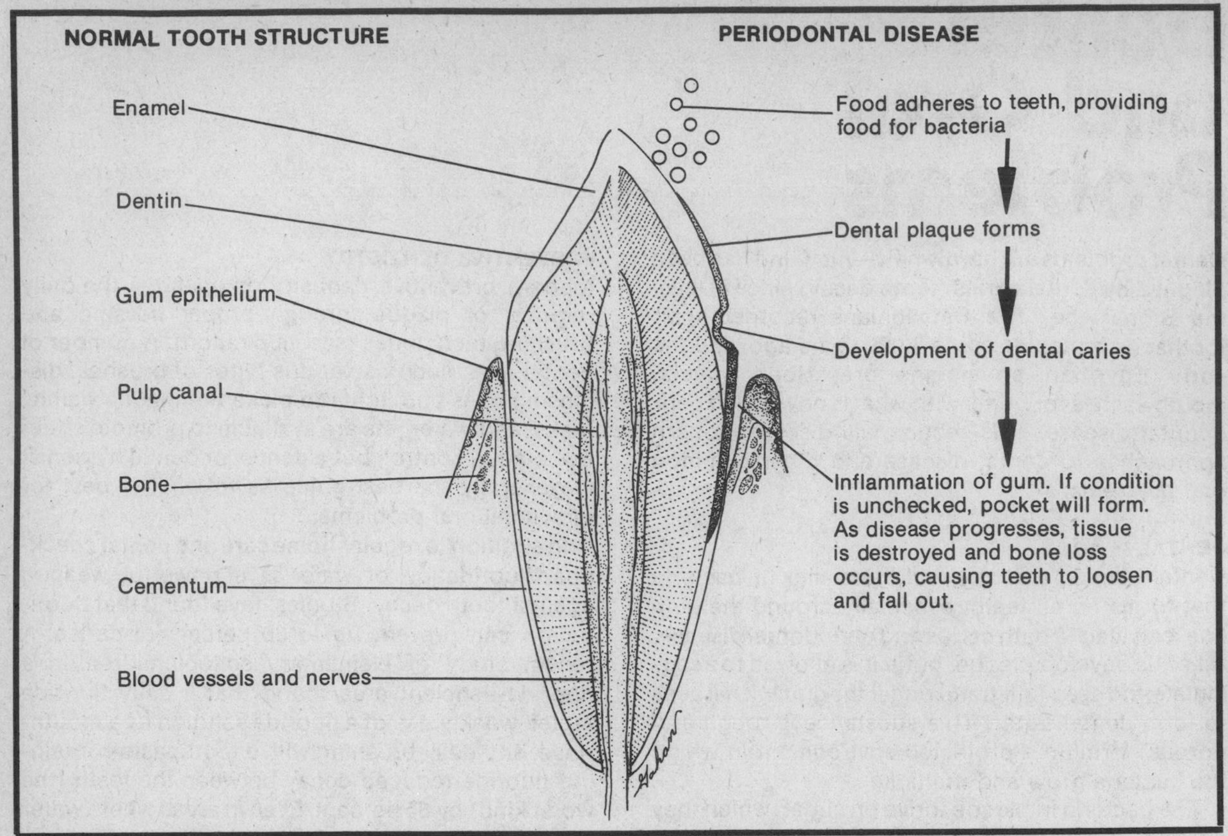

applied by either painting or spraying, has been shown to reduce decay on the first molars of six- to eight-year-old children from 53 percent to 8 percent. Such sealants can last for up to three years before needing replacement.

PERIODONTAL DISEASE

Most Americans, including two thirds of all teenagers, suffer from periodontal disease (formerly called pyorrhea), the major cause of tooth loss. It is caused primarily by bacteria but other contributing factors include poor nutrition, excessive grinding or clenching of teeth, diabetes, and certain other chronic diseases.

Prevention is the key: The two chief means for this are home plaque removal and the dentist's regular removal of tartar, which will form despite the best home care. If plaque is allowed to accumulate, it results in mild inflammation (gingivitis) of the gums. Symptoms are puffy, red gums, especially along the gum line, that bleed easily.

As the plaque and tartar build up, dental pockets are formed below the gum line. These pockets harbor the bacteria that cause plaque, and as they grow deeper along the tooth roots, the delicate fibers that hold teeth to jawbone are gradually destroyed. The supporting bone begins to erode, causing teeth to loosen and eventually fall out.

Treatment is essentially surgical. Mild cases can be treated by removal of tartar and the scraping of the root surfaces to secure gum reattachment. More advanced cases may require surgical removal of gum tissue to eliminate the pockets. Recurrence is prevented through individually prescribed home care methods, similar to those used for daily removal of plaque, but more extensive.

MISCELLANEOUS ORAL DISEASES

Trench Mouth

Vincent's infection or trench mouth is an acute infection in which the gums are ulcerated, very inflamed, and exquisitely painful. This infection, caused by two different kinds of bacteria, often occurs at time of severe stress, such as that occasionally seen in students and soldiers. Treatment is necessary and involves removal of dead tissue, plaque, and tartar; institution of home care; and specially prescribed oxygenated mouthwashes. Antibiotics may be prescribed in some cases.

Lip and Oral Sores and Ulcers

Various conditions can produce sores and ulcers on lips and mouth tissues. These vary widely in their seriousness, troublesomeness, cause, and treatment.

Fever Blisters Also known as cold sores, fever blisters commonly affect the lips. They are caused by a herpes simplex virus, which is believed to infect the individual at an early age and remain latent thereafter, with periodic flare-ups. Victims suffer attacks of these blisters when physical resistance is lowered by, say, an illness (particularly an upper respiratory infection), and often one accompanied by a fever (hence the popular names of cold sores or fever blisters), trauma (prolonged stretching of lips during dental treatment, causing cracks), emotional stress, and in some persons, exposure to sunlight.

Cold sores start as blisters, which may be quite

sore, surrounded by some swelling. In a day or two the blister breaks and the resulting ulcer develops a yellowish scab. The condition usually heals by itself within a week or two, with no scarring. Fever blisters usually appear at the outside edges of the lip and often recur in the same spot at variable intervals (commonly ranging from once a month to once a year). The condition tends to run in families and is not curable. A mild anesthetic ointment, such as one containing benzocaine (Anbesol, Orajel, or various other brands) may be recommended to relieve the pain. A lubricating ointment to keep the crust soft and prevent painful cracking also may be helpful. Antibiotics are not used unless there is a secondary bacterial infection.

Canker Sores Canker sores, whose medical name is aphthous ulcers, are round or oval, often painful, mouth ulcers ranging in size from an eighth of an inch to an inch and a quarter. These can appear either singly or in clusters, usually healing in a week or two without scarring. They affect 20 to 50 percent of the population and women are twice as likely as men to have them. Recurrences are variable; while some people have one or two a year, others may have them almost continuously.

Although their cause is unknown, canker sores do tend to run in families but are not contagious. They often appear after physical or emotional stress (in students during examination periods, for example) or trauma (for instance, a scratch from some hard food or a toothbrush bristle). Food allergies may also be a factor; some people invariably develop the ulcers after eating certain foods. Many women suffer flare-ups during menstrual periods or, more rarely, during pregnancy.

Treatment depends on the seriousness of the problem. For an occasional canker sore, a physician or dentist may use cauterization (often with silver nitrate), a protective paste, or an anesthetic paste such as those containing benzocaine. Severe or lasting attacks may be treated with prescriptions of steroids or tetracycline antibiotics.

BAD BREATH

Bad breath that has no obvious cause, such as eating onions or garlic, may be due to a number of conditions, usually periodontal disease or poor oral hygiene. It may also be due to general systemic conditions such as nutritional deficiencies, diabetes, and certain blood disorders. Therefore, persistent bad breath that is not cleared up by regular and proper dental hygiene is a clue to consult a physician or dentist.

Mouthwashes are merely oral cosmetics, unless they are specially prescribed by physician or dentist. They provide a pleasant feeling or taste and can temporarily make breath smell better. The mouth normally contains useful bacteria, and therefore any general-purpose mouthwash should not be intended to "clear the mouth of germs." Antiseptics are of little value for the normal mouth—they may lower the bacterial count temporarily, but it will return to the original level within a few hours.

SPECIAL PRECAUTIONS

Any unexplained sore that appears in the mouth or on the lips should be regarded with suspicion, especially if it fails to heal in a few days. In these cases, it is prudent to consult a physician or dentist to rule out the possibility of oral cancer or other disease that may manifest itself with mouth sores or ulcers.

IN CONCLUSION

Dental caries are virtually universal, while periodontal disease affects more than two thirds of the adult population. Preventive measures based on good oral hygiene can prevent many if not most of these problems. Other common oral problems include cold sores, fever blisters, bad breath, and other miscellaneous complaints. The following drug charts cover the nonprescription products for various mouth sores, as well as mouthwashes. Toothpastes and powders are not included; labels on these products will indicate whether they contain fluoride or are special formulations for pain-sensitive teeth.

Product	Ingredients	Actions
Anbesol (Whitehall) **Dosage** Apply freely to affected area	Benzocaine	Anesthetic
	Iodine	Antiseptic
	Glycerin	Soothing agent
	40% Alcohol	Antiseptic
Baby Orajel (Commerce) **Dosage** Apply small amount with fingertip or cotton applicator on affected area	Benzocaine	Anesthetic
	Viscous water-soluble base	
Benzodent (Vicks) **Dosage** Apply to inner surface of dentures; squeeze ¼-inch strips in area corresponding to sore spots	20% Benzocaine	Anesthetic
	0.4% Eugenol	Anesthetic and antiseptic
	0.1 Hydroxyquinoline sulfate	Antiseptic
	Denture adhesive-like base	
Betadine Mouthwash/Gargle (Purdue Frederick) **Dosage** Can be diluted with 2 parts water or used full strength as a mouthwash, gargle, or rinse	0.5% Povidone-iodine	Antiseptic
	8.8% Alcohol	Antiseptic
Blistex Ointment (Blistex) **Dosage** Apply to cold sore as needed	0.4% Phenol	Antiseptic
	1% Camphor	Anesthetic and antiseptic
	Ammonia	Counterirritant
	Mineral oil	Emollient
	Lanolin	Emollient
	Petrolatum	Emollient
	Paraffin	Emollient
	Sodium borate	Antiseptic, detergent, and astringent
	Alcohol	Antiseptic
	Peppermint oil	Flavor
	Ammonium carbonate	Counterirritant
	Beeswax	Ointment base hardener
	Polyglyceryl-3	Soothing agent, cream base
	Diisostearate	Dispersing agent
	Fragrance	

Table continued on following page

Product	Ingredients	Actions
Cold Sore Lotion (Pfeiffer) **Dosage** Apply to the lips 2 times daily or as needed	3.6% Camphor	Anesthetic and antiseptic
	4.2% Gum benzoin	Topical protectant
	0.3% Phenol	Antiseptic and anesthetic
	0.3% Menthol	Anesthetic and antiseptic
	85% Alcohol	Antiseptic
	Thymol	Antiseptic
	Peruvian balsam	Protectant
Kank-a (Blistex) **Dosage** Apply to cold sore as neeeded	Alcohol	Antiseptic
	Myrrh	Astringent
	Benzoin storax	Soothing agent
	Balsa tolu	Antiseptic and flavor
	Aloe	Soothing agent
Numzident (Purepac) **Dosage** Apply with cotton directly to affected gum area	Benzocaine	Anesthetic
	Eugenol	Anesthetic and antiseptic
	Peppermint oil	Flavor
	Polyethylene glycol-like base	
Numzit (Purepac) **Dosage** Apply with fingertip directly to affected gum area	Glycerin	Soothing agent
	10% Alcohol	Antiseptic
	Gel vehicle	
Orabase Plain (Hoyt) **Dosage** Press small dabs into place until affected area is coated with thin film of paste	Pectin	Protectant
	Gelatin	Suspending agent
	Carboxymethylcellulose sodium	Suspending agent
	Polyethylene glycol	Soothing agent
	Mineral oil	Emollient
Orabase with Benzocaine (Hoyt) **Dosage** Press small dabs into place until affected area is coated with thin film of paste	Benzocaine	Anesthetic
	Pectin	Protectant
	Gelatin	Suspending agent
	Carboxymethylcellulose sodium	Suspending agent
	Polyethylene glycol	Soothing agent
	Mineral oil	Emollient

Table continued on following page

Product	Ingredients	Actions
Orajel (Commerce) **Dosage** Squeeze small amount directly into cavity and around gum surrounding the teeth	Benzocaine	Anesthetic
	Polyethylene glycol-like base	
Orajel-D (Commerce) **Dosage** Clean and dry denture. Apply directly to gums and portions of denture which come into contact with gum areas that are tender, sore, or painful. Repeat when necessary	Benzocaine	Anesthetic
	Clove oil	Anesthetic
	Benzyl alcohol	Anesthetic and antiseptic
	Adhesive base	
Tanac (Commerce) **Dosage** Apply full strength to affected area as needed	Benzalkonium chloride	Antiseptic
	Tannic acid	Astringent
Toothache Drops (DeWitt) **Dosage** For tooth cavities only—insert one cotton pellet into cavity with applicator, which is attached to cap	5.01% Benzocaine	Anesthetic
	9.98% Clove oil	Anesthetic and antiseptic
	4.83% Beechwood creosote	Anesthetic
	20% Alcohol	Antiseptic
	Flexible collodion base	

Product	Ingredients	Actions
Cepacol (Merrell-National) **Dosage** Rinse mouth thoroughly whenever desired or as directed by physician or dentist	14% Alcohol	Antiseptic
	1:2000 Cetylpyridinium chloride	Antiseptic
	Phosphate buffer	Protectorant
	Fragrance	
Cepastat (Merrell-National) **Dosage** Gargle for not more than 15 seconds, then expel. Repeat every 2 hours as needed	1.4% Phenol	Anesthetic and antiseptic
	Eugenol	Flavor and anesthetic
	Menthol	Flavor, anesthetic, and antiseptic
	Glycerin	Soothing agent
Cherry Chloraseptic Mouthwash and Gargle (Norwich-Eaton) **Dosage** *Minor sore throat irritations and sore throat due to colds:* Use full strength. Spray 5 times (children 6–12 years, spray 3 times) and swallow. Repeat every 2 hours if necessary. Or use full strength—gargle deeply *Minor mouth and gum irritations:* Use full strength. Rinse affected area for 15 seconds, then expel remainder. Repeat every 2 hours if necessary *Daily deodorizing mouthwash and gargle:* Spray full strength or dilute with equal parts of water and rinse thoroughly, then expel remainder	1.4% Phenol	Antiseptic
	Sodium phenolate	Antiseptic and anesthetic
Cloraseptic Mouthwash (Norwich-Eaton) **Dosage** Same as for Cherry Chloraseptic	1.4% Phenol	Antiseptic
	Sodium phenolate	Antiseptic and anesthetic
Fluorigard (Colgate-Palmolive) **Dosage** Use 2 tsp, rinse, then expel, once daily after thoroughly brushing teeth	0.05% Sodium fluoride	Prevents dental caries
Greenmint Mouthwash (Block) **Dosage** May be used full strength or diluted	Alcohol	Antiseptic
	Chlorophyll	Reduces odor
	Sorbitol	Sweetener
	Surfactant	Detergent
	Flavors	

Table continued on following page

Product	Ingredients	Actions
Lavoris (Vicks) **Dosage** Use in morning and evening, and before social engagements	Alcohol	Antiseptic
	Clove oil	Anesthetic and antiseptic
	Zinc chloride	Astringent
	Glycerin	Soothing agent
	Polysorbate 80	Emulsifier and dispersing agent
	Citric acid	Acidifier
	Polaxamer 407	Detergent
	Flavors	
Listerine (Warner-Lambert) **Dosage** Use 2/3 oz for 30 seconds, morning and night	Alcohol	Antiseptic
	Benzoic acid	
	Menthol	Anesthetic and antiseptic
	Methyl salicylate	Flavor
	Eucalyptol	Flavor
	Thymol	Antiseptic
	Polaxamer 407	Detergent
	Caramel	Coloring agent
Oral Pentacresol (Upjohn) **Dosage** Dilute with 1 to 3 parts water for mouthwash, gargle, or throat spray, 2 to 3 parts for nasal douche. Do not use for more than 2 days, or for children under 3 years of age, unless directed by physician or dentist	1 mg/ml Secondary amyltricresols	Antiseptic
	30% Alcohol	Antiseptic
	8.61 mg/ml Sodium chloride	Unspecified
	0.33 mg/ml Calcium chloride	Unspecified
	0.299 mg/ml Potassium chloride	Unspecified
Scope (Procter & Gamble) **Dosage** Use 1 oz for 20 seconds, after meals or whenever desired	Cetylpyridinium chloride	Antiseptic
	0.005% Domiphen bromide	Antiseptic
	18.5% Alcohol	Antiseptic
	Glycerin	Soothing agent
	Saccharin	Sweetener
	Polysorbate 80	Emulsifier and denaturant
	Flavor	

Gastrointestinal Disorders

Heartburn, Indigestion, and Ulcers,

Everything that we eat travels the same twenty-five to thirty feet of the gastrointestinal tract during the digestive processes. This gastrointestinal (GI) tract, also called the alimentary tract or canal, extends from the top of the esophaghus to the anus. This section will discuss common problems affecting the upper part of the gastrointestinal tract, while problems affecting the lower portions are covered in the following sections of this chapter.

ANATOMICAL OVERVIEW

The GI tract is lined throughout by mucous membrane that protects the underlying tissues from gastric acids and other substances. Twin sets of muscles, one circular and the other longitudinal, extending from the throat to the rectum, help move the food in its various stages of digestion through the GI tract. These muscles are regulated and coordinated by the autonomic nervous system, which regulates body functions not consciously controlled. The particular nerve involved in digestion is the vagus (the wanderer), which travels from the skull into the neck, branches into the larynx, whence it gives off further branches to the bronchi, heart, esophagus, stomach, and small intestine.

Because of the intimate relationship that the vagus nerve creates between the heart and the stomach, indigestion is sometimes perceived as the onset of a heart attack, or the first symptom of a heart attack may be interpreted by the victim as indigestion. Moreover, because the vagus nerve in all its ramifications is activated by emotional stress, such feelings as fear, anxiety, anger, and excited anticipation often have a devastating effect on digestion. This activation of the vagus nerve causes the churning of the stomach and the eventual release of the gastric juice containing hydrochloric acid and digestive enzymes.

While this "hyperacidity" in and of itself is not a direct cause of such disorders as heartburn, indigestion, or ulcers, gastric acid is a prominent factor in all of them.

HEARTBURN

At one time or another, practically everyone has experienced the unpleasant burning sensation in the lower esophagus commonly called heartburn. The pain occurs in the region of the heart, but is in no way related to that organ. Instead, the direct cause of the discomfort is a backflow of some of the irritating acid contents of the stomach into the lower end of the esophagus, a condition referred to as reflux esophagitis.

The esophagus, also called the gullet or food pipe, is a muscular, tubular channel approximately ten inches long that carries food from the mouth to the stomach. It extends from the pharynx through the chest and joins the stomach just below the diaphragm. Under normal circumstances, the stomach is prevented from pushing up into the chest cavity because the opening (hiatus) in the diaphragm fits snugly around the esophagus.

Causes of Heartburn

Several structural defects as well as overindulgence or stress may cause heartburn. For example, when the muscles around the opening of the esophagus become chronically weakened or stretched, some of the stomach contents may be forced back into the esophagus. This condition, known as hiatus hernia, may be caused by the chronic stress of obesity, frequent overeating, or the extra pressure of pregnancy. Chronic reflux also may be caused by a weakening of the muscular ring or sphincter at the lower end of the esophagus itself, thereby permitting an excess of acidic juices to back up into the esophagus instead of staying in the stomach.

An occasional incident of heartburn may be directly attributable to overindulgence in an unusually heavy meal, too much alcohol, or emotional upset. The discomfort, which is exacerbated by lying down, often interferes with sleep. Under these circumstances, a mild antacid before bedtime helps neutralize the acid in the reflux, thus minimizing the irritation of the esophagus.

Preventive Measures

Recurrent bouts of heartburn often can be prevented by simple, practical measures, such as losing weight if obesity is a factor; foregoing heavy meals, especially in the evening; and avoiding foods or beverages that seem to trigger an attack. Smoking also may be a contributing factor. It may prove worthwhile to keep track of particular foods or food combinations that invariably cause discomfort. Constricting belts, girdles, or excessively tight pants may exacerbate the condition, as can lying down too soon after eating. If attacks invariably occur at night, avoiding large evening meals and sleeping with the head of the bed raised may be a partial cure.

When heartburn persists as a chronic problem despite sensible self-medication with antacids and self-discipline regarding controllable causes, a physician should be consulted. If surgery is recommended—as it might be in the case of a hiatus hernia—a second opinion is a good idea.

INDIGESTION

Indigestion, also called dyspepsia, is a catchall term indicating a difficulty or faultiness in the digestive process, leading to a variety of symptoms that may include heartburn, an unpleasant taste in the mouth, belching, a feeling of heaviness in the chest, cramps, nausea, vomiting, flatulence, and diarrhea.

Causes of Indigestion

Indigestion may be caused by overloading the stomach or eating too rapidly; not chewing food properly; or eating food that is too fatty, poorly prepared, or spoiled (when in doubt, discard leftovers). Anger and stress can lead to indigestion, as can eating when body and spirit are so exhausted that no anticipatory pleasure stimulates the digestive juices. Actually, digestion begins in the mouth with proper chewing and mixing the food with saliva and other substances. The salivary glands should be stimulated by the sight, smell, and thought of an attractively prepared meal. A good appetite usually means good digestion.

In some persons, allergies to certain foods may be a factor. Often foods such as onions, curries or other hot spices, or corn on the cob may lead to indigestion. Some diseases, such as an inflamed gallbladder or systemic bacterial or viral infection, may cause an "upset stomach."

There are also a number of drugs, ranging from aspirin to medications commonly prescribed for rheumatoid arthritis, anxiety, or depression, that may cause gastrointestinal side effects, including indigestion. Some antibiotics cause nausea or vomiting; others may cause diarrhea or cramps. The cancer chemotherapy drugs often cause severe nausea and vomiting. (See the individual drug charts for listing of potential gastrointestinal side effects.) If these effects prove troublesome, they should be discussed with the prescribing physician, who can often alter the medication or take other steps to minimize the GI effects.

When the major symptom is a feeling of bloating

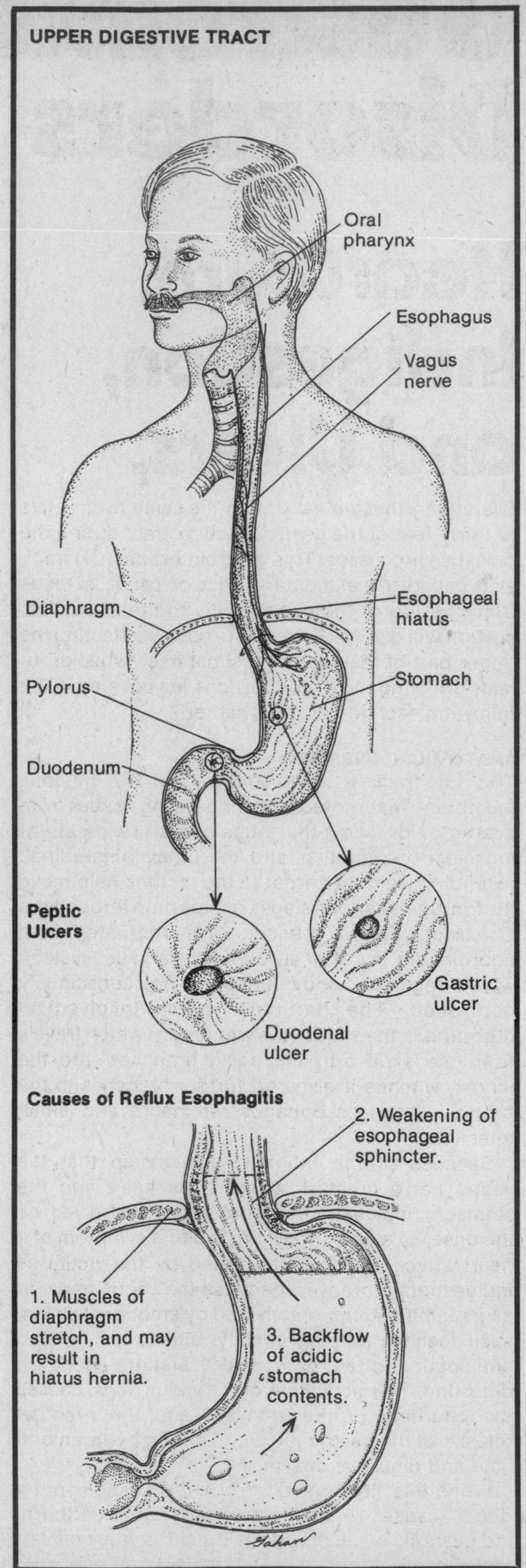

accompanied by constant belching or "gas," the problem is likely to result from swallowing air (aerophagia). Eating too quickly, inadequate chewing, stress, talking with a full mouth, chewing gum, and drinking excessive amounts of carbonated beverages are common causes of air swallowing. In addition, some people mistakenly think they are solving the problem of "gas" by inducing belching, when, in fact, this leads to swallowing even more air.

Indigestion accompanied by flatulence usually can be attributed to eating a particular food or combination of foods. A certain amount of gas is always present in the intestines as a result of the digestive process itself and the action of intestinal bacteria on certain foodstuffs. Some foods produce more gas than others—for example, beans of all kinds, including soybeans and soybean products; wheat germ and bran; and a variety of vegetables and fruits, including cabbage, broccoli, brussels sprouts, onions, and apples. If a certain food or group of foods invariably produces flatulence, avoiding these foods is an obvious solution.

Preventive Measures

An occasional bout of indigestion might be anticipated after a festive occasion involving too much food, alcohol, and excitement. Taking a mild nonprescription antacid before retiring frequently avoids problems. But chronic indigestion should not go undiagnosed, nor should one get caught up in a constant routine of unsupervised self-medication. In addition, certain gastrointestinal symptoms should alert one to see a physician. These include persistent nausea, loss of appetite, weight loss, excessive belching, burning sensations in the abdominal area, cramps, or diarrhea. Immediate medical attention is advisable if bowel movements are tarry in appearance or blood-streaked, or if stomach cramps are accompanied by a rise in temperature.

In discussing the symptoms of indigestion with a doctor over the telephone or in person, it is particularly helpful to localize the area and the nature of the discomfort, since gastrointestinal disturbances produce different kinds of pain: steady vs. intermittent; localized vs. generalized; mild vs. agonizing. What the patient describes as an attack of acute indigestion may, in fact, be the onset of a heart attack. A sharp pain seeming to emanate from the lower borders of the ribs or the bottom of the stomach may actually be a symptom of pleurisy, involving the base of a lung.

As a first step in dealing with chronic acid indigestion, review eating and drinking habits, as well as such factors as occupational or personal stress. Smoking should be stopped completely or at least reduced. Strong tea, coffee, cola beverages, and artifically carbonated beer should be rare indulgences. Cooked fruit and vegetables are less likely to cause digestive problems than raw ones. If raw fruit is eaten, it should be ripe. Discretion should be exercised about foods that are fatty or fried. If ill-fitting dentures or missing teeth cause inadequate chewing, a dental checkup should be scheduled.

ULCERS

An ulcer is any open sore that exposes the tissues below the mucous membrane or skin. While ulcers commonly occur along the gums (because of bacterial action), on varicose veins (because of inadequate blood supply), and on other surfaces, the term itself has become almost synonymous with peptic ulcers.

There are two types of peptic ulcer: gastric, which occurs in the lining of the stomach, and duodenal, which occurs in the duodenum, the first section of the small intestines. About one in every ten Americans has had a peptic ulcer at one time or another, with duodenal ulcers accounting for about 80 percent of the total. While both types come under the heading of peptic ulcers, they are now increasingly viewed as different disorders, with many underlying causes, some still unknown.

Recent research has dispelled many myths about ulcers and their treatment. Contrary to popular belief, there is no such thing as a typical ulcer patient. The disorder is increasingly common among women and is as likely to occur in a child or a housewife as in a hard-driving corporate executive. Milk is no longer looked upon as the panacea for assuaging the pain of an ulcer, and a bland diet for life is no longer considered necessary. The development of effective medication has resulted in fewer ulcer operations.

Many ulcers are asymptomatic; when symptoms do exist, they almost always involve a steady burning or gnawing pain in the area just above the navel. The pain usually sets in about two hours after eating, and may be intense enough to interrupt sleep. While milder cases may be relieved by taking an alkalizer and something to eat, it should be remembered that some ulcers give only the slightest warnings before they become medical emergencies.

While duodenal ulcers are thought to result from the excessive production of stomach acid, which leads to a breakdown in the intestinal wall membranes, gastric ulcers are caused by an inhererent weakness in the stomach wall itself. It is known, for example, that with all other variables taken into account, persons with O-type blood are more vulnerable to the disorder, and that ulcers are three times more common among blood relatives of ulcer patients than they are among the general population. It also appears that stress in and of itself does not trigger the excessive flow of gastric acid; instead, the key factor is how a particular individual responds to the stress.

Treatment of Ulcer

Peptic ulcers are treated by neutralizing the gastric (hydrochloric) acid and/or reducing its secretion. Regular use of antacids, as well as frequent small meals of foods unlikely to cause further irritation usually will accomplish the first objective. Until the latter part of the 1970s, the major antisecretory drugs used to treat peptic ulcer were the anticholinergics or antispasmodic agents, which usually contain phenobarbital, belladonna alkaloids, or similar compounds. In 1977, however, the approach to treating peptic ulcer was vastly changed by the introduction of cimetidine (Tagamet), an antisecretory drug that acts by reducing the histamine activity which promotes secretion of gastric acid. Studies have found that this drug markedly inhibits the secretion of gastric acid for about six hours. Its use may be combined with acid neutralizers or antispasmodic drugs; since the latter usually contain opiates or their derivatives and therefore may lead to problems of drug dependence, they usually are prescribed with caution.

A Word About Self-Medication

Many persons who suffer from recurrent bouts of heartburn, indigestion, or abdominal pain tend to treat themselves with a variety of nonprescription antacids. These medications often provide temporary relief—which is frequently all that is needed. If the problem is chronic, however, and accompanied by the symptoms reviewed earlier, this may be a dangerous course. In addition, certain antacids may interact with or block the action of other drugs, such as the tetracycline antibiotics. Therefore, before receiving a prescription, the patient should inform the physician of all other medications in use, including nonprescription drugs.

IN CONCLUSION

Heartburn, indigestion, and peptic ulcer are among the most common gastrointestinal disorders. In many instances, heartburn and indigestion can be controlled by altered eating habits and life-style changes, such as reducing emotional stress, especially at mealtimes. Peptic ulcer may develop into a medical emergency; therefore its symptoms, however minor, should not be ignored. It should be noted, however, that many peptic ulcers are asymptomatic, while others appear to heal without treatment.

The following charts cover the major drugs, both prescription and nonprescription, to treat these disorders. If diarrhea or nausea are among the symptoms of indigestion, specific drugs to treat these manifestations are in the sections covering these disorders.

AZULFIDINE (Sulfasalazine) Pharmacia

Tabs: 500 mg **Tabs (enteric-coated):** 500 mg

INDICATIONS	ORAL DOSAGE
Mild to moderate ulcerative colitis **Severe ulcerative colitis** (adjunctive therapy)	**Adult:** 3–4 g/day div (preferably after meals and at night) until satisfactory improvement is confirmed by endoscopic examination, then 500 mg qid for maintenance **Child:** 40–60 mg/kg/24 h in 3–6 divided doses until satisfactory improvement is confirmed by endoscopic examination, then 30 mg/kg/24 h in 4 divided doses for maintenance

ADMINISTRATION/DOSAGE ADJUSTMENTS

Unsatisfactory response with initial dose	Increase adult dosage up to 8 g/day, but consider the increased risk of toxicity
Gastric irritation with initial dose	Reduce adult dosage to 1–2 g/day to start
Gastric intolerance after first few doses	May be alleviated by distributing the total daily dose more evenly over the day or by giving enteric-coated tablets; if symptoms continue, stop treatment for 5–7 days, then reinstitute at a lower daily dose

CONTRAINDICATIONS

Hypersensitivity to sulfonamides or salicylates ●	Intestinal or urinary obstruction ●	Porphyria ●

WARNINGS/PRECAUTIONS

Blood dyscrasias	May occur and can be fatal (see ADVERSE REACTIONS); obtain frequent complete blood counts and watch for early signs (eg, sore throat, fever, pallor, purpura, jaundice) of serious blood disorders
Hypersensitivity reactions	May occur and can be fatal (see ADVERSE REACTIONS); use with caution in patients allergic to some goitrogens, diuretics, and oral hypoglycemic agents. Discontinue treatment immediately if reactions occur and do not reinstitute.
Renal damage	May occur (see ADVERSE REACTIONS); perform frequent urinalyses with careful microscopic examination
Crystalluria, urinary calculi	May be prevented by maintaining adequate fluid intake
Liver damage, irreversible neuromuscular and CNS changes, fibrosing alveolitis	May occur and can be fatal; observe patients closely during prolonged therapy. Discontinue treatment immediately if toxic reactions occur.
Hemolytic anemia	May be precipitated in patients with G6PD deficiency; reaction is dose-related
Special-risk patients	Use with caution in patients with impaired renal or hepatic function, blood dyscrasias, severe allergy, or bronchial asthma
Cross-sensitivity	May occur with goitrogens, acetazolamide, thiazide diuretics, and oral hypoglycemics

ADVERSE REACTIONS	Frequent reactions are italicized
Hematological	Agranulocytosis, aplastic anemia, thrombocytopenia, leukopenia, hemolytic anemia, Heinz body anemia, purpura, hypoprothrombinemia, cyanosis, methemoglobinemia
Hypersensitivity	Generalized skin eruptions, erythema multiforme (Stevens-Johnson syndrome), parapsoriasis varioliformis acuta (Mucha-Haberman syndrome), exfoliative dermatitis, epidermal necrolysis (Lyell's syndrome) with corneal damage, pruritus, urticaria, photosensitization, anaphylaxis, serum sickness syndrome, chills, drug fever, periorbital edema, conjunctival and scleral injection, arthralgia, transient pulmonary changes with eosinophilia and decreased pulmonary function, allergic myocarditis, polyarteritis nodosa, lupus erythematosus phenomenon, hepatitis with immune complexes
Gastrointestinal	*Anorexia, nausea, vomiting, abdominal pains,* diarrhea, bloody diarrhea, impaired folic acid absorption, stomatitis, pancreatitis, hepatitis
Central nervous system	Headache, vertigo, tinnitus, hearing loss, peripheral neuropathy, transient lesions of posterior spinal column, transverse myelitis, ataxia, convulsions, insomnia, mental depression, hallucinations, drowsiness

Table continued on following page

AZULFIDINE continued

ADVERSE REACTIONS continued

Renal	Crystalluria, hematuria, proteinuria, nephrotic syndrome, toxic nephrosis with oliguria and anuria, orange-yellow discoloration of alkaline urine, diuresis (rare)
Other	Alopecia, reduction in sperm count and viability, skin discoloration, goiter (rare)

OVERDOSAGE

Signs and symptoms	See ADVERSE REACTIONS
Treatment	Induce emesis or use gastric lavage to empty stomach; administer a cathartic. Alkalinize the urine. Force fluids if renal function is normal. If anuria is present, restrict fluids and salt, and treat for renal failure. For complete renal blockage by crystals, catheterization of the ureters may be indicated. For agranulocytosis, discontinue medication, hospitalize the patient, and institute appropriate therapy. For sensitivity reactions, discontinue drug immediately. Control urticaria, other skin rashes, and serum sickness with antihistamines and, if necessary, systemic corticosteroids.

DRUG INTERACTIONS

Methotrexate	⇧ Methotrexate serum level
Digoxin	⇩ Absorption of digoxin

ALTERED LABORATORY VALUES

Blood/serum values	⇩ PBI ⇩ ^{131}I thyroid uptake ⇩ Glucose (rare)
Urinary values	⇧ Protein

Use in children

See INDICATIONS; contraindicated for use in infants under 2 yr of age

Use in pregnancy or nursing mothers

Safe use has not been established during pregnancy; contraindicated at term and in nursing mothers. Sulfonamides cross the placental barrier, are excreted in breast milk, and may cause kernicterus.

BELLADENAL/BELLADENAL-S (Belladonna alkaloids and phenobarbital) Sandoz

Tabs: 0.25 mg belladonna alkaloids and 50 mg phenobarbital **Tabs (sust rel):** 0.25 mg belladonna alkaloids and 50 mg phenobarbital

INDICATIONS	ORAL DOSAGE
Peptic ulcer (adjunctive therapy)[1] **Irritable bowel syndrome** (irritable colon, spastic colon, mucous colitis)[1] **Acute enterocolitis**[1]	**Adult:** 2–4 tabs/day in 4–16 divided doses; sust-rel tabs: 1 tab bid in AM and PM **Child:** ¼–½ tab qd to qid

CONTRAINDICATIONS

Glaucoma ●

Increased intraocular pressure ●

Hypersensitivity to belladonna alkaloids or phenobarbital ●

Advanced hepatic or renal disease ●

WARNINGS/PRECAUTIONS

Habit-forming	Psychic and/or physical dependence and tolerance may develop, especially in addiction-prone individuals
Special-risk patients	Use with caution in the elderly
Drowsiness	Performance of potentially hazardous activities may be impaired; caution patients accordingly

ADVERSE REACTIONS

Central nervous system	Drowsiness
Gastrointestinal	Dry mouth
Ophthalmic	Blurred vision
Cardiovascular	Flushing
Genitourinary	Urinary retention

OVERDOSAGE

Signs and symptoms	*Phenobarbital-related effects:* drowsiness, confusion, coma, respiratory depression, hypotension, shock; *belladonna alkaloid-related effects:* dry mouth and throat, blurred vision, urinary retention, CNS excitation, restlessness, confusion, delirium, convulsions, stupor, and coma, leading to death
Treatment	Induce emesis or use gastric lavage to empty stomach, followed by activated charcoal. Maintain adequate pulmonary ventilation, correct hypotension, and control convulsions, if present. Force diuresis, alkalinize urine, and use catheterization to prevent urinary retention. Maintain body temperature. Hemodialysis or peritoneal dialysis may be useful.

DRUG INTERACTIONS

Alcohol, tranquilizers, sedative-hypnotics, and other CNS depressants	⇧ CNS depression
Coumarin anticoagulants	⇩ Anticoagulant effect
Amantadine	⇧ Atropine-like effects ⇧ CNS depression
Antihistamines, antimuscarinics	⇧ Atropine-like effects ⇧ CNS depression
Haloperidol, phenothiazines	⇧ Atropine-like effects ⇧ CNS depression ⇩ Antipsychotic effects
Antacids, antidiarrheal suspensions[2]	⇩ Belladonna alkaloid effects ⇩ Barbiturate effects
Corticosteroids	⇩ Corticosteroid effects
Digitalis, digitoxin	⇩ Digitalis or digitoxin effects
Griseofulvin	⇩ Griseofulvin effects
Tetracyclines, particularly doxycycline	⇩ Antimicrobial effect
Anticonvulsants	Change in pattern of epileptiform seizures
MAO inhibitors	⇧ Atropine-like effects ⇧ CNS effects
Tricyclic antidepressants	⇧ Atropine-like effects ⇩ Antidepressant effect

[1]Possibly effective
[2]When administered <1 h apart

Table continued on following page

ALTERED LABORATORY VALUES

Blood/serum values ——— ⇧ Sulfobromophthalein retention ⇩ Bilirubin

No clinically significant alterations in urinary values occur at therapeutic dosages

Use in children

See INDICATIONS.

Use in pregnancy or nursing mothers

General guidelines not established. Neonatal withdrawal syndrome has been associated with the use of phenobarbital during pregnancy.[1]

[1]Avery GS (ed): *Drug Treatment: Principles and Practice of Clinical Pharmacology and Therapeutics*, Littleton, Mass: Publishing Sciences Group Inc, 1976; Tuchmann-Duplesis H: *Drug Effects on Fetus: Monographs on Drugs*, vol 2, Acton, Mass: Publishing Sciences Group Inc, 1975

BELLERGAL/BELLERGAL-S (Phenobarbital, ergotamine tartrate, and belladonna alkaloids) Dorsey

Tabs: 20 mg phenobarbital, 0.3 mg ergotamine tartrate, and 0.1 mg belladonna alkaloids **Tabs (sust rel):** 40 mg phenobarbital, 0.6 mg ergotamine tartrate, and 0.2 mg belladonna alkaloids

INDICATIONS	ORAL DOSAGE
Gastrointestinal disorders (hypermotility, hypersecretion, nervous stomach, diarrhea, constipation) **Menopausal disorders** (hot flashes, sweats, restlessness, insomnia) **Cardiovascular disorders** (palpitations, tachycardia, chest oppression, vasomotor disturbances) **Genitourinary disorders** (uterine cramps) **Premenstrual tension** **Recurrent, throbbing headache**	**Adult:** 4 tabs/day (1 in AM, 1 at noon, and 2 at bedtime); sust-rel tabs: 2 tabs/day (in AM and PM)

ADMINISTRATION/DOSAGE ADJUSTMENTS

Refractory patients	Begin with 6 tabs/day of Bellergal and gradually reduce dosage at weekly intervals, according to response

CONTRAINDICATIONS

Peripheral vascular disease ●	Impaired hepatic or renal function ●	Hypersensitivity to phenobarbital, ergotamine tartrate, or belladonna alkaloids ●
Coronary artery disease ●	Sepsis ●	
Hypertension ●	Glaucoma ●	

WARNINGS/PRECAUTIONS

Habit-forming	Psychic and/or physical dependence and tolerance may develop, especially in addiction-prone individuals
Drowsiness	Performance of potentially hazardous activities may be impaired; caution patients accordingly
Peripheral vascular complications	May develop with large or prolonged doses in patients highly sensitive to ergotamine tartrate

ADVERSE REACTIONS

Central nervous system	Drowsiness (rare)
Ophthalmic	Blurred vision (rare)
Cardiovascular	Flushing (rare)
Gastrointestinal	Dry mouth (rare)

OVERDOSAGE

Signs and symptoms	*Phenobarbital-related effects:* drowsiness, confusion, coma, respiratory depression, hypotension, shock; *ergotamine-related effects:* vomiting, numbness, tingling, pain and cyanosis of extremities with diminished or absent peripheral pulses, hypertension or hypotension, drowsiness, stupor, coma, convulsions, shock; *belladonna alkaloid-related effects:* dry mouth and throat, blurred vision, urinary retention, CNS excitation, restlessness, confusion, delirium, convulsions, stupor, and coma, leading to death
Treatment	Induce emesis or use gastric lavage to empty stomach, followed by activated charcoal. Maintain adequate pulmonary ventilation, correct hypotension, and control convulsions, if present. Force diuresis, alkalinize urine, and use catheterization to prevent urinary retention. Maintain body temperature. Treat peripheral vasospasm with warmth *(not heat)*, and protect ischemic limbs from cold. Hemodialysis or peritoneal dialysis may be useful.

Table continued on following page

BELLERGAL/BELLERGAL-S continued

DRUG INTERACTIONS

Alcohol, tranquilizers, sedative-hypnotics, and other CNS depressants	⇧ CNS depression
Coumarin anticoagulants	⇩ Anticoagulant effect
Amantadine	⇧ Atropine-like effects ⇧ CNS depression
Antihistamines, antimuscarinics	⇧ Atropine-like effects ⇧ CNS depression
Haloperidol, phenothiazines	⇧ Atropine-like effects ⇧ CNS depression ⇩ Antipsychotic effects
Antacids, antidiarrheal suspensions[1]	⇩ Belladonna alkaloid effects ⇩ Barbiturate effects
Corticosteroids	⇩ Corticosteroid effects
Digitalis, digitoxin	⇩ Digitalis or digitoxin effects
Griseofulvin	⇩ Griseofulvin effects
Tetracyclines, particularly doxycycline	⇩ Antimicrobial effect
Anticonvulsants	Change in pattern of epileptiform seizures
MAO inhibitors	⇧ Atropine-like effects ⇧ CNS effects
Tricyclic antidepressants	⇧ Atropine-like effects ⇩ Antidepressant effect

ALTERED LABORATORY VALUES

Test	Effect
Blood/serum values	⇧ Sulfobromophthalein retention ⇩ Bilirubin

No clinically significant alterations in urinary values occur at therapeutic dosages

Use in children

General guidelines not established

Use in pregnancy or nursing mothers

Contraindicated during third trimester. Neonatal withdrawal syndrome has been associated with the use of phenobarbital during pregnancy.[1] General guidelines not established

[1]Avery GS (ed): *Drug Treatment: Principles and Practice of Clinical Pharmacology and Therapeutics*, Littleton, Mass: Publishing Sciences Group Inc, 1976; Tuchmann-Duplesis H: *Drug Effects on Fetus: Monographs on Drugs*, vol 2, Acton, Mass: Publishing Sciences Group Inc, 1975

[1]When administered <1 h apart

BENTYL (Dicyclomine hydrochloride) Merrell-National

Caps: 10 mg **Tabs:** 20 mg **Syrup:** 10 mg/5 ml **Amps:** 10 mg/ml (2 ml) **Vial:** 10 mg/ml (10 ml) **Syringe:** 10 mg/ml (2 ml)

INDICATIONS	ORAL DOSAGE	PARENTERAL DOSAGE
Irritable bowel syndrome (irritable colon, spastic colon, mucous colitis)[1] **Acute enterocolitis**[1]	**Adult:** 10–20 mg or 5–10 ml (1–2 tsp) tid or qid **Child:** 10 mg or 5 ml (1 tsp) tid or qid	**Adult:** 20 mg IM q4–6h
Infant colic[1]	**Infant:** 2.5 ml (½ tsp) tid or qid	—

CONTRAINDICATIONS

Obstructive uropathy ●

Obstructive GI disease (eg, achalasia, pyloroduodenal stenosis) ●

Paralytic ileus ●

Intestinal atony in elderly or debilitated patients ●

Unstable cardiovascular status in acute hemorrhage ●

Severe ulcerative colitis ●

Toxic megacolon, complicating ulcerative colitis ●

Myasthenia gravis ●

WARNINGS/PRECAUTIONS

Mental impairment, reflex-slowing	Performance of potentially hazardous activities may be impaired; caution patients accordingly
Ulcerative colitis	Large doses may suppress intestinal motility and lead to paralytic ileus or precipitate or aggravate toxic megacolon
Special-risk patients	Use with caution in patients with glaucoma, prostatic hypertrophy, autonomic neuropathy, hepatic or renal disease, hyperthyroidism, coronary heart disease, congestive heart failure, cardiac arrhythmias, tachycardia (atropine-like drugs may increase heart rate), hypertension, and hiatal hernia associated with reflux esophagitis (may be aggravated)
Biliary-tract disease complications	Drug may be ineffective
Fever and heat stroke	May occur in high environmental temperatures as a result of anaphoresis
Incomplete intestinal obstruction	May be manifested by diarrhea, especially in ileostomy or colostomy patients; use may be harmful under these circumstances

ADVERSE REACTIONS

Gastrointestinal	Dry mouth, nausea, vomiting, constipation
Genitourinary	Urinary hesitancy and retention, impotence
Endocrinological	Lactation suppression
Central nervous system	Headache, nervousness, drowsiness, weakness, dizziness, insomnia, confusion and/or excitement (especially in the elderly), temporary lightheadedness (with IM form)
Cardiovascular	Palpitations, tachycardia
Ophthalmic	Blurred vision, mydriasis, cycloplegia, increased ocular tension
Dermatological	Urticaria
Other	Loss of sense of taste, allergic or idiosyncratic reactions (including anaphylaxis), a bloated feeling, anaphoresis, local irritation at injection site

OVERDOSAGE

Signs and symptoms	Headache, nausea, vomiting, blurred vision, mydriasis, hot, dry skin, dizziness, dry mouth, labored swallowing, CNS stimulation, curare-like effects (neuromuscular blockade, leading to muscle weakness and possible paralysis)
Treatment	Induce emesis or use gastric lavage, followed by activated charcoal. For sedation, administer barbiturates, orally or IM.

DRUG INTERACTIONS

No clinically significant drug interactions have been observed

ALTERED LABORATORY VALUES

No clinically significant alterations in blood/serum or urinary values occur at therapeutic dosages

Use in children

See INDICATIONS

Use in pregnancy or nursing mothers

General guidelines not established for use in pregnancy. May inhibit lactation in nursing mothers.

[1]Probably effective

Table continued on following page

BENTYL with PHENOBARBITAL (Dicyclomine hydrochloride and phenobarbital) Merrell-National

Caps, syrup (per 5 ml): 10 mg dicyclomine hydrochloride and 15 mg phenobarbital **Tabs:** 20 mg dicyclomine hydrochloride and 15 mg phenobarbital

INDICATIONS	ORAL DOSAGE
Irritable bowel syndrome (irritable colon, mucous colitis)[1] **Acute enterocolitis**[1]	**Adult:** 1–2 caps, 1 tab, or 5–10 ml (1–2 tsp) tid or qid **Infant:** 2.5 ml (½ tsp) tid or qid **Child:** 1 cap or 5 ml (1 tsp) tid or qid
Infant colic[1]	**Infant:** same as for acute enterocolitis

CONTRAINDICATIONS

Obstructive uropathy ●

Obstructive GI disease (eg, achalasia, pyloroduodenal stenosis) ●

Paralytic ileus ●

Intestinal atony in elderly or debilitated patients ●

Unstable cardiovascular status in acute hemorrhage ●

Severe ulcerative colitis ●

Toxic megacolon complicating ulcerative colitis ●

Myasthenia gravis ●

Acute intermittent porphyria ●

Hypersensitivity to phenobarbital ●

WARNINGS/PRECAUTIONS

Habit-forming	Psychic and/or physical dependence or tolerance may develop, especially in addiction-prone individuals
Ulcerative colitis	Large doses may suppress intestinal motility and lead to paralytic ileus or precipitate or aggravate toxic megacolon
Special-risk patients	Use with caution in patients with glaucoma, prostatic hypertrophy, autonomic neuropathy, hepatic or renal disease, hyperthyroidism, coronary heart disease, congestive heart failure, cardiac arrhythmias, tachycardia (atropine-like drugs may increase heart rate), hypertension, and hiatal hernia associated with reflux esophagitis (may be aggravated)
Biliary-tract disease complications	Drug may be ineffective
Fever and heat stroke	May occur in high environmental temperatures as a result of anaphoresis
Mental impairment, reflex-slowing	Performance of potentially hazardous activities may be impaired; caution patients accordingly
Incomplete intestinal obstruction	May be manifested by diarrhea, especially in ileostomy or colostomy patients; use may be harmful under these conditions

ADVERSE REACTIONS

Gastrointestinal	Dry mouth, nausea, vomiting, constipation
Genitourinary	Urinary hesitancy and retention, impotence
Endocrinological	Lactation suppression
Central nervous system and neuromuscular	Headache, nervousness, drowsiness, weakness, dizziness, insomnia, confusion and/or excitement (especially in the elderly), delirium or convulsions following abrupt withdrawal in patients habituated to barbiturates, muscular pain
Cardiovascular	Palpitations, tachycardia
Ophthalmic	Blurred vision, mydriasis, cycloplegia, increased ocular tension
Dermatological	Urticaria
Other	Loss of sense of taste, allergic or idiosyncratic reactions (including anaphylaxis), a bloated feeling, anaphoresis

OVERDOSAGE

Signs and symptoms	Headache, nausea, vomiting, blurred vision, mydriasis, hot, dry skin, dizziness, dry mouth, labored swallowing, CNS stimulation, curare-like effects (neuromuscular blockade leading to muscle weakness and possible paralysis)

[1]Possibly effective

Table continued on following page

OVERDOSAGE continued

Treatment	Induce emesis and use gastric lavage to empty stomach, followed by activated charcoal. If indicated, administer parenteral cholinergic agents (eg, bethanechol chloride).

DRUG INTERACTIONS

Alcohol, tranquilizers, sedative-hypnotics, and other CNS depressants	⇧ CNS depression
Coumarin anticoagulants	⇩ Anticoagulant effect
Amantadine	⇧ CNS depression
Antihistamines, antimuscarinics	⇧ CNS depression
Haloperidol, phenothiazines	⇧ CNS depression ⇩ Antipsychotic effects
Antacids, antidiarrheal suspensions[1]	⇩ Barbiturate effects
Corticosteroids	⇩ Corticosteroid effects
Digitalis, digitoxin	⇩ Digitalis or digitoxin effects
Griseofulvin	⇩ Griseofulvin effects
Tetracyclines, particularly doxycycline	⇩ Antimicrobial effects
Anticonvulsants	Change in pattern of epileptiform seizures
MAO inhibitors	⇧ CNS effects
Tricyclic antidepressants	⇩ Antidepressant effect

ALTERED LABORATORY VALUES

Blood/serum values	⇩ Bilirubin

No clinically significant alterations in urinary values occur at therapeutic dosages

Use in children

See INDICATIONS

Use in pregnancy or nursing mothers

General guidelines not established for use in pregnancy. Neonatal withdrawal syndrome has been associated with the use of phenobarbital during pregnancy.[1] Lactation may be inhibited in nursing mothers.

[1]Avery GS (ed): *Drug Treatment: Principles and Practice of Clinical Pharmacology and Therapeutics*, Littleton, Mass: Publishing Sciences Group, Inc, 1976; Tuchmann-Duplessis H: *Drug Effects on Fetus: Monographs on Drugs*, vol 2, Acton, Mass: Publishing Sciences Group, Inc, 1975

[1]When administered <1 h apart

COMBID (Prochlorperazine maleate and isopropamide iodide) Smith Kline & French

Caps: 10 mg prochlorperazine maleate and 5 mg isopropamide iodide

INDICATIONS	ORAL DOSAGE
Peptic ulcer (adjunctive therapy)[1] **Irritable bowel syndrome** (irritable colon, spastic colon, mucous colitis)[1] **Functional diarrhea**[1]	**Adult:** 1 cap bid

CONTRAINDICATIONS

Hypersensitivity to prochlorperazine or isopropamide iodide ●

CNS depression (drug-induced) ●

Glaucoma ●

Pyloric obstruction ●

Prostatic hypertrophy ●

Bladder-neck obstruction ●

Obstructive intestinal lesions and/or ileus ●

Bone-marrow depression ●

Jaundice ●

Hepatic disease ●

Blood dyscrasias ●

Intestinal obstruction or brain tumor believed to be manifested by nausea and vomiting ●

WARNINGS/PRECAUTIONS

Mental impairment, reflex-slowing	Performance of potentially hazardous activities may be impaired; caution patients accordingly
Special-risk patients	Use cautiously in patients with a past history of jaundice, hepatic abnormality, and blood dyscrasias, in the elderly, in patients with mitral insufficiency or pheochromocytoma, and in those who have shown a sensitivity reaction to other drugs
Pregnancy tests	False-positives may occur

ADVERSE REACTIONS[2]

Neuromuscular	Opisthotonos, oculogyric crisis, hyperreflexia, dystonia, akathisia, dyskinesia, pseudo-parkinsonism, tardive dyskinesia
Central nervous system	Drowsiness, dizziness, convulsions, altered cerebrospinal fluid proteins, cerebral edema, headache, reactivated psychotic processes, catatonia
Gastrointestinal	Dry mouth, constipation, nausea, dysphagia, obstipation, adynamic ileus
Cardiovascular	Tachycardia, palpitations, ECG changes, hypotension (sometimes fatal), cardiac arrest, peripheral edema
Hepatic	Jaundice, biliary stasis
Genitourinary	Urinary hesitancy and retention, inhibited ejaculation
Ophthalmic	Mydriasis, cycloplegia, blurred vision, pigmentary retinopathy, lenticular and corneal deposits
Hematological	Pancytopenia, thrombocytopenic purpura, leukopenia, agranulocytosis, eosinophilia
Endocrinological	Lactation suppression, galactorrhea, gynecomastia, menstrual irregularities
Dermatological	Photosensitivity, itching, erythema, urticaria, eczema, exfoliative dermatitis, skin pigmentation, epithelial keratopathy
Allergic	Asthma, laryngeal edema, angioneurotic edema, anaphylactoid reactions
Other	Bloated feeling, fever, nasal congestion, SLE-like syndrome

OVERDOSAGE

Signs and symptoms	*Isopropamide-related effects:* dry mouth, dysphagia, thirst, blurred vision, mydriasis, photophobia, fever, rapid pulse and respiration, disorientation, depression, circulatory collapse; *prochlorperazine-related effects:* extrapyramidal effects (see ADVERSE REACTIONS), CNS depression, coma, agitation, restlessness, convulsions, fever, hypotension, dry mouth, ileus

[1]Possibly effective
[2]Including reactions related to both phenothiazines in general (but not necessarily prochlorperazine) and isopropamide

Table continued on following page

OVERDOSAGE continued

Treatment	Empty stomach by gastric lavage, repeated several times. *Do not induce emesis.* For respiratory depression, administer oxygen and, if needed, perform a tracheostomy, and assist ventilation. For extrapyramidal reactions, keep patient under observation and maintain open airway. Treat extrapyramidal symptoms with antiparkinsonism drugs (except levodopa), barbiturates, or diphenhydramine. For hypotension, employ standard measures. If a vasoconstrictor is indicated, use levarterenol or phenylephrine; other pressor agents may lower blood pressure further. Treat hyperpyrexia with physical cooling measures. Force fluids by mouth or give IV. For photophobia, keep patient in a darkened room. Use saline cathartics to hasten evacuation of pellets that have not already released medication. Continue supportive therapy for as long as overdosage symptoms remain.

DRUG INTERACTIONS

Alcohol, tranquilizers, sedative-hypnotics, and other CNS depressants	⇧ CNS depression
Antimuscarinics	⇧ Atropine-like effects
Antacids, antidiarrheal suspensions[3]	⇩ Prochlorperazine absorption
Anticonvulsants	⇩ Convulsion threshold
MAO inhibitors	⇧ Atropine-like effects ⇧ CNS depression
Tricyclic antidepressants	⇧ Atropine-like effects ⇧ CNS depression
Amphetamines	⇩ Amphetamine effect
Epinephrine	Severe hypotension
Guanethidine, related compounds	⇩ Antihypertensive effects
Levodopa	⇩ Antiparkinson effect

ALTERED LABORATORY VALUES

Blood/serum values	⇧ PBI ⇩ ^{131}I thyroid uptake
Urinary values	⇧ Bilirubin

Use in children

Contraindicated for use in children under 12 yr of age

Use in pregnancy or nursing mothers

Safe use not established. May inhibit lactation in nursing mothers.

[3]When administered <1 hr apart

DONNATAL/DONNATAL EXTENTABS (Phenobarbital, hyoscyamine sulfate, atropine sulfate, and hyoscine hydrobromide) **Robins**

Tabs, caps, elixir (per 5 ml): 16.2 mg phenobarbital, 0.1037 mg hyoscyamine sulfate, 0.0194 mg atropine sulfate, and 0.0065 mg hyoscine hydrobromide **No. 2 tabs:** 32.4 mg phenobarbital and the same amount of belladonna alkaloids **Tabs (sust rel):** 48.6 mg phenobarbital, 0.3111 mg hyoscyamine sulfate, 0.0582 mg atropine sulfate, and 0.0195 mg hyoscine hydrobromide

INDICATIONS	ORAL DOSAGE
Peptic ulcer (adjunctive therapy)[1] **Irritable bowel syndrome** (irritable colon, spastic colon, mucous colitis)[1] **Acute enterocolitis**[1]	**Adult:** 1-2 tabs or caps tid or qid, 5-10 ml (1-2 tsp) tid or qid, or 1-2 No. 2 tabs tid; sust-rel tabs: 1 tab q8-12h **Child (10 lb):** 0.5-0.75 ml q4-6h **Child (20 lb):** 1.25-2.0 ml q4-6h **Child (30 lb):** 2.5 ml (½ tsp) q4-6h **Child (50 lb):** 3.75-5.0 ml (¾-1 tsp) q4-6h **Child (75-80 lb):** 5.0-7.5 ml (1-1½ tsp) q4-6h

CONTRAINDICATIONS

Glaucoma ●	Obstructive uropathy ●
Renal or hepatic disease ●	Hypersensitivity to components ●

WARNINGS/PRECAUTIONS

Habit-forming	Psychic and/or physical dependence and tolerance may develop, especially in addiction-prone individuals

ADVERSE REACTIONS

Gastrointestinal	Dry mouth
Ophthalmic	Blurred vision
Dermatological	Dry skin, flushing
Genitourinary	Urinary hesitancy or retention

OVERDOSAGE

Signs and symptoms	*Phenobarbital-related effects:* drowsiness, confusion, coma, respiratory depression, hypotension, shock; *belladonna alkaloid-related effects:* dry mouth and throat, blurred vision, urinary retention, CNS excitation, restlessness, confusion, delirium, convulsions, stupor, and coma, leading to death
Treatment	Induce emesis or use gastric lavage to empty stomach, followed by activated charcoal. Maintain adequate pulmonary ventilation, correct hypotension, and control convulsions, if present. Force diuresis, alkalinize urine, and use catheterization to prevent urinary retention. Maintain body temperature. Hemodialysis or peritoneal dialysis may be useful.

DRUG INTERACTIONS

Alcohol, tranquilizers, sedative-hypnotics, and other CNS depressants	⇧ CNS depression
Coumarin anticoagulants	⇩ Anticoagulant effect
Amantadine	⇧ Atropine-like effects ⇧ CNS depression
Antihistamines, antimuscarinics	⇧ Atropine-like effects ⇧ CNS depression
Haloperidol, phenothiazines	⇧ Atropine-like effects ⇧ CNS depression ⇩ Antipsychotic effects
Antacids, antidiarrheal suspensions[2]	⇩ Belladonna alkaloid effects ⇩ Barbiturate effects
Corticosteroids	⇩ Corticosteroid effects
Digitalis, digitoxin	⇩ Digitalis or digitoxin effects
Griseofulvin	⇩ Griseofulvin effects
Tetracyclines, particularly doxycycline	⇩ Antimicrobial effect
Anticonvulsants	Change in pattern of epileptiform seizures
MAO inhibitors	⇧ Atropine-like effects ⇧ CNS effects
Tricyclic antidepressants	⇧ Atropine-like effects ⇩ Antidepressant effect

[1]Possibly effective
[2]When administered <1 h apart

Table continued on following page

DONNATAL/DONNATAL EXTENTABS continued

ALTERED LABORATORY VALUES

Blood/serum values —————— ⇧ Sulfobromophthalein retention ⇩ Bilirubin

No clinically significant alterations in urinary values occur at therapeutic dosages

Use in children

See INDICATIONS.

Use in pregnancy or nursing mothers

General guidelines not established for use during pregnancy. Neonatal withdrawal syndrome has been associated with the use of phenobarbital during pregnancy.[1] Atropine inhibits lactation and may cause toxicity in infants.[2]

[1]Avery GS (ed): *Drug Treatment: Principles and Practice of Clinical Pharmacology and Therapeutics*, Littleton, Mass: Publishing Sciences Group, Inc, 1976;: Tuchmann-Duplessis H: *Drug Effects on Fetus: Monographs on Drugs*, vol 2, Acton, Mass: Publishing Sciences Group, Inc, 1975

[2]Knowles JA: *J Pediatr* 66:1068, 1965; Speika N: *J Obstet Gynaecol Br Commonw* 54:426, 1947; Takyi BE: *J Hosp Pharm* 28:317, 1970

KINESED (Belladonna alkaloids and phenobarbital) Stuart

Tabs: 16 mg phenobarbital, 0.1 mg hyoscyamine sulfate, 0.02 mg atropine sulfate, and 0.007 mg scopolamine hydrobromide

INDICATIONS	ORAL DOSAGE
Peptic ulcer (adjunctive therapy)[1] **Irritable bowel syndrome** (irritable colon, spastic colon, mucous colitis)[1] **Acute enterocolitis**[1]	**Adult:** 1–2 tabs, tid or qid, chewed or swallowed with liquid **Child (2–12 yr):** ½–1 tab, tid or qid, chewed or swallowed with liquid

CONTRAINDICATIONS

Hypersensitivity to belladonna alkaloids or barbiturates ●	Glaucoma ●	Advanced hepatic or renal disease ●

WARNINGS/PRECAUTIONS

Special-risk patients	Use with caution in patients with incipient glaucoma, bladder-neck obstruction, or urinary bladder atony
Habituation	May result from prolonged use of barbiturates

ADVERSE REACTIONS

Ophthalmic	Blurred vision (rare)
Gastrointestinal	Dry mouth (rare)
Genitourinary	Difficult urination (rare)

OVERDOSAGE

Signs and symptoms	*Phenobarbital-related effects:* drowsiness, confusion, coma, respiratory depression, hypotension, shock; *belladonna alkaloid-related effects:* dry mouth and throat, blurred vision, urinary retention, CNS excitation, restlessness, confusion, delirium, convulsions, stupor, and coma, leading to death
Treatment	Induce emesis or use gastric lavage to empty stomach, followed by activated charcoal. Maintain adequate pulmonary ventilation, correct hypotension, and control convulsions, if present. Force diuresis, alkalinize urine, and use catheterization to prevent urinary retention. Maintain body temperature. Hemodialysis or peritoneal dialysis may be useful.

DRUG INTERACTIONS

Alcohol, tranquilizers, sedative-hypnotics, and other CNS depressants	⇧ CNS depression
Coumarin anticoagulants	⇩ Anticoagulant effect
Amantadine	⇧ Atropine-like effects ⇧ CNS depression
Antihistamines, antimuscarinics	⇧ Atropine-like effects ⇧ CNS depression
Haloperidol, phenothiazines	⇧ Atropine-like effects ⇧ CNS depression ⇩ Antipsychotic effects
Antacids, antidiarrheal suspensions[2]	⇩ Belladonna alkaloid effects ⇩ Barbiturate effects
Corticosteroids	⇩ Corticosteroid effects
Digitalis, digitoxin	⇩ Digitalis or digitoxin effects
Griseofulvin	⇩ Griseofulvin effects
Tetracyclines, particularly doxycycline	⇩ Antimicrobial effect
Anticonvulsants	Change in pattern of epileptiform seizures
MAO inhibitors	⇧ Atropine-like effects ⇧ CNS effects
Tricyclic antidepressants	⇧ Atropine-like effects ⇩ Antidepressant effect

[1]Possibly effective
[2]When administered <1 h apart

Table continued on following page

KINESED continued

ALTERED LABORATORY VALUES

Blood/serum values ⇧ Sulfobromophthalein retention ⇩ Bilirubin

No clinically significant alterations in urinary values occur at therapeutic dosages

Use in children

See INDICATIONS

Use in pregnancy or nursing mothers

General guidelines not established for use during pregnancy. Neonatal withdrawal syndrome has been associated with the use of phenobarbital during pregnancy.[1] Atropine inhibits lactation and may cause toxicity in infants.[2]

[1] Avery GS (ed): *Drug Treatment: Principles and Practice of Clinical Pharmacology and Therapeutics*, Littleton, Mass: Publishing Sciences Group Inc, 1976; Tuchmann-Duplesis H: *Drug Effects on Fetus: Monographs on Drugs*, vol 2, Acton, Mass: Publishing Sciences Group Inc, 1975

[2] Knowles JA: *J Pediatr* 66:1068, 1965; Speika N: *J Obstet Gynaecol Br Commonw* 54:426, 1947; Takyi BE: *J Hosp Pharm* 28:317, 1970

LIBRAX (Chlordiazepoxide hydrochloride and clidinium bromide) Roche

Caps: 5 mg chlordiazepoxide hydrochloride and 2.5 mg clidinium bromide

INDICATIONS	ORAL DOSAGE
Peptic ulcer (adjunctive therapy)[1] **Irritable bowel syndrome** (irritable colon, spastic colon, mucous colitis)[1] **Acute enterocolitis**[1]	**Adult:** 1–2 caps tid or qid, before meals and at bedtime

ADMINISTRATION/DOSAGE ADJUSTMENTS

Discontinuation of therapy	Withdraw gradually following prolonged high dosages; sudden withdrawal may produce anorexia, anxiety, insomnia, vomiting, ataxia, tremors, muscle twitching, confusion, and (rarely) convulsive seizures

CONTRAINDICATIONS

Glaucoma ●	Bladder-neck obstruction ●	Hypersensitivity to chlordiazepoxide or clidinium ●
Prostatic hypertrophy ●		

WARNINGS/PRECAUTIONS

Habit-forming	Psychic and/or physical dependence and tolerance may develop, especially in addiction-prone individuals
Mental impairment, reflex-slowing	Performance of potentially hazardous activities may be impaired; caution patients accordingly
Paradoxical reactions	Observe for excitement, stimulation, and acute rage in psychiatric patients
Impaired renal or hepatic function	Administer with caution and observe for signs of excessive drug accumulation

ADVERSE REACTIONS

Central nervous system and neuromuscular	Drowsiness, confusion, EEG changes, extrapyramidal symptoms
Gastrointestinal	Nausea, constipation, dry mouth
Cardiovascular	Ataxia, edema, syncope
Ophthalmic	Blurred vision
Dermatological	Skin eruptions
Endocrinological	Minor menstrual irregularities, lactation suppression, increased or decreased libido
Hematological	Blood dyscrasias, including agranulocytosis
Hepatic	Jaundice, functional impairment
Genitourinary	Urinary hesitancy

OVERDOSAGE

Signs and symptoms	*Toxic effects primarily attributable to clidinium bromide:* dry mouth, blurred vision, urinary hesitancy, constipation; *chlordiazepoxide-related effects:* somnolence, confusion, coma, diminished reflexes, cardiac and respiratory depression
Treatment	Employ supportive measures, along with gastric lavage. Administer 0.5–2.0 mg physostigmine at a rate of no more than 1 mg/min. For recurring arrhythmias, convulsions, or deep coma, repeat in 1- to 4-mg doses. Administer IV fluids and maintain adequate airway. For hypotension, use levarterenol or metaraminol. Dialysis is of limited value. Do *not* use barbiturates to combat excitation.

DRUG INTERACTIONS

Alcohol, tranquilizers, sedative-hypnotics, and other CNS depressants	⇧ CNS depression
Tricyclic antidepressants	⇧ Antidepressant effect

[1]Possibly effective

Table continued on following page

LIBRAX continued

ALTERED LABORATORY VALUES

No clinically significant alterations in blood/serum or urinary values occur at therapeutic dosages

Use in children	Use in pregnancy or nursing mothers
General guidelines not established	Drug should almost always be avoided during pregnancy. An increased risk of congenital malformations during the first trimester has been associated with minor tranquilizers, including chlordiazepoxide. Clidinium component may inhibit lactation; patient should stop nursing if drug is prescribed.

PATHIBAMATE (Tridihexethyl chloride and meprobamate) Lederle

Tabs: 25 mg tridihexethyl chloride and 200 mg meprobamate (Pathibamate-200); 25 mg tridihexethyl chloride and 400 mg meprobamate (Pathibamate-400)

INDICATIONS	ORAL DOSAGE
Peptic ulcer (adjunctive therapy)[1] **Irritable bowel syndrome** (irritable colon, spastic colon, mucous colitis, functional GI disturbances)[1]	**Adult:** 1 Pathibamate-400 tab tid, with meals, and 2 Pathibamate-400 tabs at bedtime; for greater anticholinergic effect, 2 Pathibamate-200 tabs tid, with meals, and 2 Pathibamate-200 tabs at bedtime

ADMINISTRATION/DOSAGE ADJUSTMENTS

Discontinuation of therapy	Withdraw gradually over a 1- to 2-wk period following prolonged high dosages; sudden withdrawal may produce anorexia, anxiety, insomnia, vomiting, ataxia, tremors, muscle twitching, confusion, and (rarely) convulsive seizures; alternatively, substitute a short-acting barbiturate, then gradually withdraw medication

CONTRAINDICATIONS

Obstructive uropathy (eg, urinary bladder-neck obstructions due to prostatic hypertrophy) ●	Acute intermittent porphyria ●	Allergic or idiosyncratic reactions to meprobamate, tridihexethyl chloride, or related compounds ●
Obstructive disease of the GI tract ●	Unstable cardiovascular status in acute hemorrhage ●	Severe ulcerative colitis ●
Glaucoma ●	Myasthenia gravis ●	Toxic megacolon complicating ulcerative colitis ●
	Intestinal atony in elderly or debilitated patients ●	

WARNINGS/PRECAUTIONS

Habit-forming	Psychic and/or physical dependence and tolerance may develop, especially in addiction-prone individuals
Mental impairment, reflex-slowing	Performance of potentially hazardous activities may be impaired; caution patients accordingly
Oversedation	Use lowest effective dose in elderly or debilitated patients
Potentially suicidal patients	Should not have access to large quantities of meprobamate-containing compounds; prescribe smallest amount feasible at any one time
Impaired renal or hepatic function	Administer with caution and observe for signs of excessive drug accumulation
Seizures	May be precipitated in epileptic patients
Toxic megacolon	May be precipitated or aggravated in patients with ulcerative colitis
Heat and fever stroke	May occur in high environmental temperatures as a result of anaphoresis
Incomplete intestinal obstruction	May be manifested by diarrhea, especially in ileostomy or colostomy patients; use may be harmful under these circumstances
Special-risk patients	Use with caution in patients with autonomic neuropathy, hepatic or renal disease, early evidence of ileus (as in peritonitis), hyperthyroidism, coronary heart disease, congestive heart failure, cardiac arrhythmias, hypertension, nonobstructing prostatic hypertrophy, or hiatal hernia associated with reflux esophagitis
Gastric ulcer	Gastric emptying time may be delayed, complicating treatment by producing antral stasis
Biliary-tract-disease complications	Drug may be ineffective
Curare-like action	May occur with overdosage

ADVERSE REACTIONS

Cardiovascular	Tachycardia, palpitations, various forms of arrhythmia, transient ECG changes, syncope, hypotensive crises (one fatal case)

[1]Possibly effective

Table continued on following page

ADVERSE REACTIONS continued

Central nervous system	Headache, nervousness, drowsiness, weakness, dizziness, insomnia, some degree of mental confusion and/or excitement (especially in elderly patients), slurred speech, vertigo, paresthesias, euphoria, overstimulation, paradoxical excitement, fast EEG activity
Gastrointestinal	Dry mouth, nausea, vomiting, constipation, diarrhea
Ophthalmic	Blurred vision, mydriasis, cycloplegia, increased ocular tension, impairment of visual accommodation
Endocrinological	Suppression of lactation
Hematological	Agranulocytosis, aplastic anemia, thrombocytopenic purpura (rare)
Genitourinary	Urinary hesitancy and retention
Allergic or idiosyncratic	*Mild:* itchy, urticarial or erythematous maculopapular rash (generalized or confined to groin), leukopenia, acute nonthrombocytopenic purpura, petechiae, ecchymoses, eosinophilia, peripheral edema, adenopathy, fever, fixed drug eruption with cross-reaction to carisoprodol and cross-sensitivity between meprobamate/mebutamate and meprobamate/carbromal; *severe (rare):* hyperpyrexia, chills, angioneurotic edema, bronchospasm, oliguria, anuria, anaphylaxis, erythema multiforme, exfoliative dermatitis, stomatitis, proctitis, Stevens-Johnson syndrome, bullous dermatitis
Other	Loss of taste, impotence, bloated feeling, exacerbation of porphyric symptoms, decreased sweating

OVERDOSAGE

Signs and symptoms	*Toxic effects primarily attributable to tridihexethyl chloride:* dry mouth, labored swallowing, thirst, blurred vision, photophobia, flushed, hot, dry skin, rash, hyperthermia, palpitations, tachycardia, weak pulse, hypertension, urinary urgency with difficult micturition, abdominal distention, restlessness, confusion, delirium, and other signs of acute organic psychoses; *meprobamate-related effects:* drowsiness, lethargy, stupor, ataxia, coma, shock, vasomotor and respiratory collapse, leading to death; meprobamate blood levels of 3–10 mg/dl usually correspond to mild to moderate symptoms (stupor or light coma) and 10–20 mg/dl with deeper coma, requiring more intensive treatment
Treatment	Administer supportive measures, along with gastric lavage, followed by activated charcoal. For compromised respiration or blood pressure, cautiously administer respiratory assistance, CNS stimulants, and pressor agents, as indicated. Diuresis, osmotic (mannitol) diuresis, peritoneal dialysis, or hemodialysis may be successful. Monitor urinary output to avoid overhydration. Incomplete gastric emptying and delayed absorption can lead to relapse and death.

DRUG INTERACTIONS

Alcohol, tranquilizers, sedative-hypnotics, and other CNS depressants	⇧ CNS depression
Digoxin	⇧ Serum digoxin level
MAO inhibitors, tricyclic antidepressants	⇧ CNS depression ⇧ Antidepressant effect

ALTERED LABORATORY VALUES

Urinary values	⇧ 17-Ketosteroids, 17-ketogenic steroids, and 17-hydroxycorticosteroids (methodologic interference)

No clinically significant alterations in blood/serum values occur at therapeutic dosages

Use in children

Contraindicated for use in children under 12 yr of age

Use in pregnancy or nursing mothers

Drug should almost always be avoided during pregnancy. An increased risk of congenital malformations during the first trimester has been associated with minor tranquilizers, including meprobamate. Meprobamate crosses the placental barrier and appears in umbilical cord blood at or near maternal plasma levels. Meprobamate also appears in breast milk at concentrations two to four times that of maternal plasma; patient probably should stop nursing if drug is prescribed.

Note: Tridihexethyl chloride and meprobamate also marketed as **MILPATH** (Wallace).

PRO-BANTHINE (Propantheline bromide) Searle

Tabs: 7.5, 15 mg **Vial:** 30 mg/2 ml (2 ml)

INDICATIONS	ORAL DOSAGE	PARENTERAL DOSAGE
Peptic ulcer (adjunctive therapy)	**Adult:** 15 mg ½ h before meals and 30 mg at bedtime (75 mg/day)	**Adult:** 30 mg IM or IV q6h to start, then 15 mg IM or IV q6h
Reduction of duodenal motility to facilitate diagnostic radiologic procedures, hypotonic duodenography	—	**Adult:** 30–60 mg IM 5–10 min before procedure or 30–60 mg IV (6 mg/min) immediately before procedure

PRO-BANTHINE P.A. (Propantheline bromide) Searle

Tabs (sust rel): 30 mg

INDICATIONS	ORAL DOSAGE
Peptic ulcer (adjunctive therapy)	**Adult:** 30 mg bid, in AM and at bedtime; some patients may require 30 mg q8h

ADMINISTRATION/DOSAGE ADJUSTMENTS

Mild cases, elderly patients, patients of small stature	Administer 7.5 mg tid orally

CONTRAINDICATIONS

Glaucoma ●	Intestinal atony ●	Hiatal hernia associated with reflux esophagitis ●
Obstructive uropathy ●	Severe ulcerative colitis ●	Toxic megacolon exacerbating ulcerative colitis ●
Obstructive GI disease (eg, achalasia, pyloroduodenal stenosis) ●	Unstable cardiovascular status in acute hemorrhage ●	
Paralytic ileus ●	Myasthenia gravis ●	

WARNINGS/PRECAUTIONS

Drowsiness, blurred vision	Performance of potentially hazardous activities may be impaired; caution patients accordingly
Urinary hesitancy	May occur in patients with prostatic hypertrophy
Ulcerative colitis	Large doses may suppress intestinal motility and lead to paralytic ileus or precipitate or aggravate toxic megacolon
Special-risk patients	Use with caution in the elderly and in those with autonomic neuropathy, hepatic or renal disease, hyperthyroidism, coronary heart disease, congestive heart failure, cardiac arrhythmias, hypertension
Fever and heat stroke	May occur in high environmental temperatures as a result of anaphoresis
Incomplete intestinal obstruction	May be manifested by diarrhea, especially in ileostomy or colostomy patients; therapy may be harmful under these circumstances

ADVERSE REACTIONS

Gastrointestinal	Dry mouth, nausea, vomiting, constipation
Genitourinary	Urinary hesitancy and retention, impotence
Endocrinological	Lactation suppression
Central nervous system	Headache, nervousness, confusion, drowsiness, weakness, dizziness, insomnia
Cardiovascular	Palpitations, tachycardia
Ophthalmic	Blurred vision, mydriasis, cycloplegia, increased ocular tension
Dermatological	Urticaria
Other	Loss of sense of taste, allergic or idiosyncratic reactions (including anaphylaxis), a bloated feeling, anaphoresis, local irritation at injection site

Table continued on following page

PRO-BANTHINE/PRO-BANTHINE P.A. continued

OVERDOSAGE

Signs and symptoms	Intensification of usual side effects, CNS disturbances (restlessness, excitement, psychotic behavior), circulatory changes (flushing, decrease in blood pressure, circulatory failure), respiratory failure, curare-like effects (neuromuscular blockade, leading to muscle weakness and possible paralysis), and coma
Treatment	Immediately empty stomach by gastric lavage, and inject physostigmine, 0.5–2.0 mg IV, up to 5 mg as needed. Treat fever symptomatically (ice, alcohol). Manage excessive excitement with 2% sodium thiopental IV (slowly) or 100–200 ml of 2% chloral hydrate via rectal infusion. For paralysis of respiratory muscles, institute artificial respiration.

DRUG INTERACTIONS

Digoxin	⇧ Serum digoxin level
Belladonna alkaloids	⇧ Cholinergic blockade
Anticholinergic agents	⇧ Cholinergic blockade
Phenothiazines	⇧ Cholinergic blockade
Tricyclic antidepressants	⇧ Cholinergic blockade
Quinidine	⇧ Cholinergic blockade
Antihistamines	⇧ Cholinergic blockade
Procainamide	⇧ Cholinergic blockade

ALTERED LABORATORY VALUES

No clinically significant alterations in blood/serum or urinary values occur at therapeutic dosages

Use in children

Safe use not established

Use in pregnancy or nursing mothers

Safe use not established during pregnancy or in nursing mothers. Limited, uncontrolled data suggest no significant excretion in breast milk; may inhibit lactation.

TAGAMET (Cimetidine) Smith Kline & French

Tabs: 200, 300 mg **Liq:** 300 mg/5 ml **Vials:** 300 mg/2 ml (2, 8 ml)

INDICATIONS	ORAL DOSAGE	PARENTERAL DOSAGE
Active duodenal ulcer	**Adult:** 300 mg or 5 ml (1 tsp) qid, with meals and at bedtime, for 6–8 wk (unless healing has been demonstrated endoscopically)	**Adult:** 300 mq IM or IV q6h (see ADMINISTRATION/DOSAGE ADJUSTMENTS)
Prevention of recurrent duodenal ulcer in patients likely to require surgery or when surgery carries a greater than usual risk due to comcomitant illness	**Adult:** 400 mg at bedtime	—
Pathological hypersecretory conditions (eg, Zollinger-Ellison syndrome, systemic mastocytosis, and multiple adenomas)	**Adult:** 300 mg or 5 ml (1 tsp) qid, with meals and at bedtime, as long as clinically indicated; some patients may require higher or more frequent doses, up to 2,400 mg/day	**Adult:** same as above

ADMINISTRATION/DOSAGE ADJUSTMENTS

Intravenous injection	Dilute 300 mg of cimetidine in 0.9% Sodium Chloride Injection or other compatible IV solution to a total volume of 20 ml and inject over a period of not less than 2 min
Intermittent intravenous infusion	Dilute 300 mg of cimetidine in 100 ml of Dextrose Injection (5%) or other compatible IV solution and administer over a period of 15–20 min; some patients may require more frequent dosing, up to 2,400 mg/day
Concomitant antacid therapy	In treating active duodenal ulcers, antacids should be given as needed for relief of pain
Patients with severely impaired renal function	Although experience is limited, such patients may be given 300 mg q12h orally or IV; if necessary, the dosage frequency may be increased to q8h or further, with caution. For patients on hemodialysis, schedule the dose to coincide with the end of a dialysis period.

CONTRAINDICATIONS

None

WARNINGS/PRECAUTIONS

Mild gynecomastia	Has been observed in 4% of patients treated for pathological hypersecretory states and 0.3–1.0% of other patients. The condition, which is seen after 1 mo or more of treatment, may be related to a mild antiandrogenic effect manifested in animals by a reduction in prostate and seminal vesicle weights without impairment of fertility or mating performance.
Effect on human spermiogenesis	A reversible decrease in sperm count has been reported in seven patients taking 300 mg qid for 9 wk
Leydig-cell tumors	An increased incidence of benign tumors has been observed in rats treated with 9–56 times the recommended human dose of cimetidine
Mental confusion	May occur, especially in elderly and/or severely ill patients; the condition generally clears within 48 h of discontinuing therapy
Gastric malignancy	May be present, despite symptomatic response to cimetidine therapy

ADVERSE REACTIONS

Frequent reactions are italicized

Central nervous system and neuromuscular	*Dizziness, muscular pain,* confusion; headache with dizziness and tremor (one case)
Gastrointestinal	*Mild and transient diarrhea;* rarely, hepatitis and pancreatitis; periportal hepatic fibrosis (one case)
Dermatological	*Rash*
Hematological	*Neutropenia;* rarely, agranulocytosis, thrombocytopenia, and aplastic anemia
Other	Mild gynecomastia; rarely, interstitial nephritis, fever, cardiac arrhythmias and hypotension (following rapid IV bolus injection)

Table continued on following page

TAGAMET continued

OVERDOSAGE

Signs and symptoms	Potential respiratory failure and tachycardia (experience with gross overdosage in humans is limited; in the few reported cases, doses of up to 10 g have not been associated with untoward effects)
Treatment	Induce emesis or use gastric lavage, followed by activated charcoal. Monitor patient and provide supportive therapy, as needed. For respiratory failure and tachycardia, provide assisted respiration and administer a beta-blocking agent, such as propranolol.

DRUG INTERACTIONS

Coumarin anticoagulants	⇧ Risk of hypoprothrombinemia

ALTERED LABORATORY VALUES

Blood/serum values	⇧ Creatinine ⇧ SGOT ⇧ SGPT

No clinically significant alterations in urinary values occur at therapeutic dosages

Use in children

Not recommended for children under 16 yr of age unless anticipated benefits outweigh potential risks. In a few instances, doses of 20–40 mg/kg/day have been used.

Use in pregnancy or nursing mothers

Safe use not established during pregnancy. Cimetidine is excreted in human milk; as a rule, nursing should not be attempted while a patient is taking it.

Product (Manufacturer)	Ingredients	Actions
Aludrox (Wyeth) Suspension **Dosage** **Adult:** 10 ml (2 tsp) every 4 h, as needed	307 mg Aluminum hydroxide per 5 ml	Antacid
	103 mg Magnesium hydroxide per 5 ml	Antacid
	1.1 mg Sodium per 5 ml*	
Amphojel (Wyeth) Tablets **Dosage** **Adult:** 0.6 g 5-6 times/day, between meals and at bedtime	0.3 (or 0.6) g Aluminum hydroxide	Antacid
	1.4 (or 2.8) mg Sodium*	
Amphojel (Wyeth) Suspension **Dosage** **Adult:** 10 ml (2 tsp) 5-6 times/day, between meals and at bedtime	320 mg Aluminum hydroxide per 5 ml	Antacid
	6.9 mg Sodium per 5 ml*	
A-M-T (Wyeth) Tablets **Dosage** **Adult:** 2 tabs, as needed, 5-6 times/day, up to 12 tabs/24 h	162 mg Aluminum hydroxide	Antacid
	250 mg Magnesium trisilicate	Antacid
	3.5 mg Sodium*	
Basaljel (Wyeth) Capsules **Dosage** **Adult:** 2 caps as often as every 2 h, up to 12 times daily	Aluminum carbonate (equivalent to 500 mg aluminum hydroxide)	Antacid
	2.4 mg Sodium per 5 ml*	
Basaljel (Wyeth) Tablets **Dosage** **Adult:** 2 tabs as often as every 2 h, up to 12 times daily	Aluminum carbonate (equivalent to 500 mg aluminum hydroxide)	Antacid
	2.1 Sodium*	
Basaljel (Wyeth) Suspension **Dosage** **Adult:** 10 ml (2 tsp) in water or juice taken as often as every 2 h, up to 12 times daily	Aluminum carbonate (equivalent to 400 mg aluminum hydroxide per 5 ml)	Antacid
	2.4 Sodium per 5 ml*	
Camalox (Rorer) Tablets (chewable) **Dosage** **Adult:** 2-4 tabs (well chewed) ½-1 h after meals and at bedtime, up to l6 tabs/24 h for up to 2 wk	200 mg Magnesium hydroxide	Antacid
	225 mg Aluminum hydroxide	Antacid
	250 mg Calcium carbonate	Antacid
	1.5 mg Sodium*	
Camalox (Rorer) Suspension **Dosage** **Adult:** 10-20 ml (2-4 tsp) 4 times daily, ½ h after meals and at bedtime, up to 80 ml (16 tsp)/24 h for up to 2 wk	200 mg Magnesium hydroxide per 5 ml	Antacid
	225 mg Aluminum hydroxide per 5 ml	Antacid
	250 mg Calcium carbonate per 5 ml	Antacid
	2.5 mg Sodium per 5 ml*	

Table continued on following page

Product (Manufacturer)	Ingredients	Actions
Creamalin (Winthrop) Tablets (chewable) **Dosage** **Adult:** 2-4 tabs, as needed, up to 16 tabs/day **Child (>6 yr):** same as adult	248 mg Aluminum hydroxide	Antacid
	75 mg Magnesium hydroxide	Antacid
	26–41 mg Sodium*	
Dicarbosil (Norcliff Thayer) Tablets (chewable) **Dosage** **Adult:** 1-4 tabs, as needed, up to 16 tabs/24 h for up to 2 wk	500 mg Calcium carbonate	Antacid
	Approx. 1% sodium*	
Di-Gel (Plough) Tablets **Dosage** **Adult:** 2 tabs every 2 h, or after or between meals and at bedtime, up to 20 tabs/day	25 mg Simethicone	Antiflatulent
	282 mg Aluminum hydroxide and magnesium carbonate	Antacid
	85 mg Magnesium hydroxide	Antacid
	10.6 mg Sodium*	
Di-Gel (Plough) Liquid **Dosage** **Adult:** 10 ml (2 tsp) every 2 h, or after or between meals and at bedtime, up to 100 ml (20 tsp)/day	25 mg Simethicone per 5 ml	Antiflatulent
	282 mg Aluminum hydroxide per 5 ml	Antacid
	87 mg Magnesium hydroxide per 5 ml	Antacid
	8.5 mg Sodium per 5 ml*	
Estomul-M Tablets (Riker) Tablets **Dosage** **Adult:** 1-2 tabs 3 times daily, up to 6 tabs/24 h	500 mg Aluminum hydroxide and magnesium carbonate	Antacid
	45 mg Magnesium oxide	Antacid
	16 mg Sodium*	
Estomul-M Suspension (Riker) Suspension **Dosage** **Adult:** 15-30 ml (1-2 tbsp) 3 times daily, up to 90 ml (6 tbsp)/24 h	918 mg Aluminum hydroxide and magnesium carbonate per 15 ml	Antacid
	35.1 mg Sodium per 15 ml*	
Gaviscon (Marion) Tablets (chewable) **Dosage** **Adult:** 2-4 tabs 4 times daily, chewed after meals and at bedtime (or as needed), followed by ½ glass of water, up to 16 tabs/24 h for up to 2 wk; tablets should not be swallowed whole	80 mg Aluminum hydroxide	Antacid
	20 mg Magnesium trisilicate	Antacid
	19.17 mg Sodium*	
Gaviscon (Marion) Liquid **Dosage** **Adult:** 15-30 ml (1-2 tbsp) 4 times daily, after meals and at bedtime (or as needed), followed by ½ glass of water, up to 120 ml (8 tbsp)/24 h for up to 2 wk	160 mg Aluminum hydroxide per 15 ml	Antacid
	40 mg Magnesium trisilicate per 15 ml	Antacid
	79.4 mg Sodium per 15 ml*	

Table continued on following page

Product (Manufacturer)	Ingredients	Actions
Gaviscon-2 (Marion) Tablets (chewable) **Dosage** **Adult:** 1-2 tabs 4 times daily, chewed after meals and at bedtime (or as needed), followed by ½ glass of water, up to 8 tabs/24 h for up to 2 wk; tablets should not be swallowed whole	160 mg Aluminum hydroxide	Antacid
	40 mg Magnesium trisilicate	Antacid
	38.34 mg Sodium*	
Gelusil (Parke-Davis) Tablets (chewable) **Dosage** **Adult:** 2 or more tabs 1 h after meals and at bedtime, up to 12 tabs/24 h for up to 2 wk	200 mg Aluminum hydroxide	Antacid
	200 mg Magnesium hydroxide	Antacid
	25 mg Simethicone	Antiflatulent
	0.8 mg Sodium*	
Gelusil (Parke-Davis) Suspension **Dosage** **Adult:** 10 ml (2 tsp) or more, 1 h after meals and at bedtime, up to 60 ml (12 tsp)/24 h for up to 2 wk	200 mg Aluminum hydroxide per 5 ml	Antacid
	200 mg Magnesium hydroxide per 5 ml	Antacid
	25 mg Simethicone per 5 ml	Antiflatulent
	0.7 mg Sodium per 5 ml*	
Gelusil-M (Parke-Davis) Tablets (chewable) **Dosage** **Adult:** 2 or more tabs 1 h after meals and at bedtime, up to 10 tabs/24 h for up to 2 wk	300 mg Aluminum hydroxide	Antacid
	200 mg Magnesium hydroxide	Antacid
	25 mg Simethicone	Antiflatulent
	1.3 mg Sodium*	
Gelusil-M (Parke-Davis) Suspension **Dosage** **Adult:** 10 ml (2 tsp) or more, 1 h after meals and at bedtime, up to 50 ml (10 tsp)/24 h for up to 2 wk	300 mg Aluminum hydroxide per 5 ml	Antacid
	200 mg Magnesium hydroxide per 5 ml	Antacid
	25 mg Simethicone per 5 ml	Antiflatulent
	1.2 mg Sodium per 5 ml*	
Gelusil-II (Parke-Davis) Tablets (chewable) **Dosage** **Adult:** 2 or more tabs 1 h after meals and at bedtime, up to 8 tabs/24 h for up to 2 wk	400 mg Aluminum hydroxide	Antacid
	400 mg Magnesium hydroxide	Antacid
	30 mg Simethicone	Antiflatulent
	2.1 mg Sodium*	
Gelusil-II (Parke-Davis) Suspension **Dosage** **Adult:** 10 ml (2 tsp) or more, 1 h after meals and at bedtime, up to 40 ml (8 tsp)/24 h for up to 2 wk	400 mg Aluminum hydroxide per 5 ml	Antacid
	400 mg Magnesium hydroxide per 5 ml	Antacid
	30 mg Simethicone per 5 ml	Antiflatulent
	1.3 mg Sodium per 5 ml*	
Kolantyl (Merrell-National) Wafer **Dosage** **Adult:** 1-4 wafers every 4 h, up to 12 wafers/24 h for up to 2 wk	180 mg Aluminum hydroxide	Antacid
	170 mg Magnesium hydroxide	Antacid
	2.7 mg Sodium*	

Table continued on following page

Product (Manufacturer)	Ingredients	Actions
Kolantyl (Merrell-National) Gel **Dosage** **Adult:** 5–20 ml (1–4 tsp) every 4 h, up to 60 ml (12 tsp)/24 h for up to 2 wk	150 mg Aluminum hydroxide per 5 ml	Antacid
	150 mg Magnesium hydroxide per 5 ml	Antacid
	2.6 mg Sodium per 5 ml*	
Kolantyl (Merrell-National) Tablets (chewable) **Dosage** **Adult:** 1–2 tabs every 4 h, up to 12 tabs/24 h for up to 2 wk	300 mg Aluminum hydroxide	Antacid
	185 mg Magnesium oxide	Antacid
	20 mg Sodium*	
Maalox (Rorer) Tablets (No. 1) **Dosage** **Adult:** 2–4 tabs (well chewed or swallowed with water or milk) 20–60 min after meals and at bedtime, up to 16 tabs/24 h for up to 2 wk	200 mg Magnesium hydroxide	Antacid
	200 mg Aluminum hydroxide	Antacid
	0.84 mg Sodium*	
Maalox (Rorer) Tablets (No. 2) **Dosage** **Adult:** 1–2 tabs (well chewed) 20–60 min after meals and at bedtime, up to 8 tabs/24 h for up to 2 wk	400 mg Magnesium hydroxide	Antacid
	400 mg Aluminum hydroxide	Antacid
	1.8 mg Sodium*	
Maalox (Rorer) Suspension **Dosage** **Adult:** 10–20 ml (2–4 tsp) 4 times daily, 20–60 min after meals and at bedtime, up to 80 ml (16 tsp)/24 h for up to 2 wk	200 mg Magnesium hydroxide per 5 ml	Antacid
	225 mg Aluminum hydroxide per 5 ml	Antacid
	2.5 mg Sodium per 5 ml*	
Maalox Plus (Rorer) Tablets (chewable) **Dosage** **Adult:** 2–4 tabs (well chewed) 4 times daily, 20–60 min after meals and at bedtime, up to 16 tabs/24 h for up to 2 wk	200 mg Magnesium hydroxide	Antacid
	200 mg Aluminum hydroxide	Antacid
	25 mg Simethicone	Antiflatulent
	1.4 mg Sodium*	
Maalox Plus (Rorer) Suspension **Dosage** **Adult:** 10–20 ml (2–4 tsp) 4 times daily, 20–60 min after meals and at bedtime, up to 80 ml (16 tsp)/24 h for up to 2 wk	200 mg Magnesium hydroxide per 5 ml	Antacid
	225 mg Aluminum hydroxide per 5 ml	Antacid
	25 mg Simethicone per 5 ml	Antiflatulent
	2.5 mg Sodium per 5 ml*	
Maalox Therapeutic Concentrate (Rorer) Suspension **Dosage** **Adult:** 5–10 ml (1–2 tsp), as needed, between meals and at bedtime, up to 40 ml (8 tsp)/24 h for up to 2 wk; for active peptic ulcer disease, higher doses may be taken under direct medical supervision	300 mg Magnesium hydroxide per 5 ml	Antacid
	600 mg Aluminum hydroxide per 5 ml	Antacid
	1.25 mg Sodium per 5 ml*	

Table continued on following page

Product (Manufacturer)	Ingredients	Actions
Milk of Magnesia (various manufacturers) Tablets **Dosage** **Adult:** 2–4 tabs 1–4 times daily **Child (7–14 yr):** 1 tab 1–4 times daily	325 mg Magnesium hydroxide	Antacid
Milk of Magnesia (various manufacturers) Liquid **Dosage** **Adult:** 5–15 ml (1–3 tsp) 1–4 times daily **Child (1–12 yr):** 1.25 ml (¼ tsp) to 7.5 ml (1½ tsp) 1–4 times daily	2.27–2.62 g Magnesium hydroxide per 30 ml	Antacid
Mylanta (Stuart) Tablets (chewable) **Dosage** **Adult:** 1–2 tabs (well chewed) every 2–4 h, between meals and at bedtime	200 mg Aluminum hydroxide	Antacid
	200 mg Magnesium hydroxide	Antacid
	20 mg Simethicone	Antiflatulent
	0.77 mg Sodium*	
Mylanta (Stuart) Liquid **Dosage** **Adult:** 5–10 ml (1–2 tsp) every 2–4 h, between meals and at bedtime	200 mg Aluminum hydroxide per 5 ml	Antacid
	200 mg Magnesium hydroxide per 5 ml	Antacid
	20 mg Simethicone per 5 ml	Antiflatulent
	0.68 mg Sodium per 5 ml*	
Mylanta-II (Stuart) Tablets (chewable) **Dosage** **Adult:** 1–2 tabs (well chewed) between meals and at bedtime	400 mg Aluminum hydroxide	Antacid
	400 mg Magnesium hydroxide	Antacid
	30 mg Simethicone	Antiflatulent
	1.3 mg Sodium*	
Mylanta-II (Stuart) Liquid **Dosage** **Adult:** 5–10 ml (1–2 tsp) between meals and at bedtime	400 mg Aluminum hydroxide per 5 ml	Antacid
	400 mg Magnesium hydroxide per 5 ml	Antacid
	30 mg Simethicone per 5 ml	Antiflatulent
	1.14 mg Sodium per 5 ml*	
Mylicon (Stuart) Tablets (chewable) **Dosage** **Adult:** 1–2 tabs 4 times daily, after meals and at bedtime	40 mg Simethicone	Antiflatulent
	No Sodium	
Mylicon (Stuart) Drops **Dosage** **Adult:** 0.6 ml 4 times daily, after meals and at bedtime	40 mg Simethicone per 0.6 ml	Antiflatulent
	2 mg Sodium per 0.6 ml*	
Mylicon-80 (Stuart) Tablets (chewable) **Dosage** **Adult:** 1 tab 4 times daily, after meals and at bedtime	80 mg Simethicone	Antiflatulent
	No Sodium	

Table continued on following page

NONPRESCRIPTION HEARTBURN/ULCER MEDICATIONS

Product (Manufacturer)	Ingredients	Actions
Riopan (Ayerst) Tablets (chewable or plain) **Dosage** **Adult:** 1–2 tabs (swallowed with water or chewed, depending on formulation) between meals and at bedtime, up to 20 tabs/24 h for up to 2 wk	480 mg Magaldrate	Antacid
	≤0.3 mg Sodium*	
Riopan (Ayerst) Suspension **Dosage** **Adult:** 5–10 ml (1–2 tsp) between meals and at bedtime, up to 100 ml (20 tsp)/24 h for up to 2 wk	480 mg Magaldrate per 5 ml	Antacid
	≤0.3 mg Sodium per 5 ml*	
Riopan Plus (Ayerst) Tablets (chewable) **Dosage** **Adult:** 1–2 tabs (well chewed) between meals and at bedtime, up to 20 tabs/24 h for up to 2 wk	480 mg Magaldrate	Antacid
	20 mg Simethicone	Antiflatulent
	≤0.3 mg Sodium*	
Riopan Plus (Ayerst) Suspension **Dosage** **Adult:** 5–10 ml (1–2 tsp) between meals and at bedtime, up to 100 ml (20 tsp)/24 h for up to 2 wk	480 mg Magaldrate per 5 ml	Antacid
	20 mg Simethicone per 5 ml	Antiflatulent
	≤0.3 mg Sodium per 5 ml*	
Robalate (Robins) Tablets (chewable) **Dosage** **Adult:** 2–4 tabs 4 times daily, between meals and at bedtime	0.5 g Dihydroxyaluminum aminoacetate	Antacid
	<1 mg Sodium*	
Rolaids (Warner-Lambert) Tablets (chewable) **Dosage** **Adult:** 1–2 tabs, as needed, up to 24 tabs/24 h for up to 2 wk	334 mg Dihydroxyaluminum sodium carbonate	Antacid
	53 mg Sodium*	
Silain-Gel (Robins) Liquid **Dosage** **Adult:** 5–10 ml (1–2 tsp) after or between meals and at bedtime, as needed	282 mg Aluminum hydroxide per 5 ml	Antacid
	285 mg Magnesium hydroxide per 5 ml	Antacid
	25 mg Simethicone per 5 ml	Antiflatulent
	4.8 mg Sodium per 5 ml	
Sodium Bicarbonate (various manufacturers) Tablets **Dosage** **Adult:** 0.3–2 g, as needed, 1–4 times daily	325, 487.5, 520, 650 mg Sodium bicarbonate	Antacid
	27% Sodium*	
Titralac (Riker) Tablets **Dosage** **Adult:** 0.84 g (2 tabs) 1 h after meals, up to 10 tabs/24 h for up to 2 wk	0.42 mg Calcium carbonate	Antacid
	0.3 mg Sodium*	
Titralac (Riker) Liquid **Dosage** **Adult:** 5 ml (1 tsp) 1 h after meals, up to 40 ml (8 tsp)/24 h for up to 2 wk	1 g Calcium carbonate per 5 ml	Antacid
	11 mg Sodium per 5 ml*	

Table continued on following page

Product (Manufacturer)	Ingredients	Actions
Trisogel (Lilly) Capsules **Dosage** **Adult:** 4 caps 4 times daily	4½ gr Magnesium trisilicate	Antacid
	1½ gr Aluminum hydroxide	Antacid
	<1 mg Sodium	
Trisogel (Lilly) Liquid **Dosage** **Adult:** 10 ml (2 tsp) 4 times daily with water	9 gr Magnesium trisilicate per 5 ml	Antacid
	2.3 gr Aluminum hydroxide per 5 ml	Antacid
	22 mg Sodium per /5 ml*	
Tums (Norcliff Thayer) Tablets (chewable) **Dosage** **Adult:** 1–2 tabs, as needed, up to 16 tabs/24 h for up to 2 wk	500 mg Calcium carbonate	Antacid
	2.7 mg Sodium*	
WinGel (Winthrop) Tablets (chewable) **Dosage** **Adult:** 1–2 tabs 1–4 times daily, up to 8 tabs/24 h for up to 2 wk **Child (6–12 yr):** same as adult	180 mg Aluminum hydroxide	Antacid
	160 mg Magnesium hydroxide	Antacid
	1.25–2.15 mg Sodium*	
WinGel (Winthrop) Liquid **Dosage** **Adult:** 5–10 ml (1–2 tsp) 1–4 times daily, up to 40 ml (8 tsp)/24 h for up to 2 wk **Child (6–12 yr):** same as adult	180 mg Aluminum hydroxide per 5 ml	Antacid
	160 mg Magnesium hydroxide per 5 ml	Antacid
	1.5–3.9 mg Sodium per 5 ml*	

*Sodium is not an active ingredient in antacids, but its presence is often dictated by the other ingredients. The amount is included here to alert persons who may be on a salt-restricted diet.

Nausea and Vomiting

Nausea, the feeling of wanting to vomit or expel the contents of the stomach, is a highly unpleasant sensation. Since it is characterized by a revulsion to food, it is often a protective mechanism that decreases food intake. Nausea generally precedes or accompanies vomiting, although the two may occur independently.

In vomiting, the lower (pyloric) region of the stomach contracts sharply while the pyloric sphincter—the valve that opens into the duodenum (uppermost section of the small intestine)—closes, forcing the contents of the stomach upward. The signal to vomit is transmitted through an area of the brain known as the true vomiting center. The exact mechanisms are unknown, but signals originating in the gastrointestinal tract, inner ear, cerebrum, heart, or a center in the brain known as the chemoreceptor trigger zone, all may produce vomiting.

CAUSES OF NAUSEA AND VOMITING

Nausea and vomiting may be produced by motion sickness, pregnancy, other chemical or physical stimuli, or emotional distress. Persistent nausea may be symptomatic of gastrointestinal or gallbladder disease or bacterial infection. The most common causes of nausea and vomiting and their treatments will be reviewed in this section. If the cause of nausea is not immediately apparent, a physician should be consulted.

Motion Sickness and Vertigo

Motion sickness, a primary cause of nausea, may be precipitated by any mode of travel. The nausea of motion sickness is often preceded by a feeling of fatigue and may progress to retching and vomiting. It is common for the skin to feel clammy; the victim also may feel dizzy and disoriented and may experience blurred vision.

Pitching, rolling, or yawing movements stimulate the three semicircular canals in each ear, and the multiple stimulations may cause conflicting sensations of orientation (vertigo). These conflicting sensations often intensify if visual contact with the horizon is lost (see the section on *Ear Disorders*, page 178). Motion sickness is also aggravated by odors, and the susceptible person should be in as

MECHANISM OF VOMITING

Sources of Vomiting Stimuli

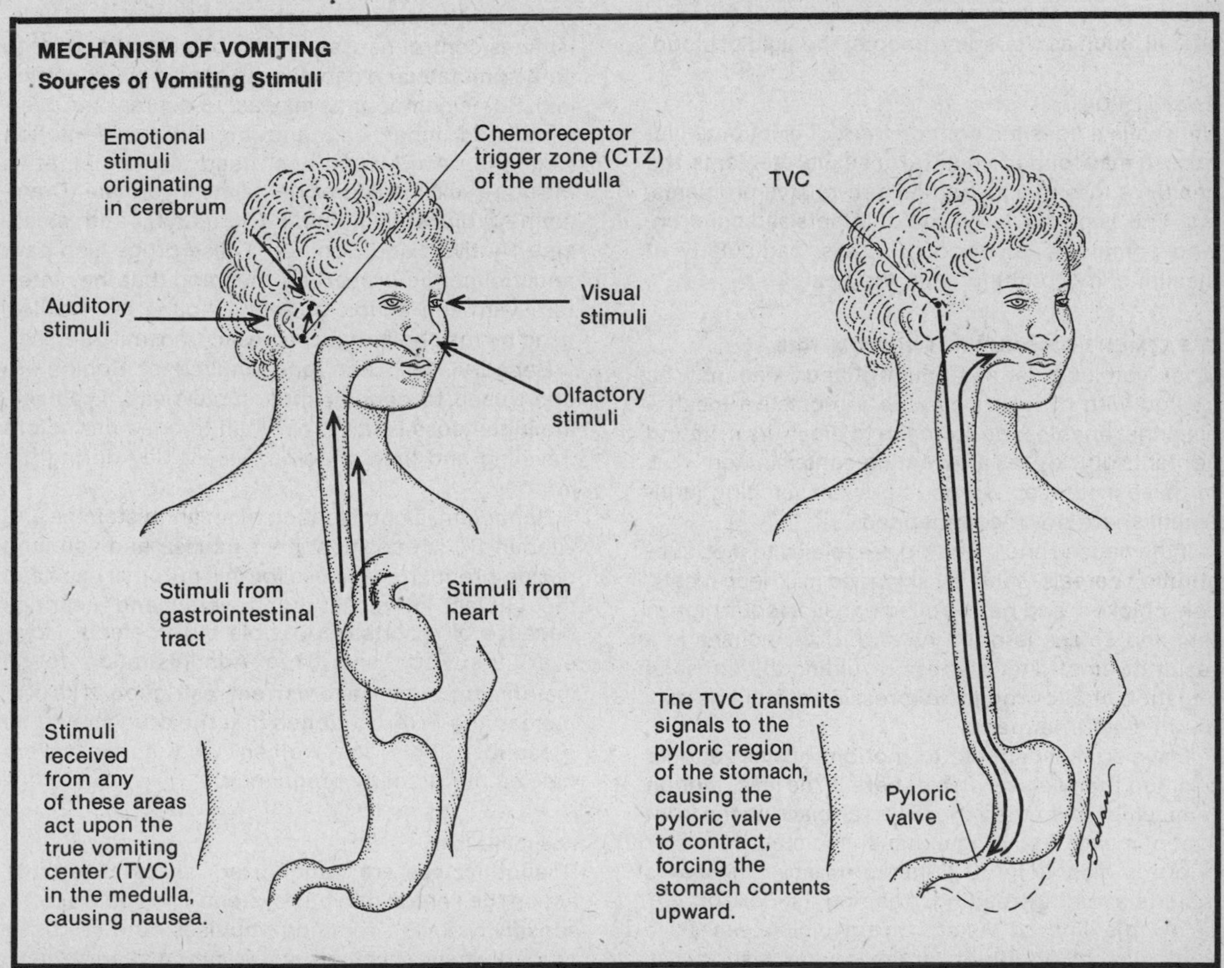

odor-free an environment as possible. The person prone to seasickness may do best in fresh air. Car sickness can sometimes be avoided by sitting in the front seat and looking out the front window.

Nausea in Pregnancy

Nausea is common during the first trimester of pregnancy. It also may be experienced during the early months of oral contraceptive use. Although it is often called "morning sickness," it can occur at any time of day or, in some instances, may recur at a regular time each day. Fatty or fried foods may aggravate nausea and should be avoided. Large amounts of fluids, especially with meals, have also been identified as contributing to nausea. Avoiding fluids for one to two hours before and after meals and consuming dry breads and crackers at two-hour intervals may bring relief to women suffering from nausea associated with pregnancy.

Physical and Chemical Stimulants

A number of physical and chemical agents may induce nausea and vomiting. Narcotics such as morphine and meperidine (Demerol) and toxic dosages of digitalis cause vomiting. Nauseous reactions to anesthetics used during surgery are also common, and nausea and vomiting are common side effects in cancer chemotherapy and radiotherapy.

Greasy or fatty foods, alcohol, and unpleasant odors may provoke nausea, as may certain visual stimuli, such as (for some people) the sight of blood.

Emotional Distress

Nausea is a possible concomitant of emotional distress. It may relate to marital or sexual problems, the health or loss of a loved one, job-related problems, etc. This is particularly true of infants and children, who commonly respond to stress, particularly at mealtime, by vomiting what they eat.

TREATMENT OF NAUSEA AND VOMITING

Most vomiting is self-limiting and need not be treated with drugs. It may be a protective mechanism that enables the stomach to empty its irritating contents quickly, as after eating contaminated food. In these instances, drugs to prevent vomiting (antiemetics) are not recommended.

If the nausea and vomiting are related to diet, substituting cereals, saltines, skimmed milk, lean meats, fish, chicken, and hard-boiled eggs for foods high in fats and spices is often helpful. If the nausea is a result of emotional distress, avoiding the stressful situation or allowing the expression of feelings may be the best treatment.

Travelers susceptible to motion sickness should position themselves where there is the least motion (amidships, over the wings in an airplane, in the front seat of a car). Avoiding exhaust and other fumes or odors is also helpful. Other preventive measures include avoiding reading, keeping the horizon 45° below the line of vision, and avoiding excessive food, alcohol, and fluids. If the journey is short, it is wise to postpone eating and drinking until arrival.

Nausea during pregnancy is also self-limiting, usually confined to the first trimester. All self-medication should be avoided during this period unless specifically recommended or approved by a physician. Some women find it helpful to prevent a completely empty stomach by eating dry crackers or toast every few hours. If the vomiting occurs upon arising in the morning, eating a couple of crackers before getting out of bed may help.

Victims of nausea often find comfort lying perfectly still and as flat as possible, but with a pillow under the knees to relax the abdomen. Others prefer the warmth and pressure of lying on the abdomen. A heating pad or hot-water bottle at the feet or on the abdomen may be comforting, as may a cool cloth on the forehead.

Persistent or prolonged vomiting can lead to electrolyte imbalance or dehydration and should be treated with antiemetics. These drugs are also sometimes given with presurgical anesthesia to reduce postoperative vomiting. Medications are often given by mouth before vomiting begins, but must be administered by suppository or parenterally once there is vomiting. Prescription antiemetics are usually either antihistamines or phenothiazines, which are tranquilizing and/or sedative agents.

Antihistamines

Although the precise mechanism by which antihistamines control nausea is unknown, they appear to both stimulate and depress the central nervous system. Some compounds may act to depress the overstimulated inner ear, and thereby ease motion sickness. Antihistamines used as antiemetics include cyclizine (Marezine), dimenhydrinate (Dramamine), diphenhydramine (Benadryl), and meclizine (Antivert and Bonine). These drugs also have anticholinergic properties, meaning that they interfere with the action of acetylcholine, a chemical used by the cholinergic nerves to transmit impulses.

Benadryl, Marezine, and Antivert or Bonine are often used to counter motion sickness. Typically, the initial dose is taken one-half to one hour before traveling and then once or twice a day during the journey.

Bendectin, a combination of an antihistamine and vitamin B_6, is specifically for nausea and vomiting during pregnancy. Its use for this purpose has been the subject of recent controversy and hearings because of reports of possible birth defects. However, the Food and Drug Administration found insufficient evidence to warrant restriction of its use. Instead the FDA cautioned that the drug should be prescribed only for women who suffer severe nausea during early pregnancy.

Phenothiazines

Phenothiazines are tranquilizers or sedatives that act on the central nervous system. They depress the sensitivity to the vomiting impulses, and are used primarily to treat nausea and vomiting after surgery, radiation therapy, or cancer chemotherapy. They also may be prescribed for nausea and vomiting associated with cancer or uremia (kidney failure). They should be used with caution, however, since they may mask the symptoms of undiagnosed conditions such as intestinal obstruction, brain tumor, Reye's syndrome, and other diseases. Antinauseants and antiemetics containing phenothiazines include prochlorperazine (Compazine), chlorpromazine (Thorazine), promethazine (Phenergan), perphenazine (Trilafon), and triflupromazine (Vesprin). These drugs have sedating properties and are often used to treat psychotic disorders; their most frequent use as antinauseants is for persons undergoing general anesthesia or cancer chemotherapy.

Control of Postoperative Nausea

Barbiturates possess antinauseant and antiemetic properties, and are sometimes administered with preoperative general anesthesia to reduce postoperative nausea. They help contol nausea by their sedating and antihistamine actions, as well as by suppressing the true vomiting center in the brain. A drug such as trimethobenzamide hydrochloride (Tigan) may be prescribed in suppository form to relieve postoperative nausea and vomiting. Other drugs used for this purpose include benzquinamide hydrochloride (Emete-con), administered by injection or intravenously; and diphenidol (Vontrol), used only in hospitalized patients.

Other Drugs

Several drugs to control nausea and vomiting are available without prescription. These include dimenhydrinate (Dramamine), used for motion sickness, and Emetrol, a compound of levulose, dextrose, and orthophosphoric acid, which controls nausea and vomiting by acting directly on the gastrointestinal tract.

Recent studies have found that tetrahydrocannabinol (THC), the hallucinogenic ingredient in marijuana, may be useful in controlling the nausea and vomiting that often accompany cancer chemotherapy. THC is now being used experimentally in several centers to further test its usefulness for this purpose.

IN CONCLUSION

Most episodes of nausea and vomiting are self-limiting or can be lessened by avoiding precipitating factors. The nausea and vomiting associated with surgery, certain drugs, and illnesses usually can be controlled by the use of drugs. The following charts cover the major drugs in this category.

ANTIVERT (Meclizine hydrochloride) **Roerig**

Tabs: 12.5, 25 mg **Chewable tabs:** 25 mg

INDICATIONS	ORAL DOSAGE
Nausea, vomiting, and dizziness associated with motion sickness	**Adult:** 25-50 mg 1 h before anticipated exposure to motion, repeated q24h, as needed
Vertigo associated with diseases affecting the vestibular system[1]	**Adult:** 25-100 mg/day div

CONTRAINDICATIONS

Hypersensitivity to meclizine

WARNINGS/PRECAUTIONS

Drowsiness	Performance of potentially hazardous activities may be impaired; caution patients accordingly

ADVERSE REACTIONS

Central nervous system	Drowsiness
Other	Dry mouth, blurred vision

OVERDOSAGE

Signs and symptoms	Sedation, possible anticholinergic effects (eg, dry mouth, blurred vision, others)
Treatment	Treat symptomatically

DRUG INTERACTIONS

No clinically significant drug interactions have been observed

ALTERED LABORATORY VALUES

No clinically significant alterations in blood/serum or urinary values occur at therapeutic dosages

Use in children

Not recommended; safety and effectiveness have not been established

Use in pregnancy or nursing mothers

Contraindicated during pregnancy, owing to reported teratogenicity in rats; general guidelines not established for use in nursing mothers

Note: Meclizine also marketed as **BONINE** (Pfipharmecs).

BENADRYL (Diphenhydramine hydrochloride) **Parke Davis**

Caps: 25, 50 mg **Elixir:** 12.5 mg/5 ml[1] **Vials:** 10 mg/ml (10, 30 ml) **Amps:** 50 mg/ml (1 ml) **Syringe:** 50 mg/ml (1 ml)

INDICATIONS	ORAL DOSAGE	PARENTERAL DOSAGE
Motion sickness	**Adult:** same as above, 30 min before anticipated travel, before meals, and before bedtime **Child:** same as above, 30 min before exposure to motion, before meals, and before bedtime	**Adult:** same as above, 30 min before exposure to motion, before meals, and before bedtime **Child:** same as above, 30 min before exposure to motion, before meals, and before bedtime
Seasonal and perennial **allergic rhinitis; vasomotor rhinitis; allergic conjunctivitis** due to inhalant allergens and foods; mild, uncomplicated **urticaria** and **angioedema;** and **dermatographism**	**Adult:** 50 mg or 20 ml (4 tsp) tid or qid **Child:** 5 mg/kg/day or 150 mg/m²/day, up to 300 mg/day **Child (>20 lb):** 12.5–25 mg tid or qid	—
Allergic reactions to blood or plasma and in **anaphylactic reactions,** as an adjunct to epinephrine and other standard measures after acute symptoms have been controlled	**Adult:** same as above **Child:** same as above	**Adult:** 10–50 mg IM (deeply) or IV (100 mg, if needed), up to 400 mg/day **Child:** 5 mg/kg/day or 150 mg/m²/day, up to 300 mg/day, IM (deeply) or IV, divided into 4 doses
Uncomplicated, **immediate-type allergic reactions,** when oral therapy is impossible or contraindicated	—	**Adult:** same as above **Child:** same as above
Parkinsonism (including drug-induced extrapyramidal symptoms) in elderly patients unable to tolerate more potent agents, and in other age groups for mild symptoms or in combination with centrally acting anticholinergic agents	**Adult:** same as above **Child:** same as above	—
Parkinsonism (as above), when oral therapy is impossible or contraindicated	—	**Adult:** same as above **Child:** same as above

Note: Full chart appears on page 920

BENDECTIN (Doxylamine succinate and pyridoxine hydrochloride) Merrell-National

Tabs: 10 mg doxylamine succinate and 10 mg pyridoxine hydrochloride

INDICATIONS	ORAL DOSAGE
Nausea and vomiting associated with pregnancy	**Adult:** 2 tabs at bedtime; for severe cases or daytime nausea, 1 tab in AM, 1 in midafternoon, and 2 at bedtime

CONTRAINDICATIONS

None

WARNINGS/PRECAUTIONS

Drowsiness — Performance of potentially hazardous activities may be impaired; caution patients accordingly

ADVERSE REACTIONS

Central nervous system — Drowsiness, vertigo, nervousness, headache, disorientation, irritability

Gastrointestinal — Epigastric pain, diarrhea

Cardiovascular — Palpitations

OVERDOSAGE

Signs and symptoms — CNS excitation or sedation

Treatment — Treat symptomatically; institute supportive measures, as indicated

DRUG INTERACTIONS

No clinically significant drug interactions have been observed

ALTERED LABORATORY VALUES

No clinically significant alterations in blood/serum or urinary values occur at therapeutic dosages

Use in children

No appropriate indication exists in children

Use in pregnancy or nursing mothers

Animal reproductive studies and epidemiological studies in women have shown no increase in fetal abnormalities; nevertheless, drug should be prescribed only when clearly indicated, especially during the first trimester. Drug is not indicated for any use other than during pregnancy.

COMPAZINE (Prochlorperazine) Smith Kline & French

Tabs. 5, 10, 25 mg **Caps (sust rel):** 10, 15, 30, 75 mg **Amps:** 5 mg/ml (2 ml) **Vial:** 5 mg/ml (10 ml) **Syringe:** 5 mg/ml (2 ml)
Supp: 2½, 5, 25 mg **Syrup:** 5 mg/5 ml **Conc:** 10 mg/ml

INDICATIONS	ORAL DOSAGE	PARENTERAL DOSAGE
Severe nausea and vomiting, excessive anxiety in adults	**Adult:** 5-10 mg tid or qid; sust rel caps: 15 mg on arising or 10 mg q12h **Child (20-29 lb):** 2.5 mg qd or bid, or up to 7.5 mg/day **Child (30-39 lb):** 2.5 mg bid or tid, or up to 10 mg/day **Child (40-85 lb):** 2.5 mg tid or 5 mg bid, or up to 15 mg/day	**Adult:** 5-10 mg IM to start, repeated q3-4h, as needed, up to 40 mg/day **Child:** 0.06 mg/lb IM
Severe nausea and vomiting associated with anesthesia and surgery	—	**Adult:** 5-10 mg IM 1-2 h before induction of anesthesia (repeat once in 30 min, if needed), as well as during or after surgery, if needed (may be repeated once); 5-10 mg IV 15-30 min before anesthesia, as well as during or after surgery, if needed (may be repeated once); or 20 mg/liter of isotonic solution added to IV infusion 15-30 min before anesthesia
Relatively mild psychiatric conditions	**Adult:** 5-10 mg tid or qid	—
Moderate to severe psychiatric conditions, in hospitalized or supervised patients	**Adult:** 10 mg tid or qid; increase dosage in small increments every 2-3 days until symptoms are controlled or side effects become disturbing; some patients respond to 50-75 mg/day	—
Severe psychiatric conditions	**Adult:** 100-150 mg/day	**Adult:** 10-20 mg IM to start, repeated q2-4h (or in resistant cases every hour), as needed; prolonged therapy: 10-20 mg IM q4-6h
Pediatric psychiatric conditions	**Child (2-12 yr):** 2.5 mg bid or tid, up to 10 mg on 1st day, followed by increases in dosage up to 20 mg/day (2-5 yr) or 25 mg/day (6-12 yr), as needed	**Child (<12 yr):** 0.06 mg/lb IM

Note: Full chart appears on page 785

DRAMAMINE (Dimenhydrinate) Searle

Tabs: 50 mg **Liq:** 12.5 mg/4 ml **Amps:** 50 mg/ml (1 ml) **Vial:** 50 mg/ml (5 ml) **Supp:** 100 mg

DRAMAMINE JUNIOR (Dimenhydrinate) Searle

Liq: 12.5 mg/4 ml

INDICATIONS	ORAL DOSAGE	PARENTERAL DOSAGE
Nausea, vomiting, and vertigo of motion sickness	**Adult:** 50–100 mg q4–6h, up to 400 mg/24 h, or 16–32 ml (4–8 tsp) q4–6h, up to 128 ml (32 tsp)/24 h **Child (2–6 yr):** 12.5–25 mg q6–8h, up to 75 mg/24 h, or 4–8 ml (1–2 tsp) q6–8h, up to 24 ml (6 tsp)/24 h **Child (6–12 yr):** 25–50 mg q6–8h, up to 150 mg/24 h, or 8–16 ml (2–4 tsp) q6–8h, up to 48 ml (12 tsp)/24 h	**Adult:** 50 mg IM or IV (slowly), as needed **Child:** 1.25 mg/kg or 37.5 mg/m² qid, up to 300 mg/day

ADMINISTRATION/DOSAGE ADJUSTMENTS

Intravenous administration — Dilute 50 mg (1 ml) in 10 ml of Sodium Chloride Injection and inject over 2-min period

Rectal use — For adults, administer 100 mg qd or bid

CONTRAINDICATIONS

Asthma ● Glaucoma ● Prostatic enlargement ●

WARNINGS/PRECAUTIONS

Antibiotic ototoxicity — May be masked; use with caution with aminoglycoside antibiotics

Drowsiness — Performance of potentially hazardous activities may be impaired; caution patients accordingly and to avoid alcoholic beverages

ADVERSE REACTIONS

Central nervous system — Drowsiness

OVERDOSAGE

Signs and symptoms — Atropine-like symptoms, sedation, mydriasis, excitation, hallucinations, confusion, convulsions, coma, respiratory failure, cardiovascular collapse

Treatment — Maintain patent airway and institute supportive measures, as indicated. Gastric lavage may be helpful. Treat symptomatically. Limit external stimulation to minimize CNS excitation.

DRUG INTERACTIONS

Alcohol, tranquilizers, sedative-hypnotics, and other CNS depressants — ⇧ CNS depression

ALTERED LABORATORY VALUES

No clinically significant alterations in blood/serum or urinary values occur at therapeutic dosages

Use in children

See INDICATIONS; not recommended for frequent or prolonged use. General guidelines not established for dosage in children under 2 yr of age.

Use in pregnancy or nursing mothers

General guidelines not established

EMETE-CON (Benzquinamide hydrochloride) Roerig

Vial: 50 mg

INDICATIONS	PARENTERAL DOSAGE
Nausea and vomiting associated with anesthesia and surgery	**Adult:** 50 mg IM or 25 mg IV (slowly) to start; IM dose only may be repeated in 1 h and then q3–4h, as needed

ADMINISTRATION/DOSAGE ADJUSTMENTS

Intramuscular administration	Inject deeply into large muscle mass 15 min prior to anesthesia to prevent nausea and vomiting
Intravenous administration to elderly or debilitated patients	Administer slowly (0.5 ml/min) and decrease dosage to ~0.5 mg/kg
Patients receiving epinephrine or other vasopressors	Reduce dosage and monitor blood pressure during administration

CONTRAINDICATIONS

Hypersensitivity to benzquinamide

WARNINGS/PRECAUTIONS

Disease, drug toxicity	Antiemetic effects may mask signs of overdosage and obscure diagnosis of such conditions as intestinal obstruction and brain tumor
Sudden hypertension and transient arrhythmias	Have been reported with IV administration; IM use is preferred; do not use IV route in the presence of cardiovascular disease or in patients receiving pre-anesthetic or cardiovascular drugs

ADVERSE REACTIONS

Autonomic nervous system	Dry mouth, shivering, sweating, hiccoughs, flushing, salivation, blurred vision
Cardiovascular	Hypertension, hypotension, dizziness, atrial fibrillation, premature auricular and ventricular contractions
Central nervous system and neuromuscular	Drowsiness, insomnia, restlessness, headache, excitement, nervousness, twitching, shaking/tremors, weakness
Gastrointestinal	Anorexia, nausea
Dermatological	Hives, rash
Allergic	Pyrexia and urticaria (one case)
Other	Fatigue, chills, hyperpyrexia

OVERDOSAGE

Signs and symptoms	CNS stimulation or depression may be anticipated, based on animal toxicology studies
Treatment	Institute supportive measures, as indicated; atropine may be helpful. Dialysis is not likely to be of value, owing to extensive protein binding.

DRUG INTERACTIONS

Epinephrine and other pressor agents	⇧ Hypertensive effect

ALTERED LABORATORY VALUES

No clinically significant alterations in blood/serum or urinary values occur at therapeutic dosages

Use in children

Not recommended

Use in pregnancy or nursing mothers

Not recommended during pregnancy; general guidelines not established for use in nursing mothers

EMETROL (Levulose, dextrose, and orthophosphoric acid) Rorer

Oral sol: "balanced amounts" of ingredients

INDICATIONS	ORAL DOSAGE
Nausea and vomiting due to functional causes, drug therapy, or inhalation anesthesia; **motion sickness**	**Adult:** 15–30 ml (1–2 tbsp) at 15-min intervals until vomiting ceases; if first dose is rejected, resume dosage schedule in 5 min **Infant:** 5–10 ml (1–2 tsp) at 15-min intervals until vomiting ceases; if first dose is rejected, resume dosage schedule in 5 min **Child:** same as for infant
Regurgitation in infants	**Infant:** 5–10 ml (1–2 tsp) 10–15 min before feeding; refractory cases: 10–15 ml (2–3 tsp) ½ h before feeding
"Morning sickness"	**Adult:** 15–30 ml (1–2 tbsp) on arising, repeated q3h or whenever nausea threatens

ADMINISTRATION/DOSAGE ADJUSTMENTS

Administer undiluted	Do not dilute solution or permit oral fluids immediately before or for at least 15 min after dose

CONTRAINDICATIONS

None

WARNINGS/PRECAUTIONS

None

ADVERSE REACTIONS

None

OVERDOSAGE

No toxicity has been reported in clinical use

DRUG INTERACTIONS

No clinically significant drug interactions have been observed

ALTERED LABORATORY VALUES

No clinically significant alterations in blood/serum or urinary values occur at therapeutic dosages

Use in children

See INDICATIONS

Use in pregnancy or nursing mothers

General guidelines not established

PHENERGAN (Promethazine hydrochloride) Wyeth

Tabs: 12.5, 25, 50 mg **Syrup:** 6.25 mg/5 ml,[1] 25 mg/5 ml[1] **Supp:** 12.5, 25, 50 mg

INDICATIONS	ORAL DOSAGE	RECTAL DOSAGE
Nausea and vomiting associated with anesthesia and surgery	**Adult:** for treatment, 25 mg to start, followed by 12.5–25 mg q4–6h, as needed; for prophylaxis, 25 mg q4–6h **Child:** adjust dosage based on child's weight and age and on the severity of the condition	**Adult:** for treatment, 12.5–25 mg q4–6h, as needed; for prophylaxis, 25 mg q4–6h **Child:** adjust dosage based on child's weight and age and on the severity of the condition
Motion sickness	**Adult:** 25 mg ½–1 h before anticipated travel, repeated 8–12 h later, if necessary; then 25 mg on arising in AM and again before evening meal **Child:** 12.5–25 mg bid	**Child:** 12.5–25 mg bid
Sedation	**Adult:** 25–50 mg at bedtime **Child:** 12.5–25 mg at bedtime	**Adult:** 25–50 mg at bedtime **Child:** 12.5–25 mg at bedtime
Preoperative medication	**Adult:** 50 mg with an equal amount of meperidine and the required amount of belladonna alkaloids **Child:** 0.5 mg/lb with an equal dose of meperidine and the appropriate dose of an atropine-like drug	**Child (<3 yr):** 25 mg **Child (3–12 yr):** 50 mg
Postoperative pain, as an adjunct to analgesia, and for **postoperative sedation**	**Adult:** 25–50 mg, as needed **Child:** 12.5–25 mg, as needed	—
Seasonal and perennial **allergic rhinitis; vasomotor rhinitis; allergic conjunctivitis** due to inhalant allergens and foods; mild, uncomplicated **urticaria** and **angioedema; dermatographism;** and in **anaphylactic reactions,** as an adjunct to epinephrine and other standard measures after acute symptoms have been controlled	**Adult:** 25 mg at bedtime or 12.5 mg before meals and at bedime, if necessary **Child:** 25 mg before bedtime or 6.25–12.5 mg tid	**Adult:** 25 mg, repeated 2 h later if necessary **Child:** same as adult
Allergic reactions to blood or plasma	**Adult:** 25 mg, as needed **Child:** 25 mg, as needed	—

Note: Full chart appears on page 932

[1]Contains 1.5% alcohol

RU-VERT (Pentylenetetrazol, pheniramine maleate, and nicotinic acid) **Boots**

Tabs: 25 mg pentylenetetrazol, 12.5 mg pheniramine maleate, and 50 mg nicotinic acid

INDICATIONS	ORAL DOSAGE
Idiopathic vertigo **Peripheral vestibular disorders** associated with Meniere's syndrome, labyrinthitis, and fenestration procedures	**Adult:** 1-2 tabs tid

CONTRAINDICATIONS

Hypersensitivity to any component ●	Arterial hypotension ●

WARNINGS/PRECAUTIONS

Special-risk patients	Use with caution in patients with epilepsy or a low convulsive threshold

ADVERSE REACTIONS

Central nervous system	Sedation
Cardiovascular	Flushing, sensation of warmth
Other	Gastrointestinal effects (rare)

OVERDOSAGE

Signs and symptoms	*Pentylenetetrazol-related effects:* epileptiform seizures, respiratory depression; *pheniramine-related effects:* vary from CNS depression (drowsiness, sedation, diminished mental alertness, apnea, cardiovascular collapse) to CNS stimulation (insomnia, excitement, hallucinations, ataxia, incoordination, athetosis, tremors, convulsions) and may include dizziness, tinnitus, blurred vision, and hypotension; CNS stimulation, followed by postictal depression, and atropine-like symptoms (dry mouth; fixed, dilated pupils; fever; flushing; GI disturbances) are particularly likely in children; *nicotinic acid-related effects:* hepatic damage, impaired glucose tolerance, toxic amblyopia, hyperuricemia
Treatment	If patient is conscious, induce emesis with syrup of ipecac, even though vomiting may have occurred spontaneously. If vomiting is unsuccessful or contraindicated, perform gastric lavage with isotonic or ½ isotonic saline solution. Remove any remaining drug in the stomach by instillation of activated charcoal. Administer a saline cathartic to rapidly dilute bowel content. Treatment is symptomatic and supportive. If breathing is significantly impaired, maintain an adequate airway and provide mechanically assisted ventilation; *do not use analeptics.* Vasopressors (eg, levarterenol) may be used for significant hypotension. Treat hyperpyrexia by sponging with tepid water or use of ice packs or a hypothermal blanket. For seizures, administer a short-acting barbiturate, diazepam, or paraldehyde.

DRUG INTERACTIONS

No clinically significant drug interactions have been observed

ALTERED LABORATORY VALUES

No clinically significant alterations in blood/serum or urinary values occur at therapeutic dosages

Use in children	Use in pregnancy or nursing mothers
General guidelines not established	General guidelines not established

THORAZINE (Chlorpromazine hydrochloride) **Smith Kline & French**

Tabs: 10, 25, 50, 100, 200 mg **Caps (sust rel):** 30, 75, 150, 200, 300 mg **Syrup:** 10 mg/5 ml **Supp:** 25, 100 mg
Conc: 30, 100 mg/ml **Amps:** 25 mg/ml (1,2 ml) **Vial:** 25 mg/ml (10 ml)

INDICATIONS	ORAL DOSAGE	PARENTERAL DOSAGE
Nausea and vomiting	**Adult:** 10–25 mg q4–6h, as needed; increase dosage, if necessary **Child:** 0.25 mg/lb q4–6h	**Adult:** 25 mg IM to start; if no hypotension occurs, 25–50 mg q3–4h, as needed, until vomiting ceases; follow with oral regimen **Child (< 5 yr or 50 lb):** 0.25 mg/lb IM q6–8h, up to 40 mg/day, if needed **Child (5–12 yr or 50–100 lb):** 0.25 mg/lb IM q6–8h, up to 75 mg/day, if needed
Nausea and vomiting during surgery	—	**Adult:** 12.5 mg IM; repeat in ½ h, if needed and if no hypotension occurs; alternative regimen: 2 mg/fractional IV injection every 2 min, up to 25 mg; dilute to 1 mg/ml for IV administration **Child:** 0.125 mg/lb IM; repeat in ½ h, if needed and if no hypotension occurs; alternative regimen: 1 mg/fractional IV injection every 2 min, up to 0.125 mg/lb; dilute to 1 mg/ml for IV administration

Note: Full chart appears on page 802

TIGAN (Trimethobenzamide hydrochloride) Beecham

Caps: 100, 250 mg **Amps:** 100 mg/ml (2 ml) **Vial:** 100 mg/ml (20 ml) **Syringe:** 100 mg/ml (2 ml)
Supp: 200 mg trimethobenzamide and 2% benzocaine **Ped supp:** 100 mg trimethobenzamide and 2% benzocaine

INDICATIONS	ORAL DOSAGE	RECTAL DOSAGE
Nausea and vomiting	**Adult:** 250 mg tid or qid **Child (30-90 lb):** 100-200 mg tid or qid	**Adult:** 200 mg (1 supp) tid or qid **Child (<30 lb):** 100 mg (½ supp or 1 ped supp) tid or qid **Child (30-90 lb):** 100-200 mg (½-1 supp or 1-2 ped supps) tid or qid

ADMINISTRATION/DOSAGE ADJUSTMENTS

Parenteral use — Usual adult dosage, 200 mg IM tid or qid; intramuscular injection may cause pain, stinging, burning, redness, and swelling at injection site; effects may be minimized by deep injection into upper outer quadrant of gluteal region and by avoiding escape of solution along route

CONTRAINDICATIONS

Hypersensitivity to trimethobenzamide or benzocaine (if suppositories are used)

WARNINGS/PRECAUTIONS

Drowsiness — Performance of potentially hazardous activities may be impaired; caution patients accordingly

Reye's syndrome — Centrally acting antiemetics may, in the presence of viral infections, cause or contribute to development of syndrome

Drug-induced extrapyramidal symptoms and other CNS reactions — May mask signs of undiagnosed primary diseases with CNS manifestations

Special-risk patients — Use with caution in patients with acute febrile illness, encephalitis, gastroenteritis, dehydration, and electrolyte imbalances (especially in children, the elderly, or debilitated patients); direct primary attention to restoring body fluids and electrolyte balance, relieving fever, and correction of underlying disease process

Drug toxicity — Antiemetic effect may mask signs of overdosage of other drugs

ADVERSE REACTIONS

Central nervous system — Parkinsonian-like symptoms, coma, convulsions, mood depression, disorientation, dizziness, drowsiness, headache, opisthotonos

Ophthalmic — Blurred vision

Cardiovascular — Hypotension

Hematological — Blood dyscrasias

Gastrointestinal — Diarrhea

Hypersensitivity — Allergic-type skin reactions

Other — Jaundice, muscle cramps

OVERDOSAGE

Signs and symptoms — See ADVERSE REACTIONS

Treatment — Discontinue use of drug; treat symptomatically

DRUG INTERACTIONS

No clinically significant drug interactions have been observed

ALTERED LABORATORY VALUES

No clinically significant alterations in blood/serum or urinary values occur at therapeutic dosages

Use in children

See INDICATIONS; use should be limited to prolonged vomiting of known etiology. Injectable form is contraindicated for use in children. Suppositories are contraindicated in premature or newborn infants.

Use in pregnancy or nursing mothers

Safe use not established

TORECAN (Thiethylperazine maleate) Boehringer Ingelheim

Tabs: 10 mg **Supp:** 10 mg **Amps:** 10 mg/2 ml (2 ml) for IM use only

INDICATIONS	ORAL DOSAGE	PARENTERAL DOSAGE
Nausea and vomiting **Vertigo**[1]	**Adult:** 10 mg 1-3 time/day	**Adult:** 10 mg IM 1-3 times/day

ADMINISTRATION/DOSAGE ADJUSTMENTS

Postoperative nausea and vomiting associated with anesthesia and surgery	Administer by deep IM injection, at or shortly before termination of anesthesia
Rectal use	For adults, administer 1 suppository 1-3 times/day

CONTRAINDICATIONS

Hypersensitivity to phenothiazines ● Severe CNS depression ● Comatose states ●

WARNINGS/PRECAUTIONS

Postoperative use	Possible complications due to phenothiazine effects must be considered (see ADVERSE REACTIONS). Restlessness and CNS depression may occur during anesthesia recovery. Use in intracardiac or intracranial surgery has not been studied.
Postural hypotension	May occur, especially after initial parenteral dose. If vasoconstrictors are required, use levarterenol or phenylephrine; do not use epinephrine. Intravenous use may result in severe hypotension and, therefore, is contraindicated.
Mental impairment, reflex-slowing	Performance of potentially hazardous activities may be impaired; warn patients
Extrapyramidal symptoms	May occur, especially in young adults and children, requiring reduction in dosage or discontinuation of drug (see ADVERSE REACTIONS)
Tartrazine sensitivity	Presence of FD&C Yellow No. 5 (tartrazine) in tablets may cause allergic-type reactions

ADVERSE REACTIONS[2]

Central nervous system	Convulsions, extrapyramidal reactions (including dystonia, torticollis, oculogyric crises, akathisia, gait disturbances, agitation, motor restlessness, dystonic reactions, trismus, opisthotonos, tremor, muscle rigidity, and akinesia), dizziness, headache, restlessness, drowsiness, excitement, bizarre dreams, aggravation of psychoses, toxic confusional states
Autonomic nervous system	Dry mouth and nose, blurred vision, tinnitus, sialorrhea, altered sense of taste, miosis, obstipation, anorexia, paralytic ileus
Endocrinological	Peripheral edema of the arms, hands, and face; menstrual irregularities; altered libido; gynecomastia; weight gain
Hematological	Agranulocytosis, leukopenia, thrombocytopenia, aplastic anemia, pancytopenia, eosinophilia, leukocytosis
Dermatological	Erythema, exfoliative dermatitis, contact dermatitis
Hepatic	Cholestatic jaundice, biliary stasis, jaundice
Cardiovascular	Hypotension, rarely leading to cardiac arrest; ECG changes
Hypersensitivity	Fever, laryngeal edema, angioneurotic edema, asthma
Other	Cerebral vascular spasm, trigeminal neuralgia, urinary retention or incontinence, hyperpyrexia, progressive pigmentation of skin or conjunctiva accompanied by **discoloration of exposed sclera and cornea, irregular or stellate opacities of anterior lens and cornea**

OVERDOSAGE

Signs and symptoms	See ADVERSE REACTIONS
Treatment	Discontinue medication; treat symptomatically and institute supportive measures

DRUG INTERACTIONS

Alcohol, opiates, anesthetics, and other CNS depressants	⇧ CNS depression
Atropine	⇧ Antimuscarinic effects
Epinephrine	Severe hypotension

ALTERED LABORATORY VALUES

Urinary values	False-positive pregnancy tests

No clinically significant alterations in blood/serum values occur at therapeutic dosages

Use in children

Safe use not established in children under 12 yr of age

Use in pregnancy or nursing mothers

Contraindicated during pregnancy; patient should stop nursing if drug is prescribed

[1]Possibly effective
[2]Includes reactions common to phenothiazines in general

VESPRIN (Triflupromazine hydrochloride) Squibb

Tabs: 10, 25, 50 mg **Susp:** 10 mg/ml (120 ml) **Syringe:** 10 mg/ml (1 ml) **Vials:** 20 mg/ml (1 ml), 10 mg/ml (10 ml)

INDICATIONS	ORAL DOSAGE	PARENTERAL DOSAGE
Severe nausea and vomiting	**Adult:** 20–30 mg/day **Child (2½–12 yr):** 0.2 mg/kg, up to 10 mg/day in 3 divided doses	**Adult:** 1 mg IV, up to 3 mg/day, or 5–15 mg IM as a single dose repeated q4h, up to 60 mg/day **Child (2½–12 yr):** 0.2–0.25 mg/kg IM, up to 10 mg/day
Manifestations of **psychotic disorders,** excluding depressive reactions	**Adult:** 100 mg to start, up to 150 mg/day; for maintenance, 30–150 mg/day **Child (2½–12 yr):** 2 mg/kg, up to 150 mg/day div	**Adult:** 60 mg IM, up to 150 mg/day, until symptoms are controlled **Child (2½–12 yr):** 0.2–0.25 mg/kg IM, up to 10 mg/day

ADMINISTRATION/DOSAGE ADJUSTMENTS

Elderly or debilitated patients — For severe nausea and vomiting, 2.5 mg IM, up to 15 mg/day

CONTRAINDICATIONS

Known or suspected subcortical brain damage with or without hypothalamic damage ●

Severe CNS depression ●

High-dose hypnotic therapy ●

Hepatic damage ●

Blood dyscrasias ●

Comatose states ●

WARNINGS/PRECAUTIONS

Extrapyramidal symptoms — May mask signs of undiagnosed primary disease; do not use in children or adolescents with suspected Reye's syndrome or other encephalopathy

Mental impairment, reflex-slowing — Performance of potentially hazardous activities may be impaired; caution patients accordingly, as well as about the additive effect of alcohol

Cross-sensitivity — Use with caution in patients with a history of phenothiazine-related cholestatic jaundice, dermatoses, or other allergic reactions

Surgical patients — Monitor psychotic patients on high-dose phenothiazine therapy closely for hypotensive phenomena; administer reduced amounts of anesthetics or CNS depressants

Antiemetic effect — May mask signs and symptoms of overdosage of other drugs or such conditions as intestinal obstruction, brain tumor, or Reye's syndrome

Grand mal convulsions — May occur in patients with a history of convulsive disorders; use with caution

Special-risk patients — Use with caution in patients with mitral insufficiency, pheochromocytoma, or a history of idiosyncratic reaction to centrally acting drugs

Renal and hepatic function — Should be evaluated periodically; discontinue medication if BUN becomes abnormal

Silent pneumonia — May develop

Mammary neoplasms — Have been reported in rodents following chronic administration of antipsychotics that increase prolactin secretion; clinical significance is at present unknown

Blood dyscrasias — Leukopenia, agranulocytosis, thrombocytopenic or nonthrombocytopenic purpura, eosinophilia, and pancytopenia have occurred with phenothiazine therapy; discontinue medication if soreness of the mouth, gums, or throat occurs, or if symptoms of upper respiratory infection and confirmatory leukocyte counts indicate bone-marrow depression

Sudden death — Has occurred in patients on phenothiazine therapy

Prolonged therapy — May cause liver damage, pigmentary retinopathy, lenticular and corneal deposits, and irreversible dyskinesia; monitor patients carefully

Postural hypotension — May occur with parenteral administration; to minimize its occurrence, keep patients in recumbent position under close supervision

Tartrazine sensitivity — Presence of FD&C Yellow No.5 (tartrazine) in 25- and 50-mg tablets may cause allergic-type reactions, including bronchial asthma, in susceptible individuals

Table continued on following page

VESPRIN continued

ADVERSE REACTIONS[1]

Central nervous system	Extrapyramidal symptoms, including pseudoparkinsonism, dystonia, dyskinesia, akathisia, oculogyric crises, opisthotonos, and hyperreflexia; persistent tardive dyskinesia; drowsiness; lethargy; catatonic-like states; restlessness; excitement; bizarre dreams; reactivation of psychotic processes; cerebral edema; EEG changes
Cardiovascular	Hypertension, hypotension (rare), fluctuations in blood pressure, tachycardia, ECG changes
Autonomic nervous system	Nausea, loss of appetite, salivation, polyuria, perspiration, dry mouth, headache, constipation, blurred vision, glaucoma, bladder paralysis, fecal impaction, paralytic ileus, nasal congestion
Metabolic and endocrinological	Weight change, peripheral edema, abnormal lactation, gynecomastia, menstrual irregularities, false pregnancy tests, impotence, increased libido (in women)
Allergic	Itching, erythema, urticaria, seborrhea, photosensitivity, eczema, exfoliative dermatitis, anaphylactoid reactions
Hematological	Leukopenia, agranulocytosis, thrombocytopenic or nonthrombocytopenic purpura, eosinophilia, pancytopenia
Other	Cholestatic jaundice, biliary stasis, sudden death, asthma, increased sensitivity to heat and phosphorous insecticides, laryngeal edema, angioneurotic edema, pigmentary retinopathy

OVERDOSAGE

Signs and symptoms	See ADVERSE REACTIONS
Treatment	Discontinue medication; treat symptomatically and institute supportive measures, as required. Combat hypotension with levarterenol. *Do not use epinephrine.* Treat extrapyramidal reactions with antiparkinsonism agents other than levodopa (such as benztropine mesylate).

DRUG INTERACTIONS

Alcohol, anesthetics, barbiturates, narcotics, and other CNS depressants	⇧ CNS depression
Anticonvulsants	⇩ Convulsion threshold
Epinephrine	Severe hypotension
Guanethidine	⇩ Antihypertensive effect
Antimuscarinics	⇧ Atropine-like effect
Amphetamines	⇩ Amphetamine effect
Antacids containing aluminum or magnesium ions	⇩ Absorption of triflupromazine
Levodopa	⇩ Antiparkinsonism effect
MAO inhibitors, tricyclic antidepressants	⇧ Sedation and antimuscarinic effects

ALTERED LABORATORY VALUES

Urinary values	⇧ Bilirubin (false elevation)

No clinically significant alterations in blood/serum values occur at therapeutic dosages

Use in children

See INDICATIONS; not recommended for use in children under 2½ yr of age

Use in pregnancy or nursing mothers

Safe use not established during pregnancy; general guidelines not established for use in nursing mothers

[1]Other reactions common to phenothiazines in general may occur but have not been specifically reported with triflupromazine

WANS (Pyrilamine maleate and pentobarbital sodium) Webcon

Supp: 50 mg pyrilamine maleate and 50 mg pentobarbital sodium (WANS No. 1); 50 mg pyrilamine maleate and 100 mg pentobarbital sodium (WANS No. 2) **Pediatric supp:** 25 mg pyrilamine maleate and 30 mg pentobarbital sodium

INDICATIONS	RECTAL DOSAGE
Nausea and vomiting	**Adult:** for mild nausea and/or vomiting, 1 No. 1 supp q4–6h, as needed, up to 4 doses/24 h; for pernicious vomiting, 1 No. 2 supp q4–6h, as needed, up to 4 doses/24 h **Child (6 mo to 2 yr or <15 kg):** up to ½ child's dosage below **Child (2–12 yr or >15 kg):** 1 ped supp q6–8h, as needed, up to 3 doses/24 h

ADMINISTRATION/DOSAGE ADJUSTMENTS

Rectal use	Moisten finger and suppository with water prior to insertion

CONTRAINDICATIONS

Hypersensitivity to barbiturates or antihistamines ●	Acute intermittent porphyria ●	Senility ●
Prior barbiturate addiction ●	Severe hepatic impairment ●	Uncontrolled pain ●
Acute head injury associated with vomiting or other signs of CNS injury ●		

WARNINGS/PRECAUTIONS

Habit-forming	Psychic and/or physical dependence may develop, especially in addiction-prone individuals (see CONTRAINDICATIONS)
Pre-existing psychological disturbances	Confusion and/or delirium may occur; symptoms may be accentuated
Mental impairment, reflex-slowing	Performance of potentially hazardous tasks may be impaired; caution patients accordingly and about potentiating effect of alcohol and other CNS depressants
Special-risk patients	Use with caution in patients with a history of drug dependence or suicidal tendencies, known acute or chronic hepatic disease (see CONTRAINDICATIONS), fever, hyperthyroidism, diabetes mellitus, severe anemia, or congestive heart failure

ADVERSE REACTIONS

Central nervous system	Drowsiness, sedation, fatigue, vertigo, incoordination, tremor, muscle weakness, excitation, euphoria, insomnia, nervousness, lethargy, paradoxical restlessness or excitement, delirium, lassitude
Autonomic nervous system	Dry mouth, nose, and throat; tinnitus; pupillary dilatation; blurred vision; urinary retention
Gastrointestinal	Epigastric and intestinal pain, anorexia, nausea, vomiting, diarrhea
Cardiovascular	Palpitations, tachycardia, hypotension
Hypersensitivity	Allergic dermatitis, urticaria, exfoliative dermatitis (rare)
Other	Impotence, blood dyscrasias, respiratory depression, coma, renal or hepatic dysfunction (rare)

OVERDOSAGE

Signs and symptoms	Varies from CNS depression (drowsiness, sedation, diminished mental alertness, apnea, cardiovascular collapse) to CNS stimulation (insomnia, excitement, hallucinations, ataxia, incoordination, athetosis, tremors, convulsions) and may include dizziness, tinnitus, blurred vision, and hypotension; CNS stimulation, followed by postictal depression, and atropine-like symptoms (dry mouth; fixed, dilated pupils; fever; flushing; GI disturbances) are particularly likely in children
Treatment	Following acute ingestion, induce emesis with syrup of ipecac, if patient is conscious, even though vomiting may have occurred spontaneously. If vomiting is unsuccessful or contraindicated, perform gastric lavage with isotonic or ½ isotonic saline solution. Remove any remaining drug in the stomach by instillation of activated charcoal. Administer a saline cathartic to rapidly dilute bowel content. Treatment is symptomatic and supportive. If breathing is significantly impaired, maintain an adequate airway and provide mechanically assisted ventilation; *do not use analeptics.* Vasopressors (eg, levarterenol) may be used for significant hypotension. Treat hyperpyrexia by sponging with tepid water or use of ice packs or a hypothermal blanket. For seizures, administer a short-acting barbiturate, diazepam, or paraldehyde.

Table continued on following page

WANS continued

DRUG INTERACTIONS

Sedative-hypnotics, narcotics, alcohol, and other CNS depressants	⇧ CNS depression
Oral anticoagulants	⇩ Prothrombin time
Corticosteroids, cardiac glycosides, tricyclic antidepressants	⇩ Plasma drug levels due to enhanced metabolism

ALTERED LABORATORY VALUES

Blood/serum values	⇧ Bilirubin

No clinically significant alterations in urinary values occur at therapeutic dosages

Use in children

Contraindicated in infants under 6 mo of age. Use in children is limited to prolonged vomiting of known etiology. Do not exceed recommended dosage; excessive dosage may cause convulsions in infants, or toxic encephalopathy (characterized by a depressed level of consciousness, marked irritability, and ataxia) in infants and children.

Use in pregnancy or nursing mothers

Safe use during pregnancy not established; general guidelines not established for use in nursing mothers

Diarrhea

Diarrhea is defined as the passage of unformed stools with marked or excessive frequency. The stools may be watery and may sometimes contain blood and mucus. In some cases, abdominal cramps, nausea, and vomiting may accompany the diarrhea. All age groups are affected, including infants; indeed, uncontrolled diarrhea remains a significant cause of infant death. Common causes of diarrhea and its prevention or treatment will be reviewed in this section.

CAUSES OF DIARRHEA

There are two major forms of diarrhea: osmotic, when there is an excess of substances that retain water in the bowel, and secretory, when the large bowel secretes rather than absorbs water and electrolytes, particularly salt. Osmotic diarrhea is frequently seen in persons who cannot tolerate lactose (milk sugar) and other sugars, while the secretory diarrheas commonly result from the presence of poisonous by-products of bacteria (bacterial toxins), unabsorbed fats, and certain drugs.

In adults, acute diarrhea most often results from emotional or physical stress or from intestinal infections caused by the ingestion of food or water contaminated with bacteria, intestinal parasites, or other disease-causing microorganisms, as well as bacterial toxins. The remaining acute diarrheas may be traced to such intestinal disorders as irritable bowel syndrome, ulcerative colitis, regional enteritis (an inflammation of segments of the intestines, also known as Crohn's disease), partial intestinal obstruction, or, occasionally, to diverticular disease—a disorder in which small areas of the intestinal wall balloon out in little sacs.

Sometimes diarrhea is a result of an allergy to certain foods, often food additives or very ordinary foods, harmless except to the allergic patient. The diarrhea usually disappears as soon as the offending food has been digested and eliminated from the body. This type of diarrhea usually is not accompanied by a loss of appetite or a feeling of weakness, as is common in other types of diarrhea.

The presence of blood in the stools is always a signal to consult a physician promptly. If the bloody diarrhea is associated with fever, weakness, or other systemic signs, the cause may be shigellosis or amebiasis—both parasitic infections—or ulcerative colitis. If no other symptoms are present, bloody diarrhea may be a manifestation of polyps of the colon, early colon cancer, or inflammation of the rectum with ulcer formation.

Diarrhea in Infants and Children

In the infant, mild diarrhea can be caused by formula that is too concentrated or rich in carbohydrates, or by overfeeding. Severe diarrhea, on the other hand, ordinarily results from a bacterial infection. Food allergy, usually to milk or a newly introduced food, may also be responsible for severe diarrhea. In these infants, a milk-free formula may be necessary; if other foods are the cause, they should be avoided in the baby's diet.

Dehydration, a severe loss of body fluids, is a dangerous consequence of diarrhea in both adults and children, and can become extremely serious very quickly in infants and young children. An abrupt weight change indicates a dangerous fluid loss and a physician should be called at once so that proper fluid replacement can be prescribed immediately. In the adult, a weight loss of 5 percent (for example, seven or eight pounds in a 150-pound man) signals the need for prompt medical attention.

Diarrhea from Food Poisoning

Food poisoning results from eating food or drinking water contaminated with bacteria, bacterial toxins, or other microorganisms. Food poisoning is more common in warm weather, when foods, particularly eggs and products containing eggs, like mayonnaise and custards, are not properly refrigerated. The common causative organisms are the *Salmonella* species, *Staphylococcus* enterotoxins, *Escherichia coli*, and *Clostridium perfringens* type A.

Outbreaks of food poisoning from the *Salmonella* species can usually be traced to contaminated poultry or poultry products, although the source may be contaminated dried or whole milk, pork, shellfish, smoked or uncooked fish, eggs, and even water. Symptoms develop within eight to forty-eight hours after eating the contaminated food and include diarrhea, headache, abdominal distress, and fever. The diarrhea may be watery, often profuse, and may contain both blood and mucus.

Infection with the *Shigella* species is always an important health problem wherever people live under crowded conditions. In the United States, shigellosis most commonly occurs in children one to four years old. The incidence is highest in late summer and early fall. The incubation period is one to five days after exposure to the organism. The first symptom is abdominal pain, followed by diarrhea, bloody mucoid stools, and fever. Abdominal pain ordinarily appears within forty-eight hours, diarrhea after about seventy-two hours, and bloody stools with mucus within four to six days.

In food poisoning from the *Staphylococcus* enterotoxin, diarrhea is the principal symptom, but nausea, vomiting, abdominal cramps, and sometimes fever and headache may also occur. *E. coli* is sometimes responsible for outbreaks of diarrhea in adults, especially persons traveling abroad, and there have been reports of sporadic epidemics resulting from imported cheese contaminated with this organism.

About one third of the cases of food poisoning reported in the United States and Great Britain can be attributed to *Clostridium perfringens* type A. The contaminated food is usually a meat or poultry dish that was not cooked through to a temperature high enough to kill the spores of the organism, and then was served either cold or merely warmed up. Diarrhea and cramping abdominal pain develop about eight to twelve hours after eating the contaminated food. The diarrhea is liquid, but it does not contain either blood or mucus. The duration of illness is about twenty-four hours, or less.

Parasitic infections, especially among persons who have visited or lived in the tropics and certain other regions of the world, are another cause of diarrhea. (See *Parasitic Infections*, page 469, for a more detailed discussion.)

Diarrhea Caused by Organic Intestinal Disorders

Irritable bowel syndrome is said to be the intestinal disorder most commonly encountered by physicians specializing in gastroenterology. Both diarrhea and constipation are symptoms of an irritable bowel, and usually the diarrhea alternates with constipation, although one symptom ordinarily predominates. Abdominal pain is also a feature. Most patients are between the ages of twenty and fifty years, with women more often affected than men.

Ulcerative colitis, an inflammatory disease of the colon, is characterized by loose, bloody stools. The patient is usually a young adult (the average age at onset is twenty-three years), but the disease has been found in infants and children. Often ulcerative colitis begins insidiously, but in some cases the onset is abrupt. Prompt diagnosis and treatment are necessary to avoid potentially severe complications.

Regional enteritis, or Crohn's disease, is an often serious intestinal inflammatory disease with diarrhea and abdominal cramps as symptoms. The classic patient is a person in the late teens or early twenties who has experienced occasional bouts of diarrhea and abdominal cramps, which now become more persistent. There is no specific therapy for this disorder; treatment must be individualized for each patient.

Diverticular disease of the colon, in which weakened portions of the intestinal wall form pockets or outpouches, is a common ailment in all of the developed countries of the world. Its cause is unknown, although it has been associated with consumption of a low-fiber diet and chronic constipation. The principal complaints are vague lower abdominal discomfort and occasional episodes of diarrhea associated with increasing constipation. Bleeding from the colon, pain, cramping, and fever also occur with considerable frequency. Treatment may be either medical or surgical; surgical treatment becomes necessary when complications such as intestinal obstruction develop.

TREATMENT OF DIARRHEA

Diarrhea not attributable to a specific cause, such as infection, an intestinal disorder, or allergy, is called nonspecific diarrhea. Very often nonspecific diarrhea can be relieved by simple home remedies and nonprescription preparations.

Management of Nonspecific Diarrhea

A period of fasting is a highly effective way of stopping an attack of nonspecific diarrhea. Both food and fluid should be avoided for at least two hours after the onset of diarrhea. If nausea and vomiting are accompanying symptoms, the fasting period may be extended to four hours after they have ceased. One frequently recommended approach involves gradual resumption of food and fluids, starting with slightly cooled or room-temperature ginger ale. If a small serving, sipped slowly, brings no return of symptoms, small servings of ginger ale, fruit juice, weak teas, or clear broth at frequent intervals may be continued until at least six hours after the last episode of diarrhea. Soft, bland food may then be tried, but a normal diet should not be resumed for a minimum of another twenty-four hours.

Many antidiarrheal preparations contain binding agents such as aluminum hydroxide gel, kaolin, pectin, and bismuth, alone or in various combinations. Kaopectate and Pargel contain only kaolin and pectin and do not require a prescription. Both are contraindicated in patients with obstructive bowel lesions. Use of these preparations for more than two days, especially if fever is present, is not recommended except on the advice of a physician. Patients taking digitalis preparations or receiving the antibiotic Lincocin should consult their physicians before taking kaolin or pectin because the latter agents absorb digitalis and Lincocin.

Paregoric or powdered opium is sometimes included in some formulations (as in Parepectolin and Donnagel PG, respectively) and therefore in some states may require a prescription. The dosage of paregoric should be reduced by one-half to two-thirds in persons with advanced liver or kidney disease and in infants with mild diarrhea, and should be used with caution in patients with acute ulcerative colitis. These same precautions should be observed with Donnagel PG. Other preparations available, without paregoric, include Pepto-Bismol and Lactinex.

Some antidiarrheal agents, such as Lomotil—sold with or without a prescription depending upon the state—produce a marked constipating effect. If an intestinal infection is suspected, Lomotil should be withheld until infection is ruled out because there is some evidence that salmonellosis and shigellosis can be thereby prolonged. Lomotil should not be taken in combination with the barbiturate drugs, tranquilizers, or alcohol, all of which act to diminish its effectiveness. Lomotil may precipitate a hypertensive crisis in patients on therapy with MAO inhibitors.

Treatment of Intestinal Infections

Infections with *Salmonella* species are managed mainly by supportive treatment, that is, bed rest, rapid replacement of body fluid lost through the severe diarrhea, fever reduction, and relief of abdominal pain. Antibiotics are often prescribed but do not always speed up elimination of the microorganisms.

Shigellosis is usually a mild, self-limiting disease, and antibiotic therapy is prescribed mainly to shorten the clinical course of the infection. The antibiotics of choice are the ampicillins or tetracyclines. Severe food poisoning also may be treated with an antibiotic, although these drugs are of no value in treating diarrhea caused by bacterial byproducts or toxins.

Treatment of Ulcerative Colitis

Various medications are used to control the diarrhea associated with ulcerative colitis—these include deodorized tincture of opium, paregoric, codeine, Imodium, and Lomotil. The mainstay of specific therapy for the ulcerative colitis itself is one of the sulfa drugs, sulfasalazine (Azulfidine). The principal contraindications are intestinal or urinary obstruction. In the patient ill enough to be hospitalized, a corticosteroid may be used to induce remission. This is a short-term measure, however, and these agents are not used for maintenance therapy.

TRAVELER'S DIARRHEA

No discussion of diarrhea is complete without a few words about traveler's diarrhea. Some recent studies have found that taking large amounts of liquid Pepto-Bismol several times a day has a preventive effect, but many travelers find it difficult or inconvenient to carry a sufficient supply of the drug. At any rate, travelers to certain foreign countries should probably take along with them an antidiarrheal remedy, such as Kaopectate or a preparation recommended by their physicians. Use of bottled drinking water (even for brushing the teeth) and avoidance of raw fruit or vegetables as well as undercooked meat, fish, or poultry are warranted in many foreign countries, especially Central and South America, parts of Asia, and the tropics. Immunization against diseases such as cholera is desirable before traveling in areas of the world where these diseases are endemic.

IN CONCLUSION

Diarrhea is a common problem that very often can be controlled with simple home treatment and nonprescription drugs. Caution should be used, however, when it occurs in infants and young children, or is prolonged in adults, since it can lead to life-threatening dehydration. If the diarrhea is accompanied by a fever, blood in the stools, or other unusual symptoms, a physician should be consulted.

The following charts cover the major drugs, both prescription and nonprescription, used to treat diarrhea. If the diarrhea is caused by an intestinal infection or parasites, antimicrobial drugs may be prescribed. These are included in the sections on *Bacterial Infections* (page 339) and *Parasitic Infections* (page 469).

DONNAGEL (Kaolin, pectin, hyoscyamine sulfate, atropine sulfate, and hyoscine hydrobromide)
Robins

Susp: 6 g kaolin, 142.8 mg pectin, 0.1037 mg hyoscyamine sulfate, 0.0194 mg atropine sulfate, and 0.0065 mg hyoscine hydrobromide per 30 ml[1]

INDICATIONS	ORAL DOSAGE
Nonspecific diarrhea	**Adult:** 30 ml (2 tbsp) to start, followed by 15–30 ml (1–2 tbsp) after each stool **Child (10 lb):** 30 minims or 2.5 ml (½ tsp) after each stool **Child (20 lb):** 5 ml (1 tsp) after each stool **Child (≥30 lb):** 5–10 ml (1–2 tsp) after each stool
Gastritis, enteritis, colitis, and associated symptoms of nausea and GI upset	**Adult:** 15 ml (1 tbsp) q3h, as needed **Child:** same as above

CONTRAINDICATIONS

Glaucoma ●	Advanced hepatic or renal disease ●	Hypersensitivity to components ●

WARNINGS/PRECAUTIONS

Bladder-neck obstruction due, eg, to prostatic hypertrophy	Use with caution; urinary retention may occur
Incipient glaucoma	Use with caution; mydriatic effect may precipitate attack

ADVERSE REACTIONS

Ophthalmic	Blurred vision
Dermatological	Flushing, dry skin
Other	Dry mouth, difficult urination

OVERDOSAGE

Signs and symptoms	Dryness of skin and mucous membranes, hyperthermia, tachycardia leading to lethargy or coma, flushing, hypotonic reflexes, pinpoint pupils, nystagmus, and respiratory depression leading to death
Treatment	Induce emesis or use gastric lavage, followed by activated charcoal. For respiratory depression, give naloxone. Monitor patient for recurrence of drug-overdose symptoms for minimum of 24 h after last dose of naloxone.

DRUG INTERACTIONS

Digoxin	⇩ Absorption of digoxin
Lincomycin	⇩ Absorption of lincomycin

ALTERED LABORATORY VALUES

No clinically significant alterations in blood/serum or urinary values occur at therapeutic dosages

Use in children

See INDICATIONS

Use in pregnancy or nursing mothers

General guidelines not established for use in pregnancy or nursing mothers; atropine is excreted in breast milk[1]

[1]Knowles JA: *J Pediatr* 66:1068, 1965; Speika N: *J Obstet Gynaecol Br Commonw* 54:426, 1947; Takyi BE: *J Hosp Pharm* 28:317, 1970

[1]Contains 3.8% alcohol

DONNAGEL-PG (Opium, kaolin, pectin, hyoscyamine sulfate, atropine sulfate, and hyoscine hydrobromide) Robins

Susp: 24 mg opium, 6 g kaolin, 142.8 mg pectin, 0.1037 mg hyoscyamine sulfate, 0.0194 mg atropine sulfate, and 0.0065 mg hyoscine hydrobromide per 30 ml[1] *C-V*

INDICATIONS	ORAL DOSAGE
Acute nonspecific diarrhea	**Adult:** 30 ml (2 tbsp) q3h, or as needed **Child (10 lb):** 30 minims or 2.5 ml (½ tsp) after each stool **Child (20 lb):** 5 ml (1 tsp) after each stool **Child (≥30 lb):** 5–10 ml (1–2 tsp) after each stool

CONTRAINDICATIONS

Glaucoma● | Advanced hepatic or renal disease● | Hypersensitivity to components●

WARNINGS/PRECAUTIONS

Habit-forming	Psychic and/or physical dependence and tolerance may develop, especially in addiction-prone individuals
Bladder-neck obstruction due, eg, to prostatic hypertrophy	Use with caution; urinary retention may occur
Incipient glaucoma	Use with caution; mydriatic effect may precipitate attack
Toxic megacolon	May occur in patients with inflammatory bowel disease; stop therapy if abdominal distention or other untoward symptoms develop[2]

ADVERSE REACTIONS

Ophthalmic	Blurred vision
Dermatological	Flushing, dry skin
Other	Dry mouth, difficult urination

OVERDOSAGE

Signs and symptoms	Dryness of skin and mucous membranes, hyperthermia, tachycardia leading to lethargy or coma, flushing, hypotonic reflexes, pinpoint pupils, nystagmus, and respiratory depression, leading to death
Treatment	Induce emesis or use gastric lavage, followed by activated charcoal. For respiratory depression, give naloxone. Monitor patient for recurrence of drug overdose symptoms for minimum of 24 h after last dose of naloxone.

DRUG INTERACTIONS

Digoxin	⇩ Absorption of digoxin
Lincomycin	⇩ Absorption of lincomycin

ALTERED LABORATORY VALUES

No clinically significant alterations in blood/serum or urinary values occur at therapeutic dosages

Use in children

See INDICATIONS

Use in pregnancy or nursing mothers

General guidelines not established for use in pregnancy or nursing mothers; atropine is excreted in breast milk[1]

[1]Knowles JA: *J Pediatr* 66:1068, 1965; Speika N: *J Obstet Gynaecol Br Commonw* 54:426, 1947; Takyi BE: *J Hosp Pharm* 28:317, 1970

[1]Contains 5.0% alcohol
[2]Sleisenger MH, Fordtran JS: *Gastrointestinal Disease: Pathophysiology, Diagnosis, Management*, ed. 2. Philadelphia, W.B. Saunders, 1978, p 1630

IMODIUM (Loperamide hydrochloride) Ortho

Caps: 2 mg *C-V*

INDICATIONS	ORAL DOSAGE
Acute nonspecific diarrhea	**Adult:** 4 mg to start, followed by 2 mg after each unformed stool, up to 16 mg/day for no more than 48 h if no clinical improvement is observed
Chronic diarrhea due to inflammatory bowel disease, or to reduce volume of discharge after ileostomy	**Adult:** same as for acute diarrhea, up to 16 mg/day, as needed; usual maintenance dosage, 4-8 mg/day

CONTRAINDICATIONS

Hypersensitivity to loperamide

Patients in whom constipation must be avoided

Infectious diarrhea — Caused by toxigenic *Escherichia coli, Salmonella, Shigella,* or other invasive organisms

Pseudomembranous colitis — Resulting from use of broad-spectrum antibiotics

WARNINGS/PRECAUTIONS

Toxic megacolon — May occur in patients with acute ulcerative colitis; stop therapy if abdominal distention or other untoward symptoms develop

Physical dependence — May occur, based on studies with monkeys; however, this has not been observed clinically

ADVERSE REACTIONS

Gastrointestinal — Abdominal pain, distention, discomfort, constipation, dry mouth, nausea, vomiting

Central nervous system — Drowsiness, dizziness, fatigue

Hypersensitivity — Skin rash

OVERDOSAGE

Signs and symptoms — Constipation, CNS depression, GI irritation, nausea, vomiting

Treatment — Empty stomach by gastric lavage, followed by activated charcoal, if vomiting has not occurred spontaneously. For CNS depression, administer naloxone. Monitor patient for recurrence of drug overdose symptoms for minimum of 24 h after last dose of naloxone.

DRUG INTERACTIONS

No clinically significant drug interactions have been observed

ALTERED LABORATORY VALUES

No clinically significant alterations in blood/serum or urinary values occur at therapeutic dosages

Use in children	Use in pregnancy or nursing mothers
Not recommended for use in children under 12 yr of age	Safe use not established

KAOPECTATE (Kaolin and pectin) Upjohn

Liq: 90 gr kaolin and 2 gr pectin per 30 ml

INDICATIONS	ORAL DOSAGE
Nonspecific diarrhea	**Adult:** 60-120 ml (4-8 tbsp) after each bowel movement or as needed **Child (<3 yr):** at discretion of physician **Child (3-6 yr):** 15-30 ml (1-2 tbsp) after each bowel movement or as needed **Child (6-12 yr):** 30-60 ml (2-4 tbsp) after each bowel movement or as needed **Child (>12 yr):** 60 ml (4 tbsp) after each bowel movement or as needed

KAOPECTATE CONCENTRATE (Kaolin and pectin) Upjohn

Liq: 135 gr kaolin and 3 gr pectin per 30 ml

INDICATIONS	ORAL DOSAGE
Same as Kaopectate	**Adult:** 45-90 ml (3-6 tbsp) after each bowel movement or as needed **Child (<3 yr):** at discretion of physician **Child (3-6 yr):** 15 ml (1 tbsp) after each bowel movement or as needed **Child (6-12 yr):** 30 ml (2 tbsp) after each bowel movement or as needed **Child (>12 yr):** 45 ml (3 tbsp) after each bowel movement or as needed

CONTRAINDICATIONS

Obstructive bowel lesions

WARNINGS/PRECAUTIONS

Persistent diarrhea — Patient should consult physician if diarrhea continues for more than 2 days or is accompanied by high fever

ADVERSE REACTIONS

None

OVERDOSAGE

Signs and symptoms — Constipation

Treatment — Stop medication

DRUG INTERACTIONS

Digoxin — ⇩ Digoxin absorption

Lincomycin — ⇩ Lincomycin absorption

ALTERED LABORATORY VALUES

No clinically significant alterations in blood/serum or urinary values occur at therapeutic dosages

Use in children

See INDICATIONS

Use in pregnancy or nursing mothers

General guidelines not established

LACTINEX *(Lactobacillus acidophilus* and *L bulgaricus)* **Hynson, Westcott & Dunning**

Tabs: 250 mg **Granules:** 1-g pkt

INDICATIONS	ORAL DOSAGE
Nonspecific diarrhea and as aid in restoring normal intestinal flora following intestinal antisepsis prior to surgery	**Adult:** 4 tabs or 1 pkt tid or qid with milk, juice, or water **Child (3-12 yr):** same as for adult
Fever blisters, canker sores	**Adult:** 4 tabs or 1 pkt tid or qid, chewed and swallowed, followed by a small amount of milk, fruit juice, or water **Child (3-12 yr):** same as for adult

CONTRAINDICATIONS

None

WARNINGS/PRECAUTIONS

Must be kept refrigerated

Do not use for preparation of *acidophilus* or *bulgaricus* milk

ADVERSE REACTIONS

None

OVERDOSAGE

Toxicity of *Lactobacillus* cultures in man has not been reported

DRUG INTERACTIONS

No clinically significant drug interactions have been observed

ALTERED LABORATORY VALUES

No clinically significant alterations in blood/serum or urinary values occur at therapeutic dosages

Use in children

See INDICATIONS

Use in pregnancy or nursing mothers

General guidelines not established

Note: *Lactobacillus acidophilus* also marketed as **BACID** (Fisons).

LOMOTIL (Diphenoxylate hydrochloride and atropine sulfate) Searle

Tabs, liq (per 5 ml): 2.5 mg diphenoxylate hydrochloride and 0.025 mg atropine sulfate *C-V*

INDICATIONS	ORAL DOSAGE
Diarrhea (adjunctive therapy)	**Adult:** 2 tabs or 10 ml (2 tsp) qid, until diarrhea is controlled; then reduce dosage **Child:** 0.3–0.4 mg/kg/day div, or as follows: **Child (2–5 yr):** 4 ml tid until diarrhea is controlled; then reduce dosage **Child (5–8 yr):** 4 ml qid until diarrhea is controlled; then reduce dosage **Child (8–12 yr):** 4 ml 5 times/day until diarrhea is controlled; then reduce dosage

CONTRAINDICATIONS	
Obstructive jaundice	
Hypersensitivity to diphenoxylate or atropine	
Infectious diarrhea	Caused by toxigenic *Escherichia coli*, *Salmonella*, *Shigella*, or other invasive organisms
Pseudomembranous colitis	Resulting from use of broad-spectrum antibiotics

WARNINGS/PRECAUTIONS	
Habit-forming	Psychic and/or physical dependence and tolerance may develop, especially in addiction-prone individuals
Severe dehydration, electrolyte imbalance	Withhold antidiarrheal therapy until appropriate corrective measures have been initiated
Toxic megacolon	May be induced in patients with acute ulcerative colitis; stop therapy if abdominal distention or other untoward symtoms develop
Hepatic coma	May be precipitated in patients with advanced hepatorenal disease or abnormal liver-function tests; use with extreme caution

ADVERSE REACTIONS	
Gastrointestinal	Anorexia, nausea, vomiting, abdominal discomfort, paralytic ileus, toxic megacolon
Central nervous system	Dizziness, drowsiness/sedation, headache, malaise/lethargy, restlessness, euphoria, depression, coma
Cardiovascular	Flushing, tachycardia
Allergic	Pruritus, swelling of the gums, giant urticaria, angioneurotic edema
Other	Hyperthermia, urinary retention, dryness of skin and mucous membranes, numbness in the extremities, respiratory depression

OVERDOSAGE	
Signs and symptoms	Dryness of skin and mucous membranes, flushing, hyperthermia, and tachycardia leading to lethargy or coma, hypotonic reflexes, nystagmus, pinpoint pupils, and respiratory depression
Treatment	Establish a patent airway and institute mechanically assisted ventilation, if indicated. If patient is conscious, induce emesis or use gastric lavage to empty stomach, followed by activated charcoal. For respiratory depression, administer naloxone (0.4 mg IV in adults, 0.01 mg/kg IV in children); the dose may be repeated, as needed, at 2- to 3-min intervals. Monitor patient for recurrence of drug overdose symptoms for minimum of 48 h after last dose of naloxone.

DRUG INTERACTIONS	
MAO inhibitors	May precipitate hypertensive crisis
Antimuscarinics	⇧ Risk of paralytic ileus
Barbiturates, alcohol, tranquilizers, and other CNS depressants	⇧ CNS depression

Table continued on following page

LOMOTIL continued

ALTERED LABORATORY VALUES

Blood/serum values ——— ⇧ Amylase

No clinically significant alterations in urinary values occur at therapeutic dosages

Use in children

Use liquid only in children up to 12 yr of age; contraindicated n children under 2 yr of age. Signs of atropinism may occur even at recommended doses, especially in children with Down's syndrome. Use with particular caution in young children because of variability of response. Dehydration increases variability and may predispose to diphenoxylate intoxication.

Use in pregnancy or nursing mothers

Safe use not established during pregnancy. Both diphenoxylate and atropine are excreted in breast milk and may affect nursing infants.

PAREGORIC (Camphorated tincture of opium) Lilly, Parke-Davis

Liq: 2 mg morphine equiv/5 ml *C-III*

INDICATIONS	ORAL DOSAGE
Nonspecific diarrhea	**Adult:** 5–10 ml (1–2 tsp), up to 4 times/day until diarrhea is controlled **Child:** 0.25–0.5 ml/kg, up to 4 times/day until diarrhea is controlled

CONTRAINDICATIONS

Advanced hepatic or renal disease

Infectious diarrhea — Caused by toxigenic *Escherichia coli*, *Salmonella*, *Shigella*, or other invasive organisms

Pseudomembranous colitis — Resulting from use of broad-spectrum antibiotics

WARNINGS/PRECAUTIONS

Habit-forming — Psychic and/or physical dependence and tolerance may develop, especially in addiction-prone individuals

Toxic megacolon — May be induced in patients with acute ulcerative colitis; stop therapy if abdominal distention or other untoward symptoms develop

ADVERSE REACTIONS

Gastrointestinal — Nausea, vomiting, constipation, abdominal pain, distention, discomfort, dry mouth

Central nervous system — Mental confusion

Other — Allergic manifestations

OVERDOSAGE

Signs and symptoms — Constipation, CNS depression

Treatment — Maintain patent airway; institute artificial respiration, if indicated. If patient is conscious, induce emesis or use gastric lavage to empty stomach, followed by activated charcoal. For respiratory depression, administer naloxone (0.4 mg IV in adults, 0.01 mg/kg IV in children); repeat dose, as needed, at 2- to 3-min intervals. Observe patient for recurrence of drug overdose symptoms for minimum of 48 h after last dose of naloxone.

DRUG INTERACTIONS

No clinically significant drug interactions have been observed

ALTERED LABORATORY VALUES

No clinically significant alterations in blood/serum or urinary values occur at therapeutic dosages

Use in children

See INDICATIONS

Use in pregnancy or nursing mothers

Safe use not established

Note: Paregoric with pectin and kaolin is marketed as **PAREPECTOLIN** (Rorer).

PEPTO-BISMOL (Bismuth subsalicylate) **Norwich-Eaton**

Tabs: 300 mg **Liq:** 1.75% bismuth subsalicylate *sugar-free*

INDICATIONS	ORAL DOSAGE
Diarrhea, indigestion, and nausea	**Adult:** 600 mg or 30 ml (2 tbsp) q½–1h, up to 8 doses/day, if needed **Child (3–6 yr):** 150 mg or 5 ml (1 tsp) q½–1h, up to 8 doses/day, if needed **Child (6–10 yr):** 300 mg or 10 ml (2 tsp) q½–1h, up to 8 doses/day, if needed **Child (10–14 yr):** 600 mg or 20 ml (4 tsp) q½–1h, up to 8 doses/day, if needed

CONTRAINDICATIONS

None

WARNINGS/PRECAUTIONS

Persistent diarrhea — Patient should consult physician if diarrhea continues for more than 2 days or is accompanied by high fever

ADVERSE REACTIONS

Gastrointestinal — Temporary darkening of stool and tongue

OVERDOSAGE

Toxicity of bismuth subsalicylate in humans has not been reported

DRUG INTERACTIONS

No clinically significant drug interactions have been observed

ALTERED LABORATORY VALUES

No clinically significant alterations in blood/serum or urinary values occur at therapeutic dosages

Use in children

See INDICATIONS

Use in pregnancy or nursing mothers

General guidelines not established

Constipation

When bowel movements occur less frequently than expected, or if stools are difficult to pass, a person may complain of being constipated. Constipation, however, is more of a subjective symptom than a disease, and as such, is difficult to define.

Many people are under the misconception that a daily bowel movement is normal and desirable and are upset if they have fewer. Many factors, including diet, exercise, and general health, determine a bowel movement pattern, so that one, two, or more movements every day may be normal for some persons, while others with equally healthy bowel habits may require only one or two movements a week. In general, constipation is defined as small, compacted stools that are difficult to pass. In this section, common causes of constipation, remedies, and the use of laxatives will be discussed.

CAUSES OF CONSTIPATION

In some rare instances, constipation may have organic causes, such as an intestinal obstruction or tumor. More frequently, there is no such organic cause; instead, the cause may range from weakened nervous system reflex to the bowel—often the result of voluntarily delayed bowel movements—to a change in diet or activity level, such as confinement in bed or travel. Constipation also may have an emotional basis.

In many instances, simple changes in life-style may be sufficient to control the problem. An appropriate diet, exercise, increased fluid intake, and an attempt to relax and achieve better bowel habits may be enough to control even chronic constipation. In other cases, an occasional laxative may be needed; however, laxatives should never be used indiscriminately because they can induce a laxative habit, in which the body's natural reflexes become sluggish from disuse. Too-frequent use of harsh laxatives can also lead to the development of irritable colon syndrome.

TREATMENT OF CONSTIPATION

Dietary Approaches

The relationship between dietary fiber or roughage and constipation has gained increased attention in recent years. In general, a diet that contains several daily servings of fresh or lightly processed fruits and vegetables, fresh green salads, and whole-grain breads and cereals will provide adequate fiber. If not, a bran cereal or small amounts of miller's bran can be added. It should be noted, however, that excessive bran can cause its own set of nutritional and digestive problems, such as failure to absorb all of the essential nutrients in food. It is preferable to eat bran in the form of whole-grain products, and to increase roughage by not peeling or overprocessing fruits and vegetables, where appropriate.

Adequate fluid intake is also important to avoid or control constipation. At least eight glasses of water (or other fluids such as tea, juice, coffee, etc.) should be consumed daily.

Life-Style Changes to Prevent Constipation

The pressures of work and a hurried pace of life can disrupt normal patterns of digestion. Since bowel movements are highly sensitive to timing, the person attempting to break the cycle of constipation should establish a schedule that allows adequate time for a bathroom visit, usually around the same time each day. A half hour or so after breakfast is an ideal time because ingestion of food on an empty stomach stimulates peristalsis. It is also important to respond promptly, if at all possible, to the urge to have a bowel movement. Delay results in a more compacted stool, and a pattern of ignoring the defecatory urge can lead to chronic constipation.

USE OF LAXATIVES

There are times when the use of a laxative is indicated. Some drugs, such as those containing codeine, may cause constipation, and concomitant use of a laxative is often recommended. Similarly, persons who are confined to bed after surgery or an accident may suffer temporary constipation and need a laxative. Constipation frequently accompanies depression, particularly in the older person, no longer physically active, who has become preoccupied with bowel movements.

In most instances, laxatives should be used for only brief periods—a few days or a week. Some laxatives, particularly the saline types, produce watery stools that may deplete the body of important electrolytes (e.g., sodium and potassium) and minerals. Some laxatives also may interfere with the absorption of various medications. Most laxatives should not be taken when there is abdominal pain, nausea, or vomiting, or other symptoms that may indicate appendicitis or other intestinal disease.

Laxatives fall into four general categories: (a) stimulants (b) lubricants (c) bulk-forming laxatives, and (d) saline laxatives. All laxatives discussed here can be purchased without a prescription with the exception of lactulose (Chronulac), which is a prescription drug.

Stimulant Laxatives

The stimulant laxatives act by irritating the intestine, literally whipping the muscles into activity to restore the intestinal waves that move the stool downwards (peristalsis). Their major disadvantage is their irritating effect, which may cause cramps until evacuation is complete. In general, these stimulant laxatives, with the possible exception of castor oil, are particularly useful in older persons and others whose peristaltic reflexes are reduced. They should be avoided by nursing mothers because they may produce diarrhea in the infant.

Many of the popular stimulant laxatives contain at least one of the following ingredients: bisacodyl, casanthranol, cascara sagrada, castor oil, danthron, phenolphthalein (yellow or white), and senna.

Castor oil is the most rapid-acting of the stimulant

laxatives, working within three to four hours. It has an unpleasant taste, but this can be masked by mixing it with fruit juices.

Phenolphthalein (contained in a variety of laxatives, including Agoral, Alophen Pills, Feen-A-Mint, Ex-Lax, Correctol, and Evac-Q-Gen) comes in two types, white and yellow. In general, the yellow type is more active than the white. It acts within six to eight hours and is generally considered to be nontoxic. On rare occasions, however, its laxative action may continue for several days. In about 5 percent of users, phenolphthalein may cause a rash.

Bisacodyl (in Dulcolax and Carter's Little Pills) acts within six to eight hours. The manufacturer of Carter's Little Pills warns that the product can cause a variety of minor symptoms such as abdominal discomfort, faintness, and rectal burning. The manufacturer recommends that Carter's Little Pills should not be taken within one hour before or after drinking milk or using an antacid.

Cascara sagrada (in Cas-Evac), danthron (in Doxidan, Dorbantyl Forte and Modane Tablets and Liquid), and senna (in Fletcher's Castoria, Senokot, and X-Prep) all produce a defecation stimulus within six to twenty-four hours. Stimulant laxatives containing senna or danthron may give the urine a slightly pinkish color; however, this is a harmless reaction.

Lubricant Laxatives

Lubricant laxatives work by softening intestinal contents to facilitate evacuation. Drugs in this category generally contain mineral oil or other softeners.

Mineral oil (in Agoral, Fleet enema oil, Tucks Saf Tip Oil Retention Enema, Neo-Cultol), taken orally or via enema, acts by mixing with the intestinal contents to soften them. The stool becomes coated with oil and is more easily expelled. For most purposes, mineral oil should be used as a laxative only in combination with other ingredients, rather than as pure mineral oil. Otherwise there may be some anal leaking of the mineral oil, because it is not absorbed. Mineral oil also may interfere with the absorption of fat-soluble vitamins, such as A and E.

The major fecal softeners are dioctyl sodium sulfosuccinate, called DOSS (combined in a variety of laxatives, including Colace and Dialose), and dioctyl calcium sulfosuccinate (in Doxidan and Surfak). These fecal softeners act much like detergents, increasing the "wetting" ability of water. They break down surface barriers and allow water and fats to penetrate the fecal matter, thereby softening it and increasing its bulk. This increased bulk stimulates the urge to defecate, and the softened stool eases passage.

When using fecal softeners, a person should drink several glasses of water a day to provide enough water in the lower intestine to mix with the food residues.

Stool softeners are preferable to stimulant laxatives for those who have sufficient muscle tone and peristaltic action. These products also are recommended for use in some postoperative patients and those with myocardial infarction who must avoid straining at stool, and thus may require laxatives.

Bulk-Forming Laxatives

The larger the stool, the greater the defecatory response. Therefore, a bowel filled with bulk (or water, as with the saline laxatives or enemas) triggers the reflex that stimulates the passage of stool. Bulk laxatives contain natural or synthetic substances that swell in water, forming a gelatinous mass that is neither digestible nor absorbed, but which remains in the lower intestine until it is expelled. Bulk-forming laxatives, such as psyllium seed derivatives, are among the safest products for promoting stool elimination. They must be taken with adequate water, however, to avoid obstruction in the alimentary canal. These laxatives should not be used when there is obstruction or fecal impaction. Otherwise, bulk laxatives are safe and do not lead to the laxative dependency that the other irritant laxatives sometimes do.

Bulking agents include products made of natural psyllium seed (in Metamucil and Effersyllium), malt soup extract (in Maltsupex), and products containing a form of methylcellulose (such as in Dialose and Serutan). Many bulk laxatives—some psyllium products, like Metamucil, and calcium polycarbophil products, like Mitrolan—can be used in conditions in which constipation alternates with diarrhea, such as in irritable colon syndrome and diverticulitis, a disorder characterized by weakened, inflamed pouches in the intestinal walls.

Saline Laxatives

Saline laxatives—like all salts—are freely soluble in water. They prevent the intestine from absorbing water, and thus fill the colon with fluid, which triggers a stool reflex. Saline laxatives act quickly, usually within three hours, depending on the dose. The stools are usually more copious than with stimulating laxatives, but most of this is water.

Saline laxatives usually contain either magnesium sulfate (better known as Epsom salt), citrate of magnesium solution, or sodium sulfate. Disposable enemas usually contain sodium phosphate solution.

Milk of magnesia (magnesium hydroxide), in Phillips' Milk of Magnesia and Haley's MO, acts more slowly and less vigorously than the other saline laxatives, and many persons prefer it for its smooth laxative effect. Essentially, milk of magnesia is both a laxative and an antacid; however, when taken in dosages large enough to help ulcer patients, it causes diarrhea. Its major side effect is that it may cause magnesium ions to accumulate in the bloodstream faster than they can be excreted by the kidneys. The resulting high blood level of magnesium may depress respiration or lower blood pressure. Milk of magnesia should therefore be avoided by persons with kidney disease.

There is some absorption of the sodium in saline laxatives; therefore, persons with restricted salt intake, such as those with edema or high blood pressure, should not use this type of laxative. If a saline laxative is used in these circumstances, magnesium sulfate is the safest.

Other Laxatives
A recently introduced laxative that does not fit into the traditional categories is lactulose (Chronulac) syrup, which requires a physician's prescription. Chronulac is reported to restore bowel function within twenty-four to forty-eight hours; thus it should avoid the potentially harmful effects of repeated laxative use. Since it contains galactose, Chronulac should not be used by people who require a low-galactose diet.

IN CONCLUSION

Constipation is a frequent complaint, but in many instances, persons who feel they are constipated have perfectly normal bowel function. If chronic constipation does exist, dietary or life-style changes can usually solve the problem. When a laxative is indicated, it should be used as briefly as possible, to avoid development of a laxative habit. There are literally hundreds of laxatives on the market; the following charts cover the major nonprescription products in each of the four categories discussed earlier, as well as the recently introduced prescription laxative, lactulose (Chronulac).

CHRONULAC (Lactulose) **Merrell-National**

Syrup: 10 g/15 ml

INDICATIONS	ORAL DOSAGE
Constipation	**Adult:** 15–30 ml (1–2 tbsp)/day, with water, milk, or juice, if desired; up to 60 ml/day, if needed

ADMINISTRATION/DOSAGE ADJUSTMENTS

Onset of action	Up to 24–48 h may be required to produce a normal bowel movement

CONTRAINDICATIONS

Low-galactose diet

WARNINGS/PRECAUTIONS

Elderly, debilitated patients	Measure serum electrolytes periodically if drug is prescribed for more than 6 mo
Diabetics	Use with caution since drug contains galactose ($<$2.2 g/15 ml) and lactose ($<$1.2 g/15 ml)

ADVERSE REACTIONS

Gastrointestinal	Flatulence, cramps, nausea

OVERDOSAGE

Signs and symptoms	Diarrhea, abdominal cramps
Treatment	Stop medication

DRUG INTERACTIONS

No clinically significant drug interactions have been reported

ALTERED LABORATORY VALUES

No clinically significant alterations in blood/serum or urinary values occur at therapeutic dosages

Use in children

Safe use not established

Use in pregnancy or nursing mothers

Safe use not established

Product (Manufacturer)	Ingredients	Actions
Agoral (Parke-Davis) Emulsion **Dosage** **Adult:** 7.5–15 ml (½–1 tbsp) at bedtime **Child (over 6 yr):** 5–10 ml (1–2 tsp) at bedtime	4.2 g Mineral oil per 15 ml	Bowel lubricant
	0.2 g Phenolphthalein per 15 ml	Intestinal stimulant
	Agar	Bulk-forming agent
	Tragacanth	Bulk-forming agent
	Acacia	Bulk-forming agent
	Egg albumin	Emulsifier
	Glycerin	Intestinal stimulant
Agoral Plain (Parke-Davis) Emulsion **Dosage** **Adult:** 15–30 ml (1–2 tbsp) at bedtime **Child (over 6 yr):** 10–20 ml (2–4 tsp) at bedtime	4.2 g Mineral oil per 15 ml	Bowel lubricant
	Agar	Bulk-forming agent
	Tragacanth	Bulk-forming agent
	Acacia	Bulk-forming agent
	Egg albumin	Emulsifier
	Glycerin	Intestinal stimulant
Caroid Laxative Tablets (Winthrop) Tablets **Dosage** **Adult:** 2 tabs 2 h after breakfast, repeated, if needed, at bedtime	50 mg Cascara sagrada extract	Intestinal stimulant
	32.4 mg Phenolphthalein	Intestinal stimulant
Cas-Evac (Parke-Davis) Liquid (4,16 oz) **Dosage** **Adult:** 1.25–2.5 ml (¼–½ tsp) twice daily or 2.5–5 ml (½–1 tsp) at bedtime	2 mg Cascara sagrada per ml	Intestinal stimulant
	18% Alcohol	Vehicle
Colace (Mead Johnson) Capsules **Dosage** **Adult:** 50–200 mg/day, as needed **Child (6–12):** 40–120 mg/day, as needed	50, 100 mg Dioctyl sodium sulfosuccinate	Bowel lubricant
Colace (Mead Johnson) Solution **Dosage** **Adult:** 50–200 mg/day, with milk or fruit juice, if desired, as needed **Child (under 3 yr):** 10–40 mg/day, with milk, fruit juice, or infant formula, if desired, as needed **Child (3–6 yr):** 20–60 mg/day, with milk or fruit juice, if desired, as needed **Child (6–12 yr):** 40–120 mg/day, with milk or fruit juice, if desired, as needed **In enemas:** Add 50–100 mg (5–10 ml of solution) to retention of flushing enema	10 mg Dioctyl sodium sulfosuccinate per ml	Bowel lubricant

Table continued on following page

Product (Manufacturer)	Ingredients	Actions
Colace (Mead Johnson) Syrup **Dosage** **Adult:** 50–200 mg/day, with milk or fruit juice, if desired, as needed **Child (under 3 yr):** 10–40 mg/day, with milk, fruit juice, or infant formula, if desired, as needed **Child (3–6 yr):** 20–60 mg/day, with milk or fruit juice, if desired, as needed **Child (6–12 yr):** 40–120 mg/day, with milk or fruit juice, if desired, as needed	4 mg Dioctyl sodium sulfosuccinate per ml	Bowel lubricant
Cologel (Lilly) Liquid (16 oz) **Dosage** **Adult:** 50–20 ml (1–4 tsp) 3 times daily with 8 oz water	90 mg Methylcellulose per ml	Bulk-forming agent
	5% Alcohol	Vehicle
Dialose (Stuart) Capsules **Dosage** **Adult:** 1 cap with 8 oz water 3 times daily to start; then adjust dosage as needed **Child (over 6 yr):** 1 cap at bedtime	100 mg Dioctyl potassium sulfosuccinate	Bowel lubricant
Dialose Plus (Stuart) Capsules **Dosage** **Adult:** 1 cap with 8 oz water twice daily to start; then adjust dosage as needed	100 mg Dioctyl potassium sulfosuccinate	Bowel lubricant
	30 mg Casanthranol	Intestinal stimulant
Dorbantyl (Riker) Capsules **Dosage** **Adult:** 2 caps at bedtime; repeat if needed **Child (6–12 yr):** 1 cap at bedtime; repeat if needed	25 mg Danthron	Intestinal stimulant
	50 mg Docusate sodium	Bowel lubricant
Dorbantyl Forte (Riker) Capsules **Dosage** **Adult:** 1 cap at bedtime; repeat if needed	50 mg Danthron	Intestinal stimulant
	100 mg Docusate sodium	Bowel lubricant
Doxan (Hoechst-Roussel) Tablets **Dosage** **Adult:** 1–2 tabs at bedtime with 8 oz water	60 mg Docusate sodium	Bowel lubricant
	50 mg Danthron	Intestinal stimulant
Doxidan (Hoechst-Roussel) Capsules **Dosage** **Adult:** 1–2 caps/day **Child (6–12 yr):** 1 cap/day at bedtime	60 mg Docusate calcium	Bowel lubricant
	50 mg Danthron	Intestinal stimulant
Doxinate (Hoechst-Roussel) Capsules **Dosage** **Adult:** 240 mg/day for several days or until bowel movements are normal; for mild cases, 60 mg/day **Child (over 6 yr):** 60–120 mg/day	60, 240 mg Docusate sodium	Bowel lubricant

Table continued on following page

Product (Manufacturer)	Ingredients	Actions
Doxinate (Hoechst-Roussel) Solution **Dosage** **Adult:** 2.5–5 ml (½–1 tsp)/day, with milk or juice if desired, for several days or until bowel movements are normal **Child (3–6 yr):** 1–2 ml (1/5–2/5 tsp)/day, with milk or juice if desired **Child (over 6 yr):** 2.5–5 ml (½–1 tsp)/day, with milk or juice if desired	50 mg Docusate sodium per ml	Bowel lubricant
	5% Alcohol	Vehicle
Effersyllium (Stuart) Powder **Dosage** **Adult:** 1 rounded tsp (1 packet) in 8 oz water 1–3 times daily **Child (over 6 yr):** 1 level tsp or ½ packet in 4 oz water at bedtime To avoid caking, powder should be removed from packet with dry spoon and placed in dry glass.	3 g Psyllium hydrocolloid per 7-g packet	Bulk-forming agent
Ex-Lax (Ex-Lax) Unflavored or chocolate tablets **Dosage** **Adult:** 1–2 tabs with 8 oz water, or 1–2 chewable tabs, at bedtime; adjust dosage as needed **Child (over 6 yr):** 1 tab or ½–1 chewable tab	90 mg Yellow phenolphthalein	Intestinal stimulant
Fleet Bisacodyl Enema (Fleet) Enema (1¼ oz) **Dosage** **Adult:** 1¼ fl oz; patient should preferably lie on left side with left knee slightly bent and right leg drawn up, or in chest-knee position	10 mg Bisacodyl per 30 ml	Intestinal stimulant
Fleet Enema (Fleet) Enema (2¼, 4¼ oz) **Dosage** **Adult:** 4 fl oz **Child (over 2 yr):** 2 fl oz; patient should preferably lie on left side with left knee slightly bent and right leg drawn up, or in chest-knee position	7 g Sodium phosphate per 118 ml	Saline (water-forming)
	19 g Sodium biphosphate per 118 ml	Saline (water-forming)
Fleet Mineral Oil Enema (Fleet) Enema (4½ oz) **Dosage** **Adult:** 4 fl oz **Child (over 2 yr):** 1–2 fl oz	133 ml Mineral oil	Bowel lubricant
Glycerin Suppositories (Squibb) Suppositories, pediatric suppositories **Dosage** **Adult:** Insert 1 supp and retain for 15 min **Child:** Insert 1 ped supp and retain for 15 min	85% Glycerin	Intestinal stimulant
	10% Sodium stearate	Emulsifier and stiffening agent

Table continued on following page

Product (Manufacturer)	Ingredients	Actions
Instant Mix Metamucil (Searle) Powder **Dosage** **Adult:** 3.5 g (1 packet) 1-3 times daily in 8 oz water. For best results, drink an additional 8 oz water.	3.5 g Psyllium hydrophilic mucilloid per packet	Bulk-forming agent
	Citric acid	Effervescent base
	Sodium bicarbonate (equiv to 250 mg sodium)	Effervescent base
	Sucrose	Dispersant
Maltsupex (Wallace) Tablets **Dosage** **Adult:** 2-3 tabs with meals and at bedtime for 4 days, then 2-4 tabs at bedtime, as needed	750 mg Malt soup extract	Bulk-forming agent
Maltsupex (Wallace) Powder, liquid **Dosage** **Adult:** 2 tbsp twice daily for 3-4 days, then 1-2 tbsp at bedtime **Infant (over 1 mo):** *bottle-fed*: ½-2 tbsp/day added to feedings; for prevention of constipation, 1-2 tsp/day added to feedings; *breast-fed*: 1-2 tsp in 2-4 oz water or juice once or twice daily before feedings **Child:** 1-2 tbsp in milk or on cereal once or twice daily	16 g Malt soup extract per tbsp	Bulk-forming agent
Metamucil (Searle) Powder (7, 14, 21 oz) **Dosage** **Adult:** 7 g (1 tsp) 1-3 times daily, as needed, in 8 oz liquid. For best results, drink an additional 8 oz of liquid. May require continuing use for 2-3 days to provide optimal benefit.	50% Psyllium hydrophilic mucilloid	Bulk-forming agent
	50% Dextrose	Dispersant
Milk of Magnesia (various manufacturers) Suspension **Dosage** **Adult:** 30-60 ml (2-4 tbsp)/day, followed by a glass of water **Child (over 1 yr):** 5 ml (1 tsp)/day **Child (under 1 yr):** 7.5-30 ml (½-2 tbsp)/day, depending on age	0.078 g Magnesium hydroxide per ml	Saline (water-forming)
Mineral Oil (various manufacturers) Liquid (30 ml, 8, 16, 32 oz, 1, 5 gal) **Dosage** **Adult:** 15-30 ml (1-2 tbsp) at bedtime **Child:** 5-15 ml (1-3 tsp) at bedtime	Mineral oil	Bowel lubricant

Table continued on following page

Product (Manufacturer)	Ingredients	Actions
Mitrolan (Robins) Tablets (chewable) **Dosage** **Adult:** 2 tabs 4 times daily, or as needed, up to 12 tabs/24 h, to be chewed before swallowing **Child (3–5 yr):** 1 tab twice daily, or as needed, up to 3 tabs/24 h, to be chewed before swallowing **Child (6–11 yr):** 1 tab three times daily, or as needed, up to 6 tabs/24 h, to be chewed before swallowing	500 mg Calcium polycarbophil	Bulk-forming agent
Modane (Warren-Teed) Tablets **Dosage** **Adult:** 37.5–75 mg with evening meal **Child (6–12 yr):** 37.5 mg with evening meal	37.5, 75 mg Danthron	Intestinal stimulant
Modane (Warren-Teed) Liquid **Dosage** **Adult:** 5–10 ml (1–2 tsp) with evening meal **Infant (6–12 mo):** 1–1.25 ml (1/5–¼ tsp) with evening meal **Child (1–6 yr):** 1.25–5 ml (¼–1 tsp) with evening meal **Child (6–12 yr):** 5 ml (1 tsp) with evening meal	7.5 Danthron per ml	Intestinal stimulant
	5% Alcohol	Vehicle
Perdiem (Rorer) Granules **Dosage** **Adult:** 1–2 rounded tsp before breakfast and after dinner, swallowed with 8 oz liquid, to start, followed after drug takes effect by a reduction in each dose to 1 rounded tsp **Child (7–11 yr):** 1 rounded tsp once or twice daily **Obstinate cases:** dosage may be increased up to 2 rounded tsp every 6 h with liquid **Patients habituated to strong purgatives:** 2 rounded tsp in AM and PM with liquid, along with ½ usual dose of purgative being used; discontinue purgative as soon as possible and reduce dosage of Perdiem when and if bowel tone shows lessened laxative dependence **Colostomy patients:** take 1–2 rounded tsp in PM with warm liquid to ensure formed stools **During pregnancy:** take 1–2 rounded tsp in PM with liquid **Inactive, bedridden, and cardiovascular disease patients:** take 1 rounded tsp once or twice daily with glass of liquid	3.3 g Psyllium per 5 ml	Bulk-forming agent
	0.46 g Senna per 5 ml	Intestinal stimulant
Peri-Colace (Mead Johnson) Capsules **Dosage** **Adult:** 1–2 caps at bedtime	30 mg Casanthranol	Intestinal stimulant
	100 mg Dioctyl sodium sulfosuccinate	Bowel lubricant

Table continued on following page

Product (Manufacturer)	Ingredients	Actions
Peri-Colace (Mead Johnson) Syrup **Dosage** **Adult:** 15–30 ml (1–2 tbsp) at bedtime **Child:** 5–15 ml (1–3 tsp) at bedtime	30 mg Casanthranol per 15 ml	Intestinal stimulant
	60 mg Dioctyl sodium sulfosuccinate per 15 ml	Bowel lubricant
	10% Alcohol	Vehicle
Phospho-Soda (Fleet) Solution (1.5, 2.5, 6, 16 oz) **Dosage** **Constipation:** **Adult:** 20 ml (4 tsp) mixed with 4 oz cold water and followed by 8 oz water, on rising, at least 30 min before a meal, or at bedtime **Child (5–10 yr):** 5 ml (1 tsp), diluted and administered as above **Child (over 10 yr):** 10 ml (2 tsp), diluted and administered as above **Bowel evacuation prior to examination or surgery:** **Adult:** 40 ml (8 tsp) mixed with 4 oz cold water and followed by 8 oz water, on rising, at least 30 min before a meal, or at bedtime **Child (5–10 yr):** 10 ml (2 tsp), diluted and administered as above **Child (over 10 yr):** 20 ml (4 tsp), diluted and administered as above	0.18 g Sodium phosphate per ml	Saline (water-forming)
	0.48 g Sodium biphosphate per ml	Saline (water-forming)
Rectalad Enema (Wallace) Enema **Dosage** **Adult:** 5 ml **Child:** 2 ml	76% Glycerin	Intestinal stimulant
	5% Dioctyl potassium sulfosuccinate	Bowel lubricant
	10% Soft soap	Intestinal stimulant
Saf-Tip Oil Retention Enema (Parke-Davis) Enema **Dosage** **Adult:** 60–120 ml/day **Child (over 2 yr):** 60 ml/day	135 ml Light mineral oil	Bowel lubricant
Saf-Tip Phosphate Enema (Parke-Davis) Enema 4 oz **Dosage** **Adult:** 120 ml/day **Child (over 2 yr):** 60 ml/day	19 g Sodium biphosphate per 120 ml	Saline (water-forming)
	7 g Sodium phosphate	Saline (water-forming)
Sal Hepatica (Bristol-Myers) Granules (90, 210, 336 g) **Dosage** **Adult:** 5–10 ml (1–2 tsp) in water	Monosodium phosphate	Saline (water-forming)
Senokap DSS (Purdue Frederick) Capsules **Dosage** **Adult:** 1–2 caps at bedtime with with 8 oz water	163 mg Senna concentrate	Intestinal stimulant
	50 mg Dioctyl sodium sulfosuccinate	Bowel lubricant

Table continued on following page

Product (Manufacturer)	Ingredients	Actions
Senokot (Purdue Frederick) Tablets **Dosage** **Adult:** 2 tabs at bedtime or up to 4 tabs twice daily **Child (over 60 lb):** 1 tab at bedtime or up to 2 tabs twice daily	187 mg Senna concentrate	Intestinal stimulant
Senokot (Purdue Frederick) Granules (2, 6, 12 oz) **Dosage** **Adult:** 1 tsp at bedtime or up to 2 tsp granules twice daily **Child (over 60 lb):** ½ tsp at bedtime or up to 1 tsp granules twice daily	326 mg Senna concentrate per 5 ml	Intestinal stimulant
Senokot (Purdue Frederick) Suppositories **Dosage** **Adult:** 1 supp at bedtime **Child (over 60 lb):** ½ supp at bedtime	652 mg Senna concentrate	Intestinal stimulant
Senokot (Purdue Frederick) Syrup (2, 8 oz) **Dosage** **Adult:** 10–15 ml (2–3 tsp) at bedtime or up to 15 ml (3 tsp) twice daily **Child (1 mo–1 yr):** 1.25–2.50 ml (¼–½ tsp) at bedtime or up to 2.50 ml (½ tsp) twice daily **Child (1–5 yr):** 2.5–5 ml (½–1 tsp) at bedtime or up to 5 ml (1 tsp) twice daily **Child (5–15 yr):** 5–10 ml (1–2 tsp) at bedtime or up to 10 ml (2 tsp) twice daily **Elderly or debilitated patients:** ½ the usual adult dosage **Refractory constipation:** if comfortable bowel movement is not achieved by the second day, daily dosage should be decreased or increased in increments of ½ the starting dose until optimum dosage is established	218 mg Senna extract per 5 ml	Intestinal stimulant
	7% Alcohol	Vehicle
Senokot-S (Purdue Frederick) Tablets **Dosage** **Adult:** 2 tabs at bedtime or up to 4 tabs twice daily **Child (over 60 lb):** 1 tab at bedtime	187 mg Senna concentrate	Intestinal stimulant
	50 mg Dioctyl sodium sulfosuccinate	Bowel lubricant
Surfak (Hoechst-Roussel) Capsules **Dosage** **Adult:** 240 mg/day for several days or until bowel movements are normal; for mild cases, 50–150 mg/day **Child (over 6 yr):** 50–150 mg/day	50, 240 mg Docusate calcium	Bowel lubricant
X-Prep (Gray) Liquid **Dosage** **Adult:** 75 ml taken between 2 and 4 PM on day prior to x-ray procedure	75 mg Senna extract	Intestinal stimulant
	7% Alcohol	Vehicle

Table continued on following page

Hemorrhoids

Hemorrhoids, commonly referred to as piles, are the single most common disorder affecting the lower gastrointestinal tract of Americans. Recent studies indicate that more than half of all Americans over the age of forty suffer to varying degrees from hemorrhoids. The disorder is seen with less frequency in younger persons, although many people in their twenties and thirties are affected.

Hemorrhoids are defined as clusters of dilated or enlarged blood vessels (varicose veins) inside and around the anus (the lower portion of the rectum). They are the result of repeated stretching of the vessel walls, which leads to weakened segments that are permanently dilated. The hemorrhoids may be either internal, meaning they are situated above the anal sphincter, or external, meaning they are below the sphincter and may protrude from the anal opening (see illustration). In fact, they can often be felt or observed by examining the anal area after a bowel movement.

External hemorrhoids are more apt to produce the painful bowel movements, itching, burning, and other symptoms associated with the condition. When they protrude from the anal opening, they are subjected to frequent irritation and squeezing as the sphincter dilates and then contracts during normal bowel function. Clots form from the pooled blood that collects in the distended veins, leading to swelling and inflammation. Blood, often bright red, may appear in the stools. In contrast, internal hemorrhoids may exist for years without causing any problems, particularly if they are situated high in the rectal canal.

CAUSES OF HEMORRHOIDS

Epidemiological studies have found that hemorrhoids are exceedingly common in industrialized Western nations, such as the United States, but rare in the less-developed countries of Africa and Asia. The development of hemorrhoids has been linked to a number of factors, including a diet low in fiber, chronic constipation, and obesity. Persons whose occupations require prolonged sitting, standing, or excessive muscle straining (e.g., lifting heavy objects) are particularly vulnerable to hemorrhoids. Many women develop hemorrhoids during the latter stages of pregnancy, but these often regress after childbirth. Pelvic tumors are yet another cause of hemorrhoids.

Several other conditions may produce symptoms resembling those of hemorrhoids; therefore, diagnosis by a physician is important. For example, blood in the stool may be caused by a tumor or other gastrointestinal disorder; anal fissures or abscesses

ANATOMY OF HEMORRHOIDS

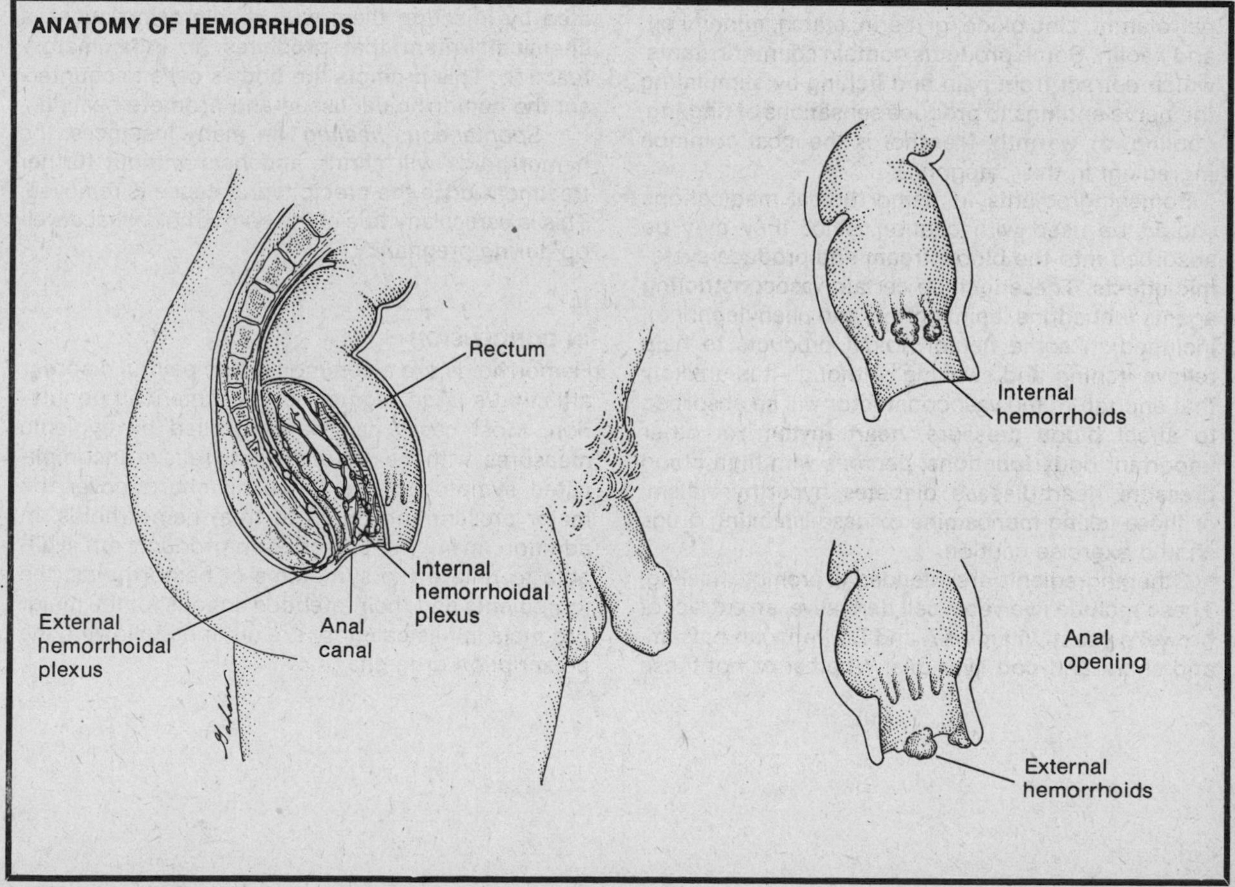

may cause discomfort, itching, or burning; and a prolapsed rectum may produce a protruding mass.

TREATMENT OF HEMORRHOIDS

Uncomplicated hemorrhoids usually can be treated by a combination of hygienic measures and medication to relieve the symptoms. If chronic constipation is a precipitating factor, dietary and other measures to overcome this are recommended. (See the preceding section on *Constipation* for a more detailed discussion.) Exercise to improve circulation, particularly among persons who stand or sit in one position for prolonged periods, is also important.

Cleanliness of the area immediately surrounding the anus is also vital to ease symptoms and prevent infection and other complications. Persons with external hemorrhoids should use moistened paper or wipes instead of dry toilet paper after bowel movements. A bidet, which facilitates cleansing the anal area with a stream of warm water, is a particularly useful bathroom fixture for a person who suffers from hemorrhoids. Warm sitz baths also help relieve symptoms and promote cleanliness.

Medications to Treat Hemorrhoids

More than 200 nonprescription preparations to treat hemorrhoids are available. Many of these contain a local anesthetic, such as benzocaine or pramoxine hydrochloride, to relieve the pain. Most are in the form of ointments, creams, or suppositories, and are intended to protect the tissue surrounding the hemorrhoids and prevent irritation. Common ingredients include calamine, cod liver or shark liver oils, lanolin, petrolatum, zinc oxide, glycerin, starch, mineral oil, and kaolin. Some products contain counterirritants, which detract from pain and itching by stimulating the nerve endings to produce sensations of tingling, cooling, or warmth. Menthol is the most common ingredient in this category.

Some ingredients in hemorrhoidal medications should be used with caution, since they may be absorbed into the bloodstream and produce systemic effects. These include certain vasoconstricting agents (ephedrine, epinephrine, and phenylephrine), included in some hemorrhoidal products to help relieve itching and swelling. Although it is unlikely that enough of the vasoconstrictor will be absorbed to affect blood pressure, heart rhythm, or other important body functions, persons with high blood pressure, heart disease, diabetes, hyperthyroidism, or those taking monoamine oxidase-inhibiting drugs should exercise caution.

Other ingredients are intended to promote healing. These include live yeast cell derivative, an extract of brewer's yeast; vitamins A and D; Peruvian balsam; and shark and cod liver oils. Whether or not these ingredients actually hasten healing is the subject of continuing controversy and study.

Still other miscellaneous ingredients in some hemorrhoidal medications include antiseptics such as boric acid or phenol, and anticholinergics, such as atropine. The multitude of microorganisms in the feces make it doubtful that topical antiseptics will have much effect. In addition, boric acid may be absorbed from the rectum and in large amounts, can lead to boric acid toxicity. Atropine also may be absorbed from the rectal tissues and result in systemic side effects.

Other Methods of Treatment

Surgery Refractory hemorrhoids may be treated surgically, either by hemorrhoidectomy, which involves removal of the hemorrhoidal tissue; or cryosurgery, which involves freezing the tissue with liquid nitrogen or nitrous oxide. The latter is a painless procedure that can be performed on an outpatient basis in a qualified physician's office. It affords quicker healing and less discomfort than hemorrhoidectomy. Within a few days, the tissue "killed" by the freezing sloughs off, leaving only small skin tabs as scars. In contrast, it may take several weeks to complete the healing process after hemorrhoidectomy, which may involve considerable discomfort.

Ligation In this procedure, a rubber band is applied to the hemorrhoid. This limits the blood flow to the tissue, causing it to shrivel and within a few days, slough off.

Injection Some hemorrhoids can be eliminated by injecting them with a sclerosing agent, a chemical irritant that produces an inflammatory reaction. This prompts the body's cells to counteract the hemorrhoidal tissue and promote healing.

Spontaneous healing In many instances, the hemorrhoids will shrink and heal without further treatment once the precipitating cause is removed. This is particularly true of the hemorrhoids that develop during pregnancy.

IN CONCLUSION

Hemorrhoids are a common, often painful disorder afflicting a large segment of the American population. Most cases can be controlled by hygienic measures, with the use of drugs to relieve uncomplicated symptoms. The following charts cover the major prescription drugs to treat hemorrhoids. In addition, many nonprescription products are available to relieve the symptoms of hemorrhoids; the ingredients and their intended actions for the major products in this category are outlined following the prescription drug charts.

ANUSOL-HC (Hydrocortisone acetate, bismuth subgallate, bismuth resorcin compound, benzyl benzoate, Peruvian balsam, and zinc oxide) Parke-Davis

Cream: 5.0 mg hydrocortisone acetate, 22.5 mg bismuth subgallate, 17.5 mg bismuth resorcin compound, 12.0 mg benzyl benzoate, 18.0 mg Peruvian balsam, 110.0 mg zinc oxide per g (1 oz) **Supp:** 10.0 mg hydrocortisone acetate, 2.25% bismuth subgallate, 1.75% bismuth resorcin compound, 1.2% benzyl benzoate, 1.8% Peruvian balsam, 11.0% zinc oxide per supp

INDICATIONS	RECTAL DOSAGE
Symptomatic relief of pain and discomfort in **external and internal hemorrhoids, proctitis, cryptitis, anal fissures, incomplete fistulas,** and following **anorectal surgery,** especially when inflammation is present (adjunctive therapy) **Pruritus ani**	**Adult:** apply cream tid or qid for 3–6 days or insert 1 supp in AM and PM for 3–6 days until inflammation subsides

ADMINISTRATION/DOSAGE ADJUSTMENTS

Use of cream — For external use, apply freely and rub in gently. For internal use, attach the plastic applicator and insert into the anus, squeezing the tube to deliver the medication.

CONTRAINDICATIONS

Hypersensitivity to any component

WARNINGS/PRECAUTIONS

Irritation — May occur; discontinue use and institute appropriate therapy

Infection — Institute appropriate antibacterial or antifungal therapy; if favorable response does not occur promptly, discontinue the corticosteroid until the infection is adequately controlled

ADVERSE REACTIONS

Dermatological — Anal irritation

Use in children

Use with caution in children and infants

Use in pregnancy or nursing mothers

Safe use not established during pregnancy; do not use unnecessarily on extensive areas, in large amounts, or for prolonged periods of time. General guidelines not established for use in nursing mothers.

PROCTOFOAM-HC (Hydrocortisone acetate) Reed & Carnick

Foam: 1% (10 g)

INDICATIONS	TOPICAL DOSAGE
Inflammatory manifestations of corticosteroid-responsive **anogenital dermatoses**	**Adult:** apply to affected areas tid or qid

ADMINISTRATION/DOSAGE ADJUSTMENTS

Rectal use	Shake foam container vigorously before use. Hold container upright and insert into opening of applicator tip with applicator plunger drawn out. Press down slowly on container cup until foam reaches fill line on applicator. Gently insert filled applicator into the anus. Once in place, push plunger to expel foam. Withdraw the applicator and wash with warm water. *Never* insert the container directly into the anus.
Perianal use	Transfer small quantity of foam to a tissue and rub in gently

CONTRAINDICATIONS

Hypersensitivity to hydrocortisone or any component of base

WARNINGS/PRECAUTIONS

Irritation	May occur; discontinue use and institute appropriate therapy
Infection	May occur; institute appropriate antifungal or antibacterial therapy. If favorable response does not occur promptly, discontinue use of foam until infection has been adequately controlled.

ADVERSE REACTIONS

Dermatological[1]	Local burning, itching, irritation, dryness, folliculitis, hypertrichosis, acneiform eruptions, hypopigmentation, allergic contact dermatitis, maceration of the skin, secondary infection, skin atrophy, striae, miliaria

Use in children

General guidelines not established

Use in pregnancy or nursing mothers

Safe use not established during pregnancy; do not use extensively, in large amounts, or for prolonged periods of time in pregnant patients. General guidelines not established for use in nursing mothers.

[1]Especially under occlusive dressings

Product (Manufacturer)	Ingredients	Actions
Anusol Ointment (Parke-Davis) Ointment **Dosage** Adult: Apply every 2–4 h. For external use, apply freely and rub in gently. For internal use, attach plastic applicator and insert into the anus, squeezing the tube to deliver the medication.	12 mg Benzyl benzoate per g	Unspecified
	18 mg Peruvian balsam per g	Astringent
	110 mg Zinc oxide per g	Astringent
	10 mg Pramoxine hydrochloride per g	Anesthetic
	Calcium phosphate	Unspecified
	Kaolin	Protectant
	Glyceryl monooleate	Protectant
	Glyceryl stearate	Protectant
	Liquid petrolatum	Protectant
	Cocoa butter	Protectant
	Polyethylene wax	Ointment base
Anusol Suppositories (Parke-Davis) Suppositories **Dosage** Adult: Insert 1 supp in AM and PM and after each bowel movement	2.25% Bismuth subgallate	Astringent
	1.75% Bismuth resorcin compound	Astringent
	1.2% Benzyl benzoate	Unspecified
	1.8% Peruvian balsam	Astringent
	11.0% Zinc oxide	Astringent
	Bismuth subiodide	Antiseptic
	Calcium phosphate	Unspecified
	Hydrogenated vegetable oil	Base
Mediconet (Medicone) Pads **Dosage** Adult: Cleanse affected area after each bowel movement; use as a compress to relieve anorectal discomfort	0.02% Benzalkonium chloride	Antiseptic
	0.5% Ethoxylated lanolin	Protectant
	0.15% Methylparaben	Antifungal preservative
	50% Hamamelis water	Astringent
	10% Glycerin	Protectant
Nupercainal (Ciba) Ointment (1, 2 oz) **Dosage** Adult: Apply freely in AM and PM and after each bowel movement. For internal use, attach plastic applicator and insert into the anus, squeezing the tube to deliver the medication.	1% Dibucaine	Anesthetic
	Lanolin	Protectant
	White petrolatum	Protectant
	Light mineral oil	Protectant
	Acetone sodium bisulfite	Antioxidant
Nupercainal (Ciba) Suppositories **Dosage** Adult: Insert 1 supp after each bowel movement	2.5 mg Dibucaine	Anesthetic
	Cocoa butter	Protectant

Product (Manufacturer)	Ingredients	Actions
Perifoam (Rowell) Foam **Dosage** Adult: Apply small amount to anorectal surface with toilet paper, cleansing tissue, cotton, or fingertip	0.1% Benzalkonium chloride	Antiseptic
	1.0% Pramoxine hydrochloride	Anesthetic
	0.3% Allantoin	Antipruritic
	0.15% Methylparaben	Antifungal preservative
	0.05% Propylparaben	Antifungal preservative
	Solubilized lanolin	Protectant
	35% Witch hazel	Astringent
	Water	
PNS (Winthrop) Suppositories **Dosage** Adult: Insert 1 supp after each bowel movement and at bedtime	10 mg Tetracaine hydrochloride	Anesthetic
	5 mg Phenylephrine hydrochloride	Vasoconstrictor
	25 mg Tyloxapol	Cleansing agent
	100 mg Bismuth surcarbonate	Astringent
Preparation H (Whitehall) Ointment (1,2 oz) **Dosage** Adult: Apply freely in AM and PM and after each bowel movement. Lubricate applicator before each application.	Live yeast cell derivative (equivalent to 2,000 units skin respiratory factor)	Wound-healing agent
	3% Shark liver oil per oz	Protectant
	Phenylmercuric nitrate 1:10,000	Preservative
Preparation H (Whitehall) Suppositories **Dosage** Adult: Insert 1 supp in AM and PM and after each bowel movement	Live yeast cell derivative (equivalent to 2,000 units skin respiratory factor)	Wound-healing agent
	3% Shark liver oil per oz	Protectant
	Phenylmercuric nitrate 1:10,000	Preservative
proctoFoam (Reed & Carnrick) Foam (15 g) **Dosage** Adult: 1 applicatorful 2 or 3 times daily and after each bowel movement. Do not use for more than 4 consecutive weeks.	1% Pramoxine hydrochloride	Anesthetic
Rectal Medicone Unguent (Medicone) Ointment (1½ oz) **Dosage** Adult: Apply liberally in AM and PM and after each bowel movement	20 mg Benzocaine per g	Anesthetic
	5 mg Oxyquinoline sulfate per g	Antiseptic
	4 mg Menthol per g	Counterirritant
	100 mg Zinc oxide per g	Astringent
	12.5 mg Balsam Peru per g	Protectant
	625 mg Petrolatum	Protectant
	210 mg Lanolin	Protectant

Product (Manufacturer)	Ingredients	Actions
Rectal Medicone Suppositories (Medicone) Suppositories **Dosage** Adult: Insert 1 supp in AM and PM and after each bowel movement	2 gr Benzocaine	Anesthetic
	¼ gr Oxyquinoline sulfate	Antiseptic
	3 gr Zinc oxide	Astringent
	⅐ gr Menthol	Counterirritant
	1 gr Balsam Peru	Protectant
Tucks (Parke-Davis) Ointment (40 g), cream (40 g) **Dosage** Adult: Apply locally 3 or 4 times daily	50% Witch hazel	Astringent
	White petrolatum	Protectant
	Anhydrous lanolin	Protectant
	Benzethonium chloride	Antiseptic
	Sorbitan monostearate	Cleansing agent
	Sorbital solution (ointment only)	Unspecified
	Polyoxyethylene stearate (cream only)	Cleansing agent and emulsifier
	Cetyl alcohol (cream only)	Emusifier
	Polysorbate 60 (cream only)	Cleansing agent
Tucks (Parke-Davis) Premoistened pads **Dosage** Adult: Apply to affected areas for 15–30 min, as needed, and use as a wipe after each bowel movement	50% Witch hazel	Astringent
	Glycerin	Protectant
	Purified water USP	
	Preservatives	
Wyanoid (Wyeth) Ointment **Dosage** Adult: Apply rectally, preferably at bedtime	5 g Zinc oxide per 100 g	Astringent
	18 g Boric acid per 100 g	Antiseptic
	0.1 g Ephedrine sulfate per 100 g	Vasoconstrictor
	2 g Benzocaine per 100 g	Anesthetic
	1 g Peruvian balsam per 100 g	Protectant
Wyanoids (Wyeth) Suppositories **Dosage** Adult: Insert 1 supp in AM and at bedtime for 6 days	15 mg Belladonna extract	Anticholinergic
	3 mg Ephedrine sulfate	Vasoconstrictor
	176 mg Zinc oxide	Astringent
	543 mg Boric acid	Antiseptic
	169 mg Bismuth subcarbonate	Astringent
	30 mg Peruvian balsam	Protectant
	Bismuth oxyiodide	Antiseptic

Hormonal Disorders

Diabetes

Diabetes is a chronic disorder of the insulin-producing cells of the pancreas that results in a derangement of carbohydrate metabolism. When the body cannot properly utilize ingested carbohydrates, blood sugar (glucose) builds up and a condition known as hyperglycemia results. Because the cells do not receive enough energy-producing glucose, the body begins to break down stored fats and proteins for energy use instead, resulting in weight loss and other symptoms.

Although there are different degrees and types of diabetes, hyperglycemia is a common characteristic. In many diabetics, the high level of blood sugar "spills over" into the urine (glycosuria). The presence of glucose in the urine was observed by the early Greek physicians, who named the disease diabetes mellitus, which means the "passing through of honey sweetness." These Greek physicians also observed that persons with diabetes often excrete excessive amounts of urine (polyuria), which is usually—but not always—sweet to the taste.

The early symptoms of diabetes are often referred to as the three "P's": polyuria (excessive urine production); polydipsia (extreme thirst and consumption of excessive amounts of water); and polyphagia (a profound feeling of hunger and excessive consumption of food often experienced because the body is, in actuality, undergoing a state of starvation).

TYPES OF DIABETES

Diabetes mellitus is unrelated to diabetes insipidus, a disorder of the pituitary gland that is characterized by increased urination but none of the other symptoms of diabetes mellitus. This discussion will focus on diabetes mellitus—a disease that afflicts as many as ten million Americans—which will be referred to simply as diabetes.

In general, there are two distinct types of diabetes: insulin-dependent (or juvenile-onset) and insulin-resistant (or maturity-onset) diabetes. Insulin-dependent diabetes is characterized by a failure of the insulin-producing (beta) cells of the pancreas to manufacture insulin. Its onset is usually in childhood, hence the term juvenile diabetes. In contrast, insulin-resistant diabetes usually manifests itself during or after the fifth decade of life. Its victims often have normal—or even above-normal—levels of insulin, yet the hormone is not effective in promoting glucose metabolism. In some cases, the disorder develops gradually, in stages. Initially, there may be no symptoms of diabetes, but blood tests will show hyperglycemia. This phase is referred to as impaired glucose tolerance and may progress to overt diabetes, in which there is hyperglycemia as well as the classic symptoms of polyuria, polydipsia, and polyphagia. There also may be glycosuria and, in women, vaginal itching and monilial vaginitis.

As a general rule, the earlier the onset of diabetes, the more pronounced the insulin deficiency. Juvenile diabetes is characterized by the sudden appearance of serious symptoms, with the child rapidly becoming severely weakened and undernourished. Ketoacidosis or diabetic coma, which can lead to death, is a manifestation of untreated or poorly controlled insulin-dependent diabetes. It is seen most often in insulin-dependent diabetes because, when glucose is not utilized for energy, the body begins to break down its own store of proteins and fats. Acidic substances called ketone bodies are produced as by-products of this process. As these ketone bodies accumulate in the blood, the acid balance of the body is altered, producing nausea, vomiting, and vague abdominal pains. These symptoms are followed by an "air hunger," or heavy, labored breathing. The breath may have a sharp, "fruity" smell, reminiscent of the acetone in nail polish remover. Urine tests during this phase show the presence of large amounts of glucose and acetone. Ketoacidosis can usually be prevented, however, by adequate control of the disease.

Long-term complications of diabetes are also of major concern and include circulatory disorders that can result in damage to the retina of the eye (diabetic retinopathy); increased risk of heart attacks; infections, particularly of the lower legs and feet; and neurological impairment, among others. However, if diabetes is treated at an early stage and is adequately controlled, these complications can be minimized.

TESTING FOR DIABETES

Diabetes often can be diagnosed by the presence of hyperglycemia along with the classic symptoms of the disease. When the diagnosis is not readily apparent, a series of at least three tests to measure blood sugar after fasting may be given. If the levels of blood sugar are consistently above normal, a diagnosis of diabetes is assumed. The glucose tolerance test—once considered the standard diagnostic procedure for diabetes—has fallen out of favor because of its highly variable results and is no longer commonly used except during pregnancy. Persons undergoing tests for diabetes should be aware that a number of factors other than eating can influence the level of blood sugar. These include alcohol consumption; the use of certain drugs, such as diuretics; pregnancy; stress; and the presence of other diseases, particularly liver disorders, Cushing's syndrome, and endocrine problems, among others.

Home Diagnostic Tests

The diagnosed diabetic must learn to perform urine tests for sugar and ketone bodies (acetone). There are many easy-to-use commercial kits available for these tests; selecting an appropriate one is a matter for discussion between the diabetic and the treating physician. It is particularly important that the patient taking insulin know how to test for ketonuria (ketone bodies in the urine), because this signals the need for adjusting diet and insulin. Proper testing of the urine for sugar is also essential because the consistent "spilling" of large quantities of sugar into the urine may signify an inadequate insulin dose, whereas a totally negative urine test for sugar may indicate too much insulin, which could lead to insulin shock or hypoglycemia. Diabetics who take insulin should have a readily available source of sugar or glucose, such as hard candy or gumdrops, handy at all times to take at the first sign of impending hypoglycemia. Symptoms of hypoglycemia include dizziness, weakness, fatigue, impaired thinking, profuse sweating, light-headedness, and flushing or pallor. Nervousness, irritability, tremors, hunger, double vision, and confusion also may be experienced, as well as numbness and chills. Later there may be hallucinations, slurred speech, and, finally, convulsions, coma, and death.

Hypoglycemia also may be precipitated by decreased food intake or by physical exercise. Most insulin-dependent diabetics are advised to decrease their insulin dosage (or increase their caloric intake) before bouts of exercise to compensate for the increased glucose utilization by the exercising muscles.

TREATMENT OF DIABETES

There are essentially three methods of treating diabetes: (1) diet alone, (2) diet and oral hypoglycemic agents, and (3) insulin and dietary regulations.

Dietary Management

Studies conducted in the U. S. and abroad have repeatedly demonstrated that 60 percent of all insulin-resistant or maturity-onset diabetics may be treated by diet alone. Obesity is a common characteristic of these patients, and, in many instances, losing weight is sufficient to restore proper insulin function. In general, the diabetic diet should provide sufficient calories for both the amount of energy expended and the maintenance of an ideal weight. It also should contain the essential nutrients necessary in any balanced diet, including carbohydrates. But extra attention may be given to the systematization of carbohydrate intake, meaning that carbohydrates should be consumed at regular intervals and in specific amounts. Since no single dietary plan is right for all patients, the diet must be individualized to meet each patient's particular needs.

The timing of food consumption is particularly important for insulin-dependent diabetics. In addition to providing adequate calories and other nutrients, meals and snacks should be spaced to avoid alternating periods of feasting and fasting with consequent high or low levels of blood glucose.

Insulin

All insulin preparations currently available must be given by injection. If taken orally, insulin, a natural protein (extracted from beef and/or pork pancreas glands), would be digested and thus rendered useless in glucose metabolism. Insulin is best injected intramuscularly, or subcutaneously where the skin is loose, and the site of injection should be changed frequently. Although many newly diagnosed diabetics are upset at the prospect of injecting themselves with insulin, most—even young children—can master this procedure in a relatively short time. Diabetic patients who require insulin are advised to carry an identification card, bracelet, or necklace stating they are diabetic—information that may be lifesaving in the event of insulin shock or diabetic coma. (These IDs are available from Medic Alert Foundation, Turlock, Calif. 95380.)

Currently, there are three types of insulin available: rapid-, intermediate-, and long-acting.

Rapid-Acting Insulin These are the regular insulins (Regular Iletin and various other brands) and the prompt insulin zinc suspension (Semilente Iletin, Semilente Insulin). The onset of action of these drugs is between one-half and one hour, with the peak effect occurring within two to seven hours; duration of action is six to sixteen hours. The regular insulin forms have a shorter duration of action than the prompt insulin zinc suspension form.

Rapid-acting insulins are used when early onset of action is desired, as in countering marked hyperglycemia, or in effecting better control of variations in blood sugar. For example, some patients may achieve the best results by taking two or three injections of regular insulin a day. For others, the rapid-acting insulin may be combined with an intermediate-acting insulin to avoid marked variations in blood sugar. In an emergency situation, such as diabetic coma, a rapid-acting insulin may be administered intravenously, as opposed to the usual intramuscular or subcutaneous injection.

Intermediate-Acting Insulin This group includes isophane insulin suspension (NPH Iletin, Isophane Insulin, and other brand names), insulin zinc suspension (Lente Iletin, Lente Insulin, and others), and globin zinc insulin (sold under that brand name). Onset of action is one to two hours, although globin zinc insulin has a slightly slower onset of action. The peak effect is between eight and sixteen hours, and the duration of action is twenty-four hours.

Long-Acting Insulin This group includes protamine zinc insulin (Protamine, Zinc and Iletin, Protamine Zinc Insulin, and other brand names) and extended insulin zinc suspension (Ultralente). The onset of action is four to eight hours, with the peak effect occurring between fourteen and twenty hours. Duration of action is up to thirty-six hours.

Stability of the diabetes is difficult to achieve with long-acting preparations; therefore they are rarely used alone and are usually combined with other forms of insulin.

Complications of Insulin Therapy

The major complication of insulin therapy is an overload of insulin, which results in insulin shock or hypoglycemia. This may occur if too much insulin is given or too little food is consumed. If symptoms of hypoglycemia occur, the diabetic can eat some sugar or candy to quickly use up the excess insulin and prevent the progression of insulin shock.

Local Reactions to Insulin Injections

Some diabetics taking insulin develop stinging or itching, followed by heat, redness, and hives at the injection site, but this usually occurs only during the initial weeks of insulin therapy. Newer forms of insulin produce fewer local reactions.

Occasionally, systemic allergic reactions such as hives, nausea, and vomiting occur; very rarely, a severe reaction (anaphylactic reaction) also may take place. On such occasions, systemic treatment with antihistamines or corticosteroids may be indicated.

In a few susceptible patients, fat tissue can become atrophied due to subcutaneous infections. This problem usually can be countered by switching to one of the newer insulin preparations.

Oral Hypoglycemic Agents

Oral hypoglycemic drugs are used to lower blood glucose levels and reduce glycosuria in maturity-onset diabetics whose disease is not controlled by diet alone. Although the mode of action of these agents is not completely understood, there is some evidence that they work, in part, by stimulating the beta cells of the islets of Langerhans in the pancreas to secrete insulin. *Oral hypoglycemic drugs are not insulin, nor are they substitutes for insulin.* Their usefulness is limited to those diabetics who produce some insulin and who have mild-to-moderate, but stable, disease. The only prescribed oral hypoglycemics in the U.S. are the sulfonylureas, which include chlorpropamide (Diabinese), acetohexamide (Dymelor), tolbutamide (Orinase) and tolazamide (Tolinase). The other major category of oral hypoglycemics—the biguanides, which include phenformin (DBI Mellitol)—has been withdrawn from general use in the U.S., although these drugs still may be prescribed for selected patients whose diabetes is not controlled by other means.

Acute toxic effects associated with oral hypoglycemic agents are relatively rare, although there is continuing controversy over possible long-term cardiovascular complications of tolbutamide. A number of drugs, particularly alcohol and salicylates (aspirin), are known to interact with some oral hypoglycemics, and beta-blocking drugs such as propranolol (Inderal) enhance their hypoglycemic effect. (See the individual drug charts for more specific information on potential drug interactions.)

The physician usually will continue a given dose for four to six weeks, and adjust dosages according to blood sugar levels and side effects, before determining whether an oral hypoglycemic agent is a success or failure.

IN CONCLUSION

As emphasized earlier, diabetes is a complex disorder that requires a multifaceted approach to treatment. Strict adherence to the physician's recommendations regarding treatment and lifestyle, including dietary suggestions, is important if serious long-range complications of the disease are to be minimized. Ongoing research in the field shows promise of a greater understanding of the disease, which may result in more effective treatments. In the meantime, most patients with diabetes can control the disease by following an individualized therapeutic regimen. The following drug charts provide more detailed information on the various oral hypoglycemic agents and forms of insulin now available.

REGULAR INSULIN **Onset:** ½–1 h **Peak:** 2–3 h **Duration:** 6 h

REGULAR ILETIN (beef and pork pancreas) **Lilly**

Vials: 40, 80, 100 units/ml (10 ml)

INSULIN (beef and pork pancreas) **Squibb**

Vials: 40, 80, 100 units/ml (10 ml)

BEEF REGULAR ILETIN (beef pancreas) **Lilly**

Vials: 100 units/ml (10 ml)

PORK REGULAR ILETIN II (pork pancreas) **Lilly**

Vials: 100 units/ml (10 ml)

REGULAR (CONCENTRATED) ILETIN II (pork pancreas) **Lilly**

Vials: 500 units/ml (20 ml)

INSULIN ZINC SUSPENSION, PROMPT **Onset:** ½–1 h **Peak:** 5–7 h **Duration:** 12–16 h

SEMILENTE ILETIN (beef and pork pancreas) **Lilly**

Vials: 40, 80, 100 units/ml (10 ml)

SEMILENTE INSULIN (beef pancreas) **Squibb**

Vials: 40, 80, 100 units/ml (10 ml)

ISOPHANE INSULIN SUSPENSION **Onset:** 1–1½ h **Peak:** 8–12 h **Duration:** 24 h

NPH ILETIN (beef and pork pancreas) **Lilly**

Vials: 40, 80, 100 units/ml (10 ml)

ISOPHANE INSULIN (beef and pork pancreas) **Squibb**

Vials: 40, 80, 100 units/ml (10 ml)

BEEF NPH ILETIN (beef pancreas) **Lilly**

Vials: 100 units/ml (10 ml)

PORK NPH ILETIN II (pork pancreas) **Lilly**

Vials: 100 units/ml (10 ml)

INSULIN ZINC SUSPENSION **Onset:** 1–1½ h **Peak:** 8–12 h **Duration:** 24 h

LENTE ILETIN (beef and pork pancreas) **Lilly**

Vials: 40, 80, 100 units/ml (10 ml)

LENTE INSULIN (beef pancreas) **Squibb**

Vials: 40, 80, 100 units/ml (10 ml)

BEEF LENTE ILETIN (beef pancreas) **Lilly**

Vials: 100 units/ml (10 ml)

PORK LENTE ILETIN II (pork pancreas) **Lilly**

Vials: 100 units/ml (10 ml)

GLOBIN ZINC INSULIN **Onset:** 2 h **Peak:** 8–16 h **Duration:** 24 h

GLOBIN ZINC INSULIN (beef and pork pancreas) **Squibb**

Vials: 40, 80, 100 units/ml (10 ml)

Table continued on following page

INSULIN continued

PROTAMINE ZINC INSULIN (PZI) **Onset:** 4–8 h **Peak:** 14–20 h **Duration:** 36 h

PROTAMINE, ZINC and ILETIN (beef and pork pancreas) **Lilly**

Vials: 40, 80, 100 units/ml (10 ml)

PROTAMINE ZINC INSULIN (beef and pork pancreas) **Squibb**

Vials: 40, 80, 100 units/ml (10 ml)

BEEF PROTAMINE, ZINC and ILETIN (beef pancreas) **Lilly**

Vials: 100 units/ml (10 ml)

PORK PROTAMINE, ZINC and ILETIN II (pork pancreas) **Lilly**

Vials: 100 units/ml (10 ml)

INSULIN ZINC SUSPENSION, EXTENDED **Onset:** 4–8 h **Peak:** 16–18 h **Duration:** 36 h

ULTRALENTE ILETIN (beef and pork pancreas) **Lilly**

Vials: 40, 80, 100 units/ml (10 ml)

ULTRALENTE INSULIN (beef pancreas) **Squibb**

Vials: 40, 80, 100 units/ml (10 ml)

INDICATIONS	PARENTERAL DOSAGE
Diabetes mellitus not controllable by diet alone	**Adult and child:** must be determined individually under direct and continuous medical supervision

ADMINISTRATION/DOSAGE ADJUSTMENTS

Timing of administration	Insulin is best administered 15–30 min before meals
Longer-acting insulins	Not suitable as a substitute for regular insulin in acidosis and emergencies; best administered before breakfast
Regular (concentrated) insulin	Subcutaneous and/or IM administration preferable, as IV injection may cause allergic or anaphylactoid reactions
Purified pork insulins	An occasional patient transferred from older Lilly pork insulin products to Iletin II may require a decrease or, less often, an increase in dosage

CONTRAINDICATIONS

Hypersensitivity to any component

WARNINGS/PRECAUTIONS

Diet	Patient should follow diet prescribed
Hypoglycemia	May occur due to excessive dosage, increased exercise, when food is not absorbed normally, or when insulin is administered too far in advance of a meal

ADVERSE REACTIONS

Cardiovascular	Hypotension
Dermatological	Local reactions (hive-like or urticarial), pruritus, redness, induration at site of injection, lipodystrophy
Gastrointestinal	Distension, nausea, vomiting, diarrhea, hunger, eructation
Cardiovascular	Bradycardia with mild hypotension, increased blood pressure, tachycardia
Central nervous system	Lethargy, lassitude, confused thinking, convulsions, coma
Other	Diaphoresis

Table continued on following page

INSULIN continued

OVERDOSAGE

Signs and symptoms	Fatigue, headache, drowsiness, lassitude, tremulousness, nausea, weakness, sweating, tremor, nervousness, delirium, mental confusion, insulin shock, coma
Treatment	Administer carbohydrate immediately; for more severe hypoglycemic reactions, give 10–20 g glucose IV promptly; carefully monitor electrolytes and treat symptomatically

DRUG INTERACTIONS

Alcohol, anabolic steroids, guanethidine, MAO inhibitors, oral hypoglycemics, salicylates (large doses)	⇧ Risk of hypoglycemia
Corticosteroids, epinephrine, oral contraceptives, phenytoin, thyroid hormones, thiazide diuretics	⇧ Blood glucose
Beta blockers	⇧ Risk of hypoglycemia and possibly hyperglycemia May mask warning signs (palpitations, tachycardia, etc) of incipient hypoglycemia

ALTERED LABORATORY VALUES

Blood/serum values	⇩ Glucose ⇩ Potassium
Urinary values	⇩ Glucose

Use in children

General guidelines not established

Use in pregnancy or nursing mothers

General guidelines not established

DIABINESE (Chlorpropamide) **Pfizer**

Tabs: 100, 250 mg

INDICATIONS	ORAL DOSAGE
Diabetes mellitus (stable, mild to moderate adult, maturity-onset, nonketotic)	**Adult:** 250 mg qd (with breakfast) to start; after 5–7 days, adjust dosage up to 500 mg/day, as needed

ADMINISTRATION/DOSAGE ADJUSTMENTS

Elderly patients	Start older diabetics on 100–125 mg/day, with breakfast
Patients receiving insulin	For patients receiving less than 40 units/day, discontinue insulin therapy abruptly and transfer directly to chlorpropamide; for patients receiving 40 units/day or more of insulin, reduce insulin dosage by 50% for a few days after starting chlorpropamide, followed by daily reductions, as response is observed. Test urine for sugar and acetone at least three times daily. Hospitalization may be advisable during the transition period.
Patients receiving acetohexamide	Transfer directly to chlorpropamide (250 mg = 500 mg acetohexamide)[1]
Patients receiving tolbutamide	Transfer directly to chlorpropamide (250 mg = 1 g tolbutamide)[1]
Patients receiving tolazamide	Transfer directly to chlorpropamide (250 mg = 250 mg tolazamide)[1]
GI disturbances	May be alleviated by dividing the total daily dose into two portions

CONTRAINDICATIONS

Juvenile or growth-onset diabetes ●

Severe or unstable ("brittle") diabetes mellitus ●

Diabetes complicated by acidosis, ketosis, coma, fever, major surgery, or severe trauma or infection (in these situations, insulin must be used) ●

Serious renal, hepatic, or thyroid dysfunction ●

WARNINGS/PRECAUTIONS

Addison's disease	May predispose to hypoglycemia; use with caution
Jaundice, incipient biliary stasis	May occur; progressive rise in serum alkaline phosphatase warrants discontinuation of drug
Alcohol, decreased caloric intake	May lead to hypoglycemia, ketosis, coma, and death
Hypoglycemia	May occur, especially when initiating therapy or transferring from insulin (may be controlled by glucose administration). Therapy should be re-evaluated. *Patient should be monitored for several days* owing to prolonged action of drug.
Edema associated with hyponatremia	May occur due to inappropriate ADH syndrome; discontinue therapy

ADVERSE REACTIONS

Idiosyncratic, hypersensitivity[2]	Jaundice (with or without low-grade fever and eosinophilia); skin eruptions, rarely progressing to exfoliative dermatitis and erythema multiforme; severe diarrhea (with or without bleeding)
Hematological	Leukopenia, thrombocytopenia, mild anemia, aplastic anemia, agranulocytosis, lymphocytosis
Gastrointestinal	Anorexia, nausea, vomiting, epigastric discomfort
Neurological[3]	Weakness, paresthesias
Other[2]	Phototoxicity, edema, hyponatremia

OVERDOSAGE

Signs and symptoms	Hypoglycemia, leading to neurological disorders (restlessness, bizarre behavior, nightmares, hallucinations, obtundation, seizures, coma and/or brain death), sympathetic hyperactivity (tachycardia precipitating myocardial ischemia, diaphoresis, tremors)
Treatment	Administer IV glucose, if indicated, in large quantities for extended time period. For possible alcoholism or malnutrition, give IV thiamine. Induce emesis or use gastric lavage, followed by activated charcoal and a cathartic. Screen urine, gastric content, and blood for other toxins. Children should be kept under close observation for 3–5 days, despite apparent recovery.

DRUG INTERACTIONS

Chloramphenicol, clofibrate, dicumarol, guanethidine, MAO inhibitors, oxyphenbutazone, phenylbutazone, probenecid, salicylates, sulfonamides	⇧ Risk of hypoglycemia

[1]Boyden T, Bressler R: *Adv Intern Med* 24:53, 1979
[2]Discontinue therapy if any of these reactions occur
[3]May be relieved by reducing dosage.

Table continued on following page.

DRUG INTERACTIONS continued

Beta blockers	⇧ Risk of hypoglycemia and possibly hyperglycemia May mask warning signs (palpitations, tachycardia, etc) of incipient hypoglycemia
Alcohol	Abdominal cramps, nausea, vomiting, intense flushing, hypoglycemia
Corticosteroids, epinephrine, phenytoin, thiazide diuretics	⇧ Blood glucose

ALTERED LABORATORY VALUES

Blood/serum values	⇩ Glucose ⇩ Sodium (SIADH) ⇧ Alkaline phosphatase
Urinary values	⇩ Glucose

Use in children

Contraindicated in juvenile or growth-onset diabetes

Use in pregnancy or nursing mothers

Contraindicated in pregnancy; may cause neonatal hypoglycemia.[1] Use with caution in women of childbearing age who may become pregnant. General guidelines not established for use in nursing mothers.

[1]Sutherland HW *et al: Arch Dis Child* 49:283, 1974; Tuchmann-Duplessis M: *Monographs on Drugs,* Vol 2, Acton, Mass, Publishing Sciences Group, Inc. 1975

DYMELOR (Acetohexamide) Lilly

Tabs: 250, 500 mg

INDICATIONS	ORAL DOSAGE
Diabetes mellitus (stable, mild adult, maturity-onset, nonketotic)	**Adult:** 250 mg to 1.5 g, given in 1 or 2 divided doses (see ADMINISTRATION/DOSAGE ADJUSTMENTS)

ADMINISTRATION/DOSAGE ADJUSTMENTS

Timing of administration	Doses of 1 g or less, give qd before morning meal; doses of 1.5 g/day, give in divided doses before morning and evening meals
Elderly patients	Start with 250 mg/day before breakfast; check blood and urine sugars during first 24 h and adjust dosage up or down, accordingly
Patients receiving insulin	For patients receiving 20 units/day or less, discontinue insulin abruptly and transfer directly to acetohexamide; for patients receiving 20-40 units/day or more, reduce insulin dosage by 25-30% daily or every other day, followed by further reduction depending upon response. Test urine for sugar and acetone at least three times daily. Hospitalization may be advisable during the transition period.
Patients receiving chlorpropamide	Transfer directly to acetohexamide (500 mg = 250 mg chlorpropamide)
Patients receiving tolbutamide	Transfer directly to acetohexamide (250 mg = 500 mg tolbutamide)
Patients receiving tolazamide	Transfer directly to acetohexamide (500 mg = 250 mg tolazamide)[1]

CONTRAINDICATIONS[2]

Hyperglycemia and glycosuria associated with primary renal disease ●	Diabetes complicated by acidosis and coma (in these situations, insulin must be used) ●

WARNINGS/PRECAUTIONS

Severe hypoglycemia	May occur, especially in elderly, malnourished, or debilitated patients and in patients with hepatic or renal disease
Fever, trauma, infection,or surgery	May necessitate a return to insulin therapy or supplementary use of insulin
Secondary failures	May occur; observe patient regularly during therapy

ADVERSE REACTIONS

Gastrointestinal	Nausea, epigastric fullness, heartburn
Central nervous system	Headache
Allergic	Pruritus; erythema; urticarial, morbilliform, or maculopapular eruptions; photosensitivity
Hematological	Leukopenia, thrombocytopenia, pancytopenia, agranulocytosis, aplastic anemia, hemolytic anemia
Hepatic	Jaundice (cholestatic and mixed hepatic)

OVERDOSAGE

Signs and symptoms	Hypoglycemia leading to neurological disorders (restlessness, bizarre behavior, nightmares, hallucinations, obtundation, seizures, coma and/or brain death), sympathetic hyperactivity (tachycardia precipitating myocardial ischemia, diaphoresis, tremors)
Treatment	Administer IV glucose, if indicated, in large quantities for extended time period. For possible alcoholism or malnutrition, give IV thiamine. Induce emesis or use gastric lavage, followed by activated charcoal and a cathartic. Screen urine, gastric content, and blood for other toxins.

DRUG INTERACTIONS

Chloramphenicol, clofibrate, dicumarol, guanethidine, MAO inhibitors, oxyphenbutazone, phenylbutazone, probenecid, salicylates, sulfonamides	⇧ Risk of hypoglycemia
Beta blockers	⇧ Risk of hypoglycemia and possibly hyperglycemia May mask warning signs (palpitations, tachycardia, etc) of incipient hypoglycemia
Alcohol	Abdominal cramps, nausea, vomiting, intense flushing, hypoglycemia
Corticosteroids, epinephrine, phenytoin, thiazide diuretics	⇧ Blood glucose

[1]Boyden T, Bressler R: *Adv Intern Med* 24:53, 1979

[2]Because acetohexamide is metabolized in part by the liver, severe hepatic disease may also be a contraindication (see WARNINGS/PRECAUTIONS)

Table continued on following page

ALTERED LABORATORY VALUES

Blood/serum values	⇩ Glucose	⇩ Uric acid
Urinary values	⇩ Glucose	⇧ Uric acid

Use in children

Not indicated for juvenile or growth-onset diabetes

Use in pregnancy or nursing mothers

Not recommended for use in pregnancy. Use with caution in women of childbearing age who may become pregnant. General guidelines not established for use in nursing mothers.

ORINASE (Tolbutamide) **Upjohn**

Tabs: 250, 500 mg

INDICATIONS	ORAL DOSAGE
Diabetes mellitus (stable, mild adult, maturity-onset, nonketotic)	**Adult:** 1-2 g/day to start, either as single dose in AM or div, followed by 0.25-2 g/day in AM or div, not to exceed 3 g/day

ADMINISTRATION/DOSAGE ADJUSTMENTS

Patients receiving insulin	For patients receiving 20 units/day or less, discontinue insulin abruptly and transfer directly to tolbutamide. For patients receiving 20-40 units/day, reduce insulin dosage by 30-50% on first day of therapy, followed by daily reductions as response is observed. For patients receiving more than 40 units/day, reduce insulin dosage by 20% on first day, followed by further reductions as response is observed. Test urine for sugar and ketone bodies at least three times daily. If ketosis or unsatisfactory control results, return patient to insulin therapy. Mild hypoglycemia may be corrected with carbohydrate and recurrences by more rapid withdrawal of insulin. Hospitalization may be advisable during the transition period for patients requiring more than 40 units of insulin daily.
Patients receiving acetohexamide	Transfer directly to tolbutamide (1 g = 500 mg acetohexamide)[1]
Patients receiving chlorpropamide	Transfer directly to tolbutamide (1 g = 250 mg chlorpropamide)[1]
Patients receiving tolazamide	Transfer directly to tolbutamide (1 g = 250 mg tolazamide)[1]
Combination therapy	Although not universally accepted, tolbutamide may be used to decrease insulin requirements in patients with maturity-onset or growth-onset diabetes; in insulin-resistant patients, use of the combination may be warranted in an effort to reduce the insulin requirement
GI disturbances	May be minimized by administering the total daily dose in divided portions after meals

CONTRAINDICATIONS[2]

Juvenile or growth-onset diabetes ● Unstable ("brittle") diabetes mellitus ●	Diabetes complicated by acidosis, ketosis, or coma (in these situations, insulin must be used) ●	Severe renal insufficiency ●

WARNINGS/PRECAUTIONS

Fever, severe trauma, infection, or surgery	May necessitate a temporary return to insulin therapy or supplementary use of insulin
Severe hypoglycemia	May occur, especially in elderly, malnourished, semistarved, or debilitated patients, and in patients with hepatic or renal impairment or adrenal or pituitary insufficiency
Secondary failures	May occur after an extended period of good control

ADVERSE REACTIONS

Gastrointestinal	Nausea, epigastric fullness, heartburn
Hepatic	Cholestatic jaundice
Central nervous system	Headache, peripheral and optic neuritis
Dermatological	Pruritus; erythema; urticarial, morbilliform, or maculopapular eruptions; photosensitivity
Hematological	Leukopenia, agranulocytosis, thrombocytopenia, hemolytic anemia, aplastic anemia, pancytopenia
Metabolic	Hepatic porphyria, porphyria cutanea tarda

OVERDOSAGE

Signs and symptoms	Hypoglycemia, leading to neurological disorders (restlessness, bizarre behavior, nightmares, hallucinations, obtundation, seizures, coma and/or brain death), sympathetic hyperactivity (tachycardia precipitating myocardial ischemia, diaphoresis, tremors)
Treatment	Administer IV glucose, if indicated, in large quantities for extended time period. For possible alcoholism or malnutrition, give IV thiamine. Induce emesis or use gastric lavage, followed by activated charcoal and a cathartic. Screen urine, gastric content, and blood for other toxins.

DRUG INTERACTIONS

Chloramphenicol, clofibrate, dicumarol, guanethidine, MAO inhibitors, oxyphenbutazone, phenylbutazone, probenecid, salicylates, sulfonamides	⇧ Risk of hypoglycemia

[1]Boyden T, Bressler R: *Adv Intern Med* 24:53, 1979
[2]Because tolbutamide is metabolized in part by the liver, severe hepatic disease may also be a contraindication (see WARNINGS/PRECAUTIONS)

Table continued on following page

DRUG INTERACTIONS continued

Beta blockers	⇧ Risk of hypoglycemia and possibly hyperglycemia May mask warning signs (palpitations, tachycardia, etc) of incipient hypoglycemia
Alcohol	Abdominal cramps, nausea, vomiting, intense flushing, hypoglycemia
Corticosteroids, epinephrine, phenytoin, thiazide diuretics	⇧ Blood glucose

ALTERED LABORATORY VALUES

Blood/serum values	⇩ Glucose ⇩ Sodium ⇩ RAI uptake
Urinary values	⇩ Glucose ⇧ Albumin (with turbidity test methods)

Use in children

Contraindicated in juvenile or growth-onset diabetes

Use in pregnancy or nursing mothers

Not recommended for use in pregnancy. Tolbutamide has been shown to have teratogenic and feticidal effects in animal studies at doses of 1,000–2,500 mg/kg/day. Tolbutamide is excreted in breast milk, although effects are insignificant with therapeutic doses.[1]

[1]Bartig B, Cohon MS: *Hosp Formul Manag* 4:27, 1969; Moiel RH, Ryan JR: *Clin Pediatr* 6:480, 1967; Takyi BE: *J Hosp Pharm* 28:317, 1970

TOLINASE (Tolazamide) Upjohn

Tabs: 100, 250, 500 mg

INDICATIONS	ORAL DOSAGE
Diabetes mellitus (stable, mild to moderate adult, maturity-onset, nonketotic)	**Adult (fasting blood sugar <200 mg/dl):** 100 mg qd, with breakfast; increase or decrease by 100–250 mg/day at weekly intervals, as needed, up to 1 g/day; divide doses over 500 mg/day **Adult (fasting blood sugar >200 mg/dl):** 250 mg qd, with breakfast; increase or decrease by 100–250 mg/day at weekly intervals, as needed, up to 1 g/day; divide doses over 500 mg/day

ADMINISTRATION/DOSAGE ADJUSTMENTS

Underweight, malnourished, or elderly patients	Administer 100 mg qd; increase dosage by 50–125 mg/day at weekly intervals, as needed
Patients receiving insulin	For patients receiving 20 units/day or less, discontinue abruptly and begin with 100 mg tolazamide qd; for patients receiving 20–40 units/day, discontinue abruptly and begin with 250 mg tolazamide qd; for patients receiving more than 40 units/day, reduce insulin dosage by 50% and begin with 250 mg tolazamide qd. Test urine for sugar and acetone at least three times daily. If significant acetonuria occurs or glucose control is unsatisfactory, return patient to insulin therapy.
Patients receiving tolbutamide	For patients receiving 1 g/day or less, discontinue tolbutamide abruptly and begin with 100 mg tolazamide qd. For patients receiving more than 1 g/day, begin with 250 mg qd.
Patients receiving chlorpropamide	Transfer directly to tolazamide (100 mg = 100 mg chlorpropamide); observe carefully for hypoglycemia during transition period (1–2 wk)
Patients receiving acetohexamide	Transfer directly to tolazamide (100 mg = 250 mg acetohexamide)

CONTRAINDICATIONS

Juvenile or growth-onset diabetes ●	Uremia ●	Diabetes complicated by acidosis, ketosis, coma, severe trauma, surgery, or infection (in these situations, insulin must be used) ●
Unstable ("brittle") diabetes mellitus ●	Hepatic, renal, or endocrine disease ●	

WARNINGS/PRECAUTIONS

Severe hypoglycemia	May occur, especially in elderly, alcoholic, malnourished, semistarved, or debilitated patients and in patients with hepatic or renal dysfunction or adrenal or pituitary insufficiency, and may mimic acute neurological disorders (eg, cerebral thrombosis)
Congestive heart failure	Can prolong duration of hypoglycemic effect and/or give rise to profound hypoglycemia secondary to hepatic congestion
Alcoholism	Increases tendency to develop profound hypoglycemia, despite absence of known liver disease

ADVERSE REACTIONS

Gastrointestinal	Nausea, vomiting, gas
Hematological	Leukopenia, thrombocytopenia, agranulocytosis, anemia
Hepatic	Altered liver-function studies, cholestatic jaundice
Dermatological	Urticaria, rash, photosensitivity
Central nervous system	Weakness, fatigue, dizziness, vertigo, malaise, headache

OVERDOSAGE

Signs and symptoms	Hypoglycemia, leading to neurological disorders (restlessness, bizarre behavior, nightmares, hallucinations, obtundation, seizures, coma and/or brain death), sympathetic hyperactivity (tachycardia precipitating myocardial ischemia, diaphoresis, tremors)
Treatment	Administer IV glucose, if indicated, in large quantities for extended time period. For possible alcoholism or malnutrition, give IV thiamine. Induce emesis or use gastric lavage, followed by activated charcoal and a cathartic. Screen urine, gastric content, and blood for other toxins.

DRUG INTERACTIONS

Chloramphenicol, clofibrate, dicumarol, guanethidine, MAO inhibitors, oxyphenbutazone, phenylbutazone, probenecid, salicylates, sulfonamides	⇧ Risk of hypoglycemia
Beta blockers	⇧ Risk of hypoglycemia and possibly hyperglycemia. May mask warning signs (palpitations, tachycardia, etc) of incipient hypoglycemia

[1]Because tolazamide is metaboized by the liver, severe hepatic disease may also be a contraindication (see WARNINGS/PRECAUTIONS)

Table continued on following page

DRUG INTERACTIONS continued

Alcohol	Abdominal cramps, nausea, vomiting, intense flushing, hypoglycemia
Corticosteroids, epinephrine, phenytoin, thiazide diuretics	⇧ Blood glucose

ALTERED LABORATORY VALUES

Blood/serum values	⇩ Glucose ⇧ Alkaline phosphatase ⇧ SGOT ⇧ SGPT ⇧ Bilirubin ⇧ Cholesterol
Urinary values	⇩ Glucose

Use in children

Contraindicated in juvenile or growth-onset diabetes

Use in pregnancy or nursing mothers

Not recommended for use in pregnancy. Use with caution in women of childbearing age who may become pregnant. General guidelines not established for use in nursing mothers.

Sex Hormones

Shortly before puberty, the "biological clock" in the brain (mediated in part by the hypothalamus), triggers the pituitary to release hormones called gonadotropins. These gonadotropins—as their name signifies—are directed to the gonads, the testes of the male and the ovaries of the female, stimulating them to begin producing the sex hormones, which regulate sexual and reproductive functions in both men and women.

With this comes the onset of puberty—a time of dramatic physical change and maturation in both boys and girls. The testes begin producing testosterone—the principal male sex hormone that is essential in the production of sperm cells. The ovaries produce estrogen and progesterone, the female sex hormones that are essential to the successful implantation and development of the fertilized egg. The levels of these hormones in the body are regulated by a delicate feedback mechanism mediated by the pituitary and hypothalamus. The pituitary manufactures the gonadotropin hormones, which stimulate the gonads to produce their respective sex hormones. When adequate levels of sex hormones have been produced, they signal the pituitary to reduce production of the gonadotropins. When the level of sex hormones falls below a certain point, the pituitary steps up production of the gonadotropins, which in turn stimulate increased production of sex hormones. The functions and medical applications of sex hormones will be reviewed in this section.

MALE SEX HORMONES

The general name for hormones that have masculinizing effects is androgens, of which testosterone, produced by the testes, is the most abundant. Despite the name "male" sex hormones, androgens are produced by the adrenal glands of both women and men, both before and after puberty; they are also produced after puberty by the ovaries, though in far smaller quantities than by the testes.

Testosterone is responsible for many of the dramatic changes that mark male puberty—the increase in muscle mass, growth of the penis, testicles, and prostate, deepening of the voice, appearance of facial and pubic hair, and secretion of seminal fluid and sperm. The production of sex hormones is initially marked by a spurt of growth, but the hormones also set in motion the epiphyseal (bone joint) closure that prevents further skeletal growth. Androgens are also responsible for growth of female pubic hair, as well as for enlargement of the female clitoris and labia majora (these analogues of the penis and scrotum have the same sensitivity to androgen stimulation). In addition, androgens provide the hormonal stimulus for the sexual drives of both men and women.

Male Hypogonadal Disorders

The therapeutic uses of androgens are essentially confined to conditions in which the body produces inadequate amounts, commonly called hypogonadal states.

Delayed puberty Various pituitary disorders may prevent the release of gonadotropins,thus hindering normal testosterone production. Or male puberty may be delayed for no discernible reason. In select cases of the latter, physicians may administer a synthetic testosterone. Often this will set the normal processes in motion and the young male's testes will start secreting testosterone themselves. In cases where there is no apparent cause of the delay—attributable perhaps to heredity—physicians traditionally have waited for the body to start pubertal changes on its own for fear of limiting the time the child will have for skeletal growth before the testosterone brings on the bone joint closure that stops growth. As noted earlier, testosterone brings on a fairly immediate growth spurt, but it is feared that treatment with the hormone might compromise ultimate height. Some reports indicate that adolescent males' heights were not limited by such treatment, though this remains an open question, and most physicians do not initiate such treatment unless the young person is very distressed by his small size and lack of sexual development.

Testosterone deficiency Certain pituitary and other disorders cause a hypogonadal state where eunuchoidal conditions result. These circumstances would include castration, which may be performed on testes that did not descend from the abdomen, or that developed malignant tumors. Such individuals must be maintained on testosterone therapy in order to preserve libido and masculine characteristics.

Low sperm count Occasionally, testosterone is used to treat low sperm count. It may have the paradoxical effect of suppresssing sperm production even more, but once treatment ceases there can be a "rebound" effect of greater numbers of sperm and greater potential for impregnation.

Male "climacteric" In rare cases of men suffering symptoms resembling those of menopause in women, including low sex drive, lassitude, "hot flashes," poor sleep—and *when* this is associated with testosterone deficiency—physicians will treat with androgens. There is controversy over the prevalence of this condition, with most experts contending it is exceptionally rare, and a few convinced it is the rule rather than the exception among older men; much discussion revolves around whether testosterone levels in the blood are a reliable indication of the amounts actually available to "prime" the sexual apparatus and contribute to stamina.

Impotence Androgen treatment in cases of impotence is indicated only when there is demonstrable androgen deficiency.

Muscle building Androgens are sometimes used (and far more often *misused* without medical supervision) as part of a dietary and exercise regimen to build muscle mass and strength. It is doubtful that they produce the desired results, and their use for this purpose is not condoned. The so-called anabolic steroids are male sex hormones, which, when taken recklessly by athletes (male or female), can have adverse, often very dangerous, effects, such as liver dysfunction. Virilism (masculinization) is a common side effect in women using these hormones.

Psychosexual behavior The male sex hormones are of considerable research interest, particularly regarding their possible relationship to psychosexual orientation, sexual behavior, and antisocial activities. Regarding the latter, suggestive evidence links aggression with high testosterone levels—higher levels being found in violent rapists and excessively aggressive athletes, among other examples. However, it is unclear whether the testosterone caused the aggressiveness, is a result of it, or is even related at all. Similarly, a number of studies have attempted to link homosexuality, as well as frequency of sexual activity, to testosterone levels, with equivocal or insignificant correlations.

FEMALE SEX HORMONES

At a somewhat earlier age in girls than in boys (usually about two years sooner), the pituitary gonadotropins—luteinizing hormones (LH) and follicle-stimulating hormones (FSH)—activate the ovaries to begin secreting the female hormone, estrogen. Following the initial breast budding—which also occurs in many prepubertal boys—the girl develops the characteristics of female adulthood. The vagina matures and develops mucosal tissue, body fat is distributed to create adult female contours, and breasts enlarge further. As mentioned, the ovaries and the adrenals also secrete small amounts of androgens, which are responsible for underarm and pubic hair growth, clitoris and labia majora enlargement, as well as increased sexual drive. The estrogens, however, keep the androgens in check to prevent the virilizing changes boys undergo, such as facial hair, deepening voice, and bulky muscles.

The estrogens also initiate the female menstrual-reproductive processes. They cause abundant growth of the cells that line the uterus (the endometrium), preparing them to receive a fertilized ovum and support a pregnancy. Under the influence of gonadotropins, each month the Graafian follicles, one of many small bodies on the ovaries which contain unripened ova, are prodded to release an egg that has matured and is ready for fertilization. (If more than one is ready and released, the woman may conceive nonidentical, or dizygotic, twins.) A small hormone-secreting body at the site of the "spent" Graafian follicle, called the corpus luteum, then secretes the other principal female hormone, progesterone (as well as minute amounts of estrogen). This hormone stops the proliferation of endometrial cells and, if the woman is not pregnant, causes them to be shed, resulting in menstruation. The oral contraceptives utilize one or both of these hormones, in varying amounts and sequences, to control this process. (See the section on *Contraception,* page 831.)

Female Hypogonadism

As in the case of boys with lack of sexual development who receive treatment with testosterone, young women who fail to develop normal changes of puberty and do not menstruate because their ovaries fail to secrete estrogen often receive treatment with estrogens. Women with pituitary conditions that result in chronic hypogonadism, and those whose ovaries must be removed for any of a variety of pelvic diseases, may be treated on a regular basis with estrogens. With supplemental estrogens, their vaginal tone and vaginal lubrication will be normal, and they will maintain a normal female appearance. Fertility, of course, depends on the nature of their condition; pituitary disorders are sometimes an aspect of genetic defects that prevent reproduction (see *Infertility,* page 875).

Menstrual Disorders

The female sex hormones are occasionally employed to correct menstrual disorders, although these are usually given in the form of birth-control pills. Women who in the past have menstruated normally but then fail to menstruate may be given progesterone. The "secretory" effect this hormone has upon the endometrial cells often succeeds in bringing about the menstrual flow. Women with abnormal menstrual-type bleeding that is not linked to a disease such as fibroids may be given progesterone. Adolescents with "primary" ovarian failure—those who have never menstruated—may be given estrogen to initiate the process.

Menopause

By far the most common use for estrogens is in the menopausal years to compensate for hormonal deficiency when the functioning of a woman's ovaries tapers off and they ultimately cease estrogen secretion entirely. Menstruation and childbearing capacity come to a halt. With estrogen no longer nourishing and maintaining the vaginal walls, they tend to atrophy. There may be itching and burning sensations within the vagina, and the dryness can make intercourse difficult and painful.

Eventually skin over much of the body begins to wrinkle because of loss of subcutaneous elasticity and some facial hair may grow, since androgens are no longer opposed by sufficient estrogens. Estrogen deprivation is also believed to be a factor in calcium loss, leading to weakening of the bones (osteoporosis) and greater susceptibility to fractures.

The most prevalent and distressing symptoms of the menopausal years, however, are emotional. While symptoms are felt acutely by the sufferers, and are very common, physicians and researchers have had great difficulty determining to what extent they are caused by "estrogen starvation" and to what extent by other changes in women's lives at this time (e.g., the "empty nest syndrome"). There is little question, however, that hormonal deprivation causes many women to experience the hot flushes or "flashes" that strike them, often at night. A sense of heat, which suffuses the head and face, and radiates down to the neck and chest, is followed by intense perspiration. At this time, many women also suffer insomnia, irritability, and depression.

Not all women suffer in these ways. In fact, perhaps half or more women adapt to diminished estrogen production and the accompanying life changes without significant distress. Obese women, for example, seem to have less trouble, because adipose tissue (in women *and* men) seems to convert androgens to estrogens.

Estrogen replacement Those women with symptoms may have estrogen replacement tailored to their specific problem. Physicians should try to use estrogens judiciously and sparingly, since their use may entail risks. Thus, women with "senile vaginitis" (the inflamed, atrophied vagina referred to earlier) or with kraurosis, a similar condition of the skin of the vulva, may be given estrogen creams to apply to the vulva or vagina, instead of oral or other forms of estrogen that affect the entire body. As it happens, estrogen creams are absorbed and also enter the bloodstream, but do not attain as high levels of concentration as oral estrogens.

Estrogen medications have been demonstrated to diminish or eliminate hot flashes and night sweats, as well as combat the bone loss of osteoporosis. There is little objective evidence that they ameliorate the insomnia, irritability, and sadness accompanying this age—although they may do so indirectly. By stopping the nighttime hot flashes and profuse perspiration, they may ease the insomnia, and this, in turn, may help ease the irritability and unhappiness.

Physicians do not engage in "wholesale" replacement therapy—giving abundant quantities to all menopausal women—because of the risks alluded to above. While there are numerous possible adverse side effects, the most alarming concern was raised by recent large studies that found a higher incidence of endometrial cancer among women who used long-term replacement estrogens for menopause. Some physicians contend that estrogens do not cause these cancers but, instead, stimulate existing cancers to proliferate and become evident. It has also been argued that women receiving estrogen treatment are examined by their physicians more regularly than other women, receiving Pap smears and cytology tests that turn up otherwise unrecognized cancers. Recent studies have also found that while there may be more tumors among the estrogen users, there is not a significant increase in mortality, suggesting that the cancers are not highly malignant. A number of gynecologists have suggested that, rather than stopping the use of estrogens, they should be used in conjunction with progesterones. The latter would arrest the tumor growth, just as in the normal menstrual cycle. This approach, they contend, would be more "physiologic"—duplicating normal physiologic processes.

While some data support the safety of replacement estrogens balanced by progesterone, a very cautious approach is advised. Physicians generally recommend using the least amount of estrogen for the shortest time necessary to eliminate symptoms of menopause. Some women are given estrogens for a brief period, while they adjust gradually to the reduced hormonal levels. Women whose senile vaginitis has been alleviated with estrogen creams are often advised that regular sexual relations can help to maintain this "rejuvenated" vaginal condition without frequent estrogen applications. All women maintained on estrogen should be watched carefully for cancer as well as adverse side effects.

OTHER MEDICAL APPLICATIONS

Estrogens and progesterones also have a number of other, less common, therapeutic applications. Estrogens are often given to men with prostate cancer, for example, in the belief that they will neutralize the male hormones that promote the cancer's spread. Estrogens may be used to prevent painful swelling of a new mother's breasts—but only if she is not going to breast-feed, since such hormones enter the mother's milk. Indeed, sex hormones are contraindicated in young children as well as pregnant women, since they can affect growth, development of the genital structure, and, possibly, other organ systems of young children and fetuses.

Much ongoing research is devoted to learning the many physiologic, as well as behavioral and psychological, effects of the male and female sex hormones. One of the more intriguing, yet least understood, areas is the role of sex hormones in the altered mood states many women experience in the course of the menstrual cycle. Also under investigation is whether fluctuating hormone levels affect human sexual desire and sexual attractiveness, perhaps through subliminally perceived pheromones (stimulus scents) as in many animals. The possible role of these hormones in heart disease and other conditions also is a subject of ongoing research.

IN CONCLUSION

Sex hormones have a profound effect on both men and women. Replacement therapy, when used judiciously, can reverse the effects of hypogonadism in both sexes. The following charts cover the major androgen and estrogen products. Hormonal drugs used to treat infertility are covered in that section (page 875) and the oral contraceptives, which contain sex hormones, are in the *Contraception* section (page 831).

ANDROID (Methyltestosterone) **Brown**

Tabs (buccal): 5 mg **Tabs:** 10, 25 mg

INDICATIONS	ORAL DOSAGE
Eunuchism, eunuchoidism **Male climacteric or impotence**	**Adult:** 10–40 mg/day div; buccal tabs: 5–20 mg/day
Postpubertal cryptorchidism with evidence of hypogonadism	**Adult:** 30 mg/day div; buccal tabs: 15 mg/day
Postpartum breast pain and engorgement	**Adult:** 80 mg/day div for 3–5 days; buccal tabs: 40 mg/day
Advanced inoperable androgen-responsive breast cancer in females (1–5 yr postmenopausal)	**Adult:** 200 mg/day div; buccal tabs: 100 mg/day

ADMINISTRATION/DOSAGE ADJUSTMENTS

Buccal tablets	Tablets should be placed in the upper or lower buccal pouch between the gum and cheek, and not swallowed. Patient should avoid eating, drinking, chewing, or smoking while the tablet is in place. Proper oral hygiene is particularly important after the use of buccal tablets.
Duration of therapy	Depends upon the response of the condition being treated and the appearance of adverse reactions

CONTRAINDICATIONS

Male breast carcinoma ●	Carcinoma of the prostate ●	Cardiac, hepatic, or renal decompensation ●
Hypercalcemia ●	Hepatic impairment ●	Prepubertal males ●
Easily stimulated patients ●		

WARNINGS/PRECAUTIONS

Hypercalcemia	May occur in immobilized patients or patients with breast cancer and bone metastases; discontinue medication
Virilization	Therapy may lead to irreversible effects, such as voice changes; closely monitor female patients
Hepatic impairment	May occur; discontinue medication if cholestatic hepatitis with jaundice occurs or liver function tests become abnormal; if reinstituted, reduce dosage
Edema	May occur in patients with cardiac, renal, or hepatic derangements, due to sodium and water retention
Priapism, excessive sexual stimulation	May develop, especially in elderly males
Oligospermia, reduced ejaculatory volume	May occur with prolonged use or excessive dosage
Hypersensitivity	May occur
Gynecomastia	May occur
Hepatocellular carcinoma, peliosis hepatitis	May occur (rarely) during prolonged androgenic-anabolic therapy

ADVERSE REACTIONS

Hypersensitivity	Skin reactions, anaphylactoid reactions
Dermatological	Acne
Endocrinological	Decreased ejaculatory volume, oligospermia, gynecomastia, priapism, virilization in females
Hepatic	Cholestatic jaundice, hepatocellular neoplasms, peliosis hepatitis
Other	Edema, hypercalcemia

Table continued on following page

ANDROID continued

OVERDOSAGE

Signs and symptoms —— See ADVERSE REACTIONS

Treatment —— Discontinue medication

DRUG INTERACTIONS

No clinically significant drug interactions have been reported

ALTERED LABORATORY VALUES

Blood/serum values —— ⇧ BSP retention ⇧ SGOT ⇩ PBI

No clinically significant alterations in urinary values occur at therapeutic dosages

Use in children

Use cautiously in young boys to avoid possible premature epiphyseal closure or precocious sexual development; general guidelines not established for specific dosages

Use in pregnancy or nursing mothers

Contraindicated during pregnancy and in nursing mothers

Note: Methyltestosterone also marketed as **METANDREN** (Ciba); **ORETON METHYL** (Schering); and **TESTRED** (ICN).

DEPO-TESTOSTERONE (Testosterone cypionate) Upjohn

Vials: 50 mg/ml (10 ml),[1] 100 mg/ml (1, 10 ml), 200 mg/ml (1, 10 ml) for IM use only

INDICATIONS	PARENTERAL DOSAGE
Eunuchism, eunuchoidism **Impotence due to testicular deficiency** **Male climacteric symptoms secondary to androgen deficiency**	**Adult:** 200–400 mg IM every 3–4 wk
Oligospermia	**Adult:** 100–200 mg IM every 3–6 wk

ADMINISTRATION/DOSAGE ADJUSTMENTS

Alternative regimen for treating oligospermia	Administer 200 mg/wk for 6–10 wk to suppress testicular function; rebound spermatogenesis may follow withdrawal of androgen therapy
Interchangeability with other testosterone preparations	Testosterone cypionate must not be used interchangeably with testosterone propionate due to differences in duration of action

CONTRAINDICATIONS

Carcinoma of the male breast ●	Cardiac, hepatic, or renal decompensation ●	Hypercalcemia ●
Known or suspected carcinoma of the prostate ●	Impairment of liver function ●	Elderly patients in whom stimulation is to be avoided ●

WARNINGS/PRECAUTIONS

Hypercalcemia	May occur in immobilized patients; discontinue use and do not reinstitute therapy
Priapism, excessive sexual stimulation	May occur; discontinue drug and, if it is restarted, use lower dosage
Special-risk patients	Use with caution in patients with organic heart disease or debilitation due to prolonged action of drug
Patients with cardiac, renal, or hepatic derangement	Discontinue use if edema develops and, if desired, reinstitute therapy at a lower dosage
Prolonged or high-dose therapy	May lead to oligospermia and reduced ejaculatory volume; discontinue use and, if therapy is restarted, use a lower dosage
Hypersensitvity, gynecomastia	May occur; discontinue use and, if therapy is restarted, use a lower dosage
Concomitant use of oral anticoagulants	Prothrombin time may rise; if indicated, reduce dosage of anticoagulant to maintain a satisfactory therapeutic hypoprothrombinemia

ADVERSE REACTIONS

Dermatological	Acne
Endocrinological	Gynecomastia, priapism, decreased ejaculatory volume
Hypersensitivity	Skin manifestations, anaphylactoid reactions
Metabolic	Edema, hypercalcemia
Other	Irritation at injection site

OVERDOSAGE

Signs and symptoms	See ADVERSE REACTIONS
Treatment	Discontinue use

DRUG INTERACTIONS

Oral anticoagulants	Hyperprothrombinemia

[1]Contains 5.4 mg/ml chlorobutanol as a preservative; this component may be habit-forming

Table continued on following page

DEPO-TESTOSTERONE continued

ALTERED LABORATORY VALUES

Blood/serum values	⇩ PBI (slightly)
Urinary values	⇩ Nitrogen ⇩ Sodium ⇩ Potassium ⇩ Chloride ⇩ Phosphorus

Use in children

Contraindicated for use in prepubertal males

Use in pregnancy or nursing mothers

No appropriate indications exist

Note: Testosterone cypionate also marketed as **T-IONATE-P.A.** (Tutag); testosterone enanthate is marketed as **DELATESTRYL** (Squibb).

DIETHYLSTILBESTROL Lilly

Tabs (enteric-coated): 0.1, 0.25, 0.5, 1, 5 mg **Tabs:** 0.1, 0.25, 0.5, 1, 5 mg

INDICATIONS	ORAL DOSAGE
Moderate to severe vasomotor symptoms associated with the menopause **Atrophic vaginitis** **Kraurosis vulvae** **Female hypogonadism** **Female castration** **Primary ovarian failure**	**Adult:** 0.2–0.5 mg/day in 28-day cycles with 3 wk on and 1 wk off; atrophic vaginitis may require up to 2 mg/day for several years of cyclic therapy
Metastatic breast cancer	**Adult:** 15 mg/day
Prostatic carcinoma	**Adult:** 1–3 mg/day to start; for advanced cases, increase dosage as needed; usual maintenance dosage: 1 mg/day

ADMINISTRATION/DOSAGE ADJUSTMENTS

Pretreatment physical examination	Obtain a complete medical and family history before initiating estrogen therapy (see WARNINGS/PRECAUTIONS). Special attention during the physical examination should be given to blood pressure, breasts, abdomen, and pelvic organs; obtain a Papanicolaou smear.
Duration of postmenopausal therapy	For vasomotor symptoms, atrophic vaginitis, and kraurosis vulvae, attempt to discontinue or taper medication at intervals of 3–6 mo

CONTRAINDICATIONS

Known or suspected breast cancer (except when used in the treatment of metastatic disease) ●

Known or suspected estrogen-dependent neoplasia ●

Known or suspected pregnancy ●

History of thrombophlebitis, thrombosis, or thromboembolism associated with prior use of estrogen (except when used in the treatment of breast or prostatic malignancy) ●

Active thrombophlebitis or thromboembolic disorders ●

Undiagnosed abnormal vaginal bleeding ●

WARNINGS/PRECAUTIONS

Malignant neoplasms	May occur with prolonged use; use with caution and closely monitor patients with a family history of breast cancer or with breast nodules, fibrocystic disease, or abnormal mammograms. Risk of endometrial carcinoma in postmenopausal women increases with duration of estrogen therapy and dose; provide close clinical surveillance and investigate all cases of undiagnosed, persistent, or recurrent abnormal vaginal bleeding for malignancy (see CONTRAINDICATIONS).
Gallbladder disease	Risk is increased 2–3 times in postmenopausal women treated with estrogens
Thromboembolic disease, thrombotic disorders, and other vascular problems	Risk is increased with dose; if feasible, discontinue medication at least 4 wk before elective surgery associated with an increased risk of thromboembolism or possibly requiring prolonged immobilization. Use with caution in patients with cerebrovascular or coronary artery disease and only when clearly needed. Large doses of estrogen (eg, 5 mg/day) have been shown to increase the risk of nonfatal myocardial infarction, pulmonary embolism, and thrombophlebitis in men.
Benign hepatic adenoma	Has occurred with use of estrogen-containing oral contraceptives, at times rupturing and resulting in intra-abdominal hemorrhage and death, and should be considered in all cases of abdominal pain and tenderness, abdominal mass, or hypovolemic shock
Hepatocellular carcinoma	Has occurred with use of estrogen-containing oral contraceptives
Hypertension	Has occurred with use of estrogen-containing oral contraceptives and may occur with menopausal use of estrogens; monitor blood pressure during therapy, especially if high doses are used
Impaired glucose tolerance	Has been observed with use of estrogen-containing oral contraceptives; closely monitor patients with diabetes
Severe hypercalcemia	May develop in patients with breast cancer and bone metastases; discontinue medication and institute appropriate measures to reduce the serum calcium level
Fluid retention	May occur; use with caution in patients with convulsive disorders, migraine, asthma, or cardiac or renal dysfunction
Excessive estrogenic stimulation	May be manifested by abnormal or excessive uterine bleeding, mastodynia, or other reactions
Mental depression	Has occurred with use of oral contraceptives; as it is unclear whether this is due to the estrogenic or progestogenic component, patients with a history of mental depression should be monitored closely during estrogen therapy

Table continued on following page

WARNINGS/PRECAUTIONS continued

Uterine leiomyomata	May increase in size
Altered cytology	Advise pathologist of estrogen therapy when submitting relevant specimens
Jaundice	Has recurred in patients with a history of jaundice with the use of estrogen-containing oral contraceptives; if jaundice develops with estrogen therapy, discontinue medication while cause is investigated
Special-risk patients	Use with caution in patients with hepatic impairment, renal insufficiency, or metabolic bone disease associated with hypercalcemia
Inappropriate indications	Diethylstilbestrol should not be used for postcoital contraception

ADVERSE REACTIONS[1]

Genitourinary	Breakthrough bleeding, spotting, change in menstrual flow, dysmenorrhea, premenstrual-like syndrome, amenorrhea during and after treatment, increase in size of uterine fibromyomata, vaginal candidiasis, change in cervical erosion and in degree of cervical secretion, cystitis-like syndrome
Endocrinological	Breast tenderness, enlargement, and secretion; altered libido
Gastrointestinal	Nausea, vomiting, abdominal cramps, bloating, cholestatic jaundice
Dermatological	Persistent chloasma or melasma, erythema multiforme, erythema nodosum, hemorrhagic eruption, loss of scalp hair, hirsutism
Ophthalmic	Steepening of corneal curvature, intolerance to contact lenses
Central nervous system	Headache, migraine, dizziness, mental depression, chorea
Other	Weight gain or loss, reduced carbohydrate tolerance, aggravation of porphyria, edema

OVERDOSAGE

Signs and symptoms	Nausea, withdrawal bleeding (see ADVERSE REACTIONS)
Treatment	Discontinue medication

DRUG INTERACTIONS

Oral anticoagulants	⇩ Anticoagulant effect
Tricyclic antidepressants	⇧ Antidepressant side effects

ALTERED LABORATORY VALUES

Blood/serum values	⇧ Alkaline phosphatase ⇧ Bilirubin ⇧ Sulfobromophthalein retention ⇧ Prothrombin ⇧ Clotting factors VII, VIII, IX, and X ⇩ Antithrombin III ⇧ PBI ⇧ Thyroxine (T_4) ⇩ Triiodothyronine (T_3) uptake ⇧ Glucose ⇧ Cortisol ⇧ Transcortin ⇧ Ceruloplasmin ⇧ Triglycerides ⇧ Phospholipids ⇩ Folic acid ⇩ Pyridoxine
Urinary values	⇩ Pregnanediol

Use in children

General guidelines not established for dosage recommendations. May cause premature epiphyseal closure; use with caution in young patients in whom bone growth is incomplete.

Use in pregnancy or nursing mothers

Contraindicated if pregnancy is known or suspected, as serious fetal damage may occur during early pregnancy. As a rule, should not be administered to nursing mothers unless clearly necessary.

[1]See WARNINGS/PRECAUTIONS regarding induction of neoplasia and increased incidence of gallbladder and thromboembolic disease

ESTRACE (Estradiol) Mead Johnson

Tabs: 1, 2 mg

INDICATIONS	ORAL DOSAGE
Moderate to severe vasomotor symptoms associated with the menopause **Atrophic vaginitis** **Kraurosis vulvae** **Female hypogonadism** **Female castration** **Primary ovarian failure**	**Adult:** 1-2 mg/day in 28-day cycles with 3 wk on and 1 wk off; adjust dosage, as necessary, to control presenting symptoms

ADMINISTRATION/DOSAGE ADJUSTMENTS

Pretreatment physical examination	Obtain a complete medical and family history before initiating estrogen therapy (see WARNINGS/PRECAUTIONS). Special attention during the physical examination should be given to blood pressure, breasts, abdomen, and pelvic organs; obtain a Papanicolaou smear.
Duration of therapy	For vasomotor symptoms, atrophic vaginitis, and kraurosis vulvae, attempt to discontinue or taper medication at intervals of 3-6 mo

CONTRAINDICATIONS

Known or suspected breast cancer thrombosis (except when used in the treatment of metastatic disease) ●	History of thrombophlebitis, thrombosis, or thromboembolism associated with prior use of estrogen (except when used in the treatment of breast or prostatic malignancy) ●	Active thrombophlebitis or thromboembolic disorders ●
Known or suspected estrogen-dependent neoplasia ●		Undiagnosed abnormal vaginal bleeding ●
Known or suspected pregnancy ●		

WARNINGS/PRECAUTIONS

Malignant neoplasms	May occur with prolonged use; use with caution and closely monitor patients with a family history of breast cancer or with breast nodules, fibrocystic disease, or abnormal mammograms. Risk of endometrial carcinoma in postmenopausal women increases with duration of estrogen therapy and dose; provide close clinical surveillance and investigate all cases of undiagnosed, persistent, or recurrent abnormal vaginal bleeding for malignancy (see CONTRAINDICATIONS).
Gallbladder disease	Risk is increased 2-3 times in postmenopausal women treated with estrogens
Thromboembolic disease, thrombotic disorders, and other vascular problems	Risk is increased with dose; if feasible, discontinue medication at least 4 wk before elective surgery associated with an increased risk of thromboembolism or during periods of prolonged immobilization. Use with caution in patients with cerebrovascular or coronary artery disease and only when clearly needed. Large doses of estrogen (eg, 5 mg/day) have been shown to increase the risk of nonfatal myocardial infarction, pulmonary embolism, and thrombophlebitis in men.
Benign hepatic adenoma	Has occurred with use of estrogen-containing oral contraceptives, at times rupturing and resulting in intra-abdominal hemorrhage and death, and should be considered in all cases of abdominal pain and tenderness, abdominal mass, or hypovolemic shock
Hepatocellular carcinoma	Has occurred with use of estrogen-containing oral contraceptives
Hypertension	Has occurred with use of estrogen-containing oral contraceptives and may occur with menopausal use of estrogens; monitor blood pressure during therapy, especially if high doses are used
Impaired glucose tolerance	Has been observed with use of estrogen-containing oral contraceptives; closely monitor patients with diabetes
Severe hypercalcemia	May develop in patients with breast cancer and bone metastases; discontinue medication and institute appropriate measures to reduce the serum calcium level
Fluid retention	May occur; use with caution in patients with convulsive disorders, migraine, asthma, or cardiac or renal dysfunction
Excessive estrogenic stimulation	May be manifested by abnormal or excessive uterine bleeding, mastodynia, and other reactions
Mental depression	Has occurred with use of oral contraceptives; as it is unclear whether this is due to the estrogenic or progestogenic component, patients with a history of mental depression should be monitored closely during estrogen therapy
Uterine leiomyomata	May increase in size
Altered cytology	Advise the pathologist of estrogen therapy when submitting relevant specimens

Table continued on following page

WARNINGS/PRECAUTIONS continued	
Jaundice	Has recurred with the use of estrogen-containing oral contraceptives in patients with a history of jaundice; if jaundice develops with estrogen therapy, discontinue medication while cause is investigated
Special-risk patients	Use with caution in patients with hepatic impairment, renal insufficiency, or metabolic bone disease associated with hypercalcemia
Tartrazine sensitivity	Presence of FD&C Yellow No. 5 (tartrazine) in 2-mg tablets may cause allergic-type reactions, including bronchial asthma, in susceptible individuals

ADVERSE REACTIONS[1]	
Genitourinary	Breakthrough bleeding, spotting, change in menstrual flow, dysmenorrhea, premenstrual-like syndrome, amenorrhea during and after treatment, increase in size of uterine fibromyomata, vaginal candidiasis, change in cervical erosion and in degree of cervical secretion, cystitis-like syndrome
Endocrinological	Breast tenderness, enlargement, and secretion; altered libido
Gastrointestinal	Nausea, vomiting, abdominal cramps, bloating, cholestatic jaundice
Dermatological	Persistent chloasma or melasma, erythema multiforme, erythema nodosum, hemorrhagic eruption, loss of scalp hair, hirsutism
Ophthalmic	Steepening of corneal curvature, intolerance to contact lenses
Central nervous system	Headache, migraine, dizziness, mental depression, chorea
Other	Weight gain or loss, reduced carbohydrate tolerance, aggravation of porphyria, edema

OVERDOSAGE	
Signs and symptoms	Nausea, withdrawal bleeding (see ADVERSE REACTIONS)
Treatment	Discontinue medication

DRUG INTERACTIONS	
Oral anticoagulants	⇩ Anticoagulant effect
Tricyclic antidepressants	⇧ Antidepressant side effects

ALTERED LABORATORY VALUES	
Blood/serum values	⇧ Alkaline phosphatase ⇧ Bilirubin ⇧ Sulfobromophthalein retention ⇧ Prothrombin ⇧ Clotting factors VII, VIII, IX, and X ⇩ Antithrombin III ⇧ PBI ⇧ Thyroxine (T_4) ⇩ Triiodothyronine (T_3) uptake ⇧ Glucose ⇧ Cortisol ⇧ Transcortin ⇧ Ceruloplasmin ⇧ Triglycerides ⇧ Phospholipids ⇩ Folic acid ⇩ Pyridoxine
Urinary values	⇩ Pregnanediol

Use in children

General guidelines not established for dosage recommendations. May cause premature epiphyseal closure; use with caution in young patients in whom bone growth is incomplete.

Use in pregnancy or nursing mothers

Contraindicated if pregnancy is known or suspected, as serious fetal damage may occur during early pregnancy. As a rule, should not be administered to nursing mothers unless clearly necessary.

[1]See WARNINGS/PRECAUTIONS regarding induction of neoplasia and increased incidence of gallbladder and thromboembolic disease

ESTROVIS (Quinestrol) **Parke-Davis**

Tabs: 100 μg

INDICATIONS	ORAL DOSAGE
Moderate to severe vasomotor symptoms associated with the menopause **Atrophic vaginitis** **Kraurosis vulvae** **Female hypogonadism** **Female castration** **Primary ovarian failure**	**Adult:** 100 μg qd for 7 days to start, followed 2 wk after initiating therapy by 100 μg/wk for maintenance; for resistant cases, increase dosage to 200 μg/wk

ADMINISTRATION/DOSAGE ADJUSTMENTS

Pretreatment physical examination	Obtain a complete medical and family history before initiating estrogen therapy (see WARNINGS/PRECAUTIONS). Special attention during the physical examination should be given to blood pressure, breasts, abdomen, and pelvic organs; obtain a Papanicolaou smear.
Duration of postmenopausal therapy	For vasomotor symptoms, atrophic vaginitis, and kraurosis vulvae, attempt to discontinue or taper medication at intervals of 3–6 mo

CONTRAINDICATIONS

Known or suspected breast cancer (except when used in the treatment of metastatic disease) ●

Known or suspected estrogen-dependent neoplasia ●

Known or suspected pregnancy ●

History of thrombophlebitis, thrombosis, or thromboembolism associated with prior use of estrogen (except when used in the treatment of breast or prostatic malignancy) ●

Active thrombophlebitis or thromboembolic disorders ●

Undiagnosed abnormal vaginal bleeding ●

WARNINGS/PRECAUTIONS

Malignant neoplasms	May occur with prolonged use; use with caution and closely monitor patients with a family history of breast cancer or with breast nodules, fibrocystic disease, or abnormal mammograms. Risk of endometrial carcinoma in postmenopausal women increases with duration of estrogen therapy and dose; provide close clinical surveillance and investigate all cases of undiagnosed, persistent, or recurrent abnormal vaginal bleeding for malignancy (see CONTRAINDICATIONS).
Gallbladder disease	Risk is increased 2–3 times in postmenopausal women treated with estrogens
Thromboembolic disease, thrombotic disorders, and other vascular problems	Risk is increased with dose; if feasible, discontinue medication at least 4 wk before elective surgery associated with an increased risk of thromboembolism or during periods of prolonged immobilization. Use with caution in patients with cerebrovascular or coronary artery disease and only when clearly needed. Large doses of estrogen (eg, 5 mg/day) have been shown to increase the risk of nonfatal myocardial infarction, pulmonary embolism, and thrombophlebitis in men.
Benign hepatic adenoma	Has occurred with use of estrogen-containing oral contraceptives, at times rupturing and resulting in intra-abdominal hemorrhage and death, and should be considered in all cases of abdominal pain and tenderness, abdominal mass, or hypovolemic shock
Hepatocellular carcinoma	Has occurred with use of estrogen-containing oral contraceptives
Hypertension	Has occurred with use of estrogen-containing oral contraceptives and may occur with menopausal use of estrogens; monitor blood pressure during therapy, especially if high doses are used
Impaired glucose tolerance	Has been observed with use of estrogen-containing oral contraceptives; closely monitor patients with diabetes
Severe hypercalcemia	May develop in patients with breast cancer and bone metastases; discontinue medication and institute appropriate measures to reduce the serum calcium level
Fluid retention	May occur; use with caution in patients with convulsive disorders, migraine, asthma, or cardiac or renal dysfunction

Table continued on following page

WARNINGS/PRECAUTIONS continued

Excessive estrogen stimulation	May be manifested by abnormal or excessive uterine bleeding, mastodynia, or other reactions; reduce dosage accordingly
Mental depression	Has occurred with use of oral contraceptives; as it is unclear whether this is due to the estrogenic or progestogenic component, patients with a history of mental depression should be monitored closely during estrogen therapy
Uterine leiomyomata	May increase in size
Altered cytology	Advise the pathologist of estrogen therapy when submitting relevant specimens
Jaundice	Has recurred with use of estrogen-containing oral contraceptives in patients with a history of jaundice; if jaundice develops with estrogen therapy, discontinue medication while cause is investigated
Special-risk patients	Use with caution in patients with hepatic impairment, renal insufficiency, or metabolic bone disease associated with hypercalcemia

ADVERSE REACTIONS[1]

Genitourinary	Breakthrough bleeding, spotting, change in menstrual flow, dysmenorrhea, premenstrual-like syndrome, amenorrhea during and after treatment, increased size of uterine fibromyomata, vaginal candidiasis, change in cervical erosion and in degree of cervical secretion, cystitis-like syndrome
Endocrinological	Breast tenderness, enlargement, and secretion; altered libido
Gastrointestinal	Nausea, vomiting, abdominal cramps, bloating, cholestatic jaundice
Dermatological	Persistent chloasma or melasma, erythema multiforme, erythema nodosum, hemorrhagic eruption, loss of scalp hair, hirsutism
Ophthalmic	Steepening of corneal curvature, intolerance to contact lenses
Central nervous system	Headache, migraine, dizziness, mental depression, chorea
Other	Weight gain or loss, reduced carbohydrate tolerance, aggravation of porphyria, edema

OVERDOSAGE

Signs and symptoms	Nausea, withdrawal bleeding (see ADVERSE REACTIONS)
Treatment	Discontinue medication

DRUG INTERACTIONS

Oral anticoagulants	⇩ Anticoagulant effect
Tricyclic antidepressants	⇧ Antidepressant side effects

ALTERED LABORATORY VALUES

Blood/serum values	⇧ Alkaline phosphatase ⇧ Bilirubin ⇧ Sulfobromophthalein retention ⇧ Prothrombin ⇧ Clotting factors VII, VIII, IX, and X ⇩ Antithrombin III ⇧ PBI ⇧ Thyroxine (T_4) ⇩ Triiodothyronine (T_3) uptake ⇧ Glucose ⇧ Cortisol ⇧ Transcortin ⇧ Ceruloplasmin ⇧ Triglycerides ⇧ Phospholipids ⇩ Folic acid ⇩ Pyridoxine
Urinary values	⇩ Pregnanediol

Use in children

General guidelines not established for dosage recommendations. May cause premature epiphyseal closure; use with caution in young patients in whom bone growth is incomplete.

Use in pregnancy or nursing mothers

Contraindicated if pregnancy is known or suspected, as serious fetal damage may occur during early pregnancy. As a rule, should not be administered to nursing mothers unless clearly necessary.

[1]See WARNINGS/PRECAUTIONS regarding induction of neoplasia and increased incidence of gallbladder and thromboembolic disease

HALOTESTIN (Fluoxymesterone) Upjohn

Tabs: 2, 5, 10 mg

INDICATIONS	ORAL DOSAGE
Eunuchism **Eunuchoidism** **Impotence due to testicular deficiency** **Male climacteric**	**Adult:** 2–10 mg/day
Panhypopituitarism related to hypogonadism **Delayed puberty in males**	Consult manufacturer
Inoperable, advanced, androgen-responsive breast cancer in females (1–5 yr postmenopausal)	**Adult:** 15–30 mg/day div for 2–3 mo
Postpartum breast pain and engorgement	**Adult:** 2.5 mg at start of active labor, followed by 5–10 mg/day div for 4–5 days

CONTRAINDICATIONS

Cardiac, hepatic, or renal decompensation ●

Hypercalcemia ●

Hepatic impairment ●

Easily stimulated patients ●

Male breast cancer ●

Carcinoma of the prostate ●

WARNINGS/PRECAUTIONS

Hepatic impairment	Discontinue medication if cholestatic hepatitis with jaundice occurs or if liver-function tests become abnormal
Hypercalcemia	May occur in immobilized patients or in patients with breast cancer and bone metastases; discontinue medication
Virilization	Therapy may lead to irreversible effects, such as voice changes; closely monitor female patients
Edema	Use with caution in patients with cardiac, renal, or hepatic disease
Priapism, excessive sexual stimulation	May develop, especially in elderly males; discontinue medication and, if reinstituted, reduce dosage
Oligospermia, reduced ejaculatory volume	May occur with prolonged use or excessive dosage; discontinue medication and, if desired, reinstitute at lower dosage
Hypersensitivity	May occur; discontinue medication and, if desired, reinstitute at lower dosage
Gynecomastia	May occur; discontinue medication and, if desired, reinstitute at lower dosage
Concomitant use of anticoagulants	Reduce dosage of oral anticoagulants to maintain satisfactory hypoprothrombinemia
Hepatocellular carcinoma, peliosis hepatitis	May occur, in rare instances, during prolonged androgenic-anabolic steroid therapy

ADVERSE REACTIONS

Dermatological	Acne, edema
Genitourinary	Decreased ejaculatory volume, priapism
Hepatic	Cholestatic jaundice, hepatocellular neoplasms (rare), peliosis hepatitis (rare)
Metabolic	Hypercalcemia
Hypersensitivity	Skin manifestations, anaphylactoid reactions
Other	Virilization (in females), gynecomastia

OVERDOSAGE

Signs and symptoms	Priapism, excessive sexual stimulation, oligospermia, reduced ejaculatory volume
Treatment	Discontinue medication; if restarted, reduce dosage

DRUG INTERACTIONS

Oral anticoagulants	⇧ Anticoagulant effect

Table continued on following page

HALOTESTIN continued

ALTERED LABORATORY VALUES

Blood/serum values	⇩ PBI (slight)
Urinary values	⇩ Nitrogen ⇩ Sodium ⇩ Potassium ⇩ Chloride ⇩ Phosphorus

Use in children

Use in prepubertal males is contraindicated

Use in pregnancy or nursing mothers

Contraindicated during pregnancy; general guidelines not established for use in nursing mothers

OGEN (Piperazine estrone sulfate) **Abbott**

Tabs: 0.75 mg (Ogen .625); 1.5 mg (Ogen 1.25); 3 mg (Ogen 2.5); 6 mg (Ogen 5)

INDICATIONS	ORAL DOSAGE
Moderate to severe vasomotor symptoms associated with the menopause **Atrophic vaginitis** **Kraurosis vulvae**	**Adult:** 0.75–6 mg/day in 28-day cycles with 3 wk on and 1 wk off
Female hypogonadism **Female castration** **Primary ovarian failure**	**Adult:** 1.5-9 mg/day for 1st 3 wk of cycle, followed by a rest period of 8-10 days; repeat course if bleeding does not occur by end of rest period; if satisfactory withdrawal bleeding does not occur, add an oral progestin during 3rd wk of cycle

ADMINISTRATION/DOSAGE ADJUSTMENTS

Pretreatment physical examination	Obtain a complete medical and family history before initiating estrogen therapy (see WARNINGS/PRECAUTIONS). Special attention during the physical examination should be given to blood pressure, breasts, abdomen, and pelvic organs; obtain a Papanicolaou smear
Duration of postmenopausal therapy	For vasomotor symptoms, atrophic vaginitis, and kraurosis vulvae, attempt to discontinue or taper medication at intervals of 3–6 mo

CONTRAINDICATIONS

Known or suspected breast cancer (except when used in the treatment of metastatic disease) ●	History of thrombophlebitis, thrombosis, or thromboembolism associated with prior use of estrogen (except when used in the treatment of breast or prostatic malignancy) ●	Active thrombophlebitis or thromboembolic disorders ●
Known or suspected estrogen-dependent neoplasia ●		Undiagnosed abnormal vaginal bleeding ●
Known or suspected pregnancy ●		

WARNINGS/PRECAUTIONS

Malignant neoplasms	May occur with prolonged use; use with caution and closely monitor patients with a family history of breast cancer or with breast nodules, fibrocystic disease, or abnormal mammograms. Risk of endometrial carcinoma in postmenopausal women increases with duration of estrogen therapy and dose; provide close clinical surveillance and investigate all cases of undiagnosed, persistent, or recurrent abnormal vaginal bleeding for malignancy (see CONTRAINDICATIONS).
Gallbladder disease	Risk is increased 2–3 times in postmenopausal women treated with estrogens
Thromboembolic disease, thrombotic disorders, and other vascular problems	Risk is increased with dose; if feasible, discontinue medication at least 4 wk before elective surgery associated with an increased risk of thromboembolic disease or during periods of prolonged immobilization. Use with caution in patients with cerebrovascular or coronary artery disease and only when clearly needed. Large doses of estrogen (eg, 5 mg/day) have been shown to increase the risk of nonfatal myocardial infarction, pulmonary embolism, and thrombophlebitis in men.
Benign hepatic adenoma	Has occurred with use of estrogen-containing oral contraceptives, at times rupturing and resulting in intra-abdominal hemorrhage and death, and should be considered in all cases of abdominal pain and tenderness, abdominal mass, or hyprovolemic shock
Hepatocellular carcinoma	Has occurred with use of estrogen-containing oral contraceptives
Hypertension	Has occurred with use of estrogen-containing oral contraceptives and may occur with menopausal use of estrogens; monitor blood pressure during therapy, especially if high doses are used
Impaired glucose tolerance	Has been observed with use of estrogen-containing oral contraceptives; closely monitor patients with diabetes
Severe hypercalcemia	May develop in patients with breast cancer and bone metastases; discontinue medication and institute appropriate measures to reduce the serum calcium level
Fluid retention	May occur; use with caution in patients with convulsive disorders, migraine, asthma, or cardiac, or renal dysfunction

Table continued on following page

OGEN continued

WARNINGS/PRECAUTIONS continued

Excessive estrogenic stimulation	May be manifested by abnormal or excessive uterine bleeding, mastodynia, or other reactions
Mental depression	Has occurred with use of oral contraceptives; as it is unclear whether this is due to the estrogenic or progestogenic component, patients with a history of mental depression should be monitored closely during estrogen therapy
Uterine leiomyomata	May increase in size
Altered cytology	Advise the pathologist of estrogen therapy when submitting relevant specimens
Jaundice	Has recurred with the use of estrogen-containing oral contraceptives in patients with a history of jaundice; if jaundice develops with estrogen therapy, discontinue medication while cause is investigated
Special-risk patients	Use with caution in patients with hepatic impairment, renal insufficiency, or metabolic bone disease associated with hypercalcemia

ADVERSE REACTIONS[1]

Genitourinary	Breakthrough bleeding, spotting, change in menstrual flow, dysmenorrhea, premenstrual-like syndrome, amenorrhea during and after treatment, increased size of uterine fibromyomata, vaginal candidiasis, change in cervical erosion and in degree of cervical secretion, cystitis-like syndrome
Endocrinological	Breast tenderness, enlargement, and secretion; altered libido
Gastrointestinal	Nausea, vomiting, abdominal cramps, bloating, cholestatic jaundice
Dermatological	Persistent chloasma or melasma, erythema multiforme, erythema nodosum, hemorrhagic eruption, loss of scalp hair, hirsutism
Ophthalmic	Steepening of corneal curvature, intolerance to contact lenses
Central nervous system	Headache, migraine, dizziness, mental depression, chorea
Other	Weight gain or loss, reduced carbohydrate tolerance, aggravation of porphyria, edema

OVERDOSAGE

Signs and symptoms	Nausea, withdrawal bleeding (see ADVERSE REACTIONS)
Treatment	Discontinue medication

DRUG INTERACTIONS

Oral anticoagulants	⇩ Anticoagulant effect
Tricyclic antidepressants	⇧ Antidepressant side effects

ALTERED LABORATORY VALUES

Blood/serum values	⇧ Alkaline phosphatase ⇧ Bilirubin ⇧ Sulfobromophthalein retention ⇧ Prothrombin ⇧ Clotting factors VII, VIII, IX, and X ⇩ Antithrombin III ⇧ PBI ⇧ Thyroxine (T_4) ⇩ Triiodothyronine (T_3) uptake ⇧ Glucose ⇧ Cortisol ⇧ Transcortin ⇧ Ceruloplasmin ⇧ Triglycerides ⇧ Phospholipids ⇩ Folic acid ⇩ Pyridoxine
Urinary values	⇩ Pregnanediol

Use in children

General guidelines not established for dosage adjustments. May cause premature epiphyseal closure; use with caution in young patients in whom bone growth is incomplete.

Use in pregnancy or nursing mothers

Contraindicated if pregnancy is known or suspected, as serious fetal damage may occur during early pregnancy. Estrogens are excreted in breast milk.

[1]See WARNINGS/PRECAUTIONS regarding induction of neoplasia and increased incidence of gallbladder and thromboembolic disease

ORTHO Dienestrol Cream (Dienestrol) Ortho

Cream: 0.01% (78 g)

INDICATIONS	INTRAVAGINAL DOSAGE
Atrophic vaginitis **Kraurosis vulvae**	**Adult:** 1-2 applicatorsful/day for 1-2 wk, followed by a gradual reduction in dosage to ½-1 applicatorful/day for 1-2 wk, then repeat cycle; usual maintenance dosage: 1 applicatorful 1-3 times/wk

ADMINISTRATION/DOSAGE ADJUSTMENTS

Pretreatment physical examination	Obtain a complete medical and family history before initiating estrogen therapy (see WARNINGS/PRECAUTIONS). Special attention during the physical examination should be given to blood pressure, breasts, abdomen, and pelvic organs; obtain Papanicolaou smear.
Duration of therapy	Attempt to discontinue or taper medication at intervals of 3-6 mo

CONTRAINDICATIONS

Known or suspected breast cancer ●	History of thrombophlebitis, thrombosis, or thromboembolism associated with prior use of estrogen ●	Active thrombophlebitis or thromboembolic disorders ●
Known or suspected estrogen-dependent neoplasia ●		Undiagnosed abnormal vaginal bleeding ●
Known or suspected pregnancy ●		

WARNINGS/PRECAUTIONS

Malignant neoplasms	May occur with prolonged use; use with caution and closely monitor patients with a family history of breast cancer or with breast nodules, fibrocystic disease, or abnormal mammograms. Risk of endometrial carcinoma in postmenopausal women increases with duration of estrogen therapy and dose; provide close clinical surveillance and investigate all cases of undiagnosed, persistent, or recurrent abnormal vaginal bleeding for malignancy (see CONTRAINDICATIONS).
Gallbladder disease	Risk is increased 2-3 times in postmenopausal women treated with estrogens
Thromboembolic disease, thrombotic disorders, and other vascular problems	Risk is increased with dose; if feasible, discontinue medication at least 4 wk before elective surgery associated with an increased risk of thromboembolism or during periods of prolonged immobilization. Use with caution in patients with cerebrovascular or coronary artery disease and only when clearly needed. Large doses of estrogen (eg, 5 mg/day) have been shown to increase the risk of nonfatal myocardial infarction, pulmonary embolism, and thrombophlebitis in men.
Benign hepatic adenoma	Has occurred with use of estrogen-containing oral contraceptives, at times rupturing and resulting in intra-abdominal hemorrhage and death, and should be considered in all cases of abdominal pain and tenderness, abdominal mass, or hypovelmic shock
Hypertension	Has occurred with use of estrogen-containing oral contraceptives and may occur with menopausal use of estrogen; monitor blood pressure during therapy, especially if high doses are used
Impaired glucose tolerance	Has been observed with use of estrogen-containing oral contraceptives; closely monitor patients with diabetes
Severe hypercalcemia	May develop in patients with breast cancer and bone metastases; discontinue medication and institute appropriate measures to reduce the serum calcium level
Fluid retention	May occur; use with caution in patients with convulsive disorders, migraine, asthma, or cardiac or renal dysfunction
Excessive estrogenic stimulation	May be manifested by abnormal or excessive uterine bleeding, mastodynia, or other reactions
Mental depression	Has occurred with use of oral contraceptives; as it is unclear whether this is due to the estrogenic or progestogenic component, patients with a history of mental depression should be monitored closely during estrogen therapy

Table continued on following page

WARNINGS/PRECAUTIONS continued

Uterine leiomyomata	May increase in size
Altered cytology	Advise the pathologist of estrogen therapy when submitting relevant specimens
Jaundice	Has recurred with the use of estrogen-containing oral contraceptives in patients with a history of jaundice; if jaundice develops with estrogen therapy, discontinue medication while cause is investigated
Special-risk patients	Use with caution in patients with hepatic impairment, renal insufficiency, or metabolic bone disease associated with hypercalcemia
Premature epiphyseal closure	Use with caution in young patients in whom bone growth is not complete

ADVERSE REACTIONS[1]

Genitourinary	Breakthrough bleeding, spotting, change in menstrual flow, dysmenorrhea, premenstrual-like syndrome, amenorrhea during and after treatment, increased size of uterine fibromyomata, vaginal candidiasis, change in cervical erosion and in degree of cervical secretion, cystitis-like syndrome
Endocrinological	Breast tenderness, enlargement, and secretion; altered libido
Gastrointestinal	Nausea, vomiting, abdominal cramps, bloating, cholestatic jaundice
Dermatological	Persistent chloasma or melasma, erythema multiforme, erythema nodosum, hemorrhagic eruption, loss of scalp hair, hirsutism
Ophthalmic	Steepening of corneal curvature, intolerance to contact lenses
Central nervous system	Headache, migraine, dizziness, mental depression, chorea
Other	Weight gain or loss, reduced carbohydrate tolerance, aggravation of porphyria, edema

DRUG INTERACTIONS

Oral anticoagulants	⇩ Anticoagulant effect
Tricyclic antidepressants	⇧ Antidepressant side effects

ALTERED LABORATORY VALUES

Blood/serum values	⇧ Alkaline phosphatase ⇧ Bilirubin ⇧ Sulfobromophthalein retention ⇧ Prothrombin ⇧ Clotting factors VII, VIII, IX, and X ⇩ Antithrombin III ⇧ PBI ⇧ Thyroxin (T_4) ⇩ Triiodothyronine (T_3) uptake ⇧ Glucose ⇧ Cortisol ⇧ Transcortin ⇧ Ceruloplasmin ⇧ Triglycerides ⇧ Phospholipids ⇩ Folic acid ⇩ Pyridoxine
Urinary values	⇩ Pregnanediol

Use in children

General guidelines not established for dosage recommendations. May cause premature epiphyseal closure; use with caution in young patients in whom bone growth is incomplete.

Use in pregnancy or nursing mothers

Contraindicated if pregnancy is known or suspected, as serious fetal damage may occur during early pregnancy. As a rule, should not be administered to nursing mothers unless clearly necessary.

[1]See WARNINGS/PRECAUTIONS regarding induction of neoplasia and increased incidence of gallbladder and thromboembolic disease

PREMARIN (Conjugated estrogens) Ayerst

Tabs: 0.3, 0.625, 1.25, 2.5 mg

INDICATIONS	ORAL DOSAGE
Moderate to severe vasomotor symptoms associated with the menopause	**Adult:** 1.25 mg/day in 28-day cycles with 3 wk on and 1 wk off, starting on the 5th day of bleeding if the patient is menstruating or arbitrarily if the patient has not menstruated for at least 2 mo
Atrophic vaginitis **Kraurosis vulvae**	**Adult:** 0.3-1.25 mg/day in 28-day cycles with 3 wk on and 1 wk off
Female hypogonadism	**Adult:** 2.5-7.5 mg/day div for 20 days, followed by a rest period of 10 days off; if bleeding occurs before the end of the 10-day rest period, add an oral progestin during the last 5 days of the next cycle
Female castration and primary ovarian failure	**Adult:** 1.25 mg/day in 28-day cycles with 3 wk on and 1 wk off; adjust dosage in accordance with patient response
Breast cancer in appropriately selected men and postmenopausal women with metastatic disease	**Adult:** 10 mg tid for at least 3 mo
Prostatic carcinoma	**Adult:** 1.25-2.5 mg tid
Postpartum breast engorgement	**Adult:** 3.75 mg q4h for 5 doses, or 1.25 mg q4h for 5 days
Estrogen-deficiency osteoporosis in conjunction with other therapeutic measures, such as diet, calcium administration, and physiotherapy[1]	**Adult:** 1.25 mg/day in 28-day cycles with 3 wk on and 1 wk off

ADMINISTRATION/DOSAGE ADJUSTMENTS

Pretreatment physical examination	Obtain a complete medical and family history before initiating estrogen therapy (see WARNINGS/PRECAUTIONS). Special attention during the physical examination should be given to blood pressure, breasts, abdomen, and pelvic organs; obtain Papanicolaou smear.
Duration of postmenopausal therapy	For vasomotor symptoms, atrophic vaginitis, and kraurosis vulvae, attempt to discontinue or taper medication at intervals of 3-6 mo

CONTRAINDICATIONS

Known or suspected breast cancer (except when used in the treatment of metastatic disease) •

Known or suspected estrogen-dependent neoplasia •

Known or suspected pregnancy •

History of thrombophlebitis, thrombosis, or thromboembolism associated with prior use of estrogen (except when used in the treatment of breast or breast or prostatic malignancy) •

Active thrombophlebitis or thromboembolic disorders •

Undiagnosed abnormal vaginal bleeding •

WARNINGS/PRECAUTIONS

Malignant neoplasms	May occur with prolonged use; use with caution and closely monitor patients with a family history of breast cancer or with breast nodules, fibrocystic disease, or abnormal mammograms. Risk of endometrial carcinoma in postmenopausal women increases with duration of estrogen therapy and dose; provide close clinical surveillance and investigate all cases of undiagnosed, persistent, or recurrent abnormal vaginal bleeding for malignancy (see CONTRAINDICATIONS).
Gallbladder disease	Risk is increased 2-3 times in postmenopausal women treated with estrogens
Thromboembolic disease, thrombotic disorders, and other vascular problems	Risk is increased with dose; if feasible, discontinue medication at least 4 wk before elective surgery associated with an increased risk of thromboembolism or during periods of prolonged immobilization. Use with caution in patients with cerebrovascular or coronary artery disease and only when clearly needed. Large doses of estrogen (eg, 5 mg/day) have been shown to increase the risk of nonfatal myocardial infarction, pulmonary embolism, and thrombophlebitis in men.
Benign hepatic adenoma	Has occurred with use of estrogen-containing oral contraceptives, at times rupturing and resulting in intra-abdominal hemorrhage and death, and should be considered in all cases of abdominal pain and tenderness, abdominal mass, or hypovolemic shock

[1]Probably effective

Table continued on following page

WARNINGS/PRECAUTIONS continued	
Hepatocellular carcinoma	Has occurred with use of estrogen-containing oral contraceptives
Hypertension	Has occurred with use of estrogen-containing oral contraceptives and may occur with menopausal use of estrogen; monitor blood pressure during therapy, especially if high doses are used
Impaired glucose tolerance	Has been observed with use of estrogen-containing oral contraceptives; closely monitor patients with diabetes
Severe hypercalcemia	May develop in patients with breast cancer and bone metastases; discontinue medication and institute appropriate measures to reduce the serum calcium level
Fluid retention	May occur; use with caution in patients with convulsive disorders, migraine, asthma, or in those with cardiac or renal dysfunction
Excessive estrogenic stimulation	May be manifested by abnormal or excessive uterine bleeding, mastodynia, or other reactions; reduce dosage accordingly
Mental depression	Has occurred with use of oral contraceptives; as it is unclear whether this is due to the estrogenic or progestogenic component, patients with a history of mental depression should be monitored closely during estrogen therapy
Uterine leiomyomata	May increase in size
Altered cytology	Advise the pathologist of estrogen therapy when submitting relevant specimens
Jaundice	Has recurred with the use of estrogen-containing oral contraceptives in patients with a history of jaundice; if jaundice develops with estrogen therapy, discontinue medication while cause is investigated
Special-risk patients	Use with caution in patients with hepatic impairment, renal insufficiency, or metabolic bone disease associated with hypercalcemia
ADVERSE REACTIONS[2]	
Genitourinary	Breakthrough bleeding, spotting, change in menstrual flow, dysmenorrhea, premenstrual-like syndrome, amenorrhea during and after treatment, increased size of uterine fibromyomata, vaginal candidiasis, change in cervical erosion and in degree of cervical secretion, cystitis-like syndrome
Endocrinological	Breast tenderness, enlargement, and secretion; altered libido
Gastrointestinal	Nausea, vomiting, abdominal cramps, bloating, cholestatic jaundice
Dermatological	Persistent chloasma or melasma, erythema multiforme, erythema nodosum, hemorrhagic eruption, loss of scalp hair, hirsutism
Ophthalmic	Steepening of corneal curvature, intolerance to contact lenses
Central nervous system	Headache, migraine, dizziness, mental depression, chorea
Other	Weight gain or loss, reduced carbohydrate tolerance, aggravation of porphyria, edema
OVERDOSAGE	
Signs and symptoms	Nausea, withdrawal bleeding (see ADVERSE REACTIONS)
Treatment	Discontinue medication; treat symptomatically
DRUG INTERACTIONS	
Oral anticoagulants	⇩ Anticoagulant effect
Tricyclic antidepressants	⇧ Antidepressant side effects

[2]See WARNINGS/PRECAUTIONS regarding induction of neoplasia and increased incidence of gallbladder and thromboembolic disease

Table continued on following page

ALTERED LABORATORY VALUES

Blood/serum values	⇧ Alkaline phosphatase ⇧ Bilirubin ⇧ Sulfobromophthalein retention ⇧ Prothrombin ⇧ Clotting factors VII, VIII, IX, and X ⇩ Antithrombin III ⇧ PBI ⇧ Thyroxine (T_4) ⇩ Triiodothyronine (T_3) uptake ⇧ Glucose ⇧ Cortisol ⇧ Transcortin ⇧ Ceruloplasmin ⇧ Triglycerides ⇧ Phospholipids ⇩ Folic acid ⇩ Pyridoxine
Urinary values	⇩ Pregnanediol

Use in children

General guidelines not established for dosage requirements. May cause premature epiphyseal closure; use with caution in young patients in whom bone growth is incomplete.

Use in pregnancy or nursing mothers

Contraindicated if pregnancy is known or suspected, as serious fetal damage may occur during early pregnancy. As a rule, should not be administered to nursing mothers unless clearly necessary.

PREMARIN Vaginal Cream (Conjugated estrogens) **Ayerst**

Cream: 0.625 mg/g (42.5 g)

INDICATIONS	INTRAVAGINAL AND TOPICAL DOSAGE
Atrophic vaginitis **Kraurosis vulvae**	**Adult:** 2–4 g/day in 28-day cycles with 3 wk on and 1 wk off

ADMINISTRATION/DOSAGE ADJUSTMENTS

Pretreatment physical examination	Obtain a complete medical and family history before initiating estrogen therapy (see WARNINGS/PRECAUTIONS). Special attention during the physical examination should be given to blood pressure, breasts, abdomen, and pelvic organs; obtain a Papanicolaou smear.
Duration of therapy	Attempt to discontinue or taper medication at intervals of 3–6 mo

CONTRAINDICATIONS

Known or suspected breast cancer ●	History of thrombophlebitis, thrombosis, or thromboembolism associated with prior use of estrogen ●	Active thrombophlebitis or thromboembolic disorders ●
Known or suspected estrogen-dependent neoplasia ●		Undiagnosed abnormal vaginal bleeding ●
Known or suspected pregnancy ●		

WARNINGS/PRECAUTIONS

Malignant neoplasms	May occur with prolonged use; use with caution and closely monitor patients with a family history of breast cancer or with breast nodules, fibrocystic disease, or abnormal mammograms. Risk of endometrial carcinoma in postmenopausal women increases with duration of estrogen therapy and dose; provide close clinical surveillance and investigate all cases of undiagnosed, persistent, or recurrent abnormal vaginal bleeding for malignancy (see CONTRAINDICATIONS).
Gallbladder disease	Risk is increased 2–3 times in postmenopausal women treated with estrogens
Thromboembolic disease, thrombotic disorders, and other vascular problems	Risk is increased with dose; if feasible, discontinue medication at least 4 wk before elective surgery associated with an increased risk of thromboembolism or during periods of prolonged immobilization. Use with caution in patients with cerebrovascular or coronary artery disease and only when clearly needed. Large doses of estrogen (eg, 5 mg/day), have been shown to increase the risk of nonfatal myocardial infarction, pulmonary embolism, and thrombophlebitis in men.
Benign hepatic adenoma	Has occurred with use of estrogen-containing oral contraceptives, at times rupturing and resulting in intra-abdominal hemorrhage and death, and should be considered in all cases of abdominal pain and tenderness, abdominal mass, or hypovolemic shock
Hepatocellular carcinoma	Has occurred with use of estrogen-containing oral contraceptives
Hypertension	Has occurred with use of estrogen-containing oral contraceptives and may occur with menopausal use of estrogen; monitor blood pressure during therapy, especially if high doses are used
Impaired glucose tolerance	Has been observed with use of estrogen-containing oral contraceptives; closely monitor patients with diabetes
Severe hypercalcemia	May develop in patients with breast cancer and bone metastases; discontinue medication and institute appropriate measures to reduce the serum calcium level
Fluid retention	May occur; use with caution in patients with convulsive disorders, migraine, asthma, or cardiac or renal dysfunction

WARNINGS/PRECAUTIONS continued

Excessive estrogenic stimulation	May be manifested by abnormal or excessive uterine bleeding, mastodynia, or other reactions
Mental depression	Has occurred with use of oral contraceptives; as it is unclear whether this is due to the estrogenic or progestogenic component, patients with a history of mental depression should be monitored closely during estrogen therapy
Uterine leiomyomata	May increase in size
Altered cytology	Advise the pathologist of estrogen therapy when submitting relevant specimens
Jaundice	Has recurred with the use of estrogen-containing oral contraceptives in patients with a history of jaundice; if jaundice develops with estrogen therapy, discontinue medication while cause is investigated
Special-risk patients	Use with caution in patients with hepatic impairment, renal insufficiency, or metabolic bone disease associated with hypercalcemia

Table continued on following page

ADVERSE REACTIONS[1]

Genitourinary	Breakthrough bleeding, spotting, change in menstrual flow, dysmenorrhea, premenstrual-like syndrome, amenorrhea during and after treatment, increased size of uterine fibromyomata, vaginal candidiasis, change in cervical erosion and in degree of cervical secretion, cystitis-like syndrome
Endocrinological	Breast tenderness, enlargement, and secretion; altered libido
Gastrointestinal	Nausea, vomiting, abdominal cramps, bloating, cholestatic jaundice
Dermatological	Persistent chloasma or melasma, erythema multiforme, erythema nodosum, hemorrhagic eruption, loss of scalp hair, hirsutism
Ophthalmic	Steepening of corneal curvature, intolerance to contact lenses
Central nervous system	Headache, migraine, dizziness, mental depression, chorea
Other	Weight gain or loss, reduced carbohydrate tolerance, aggravation of porphyria, edema

DRUG INTERACTIONS

Oral anticoagulants	⇩ Anticoagulant effect
Tricyclic antidepressants	⇧ Antidepressant side effects

ALTERED LABORATORY VALUES

Blood/serum values	⇧ Alkaline phosphatase ⇧ Bilirubin ⇧ Sulfobromophthalein retention ⇧ Prothrombin ⇧ Clotting factors VII, VIII, IX, and X ⇩ Antithrombin III ⇧ PBI ⇧ Thyroxine (T_4) ⇩ Triiodothyronine (T_3) uptake ⇧ Glucose ⇧ Cortisol ⇧ Transcortin ⇧ Ceruloplasmin ⇧ Triglycerides ⇩ Folic acid ⇩ Pyridoxine ⇧ Phospholipids
Urinary values	⇩ Pregnanediol

Use in children

General guidelines not established for dosage recommendations. May cause premature epiphyseal closure; use with caution in young patients in whom bone growth is incomplete.

Use in pregnancy or nursing mothers

Contraindicated if pregnancy is known or suspected, as serious fetal damage may occur during early pregnancy. As a rule, should not be administered to nursing mothers unless clearly necessary.

PROVERA (Medroxyprogesterone acetate) Upjohn

Tabs: 2.5, 10 mg

INDICATIONS	ORAL DOSAGE
Secondary amenorrhea	**Adult:** 5–10 mg/day for 5–10 days; to induce optimum secretory transformation of an adequately primed endometrium, 10 mg/day for 10 days, beginning at any time
Abnormal uterine bleeding due to hormonal imbalance in the absence of organic pathology	**Adult:** 5–10 mg/day for 5–10 days beginning on the 16th or 21st day of menstrual cycle; to induce optimum secretory transformation of an adequately primed endometrium, 10 mg/day for 10 days, beginning on the 16th day of menstrual cycle

ADMINISTRATION/DOSAGE ADJUSTMENTS

Pretreatment physical examination	Should include examination of the breasts and pelvic organs as well as a Papanicolaou smear
Withdrawal bleeding	Usually occurs within 3–7 days after discontinuing therapy

CONTRAINDICATIONS

Past or present thrombophlebitis, thromboembolic disorders, or cerebral apoplexy ●

Hepatic dysfunction or disease ●

Known or suspected malignancy of breast or genital organs ●

Undiagnosed vaginal bleeding ●

Missed abortion ●

Hypersensitivity to medroxyprogesterone ●

WARNINGS/PRECAUTIONS

Thrombotic disorders	May occur; discontinue medication at earliest manifestations of thrombophlebitis, cerebrovascular disorders, pulmonary embolism, or retinal thrombosis
Visual impairment	Discontinue medication if patient develops complete or partial visual loss, proptosis, diplopia, migraine of sudden onset, papilledema, or retinal vascular lesions
Mammary nodules	Have appeared in medroxyprogesterone-treated dogs, including some breast malignancies with metastases; clinical relevance has not been established
Fluid retention	May occur; use with caution in patients with epilepsy, migraine, asthma, or cardiac or renal dysfunction
Mental depression	May be exacerbated; closely monitor patients with a history of psychic depression; discontinue medication if depression becomes severe
Impaired glucose tolerance	Has been observed with use of estrogen-progestin combination drugs; closely monitor patients with diabetes
Abnormal vaginal bleeding	Consider nonfunctional causes; take adequate diagnostic measures
Prolonged use	Long-term effect on pituitary, ovarian, adrenal, hepatic, or uterine function has not been established
Climacteric	May be masked
Altered cytology	Advise the pathologist of progestin therapy when submitting relevant specimens

ADVERSE REACTIONS[1]

Endocrinological	Breakthrough bleeding, spotting, altered menstrual flow, amenorrhea, changes in cervical erosion and cervical secretions, premenstrual-like syndrome, altered libido, breast tenderness (rare), galactorrhea (rare)
Dermatological	Urticaria, pruritus, edema, generalized rash, acne, alopecia, hirsutism, erythema multiforme, erythema nodosum, hemorrhagic eruption, itching
Thromboembolic	Thrombophlebitis, pulmonary embolism, cerebral thrombosis and embolism
Genitourinary	Cystitis-like syndrome
Other	Weight gain or loss, cholestatic jaundice, mental depression, neuro-ocular lesions (causal relationship not established)

[1]Other adverse reactions have been observed with combination oral contraceptives but have not been reported in women taking progestins alone

Table continued on following page

OVERSDOSAGE

Signs and symptoms	See ADVERSE REACTIONS
Treatment	Discontinue medication; treat symptomatically

DRUG INTERACTIONS

No clinically significant drug interactions have been observed

ALTERED LABORATORY VALUES

Blood/serum values	⇧ Bilirubin ⇧ SGOT ⇧ SGPT ⇧ Sulfobromopthalein retention ⇧ Clotting factors VII, VIII, IX, and X ⇧ PBI ⇧ Butanol-extractable PBI ⇩ Triiodothyronine (T_3) uptake
Urinary values	⇩ Pregnanediol

Use in children

General guidelines not established

Use in pregnancy or nursing mothers

Not recommended for use during the first 4 mo of pregnancy, as fetal damage may occur during this period. Safe use has not been established in nursing mothers.

Note: Medroxyprogesterone acetate also marketed as **CURRETAB** (Reid-Provident) and **DEPO-PROVERA** (Upjohn).

TACE (Chlorotrianisene) **Merrell-National**

Caps: 12, 25, 72 mg

INDICATIONS	ORAL DOSAGE
Postpartum breast engorgement	**Adult:** 12 mg qid for 7 days, or 50 mg q6h for 6 doses; alternative regimen: 72 mg bid for 2 days; give first dose within 8 h after delivery
Inoperable progressing **prostatic carcinoma**	**Adult:** 12–25 mg/day
Moderate to severe **vasomotor symptoms** associated with menopause	**Adult:** 12–25 mg/day for 30 days, followed by repeated courses, as necessary
Atrophic vaginitis **Kraurosis vulvae**	**Adult:** 12–25 mg/day for 30–60 days
Female hypogonadism	**Adult:** 12–25 mg/day in 21-day cycles; if desired, give 100 mg IM progesterone immediately after the cycle or add an oral progestin during the last 5 days of the cycle; begin the next course on the 5th day of induced uterine bleeding

ADMINISTRATION/DOSAGE ADJUSTMENTS

Pretreatment physical examination	Obtain a complete medical and family history before initiating estrogen therapy (see WARNINGS/PRECAUTIONS). Special attention during the physical examination should be given to blood pressure, breasts, abdomen, and pelvic organs; obtain a Papanicolaou smear.
Duration of postmenopausal therapy	For vasomotor symptoms, atrophic vaginitis, and kraurosis vulvae, attempt to discontinue or taper medication at intervals of 3–6 mo

CONTRAINDICATIONS

Known or suspected breast cancer (except when used in the treatment of metastatic disease) ●

Known or suspected estrogen-dependent neoplasia ●

Known or suspected pregnancy ●

History of thrombophlebitis, thrombosis, or thromboembolism associated with prior use of estrogen (except when used in the treatment of breast or prostatic malignancy) ●

Active thrombophlebitis or thromboembolic disorders ●

Undiagnosed abnormal vaginal bleeding ●

WARNINGS/PRECAUTIONS

Malignant neoplasms	May occur with prolonged use; use with caution and closely monitor patients with a family history of breast cancer or with breast nodules, fibrocystic disease, or abnormal mammograms. Risk of endometrial carcinoma in postmenopausal women increases with duration of estrogen therapy and dose; provide close clinical surveillance and investigate all cases of undiagnosed, persistent, or recurrent abnormal vaginal bleeding for malignancy (see CONTRAINDICATIONS).
Gallbladder disease	Risk is increased 2-3 times in postmenopausal women treated with estrogens
Thromboembolic disease, thrombotic disorders, and other vascular problems	Risk is increased with dose; if feasible, discontinue medication at least 4 wk before elective surgery associated with an increased risk of thromboembolism or during periods of prolonged immobilization. Use with caution in patients with cerebrovascular or coronary artery disease and only when clearly needed. Large doses of estrogen (eg, 5 mg/day) have been shown to increase the risk of nonfatal myocardial infarction, pulmonary embolism, and thrombophlebitis in men.
Benign hepatic adenoma	Has occurred with use of estrogen-containing oral contraceptives, at times rupturing and resulting in intra-abdominal hemorrhage and death, and should be considered in all cases of abdominal pain and tenderness, abdominal mass, or hypovolemic shock
Hepatocellular carcinoma	Has occurred with use of estrogen-containing oral contraceptives
Hypertension	Has occurred with use of estrogen-containing oral contraceptives and may occur with menopausal use of estrogens; monitor blood pressure during therapy, especially if high doses are used
Impaired glucose tolerance	Has been observed with use of estrogen-containing oral contraceptives; closely monitor patients with diabetes
Severe hypercalcemia	May develop in patients with breast cancer and bone metastases; discontinue medication and institute appropriate measures to reduce the serum calcium level
Fluid retention	May occur; use with caution in patients with convulsive disorders, migraine, asthma, or cardiac or renal dysfunction

Table continued on following page

TACE continued

WARNINGS/PRECAUTIONS continued

Excessive estrogen stimulation	May be manifested by abnormal or excessive uterine bleeding, mastodynia, or other reactions; reduce dosage accordingly
Mental depression	Has occurred with use of oral contraceptives; as it is unclear whether this is due to the estrogenic or progestogenic component, patients with a history of mental depression should be monitored closely during estrogen therapy
Uterine leiomyomata	May increase in size
Altered cytology	Advise the pathologist of estrogen therapy when submitting relevant specimens
Jaundice	Has recurred with use of estrogen-containing oral contraceptives in patients with a history of jaundice; if jaundice develops with estrogen therapy, discontinue medication while cause is investigated
Special-risk patients	Use with caution in patients with hepatic impairment, renal insufficiency, or metabolic bone disease associated with hypercalcemia
Tartrazine sensitivity	Presence of FD&C Yellow No. 5 (tartrazine) may cause allergic-type reactions, including bronchial asthma, in susceptible individuals

ADVERSE REACTIONS[1]

Genitourinary	Breakthrough bleeding, spotting, change in menstrual flow, dysmenorrhea, premenstrual-like syndrome, amenorrhea during and after treatment, increased size of uterine fibromyomata, vaginal candidiasis, change in cervical erosion and in degree of cervical secretion, cystitis-like syndrome
Endocrinological	Breast tenderness, enlargement, and secretion; altered libido and/or potency
Gastrointestinal	Nausea, vomiting, abdominal cramps, bloating, cholestatic jaundice
Dermatological	Persistent chloasma or melasma, erythema multiforme, erythema nodosum, hemorrhagic eruption, loss of scalp hair, hirsutism, urticaria
Ophthalmic	Steepening of corneal curvature, intolerance to contact lenses
Central nervous system	Headache, migraine, dizziness, mental depression, chorea
Other	Weight gain or loss, reduced carbohydrate tolerance, aggravation of porphyria

OVERDOSAGE

Signs and symptoms	Nausea, withdrawal bleeding (see ADVERSE REACTIONS)
Treatment	Discontinue medication

DRUG INTERACTIONS

Oral anticoagulants	⇩ Anticoagulant effect
Tricyclic antidepressants	⇧ Antidepressant side effects

ALTERED LABORATORY VALUES

Blood/serum values	⇧ Alkaline phosphatase ⇧ Bilirubin ⇧ Sulfobromophthalein retention ⇧ Prothrombin ⇧ Clotting factors VII, VIII, IX, and X ⇩ Antithrombin III ⇧ PBI ⇧ Thyroxine (T_4) ⇩ Triiodothyronine (T_3) uptake ⇧ Glucose ⇧ Cortisol ⇧ Transcortin ⇧ Ceruloplasmin ⇧ Triglycerides ⇧ Phospholipids ⇩ Folic acid ⇩ Pyridoxine
Urinary values	⇩ Pregnanediol

Use in children

General guidelines not established for dosage recommendations. May cause premature epiphyseal closure; use with caution in young patients in whom bone growth is incomplete.

Use in pregnancy or nursing mothers

Contraindicated if pregnancy is known or suspected, as serious fetal damage may occur during early pregnancy. As a rule, should not be administered to nursing mothers unless clearly necessary.

[1]See WARNINGS/PRECAUTIONS regarding induction of neoplasia and increased incidence of gallbladder and thromboembolic disease

Thyroid Disorders

The normal thyroid gland, located in the front of the neck, is a butterfly-shaped structure consisting of two elongated lobes, one on each side of the trachea, connected by a bridge of thyroid tissue. Two hormones, thyroxine and triiodothyronine, originate in the thyroid gland and are essential for normal growth and development, as well as for regulating metabolism and other body functions. These hormones contain organic iodide, and adequate amounts of iodine are essential in their production. Thyroid disorders stem either from a deficiency or surplus of thyroid hormones. If there is a deficiency, the disorder is termed hypothyroidism, while conditions resulting from an excess are termed hyperthyroidism, or thyrotoxicosis.

HYPERTHYROIDISM

Women are about five times more likely to suffer hyperthyroidism than men, with the highest incidence in persons thirty to fifty years old. Hyperthyroidism takes two major forms: diffuse toxic goiter and nodular goiter.

Diffuse Toxic Goiter

More commonly referred to as Graves' disease, diffuse toxic goiter is characterized by an enlarged thyroid gland, an increased basal metabolic rate, and very often an eye complication known as exophthalmos, in which the eyes appear to bulge out. Fatigue, insomnia, loss of weight, and tremulousness are common symptoms. The skin may become thin and fine-textured, and is often moist; indeed, the patient may perspire profusely. Many patients are better able to tolerate cold, but suffer in moderate heat. Double or blurred vision, burning, and tearing may be noted, as well as decreases in visual acuity. In some patients, a complication known as pretibial myxedema occurs, in which reddish nodules appear over the side or front of the legs, just above the ankles. Sometimes, instead of nodules there is a bulging over this area of the legs and the skin takes on a shiny appearance similar to that of an orange peel.

In menstruating women with Graves' disease, the menstrual cycle may be shortened, periods may be scanty or occasionally missed, and fertility is usually decreased.

Nodular Goiter

In nodular goiter, also known as Plummer's disease, there is an increased, and often excessive, production of thyroid hormone by one or more of

THYROID GLAND AND DISORDERS

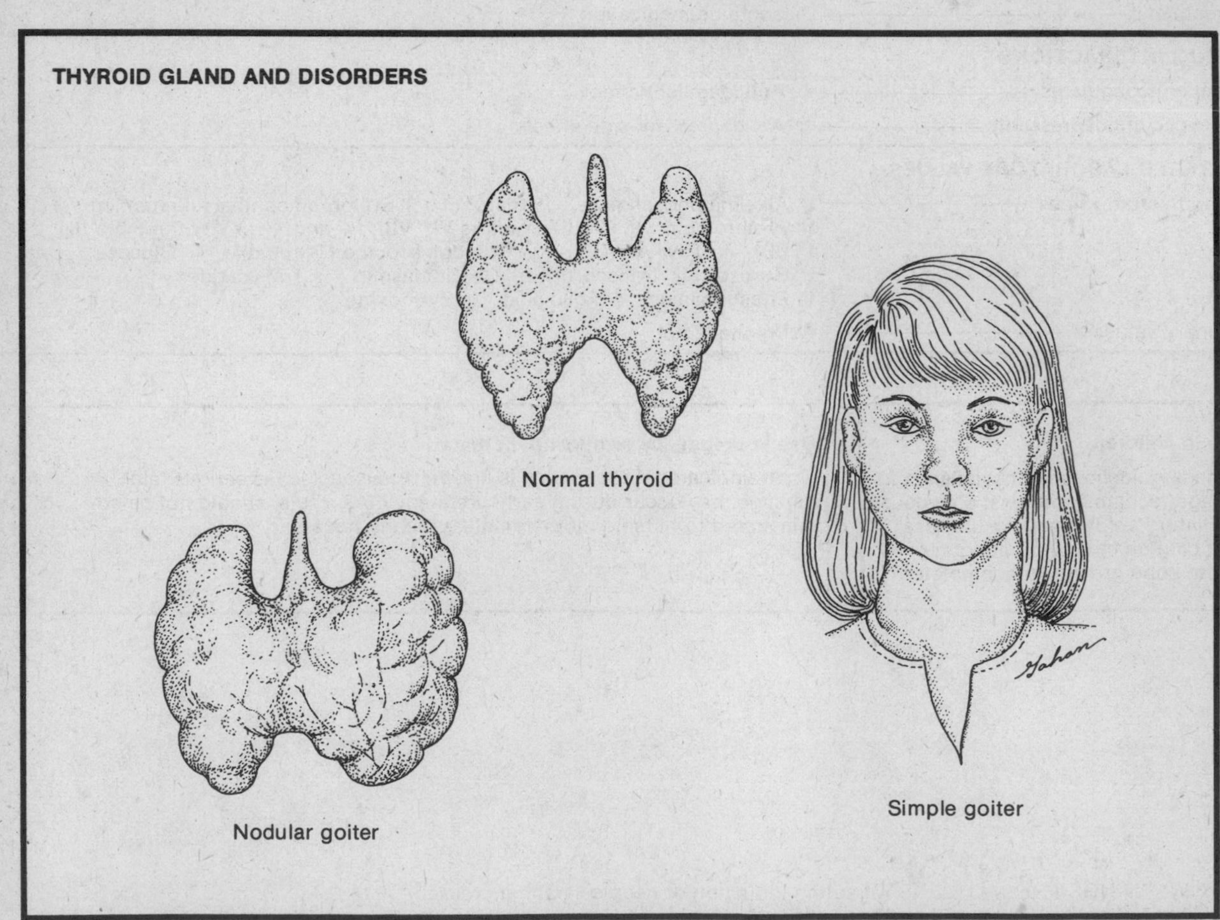

the nodules that have formed on the thyroid gland. This condition is more common in older persons, and it frequently carries no symptoms. It may be detected by palpating the thyroid gland, but the gland itself is rarely enlarged as in Graves' disease. When symptoms do occur, they resemble those of Graves' disease, with the exception of eye problems, which do not occur.

TREATMENT OF HYPERTHYROIDISM

Several measures may be employed to suppress the production of excess thyroid hormone. These include surgery to remove a portion of the thyroid gland, the use of radioactive iodine to destroy all or part of the gland, and treatment with antithyroid drugs, usually propylthiouracil (PTU) or methimazole (Tapazole).

In patients with nodular goiter, antithyroid drugs are not ordinarily employed; instead, radioactive iodine or surgery is usually the preferred treatment because, unlike Graves' disease, spontaneous remissions occur seldom if ever.

Antithyroid drugs act by blocking the production of thyroid hormone. Dosage must be individually adjusted and taken frequently because of the drugs' relatively short duration of action. Normal thyroid function may be achieved after several months of treatment, but 20 to 30 percent of all patients will require continuous use of these drugs for prolonged periods or even years. However, the patient should undergo periodic checkups and be alert for signs of recurring hyperthyroidism.

Use of Iodine

Before the advent of the modern antithyroid drugs, iodine — usually in the form of iodide salts — was the sole medication available to treat hyperthyroidism. Iodine inhibits the release of some thyroid hormone, thus helping to control the symptoms of hyperthyroidism. The therapeutic effect is seen within 24 hours and the basal metabolic rate may fall to a level usually seen only after thyroid surgery. Since surgery or modern antithyroid drugs are more certain in their effect, the present indications for iodide therapy are limited; they include preoperative preparation for thyroid surgery, use in conjunction with the antithyroid drugs, and thyroid crisis or thyroid storm.

From 1950 until recent years, radioactive iodine (^{131}I), which acts by destroying part or all of the thyroid tissue, was widely used in the treatment of hyperthyroidism in adults. (It is contraindicated in children and in pregnant women.) Radioactive iodine is still frequently used for patients over forty years of age who have Graves' disease, particularly those with heart disease. Persons with Graves' disease frequently recover after a single-dose administration of ^{131}I, although one third to half may require two or more doses.

The major disadvantage is the high incidence (about 40 to 70 percent) of drug-induced hypothyroidism in patients who have received radioactive iodine. The hypothyroidism can be readily treated with thyroid hormone, but the patient must be careful to take the thyroid hormone on the prescribed schedule for life.

In some patients, beta-blocking drugs such as propranolol (Inderal) may be given along with antithyroid drugs to help reduce the fast heart rate, tremor, and stare characteristic of exophthalmos. These drugs are most commonly used in the period before antithyroid drugs take full effect, usually a few days to two weeks.

Thyroid Storm

An emergency condition known as thyroid storm or thyroid crisis occasionally develops as a result of excessive buildup of thyroid hormones in the hyperthyroid patient. It is seen most often following surgery, but also may be triggered by infection, unusual emotional stress, pulmonary embolism, and diabetic acidosis. The typical patient is a middle-aged woman with a long history of moderate to severe hyperthyroidism.

When thyroid storm appears, all the symptoms of hyperthyroidism, including fever and an extremely fast heart rate, are exacerbated. In addition to therapy designed to suppress the production and release of thyroid hormone, Inderal has been found to be extremely useful in this rare complication.

HYPOTHYROIDISM

When the supply of thyroid hormone is inadequate to meet the metabolic needs of the body, hypothyroidism exists. True hypothyroidism most often follows the use of radioactive iodine or surgical therapy for hyperthyroidism. Symptoms include weakness, fatigue, weight gain, constipation, numbness in the extremities, and an increasing intolerance to cold. The voice may be hoarse, the skin dry, and the face puffy. Hypertension and bradycardia (very slow pulse rate) may be present.

In certain areas of the country, there is a deficiency of iodine in the soil, causing local foods to lack sufficient iodine. In those areas, up to 10 percent of the population may exhibit goiter—an enlargement of the thyroid gland. Cretinism, a severe form of mental and physical underdevelopment, is a result of hypothyroidism in infants. A severe to total lack of thyroid hormone is known as myxedema, a potentially fatal condition.

Simple Goiter

Simple goiter is particularly apt to appear at puberty and during pregnancy. Only rarely is simple goiter large enough to warrant removal, except for cosmetic purposes or when the enlarged thyroid presses on adjoining structures. A number of thyroid hormone replacement drugs, such as desiccated thyroid (Armour Thyroid) or levothyroxine sodium (Levothroid or Synthroid), are available to treat hypothyroidism. Very often, iodized salt is used to prevent endemic goiter.

Cretinism and Juvenile Hypothyroidism

Cretinism can result from a deficiency of thyroid

hormone during fetal life or early in the neonatal period. In these children, the thyroid gland is totally absent at birth or greatly reduced in size. Prolonged iodine deficiency, as may be seen in the endemic goiter regions, also may lead to this form of hypothyroidism.

In cretinism, both physical and mental development are retarded, and ossification of bones and union of the epiphyses at joints are delayed. The skin of these children is often thick, wrinkled, dry, and sallow. The lips may be thick and the tongue enlarged, so that the mouth remains open and allows drooling. Puffiness may be noted in the feet and hands, and frequently the hands will assume a spade shape. The face is broad and the nose flat.

In infancy, the cretin child appears apathetic and dull, the body temperature is usually subnormal, and constipation may be a problem. Profound, irreversible mental retardation is the outcome unless the hypothyroidism is recognized and treated early in life.

Juvenile hypothyroidism occurs in infants and children who were previously normal. This disorder is thought to be due to inflammation of the thyroid gland.

Therapy for both cretinism and juvenile hypothyroidism most often consists of desiccated thyroid or levothyroxine sodium, as in simple goiter. Once the diagnosis is made, therapy is started promptly and the child is monitored at regular intervals by the physician. In addition, the diet must contain adequate amounts of iodine, usually in the form of iodized salt.

Myxedema

Myxedema is a total or near total lack of thyroid hormone. The causes include radioactive iodine for previously existing hyperthyroidism, surgical removal of the thyroid gland (thyroidectomy), primary shrinking of the thyroid gland, or malfunctioning of the anterior lobe of the pituitary gland.

The myxedematous patient is easy to distinguish because of the characteristic facial changes, including enlarged tongue, thickened and swollen skin, puffiness (particularly about the eyelids), and scanty or absent eyebrows and scalp hair. In addition, speech becomes slow and the voice deep-toned, mental apathy and drowsiness are noted, and constipation is common. When myxedema develops in girls before puberty, menstruation may be absent. In myxedema occurring in girls after puberty, menorrhagia (excessively heavy menstrual flow) is a frequent complaint.

Treatment is with replacement thyroid hormones, which must be continued for life. In elderly patients with heart disease, thyroid replacement should begin slowly, with gradually increasing doses until the proper level is reached. If the patient has angina pectoris, the dosage must be reached even more slowly.

Myxedema Coma

Occasionally, patients with severe myxedema will go into coma, which is always a medical emergency requiring immediate treatment. In this situation, large doses of levothyroxine sodium given intravenously are the usual treatment, although in some instances, liothyronine (Cytomel), which is said to have a quicker action, is preferred. Fortunately, increased recognition and treatment of hypothyroidism have made myxedema coma increasingly rare.

Thyroiditis

Thyroiditis, which also may cause hypothyroidism, takes one of three forms—chronic, acute, and subacute. The most common chronic form is Hashimoto's thyroiditis, in which varying amounts of thyroid tissue are replaced by lymphocytes, leading to goiter and thyroid hormone insufficiency. Patients may complain of a sense of fullness in the throat, difficulty in swallowing, or, occasionally, episodes of choking.

Although Hashimoto's thyroiditis may occur even in young children, it is most often seen in adults thirty to fifty years old. The incidence in women is twenty times that of men. In some middle-aged women, in whom thyroid function is apparently normal, a diffuse and symptomless enlargement of the thyroid gland indicates the presence of Hashimoto's thyroiditis.

Thyroid hormones or levothyroxine sodium, both given orally, will usually shrink the goiter. A corticosteroid such as prednisone may also be given briefly to counter inflammation. Since spontaneous remissions do not occur in Hashimoto's thyroiditis, thyroid therapy must be continued for life.

Acute thyroiditis is caused by a bacterial infection. The initial symptoms are usually fever, a painful neck, and a mass in the thyroid area. Treatment is with antimicrobial agents, and ordinarily the process subsides very quickly with appropriate therapy.

Subacute thyroiditis is an inflammatory process that may last for weeks or months. It is thought to be viral in origin because it sometimes develops following a viral upper respiratory infection or after mumps. The symptoms are neck pain that may radiate to the jaws, arms, or chest. Hypothyroidism is a feature, but it is rarely permanent. Full recovery after several weeks or a few months is the rule.

IN CONCLUSION

The thyroid hormones are essential for normal growth, development, and metabolism. Hyperthyroidism can be effectively treated by administering antithyroid drugs or using surgery or radioactive iodine to reduce the amount or activity of functioning thyroid tissue. The hypothyroidism that may occur spontaneously or from treatment of hyperthyroidism is treated with replacement thyroid hormones.

It should be noted that all thyroid hormone preparations are contraindicated for weight reduction. In diabetic patients, a larger dosage of insulin may be required, but this determination should be made by a physician. Thyroid drugs can precipitate an attack of angina in persons with coronary artery disease. Indeed, because hypothyroidism can mask the presence of cardiac disease, it has been recommended that patients in whom coronary artery disease is a possibility have treadmill exercise testing before thyroid drugs are started.

The following drug charts cover the major thyroid hormone preparations as well as antithyroid drugs. Propranolol (Inderal), which is sometimes prescribed in conjunction with antithyroid drugs to treat the symptoms of thyroid storm, is included in the section on *Coronary Artery Disease* (page 15).

ARMOUR THYROID (Thyroid, desiccated) Armour

Tabs: ¼, ½, 1, 1½, 2, 3, 4, 5 gr

INDICATIONS	ORAL DOSAGE
Myxedema (PBI ≤ 2.5 μg/dl)	**Adult:** ¼ gr/day to start, followed by an increase to ½ gr/day after 2 wk and to 1 gre/day after 1 mo; assess patient 1 mo; assess patient 1 mo later and, again, after 2 mo of treatment with 1 gr/day; if necessary, increase dosage to 2 gr/day, wait 2 mo, and reassess patient; if necessary, increase dosage to 3 gr/day or more in increments of ½–1 gr/day until desired clinical and laboratory respose is achieved; usual maintenance dosage, 1–3 gr/day, but may vary from ½ to 10 gr/day
Hypothyroidism (PBI = 2.5–4.5 μg/dl)	**Adult:** 1 gr/day to start, followed by increases of 1 gr/day every 30 days until desired response is achieved; usual maintenance dosage: 1–3 gr/day
Cretinism, severe hypothyroidism in children	**Child:** same as for myxedema in adults, but increase dosage, if necessary, every 2 wk until desired response is obtained; usual maintenance dosage may be greater than in adult

CONTRAINDICATIONS

Concurrent hypothyroidism and hypoadrenalism (unless preceded by corticosteroid therapy) ●

Acute myocardial infarction without hypothyroidism ●

Thyrotoxicosis ●

WARNINGS/PRECAUTIONS

Euthyroid patients	Ineffective for weight reduction; large doses may produce serious, possibly lethal toxicity, especially when given with sympathomimetic agents
Cardiovascular disease, including hypertension	Use with caution with caution; reduce dosage if chest pain or other manifestations of cardiovascular disease develop
Coronary insufficiency	May be precipitated in thyroid-treated patients following injection of epinephrine or other catecholamines; patients with coronary-artery disease undergoing surgery should be carefully monitored for cardiac arrhythmias
Concomitant anticoagulant therapy	Reduce dosage of coumarin anticoagulants by 1/3 when initiating thyroid therapy; subsequently, readjust anticoagulant dosage based on prothrombin time
Adrenal insufficiency (Addison's disease)	May coexist as a result of hypopituitarism and should be corrected with corticosteroids before instituting thyroid therapy
Increased insulin requirements	Diabetics may require higher doses of insulin or oral hypoglycemic agents; if thyroid hormone dosage is decreased, insulin or oral hypoglycemic dosage may need to be decreased as well to avoid hypoglycemia

ADVERSE REACTIONS

Cardiovascular	Palpitations, tachycardia, arrhythmias, angina pectoris
Central nervous system	Tremor, headache, nervousness, insomnia
Metabolic	Weight loss, diaphoresis, heat intolerance, fever

OVERDOSAGE

Signs and symptoms	See ADVERSE REACTIONS
Treatment	Discontinue medication for several days and reinstitute therapy at a lower dosage. For acute poisoning, induce emesis or use gastric lavage to empty stomach. For tachycardia nd arrhythmias, administer propranolol. Institute supportive measures, as indicated. Treatment of unrecognized adrenal insufficiency should be considered.

DRUG INTERACTIONS

Oral anticoagulants	⇧ Anticoagulant effect
Insulin, oral hypoglycemics	⇩ Hypoglycemic effect
Ketamine	⇧ Blood pressure and heart rate
Phenytoin	⇧ Thyroxine blood level
Cholestyramine	⇩ Absorption of thyroid hormone
Tricyclic antidepressants	⇧ Antidepressant effect

ALTERED LABORATORY VALUES

Blood/serum values	⇧ Glucose ⇧ PBI ⇩ Cholesterol ⇩ TSH ⇩ ^{131}I thyroid uptake

No clinically significant alterations in urinary values occur at therapeutic dosages

Use in children

See INDICATIONS

Use in pregnancy or nursing mothers

General guidelines not established

CYTOMEL (Liothyronine sodium) **Smith Kline & French**

Tabs: 5, 25, 50 μg

INDICATIONS	ORAL DOSAGE
Mild hypothyroidism	**Adult:** 25 μg/day to start, followed by increases of 12.5–25 μg/day every 1–2 wk until optimum clinical response is achieved; usual maintenance dosage: 25–75 μg/day; some patients may require smaller or larger doses
Myxedema, simple (nontoxic) goiter	**Adult:** 5 μg/day to start, followed by increases of 5–10 μg/day every 1–2 wk up to a total of 25 μg/day, then by 12.5–25 μg/day every 1–2 wk until optimal clinical response is achieved; usual maintenance dosage: 50–100 μg/day for myxedema, 75 μg/day for goiter **Child:** same as adult but with increments of 5 μg/day at recommended intervals
Cretinism	**Child:** 5 μg/day to start, followed by increases of 5 μg/day every 3–4 days until desired response is achieved; usual maintenance dosage: 20 μg/day at a few months, 50 μg/ day at 1 yr, and full adult dosage in children >3 yr of age

ADMINISTRATION/DOSAGE ADJUSTMENTS

T_3 suppression test	To differentiate suspected hyperthyroidism from euthyroidism when ^{131}I thyroid uptake is in the borderline-to-high range, administer 75–100 μg/day of liothyronine for 7 days, then repeat uptake test. In the hyperthyroid patient, 24-h ^{131}I thyroid uptake will not be affected significantly; in the euthyroid patient, it will drop to 20%.
Hypothyroidism in patients with cardiovascular disease	Use only if clearly indicated; initiate therapy with 5 μg/day and increase dosage, if necessary, by no more than 5 μg/day at 2-week intervals
Elderly patients	Start with 5 μg/day and increase dosage by no more than 5 μg/day at recommended intervals until desired response is achieved
Patients taking thyroid, levothyroxine, or thyroglobulin	When transferring patient to liothyronine, initiate therapy at low dosage and increase gradually according to clinical response, bearing in mind that drug has a rapid onset of action and that residual effects of previous therapy may persist for several weeks

CONTRAINDICATIONS

Uncorrected adrenal insufficiency ● Morphological hypogonadism ● **Nephrosis** ●

WARNINGS/PRECAUTIONS

Euthyroid patients	Ineffective for weight reduction; large doses may produce serious, possibly lethal toxicity, especially when given with sympathomimetic agents
Adrenal insufficiency (Addison's disease)	May coexist as a result of hypopituitarism and should be corrected with corticosteroids before instituting thyroid therapy; supplemental corticosteroid therapy may also be needed in cases of severe, prolonged hypothyroidism

ADVERSE REACTIONS

Central nervous system	Nervousness
Cardiovascular	Cardiac arrhythmias, angina pectoris
Gastrointestinal	Diarrhea
Other	Menstrual irregularities, allergic skin reactions (rare)

OVERDOSAGE

Signs and symptoms	Headache, irritability, nervousness, sweating, tachycardia, increased bowel motility, menstrual irregularities, angina pectoris, congestive heart failure, shock; massive overdosage may produce symptoms of thyroid storm
Treatment	Discontinue medication for several days and reinstitute therapy at a lower dosage. For acute poisoning, induce emesis or use gastric lavage to empty stomach. For arrhythmias, administer propranolol. Institute supportive measures, as indicated. Treatment of unrecognized adrenal insufficiency should be considered.

DRUG INTERACTIONS

Oral anticoagulants	⇧ Anticoagulant effect
Insulin, oral hypoglycemics	⇩ Hypoglycemic effect
Ketamine	⇧ Blood pressure and heart rate
Phenytoin	⇧ Thyroxine blood level
Cholestyramine	⇩ Absorption of liothyronine
Tricyclic antidepressants	⇧ Antidepressant effect

Table continued on following page

CYTOMEL continued

ALTERED LABORATORY VALUES

Blood/serum values —————— ⇧ Glucose ⇩ Cholesterol ⇩ TSH ⇩ ^{131}I thyroid uptake ⇩ Uric acid

No clinically significant alterations in urinary values occur at therapeutic dosages

Use in children	Use in pregnancy or nursing mothers
See INDICATIONS	General guidelines not established

EUTHROID (Liotrix) **Parke-Davis**

Tabs: ½, 1, 2, 3 gr

INDICATIONS	ORAL DOSAGE
Hypothyroidism, including **myxedema** and **cretinism** **Simple (nontoxic) goiter** Subacute or chronic **thyroiditis,** including Hashimoto's disease **Goiter prophylaxis** in patients receiving thiouracil derivatives **Intolerance to thyroid preparations of animal origin**	**Adult:** start at low daily doses, followed by gradual increases every 2 wk until desired clinical response is achieved; usual maintenance dosage: 1-3 gr/day **Child:** same as for adult, but increase dosage, if necessary, every 2 wk until desired response is obtained; usual maintenance dosage may be higher than in adult

ADMINISTRATION/DOSAGE ADJUSTMENTS

Patients with cardiovascular disease	Use only if clearly indicated; start with ½-1 gr and increase dosage at 2-wk intervals, as needed

CONTRAINDICATIONS

Hypersensitivity to synthetic levothyroxine or liothyronine ●

Uncorrected adrenal insufficiency ●

Acute myocardial infarction ●

Nephrosis ●

Morphological hypogonadism ●

WARNINGS/PRECAUTIONS

Euthyroid patients	Ineffective for weight reduction; large doses may produce serious, possibly lethal toxicity, especially when given with sympathomimetic agents
Coronary insufficiency	Patients with coronary artery disease undergoing surgery should be carefully monitored for cardiac arrhythmias
Concomitant anticoagulant therapy	Prothrombin time may be altered; monitor patient closely
Adrenal insufficiency (Addison's disease)	May coexist and should be corrected with corticosteroids before instituting thyroid therapy
Severe hypothyroidism, myxedema	Patients may be unusually sensitive to thyroid hormones
Increased insulin requirements	Diabetics may require higher doses of insulin or oral hypoglycemic agents; if thyroid hormone dosage is decreased, insulin or oral hypoglycemic dosage may need to be decreased as well to avoid hypoglycemia

ADVERSE REACTIONS

Cardiovascular	Cardiac arrhythmias, angina pectoris
Central nervous system	Nervousness
Metabolic	Menstrual irregularities

OVERDOSAGE

Signs and symptoms	Headache, instability, nervousness, sweating, tachycardia, unusual bowel motility, angina pectoris, congestive heart failure, shock; massive overdosage may produce symptoms of thyroid storm
Treatment	Discontinue medication for several days and reinstitute therapy at a lower dosage. For acute poisoning, induce emesis or use gastric lavage to empty stomach. For tachycardia and arrhythmias, administer propranolol. Institute supportive measures, as indicated. Treatment of unrecognized adrenal insufficiency should be considered.

DRUG INTERACTIONS

Oral anticoagulants	⇧ Anticoagulant effect
Insulin, oral hypoglycemics	⇩ Hypoglycemic effect
Ketamine	⇧ Blood pressure and heart rate
Phenytoin	⇧ Thyroxine blood level
Cholestyramine	⇩ Absorption of liotrix
Tricyclic antidepressants	⇧ Antidepressant effect

Table continued on following page

EUTHROID continued

ALTERED LABORATORY VALUES

Blood/serum values —————— ⇧ Glucose ⇩ Cholesterol ⇩ TSH ⇩ ^{131}I thyroid uptake

No clinically significant alterations in urinary values occur at therapeutic dosages

Use in children	**Use in pregnancy or nursing mothers**
See INDICATIONS	General guidelines not established

Note: Liotrix also marketed as **THYROLAR** (Armour).

LEVOTHROID (Levothyroxine sodium) Armour

Tabs: 25, 50, 100, 150, 175, 200, 300 μg

INDICATIONS	ORAL DOSAGE
Myxedema, hypothyroidism with angina	**Adult:** 25 μg/day to start, followed by increases of 25–50 μg/day every 2–4 wk until desired response is obtained
Hypothyroidism, nontoxic goiter	**Adult:** 50 μg/day to start, followed by increases of 50 μg/day every 2–4 wk until patient is euthyroid or symptoms preclude further dosage increases; patients with no complicating endocrine or cardiovascular disease may be started immediately on full maintenance dosage (usually 100–200 μg/day)
Cretinism, severe hypothyroidism in children	**Child:** 25–50 μg/day to start, followed by increases of 50–100 μg/day every 2 wk until patient is euthyroid and laboratory values are in the normal range; usual maintenance dosage in growing children may be as high as 300–400 μg/day

CONTRAINDICATIONS

Acute myocardial infarction ● Uncorrected adrenal insufficiency ● Thyrotoxicosis ●

WARNINGS/PRECAUTIONS

Euthyroid patients	Ineffective for weight reduction; large doses may produce serious, possibly lethal toxicity, especially when given with sympathomimetic agents
Cardiovascular disease, including hypertension	Use with caution; reduce dosage if chest pain or other manifestations of cardiovascular disease develop
Coronary insufficiency	May be precipitated in thyroid-treated patients following injection of epinephrine or other catecholamines; patients with coronary-artery disease undergoing surgery should be carefully monitored for cardiac arrhythmias
Concomitant anticoagulant therapy	Reduce dosage of coumarin anticoagulants by 1/3 when initiating thyroid therapy; subsequently, readjust anticoagulant dosage based on prothrombin time
Adrenal insufficiency (Addison's disease)	May coexist as a result of hypopituitarism and should be corrected with corticosteroids before instituting thyroid therapy
Increased insulin requirements	Diabetics may require higher doses of insulin or oral hypoglycemic agents; if thyroid hormone dosage is decreased, insulin or oral hypoglycemic dosage may need to be decreased as well to avoid hypoglycemia

ADVERSE REACTIONS

Central nervous system	Nervousness, tremor, headache, insomnia
Cardiovascular	Palpitations, tachycardia, cardiac arrhythmias, angina pectoris
Metabolic	Weight loss, diaphoresis, heat intolerance, fever
Gastrointestinal	Diarrhea, abdominal cramps

OVERDOSAGE

Signs and symptoms	See ADVERSE REACTIONS
Treatment	Discontinue medication for several days and reinstitute therapy at a lower dosage. For acute poisoning, induce emesis or use gastric lavage to empty stomach. For tachycardia and arrhythmias, administer propranolol. Institute supportive measures, as indicated. Treatment of unrecognized adrenal insufficiency should be considered.

DRUG INTERACTIONS

Oral anticoagulants	⇧ Anticoagulant effect
Insulin, oral hypoglycemics	⇩ Hypoglycemic effect
Ketamine	⇧ Blood pressure and heart rate
Phenytoin	⇧ Thyroxine blood level
Cholestyramine	⇩ Absorption of levothyroxine
Tricyclic antidepressants	⇧ Antidepressant effect

Table continued on following page

LEVOTHROID continued

ALTERED LABORATORY VALUES

Blood/serum values —— ⇧ Glucose ⇧ PBI ⇩ Cholesterol ⇩ TSH ⇩ ^{131}I thyroid uptake ⇩ Uric acid

No clinically significant alterations in urinary values occur at therapeutic dosages

Use in children	**Use in pregnancy or nursing mothers**
See INDICATIONS	General guidelines not established

NOTE: Levothyroxine sodium also marketed as **SYNTHROID** (Flint).

PROLOID (Thyroglobulin) Parke-Davis

Tabs: ½, 1, 1½, 2, 3 gr (32, 65, 100, 130, 200 mg)

INDICATIONS	ORAL DOSAGE
Myxedema, hypothyroidism, simple (nontoxic) goiter, cretinism	**Adult:** ½ gr/day (32 mg/day) to start, followed by increases of ½ gr/day (32 mg/day) every 1-2 wk until desired clinical response is achieved; usual maintenance dosage: ½-3 gr (32-200 mg)/day

CONTRAINDICATIONS

Uncorrected adrenal insufficiency ● Morphological hypogonadism ● Nephrosis ●

WARNINGS/PRECAUTIONS

Euthyroid patients	Ineffective for weight reduction; large doses may produce serious, possibly lethal toxicity, especially when given with sympathomimetic agents
Cardiovascular disease	Use only if clearly indicated
Adrenal insufficiency (Addison's disease)	May coexist as a result of hypopituitarism and should be corrected with corticosteroids before instituting thyroid therapy
Myxedematous patients	May be unusually sensitive to thyroid preparations

ADVERSE REACTIONS

Cardiovascular	Cardiac arrhythmias, angina pectoris
Central nervous system	Nervousness
Other	Menstrual irregularities

OVERDOSAGE

Signs and symptoms	Headache, instability, nervousness, sweating, tachycardia, unusual bowel motility, angina pectoris, congestive heart failure, shock; massive overdosage may produce symptoms of thyroid storm
Treatment	Induce emesis or use gastric lavage to empty stomach. For tachycardia and arrhythmias, administer propranolol. Institute supportive measures, as indicated. Treatment of unrecognized adrenal insufficiency should be considered.

DRUG INTERACTIONS

Oral anticoagulants	⇧ Anticoagulant effect
Insulin, oral hypoglycemics	⇩ Hypoglycemic effect
Ketamine	⇧ Blood pressure and heart rate
Phenytoin	⇧ Thyroxine blood level
Cholestyramine	⇩ Absorption of thyroglobulin
Tricyclic antidepressants	⇧ Antidepressant effect

ALTERED LABORATORY VALUES

Blood/serum values	⇧ Glucose ⇧ PBI ⇩ Cholesterol ⇩ TSH ⇩ ^{131}I thyroid uptake

No clinically significant alterations in urinary values occur at therapeutic dosages

Use in children

General guidelines not established

Use in pregnancy or nursing mothers

General guidelines not established

PROPYLTHIOURACIL Lilly

Tabs: 50 mg

INDICATIONS	ORAL DOSAGE
Hyperthyroidism	**Adult:** 300 mg/day in 3 equally divided doses q8h to start; for severe hyperthyroidism or large goiters, 400-900 mg/day in 3 equally divided doses q8h to start; usual maintenance dosage, 100-150 mg/day div **Child (6-10 yr):** 50-150 mg/day in 3 equally divided doses q8h to start, then adjust dosage according to response **Child (≥10 yr):** 150-300 mg/day in 3 equally divided doses q8h to start, then adjust dosage according to response

CONTRAINDICATIONS

Hypersensitivity to propylthiouracil

WARNINGS/PRECAUTIONS

Blood dyscrasias	May occur (see ADVERSE REACTIONS), especially in patients receiving other agents known to cause agranulocytosis. Monitor patients for early signs (eg, sore throat, skin eruptions, fever, headache, or general malaise) of serious blood disorders and obtain WBC and differential counts if agranulocytosis is suspected.
Hypothrombinemia and bleeding	May occur; monitor prothrombin time, especially before surgery

ADVERSE REACTIONS

Dermatological	Rash, urticaria, pruritis, skin pigmentation, alopecia
Gastrointestinal	Nausea, vomiting, epigastric distress
Central nervous system and neuromuscular	Headache, drowsiness, neuritis, vertigo, arthralgia, paresthesia, myalgia
Hematological[1]	Agranulocytosis, granulopenia, thrombocytopenia, hypoprothrombinemia, bleeding
Other	Loss of taste, edema, jaundice, periarteritis, sialadenopathy, lymphadenopathy, drug fever, lupus erythematosus-like syndrome, hepatitis

OVERDOSAGE

Signs and symptoms	Nausea, vomiting, epigastric distress, headache, fever, arthralgia, pruritus, edema, hypothyroidism (with prolonged therapy), pancytopenia, agranulocytosis, exfoliative dermatitis, hepatitis, neuropathies, CNS stimulation or depression
Treatment	Discontinue therapy if agranulocytosis, pancytopenia, hepatitis, fever, or exfoliative dermatitis occurs. Institute general symptomatic therapy and supportive measures (ie, rest, analgesics, gastric lavage, IV fluids, and mild sedation). Treat bone-marrow depression with antibiotics, transfusions of fresh whole blood, and a corticosteroid, if needed. For hepatitis, rest and adequate diet and, in severe cases, a corticosteroid are indicated.

DRUG INTERACTIONS

Oral anticoagulants, heparin	⇧ Anticoagulant effect
Agranulocytosis-producing medications	⇧ Risk of agranulocytosis

[1]Of patients with untreated hyperthyroidism, 10% have leukopenia (WBC$<$4,000/mm^3), often with relative granulopenia

Table continued on following page

ALTERED LABORATORY VALUES

Blood/serum values ⇧ Prothrombin time ⇧ Alkaline phosphatase ⇧ SGOT ⇧ SGPT

No clinically significant alterations in urinary values occur at therapeutic dosages

Use in children

See INDICATIONS

Use in pregnancy or nursing mothers

Use judiciously in pregnant hyperthyroid women. Propylthiouracil crosses the placental barrier and can cause fetal goiter or cretinism; use a sufficient, but not excessive, dosage. In many pregnant hyperthyroid women, the thyroid dysfunction improves as the pregnancy proceeds; consequently, a reduction is possible, and, in some instances, the drug can be withdrawn 2–3 weeks before delivery. Concomitant administration of thyroid is recommended during propylthiouracil therapy of pregnant hyperthyroid patients to prevent hypothyroidism in the mother and fetus; administration of thyroid hormone should be continued throughout pregnancy and after delivery. Nursing should not be undertaken.

TAPAZOLE (Methimazole) Lilly

Tabs: 5, 10 mg

INDICATIONS	ORAL DOSAGE
Hyperthyroidism	**Adult:** for mild cases, 15 mg/day in 3 equally divided doses q8h to start; for moderately severe cases, 30–40 mg in 3 equally divided doses q8h to start; for severe cases, 60 mg/day in 3 equally divided doses q8h to start; for maintenance, 5–14 mg/day in 3 equally divided doses q8h **Child:** 0.4 mg/kg/day in 3 equally divided doses q8h to start, followed by ~0.2 mg/kg/day in 3 equally divided doses q8h for maintenance

CONTRAINDICATIONS

Hypersensitivity to methimazole

WARNINGS/PRECAUTIONS

Blood dyscrasias — May occur (see ADVERSE REACTIONS), especially in patients receiving other agents known to cause agranulocytosis. Monitor patients for early signs (eg, sore throat, skin eruptions, fever, headache, or general malaise) of serious blood disorders and obtain WBC and differential counts if agranulocytosis is suspected.

ADVERSE REACTIONS

Dermatological — Rash, urticaria, pruritus, skin pigmentation, alopecia

Hematological[1] — Agranulocytosis, granulopenia, thrombocytopenia, hypoprothrombinemia

Gastrointestinal — Nausea, vomiting, epigastric distress

Central nervous system and neuromuscular — Headache, drowsiness, neuritis, vertigo, arthralgia, paresthesia, myalgia

Other — Drug fever, jaundice, hepatitis, lymphadenopathy, lupus erythematosus-like syndrome, loss of taste, edema, sialadenopathy, periarteritis

OVERDOSAGE

Signs and symptoms — Nausea, vomiting, epigastric distress, headache, fever, arthralgia, pruritus, edema, hypothyroidism (with prolonged therapy), pancytopenia, agranulocytosis, exfoliative dermatitis, hepatitis, neuropathies, CNS stimulation or depression

Treatment — Discontinue therapy if agranulocytosis, pancytopenia, hepatitis, fever, or exfoliative dermatitis occurs. Institute general symptomatic therapy and supportive measures (ie, rest, analgesics, gastric lavage, IV fluids, and mild sedation). Treat bone-marrow depression with antibiotics, transfusions of fresh whole blood, and a corticosteroid, if needed. For hepatitis, rest and adequate diet and, in severe cases, a corticosteroid are indicated.

DRUG INTERACTIONS

Oral anticoagulants, heparin — ⇧ Anticoagulant effect

Agranulocytosis-producing medications — ⇧ Risk of agranulocytosis

ALTERED LABORATORY VALUES

Blood/serum values — ⇧ Bilirubin ⇧ Lactic dehydrogenase (LDH) ⇧ Prothrombin time ⇧ SGOT ⇧ SGPT ⇧ Alkaline phosphatase

No clinically significant alterations in urinary values occur at therapeutic dosages

Use in children

See INDICATIONS

Use in pregnancy or nursing mothers

Use judiciously in pregnant hyperthyroid women. Methimazole crosses the placental barrier and can cause fetal goiter or cretinism; use a sufficient, but not excessive, dosage. In many pregnant hyperthyroid women, the thyroid dysfunction improves as the pregnancy proceeds; consequently, a reduction is possible, and, in some instances, the drug can be withdrawn 2–3 weeks before delivery. Concomitant administration of thyroid is recommended during Methimazole therapy of pregnant hyperthyroid patients to prevent hypothyroidism in the mother and fetus; administration of thyroid hormone should be continued throughout pregnancy and after delivery. Nursing should not be undertaken.

[1] Of patients with untreated hyperthyroidism, 10% have leukopenia (WBC<4,000/mm^3), often with relative granulopenia

Infectious Diseases

Bacterial Infections

One of the phenomenal medical achievements of this century has been the control of infectious disease. Improved public health and preventive measures, widespread immunization programs, better nutrition, and a higher standard of living in the developed countries have greatly reduced the frequency of life-threatening and chronic debilitating infectious disease, particularly among the young and middle-aged. Potent antibiotic drugs can now control and cure almost all bacterial infections that arise in basically healthy persons. Problems do remain, however, with infectious diseases continuing to be a serious problem among the aged and persons with lowered resistance. This section will review the major types of infectious diseases and the antibiotic drugs used to treat them.

GENERAL CONSIDERATIONS

The first antibiotics, which were introduced in the mid-1930's and early 1940's, were the sulfa drugs, followed by penicillin. Since then, hundreds of different antimicrobial agents have been developed. Some of these are, like penicillin, derived from natural substances; others are completely man-made, and still others are chemical alterations of natural substances. All antibiotic drugs work by interfering with vital processes of the bacteria. For example, the penicillins kill by interfering with the production of the bacterial cell wall, the aminoglycosides (e.g., streptomycin) act by disordering protein formation in the cell protoplasm, and the sulfa drugs upset the metabolism of folic acid, an essential B vitamin. Indeed, the range of bacterial drugs is now so wide that a physician can often tailor individual therapy with considerable precision and effect. Factors that should be considered, in addition to identifying the specific infecting microorganism, include the site of infection, the concentration of antibiotic drug required to kill, the manner in which the microorganism may develop resistance to the drug, the strength of a patient's immune defenses, the route of administration (e.g., whether the drug will be destroyed by stomach acid if given orally), the length of treatment, and potential side effects. (It should be noted that antibiotics are not effective against viruses, although they are sometimes prescribed for persons with viral disease to counteract secondary bacterial infections that may derive from the primary viral infection.)

DIAGNOSIS

Diagnosis of a particular infectious disease is generally easier than identification of the specific infecting microorganism. The latter step, however, is often of pivotal importance in treating the infection because administering the wrong antibiotic or one to which the bacteria will quickly develop resistance can be counterproductive. Cultures to identify the bacteria should be taken from samples of the suspected site of infection. This usually entails analyzing specimens—depending upon the presumed diagnosis—of urine, blood, abscesses and wounds, sputum, joint fluid, spinal fluid, and penile or vaginal secretions.

The next step is to perform a Gram stain—a simple test that takes ten minutes—to determine the presence and shape of the bacteria and whether they can be stained by a certain dye. This test is immediately useful because it can act as a guide to preliminary treatment—an important consideration since the results of the culture studies may not be known for several days. If bacterial infection is suspected, medication is started immediately after the culture samples are obtained and the Gram stain has been done. A broad-range drug, or a combination of two or three antibiotics if the disease is severe, can be started and then adjusted appropriately when the specific microorganism has been identified. The drug selection can be further refined by growing several colonies of the bacteria and subjecting them to different antibiotics. It should be noted, however, that the results obtained in laboratory studies are not always duplicated in the body.

The length of treatment varies with the disease and individual considerations. In most instances, the antibiotics are administered for seven to ten days, but some infections, such as endocarditis, an infection of the heart valves, require six weeks of high-dose intravenous antibiotic therapy. Tuberculosis requires up to eighteen months of drug therapy. It is particularly important to complete the recommended course of therapy; interruption of treatment can lengthen the course of disease, promote the development of resistant strains of bacteria, and encourage relapses or complications.

COMMON INFECTIOUS DISEASES

Lung Infections

Pneumonia, the most common of man's major bacterial infections, is usually caused by the pneumonococcus, a strain of common bacteria that is generally effectively treated by penicillin, tetracycline, or erythromycin. The typical symptoms of pneumonia include high fever, cough, mucus production, chest pains, and overall weakness. Most patients respond quickly to treatment, with complete recovery. More serious pneumonias are caused by the staphylococci, a kind of bacteria that grows in clumps. These bacteria are often resistant to penicillin because of their production of penicillinase, an enzyme that can destroy penicillin's vital structure. Staphylococcal pneumonias are usually treated with synthetic penicillins (e.g., oxacillin or methicillin) that are not attacked by penicillinase. Lung infections caused by microorganisms that do not pick up the Gram dye (Gram-negative organisms) are rapidly progressive and virulent and can destroy lung tissue, leading to life-threatening shock and pulmonary failure. These cases are treated with high doses of intravenous drugs, usually in combinations that include cephalosporins, aminoglycosides, and extended-range penicillins. These pneumonias are particularly lethal to the infirm and aged.

The atypical pneumonias, which are most common in young adults, are caused by viruses or primitive bacteria that lack cell walls, and thus are not affected by penicillin. Erythromycin is the drug of choice in these pneumonias (as it is in Legionnaire's disease), but the chances of success are often poor.

Urinary Tract Infections

The bladder, kidney, and prostate are the most frequent sites of urinary tract infections. Although disease can be present without symptoms, urinary tract infections usually are signaled by some combination of fever, back or groin pain, and painful, frequent, or bloody urination. Diagnosis is established by microscopic examination of the urine and culture of the microorganism.

Kidney infections are usually treated with ampicillin—sometimes administered intravenously. Bladder infections can be treated orally with tetracycline, a sulfa drug, trimethaprim, or ampicillin. Chronic and recurrent urinary infection should be treated with long-term suppressive therapy for months or even years to prevent permanent kidney damage. Catheterization—the passing of a tube into the bladder—carries, under even the best of sterile conditions, a high risk of infection. The prostate, unfortunately, can be a haven for bacteria because its poor local blood supply results in low antibiotic penetration. Chronic or relapsing prostatic disease caused by *Escherichia coli*, a kind of intestinal bacterium, or the staphylococci, occurs frequently and treatment failure is common, necessitating the initiation of other drug regimens.

Venereal Infections

Gonorrhea is the most common venereal disease in this country. Its causal agent, the gonococcus, has gradually become increasingly resistant to penicillin, and every few years, the recommended doses of antibiotic are revised upward. Still, most cases respond to 4,800,000 units of procaine penicillin, administered in a single injection along with probenecid, a drug that keeps penicillin in the body longer. Most "resistant" cases are actually reinfections, but some gonococci produce penicillinase and must be treated with other agents, such as spectinomycin. Erythromycin can be used in patients allergic to penicillin.

Although gonorrhea does not always produce symptoms, especially in women, it is important to identify and treat all sexual partners who have been exposed to the disease. Untreated gonorrhea can be particulary serious in women, leading to pelvic inflammatory disease, an infection that may require hospitalization and high-dose medication, and which often results in tubal scarring and infertility.

Another increasingly common venereal disease is nonspecific urethritis. This infection is caused by chlamydia, a strain of primitive microorganisms. It is transmitted sexually and can produce symptoms similar to those of gonorrhea. It is treated by administering tetracycline for two weeks.

Still another venereal disease that has increased markedly in recent years is genital herpes infection, a viral disease. This disorder is characterized by painful, recurrent blisters or sores, usually in the genital area. Since the cause is a virus, antibiotics are of no help in treating it. As yet, there is no cure for genital herpes, although creams may afford some symptomatic relief. The disease itself is not a serious threat to health, except to an infant who may be exposed to it during birth. To avoid this, delivery by cesarean section is often recommended for women with an active herpes infection at the time of birth.

Syphilis, one of the most dreaded diseases of the past, is now relatively rare and is easily cured with penicillin or erythromycin. No known resistance occurs. Syphilis is diagnosed with a blood test (STS or FTA); however, since these tests may stay positive long after successful treatment, the results may be misleading.

Miscellaneous Infectious Diseases

Meningitis Fever, headache, stiff neck, and changes in personality or alertness point to the possibility of bacterial meningitis. Whenever meningitis is suspected, microscopic examination of the spinal fluid for bacteria and pus should be performed. Medication is usually begun immediately with a high intravenous dose of penicillin or chloramphenicol. A delay in treatment can result in permanent brain damage or even death. For asymptomatic carriers or persons exposed to meningitis caused by *Neisseria meningitidis,* rifampin (Rifadin)—an antibiotic used to treat tuberculosis—may help prevent its development, but is not used to treat the disease once it develops.

Tuberculosis Fortunately, tuberculosis of the kind described by Thomas Mann in *The Magic Mountain* is a thing of the past. Although the disease still occurs, it is usually seen in persons with lowered resistance, such as patients undergoing cancer treatment, chronic alcoholics, or the aged. The tuberculosis bacillus—a specific type of bacterium—usually attacks the lungs, but also may be centered in bone, the kidneys, and elsewhere. Treatment usually consists of some combination of isoniazid, rifampin, streptomycin, and ethambutol. In most cases, patients leave the hospital after several weeks of intensive therapy because the disease is no longer contagious, and their physical condition is usually vastly improved. Outpatient treatment, however, must continue for eighteen months to two years.

OVERUSE OF ANTIBIOTICS

No discussion of antibiotics is complete without a caution against the misuse and overuse of these important drugs. While antibiotics are truly lifesaving "wonder drugs," many of the common infections of everyday life do not require their use. Viral infections, upset stomachs, the usual childhood diseases (mumps, measles, and so forth), and the common cold are not affected by antibiotics. Antibiotics may be prescribed for persons with chronic lung disease, such as emphysema, when they have colds to lessen the likelihood of pneumonia or bronchitis. But healthy individuals with normal lungs will not benefit from antibiotic treatment, and in fact may suffer a more complex infection with resistant organisms or an unpleasant adverse reaction, such as an overgrowth of fungi in the mouth or vagina.

In other instances, the need for antibiotics is ambiguous, and their use is best left to the judgment of the physician. Strep throat, for example, generally requires antibiotic treatment, but 20 percent of adults carry streptococci in their mouths as harmless "normal flora." Repeated positive throat cultures in patients with minimal symptoms should signal this possibility and raise doubts as to the need for repeated treatment. Tonsillitis also usually responds to drug treatment but can often be eradicated simply with gargles of diluted hydrogen peroxide. Bacillary dysentery, caused by the shigella bacteria, with diarrhea, cramps, and fever, almost always subsides in one week by itself, but ampicillin can speed recovery if cultures (which are rarely taken in time) are positive. Minor abscesses, boils, and shallow skin infections around cuts and sutures can often be cured by cleanliness and hot soaks alone.

GUIDELINES FOR PROPER USE

When antibiotics are indicated, patients should be careful to follow instructions. Particular attention should be paid to length of treatment, the number of pills to take per day, and how to time their consumption to maintain a constant body level of the drug and avoid possible interactions with food or other drugs. Some tetracyclines, for example, should not be taken with antacids or food, particularly milk or other foods high in calcium, because they will diminish absorption of the antibiotic. The aminoglycosides and other antibiotics can increase the effectiveness of oral anticoagulant drugs used in the treatment of phlebitis and other circulatory disorders. This drug interaction may cause serious bleeding by decreasing the ability of blood to clot beyond the degree originally sought by the physician. Alcohol taken while on metronidazole therapy can produce severe nausea, vomiting, and heart palpitations. Other specific cautions and instructions for using specific drugs are included in the charts at the end of this section.

Potential Adverse Reactions

Allergic reactions, usually in the form of rash or hives, are the most frequent side effects encountered with use of antibiotics. In very rare instances, anaphylaxis, a severe allergic reaction manifested by shock and bronchospasm (asthma) occurs after injection of an antibiotic (usually penicillin). Anaphylaxis must be treated immediately—usually with an injection of epinephrine—to avoid death. The more common allergic reactions—it is estimated, for example, that 10 percent of the American population is allergic to penicillin—are treated with antihistamines and a change in drugs.

Other adverse effects fall into two categories. The first is fairly predictable and often related to the total amount of drug given. For example, damage to the kidney and the nerve structures of the ear can occur with the aminoglycosides, particularly streptomycin. Short-term effects are usually reversible with discontinuation or reduction of dosage. However, careful monitoring of total dosage and of kidney function is important.

The second type of reaction is idiosyncratic and unpredictable. Chloramphenicol, which is important in treating certain severe infections such as meningitis, causes an irreversible destruction of the bone marrow in about one of 10,000 patients. While this risk is very small, it does mandate that the drug be reserved for serious illnesses.

Fortunately, most adverse reactions are mild, and require only a change of drug. A number of side effects that are unpleasant but essentially harmless occur frequently with the use of antibiotics in general. These include gastrointestinal upset, diarrhea, overgrowth of normal vaginal organisms, worsening of acne, and nonspecific indisposition. Some persons taking tetracycline experience increased sensitivity to sunlight. These drugs also cause discoloring of youngsters' teeth when given to young children or during pregnancy.

Failure of Treatment

While antibiotics are capable of curing most

bacterial infections, especially in healthy individuals, failures do occur. For example, the antibiotic itself may change the growth environment in the patient and lead to the development of resistant microorganisms. Failure also may occur when the normal internal balance of previously harmless bacteria is upset by antibiotics, causing these microorganisms to proliferate out of control—an event referred to as "superinfection." These superinfections usually require different, more toxic, and higher doses of antibiotics. In some instances, this sets in motion a cycle of toxicity, resistance, and superinfections. This is particularly true in treating nosocomial infections, defined as those that arise in hospitalized patients, especially in the intensive and respiratory care units where patients are the most vulnerable.

Another major reason for treatment failure is that the antibiotic simply cannot do the job alone. A bacterial infection can be rampant, virulent, smoldering, or resistant, especially if the patient has impaired defenses against infection. Conditions that lower host resistance include alcoholism, drug abuse, malnutrition, the use of steroid drugs, delay in starting treatment, hereditary disorders, and such other coexisting diseases as diabetes, kidney failure, and emphysema. Cancer, especially leukemia, lowers general host resistance, and anticancer drugs may destroy or suppress the remaining body defenses. The problem is serious; patients on cancer chemotherapy are often severely infected, even by bacteria that are generally harmless in healthy people. Still, antibiotic therapy usually works, although in some cases transfusions of white blood cells may be given to bolster the patient's weakened immune system.

Finally, some infections must be treated by a combination of antibiotics and surgical drainage. Such cases include deep abscesses or disease in tightly enclosed spaces, such as tendon sheaths and muscle compartments.

IN CONCLUSION

While antibiotics have not eradicated infectious disease, as once was hoped, they have dramatically changed the treatment and prognosis of the most common bacterial infections. The use of these drugs, together with public health programs, improved nutrition, and a higher standard of living, have marvelously changed the quality and length of life. For the first time in history, most persons can achieve the Biblical allotment of threescore and ten years.

Infections are still with us, however. As the degenerative diseases, characterized by functional decline and cell systems gone awry, have increasingly become the major causes of illnesses and death, infection in these patients has become more difficult to treat. The following drug charts cover the major antibiotics now in use. They are arranged by drug classification, i.e., penicillins, aminoglycosides, etc. Nonprescription antibacterial agents are covered in the chart on Nonprescription Antibiotics.

AMIKIN (Amikacin sulfate) Bristol

Vials: 100, 500 mg (2 ml), 1 g (4 ml) **Syringe:** 500 mg (2 ml)

INDICATIONS	PARENTERAL DOSAGE
Bacteremia, septicemia, and serious respiratory-tract infections, bone and joint infections, CNS infections (including meningitis), skin and soft-tissue infections, intra-abdominal infections (including peritonitis), burn infections, and postoperative infections (including postvascular surgery) caused by susceptible strains of Gram-negative bacteria, including *Pseudomonas, Escherichia coli, Proteus, Providencia, Klebsiella-Enterobacter-Serratia,* and *Acinetobacter*	**Adult:** 7.5 mg/kg q12h or 5 mg/kg q8h IM or IV **Child:** same as adult
Neonatal sepsis, when other aminoglycosides cannot be used[1]	**Neonate:** 10 mg/kg IM or IV to start, followed by 7.5 mg/kg q12h
Uncomplicated urinary-tract infections[2]	**Adult:** 250 mg IM bid

ADMINISTRATION/DOSAGE ADJUSTMENTS

Duration of treatment	Usual duration of treatment is 7–10 days; if a longer course of therapy is required, renal and auditory functions should be monitored daily
Patients with renal impairment	Lengthen interval between doses by giving normal dose at intervals (in hours) obtained by multiplying the serum creatinine concentration by 9; alternatively, give normal loading dose followed by 12-hourly maintenance doses obtained by dividing normally recommended dose by the serum creatinine concentration
Maximum dose	Total daily dose for all routes of administration should not exceed 15 mg/kg/day or 1.5 g/day; monitor serum drug level when feasible, and avoid prolonged peak concentrations >35 μg/ml
Intravenous administration	Should be accomplished over a 30- to 60-min period; the infusion period for infants should be extended to 1–2 h

CONTRAINDICATIONS

Hypersensitivity to amikacin or other aminoglycoside antibiotics

WARNINGS/PRECAUTIONS

Lack of response	Discontinue therapy and recheck antibiotic sensitivity if no definite clinical response occurs within 3–5 days; treatment failure may indicate bacterial resistance or the presence of septic foci requiring surgical drainage
Renal impairment	Closely monitor renal and eighth-nerve function in patients with known or suspected renal impairment or in those who develop renal insufficiency during therapy
Ototoxicity, nephrotoxicity, neurotoxicity	May occur, especially at higher doses or for administration periods longer than recommended; risk is greater in patients with renal damage. Reduce dosage or discontinue therapy if renal, vestibular, or auditory function becomes impaired. Concurrent or serial use of other ototoxic or nephrotoxic agents (see DRUG INTERACTIONS) should be avoided.
Renal irritation	May be minimized by adequate hydration; increase hydration if signs of irritation appear
Renal dysfunction developing during therapy	Reduce dosage or stop treatment if azotemia increases or urinary output decreases progressively
Cross-allergenicity	Use with caution in patients demonstrating sensitivity to other aminoglycosides
Superinfection	Overgrowth of nonsusceptible organisms may occur

[1]Concomitant penicillin therapy may be indicated because of the possibility of infection due to Gram-positive organisms (eg, streptococci, pneumococci)

[2]Not recommended in initial episodes unless causative organisms are resistant to potentially less toxic antibiotics

Table continued on following page

AMIKIN continued

ADVERSE REACTIONS

Renal	Albuminuria, red and white blood cells or casts in urine, azotemia, oliguria
Gastrointestinal	Nausea, vomiting
Central nervous system and neuromuscular	Paresthesias, tremor, headache, arthralgia
Otic	Deafness, vertigo
Hematological	Eosinophilia, anemia
Cardiovascular	Hypotension
Hypersensitivity	Drug fever, skin rash

OVERDOSAGE

Signs and symptoms	Deafness, vertigo, renal dysfunction, neuromuscular blockade, respiratory paralysis
Treatment	Reduce dosage or discontinue medication; institute supportive measures. Peritoneal dialysis or hemodialysis may be used to eliminate drug from bloodstream.

DRUG INTERACTIONS

Other aminoglycoside antibiotics	⇧ Risk of ototoxicity, nephrotoxicity, and neuromuscular blockade
Cephaloridine, cephalothin	⇧ Risk of nephrotoxicity
Polymyxin antibiotics	⇧ Risk of nephrotoxicity and neuromuscular blockade
Potent diuretics (eg, ethacrynic acid, furosemide, mannitol, mercaptomerin), cisplatin, vancomycin, viomycin, capreomycin	⇧ Risk of ototoxicity and nephrotoxicity
Anesthetics, neuromuscular blocking agents	⇧ Risk of neuromuscular blockade and respiratory paralysis (reversible with calcium)

ALTERED LABORATORY VALUES

Blood/serum values	⇧ BUN ⇧ Creatinine
Urinary values	⇧ Protein ⇩ Specific gravity

Use in children

See INDICATIONS; use in infants only when other aminoglycosides are contraindicated and patient can be closely observed for evidence of ototoxicity

Use in pregnancy or nursing mothers

Safe use not established during pregnancy; patient should stop nursing if drug is prescribed

GARAMYCIN (Gentamicin sulfate) Schering

Vials: 10 mg/ml (2 ml, for pediatric use), 40 mg/ml (2, 20 ml) **Syringe:** 40 mg/ml (1.5, 2 ml) **Amps:** 2 mg/ml (2 ml) for intrathecal administration **Dermatological ointment:** 0.1% (15 g) **Dermatological cream:** 0.1% (15 g) **Ophthalmic ointment:** 3 mg/g (⅛ oz) **Ophthalmic solution:** 3 mg/ml (5 ml)

INDICATIONS	PARENTERAL DOSAGE
Neonatal sepsis, septicemia, serious CNS infections (meningitis), urinary-tract infections, respiratory-tract infections, GI-tract infections (including peritonitis), and skin, bone, and soft-tissue infections (including burn infections) caused by susceptible strains of *Pseudomonas aeruginosa, Proteus, Escherichia coli, Klebsiella-Enterobacter-Serratia, Citrobacter,* and *Staphylococcus* **Suspected or confirmed Gram-negative bacterial infections** As an adjunct to penicillin in the treatment of **endocarditis** caused by Group D streptococci **Serious staphylococcal infections** caused by susceptible strains when other potentially less toxic drugs are contraindicated **Mixed infections** caused by susceptible strains of staphylococci and Gram-negative organisms	**Adult:** 3 mg/kg/day IM or IV in 3 equal doses q8h; for life-threatening infections, up to 5 mg/kg/day IM or IV in 3–4 equally divided doses may be given, followed by 3 mg/kg/day as soon as clinically indicated **Premature infant and full-term neonate (≤1 wk):** 2.5 mg/kg q12h **Infant (>1 wk):** 2.5 mg/kg q8h **Child:** 2.0–2.5 mg/kg q8h

ADMINISTRATION/DOSAGE ADJUSTMENTS

Intermittent intravenous infusion	A single dose may be diluted in 50–200 ml (less for infants and children) of isotonic saline or 5% dextrose in water and infused over a period of 30 min to 2 h; gentamicin should not be added to solutions of other drugs
Intrathecal administration	For serious CNS infections (meningitis, ventriculitis) caused by susceptible strains of *Pseudomonas* in adults, administer 4–8 mg qd intrathecally (for infants >3 mo of age and children, reduce dosage to 1–2 mg qd) as an adjunct to systemic gentamicin therapy. Draw required dose into a 5-or 10-ml syringe. After lumbar puncture and removal of fluid for laboratory analysis, insert syringe into hub of spinal needle. Allow a small amount of CSF (~10% of estimated total CSF volume) to flow into syringe and mix with gentamicin; then inject resultant fluid over a period of 3–5 min, with bevel of needle directed upward. If CSF is grossly purulent or unobtainable, dilute gentamicin with normal saline. The solution may also be injected directly into the subdural space or intraventricularly.
Use of serum concentrations	To determine adequacy and safety of dosage, measure both peak and trough serum concentrations of gentamicin; dosage should be adjusted so that prolonged peak levels above 12 μg/ml or trough levels (measured just prior to the next dose) above 2 μg/ml are avoided
Patients with renal impairment	Dosage must be adjusted either by increasing the interval between administration of normal doses (multiply the serum creatinine level [mg/dl] by 8 to determine the dosage interval in hours) or by administering the drug more frequently (q8h) at reduced doses (after the normal initial dose, divide the normally recommended dose by the serum creatinine level); renal function should be carefully monitored, since it may change over the course of the infectious process
Patients undergoing hemodialysis	For adults, 1–1.7 mg/kg should be administered at the end of each dialysis period; for children, 2 mg/kg may be administered
Primary and secondary skin infections caused by susceptible bacteria	Apply a small amount of cream or ointment to the lesions tid or qid
Infections of the external eye and adnexa caused by susceptible bacteria	Instill 1–2 drops q4h into the affected eye; for severe infections, up to 2 drops qh may be used; or apply a small amount of ointment to the affected eye bid or tid. Do not introduce solution into the anterior chamber of the eye or inject subconjunctivally.

CONTRAINDICATIONS

Hypersensitivity or toxic reaction to other aminoglycosides (relative contraindication)	Hypersensitivity to gentamicin or to other components of the dermatological and ophthalmic formulations (absolute contraindication)

Table continued on following page

GARAMYCIN continued

WARNINGS/PRECAUTIONS	
Renal impairment	Closely monitor renal and eighth-nerve function in patients with known or suspected renal impairment (particularly the elderly) or in those who develop renal insufficiency during therapy; all patients should be well hydrated. Examine urine periodically for the presence of cells or casts, a reduction in specific gravity, and/or an increase in protein. Other signs of nephrotoxicity include a rising BUN, NPN, and serum creatinine level and oliguria. Reduce dosage or discontinue use of drug, if necessary.
Ototoxicity, nephrotoxicity, neurotoxicity	May occur, especially at higher doses or for administration periods longer than recommended; risk is greater in patients with renal damage. Concurrent or serial use of other ototoxic or nephrotoxic agents or diuretics (see DRUG INTERACTIONS) should be avoided. Serial audiograms should be obtained if patient is old enough to be tested (loss of high-frequency perception is usual initial manifestation of hearing loss); other symptoms of ototoxicity include dizziness, vertigo, tinnitus, and roaring in the ears. Neurotoxicity may be evidenced by numbness, a tingling sensation, muscle twitching, and/or convulsions. In each case, reduce dosage or discontinue use of drug, if necessary.
Long-term therapy	Usual duration of therapy is 7–10 days; if a longer course is necessary, renal, auditory, and vestibular functions should be monitored, since the risk of toxicity is increased after 10 days. Dosage should be reduced if clinically indicated.
Neuromuscular blockade and respiratory paralysis	May occur in patients receiving anesthetics, neuromuscular blocking agents, or massive transfusions of citrate-anticoagulated blood; calcium salts may reverse blockade if it occurs
Muscle weakness	May worsen in patients with neuromuscular disorders (eg, myasthenia gravis or parkinsonism) because of drug's curare-like effect on the neuromuscular junction
Superinfection	Overgrowth of nonsusceptible organisms may occur; discontinue use of dermatological preparations and institute appropriate therapy
Cross-allergenicity	Use with caution in patients demonstrating hypersensitivity to other aminoglycosides
Corneal healing	May be retarded by use of ophthalmic ointment

ADVERSE REACTIONS	
Renal	Casts, cells, or protein in the urine; oliguria
Hepatic	Transient hepatomegaly, splenomegaly
Gastrointestinal	Nausea, vomiting, increased salivation, stomatitis
Central nervous system and neuromuscular	Dizziness, vertigo, numbness, tingling sensation, muscle twitching, convulsions, lethargy, confusion, depression, visual disturbances, pseudotumor cerebri, acute organic brain syndrome, joint pain, arachnoiditis or burning at injection site (with intrathecal use)
Otic	Tinnitus, roaring in the ears, hearing loss
Hematological	Anemia, granulocytopenia, leukopenia, transient agranulocytopenia, eosinophilia, increased or decreased reticulocyte count, thrombocytopenia, purpura
Cardiovascular	Hypotension, hypertension
Respiratory	Depression, pulmonary fibrosis
Dermatological and hypersensitivity	Rash, pruritus, erythema (with dermatological use), urticaria, generalized burning sensation, laryngeal edema, anaphylactoid reactions, fever, headache, photosensitization (with dermatological use), subcutaneous atrophy and fat necrosis at injection site (rare)
Other	Decreased appetite, weight loss, alopecia, transient burning or irritation (with ophthalmic use), pain at injection site

OVERDOSAGE	
Signs and symptoms	Hearing loss, vertigo, renal dysfunction, neuromuscular blockade, respiratory paralysis
Treatment	Reduce dosage or discontinue medication; institute supportive measures, as required. Peritoneal dialysis or hemodialysis may be used to help eliminate drug from bloodstream.

Table continued on following page

GARAMYCIN continued

DRUG INTERACTIONS

Other aminoglycoside antibiotics	⇧ Risk of ototoxicity, nephrotoxicity, and neuromuscular blockade
Cephaloridine, cephalothin	⇧ Risk of nephrotoxicity
Polymyxin antibiotics	⇧ Risk of nephrotoxicity and neuromuscular blockade
Potent diuretics (eg, ethacrynic acid, furosemide), cisplatin, vancomycin, viomycin, capreomycin	⇧ Risk of ototoxicity and nephrotoxicity
Anesthetics, neuromuscular blocking agents	⇧ Risk of neuromuscular blockade and respiratory paralysis (reversible with calcium)
Carbenicillin	⇩ Gentamicin serum half-life (in patients with severe renal impairment)

ALTERED LABORATORY VALUES

Blood/serum values	⇧ BUN ⇧ NPN ⇧ Creatinine ⇧ SGOT ⇧ SGPT ⇧ Lactate dehydrogenase ⇧ Bilirubin ⇩ Calcium ⇩ Magnesium ⇩ Sodium ⇩ Potassium
Urinary values	⇧ Protein ⇩ Specific gravity

Use in children

See INDICATIONS

Use in pregnancy or nursing mothers

Safe use not established during pregnancy; general guidelines not established for use in nursing mothers

KANTREX (Kanamycin sulfate) Bristol

Caps: 500 mg **Vials:** 75 mg (2 ml, for pediatric use), 500 mg (2 ml), 1 g (3 ml) **Syringe:** 500 mg (2 ml)

INDICATIONS	ORAL DOSAGE	PARENTERAL DOSAGE
Serious infections caused by susceptible strains of *Escherichia coli*, *Proteus*, *Enterobacter aerogenes*, *Klebsiella pneumoniae*, *Serratia marcescens*, and *Acinetobacter* **Staphylococcal infections** caused by susceptible strains of *Staphylococcus aureus* and *S epidermidis* in patients allergic to other antibiotics, **mixed staphylococcal** and **Gram-negative bacterial infections,** and **severe infections** thought to be caused by either a Gram-negative bacterium or *Staphylococcus*	—	**Adult:** 7.5 mg/kg IM q12h or up to 15 mg/kg/day IM or IV (slowly) in 2-3 equally divided doses; to achieve continuously high blood levels, give 15 mg/kg/day IM in equally divided doses q6-8h, not to exceed 1.5 g/day **Child:** same as adult
Suppression of intestinal bacteria (short-term adjunctive therapy)	**Adult:** 1 g q4h, followed by 1 g q6h for 36-72 h	—
Hepatic coma (adjunctive therapy)[1]	**Adult:** 8-12 g/day div	—

ADMINISTRATION/DOSAGE ADJUSTMENTS

Duration of treatment	Usual duration of parenteral therapy is 7-10 days; when used orally as an adjunct to mechanical cleansing of the large bowel, the duration will depend on the patient's condition, whether catharsis or enemas are used and to what degree, and the customary medical routine for bowel preparation before surgery
Patients with renal impairment	Renal dysfunction may necessitate reduced frequency of administration; dosing interval in hours may be calculated by multiplying patient's serum creatinine level (mg/dl) by 9. Since renal function may alter appreciably during therapy, serum creatinine level should be checked frequently.
Intramuscular injection	Inject calculated dose deeply into the upper outer quadrant of gluteus muscle
Intravenous infusion	Dilute contents of 500-mg vial with 100-200 ml of normal saline or 5% dextrose (or contents of 1-g vial with 200-400 ml) and administer over a period of 30-60 min; for children, use sufficient diluent to infuse calculated pediatric dose over a similar period
Intraperitoneal use following exploration for established peritonitis or peritoneal contamination due to fecal spillage during surgery	Dilute contents of 500-mg vial in 20 ml of sterile distilled water and instill via a catheter sutured into the wound at closure; if possible, postpone instillation until effects of anesthesia and muscle-relaxing drugs have dissipated
Aerosol treatment	Dilute 250 mg in 3 ml of normal saline, place in a nebulizer, and administer bid to qid
Irrigating solution	Concentrations of 2.5 mg/ml may be used to irrigate abscess cavities, pleural space, and peritoneal and ventricular cavities

CONTRAINDICATIONS

Hypersensitivity or toxic reaction to kanamycin or other aminoglycosides (relative contraindication) ●	Intestinal obstruction (with oral form) ●	Long-term parenteral use ●

WARNINGS/PRECAUTIONS

Lack of response	Discontinue therapy and recheck antibiotic sensitivity if no definite clinical response occurs within 3-5 days; treatment failure may indicate bacterial resistance or the presence of septic foci requiring surgical drainage
Renal impairment	Closely monitor renal and eighth-nerve function in patients with known or suspected renal impairment or in those who develop renal insufficiency during therapy. Reduce dosage or stop treatment if azotemia increases or urinary output decreases progressively. Audiograms should be taken before initiating treatment and again periodically. Discontinue therapy if patient develops significant loss of high-frequency perception, tinnitus, or subjective hearing loss.
Ototoxicity, nephrotoxicity, neurotoxicity	May occur, especially at higher doses or for administration periods longer than recommended; risk is greater in patients with renal damage. Concurrent or serial use of other ototoxic or nephrotoxic agents or diuretics should be avoided (see DRUG INTERACTIONS). Elderly patients, patients with pre-existing tinnitus, vertigo, or known subclinical deafness, patients who have received ototoxic drugs in the past, and patients receiving a total dose of 15 g or more of kanamycin should be carefully observed for signs of eighth-nerve damage; hearing loss may occur in such patients even with normal renal function.

[1]To lower blood ammonia by suppressing ammonia-forming bacteria in the intestinal tract

Table continued on following page

KANTREX continued

WARNINGS/PRECAUTIONS continued	
Renal irritation	May be minimized by adequate hydration; increase hydration or reduce dosage if signs of irritation (eg, casts, WBC, RBC, albumin) appear
Intestinal absorption	Although absorption of oral kanamycin is usually negligible, the presence of ulcerated or denuded areas may increase absorption from the intestine
Superinfection	Overgrowth of nonsusceptible organisms, including fungi, may occur
Malabsorption syndrome	Characterized by increased fecal fat and by decreased serum carotene and xylose absorption, may occur with prolonged oral therapy
Neuromuscular blockade and respiratory paralysis	May occur in patients receiving anesthetics, neuromuscular blocking agents, or massive transfusion of citrate-anticoagulated blood; calcium salts or neostigmine may reverse blockade if it occurs
Muscle weakness	May worsen in patients with myasthenia gravis because of curare-like effect of drug on neuromuscular junction
Cross-allergenicity	Use with caution in patients demonstrating sensitivity to other aminoglycosides

ADVERSE REACTIONS[2]	
Renal	Albuminuria, red and white blood cells or granular casts in urine, azotemia, oliguria
Gastrointestinal	Nausea, vomiting, and diarrhea (with oral use)
Central nervous system and neuromuscular	Headache, paresthesias
Otic	Tinnitus, vertigo, partial to irreversible hearing loss
Hypersensitivity	Skin rash, drug fever
Other	Local irritation or pain following IM injection

OVERDOSAGE	
Signs and symptoms	Deafness, vertigo, renal dysfunction, neuromuscular blockade, respiratory paralysis
Treatment	Reduce dosage or discontinue medication; institute supportive measures. Peritoneal dialysis or hemodialysis may be used to eliminate drug from bloodstream. Newborns may, in addition, benefit from exchange transfusion.

DRUG INTERACTIONS	
Other aminoglycoside antibiotics	⇧ Risk of ototoxicity, nephrotoxicity, and neuromuscular blockade
Cephaloridine, cephalothin	⇧ Risk of nephrotoxicity
Polymyxin antibiotics	⇧ Risk of nephrotoxicity and neuromuscular blockade
Potent diuretics (eg, ethacrynic acid, furosemide, mannitol, mercaptomerin), cisplatin, vancomycin, viomycin, capreomycin	⇧ Risk of ototoxicity and nephrotoxicity
Anesthetics, neuromuscular blocking agents	⇧ Risk of neuromuscular blockade and respiratory paralysis (reversible with calcium or neostigmine)

ALTERED LABORATORY VALUES	
Blood/serum values	⇧ BUN ⇧ Creatinine
Urinary values	⇧ Protein ⇩ Specific gravity

Use in children

See INDICATIONS; infants and children generally tolerate the parenteral form as well. General guidelines not established for use of oral form in children and appropriate dosages.

Use in pregnancy or nursing mothers

Safe use not established; general guidelines not established for use in nursing mothers

[2]Side effects of oral therapy are mainly gastrointestinal; however, prolonged, high-dose oral administration in hepatic coma may result in nephrotoxicity and ototoxicity

MYCIFRADIN (Neomycin sulfate) Upjohn

Tabs: 0.5 g **Oral sol:** 125 mg/5 ml **Vial:** 250 mg/ml after reconstitution (for IM use only)

INDICATIONS	ORAL DOSAGE	PARENTERAL DOSAGE
Diarrhea caused by enteropathogenic *Escherichia coli*	**Adult:** 50 mg/kg/day div for 2–3 days **Infant and child:** same as adult	——
Bowel preparation for surgery	**Adult:** 1 g qh for 4 doses, followed by 1 g q4h for a total of 24 h, or 88 mg/kg/day (40 mg/lb/day) in 6 equally divided doses q4h for 2–3 days before surgery	——
Urinary-tract infections caused by *Pseudomonas aeruginosa, Klebsiella pneumoniae, Proteus vulgaris, Escherichia coli,* and *Enterobacter aerogenes* in hospitalized patients[1]	——	**Adult:** 15 mg/kg/day, up to 1 g/day, in 4 equally divided IM doses q6h for up to 10 days
Hepatic coma (adjunctive therapy)[2]	**Adult:** 4–12 g/day div for 5–6 days; in cases of chronic hepatic insufficiency, up to 4 g/day div indefinitely	——

CONTRAINDICATIONS

Hypersensitivity to neomycin●	Intestinal obstruction (oral use)●

WARNINGS/PRECAUTIONS

Ototoxicity, nephrotoxicity, neurotoxicity	May occur, even with conventional dosages, particularly in patients with renal impairment or prerenal azotemia; use with extreme caution in such patients. Before initiating parenteral therapy, examine the urine for albumin, casts, and cells and obtain a BUN measurement; repeat the urinalysis daily and BUN study every other day while the drug is being given. Blood and urine studies are also advisable prior to and during extended oral therapy in patients with renal and/or hepatic disease. Audiometric testing is indicated for all patients both before and during therapy. Discontinue therapy if tinnitus or other signs of auditory or renal toxicity develop. Neurotoxicity may result in respiratory paralysis. Loss of hearing may first appear several weeks after neomycin has been discontinued and may progress to complete deafness. If renal insufficiency develops, reduce dosage or discontinue use.
Concomitant therapy	Do not give concurrently or serially with other ototoxic, nephrotoxic, and/or neurotoxic drugs (see DRUG INTERACTIONS)
Superinfection	Overgrowth of nonsusceptible organisms, including fungi, may occur

ADVERSE REACTIONS

Frequent reactions to oral neomycin are italicized

Gastrointestinal	*Nausea, vomiting, diarrhea,* malabsorption syndrome (with prolonged therapy)
Dermatological	Skin rash
Other	Hypersensitivity, irreversible deafness and/or renal damage (see WARNINGS/PRECAUTIONS)

OVERDOSAGE

Signs and symptoms	Hearing loss, vertigo, renal impairment, respiratory paralysis
Treatment	Discontinue medication; treat symptomatically and institute supportive measures, as needed

DRUG INTERACTIONS

Other aminoglycoside antibiotics	⇧ Risk of ototoxicity, nephrotoxicity, and/or neurotoxicity, and neuromuscular blockade
Loop diuretics, capreomycin, cisplatin, vancomycin, viomycin	⇧ Risk of ototoxicity and/or neurotoxicity
Anesthetics, neuromuscular blocking agents	⇧ Risk of neuromuscular blockade
Polymyxin antibiotics	⇧ Risk of neurotoxicity and/or nephrotoxicity
Cephaloridine, cephalothin	⇧ Risk of nephrotoxicity

[1]Because of potential toxicity, reserve for cases in which no other antimicrobial agent is effective
[2]To lower blood ammonia by suppressing ammonia-forming bacteria in the intestinal tract

Table continued on following page

MYCIFRADIN continued

ALTERED LABORATORY VALUES

Blood/serum values —— ⇧ Creatinine ⇧ BUN ⇩ Carotene

No clinically significant alterations in urinary values occur at therapeutic dosages

Use in children

See INDICATIONS; Parenteral form is not recommended for use in infants and children.

Use in pregnancy or nursing mothers

Safe use not established during pregnancy; general guidelines not established for use in nursing mothers

NEBCIN (Tobramycin) Lilly

Amps: 80 mg/2 ml (2 ml) **Pediatric amps:** 20 mg/2 ml (2 ml) **Syringe:** 60 mg/1.5 ml (1.5 ml), 80 mg/2 ml (2 ml)

INDICATIONS	PARENTERAL DOSAGE
Septicemia, serious central-nervous-system infections (including meningitis), neonatal sepsis, serious lower respiratory infections, gastrointestinal infections (including peritonitis), serious skin, bone, and soft-tissue infections (including burn infections), and serious, recurrent urinary tract infections caused by susceptible strains of *Pseudomonas aeruginosa, Escherichia coli, Proteus, Providencia, Klebsiella-Enterobacter-Serratia, Citrobacter*, and staphylococci (including *Staphylococcus aureus)*	**Adult:** 3 mg/kg/day IM or IV in equally divided doses q8h; for life-threatening infections, up to 5 mg/kg/day may be given in 3-4 equal doses, to be reduced to 3 mg/kg/day as soon as clinically indicated **Neonate (≤1 wk):** up to 4 mg/kg/day IM or IV in equally divided doses q12h **Older infant:** same as adult **Child:** same as adult

ADMINISTRATION/DOSAGE ADJUSTMENTS

Duration of treatment	Usual duration of treatment is 7-10 days; if a longer course of therapy is required, renal, auditory, and vestibular functions should be monitored because neurotoxicity is more likely after 10 days
Serum-level monitoring	**To prevent toxicity caused by excessive blood levels, dosage should not exceed 5 mg/kg/day unless serum levels are monitored; prolonged serum levels >12 µg/ml should be avoided**
Intramuscular administration in patients with impaired renal function (creatinine clearance rate ≤70 ml/min)	Administer 1 mg/kg to start, followed by reduced doses administered at 8-h intervals (divide normally recommended dose by patient's serum creatinine level) or normal doses given at prolonged intervals (multiply patient's serum creatinine level by 6 to determine dosage frequency in hours); neither method should be used when dialysis is being performed
Intravenous infusion	Dilute required amount of tobramycin with 50-100 ml (less for children) of 0.9% sodium chloride or 5% dextrose and administer over a period of 20-60 min; do not premix with other drugs

CONTRAINDICATIONS

Hypersensitivity to tobramycin

WARNINGS/PRECAUTIONS

Renal impairment	Closely monitor renal and eighth-nerve function in patients with known or suspected renal impairment or in those who develop renal insufficiency during therapy
Ototoxicity, nephrotoxicity, neurotoxicity	**May occur, especially at higher doses or for administration periods longer than recommended; risk is greater in patients with renal damage. Reduce dosage or discontinue therapy if renal, vestibular, or auditory function becomes impaired. Concurrent or serial use of other ototoxic or nephrotoxic agents or diuretics (see DRUG INTERACTIONS) should be avoided.**
Cross-allergenicity	Use with caution in patients demonstrating sensitivity to other aminoglycosides
Superinfection	Overgrowth of nonsusceptible organisms may occur
Prolonged or secondary apnea	May occur if tobramycin is administered to anesthetized patients being treated with neuromuscular blocking agents

ADVERSE REACTIONS

Renal	Oliguria, cylindruria, increased proteinuria
Central nervous system and neuromuscular	Dizziness, headache, lethargy
Otic	**Vertigo, tinnitus, roaring sound in the ears, hearing loss**
Gastrointestinal	Nausea, vomiting
Hematological	Anemia, granulocytopenia, thrombocytopenia
Hypersensitivity	Fever, rash, itching, urticaria

Table continued on following page

NEBCIN continued

OVERDOSAGE	
Signs and symptoms	Deafness, vertigo, renal dysfunction, neuromuscular blockade, respiratory paralysis
Treatment	Reduce dosage or discontinue medication; institute supportive measures. Peritoneal dialysis or hemodialysis may be used to eliminate drug from bloodstream.

DRUG INTERACTIONS	
Other aminoglycoside antibiotics	⇧ Risk of ototoxicity, nephrotoxicity, and neuromuscular blockade
Cephaloridine, cephalothin	⇧ Risk of nephrotoxicity
Polymyxin antibiotics	⇧ Risk of nephrotoxicity and neuromuscular blockade
Potent diuretics (eg, loop diuretics), cisplatin, vancomycin, viomycin, capreomycin	⇧ Risk of ototoxicity and nephrotoxicity
Anesthetics, neuromuscular blocking agents	⇧ Risk of neuromuscular blockade and respiratory paralysis (reversible with calcium)

ALTERED LABORATORY VALUES	
Blood/serum values	⇧ BUN ⇧ NPN ⇧ Creatinine ⇧ SGOT ⇧ SGPT ⇧ Bilirubin
Urinary values	⇧ Protein ⇩ Specific gravity

Use in children

Use with caution in premature and neonatal infants because of renal immaturity; for older infants and children, see INDICATIONS

Use in pregnancy or nursing mothers

Safe use not established; general guidelines not established for use in nursing mothers

STREPTOMYCIN SULFATE (Streptomycin sulfate) Lilly

Vial: 0.5 g/ml (2, 10 ml) **Powder:** 1 g (5 ml), 5 g (30 ml)

INDICATIONS	PARENTERAL DOSAGE
Mycobacterium tuberculosis caused by susceptible organisms	**Adult:** 1 g/day IM (with one or more anti-tubercular drugs), followed by 1 g 2–3 times/wk
Tularemia	**Adult:** 1–2 g/day IM div for 7–10 days, until the patient is afebrile for 5–7 days
Plague	**Adult:** 2–4 g/day IM div until the patient is afebrile for at least 3 days
Endocarditis caused by penicillin-sensitive alpha-and nonhemolytic streptococci	**Adult:** 1 g IM bid for 1 wk, followed by 0.5 g IM bid for 1 wk, along with penicillin
Enterococcal endocarditis	**Adult:** 1 g IM bid for 2 wk, followed by 0.5 g IM bid for 4 wk, along with penicillin
Severe fulminating Gram-negative bacillary bacteremia, meningitis, and **pneumonia; brucellosis, granuloma inguinale; chancroid;** and **urinary-tract infections** (caused by susceptible organisms)	**Adult:** 2–4 g/day IM div q6–12h, along with other anti-infective agents **Child:** 20–40 mg/kg/day IM div q6–12h, along with other anti-infective agents
Less severe Gram-negative bacillary bacteremia, meningitis, and **pneumonia; brucellosis; granuloma inguinale; chancroid;** and **urinary-tract infections** (caused by highly susceptible organisms)	**Adult:** 1–2 g/day IM div q6–12h, along with other anti-infective agents **Child:** 20–40 mg/kg/day IM div q6–12h, along with other anti-infective agents

ADMINISTRATION/DOSAGE ADJUSTMENTS

Elderly patients	When treating tuberculosis, reduce daily dose in accordance with age, renal function, and eighth nerve function; when treating bacterial endocarditis, give patients over 60 yr of age 0.5 g bid for the entire 2-wk period
Duration of anti-tubercular therapy	Continue treatment for a minimum of 1 yr unless toxic symptoms appear, impending toxicity is feared, organisms become resistant, or full therapeutic effect is obtained

CONTRAINDICATIONS

Prior toxic reaction or hypersensitivity to streptomycin

WARNINGS/PRECAUTIONS

Severe nausea, vomiting, and vertigo	May occur, particularly in elderly patients and those with renal impairment, due to adverse effects on the vestibular branch of the auditory nerve; discontinue use if symptoms of ototoxicity occur
Loss of hearing	May occur with prolonged use, due to ototoxic effect on the auditory branch of the eighth nerve; when extensive, hearing loss may be permanent
Tinnitus, roaring noises, or the sense of fullness in the ears	May occur; perform audiometric examination and/or discontinue use
Prolonged therapy	Perform baseline and periodic caloric stimulation tests and audiometric examination
Skin sensitivity reactions	May occur; care should be taken by individuals handling or preparing streptomycin for injection
Superinfection	Overgrowth of nonsusceptible organisms, including fungi, may occur; institute appropriate therapy, if required

ADVERSE REACTIONS

Auditory	Ototoxicity (nausea, vomiting, vertigo), deafness
Neuromuscular	Circumoral or peripheral paresthesias, muscular weakness
Dermatological	Rash, urticaria, exfoliative dermatitis
Hematological	Eosinophilia, leukopenia, thrombocytopenia, pancytopenia, hemolytic anemia
Other	Fever, angioneurotic edema, anaphylaxis, azotemia, amblyopia, myocarditis, hepatic necrosis

OVERDOSAGE

Signs and symptoms	See ADVERSE REACTIONS
Treatment	Discontinue use and institute supportive measures, as required

Table continued on following page

DRUG INTERACTIONS

Other aminoglycoside antibiotics	⇧ Risk of ototoxicity, nephrotoxicity, and neuromuscular blockade
Cephaloridine, cephalothin	⇧ Risk of nephrotoxicity
Polymyxin antibiotics	⇧ Risk of nephrotoxicity and neuromuscular blockade
Diuretics (especially loop diuretics), cisplatin, vancomycin, viomycin, capreomycin	⇧ Risk of ototoxicity and nephrotoxicity
Anesthetics, neuromuscular blocking agents	⇧ Risk of neuromuscular blockade and respiratory paralysis (reversible with calcium)

ALTERED LABORATORY VALUES

Urinary values	⇧ Protein ⇧ Glucose (false elevation with Benedict's solution)

No clinically significant alterations in blood/serum values occur at therapeutic dosages

Use in children

See INDICATIONS; avoid excessive dosage

Use in pregnancy or nursing mothers

Use with caution during pregnancy to prevent ototoxicity in the fetus; general guidelines not established for use in nursing mothers

ANCEF (Cefazolin sodium) Smith Kline & French

Vials: 250 mg, 500 mg, 1 g **Piggyback vials:** 500 mg, 1 g **Pharmacy bulk vials:** 5, 10 g

INDICATIONS	PARENTERAL DOSAGE
Respiratory-tract infections caused by susceptible strains of *Streptococcus pneumoniae, Klebsiella, Haemophilus influenzae, Staphylococcus aureus,* and Group A beta-hemolytic streptococci **Urinary-tract infections** caused by susceptible strains of *Escherichia coli, Proteus mirabilis, Klebsiella, Enterobacter,* and enterococci **Skin-structure infections** caused by susceptible strains of *Staphylococcus aureus,* Group A beta-hemolytic streptococci, and other streptococci **Biliary-tract infections** caused by susceptible strains of *Escherichia coli,* streptococci, *Proteus mirabilis, Klebsiella,* and *Staphylococcus aureus* **Bone and joint infections** caused by susceptible strains of *Staphylococcus aureus* **Septicemia** caused by susceptible strains of *Streptococcus pneumoniae, Staphylococcus aureus, Proteus mirabilis, Escherichia coli,* and *Klebsiella* **Endocarditis** caused by susceptible strains of *Staphylococcus aureus,* and Group A beta-hemolytic streptococci **Genital infections** caused by susceptible strains of *Escherichia coli, Proteus mirabilis, Klebsiella,* and enterococci	**Adult:** for mild infections caused by susceptible Gram-positive cocci, 250–500 mg IM or IV q8h; for moderate to severe infections, 500 mg to 1 g IM or IV q6–8h; for acute uncomplicated urinary-tract infections, 1 g IM or IV q12h; for pneumococcal pneumonia, 500 mg IM or IV q12h; for life-threatening infections, such as endocarditis and septicemia, 1–1.5 g IM or IV q6h, up to 12 g/day **Infant (≥1 mo) and child:** for mild to moderately severe infections, 25–50 mg/kg/day in 3 or 4 equally divided doses; for severe infections, up to 100 mg/kg/day in 3 or 4 equally divided doses
Prevention of postoperative infection in patients undergoing contaminated or potentially contaminated procedures or when infection at the operative site would present a serious risk	**Adult:** 1 g IM or IV ½–1 h prior to surgery, followed by 0.5–1 g IM or IV during lengthy (2 h or more) procedures and q6–8h for 24 h postoperatively

ADMINISTRATION/DOSAGE ADJUSTMENTS

Adults with renal impairment	Administer an initial loading dose appropriate to the severity of infection, followed by full doses at intervals of at least 8 h when creatinine clearance rate (CCr) = 35–54 ml/min; 50% of the usual dose q12h when CCr = 11–34 ml/min; 50% of the usual dose q18–24h when CCr ≤10 ml/min
Children with renal impairment	Following the usual loading dose, administer 60% of the normal daily dose div q12h when CCr = 40–70 ml/min; 25% of the normal daily dose div q12h when CCr = 20–40 ml/min; 10% of the normal daily dose q24h when CCr = 5–20 ml/min
Intramuscular injection	Dilutions of 250 mg/2 ml, 500 mg/2 ml, or 1 g/2.5 ml of Sterile (or Bacteriostatic) Water for Injection or Sodium Chloride for Injection should be injected into a large muscle mass
Intravenous injection	Dilutions of 500 mg/10 ml or 1 g/10 ml of Sterile Water for Injection should be injected over a period of 3–5 min; administer directly into vein or through IV tubing
Intermittent intravenous infusion	Cefazolin may be administered with primary IV fluid management programs in a volume control set or in a separate secondary IV bottle; 500 mg or 1 g should be diluted in 50–100 ml of compatible IV solution
Duration of prophylaxis following surgery	Prophylactic administration may be continued for 3–5 days following surgery where infection may be particularly devastating (eg, open-heart surgery and prosthetic arthroplasty)

CONTRAINDICATIONS

Hypersensitivity to cephalosporins

Table continued on following page

ANCEF continued

WARNINGS/PRECAUTIONS	
Cross-allergenicity	Use with caution in penicillin-allergic patients
Hypersensitivity reactions	Serious acute hypersensitivity reactions may occur, most likely in patients with a history of allergy, particularly to drugs; anaphylactic reactions may require administration of epinephrine and other emergency measures
Superinfection	Overgrowth of nonsusceptible organisms may occur; careful clinical observation is essential
Renal impairment	Patients with impaired renal function may require a lower daily dosage (see ADMINISTRATION/DOSAGE ADJUSTMENTS)

ADVERSE REACTIONS	
Gastrointestinal	Nausea, anorexia, vomiting, diarrhea, oral candidiasis
Hypersensitivity	Drug fever, skin rash, vulvar pruritus, eosinophilia
Genitourinary	Genital and anal pruritus, genital moniliasis, vaginitis
Hematological	Neutropenia, leukopenia, eosinophilia, thrombocytopenia
Other	Pain on IM injection, sometimes with induration; phlebitis at injection site

OVERDOSAGE	
Signs and symptoms	See ADVERSE REACTIONS
Treatment	Discontinue medication; treat symptomatically and institute supportive measures, as required

DRUG INTERACTIONS	
Probenecid	⇧ Cefazolin blood level and/or toxicity

ALTERED LABORATORY VALUES	
Blood/serum values	⇧ Alkaline phosphatase ⇧ SGOT ⇧ SGPT ⇧ BUN + Coombs' test
Urinary values	⇧ Glucose (with Clinitest tablets)

Use in children

See INDICATIONS; not recommended for use in premature infants or in infants under 1 mo of age

Use in pregnancy or nursing mothers

Safe use not established during pregnancy; general guidelines not established for use in nursing mothers

Note: Cefazolin sodium also marketed as **KEFZOL** (Lilly).

ANSPOR (Cephradine) Smith Kline & French

Caps: 250, 500 mg **Susp:** 125 mg/5 ml, 250 mg/5 ml after reconstitution

INDICATIONS	ORAL DOSAGE
Respiratory-tract infections caused by susceptible strains of Group A beta-hemolytic streptococci and *Streptococcus pneumoniae* **Skin and soft-tissue infections** caused by susceptible strains of staphylococci	**Adult:** 250 mg q6h or 500 mg q12h; for severe or chronic infections, up to 1 g qid may be given **Infant (≥ 9 mo) and child:** 25–50 mg/kg/day in divided doses q6h or q12h; for severe or chronic infections, up to 1 g qid may be given
Urinary-tract infections caused by susceptible strains of *Escherichia coli, Proteus mirabilis,* and *Klebsiella* **Lobar pneumonia** caused by susceptible strains of *Streptococcus pneumoniae*	**Adult:** 500 mg q6h or 1 g q12h; for severe or chronic infections, up to 1 g qid may be given
Otitis media caused by susceptible strains of Group A beta-hemolytic streptococci, *Streptococcus pneumoniae, Haemophilus influenzae,* and staphylococci	**Infant (≥9 mo) and child:** 75–100 mg/kg/day in divided doses q6h or q12h; for severe or chronic infections, up to 1 g qid may be given

ADMINISTRATION/DOSAGE ADJUSTMENTS

Patients with renal impairment	Administer 500 mg q6h when creatinine clearance rate (CCr) >20 ml/min; 250 mg q6h when CCr=5–20 ml/min; 250 mg q12h when CCr<5 ml/min
Chronic intermittent hemodialysis	Administer 250 mg to start; followed by 250 mg 12 h later and 250 mg 36–48 h after initial dose
Streptococcal infection	Infections caused by Group A beta-hemolytic streptococci should be treated for at least 10 days to guard against risk of rheumatic fever or glomerulonephritis
Prostatitis	Prolonged intensive therapy is recommended

CONTRAINDICATIONS

Hypersensitivity to cephalosporins

WARNINGS/PRECAUTIONS

Cross-allergenicity	Use with caution in penicillin-allergic patients
Hypersensitivity	Serious acute hypersensitivity reactions may occur (most likely in patients with a history of allergy, asthma, hay fever, or urticaria); anaphylactic reactions may require administration of epinephrine, pressor amines, antihistamines, or corticosteroids
Impaired renal function	Patients with markedly impaired renal function should be carefully monitored during therapy, since cephradine accumulates in the serum and tissues (see ADMINISTRATION/DOSAGE ADJUSTMENTS)
Superinfection	Overgrowth of nonsusceptible organisms may occur
Chronic urinary-tract infection	Frequent bacteriological and clinical appraisal is necessary during therapy and may be required for several months afterward

ADVERSE REACTIONS

Gastrointestinal	Glossitis, nausea, vomiting, diarrhea, loose stools, abdominal pain, heartburn
Hypersensitivity	Mild urticaria, skin rash, pruritus, joint pains (see WARNINGS/PRECAUTIONS)
Hematological	Mild transient eosinophilia, leukopenia, neutropenia
Other	Dizziness, tightness in the chest, candidal vaginitis

Table continued on following page

ANSPOR continued

OVERDOSAGE

Signs and symptoms	See ADVERSE REACTIONS
Treatment	Discontinue medication; treat symptomatically and institute supportive measures, as required

DRUG INTERACTIONS

Probenecid	⇧ Cephradine blood level and/or toxicity

ALTERED LABORATORY VALUES

Blood/serum values	⇧ Alkaline phosphatase ⇧ Bilirubin ⇧ SGOT ⇧ SGPT ⇧ BUN + Coombs' test
Urinary values	⇧ Glucose (with Clinitest tablets)

Use in children

Adequate information is not available on the efficacy of bid regimens in children under 9 mo of age. Doses for older children should not exceed recommended adult dose; see INDICATIONS.

Use in pregnancy or nursing mothers

Safe use not established; cephradine appears in breast milk

Note: Cephradine also marketed as **VELOSEF** (Squibb).

CECLOR (Cefaclor) Lilly

Caps: 250, 500 mg **Susp:** 125 mg/5 ml, 250 mg/5 ml

INDICATIONS

Otitis media caused by susceptible strains of *Streptococcus pneumoniae, Haemophilus influenzae*, staphylococci, and *Streptococcus pyogenes*
Lower-respiratory-tract infections caused by susceptible strains of *Streptococcus pneumoniae, Haemophilus influenzae*, and *S pyogenes*
Upper-respiratory infections, including pharyngitis and tonsillitis, caused by susceptible strains of *Streptococcus pyogenes*
Urinary-tract infections, including pyelonephritis and cystitis, caused by susceptible strains of *Escherichia coli, Proteus mirabilis, Klebsiella*, and coagulase-negative staphylococci
Skin and skin-structure infections caused by *Staphylococcus aureus* and *Streptococcus pyogenes*

ORAL DOSAGE

Adult: 250 mg q8h; for more severe infections or those caused by less susceptible organisms, dose may be doubled, up to 4 g/day
Infant (≥1 mo) and child: 20 mg/kg/day in divided doses q8h; for more serious infections, otitis media, or infections caused by less susceptible organisms, 40 mg/kg/day is recommended, or up to 1 g/day, if needed

ADMINISTRATION/DOSAGE ADJUSTMENTS

Streptococcal infections	Infections caused by beta-hemolytic streptococci should be treated for at least 10 days

CONTRAINDICATIONS

Hypersensitivity to cephalosporins

WARNINGS/PRECAUTIONS

Cross-allergenicity	Use with caution in penicillin-allergic patients
Hypersensitivity	Allergic reactions may occur, most likely in patients with a history of allergy, particularly to drugs; anaphylactic reactions may require treatment with pressor amines, antihistamines, or corticosteroids
Superinfection	Overgrowth of nonsusceptible organisms may occur
Renal impairment	Patients with markedly impaired renal function should be carefully monitored during therapy, since safe dosage may be lower than that usually recommended

ADVERSE REACTIONS

Frequent reactions are italicized

Gastrointestinal	*Diarrhea (1.4%), nausea and vomiting (1.1%)*
Hypersensitivity	*Morbilliform eruptions (1.0%)*, pruritus, urticaria (see WARNINGS/PRECAUTIONS)
Other	*Eosinophilia (2.0%)*, genital pruritus, vaginitis

OVERDOSAGE

Signs and symptoms	See ADVERSE REACTIONS
Treatment	Discontinue medication; treat symptomatically and institute supportive measures, as required

DRUG INTERACTIONS

Probenecid	⇧ Cefaclor blood level and/or toxicity

ALTERED LABORATORY VALUES

Blood/serum values	⇧ Alkaline phosphatase ⇧ SGOT ⇧ SGPT ⇧ BUN
Urinary values	⇧ Glucose (with Clinitest tablets)

Use in children

See INDICATIONS; safe use not established in infants under 1 mo of age

Use in pregnancy or nursing mothers

Safe use not established; general guidelines not established for use in nursing mothers

CEFADYL (Cephapirin sodium) Bristol

Vials: 1, 2 g **Piggyback units:** 1, 2, 4 g **Hospital bulk package:** 20 g

INDICATIONS

Respiratory-tract infections caused by susceptible strains of *Streptococcus pneumoniae, Staphylococcus aureus, Klebsiella, Haemophilus influenzae,* and Group A beta-hemolytic streptococci
Skin and soft-tissue infections caused by susceptible strains of *Staphylococcus aureus, Escherichia coli, Proteus mirabilis, Klebsiella,* and Group A beta-hemolytic streptococci
Urinary-tract infections caused by susceptible strains of *Staphylococcus aureus, Escherichia coli, Proteus mirabilis,* and *Klebsiella*
Septicemia caused by susceptible strains of *Staphylococcus aureus, viridans*-type streptococci, *Escherichia coli, Klebsiella,* and Group A beta-hemolytic streptococci
Endocarditis caused by susceptible strains of *viridans*-type streptococci and *Staphylococcus aureus*
Osteomyelitis caused by susceptible strains of *Staphylococcus aureus, Klebsiella, Proteus mirabilis,* and Group A beta-hemolytic streptococci

PARENTERAL DOSAGE

Adult: 500 mg to 1 g IM or IV q4–6h; very serious or life-threatening infections may require up to 12 g/day, preferably IV if high doses are indicated. The IV route may also be preferable for patients with bacteremia, septicemia, or other severe or life-threatening infections who may be poor risks because of lowered resistance resulting, eg, from malnutrition, trauma, surgery, diabetes, heart failure, or malignancy, particularly if shock is present or imminent.
Infant (≥3 mo) and child: 40–80 mg/kg/day IM or IV in 4 equally divided doses

ADMINISTRATION/DOSAGE ADJUSTMENTS

Intramuscular administration	Dilute contents of 1-g vial in 2 ml of Sterile (or Bacteriostatic) Water for Injection and inject required dose deeply into the muscle mass
Intermittent intravenous infusion	For intermittent use, dilute contents of 1- or 2-g vial in 10 ml or more of diluent and inject required dose slowly over a period of 3–5 min; when administering cephapirin through a Y-type administration set, temporarily discontinue infusion of bulk IV solution
Streptococcal infections	Treatment of infections caused by beta-hemolytic streptococci should be continued for at least 10 days
Patients with renal impairment	Administer 7.5–15 mg/kg IM or IV q12h when serum creatinine level >5 mg/dl or moderately severe oliguria is present; patients with severe renal impairment who are to be dialyzed should receive the same dose immediately prior to dialysis and q12h thereafter

CONTRAINDICATIONS

Hypersensitivity to cephalosporins

WARNINGS/PRECAUTIONS

Cross-allergenicity	Use with great caution in penicillin-allergic patients
Hypersensitivity	Serious anaphylactoid reactions may occur (most likely in patients with a history of allergy, particularly to drugs), necessitating immediate emergency treatment with epinephrine, oxygen, intravenous steroids, and airway management, including intubation
Superinfection	Overgrowth of nonsusceptible organisms may occur
Renal impairment	Patients with impaired renal function should be carefully monitored during therapy (see ADMINISTRATION/DOSAGE ADJUSTMENTS)

Table continued on following page

CEFADYL continued

ADVERSE REACTIONS

Hypersensitivity	Maculopapular rash, urticaria, serum-sickness-like reactions, drug fever, eosinophilia, anaphylaxis (see WARNINGS/PRECAUTIONS)
Hematological	Neutropenia, leukopenia, anemia

OVERDOSAGE

Signs and symptoms	See ADVERSE REACTIONS
Treatment	Discontinue medication; treat symptomatically and institute supportive measures, as required

DRUG INTERACTIONS

Probenecid	⇧ Cephapirin blood level and/or toxicity

ALTERED LABORATORY VALUES

Blood/serum values	⇧ BUN ⇧ SGOT ⇧ SGPT + Coombs' test
Urinary values	⇧ Glucose (with Clinitest tablets)

Use in children

See INDICATIONS; safe use not established in children under 3 mo of age

Use in pregnancy or nursing mothers

Safe use not established during pregnancy; general guidelines not established for use in nursing mothers

DURICEF (Cefadroxil monohydrate) Mead Johnson

Caps: 500 mg

INDICATIONS	ORAL DOSAGE
Urinary-tract infections caused by susceptible strains of *Escherichia coli, Proteus mirabilis,* and *Klebsiella*	**Adult:** for uncomplicated lower urinary-tract infections (cystitis), 1-2 g/day in a single daily dose or div (bid); for all other urinary-tract infections: 1 g bid
Skin and skin-structure infections caused by susceptible strains of staphylococci and/or streptococci	**Adult:** 1 g/day in a single daily dose or div (bid)
Pharyngitis caused by Group A beta-hemolytic streptococci	**Adult:** 500 mg bid for 10 days

ADMINISTRATION/DOSAGE ADJUSTMENTS

Culture and susceptibility tests	Should be initiated prior to and during therapy
Patients with renal impairment	Administer 1 g to start, followed by 500 mg q12h when creatinine clearance rate (CCr)=25-50 ml/min; 500 mg q24h when CCr=10-25 ml/min; or 500 mg q36h when CCr≤10 ml/min
Nausea	May be diminished by administration with food

CONTRAINDICATIONS

Hypersensitivity to cephalosporins

WARNINGS/PRECAUTIONS

Cross-allergenicity	Use with caution in penicillin-allergic patients
Hypersensitivity	Serious anaphylactic reactions may occur, most likely in patients with a history of allergy, necessitating administration of epinephrine or pressor amines, antihistamines, or corticosteroids
Superinfection	Overgrowth of nonsusceptible organisms may occur
Renal impairment	Patients with markedly impaired renal function (CCr<50 ml/min) should be carefully monitored prior to and during therapy (see ADMINISTRATION/DOSAGE ADJUSTMENTS)

ADVERSE REACTIONS	Frequent reactions are italicized
Gastrointestinal	*Nausea*, diarrhea
Hypersensitivity	Rash, urticaria, angioedema
Genitourinary	Dysuria, genital pruritus, genital moniliasis, vaginitis
Other	Moderate transient neutropenia

OVERDOSAGE

Signs and symptoms	See ADVERSE REACTIONS
Treatment	Discontinue medication; treat symptomatically; institute supportive measures, as required

DRUG INTERACTIONS

Probenecid	⇧ Cefadroxil blood level and/or toxicity

ALTERED LABORATORY VALUES

Blood/serum values	⇧ Alkaline phosphatase ⇧ SGOT ⇧ SGPT + Coombs' test
Urinary values	⇧ Glucose (with Clinitest tablets)

Use in children

Safe use not established

Use in pregnancy or nursing mothers

Safe use not established; general guidelines not established for use in nursing mothers

KEFLEX (Cephalexin) Lilly

Caps: 250, 500 mg **Tabs:** 1 g **Oral susp:** 125 mg/5 ml, 250 mg/5 ml after reconstitution
Pediatric drops: 100 mg/ml after reconstitution

INDICATIONS	ORAL DOSAGE
Respiratory-tract infections caused by susceptible strains of *Streptococcus pneumoniae* and Group A beta-hemolytic streptococci **Skin and soft-tissue infections** caused by susceptible strains of staphylococci and/or streptococci **Bone infections** caused by susceptible strains of staphylococci and/or *Proteus mirabilis* **Genitourinary-tract infections** caused by susceptible strains of *Escherichia coli, Proteus mirabilis,* and *Klebsiella*	**Adult:** 1–4 g/day div (usual dosage, 250 mg q6h); if greater dosage is required, parenteral cephalosporin therapy should be considered **Infant and child:** 25–50 mg/kg/day in 4 divided doses; for severe infections, 50–100 mg/kg/day in 4 divided doses
Otitis media caused by susceptible strains of *Streptococcus pneumoniae, Haemophilus influenzae,* staphylococci, streptococci, and *Neisseria catarrhalis*	**Infant and child:** 75–100 mg/kg/day in 4 divided doses

ADMINISTRATION/DOSAGE ADJUSTMENTS

Streptococcal infection — All infections caused by beta-hemolytic streptococci should be treated for at least 10 days

CONTRAINDICATIONS

Hypersensitivity to cephalosporins

WARNINGS/PRECAUTIONS

Cross-allergenicity — Use with caution in penicillin-allergic patients

Hypersensitivity — Serious anaphylactic reactions may occur, most likely in patients with a history of allergy, necessitating administration of epinephrine, pressor amines, antihistamines, or corticosteroids

Superinfection — Overgrowth of nonsusceptible organisms may occur

Renal impairment — Patients with markedly impaired renal function should be carefully monitored during therapy, as lower than usual dosage may be required

ADVERSE REACTIONS

Frequent reactions are italicized

Gastrointestinal — *Diarrhea,* nausea, vomiting, dyspepsia, abdominal pain

Hypersensitivity — Rash, urticaria, angioedema, anaphylaxis

Genitourinary — Genital and anal pruritus, genital moniliasis, vaginitis, vaginal discharge

Central nervous system — Dizziness, fatigue, headache

Hematological — Eosinophilia, neutropenia

OVERDOSAGE

Signs and symptoms — See ADVERSE REACTIONS

Treatment — Discontinue medication; treat symptomatically and institute supportive measures, as required

DRUG INTERACTIONS

Probenecid — ⇧ Cephalexin blood level and/or toxicity

ALTERED LABORATORY VALUES

Blood/serum values — ⇧ Alkaline phosphatase ⇧ SGOT ⇧ SGPT + Coombs' test

Urinary values — ⇧ Glucose (with Clinitest tablets)

Use in children	**Use in pregnancy or nursing mothers**
See INDICATIONS	Safe use not established; general guidelines not established for use in nursing mothers

KEFLIN (Cephalothin sodium) Lilly

Vials: 1 g (10, 100 ml), 2 g (20, 100 ml), 4 g (50 ml), 20 g (200 ml)

INDICATIONS	PARENTERAL DOSAGE
Respiratory-tract infections caused by susceptible strains of *Streptococcus pneumoniae*, staphylococci, Group A beta-hemolytic streptococci, *Klebsiella*, and *Haemophilus influenzae* **Skin and soft-tissue infections,** including peritonitis, caused by susceptible strains of staphylococci, Group A beta-hemolytic streptococci, *Escherichia coli, Proteus mirabilis,* and *Klebsiella* **Genitourinary-tract infections** caused by susceptible strains of *Escherichia coli, Proteus mirabilis,* and *Klebsiella* **Septicemia,** including endocarditis, caused by susceptible strains of *Streptococcus pneumoniae,* staphylococci, Group A beta-hemolytic streptococci, *viridans*-type streptococci, *Escherichia coli, Proteus mirabilis,* and *Klebsiella* **Gastrointestinal infections** caused by susceptible strains of *Salmonella* and *Shigella* **Bone and joint infections** caused by susceptible strains of staphylococci **Meningitis** caused by susceptible strains of *Streptococcus pneumoniae,* Group A beta-hemolytic streptococci, and staphylococci[1]	**Adult: 500 mg to 1 g IM or IV q4–6h; for uncomplicated pneumonia, furunculosis with** cellulitis, and most urinary-tract infections, 500 mg q6h; in life-threatening infections, up to 2 g IM or IV q4h may be required. The IV route may be preferable for patients with bacteremia, septicemia, or other severe or life-threatening infections who may be poor risks because of lowered resistance resulting, eg, from malnutrition, trauma, surgery, diabetes, heart failure, or malignancy, particularly if shock is present or imminent. **Infant and child:** 80–160 mg/kg/day div IM or IV
Prevention of postoperative infection in patients undergoing contaminated or potentially contaminated procedures or when infection at the operative site would present a serious risk	**Adult:** 1–2 g IV ½–1 h prior to initial incision; repeat dose during surgery and q6h postoperatively for 24 h **Child:** 20–30 mg/kg IV, following the same schedule as in adults

ADMINISTRATION/DOSAGE ADJUSTMENTS

Patients with renal impairment	Administer 1–2 g IV to start, followed by up to 2 g q6h when creatinine clearance rate (CCr)=50–80 ml/min; 1.5 g q6h when CCr=25–50 ml/min; 1 g q6h when CCr=10–25 ml/min; 0.5 g q6h when CCr=2–10 ml/min; 0.5 g q8h when CCr< 2 ml/min
Intraperitoneal procedures	During peritoneal dialysis, up to 6 mg cephalothin per 100 ml of dialysis fluid may be instilled into the peritoneal space for 16–30 h; intraperitoneal administration of 0.1–4.0% cephalothin in saline may be used to treat peritonitis or a contaminated peritoneal cavity (the amount given should be considered in the total daily dose)
Streptococcal infections	All infections caused by beta-hemolytic streptococci should be treated for at least 10 days
Intramuscular administration	Dilute 1 g of cephalothin with 4 ml of Sterile Water for Injection and inject required dose into a large muscle mass, eg, the gluteus or lateral aspect of the thigh
Intermittent intravenous infusion	For intermittent use, dilute 1 g of cephalothin in 10 ml of diluent and slowly inject required dose directly into vein over a period of 3–5 min or administer through IV tubing; when administering cephalothin through a Y-type administration set, temporarily discontinue infusion of bulk IV solution
Continuous intravenous infusion	Dilute 1 or 2 g of cephalothin with 10 ml or more of Sterile Water for Injection and add to IV bottle containing compatible solution

CONTRAINDICATIONS

Hypersensitivity to cephalosporins

[1]Because only low levels of cephalothin appear in cerebrospinal fluid, the drug is not reliable in the treatment of meningitis and may be considered only for unusual circumstances in which more reliable antibiotics cannot be used

Table continued on following page

KEFLIN continued

WARNINGS/PRECAUTIONS

Cross-allergenicity	Use with caution in penicillin-allergic patients
Hypersensitivity	Serious anaphylactic reactions may occur, most likely in patients with a history of allergy, particularly to drugs, necessitating administration of epinephrine or pressor amines, antihistamines, or corticosteroids
Superinfection	Overgrowth of nonsusceptible organisms may occur
Renal impairment	Patients with impaired renal function should be carefully monitored during therapy; usual doses in such patients can result in excessive serum concentrations (see ADMINISTRATION/DOSAGE ADJUSTMENTS)
Thrombophlebitis	May occur, particularly when IV doses >6 g/day are given by infusion for periods of more than 3 days; small IV needles and larger veins should be used, and the veins may need to be alternated. The addition of 10–25 mg hydrocortisone to IV solutions of 4–6 g of cephalothin may reduce the incidence of thrombophlebitis.

ADVERSE REACTIONS

Hypersensitivity	Maculopapular rash, urticaria, serum-sickness-like reactions, anaphylaxis, drug fever, eosinophilia
Hematological	Neutropenia, thrombocytopenia, hemolytic anemia
Other	Pain, induration, tenderness, and elevated temperature with repeated IM injection; thrombophlebitis (see WARNINGS/PRECAUTIONS)

OVERDOSAGE

Signs and symptoms	See ADVERSE REACTIONS
Treatment	Discontinue medication; treat symptomatically and institute supportive measures, as required

DRUG INTERACTIONS

Aminoglycosides, ethacrynic acid, furosemide, polymyxin antibiotics	⇧ Risk of nephrotoxicity
Probenecid	⇧ Cephalothin blood level and/or toxicity

ALTERED LABORATORY VALUES

Blood/serum values	⇧ Alkaline phosphatase ⇧ BUN ⇧ SGOT ⇧ SGPT + Coombs' test
Urinary values	⇧ Glucose (with Clinitest tablets) ⇩ Creatinine clearance

Use in children

Dosage should be adjusted according to age, weight, and severity of infection; see INDICATIONS

Use in pregnancy or nursing mothers

Safe use not established; general guidelines not established for use in nursing mothers

MANDOL (Cefamandole nafate) **Lilly**

Vials: 500 mg (10 ml), 1 g (10, 100 ml), 2 g (20, 200 ml)

INDICATIONS	PARENTERAL DOSAGE
Lower-respiratory-tract infections caused by susceptible strains of *Streptococcus pneumoniae, Haemophilus influenzae, Klebsiella, Staphylococcus aureus,* beta-hemolytic streptococci, and *Proteus mirabilis* **Peritonitis** caused by susceptible strains of *Escherichia coli* and *Enterobacter* **Septicemia** caused by susceptible strains of *Escherichia coli, Staphylococcus aureus, Streptococcus pneumoniae, Streptococcus pyogenes, Haemophilus influenzae,* and *Klebsiella* **Skin and skin-structure infections** caused by susceptible strains of *Staphylococcus aureus, Streptococcus pyogenes, Haemophilus influenzae, Escherichia coli, Enterobacter,* and *Proteus mirabilis* **Bone and joint infections** caused by susceptible strains of *Staphylococcus aureus*	**Adult:** for skin-structure infections and uncomplicated pneumonia, 500 mg IM or IV q6h; for other or more serious infections, 500 mg to 1 g IM or IV q4–8h; for severe infections, 1 g IM or IV q4–6h; for life-threatening or resistant infections caused by less susceptible organisms, up to 2 g IM or IV q4h may be needed. The IV route may be preferable for patients with septicemia, localized parenchymal abscesses (eg, intra-abdominal abscess), peritonitis, or other severe or life-threatening infections who may be poor risks because of lowered resistance. **Infant (≥6 mo) and child:** 50–100 mg/kg/day IM or IV in equally divided doses q4–8h; for severe infections, up to 150 mg/kg/day IM or IV in equally divided doses q4–8h may be needed
Urinary-tract infections caused by susceptible strains of *Escherichia coli, Proteus, Enterobacter, Klebsiella,* Group D streptococci, and *Streptococcus epidermidis*	**Adult:** for uncomplicated infections, 500 mg IM or IV q8h; for more serious infections, 1 g IM or IV q8h **Infant (≥6 mo) and child:** Same as child dosage above.

ADMINISTRATION/DOSAGE ADJUSTMENTS

Duration of therapy	Treatment should be continued for at least 48–72 h after patient has become asymptomatic or bacteria have been eradicated. Infections caused by beta-hemolytic streptococci should be treated for at least 10 days to guard against the risk of rheumatic fever or glomerulonephritis. Persistent infections may require treatment for several weeks.
Intramuscular injection	Dilute 1 g of cefamandole with 3 ml of Sterile (or Bacteriostatic) Water for Injection, 0.9% sodium chloride, or Bacteriostatic Sodium Chloride Injection and inject required dose deeply into a large muscle mass (eg, the gluteus or lateral aspect of the thigh) to minimize pain
Intermittent intravenous infusion	For intermittent use, dilute 1 g of cefamandole with 10 ml of Sterile Water for Injection, 0.9% sodium chloride, or 5% dextrose and slowly inject required dose directly into a vein or administer through IV tubing; when administering cefamandole through a Y-type administration set, temporarily discontinue infusion of bulk IV solution
Continuous intravenous infusion	Dilute 1 g of cefamandole with 10 ml of Sterile Water for Injection and add to IV bottle containing compatible solution; do not mix an aminoglycoside with cefamandole in the same container
Patients with renal impairment and life-threatening infections	Administer 1–2 g IM or IV to start, followed by 2 g q4h when creatinine clearance rate (CCr)>80 ml/min; 1.5 g q4h or 2 g q6h when CCr=50–80 ml/min; 1.5 g q6h or 2 g q8h when CCr=25–50 ml/min; 1 g q6h or 1.25 g q8h when CCr=10–25 ml/min; 0.67 g q8h or 1 g q12h when CCr=2–10 ml/min; 0.5 g q8h or 0.75 g q12h when CCr<2 ml/min. Creatinine clearance may be calculated from the serum creatinine concentration by use of the following formula: CCr (in males)=[patient's weight *(kg)*×(146 – patient's age)]/[72×creatinine concentration *(mg/dl)*]; for females, multiply the value obtained by this formula by 0.9.

Table continued on following page

ADMINISTRATION/DOSAGE ADJUSTMENTS continued

Patients with renal impairment and less severe infections	Administer 1-2 g IM or IV to start, followed by 1-2 g q6h when creatinine clearance rate (CCr)>80 ml/min; 0.75-1.5 g q6h when CCr=50-80 ml/min; 0.75-1.5 g q8h when CCr=25-50 ml/min; 0.5-1 g q8h when CCr=10-25 ml/min; 0.5-0.75 g q12h when CCr= 2-10 ml/min; 0.25-0.5 g q12h when CCr<2 ml/min. Creatinine clearance may be calculated from the serum creatinine concentration by use of the formula given above.
Chronic urinary-tract infection	Frequent bacteriological and clinical appraisal is necessary during therapy and may be required for several weeks afterward

CONTRAINDICATIONS

Hypersensitivity to cephalosporins

WARNINGS/PRECAUTIONS

Cross-allergenicity	Use with caution in penicillin-allergic patients
Hypersensitivity	Serious acute hypersensitivity reactions may occur, especially in patients with a history of allergy (particularly to drugs), and may necessitate use of epinephrine and other emergency measures
Superinfection	Overgrowth of nonsusceptible organisms may occur
Renal impairment	Patients with impaired renal function should be carefully monitored during therapy and should receive a reduced dosage determined by degree of impairment, severity of infection, and susceptibility of organism (see ADMINISTRATION/DOSAGE ADJUSTMENTS)
Hypoprothrombinemia	May occur rarely, with or without bleeding, particularly in the elderly, debilitated, or otherwise compromised patients with vitamin K deficiencies; may be reversed by administration of vitamin K. Prophylactic administration of vitamin K may be indicated in such patients, especially prior to bowel preparation and/or surgery.

ADVERSE REACTIONS

Hypersensitivity	Maculopapular rash, urticaria, eosinophilia, drug fever
Hematological	Neutropenia (especially with prolonged use), thrombocytopenia (rare)
Other	Pain on IM injection, thrombophlebitis (rare)

OVERDOSAGE

Signs and symptoms	See ADVERSE REACTIONS
Treatment	Discontinue use of drug; treat symptomatically and institute supportive measures, as required

DRUG INTERACTIONS

Aminoglycoside antibiotics	⇧ Risk of nephrotoxicity

ALTERED LABORATORY VALUES

Blood/serum values	⇧ Alkaline phosphatase ⇧ BUN ⇧ Creatinine ⇧ SGOT ⇧ SGPT + Coombs' test
Urinary values	⇧ Glucose (with Clinitest tablets) ⇩ Creatinine clearance

Use in children

Safe use not established in children under 6 mo; for older children, total dose should not exceed maximum adult daily dose (see INDICATIONS)

Use in pregnancy or nursing mothers

Safe use not established during pregnancy; general guidelines not established for use in nursing mothers

MEFOXIN (Cefoxitin sodium) Merck Sharp & Dohme

Vials, infusion bottles: 1, 2 g

INDICATIONS	PARENTERAL DOSAGE
Lower-respiratory-tract infections, including pneumonia and lung abscess, caused by susceptible strains of *Streptococcus pneumoniae*, other streptococci (excluding enterococci), *Staphylococcus aureus, Escherichia coli, Klebsiella, Haemophilus influenzae*, and *Bacteroides* **Urinary-tract infections** caused by susceptible strains of *Escherichia coli, Klebsiella, Proteus mirabilis*, indole-positive *Proteus*, and *Providencia* **Intra-abdominal infections,** including peritonitis and intra-abdominal abscess, caused by susceptible strains of *Escherichia coli, Klebsiella, Bacteroides*, and *Clostridium* **Gynecological infections,** including endometritis, pelvic cellulitis, and pelvic inflammatory disease, caused by susceptible strains of *Escherichia coli, Neisseria gonorrhoeae, Bacteroides, Clostridium, Peptococcus, Peptostreptococcus*, and Group B streptococci **Septicemia** caused by susceptible strains of *Streptococcus pneumoniae, Staphylococcus aureus, Escherichia coli, Klebsiella*, and *Bacteroides* **Bone and joint infections** caused by susceptible strains of *Staphylococcus aureus* **Skin and skin-structure infections** caused by susceptible strains of *Staphylococcus aureus, S epidermidis*, streptococci (excluding enterococci), *Escherichia coli, Proteus mirabilis, Klebsiella, Bacteroides, Clostridium, Peptococcus*, and *Peptostreptococcus*	**Adult:** for uncomplicated infections in which bacteremia is absent or unlikely, 1 g IM or IV q6–8h; for moderately severe to severe infections, 1 g IV q4h or 2 g IV q6–8h; for infections commonly requiring high-dose antibiotic therapy, 2 g IV q4h or 3 g IV q6h. The IV route is preferable for patients who may be poor risks because of lowered resistance resulting, eg, from malnutrition, trauma, surgery, diabetes, heart failure, or malignancy, particularly if shock is present or imminent. **Infant (>3 mo) and child:** 80–160 mg/kg/day, up to 12 g/day, IM or IV in 4–6 equally divided doses
Uncomplicated gonorrhea caused by *Neisseria gonorrhoeae*	**Adult:** 2 g IM (with 1 g probenecid orally 0–30 min before injection)

ADMINISTRATION/DOSAGE ADJUSTMENTS

Intramuscular administration	Dilute 1 g of cefoxitin with 2 ml of Sterile Water for Injection (or, to minimize injection pain, with 2 ml of 0.5% lidocaine) and inject required dose well within the body of a relatively large muscle, such as the gluteus maximus
Intermittent intravenous administration	For intermittent use, dilute 1–2 g of cefoxitin with 10 ml of Sterile Water for Injection and inject required dose slowly over a period of 3–5 min, or administer over longer periods through IV tubing, temporarily discontinuing the administration of any other IV solutions being given at the same site
Continuous intravenous infusion	For administration of higher doses by continuous infusion, cefoxitin may be added to an IV bottle containing 5% dextrose, 0.9% sodium chloride, 5% dextrose and 0.9% sodium chloride, or 5% dextrose with 0.02% sodium bicarbonate; do not mix an aminoglycoside with cefoxitin in the same container
Streptococcal infection	Infections caused by Group A beta-hemolytic streptococci should be treated for at least 10 days to guard against the risk of rheumatic fever or glomerulonephritis

Table continued on following page

MEFOXIN continued

ADMINISTRATION/DOSAGE ADJUSTMENTS continued

Patients with renal impairment	Administer an initial loading dose of 1-2 g, followed by 1-2 g q8-12h when creatinine clearance rate (CCr)=30-50 ml/min; 1-2 g q12-24h when CCr=10-29 ml/min; 0.5-1 g q12-24h when CCr=5-9 ml/min; 0.5-1 g q24-48h when CCr<5 ml/min. Creatinine clearance may be calculated from the serum creatinine concentration by use of the following formula: CCr (in males)=[patient's weight (*kg*)×(140 − patient's age)]/[72×creatinine concentration (*mg/dl*)]; for females, multiply the value obtained by this formula by 0.85.
Patients undergoing hemodialysis	Administer 1-2 g after each dialysis treatment and adjust maintenance dosage according to renal impairment schedule

CONTRAINDICATIONS

Hypersensitivity to cefoxitin or other cephalosporins

WARNINGS/PRECAUTIONS

Cross-allergenicity	Use with caution in penicillin-allergic patients
Hypersensitivity	Serious hypersensitivity reactions may occur, especially in patients with a history of allergy (particularly to drugs), and may require the use of epinephrine and/or other emergency measures
Superinfection	Overgrowth of nonsusceptible organisms may occur
Renal insufficiency	Adjust dosage in patients with a transient or persistent reduction in urinary output due to impaired renal function, since usual dosage can produce high, prolonged serum concentrations in such individuals (see ADMINISTRATION/DOSAGE ADJUSTMENTS)

ADVERSE REACTIONS

Hypersensitivity	Rash, pruritus, eosinophilia, fever, other reactions
Gastrointestinal	Nausea, vomiting, diarrhea
Hematological	Transient eosinophilia, leukopenia, neutropenia, and hemolytic anemia
Other	Pain, induration, and tenderness at site of IM injection; thrombophlebitis with IV administration

OVERDOSAGE

Signs and symptoms	See ADVERSE REACTIONS
Treatment	Discontinue medication; treat symptomatically and institute supportive measures, as required

DRUG INTERACTIONS

Aminoglycoside antibiotics	⇧ Risk of nephrotoxicity

ALTERED LABORATORY VALUES

Blood/serum values	⇧ Alkaline phosphatase ⇧ SGOT ⇧ SGPT ⇧ Lactate dehydrogenase ⇧ BUN ⇧ Creatinine (with Jaffe reaction) + Coombs' test
Urinary values	⇧ Creatinine (with Jaffe reaction) ⇧ Glucose (with Clinitest tablets)

Use in children

See INDICATIONS; safety and efficacy have not been established in infants from birth to 3 mo of age. In children 3 mo of age and older, doses higher than those recommended are associated with an increased incidence of eosinophilia and elevation in SGOT.

Use in pregnancy or nursing mothers

Safe use not established during pregnancy; cefoxitin appears in breast milk in low concentrations

AMOXIL (Amoxicillin) Beecham

Caps: 250, 500 mg **Susp:** 125 mg/5 ml, 250 mg/5 ml after reconstitution **Pediatric drops:** 50 mg/ml after reconstitution

INDICATIONS	ORAL DOSAGE
Ear, nose, and throat infections caused by susceptible strains of streptococci, *Streptococcus pneumoniae*, nonpenicillinase-producing staphylococci, and *Haemophilus influenzae* **Genitourinary-tract infections** caused by susceptible strains of *Escherichia coli, Proteus mirabilis*, and *Streptococcus faecalis* **Skin and soft-tissue infections** caused by susceptible strains of streptococci, staphylococci, and *Escherichia coli*	**Adult:** 250 mg q8h; for severe infections, 500 mg q8h **Infant: (<6 kg):** 25 mg (0.5 ml) q8h **Infant (6-8 kg):** 50 mg (1 ml) q8h **Child (<20 kg):** 20 mg/kg/day in divided doses q8h; for severe infections, 40 mg/kg/day in divided doses q8h **Child (≥20 kg):** same as adult
Lower-respiratory-tract infections caused by susceptible strains of streptococci, *Streptococcus pneumoniae*, nonpenicillinase-producing staphylococci, and *Haemophilus influenzae*	**Adult:** 500 mg q8h **Infant (<6 kg):** 50 mg (1 ml) q8h **Infant (6-8 kg):** 100 mg (2 ml) q8h **Child (<20 kg):** 40 mg/kg/day in divided doses q8h **Child (≥20 kg):** same as adult
Gonorrhea, acute uncomplicated anogenital and urethral infections caused by *Neisseria gonorrhoeae*	**Adult:** 3 g in a single dose

ADMINISTRATION/DOSAGE ADJUSTMENTS

Duration of treatment	Continue treatment for at least 48-72 h after patient has become asymptomatic or bacteria have been eradicated; beta-hemolytic streptococcal infections should be treated for at least 10 days to prevent rheumatic fever and glomerulonephritis
Use of oral suspension in children	After reconstitution; place required dose directly on child's tongue for swallowing or add to formula, milk, fruit juice, water, ginger ale, or cold drinks; infants weighing 8 kg (18 lb) or less should be given pediatric drops

CONTRAINDICATIONS

Hypersensitivity to penicillins

WARNINGS/PRECAUTIONS

Hypersensitivity	Serious and occasionally fatal anaphylactoid reactions may occur, most likely in patients with a history of sensitivity to multiple allergens. Urticaria, other skin rashes, and serum sickness-like reactions may be controlled with antihistamines and, if necessary, systemic corticosteroids. Drug should be discontinued unless infection is life-threatening and amenable only to amoxicillin. Severe reactions may require emergency measures, such as immediate use of epinephrine, oxygen, IV corticosteroids, and airway management, including intubation; use with caution in patients who have experienced allergic reactions to cephalosporins.
Long-term therapy	Perform blood, renal, and hepatic studies periodically
Superinfection	Overgrowth of nonsusceptible organisms, including fungi, may occur
Venereal disease	If syphilis is suspected, perform dark-field examination before instituting therapy and perform serology testing monthly for at least 4 mo
Chronic urinary-tract infection	Requires frequent bacteriological and clinical appraisal during therapy, and possibly for several months afterward; do not use doses smaller than those recommended above

ADVERSE REACTIONS

Gastrointestinal	Nausea, vomiting, diarrhea
Hypersensitivity	Erythematous maculopapular rash, urticaria
Hematological	Anemia, thrombocytopenia, thrombocytopenic purpura, eosinophilia, leukopenia, agranulocytosis

OVERDOSAGE

Signs and symptoms	See ADVERSE REACTIONS
Treatment	Discontinue medication; treat symptomatically

Table continued on following page

AMOXIL continued

DRUG INTERACTIONS

Probenecid ——————— ⇧ Amoxicillin blood level and/or toxicity

ALTERED LABORATORY VALUES

Blood/serum values ——————— ⇧ SGOT

No clinically significant alterations in urinary values occur at therapeutic dosages

Use in children	**Use in pregnancy or nursing mothers**
See INDICATIONS; do not exceed adult dose	Safe use not established during pregnancy; general guidelines not established for use in nursing mothers

Note: Amoxicillin also marketed as **LAROTID** (Roche); **POLYMOX** (Bristol); and **TRIMOX** (Squibb).

BICILLIN L-A (Penicillin G benzathine) Wyeth

Vials: 300,000 units/ml (10 ml) **Cartridge-needle units:** 600,000 units/ml (1, 1.5, 2 ml) **Syringes:** 600,000 units/ml (2, 4 ml)

INDICATIONS	PARENTERAL DOSAGE
Mild to moderate nonbacteremic upper-respiratory-tract infections caused by Group A streptococci	**Adult:** 1.2 million units IM in a single dose **Infant:** 300,000-600,000 units IM in a single dose **Child (<60 lb):** 300,000-600,000 units IM in a single dose **Child (>60 lb):** 900,000 units IM in a single dose
Primary, secondary, and latent syphilis	**Adult:** 2.4 million units IM in a single dose
Tertiary syphilis and neurosyphilis	**Adult:** 2.4 million units IM at 7-day intervals for 3 doses
Congenital syphilis	**Infant (<2 yr): 50,000 units/kg IM** **Child (2-12 yr):** adjust dosage according to adult schedule
Yaws, bejel, and pinta	**Adult:** 1.2 million units IM in a single dose
Prophylaxis for rheumatic fever, chorea, rheumatic heart disease, and acute glomerulonephritis	**Adult: 1.2 million units IM once a month or 600,000 units IM every 2 wk following an acute** attack

ADMINISTRATION/DOSAGE ADJUSTMENTS

Duration of treatment for streptococcal infections	Therapy must be sufficient to eliminate the organism and prevent sequelae of streptococcal disease; cultures should be performed at completion of treatment
Intramuscular injection	Inject deeply into the upper outer quadrant of the buttock (adults) or midlateral aspect of the thigh (infants and small children); care should be taken to avoid IV or intra-arterial administration or injection into or near major peripheral nerves or blood vessels

CONTRAINDICATIONS

Hypersensitivity to penicillins

WARNINGS/PRECAUTIONS

Hypersensitivity	Serious and occasionally fatal anaphylactoid reactions may occur, most likely in patients with a history of sensitivity to multiple allergens; use with caution in patients who have experienced allergic reactions to cephalosporins. If an allergic reaction occurs, discontinue medication and employ pressor amines, antihistamines, and corticosteroids, as needed.
Superinfection	Overgrowth of nonsusceptible organisms, including fungi, may occur

ADVERSE REACTIONS

Hypersensitivity	Skin eruptions ranging from maculopapular rash to exfoliative dermatitis, urticaria, and other serum sickness-like reactions; fever; eosinophilia; laryngeal edema; anaphylaxis (see WARNINGS/PRECAUTIONS)
Hematological	Hemolytic anemia, leukopenia, and thrombocytopenia (with high parenteral doses)
Other	Jarisch-Herxheimer reaction (with syphilis treatment); neuropathy and nephropathy (with high parenteral doses)

OVERDOSAGE

Signs and symptoms	See ADVERSE REACTIONS
Treatment	Discontinue medication; treat symptomatically

DRUG INTERACTIONS

Probenecid	⇧ Penicillin blood level and/or toxicity

ALTERED LABORATORY VALUES

No clinically significant alterations in blood/serum or urinary values occur at therapeutic dosages

Use in children	Use in pregnancy or nursing mothers
See INDICATIONS	General guidelines not established

CYCLAPEN-W (Cyclacillin) Wyeth

Tabs: 250, 500 mg **Susp:** 125 mg/5 ml, 250 mg/5 ml

INDICATIONS	ORAL DOSAGE
Tonsillitis and pharyngitis caused by susceptible strains of Group A beta-hemolytic streptococci	**Adult:** 250 mg qid in equally spaced doses **Child (<20 kg):** 125 mg qid in equally spaced doses **Child (>20 kg):** same as adult
Mild or moderate bronchitis and pneumonia caused by susceptible strains of *Streptococcus pneumoniae*	**Adult:** 250 mg qid in equally spaced doses **Child:** 50 mg/kg/day in 4 equally spaced doses
Otitis media caused by susceptible strains of *Streptococcus pneumoniae* and *Haemophilus influenzae* **Skin and skin-structure infections** caused by susceptible strains of Group A beta-hemolytic streptococci and nonpenicillinase-producing staphylococci	**Adult:** 250–500 mg qid in equally spaced doses, depending on severity **Child:** 50–100 mg/kg/day in 4 equally spaced doses, depending on severity
Acute exacerbations of chronic bronchitis caused by susceptible strains of *Haemophilus influenzae*	**Adult:** 500 mg qid in equally spaced doses **Child:** 100 mg/kg/day in 4 equally spaced doses
Urinary-tract infections caused by susceptible strains of *Escherichia coli* and *Proteus mirabilis* **Chronic bronchitis and pneumonia** caused by susceptible strains of *Streptococcus pneumoniae*	**Adult:** 500 mg qid in equally spaced doses **Child:** 100 mg/kg/day in 4 equally spaced doses

ADMINISTRATION/DOSAGE ADJUSTMENTS

Cultures and susceptibility tests	Should be initiated prior to therapy and performed periodically during treatment to monitor its effectiveness and bacterial susceptibility
Duration of treatment	Continue treatment for at least 48–72 h after patient has become asymptomatic or bacteria have been eradicated; beta-hemolytic streptococcal infections should be treated for at least 10 days to prevent rheumatic fever and glomerulonephritis
Patients with renal impairment	Administer full doses q12h when creatinine clearance rate (CCr)=30–50 ml/min, q18h when CCr=15–30 ml/min, q24h when CCr=10–15 ml/min; if CCr≤10 ml/min or serum creatinine level ≥10 mg/dl, determine dosage and frequency by serum drug levels

CONTRAINDICATIONS

Hypersensitivity to penicillins

WARNINGS/PRECAUTIONS

Hypersensitivity	Serious and occasionally fatal anaphylactoid reactions may occur, most likely in patients with a history of sensitivity to multiple allergens, necessitating immediate emergency treatment with epinephrine, oxygen, IV corticosteroids, and airway management, including intubation; use with caution in patients who have experienced allergic reactions to cephalosporins
Superinfection	Overgrowth of nonsusceptible organisms may occur
Chronic urinary-tract infection	Requires frequent bacteriological and clinical appraisal during therapy, and possibly for several months afterward

ADVERSE REACTIONS

Frequent reactions are italicized

Gastrointestinal	*Diarrhea (5%), nausea and vomiting (2%),* abdominal pain
Hypersensitivity	*Skin rash (1.7%),* urticaria
Hematological	Anemia, thrombocytopenia, thrombocytopenic purpura, leukopenia, neutropenia, eosinophilia
Central nervous system	Headache, dizziness
Other	Vaginitis

Table continued on following page

CYCLAPEN-W continued

OVERDOSAGE

Signs and symptoms — See ADVERSE REACTIONS

Treatment — Discontinue medication; treat symptomatically

DRUG INTERACTIONS

No clinically significant drug interactions have been observed

ALTERED LABORATORY VALUES

Blood/serum values — ⇧ SGOT

No clinically significant alterations in urinary values occur at therapeutic dosages

Use in children

See INDICATIONS; do not exceed adult dose or use in children under 2 mo of age

Use in pregnancy or nursing mothers

Safe use not established. Drug may or may not be excreted in breast milk; use with caution if patient is nursing.

GEOCILLIN (Carbenicillin indanyl sodium) Roerig

Tabs: equiv to 382 mg carbenicillin

INDICATIONS	ORAL DOSAGE
Urinary-tract infections and asymptomatic bacteriuria caused by susceptible strains of *Escherichia coli, Proteus mirabilis, P morgani, P rettgeri, P vulgaris,* and *Enterobacter*	**Adult:** 1–2 tabs qid
Urinary-tract infections caused by susceptible strains of *Pseudomonas* and *Streptococcus faecalis* **Prostatitis** caused by susceptible strains of *Escherichia coli, Proteus mirabilis, Enterobacter,* and *Streptococcus faecalis*	**Adult:** 2 tabs qid

CONTRAINDICATIONS

Hypersensitivity to penicillins

WARNINGS/PRECAUTIONS

Hypersensitivity	Serious and occasionally fatal anaphylactoid reactions may occur, most likely in patients with a history of sensitivity to multiple allergens, and may necessitate immediate emergency treatment with epinephrine, oxygen, IV corticosteroids, and airway management, including intubation; use with caution in patients who have experienced allergic reactions to cephalosporins
Long-term therapy	Perform blood, renal, and hepatic studies periodically
Superinfection	Overgrowth of nonsusceptible organisms may occur
Renal impairment	Patients with severe impairment (creatinine clearance <10 ml/min) will not achieve therapeutic urine levels of carbenicillin

ADVERSE REACTIONS

Gastrointestinal	Nausea, vomiting, diarrhea, flatulence, dry mouth, furry tongue, abdominal cramps
Hypersensitivity	Skin rash, urticaria, pruritus
Hematological	Anemia, thrombocytopenia, leukopenia, neutropenia, eosinophilia
Other	Vaginitis

OVERDOSAGE

Signs and symptoms	See ADVERSE REACTIONS
Treatment	Discontinue medication; treat symptomatically

DRUG INTERACTIONS

Probenecid	⇧ Carbenicillin blood level and/or toxicity ⇩ Urine level

ALTERED LABORATORY VALUES

Blood/serum values	⇧ SGOT ⇧ SGPT

No clinically significant alterations in urinary values occur at therapeutic dosages

Use in children	Use in pregnancy or nursing mothers
Safe use not established	Safe use not established during pregnancy; general guidelines not established for use in nursing mothers

GEOPEN (Carbenicillin disodium) Roerig

Vials: 1, 2, 5 g **Piggyback units:** 2, 5, 10 g **Bulk pharmacy package:** 30 g

INDICATIONS	PARENTERAL DOSAGE
Urinary-tract infections caused by susceptible strains of *Pseudomonas aeruginosa, Enterobacter,* and *Streptococcus faecalis*	**Adult:** for uncomplicated infections, 1–2 g IM or IV q6h; for serious infections, 200 mg/kg/day by IV drip **Child:** 50–200 mg/kg/day IM or IV in divided doses q4–6h
Urinary-tract infections caused by susceptible strains of *Proteus* and *Escherichia coli*	**Adult:** Same as adult dosage above. **Child:** 50–100 mg/kg/day IM or IV in divided doses q4–6h
Severe systemic infections, septicemia, and **respiratory and soft-tissue infections** caused by susceptible strains of *Pseudomonas aeruginosa* and anaerobic bacteria	**Adult:** 400–500 mg/kg/day IV in divided doses or by continuous infusion **Child:** same as adult
Severe systemic infections, septicemia, and respiratory and soft-tissue infections caused by susceptible strains of *Proteus* and *Escherichia coli*	**Adult:** 300–400 mg/kg/day IV in divided doses or by continuous infusion **Child:** 300–400 mg/kg/day IM or IV in divided doses
Meningitis caused by susceptible strains of *Haemophilus influenzae* and *Streptococcus pneumoniae*	**Adult:** 400–500 mg/kg/day IV in divided doses or by continuous infusion **Child:** same as adult
Gonorrhea, acute uncomplicated anogenital and urethral infections caused by susceptible strains of *Neisseria gonorrhoeae*	**Adult:** 4 g in a single IM injection divided between two sites (with 1 g probenecid orally 30 min prior to injection)
Neonatal sepsis caused by susceptible strains of *Pseudomonas aeruginosa, Proteus, Escherichia coli, Haemophilus influenzae,* and *Streptococcus pneumoniae*	**Infant (<2 kg):** 100 mg/kg IM or IV to start; followed by 75 mg/kg IM or IV q8h during 1st wk of life and 100 mg/kg IM or IV q6h thereafter[1] **Infant (>2 kg):** 100 mg/kg IM or IV to start, followed by 75 mg/kg IM or IV q6h during first 3 days of life and 100 mg/kg IM or IV q6h thereafter[1]

ADMINISTRATION/DOSAGE ADJUSTMENTS

Intravenous infusion	Administer as slowly as possible to avoid vein irritation; to reduce irritation further, dilute to approximately 1 g/20 ml or more
Intramuscular administration	Inject not more than 2 g at once, well within the body of a relatively large muscle
Serious urinary-tract and systemic infections	**Intravenous therapy in higher doses (up to 40 g/day) may be required**
Patients with renal impairment	Administer 2 g IV q8–12h to adults with a creatinine clearance rate <5 ml/min
Dialysis patients	Administer 2 g IV q6h to adults during peritoneal dialysis or 2 g IV q4h to adults receiving hemodialysis

CONTRAINDICATIONS

Hypersensitivity to penicillins

WARNINGS/PRECAUTIONS

Hypersensitivity	Serious and occasionally fatal anaphylactoid reactions may occur, most likely in patients with a history of sensitivity to multiple allergens; use with caution in patients who have experienced allergic reactions to cephalosporins. If an allergic reaction occurs, institute appropriate therapy and consider discontinuing carbenicillin. Serious reactions may require emergency treatment with epinephrine, oxygen, and IV corticosteroids.
Long-term therapy	Perform blood, renal, and hepatic studies periodically
Superinfection	**May result from emergence of resistant organisms, such as *Klebsiella* and *Serratia***
Bleeding abnormalities	May occur in patients with renal impairment; discontinue use of carbenicillin and institute appropriate therapy

[1] Neonatal doses may be given IM or by 15-min IV infusion

Table continued on following page

GEOPEN continued

WARNINGS/PRECAUTIONS continued

Sodium overload	May occur (each gram contains 4.7 mEq of sodium); monitor electrolytes and cardiac status periodically in patients who require sodium restriction (eg, cardiac patients)
Hypokalemia	May occur with high doses; monitor serum potassium level periodically, and institute appropriate corrective measures, as needed
Venereal disease	If syphilis is suspected, perform dark-field examination before instituting therapy, and perform serology testing monthly for at least 4 mo

ADVERSE REACTIONS

Hypersensitivity	Skin rash, pruritus, urticaria, drug fever, anaphylaxis (see WARNINGS/PRECAUTIONS)
Gastrointestinal	Nausea
Hematological	Anemia, thrombocytopenia, leukopenia, neutropenia, eosinophilia
Central nervous system	Convulsions or neuromuscular irritability (with excessively high serum levels)
Other	Pain and (rarely) induration at injection site after IM and IV administration; vein irritation and phlebitis

OVERDOSAGE

Signs and symptoms	See ADVERSE REACTIONS
Treatment	Discontinue medication; treat symptomatically

DRUG INTERACTIONS

Probenecid	⇧ Carbenicillin blood level and/or toxicity ⇩ Urine level

ALTERED LABORATORY VALUES

Blood/serum values	⇧ SGOT ⇧ SGPT

No clinically significant alterations in urinary values occur at therapeutic dosages

Use in children

See INDICATIONS

Use in pregnancy or nursing mothers

Safe use not established during pregnancy; general guidelines not established for use in nursing mothers

PENTIDS (Penicillin G potassium) Squibb

Tabs: 125 mg (Pentids), 250 mg (Pentids 400), 500 mg (Pentids 800)
Syrup: 125 mg/5 ml after reconstitution (Pentids), 250 mg/5 ml after reconstitution (Pentids 400)

INDICATIONS	ORAL DOSAGE
Mild to moderately severe upper-respiratory-tract infections, skin infections, soft-tissue infections, scarlet fever, and erysipelas caused by penicillin G-sensitive streptococci in the absence of bacteremia	**Adult:** for mild infections, 125 mg tid or qid for 10 days; for moderately severe infections, 250 mg tid or 500 mg bid for 10 days **Child (< 12 yr):** 15-56 mg/kg/day in 3-6 divided doses
Otitis media and other mild to moderately severe upper-respiratory-tract infections caused by penicillin G-sensitive *Streptococcus pneumoniae*	**Adult:** 250 mg qid until patient has been afebrile for at least 2 days **Child (<12 yr):** 15-56 mg/kg/day in 3-6 divided doses
Mild skin and soft-tissue infections caused by penicillin G-sensitive staphylococci	**Adult:** 125-250 mg tid or qid until infection is cured **Child (<12 yr):** 15-56 mg/kg/day in 3-6 divided doses
Fusospirochetosis (Vincent's gingivitis and pharyngitis)	**Adult:** 250 mg tid or qid **Child (<12 yr):** 15-56 mg/kg/day in 3-6 divided doses
Continuous prophylaxis to prevent recurrence of rheumatic fever and/or chorea	**Adult:** 125 mg bid
Short-term prophylaxis to prevent bacterial endocarditis in the presence of congenital or rheumatic heart lesions **Short-term prophylaxis to prevent bacteremia following tooth extraction**	**Adult:** 750 mg 1 h prior to dental procedure or minor upper-respiratory-tract surgery or instrumentation, followed by 375 mg q6h for at least 3 days

ADMINISTRATION/DOSAGE ADJUSTMENTS

Timing of administration	**Administer ½h before or at least 2 h after meals to assure maximum absorption**
Duration of treatment for streptococcal infections	Therapy should be continued for a minimum of 10 days to prevent sequelae of streptococcal disease; cultures should be taken on completion of therapy to determine whether streptococci have been eradicated
Patients receiving prophylactic penicillin	**May harbor increased numbers of penicillin-resistant organisms; if penicillin will be used at the time or surgery, interrupt regular program 1 wk before procedure**

CONTRAINDICATIONS

Hypersensitivity to penicillins

WARNINGS/PRECAUTIONS

Hypersensitivity	Serious and occasionally fatal anaphylactoid reactions may occur, most likely in patients with a history of sensitivity to multiple allergens. Urticaria, other skin rashes, and serum sickness-like reactions may be controlled with antihistamines and, if necessary, systemic corticosteroids. Drug should be discontinued unless infection is life-threatening and amenable only to penicillin. Severe reactions may necessitate emergency measures, such as immediate use of epinephrine, aminophylline, oxygen, and IV corticosteroids; use with caution in patients who have experienced allergic reactions to cephalosporins.
Long-term therapy	Perform blood, renal, and hepatic studies periodically, particularly with high-dosage schedules
Superinfection	Overgrowth of nonsusceptible organisms, including fungi, may occur
Impaired absorption	Oral administration should not be relied on in patients with severe illness, nausea, vomiting, gastric dilatation, cardiospasm, or intestinal hypermotility (see also ADMINISTRATION/DOSAGE ADJUSTMENTS)

Table continued on following page

WARNINGS/PRECAUTIONS continued

Tartrazine sensitivity	Presence of FD&C Yellow No. 5 (tartrazine) in 500-mg tablets and both syrup formulations may cause allergic-type reactions, including bronchial asthma, in susceptible individuals
Inappropriate indications	Oral penicillin G should not be used for treatment during the acute stages of severe pneumonia, empyema, bacteremia, pericarditis, meningitis, or septic arthritis, or for prophylaxis preceding genitourinary instrumentation or surgery, lower-intestinal-tract surgery, sigmoidoscopy, or childbirth

ADVERSE REACTIONS — Frequent reactions are italicized

Gastrointestinal	*Nausea, vomiting, epigastric distress, diarrhea, black hairy tongue,* sore mouth or tongue
Hypersensitivity	Skin rashes ranging from maculopapular rashes to exfoliative dermatitis, urticaria, serum sickness-like reactions (including chills, fever, edema, arthralgia, and prostration), eosinophilia, laryngeal edema, anaphylaxis (see WARNINGS/PRECAUTIONS)
Hematological	Hemolytic anemia, leukopenia, thrombocytopenia
Other	Neuropathy and nephropathy (usually only with high-dosage parenteral therapy)

OVERDOSAGE

Signs and symptoms	See ADVERSE REACTIONS
Treatment	Discontinue medication; treat symptomatically

DRUG INTERACTIONS

Probenecid	⇧ Penicillin blood level and/or toxicity

ALTERED LABORATORY VALUES

No clinically significant alterations in blood/serum or urinary values occur at therapeutic dosages

Use in children

See INDICATIONS

Use in pregnancy or nursing mothers

General guidelines not established

PEN•VEE K (Penicillin V potassium) Wyeth

Tabs: 125, 250, 500 mg **Sol:** 125, 250 mg/5 ml after reconstitution

INDICATIONS	ORAL DOSAGE
Mild to moderately severe upper-respiratory-tract infections, scarlet fever, and erysipelas caused by penicillin G-sensitive streptococci in the absence of bacteremia	**Adult:** 125–250 mg q6–8h for 10 days
Otitis media and other mild to moderately severe respiratory-tract infections caused by penicillin G-sensitive *Streptococcus pneumoniae*	**Adult:** 250–500 mg q6h until patient has been afebrile for at least 2 days
Mild skin and soft-tissue infections caused by penicillin G-sensitive staphylococci **Fusospirochetosis** (Vincent's gingivitis and pharyngitis)	**Adult:** 250–500 mg q6–8h
Continuous prophylaxis to prevent recurrence of rheumatic fever and/or chorea	**Adult:** 125–250 mg bid
Short-term prophylaxis to prevent bacterial endocarditis in the presence of congenital and/or rheumatic heart lesions	**Adult:** 2 g 30 min to 1 h prior to dental procedure or minor upper-respiratory-tract surgery or instrumentation, followed by 500 mg q6h for 8 doses **Child (<60 lb):** use ½ the adult dose **Child (≥60 lb):** same as adult

ADMINISTRATION/DOSAGE ADJUSTMENTS

Duration of treatment for streptococcal infections	Therapy should be continued for a minimum of 10 days to prevent sequelae of streptococcal disease; cultures should be taken on completion of therapy to determine whether streptococci have been eradicated
Patients receiving prophylactic penicillin	May harbor increased numbers or penicillin-resistant organisms; if penicillin is intended for prophylactic use at the time of surgery, interrupt regular program 1 wk before procedure

CONTRAINDICATIONS

Hypersensitivity to penicillins

WARNINGS/PRECAUTIONS

Hypersensitivity	Serious and occasionally fatal anaphylactoid reactions may occur, most likely in patients with a history of sensitivity to multiple allergens; use with caution in patients who have experienced allergic reactions to cephalosporins. If an allergic reaction occurs, discontinue medication and employ epinephrine, antihistamines, and/or corticosteroids, as needed.
Superinfection	Overgrowth of nonsusceptible organisms, including fungi, may occur
Impaired absorption	Oral administration should not be relied on in patients with severe illness, nausea, vomiting, gastric dilatation, cardiospasm, or intestinal hypermotility
Inappropriate indications	Oral penicillin V should not be used for treatment during the acute stages of severe **pneumonia, empyema, bacteremia, pericarditis, meningitis, or septic arthritis, or for** prophylaxis preceding genitourinary instrumentation or surgery, lower intestinal-tract surgery, sigmoidoscopy, or childbirth

ADVERSE REACTIONS

Gastrointestinal	Nausea, vomiting, epigastric distress, diarrhea, black hairy tongue
Hypersensitivity	Skin eruptions ranging from maculopapular rash to exfoliative dermatitis, urticaria, and other serum sickness-like reactions; fever; eosinophilia; laryngeal edema; anaphylaxis (see WARNINGS/PRECAUTIONS)
Hematological	Hemolytic anemia, leukopenia, thrombocytopenia
Other	Neuropathy and nephropathy (usually only with high-dosage parenteral therapy)

Table continued on following page

OVERDOSAGE

Signs and symptoms — See ADVERSE REACTIONS

Treatment — Discontinue medication; treat symptomatically

DRUG INTERACTIONS

Probenecid — ⇧ Penicillin blood level and/or toxicity

ALTERED LABORATORY VALUES

No clinically significant alterations in blood/serum or urinary values occur at therapeutic dosages

Use in children

See INDICATIONS

Use in pregnancy or nursing mothers

General guidelines not established

Note: Penicillin V potassium also marketed as **V-CILLIN K** (Lilly); **BETAPEN-VK** (Bristol); **ROBICILLIN VK** (Robins); **SK-PENICILLIN VK** (Smith Kline & French); **UTICILLIN VK** (Upjohn); and **VEETIDS** (Squibb).

POLYCILLIN (Ampicillin) Bristol

Caps: 250, 500 mg **Susp:** 125 mg/5 ml, 250 mg/5 ml, 500 mg/5 ml after reconstitution **Pediatric drops:** 100 mg/ml

POLYCILLIN-N (Ampicillin sodium) Bristol

Vials: 125, 250, 500 mg; 1, 2 g **Piggyback units:** 500 mg; 1, 2 g **Hospital bulk package:** 10 g

INDICATIONS	ORAL DOSAGE	PARENTERAL DOSAGE
Respiratory-tract and soft-tissue infections caused by susceptible strains of *Haemophilus influenzae*, penicillin G-sensitive staphylococci, streptococci, and *Streptococcus pneumoniae*	**Adult:** 250 mg q6h **Child (<20 kg):** 50 mg/kg/day in equally divided doses q6-8h **Child (≥20 kg):** same as adult	**Adult:** 250-500 mg IM or IV q6h **Child (<40 kg):** 25-50 mg/kg/day IM or IV in equally divided doses q6-8h **Child (≥40 kg):** same as adult
Gastrointestinal- and genitourinary-tract infections caused by susceptible strains of *Shigella*, *Salmonella* (including *S typhosa*), *Escherichia coli*, *Proteus mirabilis*, enterococci, and *Neisseria gonorrhoeae* (in females)	**Adult:** 500 mg q6h; for stubborn or severe infections, higher doses may be needed, possibly for several weeks **Child (<20 kg):** 100 mg/kg/day in equally divided doses q6-8h; for stubborn or severe infections, higher doses may be needed, possibly for several weeks **Child (≥20 kg):** same as adult	**Adult:** 500 mg IM or IV q6h; for stubborn or severe infections, higher doses may be needed, possibly for several weeks **Child (<40 kg):** 50 mg/kg/day IM or IV q6-8h; for stubborn or severe infections, higher doses may be needed, possibly for several weeks **Child (≥40 kg):** same as adult
Urethritis caused by *Neisseria gonorrhoeae*	**Adult:** 3.5 g given simultaneously with 1 g probenecid	—
Urethritis in males caused by *Neisseria gonorrhoeae*	—	**Adult:** 500 mg IM or IV q8-12h for 2 doses; may be repeated or extended, if necessary
Bacterial meningitis caused by susceptible strains of *Neisseria meningitidis* and *Haemophilus influenzae* **Septicemia** caused by susceptible strains of Gram-positive and Gram-negative bacteria	—	**Adult:** 150-200 mg/kg/day in equally divided doses q3-4h, beginning by slow IV infusion (for a minimum of 3 days in treating septicemia) and followed by IM injection q3-4h **Child:** same as adult

ADMINISTRATION/DOSAGE ADJUSTMENTS

Duration of treatment	Continue treatment for at least 48-72 h after patient becomes asymptomatic or bacteria have been eradicated; beta-hemolytic streptococcal infections should be treated for at least 10 days to prevent rheumatic fever and glomerulonephritis

CONTRAINDICATIONS

Hypersensitivity to penicillins

WARNINGS/PRECAUTIONS

Hypersensitivity	Serious and occasionally fatal anaphylactoid reactions may occur, most likely in patients with a history of sensitivity to multiple allergens. Urticaria, other skin rashes, and serum sickness-like reactions may be controlled with antihistamines and, if necessary, systemic corticosteroids. Drug should be discontinued unless infection is life-threatening and amenable only to ampicillin. Severe reactions may necessitate emergency measures, such as immediate use of epinephrine, oxygen, IV corticosteroids, and airway management, including intubation; use with caution in patients who have experienced allergic reactions to cephalosporins.
Long-term therapy	Perform blood, renal, and hepatic studies periodically
Superinfection	Overgrowth of nonsusceptible organisms, including fungi, may occur
Venereal disease	If syphilis is suspected, perform dark-field examination before instituting therapy, and perform serology testing monthly for at least 4 mo
Chronic urinary-tract and intestinal infections	Require frequent bacteriological and clinical appraisal during therapy and possibly for several months afterward
Complications of gonorrheal urethritis, such as prostatitis and epididymitis	Prolonged and intensive therapy is recommended
Inappropriate indications	Ampicillin should not be used for the treatment of infectious mononucleosis; a high percentage of patients with mononucleosis develop a skin rash after receiving ampicillin

Table continued on following page

ADVERSE REACTIONS	Frequent reactions are italicized
Gastrointestinal	Glossitis, stomatitis, black hairy tongue, nausea, vomiting, enterocolitis, pseudomembranous colitis, diarrhea
Hypersensitivity	*Skin rash, urticaria,* exfoliative dermatitis, erythema multiforme, anaphylaxis (see WARNINGS/PRECAUTIONS)
Hematological	Anemia, thrombocytopenia, thrombocytopenic purpura, eosinophilia, leukopenia, agranulocytosis
OVERDOSAGE	
Signs and symptoms	See ADVERSE REACTIONS
Treatment	Discontinue medication; treat symptomatically
DRUG INTERACTIONS	
Probenecid	⇧ Ampicillin blood level and/or toxicity
ALTERED LABORATORY VALUES	
Blood/serum values	⇧ SGOT (especially in infants)
Urinary values	⇧ Glucose (with Clinitest tablets)

Use in children	**Use in pregnancy or nursing mothers**
See INDICATIONS; do not exceed adult dose	Safe use not established during pregnancy; general guidelines not established for use in nursing mothers

Note: Ampicillin also marketed as **AMCILL** (Parke-Davis); **OMNIPEN** (Wyeth); **PRINCIPEN** (Squibb); and **SK-AMPICILLIN** (Smith Kline & French). Ampicillin sodium also marketed as **PRINCIPEN/N** (Squibb); **TOTACILLIN** and **TOTACILLIN-N** (Beecham).

PROSTAPHLIN (Oxacillin sodium) Bristol

Caps: 250, 500 mg **Sol:** 250 mg/5 ml after reconstitution **Vials:** 250, 500 mg; 1, 2, 4 g **Piggyback units:** 1, 2, 4 g
Bulk pharmacy package: 10 g

INDICATIONS	ORAL DOSAGE	PARENTERAL DOSAGE
Mild to moderate upper-respiratory and localized skin and soft-tissue infections caused by susceptible strains of penicillinase-producing staphylococci[1]	**Adult:** 500 mg q4–6h for at least 5 days **Child: (<40 kg):** 50 mg/kg/day in equally divided doses q6h for at least 5 days **Child (≥40 kg):** same as adult	**Adult:** 250–500 mg IM or IV q4–6h **Premature and neonatal infants:** 25 mg/kg/day div IM or IV **Child (<40 kg):** 50 mg/kg/day IM or IV in equally divided doses q6h **Child (≥40 kg):** same as adult
Severe lower-respiratory-tract infections or disseminated infections caused by susceptible strains of penicillinase-producing staphylococci	—	**Adult:** 1 g or more IM or IV q4–6h, followed by 1 g orally q4–6h **Child (<40 kg):** 100 mg/kg/day IM or IV or more in equally divided doses q4–6h, followed by 100 mg/kg/day or more orally in equally divided doses q4–6h **Child (≥ 40 kg):** same as adult

ADMINISTRATION/DOSAGE ADJUSTMENTS

Duration of treatment	Continue treatment of serious systemic infections for at least 1–2 wk after fever has subsided and cultures are sterile; very severe infections may require very high doses and prolonged therapy, and osteomyelitis may require several months of intensive treatment. Infections caused by beta-hemolytic streptococci should be treated for at least 10 days to prevent rheumatic fever and glomerulonephritis.
Direct intravenous injection	Administer slowly over a period of approximately 10 min
Timing of oral administration	Administer 1–2 h before meals

CONTRAINDICATIONS

Hypersensitivity to penicillins

WARNINGS/PRECAUTIONS

Hypersensitivity	Serious and occasionally fatal anaphylactoid reactions may occur, most likely in patients with asthma or a history of sensitivity to multiple allergens; use caution with patients who have experienced allergic reactions to cephalosporins
Long-term therapy	Perform blood, renal, and hepatic studies periodically
Superinfection	Overgrowth of nonsusceptible organisms, including fungi, may occur
Methicillin resistance	Methicillin-resistant strains of staphylococci should be considered resistant to oxacillin as well
Impaired absorption	Oral administration should not be relied on in patients with severe illness, nausea, vomiting, gastric dilatation, cardiospasm, or intestinal hypermotility
Renal impairment	Newborns and infants receiving high doses (150–175 mg/kg/day) may develop transient hematuria, albuminuria, or azotemia and should be closely monitored

ADVERSE REACTIONS

Gastrointestinal	Glossitis, stomatitis
Hypersensitivity	Skin rashes, urticaria, serum sickness, anaphylactoid reactions, fever
Hematological	Hemolytic anemia; transient neutropenia with evidence of granulocytopenia or thrombocytopenia; eosinophilia
Renal	Oliguria, albuminuria, hematuria, pyuria, cylindruria (generally with parenteral use)
Other	Thrombophlebitis, cholestatic or nonspecific hepatitis, oral and rectal monoliasis

[1] Oxacillin sodium has been shown to be effective only in the treatment of infections caused by *Streptococcus pneumoniae*, Group A beta-hemolytic streptococci, and penicillin G-resistant and penicillin G-susceptible staphylococci

Table continued on following page

PROSTAPHLIN continued

OVERDOSAGE

Signs and symptoms	See ADVERSE REACTIONS
Treatment	Discontinue medication; treat symptomatically

DRUG INTERACTIONS

Probenecid	⇧ Oxacillin blood level and/or toxicity

ALTERED LABORATORY VALUES

Blood/serum values	⇧ SGOT ⇧ SGPT ⇧ BUN
Urinary values	⇧ Albumin

Use in children

See INDICATIONS; safe use in premature infants and newborns not established; frequent evaluation of organ system function is recommended in such cases (see WARNINGS/PRECAUTIONS)

Use in pregnancy or nursing mothers

Safe use not established during pregnancy; general guidelines not established for use in nursing mothers

PYOPEN (Carbenicillin disodium) Beecham

Vials: 1, 2, 5 g **Piggyback units:** 2, 5 g **Bulk pharmacy package:** 10 g

INDICATIONS	PARENTERAL DOSAGE
Urinary-tract infections caused by susceptible strains of *Pseudomonas aeruginosa, Enterobacter*, and *Streptococcus faecalis*	**Adult:** for uncomplicated infections, 1-2 g IM or IV q6h; for serious infections, 200 mg/kg/day by IV drip **Child:** 50-200 mg/kg/day IM or IV in divided doses q4-6h
Urinary-tract infections caused by susceptible strains of *Proteus* and *Escherichia coli*	**Adult:** same as above **Child:** 50-100 mg/kg/day IM or IV in divided doses q4-6h
Severe systemic infections, septicemia, and respiratory and soft-tissue infections caused by susceptible strains of *Pseudomonas aeruginosa* and anaerobic bacteria	**Adult:** 400-500 mg/kg/day IV in divided doses or by continuous infusion **Child:** same as adult
Severe systemic infections, septicemia, respiratory and soft-tissue infections caused by susceptible strains of *Proteus* and *Escherichia coli*	**Adult:** 250-400 mg/kg/day IV in divided doses or by continuous infusion **Child:** 250-400 mg/kg/day IM or IV in divided doses or by continuous infusion
Meningitis caused by susceptible strains of *Haemophilus influenzae*	**Adult:** 400-500 mg/kg/day IV in divided doses or by continuous infusion **Child:** same as adult
Gonorrhea, acute uncomplicated anogenital and urethral infections caused by susceptible strains of *Neisseria gonorrhoeae*	**Adult:** 4 g in a single IM injection divided between 2 sites (with 1 g probenecid orally 30 min prior to injection)
Neonatal sepsis caused by susceptible strains of *Pseudomonas aeruginosa, Proteus, Escherichia coli*, and *Haemophilus influenzae*	**Infant (<2 kg):** 100 mg/kg IM or IV to start, followed by 75 mg/kg IM or IV q8h during 1st wk of life and 100 mg/kg IM or IV q6h thereafter[1] **Infant (>2 kg):** 100 mg/kg IM or IV to start, followed by 75 mg/kg IM or IV q6h during first 3 days of life and 100 mg/kg IM or IV q6h thereafter[1]

ADMINISTRATION/DOSAGE ADJUSTMENTS

Intravenous infusion	Administer as slowly as possible to avoid vein irritation; to reduce irritation further, dilute to approximately 1 g/20 ml or more. Total daily dose may be given continuously or intermittently in 6 equally divided doses administered over a period of 30 min to 2 h.
Intramuscular administration	Inject not more than 2 g at once well within the body of a relatively large muscle
Serious urinary-tract and systemic infections	IV therapy in higher doses up to 40 g/day may be required
Concomitant therapy	Gentamicin may be used concomitantly with carbenicillin for initial therapy until results of cultures and susceptibility tests are known; however, the two antibiotics should not be mixed together in the same IV solution
Patients with renal impairment	For infections caused by *Pseudomonas aeruginosa, Proteus*, or *Escherichia coli*, administer 2 g IV q8h to adults with a creatinine clearance rate <5 ml/min
Dialysis patients	For infections caused by *Pseudomonas aeruginosa, Proteus*, or *Escherichia coli*, administer 2 g IV q6h to adults during peritoneal dialysis or 2 g IV q4h to adults receiving hemodialysis

CONTRAINDICATIONS

Hypersensitivity to penicillins

[1]Neonatal doses may be given IM or by 15-min IV infusion

Table continued on following page

PYOPEN continued

WARNINGS/PRECAUTIONS

Hypersensitivity	Serious and occasionally fatal anaphylactoid reactions may occur, most likely in patients with a history of sensitivity to multiple allergens. If a reaction occurs, drug should be discontinued unless infection is life-threatening and amenable only to carbenicillin. Severe reactions may necessitate immediate emergency treatment with epinephrine, oxygen, IV corticosteroids, and airway management, including intubation; use with caution in patients who have experienced allergic reactions to cephalosporins.
Long-term therapy	Perform blood, renal, and hepatic studies periodically
Superinfection	May result from emergence of resistant organisms, such as *Klebsiella* and *Serratia*
Abnormal bleeding	Hemorrhagic manifestations associated with abnormalities of coagulation tests, such as bleeding time and platelet aggregation, may develop, particularly in uremic patients receiving high doses (eg, 24 g/day); discontinue use of drug and institute appropriate therapy
Patients with renal impairment	Convulsions or neuromuscular excitability may occur when large doses are used
Sodium overload	May occur (each vial contains up to 6.5 mEq sodium/g of carbenicillin); monitor electrolyte and cardiac status carefully
Hypokalemia	May occur; monitor serum potassium level periodically and institute appropriate corrective measures, as needed
Venereal disease	If syphilis is suspected, perform dark-field examination before instituting therapy and perform serology testing monthly for at least 4 mo

ADVERSE REACTIONS

Hypersensitivity	Skin rash, eosinophilia, urticaria, pruritus, drug fever, anaphylaxis (see WARNINGS/PRECAUTIONS)
Gastrointestinal	Nausea, unpleasant taste
Hematological	Leukopenia, neutropenia, thrombocytopenia, hemolytic anemia
Central nervous system	Convulsions and neuromuscular excitability, especially with large doses in patients with renal impairment
Other	Pain and induration at IM injection site, vein irritation and phlebitis

OVERDOSAGE

Signs and symptoms	See ADVERSE REACTIONS
Treatment	Discontinue medication; treat symptomatically

DRUG INTERACTIONS

Probenecid	⇧ Carbenicillin blood level and/or toxicity ⇩ Urine level

ALTERED LABORATORY VALUES

Blood/serum values	⇧ SGOT ⇧ SGPT

No clinically significant alterations in urinary values occur at therapeutic dosages

Use in children

See INDICATIONS

Use in pregnancy or nursing mothers

Safe use not established during pregnancy; general guidelines not established for use in nursing mothers

TEGOPEN (Cloxacillin sodium) Bristol

Caps: 250, 500 mg **Sol:** 125 mg/5 ml after reconstitution

INDICATIONS	ORAL DOSAGE
Mild to moderate **upper-respiratory and localized skin and soft-tissue infections** caused by susceptible strains of penicillinase-producing staphylococci[1]	**Adult:** 250 mg q6h **Child (< 20 kg):** 50 mg/kg/day in equally divided doses q6h **Child (≥ 20 kg):** same as adult
Severe infections of the lower-respiratory tract or disseminated infections	**Adult:** 500 mg or higher q6h **Child (< 20 kg):** 100 mg/kg/day or higher in equally divided doses q6h **Child (≥ 20 kg):** same as adult

ADMINISTRATION/DOSAGE ADJUSTMENTS

Group A beta-hemolytic streptococcal infections	Should be treated for at least 10 days to prevent rheumatic fever and glomerulonephritis
Timing of administration	**Administer on an empty stomach, preferably 1–2 h before meals, to maximize absorption**

CONTRAINDICATIONS

Hypersensitivity to penicillins

WARNINGS/PRECAUTIONS

Hypersensitivity	Serious and occasionally fatal anaphylactoid reactions may occur, most likely in patients with a history of sensitivity to multiple allergens, and may require discontinuation of cloxacillin and treatment with pressor amines, antihistamines, and corticosteroids; use with caution in patients who have experienced allergic reactions to cephalosporins
Long-term therapy	**Perform blood, renal, and hepatic function studies periodically**
Superinfection	Overgrowth of nonsusceptible organisms, including fungi, may occur
Methicillin resistance	Methicillin-resistant strains of staphylococci should be considered resistant to cloxacillin as well

ADVERSE REACTIONS

Gastrointestinal	Nausea, epigastric discomfort, flatulence, loose stools
Hypersensitivity	Skin rashes, allergic symptoms (eg, wheezing and sneezing)
Hematological	Eosinophilia

OVERDOSAGE

Signs and symptoms	See ADVERSE REACTIONS
Treatment	Discontinue medication; treat symptomatically

DRUG INTERACTIONS

Probenecid	⇧ Cloxacillin blood level and/or toxicity

ALTERED LABORATORY VALUES

Blood/serum values	⇧ SGOT

No clinically significant alterations in urinary values occur at therapeutic dosages

Use in children	Use in pregnancy or nursing mothers
See INDICATIONS	Safe use not established during pregnancy; general guidelines not established for use in nursing mothers

[1]Cloxacillin has been shown to be effective only in the treatment of infections caused by *Streptococcus pneumoniae*, Group A beta-hemolytic streptococci, and penicillin G-resistant and penicillin G-susceptible staphylococci

TICAR (Ticarcillin disodium) Beecham

Vials: 1, 3, 6 g **Piggyback units:** 3, 6 g

INDICATIONS	PARENTERAL DOSAGE
Bacterial septicemia, skin and soft-tissue infections, and acute and chronic respiratory-tract infections caused by susceptible strains of *Pseudomonas aeruginosa, Proteus, Escherichia coli*, and anaerobic bacteria **Lower-respiratory-tract infections,** including empyema, anaerobic pneumonitis, and lung abscess, caused by susceptible anaerobic bacteria **Intra-abdominal infections,** including peritonitis and intra-abdominal abscess, caused by susceptible anaerobic bacteria **Female pelvic and genital-tract infections,** including endometritis, pelvic inflammatory disease, pelvic abscess, and salpingitis, caused by susceptible anaerobic bacteria	**Adult:** 200–300 mg/kg/day IV in divided doses q3, 4, or 6h, depending on severity **Child (<40 kg):** 200–300 mg/kg/day IV in divided doses q4–6h **Child (≥40 kg):** same as adult
Genitourinary-tract infections caused by susceptible strains of *Pseudomonas aeruginosa, Proteus, Escherichia coli, Enterobacter*, and *Streptococcus faecalis*	**Adult:** for uncomplicated infections, 1 g IM or IV q6h; for complicated infections, 150–200 mg/kg/day IV in divided doses q4–6h **Child (<40 kg):** for uncomplicated infections, 50–100 mg/kg/day IM or IV in divided doses q6–8h; for complicated infections, 150–200 mg/kg/day IV in divided doses q4–6h **Child (≥40 kg):** same as adult
Neonatal sepsis caused by susceptible strains of *Pseudomonas, Proteus*, and *Escherichia coli*	**Infant (<2 kg):** 100 mg/kg IM or IV to start, followed by 75 mg/kg IM or IV q8h during 1st wk of life; for infants over 7 days of age, 100 mg/kg IM or IV q4h[1] **Infant (>2 kg):** 100 mg/kg IM or IV to start, followed by 75 mg/kg IM or IV q4–6h during first 2 wk of life; for infants over 2 wk of age, 100 mg/kg IM or IV q4h[1]

ADMINISTRATION/DOSAGE ADJUSTMENTS

Intramuscular administration	Inject not more than 2 g at once, well within the body of a relatively large muscle
Intravenous infusion	Administer as slowly as possible to avoid vein irritation; to reduce irritation further, dilute to approximately 1 g/20 ml or more. Total daily dose may be given continuously or intermittently in 6 equally divided doses administered over a period of 30 min to 2 h.
Serious urinary-tract and systemic infections	Intravenous therapy in higher doses may be required
Patients with renal impairment	Administer in an initial (adult) loading dose of 3 g IV, followed by 3 g IV q4h when creatnine clearance rate (CCr)>60 ml/min; 2 g IV q4h when CCr=30-60 ml/min; 2 g IV q8h when CCr=10-30 ml/min; 2 g IV q12h or 1 g IM q6h when CCr<10 ml/min; 2 g IV q24h or 1 g IM q12h when CCr<10 ml/min and hepatic insufficiency exists
Dialysis patients	Administer 3 g IV q12h to adults during peritoneal dialysis or 3 g IV after each dialysis treatment to adults receiving hemodialysis

CONTRAINDICATIONS

Hypersensitivity to penicillins

[1]Neonatal doses may be given IM or by 10–20 min IV infusion

Table continued on following page

TICAR continued

WARNINGS/PRECAUTIONS

Hypersensitivity	Serious and occasionally fatal anaphylactoid reactions may occur, most likely in patients with a history of sensitivity to multiple allergens. If a reaction occurs, drug should be discontinued unless infection is life-threatening and amenable only to ticarcillin. Severe reactions may necessitate immediate emergency treatment with epinephrine, oxygen, IV corticosteroids, and airway management, including intubation; use with caution in patients who have experienced allergic reactions to cephalosporins.
Long-term therapy	Perform blood, renal, and hepatic studies periodically
Superinfection	Overgrowth of nonsusceptible organisms, including fungi, may occur
Abnormal bleeding	Hemorrhagic manifestations associated with abnormalities of coagulation tests, such as bleeding time and platelet aggregation, may develop, particularly in patients receiving high doses or in those with renal impairment; discontinue use of drug and institute appropriate therapy
Sodium overload	May occur (each vial contains up to 6.5 mEq sodium/g of ticarcillin); monitor electrolyte and cardiac status periodically
Hypokalemia	May occur; monitor serum potassium level periodically and institute appropriate corrective measures, as needed

ADVERSE REACTIONS

Gastrointestinal	Nausea, vomiting
Hypersensitivity	Skin rash, pruritus, urticaria, drug fever
Hematological	Anemia, thrombocytopenia, leukopenia, neutropenia, eosinophilia
Central nervous system	Convulsions and neuromuscular excitability (especially with high doses in patients with renal impairment)
Other	Pain and (rarely) induration at injection site, vein irritation, phlebitis

OVERDOSAGE

Signs and symptoms	See ADVERSE REACTIONS
Treatment	Discontinue medication; treat symptomatically

DRUG INTERACTIONS

Probenecid	⇧ Ticarcillin blood level and/or toxicity
Gentamicin, tobramycin	⇧ Bactericidal activity of both drugs against certain strains of *Pseudomonas aeruginosa* in vitro *(do not mix in same IV bottle)*

ALTERED LABORATORY VALUES

Blood/serum values	⇧ SGOT ⇧ SGPT

No clinically significant alterations in urinary values occur at therapeutic dosages

Use in children

See INDICATIONS; do not exceed adult dose

Use in pregnancy or nursing mothers

Safe use not established during pregnancy; general guidelines not established for use in nursing mothers

ACHROMYCIN (Tetracycline hydrochloride) Lederle

Vials: 100, 250 mg (for IM use); 250, 500 mg (for IV use)

ACHROMYCIN V (Tetracycline hydrochloride) Lederle

Caps: 250, 500 mg **Syrup:** 125 mg/5 ml

INDICATIONS	ORAL DOSAGE	PARENTERAL DOSAGE
Infections caused by rickettsiae, *Mycoplasma pneumoniae, Haemophilus ducreyi, Yersinia pestis, Francisella tularensis, Bartonella bacilliformis, Bacteroides, Vibrio comma,* and *Camplyobacter fetus,* as well as susceptible strains of *Escherichia coli, Enterobacter aerogenes, Shigella, Acinetobacter, Streptococcus,* and *S pneumoniae* **Respiratory infections** caused by susceptible strains of *Haemophilus influenzae* and *Klebsiella* **Urinary-tract infections** caused by susceptible strains of *Klebsiella* **Skin and soft-tissue infections** caused by susceptible strains of *Staphylococcus aureus* **Psittacosis, ornithosis** **Infections** caused by *Treponema pertenue, Listeria monocytogenes, Clostridium, Bacillus anthracis, Fusobacterium fusiforme,* and *Actinomyces* in penicillin-allergic patients **Lymphogranuloma venereum, granuloma inguinale** **Relapsing fever** **Trachoma** **Inclusion conjunctivitis** **Intestinal amebiasis** (adjunctive therapy)	**Adult:** 1-2 g/day in 2 or 4 equally divided doses, depending on the severity of the infection **Child (>8 yr):** 25-50 mg/kg in 2-4 equally divided doses	**Adult:** 250 mg IM q24h; 300 mg IM in divided doses q8-12h; or 250-500 mg IV q12h, or up to 500 mg IV q6h, if needed **Child (>8 yr):** 15-25 mg/kg IM, up to 250 mg/day, in a single daily dose or divided doses q8-12h; or 10-20 mg/kg/day IV, depending on the severity of the infection (usual dosage, 6 mg/kg bid)
Severe acne (adjunctive therapy)	**Adult:** Same as adult dosage above.	—
Infections caused by *Neisseria gonorrhoeae* in penicillin-allergic patients	**Adult:** 1.5 g to start, followed by 0.5 g q6h for 4 days for a total of 9 g	**Adult:** Same as adult dosage above.
Syphilis	**Adult:** 30-40 g in equally divided doses over a period of 10-15 days	—
Brucellosis	**Adult:** 500 mg qid for 3 wk (with 1 g streptomycin IM bid 1st wk and qd 2nd wk)	—

ADMINISTRATION/DOSAGE ADJUSTMENTS

Duration of treatment	Unless otherwise indicated, continue treatment for at least 24-48 h after symptoms and fever have subsided; infections caused by Group A beta-hemolytic streptococci should be treated for at least 10 days. If patient is started on parenteral therapy, institute oral therapy as soon as possible.
Intramuscular administration	Reserve for situations in which oral therapy is not feasible. Add 2 ml of Sterile Water for Injection or Sodium Chloride Injection to 100- or 250-mg vial, withdraw required dose, and inject deeply into a large muscle mass, such as the gluteus. IM administration produces lower blood levels than oral administration at recommended dosages.
Intravenous administration	Use only when rapidly attained, high blood levels are needed and oral therapy is not adequate or tolerated. Prolonged IV administration may cause thrombophlebitis. Avoid rapid administration and solutions containing calcium, as these tend to form precipitates with tetracyclines; however, Ringer's or lactated Ringer's solution may be used with caution.
Timing of oral administration	Food and some dairy products interfere with absorption; give oral forms 1 h before or 2 h after meals. In treating infants, administer syrup 1 h before feeding; do not add to milk formulas

CONTRAINDICATIONS

Hypersensitivity to tetracyclines

Table continued on following page

ACHROMYCIN/ACHROMYCIN V continued

WARNINGS/PRECAUTIONS	
Renal impairment	Usual doses may lead to excessive drug accumulation and possible hepatic toxicity. If impairment is significant, azotemia, hyperphosphatemia, and acidosis may occur due to antianabolic action of drug. Reduce dosage by lowering individual doses and/or lengthening interval between doses, monitor kidney and liver function both before and during therapy, and follow serum tetracycline levels periodically (particularly if therapy is prolonged).
Pregnant and postpartum patients with pyelonephritis	Potentially fatal hepatic failure may occur with parenteral administration; do not allow serum level to exceed 15 μg/ml, monitor liver function frequently, and avoid concomitant use of other potentially hepatotoxic drugs
Superinfection	Overgrowth of nonsusceptible organisms, including fungi, may occur
Venereal disease	If syphilis is suspected, perform dark-field examination before instituting therapy and perform serology tests monthly for at least 4 mo
Long-term therapy	Perform hemapoietic, renal, and hepatic studies periodically
Photosensitivity (exaggerated sunburn)	May occur; caution patients likely to be exposed to direct sunlight or UV light and discontinue use of tetracycline at first sign of skin erythema

ADVERSE REACTIONS	
Gastrointestinal	Anorexia, nausea, vomiting, diarrhea, glossitis, dysphagia, enterocolitis, inflammatory lesions (with monilial overgrowth) in the anogenital region
Dermatological	Maculopapular and erythematous rashes, exfoliative dermatitis (rare), photosensitivity
Hypersensitivity	Urticaria, angioneurotic edema, anaphylaxis, anaphylactoid purpura, pericarditis, exacerbation of systemic lupus erythematosus
Hematological	Hemolytic anemia, thrombocytopenia, neutropenia, eosinophilia
Other	Microscopic discoloration of thyroid glands, bulging fontanels in infants, local irritation after IM injection

OVERDOSAGE	
Signs and symptoms	See ADVERSE REACTIONS
Treatment	Discontinue medication, treat symptomatically, and institute supportive measures, as required

DRUG INTERACTIONS	
Oral anticoagulants	⇧ Prothrombin time
Penicillin	⇩ Bactericidal activity of penicillin
Antacids, iron supplements	⇩ Absorption of tetracycline
Methoxyflurane	⇧ Risk of nephrotoxicity
Sodium bicarbonate	⇩ Absorption of tetracycline

ALTERED LABORATORY VALUES	
Blood/serum values	⇧ Alkaline phosphatase ⇧ BUN ⇧ Amylase ⇧ Bilirubin ⇧ SGOT ⇧ SGPT ⇩ Prothrombin activity
Urinary values	⇧ Catecholamines (with Hingerty fluorometric method)

Use in children

Not recommended for use during infancy through 8 yr of age unless other drugs are not likely to be effective or are contraindicated; use in this age group may cause permanent discoloration of teeth or enamel hypoplasia. A reversible decrease in fibula growth rate has been observed in premature infants given oral tetracycline (100 mg/kg/day).

Use in pregnancy or nursing mothers

Use during latter half of pregnancy (fetal tooth development) may cause permanent discoloration of teeth or enamel hypoplasia. Animal studies indicate that tetracyclines cross the placental barrier, are found in fetal tissues, and can cause both embryotoxicity and fetal toxicity, including retardation of skeletal development. Tetracyclines are excreted in breast milk; general guidelines not established for use in nursing mothers.

Note: Tetracycline hydrochloride also marketed as **SUMYCIN** (Squibb).

MINOCIN (Minocycline hydrochloride) Lederle

Caps: 50, 100 mg **Syrup:** 50 mg/ml **Vials:** 100 mg

INDICATIONS	ORAL DOSAGE	PARENTERAL DOSAGE
Infections caused by rickettsiae, *Mycoplasma pneumoniae, Haemophilus ducreyi, Yersinia pestis, Francisella tularensis, Bartonella bacilliformis, Bacteroides, Vibrio comma,* and *Camplyobacter fetus,* as well as susceptible strains of *Escherichia coli, Enterobacter aerogenes, Shigella, Acinetobacter, Streptococcus,* and *S pneumoniae* **Respiratory infections** caused by susceptible strains of *Haemophilus influenzae* and *Klebsiella* **Urinary-tract infections** caused by susceptible strains of *Klebsiella* **Skin and soft-tissue infections** caused by susceptible strains of *Staphylococcus aureus* **Psittacosis, ornithosis** **Infections** caused by *Treponema pertenue, Listeria monocytogenes, Clostridium, Bacillus anthracis, Fusobacterium fusiforme,* and *Actinomyces* in penicillin-allergic patients **Lymphogranuloma venereum, granuloma inguinale** **Relapsing fever** **Trachoma** **Inclusion conjunctivitis** **Intestinal amebiasis** (adjunctive therapy)	**Adult:** 200 mg to start, followed by 100 mg q12h, or 100–200 mg to start, followed by 50 mg qid **Child (>8 yr):** 4 mg/kg to start, followed by 2 mg/kg q12h	**Adult:** 200 mg IV to start, followed by 100 mg IV q12h, or up to 400 mg/24 h if needed **Child (>8 yr):** 4 mg/kg IV to start, followed by 2 mg/kg IV q12h
Severe acne (adjunctive therapy)	**Adult:** Same as adult dosage above.	—
Infections caused by *Neisseria meningitidis* in penicillin-allergic patients	—	**Adult:** Same as adult dosage above.
Infections caused by *Neisseria gonorrhoeae* in penicillin-allergic patients	**Adult:** 200 mg to start, followed by 100 mg q12h for a minimum of 4 days	—
Infections caused by *Mycobacterium marinum*	**Adult:** 100 mg bid for 6–8 wk	—
Syphilis	**Adult:** usual dosage, for 10–15 days	—
Brucellosis	**Adult:** usual dosage, for 3 wk (with 1 g streptomycin IM bid 1st wk and qd 2nd wk)	—
Meningococcal carrier state	**Adult:** 100 mg q12h for 5 days	—

ADMINISTRATION/DOSAGE ADJUSTMENTS

Duration of treatment	Unless otherwise indicated, continue treatment for at least 24–48 h after symptoms and fever have subsided; infections caused by Group A beta-hemolytic streptococci should be treated for at least 10 days. If patient is started on parenteral therapy, institute oral therapy as soon as possible.
Intravenous administration	Use only when rapidly attained, high blood levels are needed and oral therapy is not adequate or tolerated. Prolonged IV administration may cause thrombophlebitis. Avoid rapid administration and solutions containing calcium, as these tend to form precipitates with tetracyclines; however, Ringer's or lactated Ringer's solution may be used.
Timing of oral administration	May be administered with food or milk, if desired

CONTRAINDICATIONS

Hypersensitivity to tetracyclines

Table continued on following page

MINOCIN continued

WARNINGS/PRECAUTIONS

Renal impairment	Usual doses may lead to excessive drug accumulation and possible hepatic toxicity. If impairment is significant, azotemia, hyperphosphatemia, and acidosis may occur due to antianabolic action of drug. Reduce dosage by lowering individual doses and/or lengthening interval between doses, monitor kidney and liver function both before and during therapy, and follow serum tetracycline levels periodically (particularly if therapy is prolonged).
Pregnant and postpartum patients with pyelonephritis	Potentially fatal hepatic failure may occur with parenteral administration; do not allow serum level to exceed 15 μg/ml, monitor liver function frequently, and avoid concomitant use of other potentially hepatotoxic drugs
Superinfection	Overgrowth of nonsusceptible organisms, including fungi, may occur
Venereal disease	If syphilis is suspected, perform dark-field examination before instituting therapy and perform serology testing monthly for at least 4 mo
Long-term therapy	Perform hemapoietic, renal, and hepatic studies periodically
Photosensitivity (exaggerated sunburn)	May occur; caution patients likely to be exposed to direct sunlight or UV light and discontinue use of minocycline at first sign of skin erythema
Lightheadedness, dizziness, and/or vertigo	Performance of potentially hazardous activities may be impaired; caution patients accordingly
Thrombophlebitis	May result from prolonged IV administration; switch to oral form as soon as possible

ADVERSE REACTIONS

Gastrointestinal	Anorexia, nausea, vomiting, diarrhea, glossitis, dysphagia, enterocolitis, inflammatory lesions (with monilial overgrowth) in the anogenital region
Dermatological	Maculopapular and erythematous rashes, exfoliative dermatitis (rare), photosensitivity (rare), pigmentation of skin and mucous membranes
Hypersensitivity	Urticaria, angioneurotic edema, anaphylaxis, anaphylactoid purpura, pericarditis, exacerbation of systemic lupus erythmatosus
Hematological	Hemolytic anemia, thrombocytopenia, neutropenia, eosinophilia
Central nervous system	Lightheadedness, dizziness, vertigo
Other	Microscopic discoloration of thyroid glands, bulging fontanels in infants

OVERDOSAGE

Signs and symptoms	See ADVERSE REACTIONS
Treatment	Discontinue medication; treat symptomatically and institute supportive measures, as required

DRUG INTERACTIONS

Oral anticoagulants	⇧ Prothrombin time
Penicillin	⇩ Bactericidal activity of penicillin
Antacids, iron supplements	⇩ Absorption of minocycline
Methoxyflurane	⇧ Risk of nephrotoxicity
Sodium bicarbonate	⇩ Absorption of minocycline

ALTERED LABORATORY VALUES

Blood/serum values	⇧ Alkaline phosphatase ⇧ BUN ⇧ Amylase ⇧ Bilirubin ⇧ SGOT ⇧ SGPT ⇩ Prothrombin activity
Urinary values	⇧ Catecholamines (with Hingerty fluorometric method)

Use in children

Not recommended for use during infancy through 8 yr of age unless other drugs are not likely to be effective or are contraindicated; use in this age group may cause permanent discoloration of teeth or enamel hypoplasia. A reversible decrease in fibula growth rate has been observed in premature infants given oral tetracycline (100 mg/kg/day).

Use in pregnancy or nursing mothers

Use during latter half of pregnancy (fetal tooth development) may cause permanent discoloration of teeth or enamel hypoplasia. Animal studies indicate that tetracyclines cross the placental barrier, are found in fetal tissues, and can cause both embryotoxicity and fetal toxicity, including retardation of skeletal development. Tetracyclines are excreted in breast milk; general guidelines not established for use in nursing mothers.

MYSTECLIN-F (Tetracycline hydrochloride and amphotericin B) Squibb

Caps: 125 mg tetracycline hydrochloride and 25 mg amphotericin B; 250 mg tetracycline hydrochloride and 50 mg amphotericin B
Syrup: 125 mg tetracycline hydrochloride and 25 mg amphotericin B per 5 ml

INDICATIONS	ORAL DOSAGE
Infections caused by susceptible Gram-positive and Gram-negative bacteria, spirochetes, lymphogranuloma-psittacosis-trachoma viruses, rickettsiae, and *Entamoeba histolytica* in patients susceptible to candidal overgrowth	**Adult:** 250 mg qid; for severe infections, 500 mg qid **Child:** 10–20 mg/lb/day div, or 2.5 ml (½ tsp)/20 lb (up to 80 lb) qid
Acne vulgaris (adjunctive therapy)	**Adult:** 1 g/day div to start, followed by 125–500 mg/day after 1 wk; alternate-day or intermittent therapy may be adequate in some patients for maintenance

ADMINISTRATION/DOSAGE ADJUSTMENTS

Duration of treatment	Continue treatment of most common infections for 24–48 h after symptoms and fever subside; streptococcal infections should be treated for a full 10 days to prevent rheumatic fever and glomerulonephritis. Staphylococcal infections may require prolonged high-dose therapy.
Timing of oral administration	Food and some dairy products interfere with absorption; give 1 h before or 2 h after meals. In treating infants, administer syrup 1 h before feeding; do not add to milk formulas or other food containing calcium.

CONTRAINDICATIONS

Hypersensitivity to tetracyclines or amphotericin B

WARNINGS/PRECAUTIONS

Renal impairment	Usual doses may lead to excessive accumulation and possible liver toxicity; reduce dosage and follow serum tetracycline levels periodically (particularly if therapy is prolonged)
Superinfection	Overgrowth of nonsusceptible organisms, including fungi, may occur
Long-term therapy	Perform hemapoietic, renal, and hepatic studies periodically
Photosensitivity (exaggerated sunburn)	May occur; caution patients with a history of photosensitivity and discontinue use of the drug at first sign of skin discomfort
Sensitivity reactions	Are more likely to occur in patients with a history of allergy, asthma, hay fever, or urticaria; use with caution and discontinue use of drug if an allergic or idiosyncratic reaction occurs. Cross-sensitivity among tetracyclines is common.
Venereal disease	If syphilis is suspected, perform dark-field examination before instituting therapy and perform serology tests monthly for at least 3 mo

ADVERSE REACTIONS

Gastrointestinal	Anorexia, epigastric distress, nausea, vomiting, diarrhea, bulky loose stools, glossitis, stomatitis, dysphagia, enterocolitis, proctitis, pruritus ani, peptic ulcer, bleeding, hepatic cholestasis, black hairy tongue
Dermatological	Maculopapular and erythematous rashes, exfoliative dermatitis (rare), photosensitivity (rare), onycholysis, nail discoloration
Hypersensitivity	Urticaria, serum sickness-like reactions (fever, rash, arthralgia), angioneurotic edema, anaphylactoid shock
Hematological	Hemolytic anemia, thrombocytopenic purpura, neutropenia, eosinophilia
Other	Sore throat, hoarseness, increased intracranial pressure with bulging fontanels (in infants)

OVERDOSAGE

Signs and symptoms	See ADVERSE REACTIONS
Treatment	Discontinue medication, treat symptomatically, and institute supportive measures, as required

Table continued on following page

DRUG INTERACTIONS

Oral anticoagulants	⇧ Prothrombin time
Penicillin	⇩ Bactericidal activity of penicillin
Antacids, iron supplements	⇩ Absorption of tetracycline component
Methoxyflurane	⇧ Risk of nephrotoxicity
Sodium bicarbonate	⇩ Absorption of tetracycline component
Digitalis	⇧ Digitalis toxicity secondary to hypokalemia
Urinary alkalizers	⇧ Excretion of amphotericin B component

ALTERED LABORATORY VALUES

Blood/serum values	⇧ Alkaline phosphatase ⇧ BUN ⇧ Amylase ⇧ Bilirubin ⇧ SGOT ⇧ SGPT ⇩ Prothrombin activity
Urinary values	⇧ Catecholamines (with Hingerty fluorometric method) ⇧ Nitrogen ⇧ Sodium

Use in children

Not recommended for use during infancy through 8 yr of age unless other drugs are not likely to be effective or are contraindicated; use in this age group may cause permanent discoloration of teeth or enamel hypoplasia

Use in pregnancy or nursing mothers

Use during latter half of pregnancy (fetal tooth development) may cause permanent discoloration of teeth or enamel hypoplasia; general guidelines not established for use in nursing mothers

TERRAMYCIN (Oxytetracycline) Pfizer

Tabs: 250 mg **Caps:** 125, 250 mg **Syrup:** 125 mg/5 ml **Amps:** 100 mg/2 ml, 250 mg/2 ml (2 ml)
Syringes: 100 mg/2 ml, 250 mg/2 ml (2 ml) **Vials:** 50 mg/ml (10 ml) for IM use; 250, 500 mg (for IV use)

INDICATIONS	ORAL DOSAGE	PARENTERAL DOSAGE
Infections caused by rickettsiae, *Mycoplasma pneumoniae, Haemophilus ducreyi, Yersinia pestis, Francisella tularensis, Bartonella bacilliformis, Bacteroides, Vibrio comma, Camplyobacter fetus,* as well as susceptible strains of *Escherichia coli, Enterobacter aerogenes, Shigella, Acinetobacter, Streptococcus,* and *S pneumoniae* **Respiratory infections** caused by susceptible strains of *Haemophilus influenzae* and *Klebsiella* **Urinary-tract infections** caused by susceptible strains of *Klebsiella* **Skin and soft-tissue infections** caused by susceptible strains of *Staphylococcus aureus* **Psittacosis, ornithosis** **Infections** caused by *Treponema pertenue, Listeria monocytogenes, Clostridium, Bacillus anthracis, Fusobacterium fusiforme,* and *Actinomyces* in penicillin-allergic patients **Lymphogranuloma venereum, granuloma inguinale** **Relapsing fever** **Trachoma** **Inclusion conjunctivitis** **Intestinal amebiasis** (adjunctive therapy)	**Adult:** 2 tabs (500 mg) to start, followed by 1 tab (250 mg) q6h; for severe infections, 2-4 tabs (500-1,000 mg) q6h; caps, syrup: 1-2 g/day, depending on the severity of the infection, in 4 equally divided doses **Child (>8 yr):** 25-50 mg/kg/day in 4 equally divided doses	**Adult:** 250 mg IM q24h; 300 mg/day IM in divided doses q8-12h; or 250-500 mg IV q12h, or up to 500 mg IV q6h, if needed **Child (>8 yr):** 15-25 mg/kg/day IM, up to 250 mg/day, in a single daily dose or divided doses q8-12h; or 10-20 mg/kg/day IV, depending on the severity of the infection (usual dosage, 6 mg/kg bid)
Severe acne (adjunctive therapy)	**Adult:** Same as adult dosage above.	—
Infections caused by *Neisseria meningitidis* in penicillin-allergic patients	—	**Adult:** 250-500 mg IV q12h, or up to 500 mg IV q6h, if needed **Child:** 10-20 mg/kg/day IV, depending on the severity of the infection
Infections caused by *Neisseria gonorrhoeae* in penicillin-allergic patients	**Adult:** 1.5 g to start, followed by 500 mg qid for a total of 9 g	—
Syphilis	**Adult:** 30-40 g in equally divided divided doses over a period of 10-15 days	—
Brucellosis	**Adult:** 500 mg qid for 3 wk (with 1 g streptomycin IM bid 1st wk and qd 2nd wk)	—

ADMINISTRATION/DOSAGE ADJUSTMENTS

Duration of treatment	Unless otherwise indicated, continue treatment for at least 24-48 h after symptoms and fever have subsided; infections caused by Group A beta-hemolytic streptococci should be treated for at least 10 days. If patient is started on parenteral therapy, institute oral therapy as soon as possible.
Intramuscular administration	Reserve for situations in which oral therapy is not feasible. Inject required dose well within the body of a relatively large muscle. IM administration produces lower blood levels than oral administration at recommended dosages.
Intravenous administration	Use only when rapidly attained, high blood levels are needed and oral therapy is not adequate or tolerated. Prolonged IV administration may cause thrombophlebitis. Avoid rapid administration.
Timing of oral administration	Food and some dairy products interfere with absorption; give oral forms 1 h before or 2 h after meals. In treating infants, administer syrup 1 h before feeding; do not add to milk formulas

CONTRAINDICATIONS

Hypersensitivity to tetracyclines

Table continued on following page

TERRAMYCIN continued

WARNINGS/PRECAUTIONS	
Renal impairment	Usual doses may lead to excessive drug accumulation and possible hepatic toxicity. If impairment is significant, azotemia, hyperphosphatemia, and acidosis may occur due to antianabolic action of drug. Reduce dosage by lowering individual doses and/or lengthening interval between doses, monitor kidney and liver function both before and during therapy, and follow serum tetracycline levels periodically (particularly if therapy is prolonged).
Pregnant and postpartum patients with pyelonephritis	Potentially fatal hepatic failure may occur with parenteral administration; do not allow serum level to exceed 15 μg/ml, monitor liver function frequently, and avoid concomitant use of other potentially hepatotoxic drugs
Superinfection	Overgrowth of nonsusceptible organisms, including fungi, may occur
Venereal disease	If syphilis is suspected, perform dark-field examination before instituting therapy and perform serology testing monthly for at least 4 mo
Long-term therapy	Perform hemapoietic, renal, and hepatic studies periodically
Photosensitivity (exaggerated sunburn)	May occur; caution patients likely to be exposed to direct sunlight or UV light and discontinue use of oxytetracycline at first sign of skin erythema

ADVERSE REACTIONS	
Gastrointestinal	Anorexia, nausea, vomiting, diarrhea, glossitis, dysphagia, enterocolitis, inflammatory lesions (with monilial overgrowth) in the anogenital region
Dermatological	Maculopapular and erythematous rashes, exfoliative dermatitis (rare), photosensitivity
Hypersensitivity	Urticaria, angioneurotic edema, anaphylaxis, anaphylactoid purpura, pericaditis, exacerbation of systemic lupus erythematosus
Hematological	Hemolytic anemia, thrombocytopenia, neutropenia, eosinophilia
Other	Microscopic discoloration of thyroid glands, bulging fontanels in infants, benign intracranial hypertension in adults, local irritation after IM injection

OVERDOSAGE	
Signs and symptoms	See ADVERSE REACTIONS
Treatment	Discontinue medication; treat symptomatically and institute supportive measures, as required

DRUG INTERACTIONS	
Oral anticoagulants	⇧ Prothrombin time
Penicillin	⇩ Bactericidal activity of penicillin
Antacids, iron supplements	⇩ Absorption of oxytetracycline
Methoxyflurane	⇧ Risk of nephrotoxicity
Sodium bicarbonate	⇩ Absorption of oxytetracycline

ALTERED LABORATORY VALUES	
Blood/serum values	⇧ Alkaline phosphatase ⇧ BUN ⇧ Amylase ⇧ Bilirubin ⇧ SGOT ⇧ SGPT ⇩ Prothrombin activity
Urinary values	⇧ Catecholamines (with Hingerty fluorometric method)

Use in children

Not recommended for use during infancy through 8 yr of age unless other drugs are not likely to be effective or are contraindicated; use in this age group may cause permanent discoloration of teeth or enamel hypoplasia. A reversible decrease in fibula growth rate has been observed in premature infants given oral tetracycline (100 mg/kg/day).

Use in pregnancy or nursing mothers

Use during latter half of pregnancy (fetal tooth development) may cause permanent discoloration of teeth or enamel hypoplasia. Animal studies indicate that tetracyclines cross the placental barrier, are found in fetal tissues, and can cause both embryotoxicity and fetal toxicity, including retardation of skeletal development. Tetracyclines are excreted in breast milk; general guidelines not established for use in nursing mothers.

TETREX (Tetracycline phosphate complex) Bristol

Caps: 250, 500 mg

INDICATIONS	ORAL DOSAGE
Infections caused by rickettsiae, *Mycoplasma pneumoniae, Haemophilus ducreyi, Yersinia pestis, Francisella tularensis, Bartonella bacilliformis, Bacteroides, Vibrio comma,* and *Camplyobacter fetus,* as well as susceptible strains of *Escherichia coli, Enterobacter aerogenes, Shigella, Acinetobacter, Streptococcus,* and *S pneumoniae* **Respiratory infections** caused by susceptible strains of *Haemophilus influenzae* and *Klebsiella* **Urinary-tract infections** caused by susceptible strains of *Klebsiella* **Skin and soft-tissue infections** caused by susceptible strains of *Staphylococcus aureus* **Psittacosis, ornithosis** **Infections** caused by *Treponema pertenue, Listeria monocytogenes, Clostridium, Bacillus anthracis, Fusobacterium fusiforme,* and *Actinomyces* in penicillin-allergic patients **Lymphogranuloma venereum, granuloma inguinale** **Relapsing fever** **Trachoma** **Inclusion conjunctivitis** **Intestinal amebiasis** (adjunctive therapy)	**Adult:** 500 mg bid or 250 mg qid; for severe infections, increase dosage **Child ($>$8 yr and $\leq$40 kg):** 25 mg/kg/day in 4 equally divided doses **Child ($>$8 yr and $>$40 kg):** same as adult
Severe acne (adjunctive therapy)	**Adult:** Same as adult dosage above.
Infections caused by *Neisseria gonorrhoeae* in penicillin-allergic patients	**Adult:** 1.5 g to start, followed by 500 mg qid for a total of 9 g
Syphilis	**Adult:** 30–40 g in equally divided doses over a period of 10–15 days
Brucellosis	**Adult:** 500 mg qid for 3 wk (with 1 g streptomycin IM bid 1st wk and qd 2nd wk)

ADMINISTRATION/DOSAGE ADJUSTMENTS

Duration of treatment	Unless otherwise indicated, continue treatment for at least 24–48 h after symptoms and fever have subsided; infections caused by Group A beta-hemolytic streptococci should be treated for at least 10 days.
Timing of oral administration	Food and some dairy products interfere with absorption; give 1 h before or 2 h after meals. In treating infants, administer dose 1 h before feeding; do not add contents of capsule to milk formulas.

CONTRAINDICATIONS

Hypersensitivity to tetracyclines

WARNINGS/PRECAUTIONS

Renal impairment	Usual doses may lead to excessive drug accumulation and possible hepatic toxicity. If impairment is significant, azotemia, hyperphosphatemia, and acidosis may occur due to antianabolic action of drug. Reduce dosage by lowering individual doses and/or lengthening interval between doses and follow serum tetracycline levels periodically (particularly if therapy is prolonged).
Superinfection	Overgrowth of nonsusceptible organisms, including fungi, may occur
Venereal disease	If syphilis is suspected, perform dark-field examination before instituting therapy and perform serology testing monthly for at least 4 mo

Table continued on following page

TETREX continued

WARNINGS/PRECAUTIONS continued

Long-term therapy	Perform hemapoietic, renal, and hepatic studies periodically
Photosensitivity (exaggerated sunburn)	May occur; caution patients likely to be exposed to direct sunlight or UV light and discontinue use of tetracycline at first sign of skin erythema

ADVERSE REACTIONS

Gastrointestinal	Anorexia, nausea, vomiting, diarrhea, glossitis, dysphagia, enterocolitis, inflammatory lesions (with monilial overgrowth) in the anogenital region
Dermatological	Maculopapular and erythematous rashes, exfoliative dermatitis, photosensitivity (rare)
Hypersensitivity	Urticaria, angioneurotic edema, anaphylaxis, anaphylactoid purpura, pericarditis, exacerbation of systemic lupus erythematosus
Hematological	Hemolytic anemia, thrombocytopenia, neutropenia, eosinophilia
Other	Microscopic discoloration of thyroid glands, bulging fontanels in infants

OVERDOSAGE

Signs and symptoms	See ADVERSE REACTIONS
Treatment	Discontinue medication; treat symptomatically and institute supportive measures, as required

DRUG INTERACTIONS

Oral anticoagulants	⇧ Prothrombin time
Penicillin	⇩ Bactericidal activity of penicillin
Antacids, iron supplements	⇩ Absorption of tetracycline
Methoxyflurane	⇧ Risk of nephrotoxicity
Sodium bicarbonate	⇩ Absorption of tetracycline

ALTERED LABORATORY VALUES

Blood/serum values	⇧ Alkaline phosphatase ⇧ BUN ⇧ Amylase ⇧ Bilirubin ⇧ SGOT ⇧ SGPT ⇩ Prothrombin activity
Urinary values	⇧ Catecholamines (with Hingerty fluorometric method)

Use in children

Not recommended for use during infancy through 8 yr of age unless other drugs are likely to be effective or are contraindicated; use in this age group may cause permanent discoloration of teeth or enamel hypoplasia. A reversible decrease in fibula growth rate has been observed in premature infants given oral tetracycline (100 mg/kg/day).

Use in pregnancy or nursing mothers

Use during latter half of pregnancy (fetal tooth development) may cause permanent discoloration of teeth or enamel hypoplasia. Animal studies indicate that tetracyclines cross the placental barrier, are found in fetal tissues, and can cause both embryotoxicity and fetal toxicity, including retardation of skeletal development. Tetracyclines are excreted in breast milk; general guidelines not established for use in nursing mothers.

VIBRAMYCIN (Doxycycline) Pfizer

Caps: 50, 100 mg doxycycline hyclate **Syrup:** 50 mg doxycycline calcium/5 ml **Oral susp:** 25 mg doxycycline monohydrate/5 ml after reconstitution **Vials:** doxycycline hyclate equivalent to 100 and 200 mg doxycycline (for IV use only)

INDICATIONS	ORAL DOSAGE	PARENTERAL DOSAGE
Infections caused by rickettsiae, *Mycoplasma pneumoniae, Haemophilus ducreyi, Yersinia pestis, Francisella tularensis, Bartonella bacilliformis, Bacteroides, Vibrio comma,* and *Camplyobacter fetus,* as well as susceptible strains of *Escherichia coli, Enterobacter aerogenes, Shigella, Acinetobacter, Streptococcus,* and *S pneumoniae* **Respiratory infections** caused by susceptible strains of *Haemophilus influenzae* and *Klebsiella* **Urinary-tract infections** caused by susceptible strains of *Klebsiella* **Skin and soft-tissue infections** caused by susceptible strains of *Staphylococcus aureus* **Psittacosis, ornithosis** **Infections** caused by *Treponema pertenue, Listeria monocytogenes, Clostridium, Bacillus anthracis, Fusobacterium fusiforme,* and *Actinomyces* in penicillin-allergic patients **Lymphogranuloma venereum, granuloma inguinale** **Relapsing fever** **Trachoma** **Inclusion conjunctivitis** **Intestinal amebiasis** (adjunctive therapy) **Infections** caused by *Neisseria meningitidis* in penicillin-allergic patients	**Adult:** 100 mg q12h to start, followed by 100 mg/day in a single daily dose or 2 divided doses q12h; for severe infections, 100 mg q12h **Child (>8 yr and ≤100 lb):** 2 mg/lb in 2 divided doses to start, followed by 1 mg/lb in a single daily dose or 2 divided doses; for severe infections, up to 2 mg/lb may be used after initial dose **Child (>8 yr and >100 lb):** same as adult	**Adult:** 200 mg IV in 1 or 2 infusions to start, followed by 100-200 mg/day IV, depending on the severity of the infection **Child (>8 yr and ≤100 lb):** 2 mg/lb IV in 1-2 infusions to start, followed by 1-2 mg/lb in 1-2 infusions, depending on the severity of the infection **Child (>8 yr and >100 lb):** same as adult
Severe acne (adjunctive therapy)	**Adult:** Same as adult dosage above.	—
Infections caused by *Neisseria gonorrhoeae* in penicillin-allergic patients	**Adult:** 200 mg stat and 100 mg at bedtime, followed by 100 mg bid for 3 days; alternative regimen: 300 mg stat, followed in 1 h by 300 mg	**Adult:** Same as adult dosage above.
Primary and secondary syphilis	**Adult:** 300 mg/day div for at least 10 days	**Adult:** 300 mg/day IV for at least 10 days
Brucellosis	**Adult:** usual dosage for 3 wk (with 1 g streptomycin IM bid 1st wk and qd 2nd wk)	—

ADMINISTRATION/DOSAGE ADJUSTMENTS

Duration of treatment	Unless otherwise indicated, continue treatment for at least 24-48 h after symptoms and fever have subsided; infections caused by Group A beta-hemolytic streptococci should be treated for at least 10 days. If patient is started on parenteral therapy, institute oral therapy as soon as possible.
Intravenous administration	Reserve for situations in which oral therapy is not feasible. Prolonged IV administration may cause thrombophlebitis. Avoid rapid administration; the usual duration of infusion varies from 1 to 4 h. To ensure adequate stability, the infusion must be completed within 12 h after reconstitution of the solution.
Timing of oral administration	May be administered with food, milk, or carbonated beverages, if desired

CONTRAINDICATIONS

Hypersensitivity to tetracyclines

Table continued on following page

VIBRAMYCIN continued

WARNINGS/PRECAUTIONS

Superinfection	Overgrowth of nonsusceptible organisms, including fungi, may occur
Venereal disease	If syphilis is suspected, perform dark-field examination before instituting therapy and perform serology testing monthly for at least 4 mo
Long-term therapy	Perform hemapoietic, renal, and hepatic studies periodically
Photosensitivity (exaggerated sunburn)	May occur; caution patients likely to be exposed to direct sunlight or UV light and discontinue use of doxycycline at first sign of skin erythema

ADVERSE REACTIONS

Gastrointestinal	Anorexia, nausea, vomiting, diarrhea, glossitis, dysphagia, enterocolitis, inflammatory lesions (with monilial overgrowth) in the anogenital region
Dermatological	Maculopapular and erythematous rashes, exfoliative dermatitis (rare), photosensitivity
Hypersensitivity	Urticaria, angioneurotic edema, anaphylaxis, anaphylactoid purpura, pericarditis, exacerbation of systemic lupus erythematosus
Hematological	Hemolytic anemia, thrombocytopenia, neutropenia, eosinophilia
Other	Microscopic discoloration of thyroid glands, bulging fontanels in infants, benign intracranial hypertension

OVERDOSAGE

Signs and symptoms	See ADVERSE REACTIONS
Treatment	Discontinue medication, treat symptomatically, and institute supportive measures, as required

DRUG INTERACTIONS

Oral anticoagulants	⇧ Prothrombin time
Penicillin	⇩ Bactericidal activity of penicillin
Antacids, iron supplements	⇩ Absorption of doxycycline
Methoxyflurane	⇧ Risk of nephrotoxicity
Sodium bicarbonate	⇩ Absorption of doxycycline

ALTERED LABORATORY VALUES

Blood/serum values	⇧ Alkaline phosphatase ⇧ SGOT ⇧ SGPT ⇧ BUN ⇧ Amylase ⇧ Bilirubin ⇩ Prothrombin activity
Urinary values	⇧ Catecholamines (with Hingerty fluorometric method)

Use in children

Not recommended for use during infancy through 8 yr of age unless other drugs are likely to be effective or are contraindicated; use in this age group may cause permanent discoloration of teeth or enamel hypoplasia. A reversible decrease in fibula growth rate has been observed in premature infants given oral tetracycline (100 mg/kg/day).

Use in pregnancy or nursing mothers

Use during latter half of pregnancy (fetal tooth development) may cause permanent discoloration of teeth or enamel hypoplasia. Animal studies indicate that tetracyclines cross the placental barrier, are found in fetal tissues, and can cause both embryotoxicity and fetal toxicity, including retardation of skeletal development. Tetracyclines are excreted in breast milk; general guidelines not established for use in nursing mothers.

CHLOROMYCETIN (Chloramphenicol) Parke-Davis

Caps: 250 mg **Ophthalmic ointment:** 1% (3.5 g): **Otic drops:** 5 mg/ml **Dermatological cream:** 1% (28 g)

CHLOROMYCETIN PALMITATE (Chloramphenicol palmitate) Parke-Davis

Susp: chloramphenicol palmitate equivalent to 150 mg chloramphenicol/5 ml

CHLOROMYCETIN SODIUM SUCCINATE (Chloramphenicol sodium succinate) Parke-Davis

Vial: 100 mg/ml when reconstituted (for IV use only)

INDICATIONS	ORAL DOSAGE	PARENTERAL DOSAGE
Acute infections caused by susceptible strains of *Salmonella typhi*[1] **Serious infections** caused by susceptible strains of *Salmonella*, *Haemophilus influenzae* (specifically, meningeal infections), rickettsia, lymphogranuloma-psittacosis group, and various Gram-negative bacteria, as well as other susceptible organisms resistant to all other appropriate antibiotics[2] **Cystic fibrosis** (adjunctive therapy)	**Adult:** 50 mg/kg/day in divided doses q6h; for infections caused by moderately resistant organisms, up to 100 mg/kg/day to start, followed by lower dosages as soon as possible **Newborn (<2 wk):** 25 mg/kg/day in divided doses q6h **Full-term infant (>2 wk):** up to 50 mg/kg/day in divided doses q6h **Child:** same as adult	**Adult:** 50 mg/kg/day IV in divided doses q6h **Newborn (<2 wk):** 25 mg/kg/day IV in divided doses q6h **Full-term infant (>2 wk):** up to 50 mg/kg/day IV in divided doses q6h **Child:** same as adult

ADMINISTRATION/DOSAGE ADJUSTMENTS

Infants and children with impaired metabolic processes	Reduce oral and IV dosage to 25 mg/kg/day and follow blood chloramphenicol levels by microtechniques; therapeutic level ranges from 5 to 20 μg/ml
Intravenous administration	Dilute powder supplied with 10 ml of aqueous diluent to a concentration of 100 mg/ml and inject over at least a 1-min period; replace with oral therapy as soon as possible
Superficial skin infections caused by susceptible bacteria	After cleansing, apply cream to infected area tid or qid; in all except very superficial infections, supplement topical therapy with appropriate systemic medication
Superficial infections of the external auditory canal caused by susceptible bacteria	Instill 2-3 drops of otic solution into the ear tid; in all except very superficial infections, supplement topical therapy with appropriate systemic medication
Superficial ocular infections involving the conjunctiva and/or cornea and caused by susceptible organisms	Place small amount of ophthalmic ointment into lower conjunctival sac q3h or more frequently, if necessary; continue treatment day and night for first 48 h, after which dosing interval may be increased. Continue treatment at least 48 h after eye appears normal. In all except very superficial infections, supplement topical therapy with appropriate systemic medication.

CONTRAINDICATIONS

Hypersensitivity or (for systemic use) prior toxic reaction to chloramphenicol

WARNINGS/PRECAUTIONS

Blood dyscrasias	May occur after short- or long-term oral, parenteral, or topical therapy and may be severe or even fatal (see ADVERSE REACTIONS). Obtain blood studies before starting therapy and approximately every 2 days during treatment. Discontinue use upon first sign of abnormality attributable to chloramphenicol (bone-marrow depression may not be evident prior to development of aplastic anemia).
Prolonged or repeated use	Should be avoided; treatment should not be continued longer than required to effect a cure with little or no risk of relapse
Inappropriate indications	Chloramphenicol should not be used in trivial bacterial infections, where not indicated (eg, viral infections), for prophylaxis, or when other, less potentially dangerous drugs would be effective
Hepatic or renal impairment	May result in excessive blood levels; adjust dosage accordingly or (preferably) monitor blood level at appropriate intervals
Superinfection	Overgrowth of nonsusceptible organisms, including fungi, may occur. If overgrowth occurs during topical therapy, discontinue use of chloramphenicol and institute appropriate therapeutic measures.

[1] Do not use for routine treatment of the carrier state
[2] When used for initial therapy, perform in vitro sensitivity tests to determine if infecting organism is susceptible to other, potentially less hazardous agents

Table continued on following page

CHLOROMYCETIN continued

ADVERSE REACTIONS

Hypersensitivity reactions, including bone-marrow hypoplasia	May occur with prolonged or frequent intermittent use of topical chloramphenicol
Hematological	Pancytopenia; aplastic anemia; hypoplastic anemia; thrombocytopenia; granulocytopenia; reversible bone-marrow depression characterized by vacuolization of erythroid cells, reduction in reticulocyte count, and leukopenia; paroxysmal nocturnal hemoglobinuria
Gastrointestinal	Nausea, vomiting, glossitis, stomatitis, diarrhea, enterocolitis
Central nervous system	Headache, mild depression, mental confusion, delirium, optic and peripheral neuritis (usually following long-term therapy)
Hypersensitivity	Fever, macular and vesicular rashes, angioedema, urticaria, anaphylaxis, Herxheimer reactions (during therapy for typhoid fever)
Other	"Gray syndrome" in premature and newborn infants, local irritation with itching and burning (with topical use)

OVERDOSAGE

Signs and symptoms	See ADVERSE REACTIONS
Treatment	Discontinue medication; treat symptomatically and institute supportive methods, as required

DRUG INTERACTIONS

Oral anticoagulants	⇧ Prothrombin time
Myelosuppressive agents	⇧ Risk of bone-marrow depression; do not use concomitantly
Chlorpropamide, tolbutamide	⇧ Risk of hypoglycemia
Phenytoin	⇧ Phenytoin blood level and/or toxicity

ALTERED LABORATORY VALUES

Urinary values	⇧ Glucose (with Clinitest tablets)

No clinically significant alterations in blood/serum values occur at therapeutic dosages

Use in children

See INDICATIONS; blood levels of drug should be carefully followed by microtechniques in young infants and other children with known or suspected immature metabolic processes. Toxic reactions, including fatalities, have ocurred in premature and newborn infants; follow dosage recommendations closely.

Use in pregnancy or nursing mothers

Safe use not established during pregnancy. Chloramphenicol readily crosses the placental barrier; use with particular caution at term or during labor because of potential toxic effects on the fetus ("gray syndrome"). The drug also appears in breast milk and should be used with caution in nursing mothers.

CLEOCIN HCl (Clindamycin hydrochloride) Upjohn

Caps: 75, 150 mg

CLEOCIN PEDIATRIC (Clindamycin palmitate hydrochloride) Upjohn

Granules for oral sol: clindamycin palmitate hydrochloride equivalent to 75 mg clindamycin/5 ml when reconstituted

CLEOCIN PHOSPHATE (Clindamycin phosphate) Upjohn

Amps: clindamycin phosphate equivalent to 150 mg clindamycin/ml (2, 4 ml)

INDICATIONS	ORAL DOSAGE	PARENTERAL DOSAGE
Serious infections caused by susceptible anaerobic bacteria, including serious respiratory-tract infections (eg, empyema, anaerobic pneumonitis, and lung abscesses); serious skin and soft-tissue infections; septicemia; intra-abdominal infections (eg, peritonitis, intra-abdominal abscesses); infections of the female pelvis and genital tract (eg, endometritis, nongonococcal tubo-ovarian abscesses, pelvic cellulitis, and postsurgical vaginal cuff infection) **Serious respiratory-tract infections and serious skin and soft-tissue infections** caused by susceptible strains of streptococci and staphylococci in penicillin-allergic patients **Serious respiratory-tract infections** caused by susceptible strains of *Streptococcus pneumoniae* in penicillin-allergic patients	**Adult:** 150–300 mg q6h; for severe infections, 300–450 mg q6h **Child:** 8–16 mg/kg/day in 3–4 equally divided doses; for severe infections, 16–20 mg/kg/day in 3–4 equally divided doses; **pediatric formula:** 8–12 mg/kg/day in 3–4 equally divided doses; for severe infections, 13–16 mg/kg/day in 3–4 equally divided doses; for very severe infections, 17–25 mg/kg/day in 3–4 equally divided doses	**Adult:** 600–1,200 mg/kg/day IM or IV in 2–4 equally divided doses; for severe infections, 1,200–2,700 mg/day IM or IV in 2–4 equally divided doses **Child (>1 mo):** 15–25 mg/kg/day IM or IV in 3–4 equally divided doses; for severe infections, 25–40 mg/kg/day in 3–4 equally divided doses
As an adjunct to surgical treatment of **chronic bone and joint infections** caused by susceptible bacteria	—	**Adult:** Same as adult dosage above. **Child (>1 mo):** Same as child dosage above.

ADMINISTRATION/DOSAGE ADJUSTMENTS

Dilution and infusion rates	Single IM injections of >600 mg are not recommended. Dilute clindamycin before IV administration to a minimum of 300 mg in 50 ml and infuse at a rate of 30 mg/min; do not give more than 1,200 mg in a single 1-h infusion
Esophageal irritation	May be avoided by administering each dose with a full glass of water
Minimum pediatric dose	Give at least 37.5 mg (½ tsp) orally tid to children weighing ≤10 kg; for severe infections, give no less than 300 mg/day IM or IV, regardless of body weight
High-dose parenteral therapy	In life-threatening situations, adult IV dose has been as much as 4.8 g/day
Adjunctive therapy	Perform indicated surgical procedures in conjunction with antibiotic therapy; obtain bacteriological studies to determine the causative organisms and their susceptibility to clindamycin
Beta-hemolytic streptococcal infections	Continue treatment for at least 10 days to prevent rheumatic fever and glomerulonephritis
Anaerobic infections	Use clindamycin phosphate injection initially, followed by oral therapy

CONTRAINDICATIONS

Hypersensitivity to clindamycin or lincomycin

WARNINGS/PRECAUTIONS

Inappropriate indications	Clindamycin should not be used in patients with nonbacterial infections (eg, most upper-respiratory-tract infections) or in the treatment of meningitis, since adequate diffusion into the CSF does not occur
Superinfection	May result in the overgrowth of nonsusceptible organisms, particularly yeasts

Table continued on following page

WARNINGS/PRECAUTIONS continued

Severe colitis	May occur due to enterotoxin-producing strains of *Clostridium* (particularly *C difficile).* May be characterized by severe persistent diarrhea and abdominal cramps, and may be associated with the passage of blood and mucus; endoscopic examination may reveal pseudomembranous colitis. When significant diarrhea occurs, discontinue medication or, if necessary, continue only with close observation; large bowel endoscopy is recommended. Antiperistaltic agents (eg, opiates and diphenyloxylate with atropine) may prolong and/or worsen the condition. Mild cases of colitis may respond to withdrawal of the drug alone. Moderate to severe cases should be managed by fluid and electrolyte replacement and protein supplementation. The use of systemic corticosteroids and steroid retention enemas may help relieve the colitis. Rule out other possible causes.
Special-risk patients	Use with caution in the elderly and in patients with a history of GI disease (particularly colitis), atopic individuals, or patients with very severe renal or hepatic disease accompanied by severe metabolic aberrations. Monitor serum levels during high-dose therapy; severely ill older patients should be closely followed for changes in bowel frequency.
Prolonged therapy	Perform periodic liver- and kidney-function tests and blood counts
Tartrazine sensitivity	Presence of FD&C Yellow No. 5 (tartrazine) in capsules may cause allergic-type reactions, including bronchial asthma, in susceptible individuals

ADVERSE REACTIONS

Gastrointestinal	Abdominal pain, esophagitis, nausea, vomiting, diarrhea, jaundice, abnormal liver-function tests
Dermatological	Maculopapular rash, urticaria, generalized mild to moderate morbilliform-like skin rashes, and (rarely) erythema multiforme (sometimes resembling Stevens-Johnson syndrome)
Hematological	Transient neutropenia (leukopenia) and eosinophilia, agranulocytosis, thrombocytopenia (causal relationship not established)
Musculoskeletal	Polyarthritis (rare)
Other	Hypersensitivity, anaphylactoid reactions; pain, induration, and sterile abscess (with IM use), thrombophlebitis (with IV use)

OVERDOSAGE

Signs and symptoms	See ADVERSE REACTIONS
Treatment	Discontinue medication; treat symptomatically

DRUG INTERACTIONS

General anesthetics, neuromuscular-blocking agents	⇧ Neuromuscular blockade, resulting in skeletal muscle weakness, respiratory depression, or paralysis
Antiperistaltic antidiarrheal agents	⇧ Risk and severity of diarrhea
Chloramphenicol, erythromycin	⇩ Antibacterial effect of clindamycin; do not use concomitantly
Kaolin	⇩ Absorption of clindamycin

ALTERED LABORATORY VALUES

No clinically significant alterations in blood/serum or urinary values occur at therapeutic dosages

Use in children

See INDICATIONS; monitor organ system function when treating newborns and infants

Use in pregnancy or nursing mothers

Safe use during pregnancy not established; clindamycin appears in breast milk at levels approximating maternal blood levels (0.7–3.8 μg/ml)

COLY-MYCIN M (Colistimethate sodium) Parke-Davis

Vial: colistimethate sodium equivalent to 150 mg colistin

INDICATIONS	PARENTERAL DOSAGE
Acute or chronic infections caused by susceptible strains of *Enterobacter aerogenes, Escherichia coli, Klebsiella pneumoniae,* and *Pseudomonas aeruginosa*	**Adult:** 2.5–5 mg/kg/day IM or IV in 2–4 divided doses **Child:** same as adult

ADMINISTRATION/DOSAGE ADJUSTMENTS

Intermittent intravenous infusion	Administer ½ the daily dose slowly (over 3–5 min) q12h
Continuous intravenous infusion	Slowly inject ½ the daily dose over a period of 3–5 min and administer the remaining dose as a slow infusion (5–6 mg/h) 1–2 h after the initial dose
Patients with renal impairment	Modify dosage schedule as follows: 75–115 mg bid when plasma creatinine concentration = 1.3–1.5 mg/dl; 66–150 mg bid or qd when plasma creatinine concentration = 1.6–2.5 mg/dl; 100–150 mg q36h when plasma creatinine concentration = 2.6–4 mg/dl

CONTRAINIDICATIONS

Hypersensitivity to colistimethate

WARNINGS/PRECAUTIONS

Maximum dose	Should not exceed 5 mg/kg/day
Neurological disturbances	May occur, including circumoral paresthesias; numbness, tingling, and formication of the extremities; generalized pruritus; vertigo; dizziness; and slurring of speech. Performance of potentially hazardous activities may be impaired; caution patients accordingly. Patients should be closely observed; reduction of dosage may alleviate symptoms.
Renal impairment	Use with caution, especially in elderly patients (see ADMINISTRATION/DOSAGE ADJUSTMENTS). Further impairment, acute renal insufficiency, renal shutdown, and further concentration to toxic levels can occur. Interference of nerve transmission at neuromuscular junctions may then occur and result in muscle weakness and apnea. The drug should be discontinued at the first sign of decreased urine output or rising BUN and serum creatinine concentration. In life-threatening situations, therapy may be reinstated at a lower dosage after blood levels have fallen.
Concomitant therapy	Other antibiotics with a Gram-negative antimicrobial spectrum and curariform muscle relaxants should be given only with extreme caution (see DRUG INTERACTIONS)

ADVERSE REACTIONS

Respiratory	Respiratory arrest, apnea
Neurological	Paresthesias, tingling of extremities and/or tongue, neuromuscular blockade, vertigo, slurred speech
Renal	Nephrotoxicity, decreased urine output
Gastrointestinal	Upset
Hypersensitivity	Generalized itching, urticaria, drug fever

OVERDOSAGE

Signs and symptoms	Renal insufficiency, muscular weakness, apnea, neuromuscular blockade
Treatment	Discontinue medication; institute supportive measures, including assisted respiration, oxygen therapy, and IV calcium chloride, as needed

Table continued on following page

DRUG INTERACTIONS

Kanamycin, streptomycin, polymyxin B, neomycin	⇧ Risk of neurotoxicity
Cephalothin	⇧ Risk of nephrotoxicity
Curariform muscle relaxants	⇧ Neuromuscular blockade

ALTERED LABORATORY VALUES

Blood/serum values	⇧ BUN ⇧ Creatinine
Urinary values	⇧ Protein

Use in children

See INDICATIONS

Use in pregnancy or nursing mothers

Safe use during pregnancy not established; general guidelines not established for use in nursing mothers

E.E.S. (Erythromycin ethylsuccinate) **Abbott**

Tabs: 400 mg **Tabs (chewable):** 200 mg **Oral susp:** 200 mg/5 ml (E.E.S. 200), 400 mg/5 ml (E.E.S. 400)
Oral susp granules: 200 mg/5 ml after reconstitution **Drops:** 100 mg/2.5 ml after reconstitution

INDICATIONS	ORAL DOSAGE
Acute mild to moderate **skin and soft-tissue infections** caused by susceptible strains of *Staphylococcus aureus*[1] Mild to moderate **upper- and lower-respiratory-tract, skin, and soft-tissue infections** caused by *Streptococcus pyogenes* Mild to moderate **upper- and lower-respiratory-tract infections** caused by *Streptococcus pneumoniae* and *Mycoplasma pneumoniae* As an adjunct to antitoxin for **prevention and/or elimination of carrier state** in individuals exposed to *Corynebacterium diphtheriae* **Infections** caused by *Listeria monocytogenes* **Erythrasma** caused by *Corynebacterium minutissimum*	**Adult:** 400 mg q6h; for severe infections, up to 4 g/day div **Child:** 30–50 mg/kg/day div; for severe infections, up to 60–100 mg/kg/day
Mild to moderate **upper-respiratory-tract infections** caused by susceptible strains of *Haemophilus influenzae*	**Adult:** 400 mg q6h; for severe infections, up to 4 g/day div (with appropriate sulfonamide therapy) **Child:** 30–50 mg/kg/day div; for severe infections, up to 60–100 mg/kg/day (with appropriate sulfonamide therapy)
Prophylaxis against bacterial endocarditis caused by alpha-hemolytic streptococci in penicillin-allergic patients with a history of rheumatic fever or congenital heart disease[2]	**Adult:** for continuous prophylaxis, 400 mg bid; for short-term prophylaxis, 800 mg prior to procedure, followed by 400 mg q6h for 4 doses **Child:** 30–50 mg/kg/day in 3–4 evenly spaced doses
Primary syphilis in penicillin-allergic patients	**Adult:** 48–64 g div over a 10- to 15-day period
Intestinal amebiasis caused by *Entamoeba histolytica*	**Adult:** 400 mg qid for 10–14 days **Child:** 30–50 mg/kg/day div for 10–14 days
Legionnaires' disease	**Adult:** 1.6–4 g/day div
Nasopharyngeal carriage of *Bordetella pertussis*	**Adult:** 40–50 mg/kg/day div for 5–14 days

ADMINISTRATION/DOSAGE ADJUSTMENTS

Streptococcal infections	Caused by Group A beta-hemolytic streptococci should be treated for a minimum of 10 days
Alternative dosing schedule	Half the total daily dose may be given q12h, or ⅓ the total daily dose may be given q8h
Chewable tablets	Must be chewed thoroughly

CONTRAINDICATIONS

Hypersensitivity to erythromycin

[1]Resistance may develop during treatment
[2]Unsuitable prior to genitourinary surgery if organisms are Gram-negative bacilli or belong to the enterococcus group of streptococci

Table continued on following page

E.E.S. continued

WARNINGS/PRECAUTIONS

Hepatic dysfunction	May occur, with or without jaundice, in patients receiving oral erythromycin therapy
Patients with existing hepatic impairment	Use with caution and watch for signs of excessive accumulation, since drug is excreted primarily by the liver
Concomitant theophylline therapy	**May produce elevated serum theophylline levels or theophylline toxicity; reduce theophylline dosage accordingly**
Primary syphilis	Spinal-fluid examinations should be performed before treatment and as part of follow-up therapy
Localized infections	May require surgical drainage, in addition to antibiotic therapy
Superinfection	Overgrowth of nonsusceptible bacteria or fungi may occur

ADVERSE REACTIONS

Gastrointestinal	Nausea, vomiting, abdominal cramping and discomfort, diarrhea
Hypersensitivity	Urticaria, skin rashes, anaphylaxis

OVERDOSAGE

Signs and symptoms	See ADVERSE REACTIONS
Treatment	Discontinue medication; treat symptomatically

DRUG INTERACTIONS

Lincomycin	⇩ Bactericidal action of lincomycin
Aminophylline	**⇧ Serum theophylline level**
Oxtriphylline	**⇧ Serum theophylline level**
Theophylline	⇧ Serum theophylline level

ALTERED LABORATORY VALUES

Blood/serum values	⇧ Alkaline phosphatase ⇧ Bilirubin ⇧ SGOT ⇧ SGPT
Urinary values	⇧ Catecholamines (with Hingerty fluorometric method)

Use in children

Age, weight, and severity of infection are important factors in determining the proper dosage; see INDICATIONS

Use in pregnancy or nursing mothers

Safe use not established; erythromycin crosses the placental barrier and appears in breast milk

Note: Erythromycin ethylsuccinate also marketed as **PEDIAMYCIN** (Ross).

E-MYCIN (Erythromycin) **Upjohn**

Tabs: 250 mg

INDICATIONS	ORAL DOSAGE
Acute mild to moderate **skin and soft-tissue infections** caused by susceptible strains of *Staphylococcus aureus*[1] As an adjunct to antitoxin for **prevention and/or elimination of carrier state** in individuals exposed to *Corynebacterium diphtheriae* **Infections** caused by *Listeria monocytogenes* **Erythrasma** caused by *Corynebacterium minutissimum* Mild to moderate **upper- and lower-respiratory-tract, skin, and soft-tissue infections** caused by *Streptococcus pyogenes* Mild to moderate **upper- and lower-respiratory-tract infections** caused by *Streptococcus pneumoniae* and *Mycoplasma pneumoniae*	**Adult:** 250 mg qid; for severe infections, up to 4 g/day **Child:** 30-50 mg/kg/day div; for severe infections, up to 60-100 mg/kg/day
Mild to moderate **upper-respiratory-tract infections** caused by susceptible strains of *Haemophilus influenzae*	**Adult:** 250 mg q6h; for severe infections, up to 4 g/day (with appropriate sulfonamide therapy) **Child:** 30-50 mg/kg/day div; for severe infections, up to 60-100 mg/kg/day (with appropriate sulfonamide therapy)
Acute pelvic inflammatory disease caused by *Neisseria gonorrhoeae* in penicillin-allergic patients	**Adult:** initiate treatment with erythromycin lactobionate (500 mg IV q6h for 3 days), followed by 250 mg of erythromycin orally q6h for 7 days
Prophylaxis against bacterial endocarditis caused by alpha-hemolytic streptococci in penicillin-allergic patients with a history of rheumatic fever or congenital heart disease[2]	**Adult:** for continuous prophylaxis, 250 mg bid; for short-term prophylaxis, 1 g, given 1½-2 h prior to procedure, followed by 500 mg q6h for 8 doses **Child:** 20 mg/kg, given 1½-2 h prior to procedure, followed by 10 mg/kg q6h for 8 doses
Primary syphilis in penicillin-allergic patients	**Adult:** 30-40 g div for 10-15 days
Intestinal amebiasis caused by *Entamoeba histolytica*	**Adult:** 250 mg qid for 10-14 days **Child:** 30-50 mg/kg/day div for 10-14 days
Legionnaires' disease	**Adult:** 1-4 g/day div

E-MYCIN E (Erythromycin ethylsuccinate) **Upjohn**

Susp: 200 mg/5 ml, 400 mg/5 ml

INDICATIONS	ORAL DOSAGE
Acute mild to moderate **skin and soft-tissue infections** caused by susceptible strains of *Staphylococcus aureus*[1] As an adjunct to antitoxin for **prevention and/or elimination of carrier state** in individuals exposed to *Corynebacterium diphtheriae* **Infections** caused by *Listeria monocytogenes* **Erythrasma** caused by *Corynebacterium minutissimum* Mild to moderate **upper- and lower-respiratory-tract, skin, and soft-tissue infections** caused by *Streptococcus pyogenes* Mild to moderate **upper- and lower-respiratory-tract infections** caused by *Streptococcus pneumoniae* and *Mycoplasma pneumoniae*	**Adult:** 400 mg q6h; for severe infections, up to 4 g/day **Child:** 30-50 mg/kg/day div; for severe infections, up to 60-100 mg/kg/day

[1] Resistance may develop during treatment

[2] Unsuitable prior to genitourinary surgery if organisms are Gram-negative bacilli or belong to the enterococcus group of streptococci

Table continued on following page

INDICATIONS continued	ORAL DOSAGE
Prophylaxis against bacterial endocarditis caused by alpha-hemolytic streptococci in penicillin-allergic patients with a history of rheumatic fever or congenital heart disease[2]	**Adult:** for continuous prophylaxis, 400 mg bid; for short-term prophylaxis, 800 mg, given 1½–2 h prior to procedure, followed by 400 mg q6h for 4 doses **Child:** 30–50 mg/kg/day div in 3–4 evenly spaced doses
Primary syphilis in penicillin-allergic patients	**Adult:** 48–64 g div over 10–14 days
Intestinal amebiasis caused by *Entamoeba histolytica*	**Adult:** 400 mg qid for 10–14 days **Child:** 30–50 mg/kg/day div for 10–14 days
Legionnaires' disease	**Adult:** 1–4 g/day div

ADMINISTRATION/DOSAGE ADJUSTMENTS

Streptococcal infections	Caused by Group A beta-hemolytic streptococci should be treated for a minimum of 10 days
Alternative dosing schedule	Half of the total daily dose may be given q12h; twice-a-day dosing is not recommended when daily doses exceed 1 g

CONTRAINDICATIONS

Hypersensitivity to erythromycin

WARNINGS/PRECAUTIONS

Hepatic dysfunction	May occur, with or without jaundice, in patients receiving oral erythromycin
Patients with existing hepatic impairment	Use with caution and watch for signs of excessive accumulation, since drug is excreted primarily by the liver
Concomitant theophylline therapy	May produce elevated serum theophylline levels or theophylline toxicity; reduce theophylline dosage accordingly
Venereal disease	If syphilis is suspected, perform dark-field examination before instituting therapy and perform serology testing monthly for at least 4 mo
Primary syphilis	Spinal fluid examinations should be done before treatment and as part of follow-up therapy
Hypersensitivity	Serious allergic reactions, including anaphylaxis, have been reported; eliminate unabsorbed drug promptly, and administer epinephrine, corticosteroids, and antihistamines, as indicated
Superinfection	Overgrowth of nonsusceptible bacteria or fungi may occur

ADVERSE REACTIONS

Gastrointestinal	Nausea, vomiting, abdominal cramping and discomfort, diarrhea
Hypersensitivity	Urticaria, skin rashes, anaphylaxis

OVERDOSAGE

Signs and symptoms	See ADVERSE REACTIONS
Treatment	Discontinue medication; treat symptomatically

DRUG INTERACTIONS

Lincomycin	⇩ Bactericidal action of lincomycin
Aminophylline	⇧ Serum theophylline level
Oxtriphylline	⇧ Serum theophylline level
Theophylline	⇧ Serum theophylline level

ALTERED LABORATORY VALUES

Blood/serum values	⇧ Alkaline phosphatase ⇧ Bilirubin ⇧ SGOT ⇧ SGPT
Urinary values	⇧ Catecholamines (with Hingerty fluorometric method)

Use in children

Age, weight, and severity of infection are important factors in determining proper dosage; see INDICATIONS

Use in pregnancy or nursing mothers

Safe use not established; erythromycin crosses the placental barrier, but fetal plasma levels are low. General guidelines not established for use in nursing mothers.

[2]Unsuitable prior to genitourinary surgery if organisms are Gram-negative bacilli or belong to the enterococcus group of streptococci

ERYTHROCIN LACTOBIONATE-I.V. (Erythromycin lactobionate) **Abbott**

Vials: erythromycin lactobionate equivalent to 500 mg or 1 g erythromycin

ERYTHROCIN PIGGYBACK (Erythromycin lactobionate) **Abbott**

Piggyback vial: 5 mg/ml after reconstitution (for IV use only

ERYTHROCIN STEARATE (Erythromycin stearate) **Abbott**

Tabs: 125, 250, 500 mg

INDICATIONS	ORAL DOSAGE	PARENTERAL DOSAGE
Acute mild to moderate **skin and soft-tissue infections** caused by susceptible strains of *Staphylococcus aureus*[1] As an adjunct to antitoxin for **prevention and/or elimination of carrier state** in individuals exposed to *Corynebacterium diphtheriae* **Infections** caused by *Listeria monocytogenes* **Erythrasma** caused by *Corynebacterium minutissimum* Mild to moderate **upper- and lower-respiratory-tract, skin, and soft-tissue infections** caused by *Streptococcus pyogenes* Mild to moderate **upper- and lower-respiratory-tract infections** caused by *Streptococcus pneumoniae* and *Mycoplasma pneumoniae*	**Adult:** 250 mg q6h; for severe infections, up to 4 g/day div **Child:** 30–50 mg/kg/day in 3–4 doses; for severe infections, up to 60–100 mg/kg/day	**Adult:** for severe infections, 15-20 mg/kg/day IV; for very severe infections, up to 4 g/day IV **Child:** same as adult
Mild to moderate **upper-respiratory-tract infections** caused by susceptible strains of *Haemophilus influenzae*	**Adult:** 250 mg q6h; for severe infections, up to 4 g/day div (with appropriate sulfonamide therapy) **Child:** 30–50 mg/kg/day in 3–4 doses; for severe infections, up to 60–100 mg/kg/day (with appropriate sulfonamide therapy)	—
Acute pelvic inflammatory disease caused by *Neisseria gonorrhoeae* in penicillin-allergic patients	—	**Adult:** 500 mg IV q6h for 3 days, followed by 250 mg q6h orally for 7 days
Prophylaxis against bacterial endocarditis caused by alpha-hemolytic streptococci in penicillin-allergic patients with a history of rheumatic fever or congenital heart disease[2]	**Adult:** for continuous prophylaxis, 250 mg bid; for short-term prophylaxis, 500 mg prior to procedure, followed by 250 mg q6h for 4 doses **Child:** 30–50 mg/kg/day in 3–4 evenly spaced doses	—
Primary syphilis in penicillin-allergic patients	**Adult:** 30–40 g div over 10–15 days	—
Intestinal amebiasis caused by *Entamoeba histolytica*	**Adult:** 250 mg qid for 10–14 days **Child:** 30–50 mg/kg/day div for 10–14 days	—
Legionnaires' disease	**Adult:** 1–4 g/day div	**Adult:** 1–4 g/day IV
Nasopharyngeal carriage of *Bordetella pertussis*	**Adult:** 40–50 mg/kg/day div for 5–14 days	—

ADMINISTRATION/DOSAGE ADJUSTMENTS

Streptococcal infections	Caused by Group A beta-hemolytic streptococci should be treated for a minimum of 10 days

[1] Resistance may develop during treatment
[2] Unsuitable prior to genitourinary surgery if organisms are Gram-negative bacilli or belong to the enterococcus group of streptococci

Table continued on following page

ERYTHROCIN continued

ADMINISTRATION/DOSAGE ADJUSTMENTS continued

Continuous infusion (preferable for intravenous use)	Give total daily dose slowly as a final concentration of 1 g/liter; final solution should be administered within a period of 8 h due to poor stability
Intermittent infusion	Give ¼ the total daily dose (at a concentration of 250–500 mg in 100–250 ml) over a period of 20–60 min at intervals not greater than q6h
Alternative dosing schedule	Half the total daily dose may be given q12h in the fasting state or immediately before meals

CONTRAINDICATIONS

Hypersensitivity to erythromycin

WARNINGS/PRECAUTIONS

Hepatic dysfunction	May occur, with or without jaundice, in patients receiving oral erythromycin
Patients with existing hepatic impairment	Use with caution and watch for signs of excessive accumulation, since drug is excreted by the liver
Concomitant theophylline therapy	May produce elevated serum theophylline levels or theophylline toxicity; reduce theophylline dosage accordingly
Venereal disease	If syphilis is suspected, perform dark-field examination before instituting therapy and perform serology testing monthly for at least 4 mo
Primary syphilis	Spinal-fluid examinations should be performed before treatment and as part of follow-up therapy
Localized infections	May require surgical drainage, in addition to antibiotic therapy
Superinfection	Overgrowth of nonsusceptible bacteria or fungi may occur

ADVERSE REACTIONS

Gastrointestinal	Abdominal cramping, discomfort, nausea, vomiting, and diarrhea (with oral use)
Hypersensitivity	Urticaria, skin rashes, anaphylaxis
Ototoxicity	Reversible hearing loss with IV infusions of 4 g/day or more (rare)
Other	Venous irritation with IV use (rare)

OVERDOSAGE

Signs and symptoms	See ADVERSE REACTIONS
Treatment	Discontinue medication; treat symptomatically

DRUG INTERACTIONS

Lincomycin	⇩ Bactericidal action of lincomycin
Aminophylline	⇧ Serum theophylline level
Oxtriphylline	⇧ Serum theophylline level
Theophylline	⇧ Serum theophylline level

ALTERED LABORATORY VALUES

Blood/serum values	⇧ Alkaline phosphatase ⇧ Bilirubin ⇧ SGOT ⇧ SGPT
Urinary values	⇧ Catecholamines (with Hingerty fluorometric method)

Use in children

Age, weight, and severity of infection are important factors in determining the proper dosage; see INDICATIONS

Use in pregnancy or nursing mothers

Safe use not established; erythromycin crosses the placental barrier and appears in breast milk

ILOSONE (Erythromycin estolate) Dista

Caps: 125, 250 mg **Tabs:** 500 mg **Tabs (chewable):** 125, 250 mg **Susp:** 125 mg/5 ml, 250 mg/5 ml
Susp (conc): 125 mg/5 ml after dilution **Drops:** 100 mg/ml

INDICATIONS	ORAL DOSAGE
Acute mild to moderate **skin and soft-tissue infections** caused by *Staphylococcus aureus*[1] As an adjunct to antitoxin for **prevention and/or elimination of carrier state** in individuals exposed to *Corynebacterium diphtheriae* **Infections** caused by *Listeria monocytogenes* **Erythrasma** caused by *Corynebacterium minutissimum* Mild to moderate **upper- and lower-respiratory-tract, skin, and soft-tissue infections** caused by *Streptococcus pyogenes* Mild to moderate **upper- and lower-respiratory-tract infections** caused by *Streptococcus pneumoniae* and *Mycoplasma pneumoniae*	**Adult:** 250 mg q6h; for severe infections, up to 4 g/day div **Child:** 30–50 mg/kg/day div; for severe infections, up to 60–100 mg/kg/day
Streptococcal pharyngitis and tonsillitis	**Adult:** 20–50 mg/kg/day div **Child:** same as adult
Mild to moderate **upper-respiratory-tract infections** caused by susceptible strains of *Haemophilus influenzae*	**Adult:** 250 mg q6h; for severe infections, up to 4 g/day div (with appropriate sulfonamide therapy) **Child:** 30–50 mg/kg/day div; for severe infections, up to 60–100 mg/kg/day (with appropriate sulfonamide therapy)
Prophylaxis against bacterial endocarditis caused by alpha-hemolytic streptococci in penicillin-allergic patients with a history of rheumatic fever or congenital heart disease[2]	**Adult:** for continuous prophylaxis, 250 mg bid; for short-term prophylaxis, 500 mg prior to procedure, followed by 250 mg q8h for 4 doses **Child:** 30–50 mg/kg/day in 3–4 evenly spaced doses
Primary syphilis in penicillin-allergic patients	**Adult:** 20 g div over a 10-day period
Intestinal amebiasis caused by *Entamoeba histolytica*	**Adult:** 250 mg qid for 10–14 days **Child:** 30–50 mg/kg/day div for 10–14 days
Legionnaires' disease	**Adult:** 1–4 g/day div

ADMINISTRATION/DOSAGE ADJUSTMENTS

Streptococcal infections	Caused by Group A beta-hemolytic streptococci should be treated for a minimum of 10 days
Alternative dosing schedule	Half the total daily dose may be given q12h

CONTRAINDICATIONS

Hypersensitivity to erythromycin ●	Pre-existing liver disease ●

WARNINGS/PRECAUTIONS

Reversible hepatic dysfunction, cholestatic hepatitis	May occur, with or without jaundice, generally following 1–2 wk of continuous therapy. Observe patient for malaise, nausea, vomiting, abdominal cramps, and fever; severe abdominal pain simulating an abdominal surgical emergency may also occur. Laboratory findings include abnormal liver-function tests, peripheral eosinophilia, and leukocytosis. Discontinue medication promptly.
Patients with existing hepatic impairment	Use with caution and watch for signs of excessive accumulation, since drug is excreted primarily by the liver

[1] Resistance may develop during treatment
[2] Unsuitable prior to genitourinary surgery if organisms are Gram-negative bacilli or belong to the enterococcus group of streptococci

Table continued on following page

ILOSONE continued

WARNINGS/PRECAUTIONS continued

Concomitant theophylline therapy	May produce elevated serum theophylline levels or theophylline toxicity; reduce theophylline dosage accordingly
Primary syphilis	Spinal-fluid examinations should be performed before treatment and as part of follow-up therapy
Superinfection	Overgrowth of nonsusceptible bacteria or fungi may occur

ADVERSE REACTIONS

Gastrointestinal	Nausea, vomiting, abdominal cramping and discomfort, diarrhea
Hypersensitivity	Urticaria, skin rashes, anaphylaxis

OVERDOSAGE

Signs and symptoms	See ADVERSE REACTIONS
Treatment	Discontinue medication; treat symptomatically

DRUG INTERACTIONS

Lincomycin	⇩ Bactericidal action of lincomycin
Aminophylline	⇧ **Serum theophylline level**
Oxtriphylline	⇧ **Serum theophylline level**
Theophylline	⇧ Serum theophylline level

ALTERED LABORATORY VALUES

Blood/serum values	⇧ Alkaline phosphatase ⇧ Bilirubin ⇧ SGOT ⇧ SGPT
Urinary values	⇧ Catecholamines (with Hingerty fluorometric method)

Use in children

Age, weight, and severity of infection are important factors in determining the proper dosage; see INDICATIONS

Use in pregnancy or nursing mothers

Safe use not established; **general guidelines not established** for use in nursing mothers

AZO GANTANOL (Sulfamethoxazole and phenazopyridine hydrochloride) **Roche**

Tabs: 0.5 g sulfamethoxazole and 100 mg phenazopyridine hydrochloride

INDICATIONS	ORAL DOSAGE
Painful urinary-tract infections caused by susceptible strains of *Escherichia coli, Klebsiella-Enterobacter, Staphylococcus aureus, Proteus mirabilis,* and *P vulgaris* in the absence of obstructive uropathy or foreign bodies	**Adult:** 4 tabs to start, followed by 2 tabs in AM and PM for up to 3 days; continue treatment with sulfamethoxazole alone once pain relief is obtained

ADMINISTRATION/DOSAGE ADJUSTMENTS

Therapeutic blood levels	For most infections, 5–15 mg/dl; for serious infections, 12–15 mg/dl; blood levels >20 mg/dl increase the probability of adverse reactions

CONTRAINDICATIONS

Hypersensitivity to sulfonamides ●	Glomerulonephritis ●	Severe hepatitis ●
Uremia ●	Pyelonephritis of pregnancy with GI disturbances ●	

WARNINGS/PRECAUTIONS

In vitro sulfonamide sensitivity tests	May not be reliable; coordinate test results with bacteriological and clinical responses
Blood dyscrasias	May occur and can be fatal (see ADVERSE REACTIONS); obtain CBC frequently and watch for early signs (eg, sore throat, fever, pallor, purpura, jaundice) of serious blood disorders
Hypersensitivity reactions	May occur and can be fatal (see ADVERSE REACTIONS); use with caution in patients allergic to some goitrogens, diuretics, and oral hypoglycemic agents
Renal complications	May occur (see ADVERSE REACTIONS); perform a urinalysis, with microscopic examination, frequently
Crystalluria, urinary calculi	May be prevented by maintaining adequate fluid intake
Urine discoloration	Caution patient that urine may appear reddish-orange in color
Special-risk patients	Use with caution in patients with impaired renal or hepatic function, severe allergy, bronchial asthma, G6PD deficiency, or porphyria[1]

ADVERSE REACTIONS

Hematological	Agranulocytosis, aplastic anemia, thrombocytopenia, leukopenia, hemolytic anemia, purpura, hypoprothrombinemia, methemoglobinemia
Allergic	Erythema multiforme (Stevens-Johnson syndrome), generalized skin eruptions, epidermal necrolysis, urticaria, serum sickness, pruritus, exfoliative dermatitis, anaphylactoid reactions, periorbital edema, conjunctival and scleral injection, photosensitization, arthralgia, allergic myocarditis
Gastrointestinal	Nausea, vomiting, abdominal pain, hepatitis, diarrhea, anorexia, pancreatitis, stomatitis
Central nervous system	Headache, peripheral neuritis, mental depression, convulsions, ataxia, hallucinations, tinnitus, vertigo, insomnia
Renal	Toxic nephrosis with oliguria and anuria, crystalluria, urinary calculi, diuresis (rare)
Endocrinological	Goiter (rare), hypoglycemia (rare)
Other	Drug fever, chills, periarteritis nodosa, lupus erythematosus phenomena

OVERDOSAGE

Signs and symptoms	See ADVERSE REACTIONS
Treatment	Discontinue use of drug; treat symptomatically

DRUG INTERACTIONS

Para-aminobenzoic acid	⇩ Bacteriostatic effect of sulfisoxazole
Oral anticoagulants, oral hypoglycemics, methotrexate, phenytoin, thiopental	Effects increased or prolonged ⇧ Toxicity
Methenamine	⇧ Risk of crystalluria
Methotrexate	⇧ Methotrexate serum level

[1] *United States Pharmacopeia Dispensing Information 1980.* Rockville, Md., United States Pharmacopeial Convention, Inc., 1980

Table continued on following page

AZO GANTANOL continued

ALTERED LABORATORY VALUES

Blood/serum values	⇩ PBI ⇩ ^{131}I thyroid uptake
Urinary values	⇧ Glucose (with Clinitest tablets) ⇧ Protein (with sulfosalicylic acid method)

Use in children

Contraindicated for use in children under 12 yr of age

Use in pregnancy or nursing mothers

Safe use not established during pregnancy; the drug is contraindicated at term and in nursing mothers. Sulfonamides cross the placental barrier, are excreted in breast milk, and may cause kernicterus.

AZO GANTRISIN (Sulfisoxazole and phenazopyridine hydrochloride) Roche

Tabs: 0.5 g sulfisoxazole and 50 mg phenazopyridine hydrochloride

INDICATIONS	ORAL DOSAGE
Painful urinary-tract infections caused by susceptible strains of *Escherichia coli, Klebsiella-Enterobacter, Staphylococcus aureus, Proteus mirabilis,* and *P vulgaris* in the absence of obstructive uropathy or foreign bodies	**Adult:** 4–6 tabs to start, followed by 2 tabs qid for up to 3 days; continue treatment with sulfisoxazole alone once pain relief is obtained

ADMINISTRATION/DOSAGE ADJUSTMENTS

Therapeutic blood levels	For most infections, 5–15 mg/dl; for serious infections, 12–15 mg/dl; blood levels >20 mg/dl increase the probability of adverse reactions

CONTRAINDICATIONS

Hypersensitivity to sulfonamides ●	Glomerulonephritis ●	Severe hepatitis ●
Uremia ●	Pyelonephritis of pregnancy with GI disturbances ●	

WARNINGS/PRECAUTIONS

In vitro sulfonamide sensitivity tests	May not be reliable; coordinate test results with bacteriological and clinical responses
Blood dyscrasias	May occur and can be fatal (see ADVERSE REACTIONS); obtain CBC frequently and watch for early signs (eg, sore throat, fever, pallor, purpura, jaundice) of serious blood disorders
Hypersensitivity reactions	May occur and can be fatal (see ADVERSE REACTIONS); use with caution in patients allergic to some goitrogens, diuretics, and oral hypoglycemic agents
Renal complications	May occur (see ADVERSE REACTIONS); perform a urinalysis, with microscopic examination, frequently
Crystalluria, urinary calculi	May be prevented by maintaining adequate fluid intake
Urine discoloration	Caution patient that urine may appear reddish-orange in color
Special-risk patients	Use with caution in patients with impaired renal or hepatic function, severe allergy, bronchial asthma, G6PD deficiency, or porphyria[1]

ADVERSE REACTIONS

Hematological	Agranulocytosis, aplastic anemia, thrombocytopenia, leukopenia, hemolytic anemia, purpura, hypoprothrombinemia, methemoglobinemia
Allergic	Erythema multiforme (Stevens-Johnson syndrome), generalized skin eruptions, epidermal necrolysis, urticaria, serum sickness, pruritus, exfoliative dermatitis, anaphylactoid reactions, periorbital edema, conjunctival and scleral injection, photosensitization, arthralgia, allergic myocarditis
Gastrointestinal	Nausea, vomiting, abdominal pain, hepatitis, diarrhea, anorexia, pancreatitis, stomatitis
Central nervous system	Headache, peripheral neuritis, mental depression, convulsions, ataxia, hallucinations, tinnitus, vertigo, insomnia
Renal	Toxic nephrosis with oliguria and anuria, crystalluria, urinary calculi, diuresis (rare)
Endocrinological	Goiter (rare), hypoglycemia (rare)
Other	Drug fever, chills, periarteritis nodosa, lupus erythematosus phenomena

OVERDOSAGE

Signs and symptoms	See ADVERSE REACTIONS
Treatment	Discontinue use of drug; treat symptomatically

DRUG INTERACTIONS

Para-aminobenzoic acid	⇩ Bacteriostatic effect of sulfisoxazole
Oral anticoagulants, oral hypoglycemics, methotrexate, phenytoin, thiopental	Effects increased or prolonged ⇧ Toxicity
Methenamine	⇧ Risk of crystalluria
Methotrexate	⇧ Methotrexate serum level

[1] *United States Pharmacopeia Dispensing Information 1980.* Rockville, Md., United States Pharmacopeial Convention, Inc., 1980

Table continued on following page

AZO GANTRISIN continued

ALTERED LABORATORY VALUES

Blood/serum values	⇩ PBI ⇩ ^{131}I thyroid uptake
Urinary values	⇧ Glucose (with Clinitest tablets) ⇧ Protein (with sulfosalicylic acid method)

Use in children

Contraindicated for use in children under 12 yr of age

Use in pregnancy or nursing mothers

Safe use not established during pregnancy; the drug is contraindicated at term and in nursing mothers. Sulfonamides cross the placental barrier, are excreted in breast milk, and may cause kernicterus.

BACTRIM (Trimethoprim and sulfamethoxazole) Roche

Tabs: 80 mg trimethoprim and 400 mg sulfamethoxazole **Susp, pediatric susp:** 40 mg trimethoprim and 200 mg sulfamethoxazole per 5 ml

BACTRIM DS (Trimethoprim and sulfamethoxazole) Roche

Tabs: 160 mg trimethoprim and 800 mg sulfamethoxazole

INDICATIONS	ORAL DOSAGE
Urinary-tract infections caused by susceptible strains of *Escherichia coli, Klebsiella-Enterobacter, Proteus mirabilis, P vulgaris,* and *P morganii*[1]	**Adult:** 2 Bactrim tabs, 1 Bactrim DS tab, or 20 ml (4 tsp) q12h for 10–14 days **Child:** 4 mg/kg trimethoprim and 20 mg/kg sulfamethoxazole q12h for 10 days, or as follows: **Child (10 kg or 22 lb):** ½ Bactrim tab or 5 ml (1 tsp) q12h for 10 days **Child (20 kg or 44 lb):** 1 Bactrim tab or 10 ml (2 tsp) q12h for 10 days **Child (30 kg or 66 lb):** 1½ Bactrim tabs or 15 ml (3 tsp) q12h for 10 days **Child (40 kg or 88 lb):** 2 Bactrim tabs, 1 Bactrim DS tab, or 20 ml (4 tsp) q12h for 10 days
Acute otitis media caused by susceptible strains of *Haemophilus influenzae* or *Streptococcus pneumoniae*[2]	**Child:** same as child's dosage above
Acute exacerbations of chronic bronchitis caused by susceptible strains of *Haemophilus influenzae* or *Streptococcus pneumoniae*	**Adult:** same as adult's dosage above
Enteritis caused by susceptible strains of *Shigella flexneri* and *S sonnei*	**Adult:** same as adult's dosage above for 5 days **Child:** same as child's dosage above for 5 days
***Pneumocystis carinii* pneumonitis**	**Adult:** 5 mg/kg trimethoprim and 25 mg/kg sulfamethoxazole q6h for 14 days **Child:** same as for adult, or as follows: **Child (8 kg or 18 lb):** ½ Bactrim tab or 5 ml (1 tsp) q6h for 14 days **Child (16 kg or 35 lb):** 1 Bactrim tab or 10 ml (2 tsp) q6h for 14 days **Child (24 kg or 53 lb):** 1½ Bactrim tabs or 15 ml (3 tsp) q6h for 14 days **Child (32 kg or 70 lb):** 2 Bactrim tabs, 1 Bactrim DS tab, or 20 ml (4 tsp) q6h for 14 days **Child (36 kg or 80 lb):** 1 Bactrim DS tab q6h for 14 days

ADMINISTRATION/DOSAGE ADJUSTMENTS

Patients with renal impairment	Follow the usual dosage regimen if creatinine clearance rate (CCr) >30 ml/min. Administer half the usual dosage if CCr=15–30 ml/min. Use is not recommended if CCr<15 ml/min.

CONTRAINDICATIONS

Hypersensitivity to trimethoprim or sulfonamides

WARNINGS/PRECAUTIONS

Group A beta-hemolytic streptococcal pharyngitis	Sulfonamides have no place in the treatment of such infections, as they will neither eradicate the causative organism from the tonsillopharyngeal area nor prevent complications
Blood dyscrasias	May occur and can be fatal (see ADVERSE REACTIONS); obtain CBC frequently and watch for early signs (eg, sore throat, fever, pallor, purpura, jaundice) of serious blood disorders. Discontinue treatment if count of any formed blood element falls significantly.
Hypersensitivity reactions	May occur and can be fatal (see ADVERSE REACTIONS); use with caution in patients allergic to some goitrogens, diuretics, and oral hypoglycemic agents
Renal complications	May occur (see ADVERSE REACTIONS); perform a urinalysis, with careful microscopic examination, during therapy, particularly if renal function is impaired
Crystalluria, urinary calculi	May be prevented by maintaining adequate fluid intake
Special-risk patients	Use with caution in patients with impaired renal or hepatic function, folate deficiency, severe allergy, bronchial asthma, G6PD deficiency, or porphyria[3] and in elderly patients being treated with certain diuretics, particularly thiazides

[1]Initial episodes of uncomplicated infections should be treated with a single, effective antibacterial agent, rather than a combination
[2]Not indicated for prophylaxis or prolonged administration
[3]*United States Pharmacopeia Dispensing Information 1980.* Rockville, Md., United States Pharmacopeial Convention, Inc., 1980

Table continued on following page

BACTRIM/BACTRIM DS continued

ADVERSE REACTIONS[4]

Hematological	Agranulocytosis, aplastic anemia, megaloblastic anemia, thrombopenia, leukopenia, hemolytic anemia, purpura, hypoprothrombinemia, methemoglobinemia
Allergic	Erythema multiforme (Stevens-Johnson syndrome), generalized skin eruptions, epidermal necrolysis, urticaria, serum sickness, pruritus, exfoliative dermatitis, anaphylactoid reactions, periorbital edema, conjunctival and scleral injection, photosensitization, arthralgia, allergic myocarditis
Gastrointestinal	Glossitis, stomatitis, nausea, vomiting, abdominal pain, hepatitis, diarrhea, pancreatitis
Central nervous system	Headache, peripheral neuritis, mental depression, convulsions, ataxia, hallucinations, tinnitus, vertigo, insomnia, apathy, fatigue, muscle weakness, nervousness
Renal	Toxic nephrosis with oliguria and anuria, crystalluria, urinary calculi, diuresis (rare)
Endocrinological	Goiter (rare), hypoglycemia (rare)
Other	Drug fever, chills, periarteritis nodosa, lupus erythematosus phenomena

OVERDOSAGE

Signs and symptoms	See ADVERSE REACTIONS
Treatment	Discontinue use of drug; treat symptomatically

DRUG INTERACTIONS

Diuretics (especially thiazides)	⇧ Risk of thrombopenia with purpura in elderly patients
Para-aminobenzoic acid	⇩ Bacteriostatic effect of sulfamethoxazole
Warfarin	⇧ Prothrombin time
Oral hypoglycemics, methotrexate, phenytoin, thiopental	Effects increased or prolonged ⇧ Toxicity
Methenamine	⇧ Risk of crystalluria

ALTERED LABORATORY VALUES

Blood/serum values	⇩ PBI ⇩ ^{131}I thyroid uptake

No clinically significant alterations in urinary values occur at therapeutic dosages

Use in children

See INDICATIONS. Data on the safety of repeated use in children under 2 yr of age are limited; contraindicated for infants under 2 mo of age.

Use in pregnancy or nursing mothers

Contraindicated during pregnancy and in nursing mothers

[4]Includes reactions common to sulfonamides in general

FURADANTIN (Nitrofurantoin) Norwich-Eaton

Tabs: 50, 100 mg **Susp:** 25 mg/5 ml

INDICATIONS	ORAL DOSAGE
Urinary-tract infections caused by susceptible strains of *Escherichia coli*, enterococci, and *Staphylococcus aureus*,[1] and certain susceptible strains of *Klebsiella, Enterobacter*, and *Proteus*	**Adult:** 50–100 mg qid **Child:** 5–7 mg/kg/24 h in 4 divided doses, or as follows: **Child (15–26 lb):** 2.5 ml (½ tsp) qid **Child (27–46 lb):** 5 ml (1 tsp) qid **Child (47–68 lb):** 7.5 ml (1½ tsp) qid **Child (69–91 lb):** 10 ml (2 tsp) qid

ADMINISTRATION/DOSAGE ADJUSTMENTS

Cultures and susceptibility tests	Should be obtained prior to and during therapy
Gastric irritation	May be minimized by administering with food or milk
Duration of therapy	Continue treatment for a minimum of 1 wk and at least 3 days after urine becomes sterile

CONTRAINDICATIONS

Anuria or oliguria ●	Significantly impaired renal function ●	Hypersensitivity to nitrofurantoin ●

WARNINGS/PRECAUTIONS

Pulmonary reactions	May occur and can be fatal; discontinue drug and take appropriate measures
Long-term therapy	May lead to insidious onset of diffuse interstitial pneumonitis and/or pulmonary fibrosis; monitor patients closely and consider reduction in dosage
Hemolytic anemia of the primaquine-sensitivity type	May be induced in patients with G6PD deficiency; discontinue therapy
Superinfection	May occur, caused primarily by *Pseudomonas*
Severe or irreversible peripheral neuropathy	May occur and can be fatal; administer with caution to patients with renal impairment, anemia, diabetes, electrolyte imbalance, vitamin B deficiency, or debilitating disease

ADVERSE REACTIONS

	Frequent reactions are italicized
Gastrointestinal	*Anorexia, nausea, vomiting,* abdominal pain, diarrhea
Dermatological	Maculopapular, erythematous, or eczematous eruption; pruritus, urticaria, angioedema
Hematological	Hemolytic anemia, granulocytopenia, leukopenia, eosinophilia, megaloblastic anemia
Central nervous system	Peripheral neuropathy, headache, dizziness, nystagmus, drowsiness
Acute hypersensitivity[2]	Fever, chills, cough, chest pain, dyspnea, pulmonary infiltration with consolidation or pleural effusion on x-ray, eosinophilia
Chronic hypersensitivity[3]	Malaise, dyspnea on exertion, cough, altered pulmonary function, diffuse interstitial pneumonitis and/or fibrosis, fever (rarely prominent)
Other sensitivity reactions	Anaphylaxis, asthmatic attack (in patients with a history of asthma), cholestatic jaundice, drug fever, arthralgia
Other	Transient alopecia, genitourinary superinfection, hepatitis (rare)

OVERDOSAGE

Signs and symptoms	See ADVERSE REACTIONS
Treatment	Discontinue therapy; treat symptomatically

DRUG INTERACTIONS

Nalidixic acid	⇩ Effect of nitrofurantoin
Probenecid, sulfinpyrazone	⇧ Nitrofurantoin serum level and/or toxicity

ALTERED LABORATORY VALUES

Urinary values	⇧ Glucose (with Clinitest tablets)

No clinically significant alterations in blood/serum values occur at therapeutic dosages

Use in children	Use in pregnancy or nursing mothers
Contraindicated in infants under 1 mo of age because of the risk of hemolytic anemia due to glutathione instability	Contraindicated at term; safe use not established during pregnancy or in nursing mothers

[1]Not indicated for associated renal cortical or perinephric abscesses
[2]Usually occurs within the first week of treatment and is reversible with cessation of therapy; if drug is not withdrawn, symptoms may worsen
[3]Usually occurs after the first 6 mo of continuous treatment; permanent impairment of pulmonary function may remain even after drug is discontinued

Table continued on following page

GANTANOL (Sulfamethoxazole) **Roche**

Tabs: 0.5 g **Susp:** 0.5 g/5 ml

GANTANOL DS (Sulfamethoxazole) **Roche**

Tabs: 1 g

INDICATIONS	ORAL DOSAGE
Acute, recurrent, or chronic urinary-tract infections caused by susceptible strains of *Escherichia coli*, *Klebsiella-Enterobacter*, staphylococci, *Proteus mirabilis*, and *P vulgaris* in the absence of obstructive uropathy and foreign bodies **Prophylaxis of meningococcal meningitis** caused by sulfonamide-sensitive Group A strains **Acute otitis media** caused by *Haemophilus influenzae* when used concomitantly with penicillin **Trachoma, inclusion conjunctivitis, nocardiosis, chancroid** **Toxoplasmosis** (adjunctive therapy) **Malaria** caused by chloroquine-resistant strains of *Plasmodium falciparum* (adjunctive therapy)	**Adult:** 2 g or 20 ml (4 tsp) to start, followed by 1 g or 10 ml (2 tsp) bid (mild to moderate infections) or tid (severe infections) **Child:** 50–60 mg/kg to start, followed by 25–30 mg/kg bid (up to 75 mg/kg/24 h), or as follows: **Infant (20 lb):** 0.5 g or 5 ml (1 tsp) to start, followed by 0.25 g or 2.5 ml (½ tsp) bid **Child (40 lb):** 1 g or 10 ml (2 tsp) to start, followed by 0.5 g or 5 ml (1 tsp) bid **Child (60 lb):** 1.5 g or 15 ml (3 tsp) to start, followed by 0.75 g or 7.5 ml (1½ tsp) bid **Child (80 lb):** 2 g or 20 ml (4 tsp) to start, followed by 1 g or 10 ml (2 tsp) bid

ADMINISTRATION/DOSAGE ADJUSTMENTS

Therapeutic blood levels	For most infections, 5–15 mg/dl; for serious infections, 12–15 mg/dl; blood levels >20 mg/dl increase the probability of adverse reactions

CONTRAINDICATIONS

Hypersensitivity to sulfonamides

WARNINGS/PRECAUTIONS

Group A beta-hemolytic streptococcal infections	Sulfonamides have no place in the treatment of such infections, as they will neither eradicate the causative organism nor prevent complications
In vitro sulfonamide sensitivity tests	May not be reliable; coordinate test results with bacteriological and clinical response
Blood dyscrasias	May occur and can be fatal (see ADVERSE REACTIONS); obtain CBC frequently and watch for early signs (eg, sore throat, fever, pallor, purpura, jaundice) of serious blood disorders
Hypersensitivity reactions	May occur and can be fatal (see ADVERSE REACTIONS); use with caution in patients allergic to some goitrogens, diuretics, and oral hypoglycemic agents
Renal complications	May occur (see ADVERSE REACTIONS); perform a urinalysis, with microscopic examination, frequently
Crystalluria, urinary calculi	May be prevented by maintaining adequate fluid intake
Special-risk patients	Use with caution in patients with impaired renal or hepatic function, severe allergy, bronchial asthma, G6PD deficiency, or porphyria[1]

ADVERSE REACTIONS

Hematological	Agranulocytosis, aplastic anemia, thrombocytopenia, leukopenia, hemolytic anemia, purpura, hypoprothrombinemia, methemoglobinemia
Allergic	Erythema multiforme (Stevens-Johnson syndrome), generalized skin eruptions, epidermal necrolysis, urticaria, serum sickness, pruritus, exfoliative dermatitis, anaphylactoid reactions, periorbital edema, conjunctival and scleral injection, photosensitization, arthralgia, allergic myocarditis
Gastrointestinal	Nausea, vomiting, abdominal pain, hepatitis, diarrhea, anorexia, pancreatitis, stomatitis
Central nervous system	Headache, peripheral neuritis, mental depression, convulsions, ataxia, hallucinations, tinnitus, vertigo, insomnia

[1] *United States Pharmacopeia Dispensing Information 1980.* Rockville, Md., United States Pharmacopeial Convention, Inc., 1980

Table continued on following page

GANTANOL/GANTANOL DS continued

ADVERSE REACTIONS continued

Renal	Toxic nephrosis with oliguria and anuria, crystalluria, urinary calculi, diuresis (rare)
Endocrinological	Goiter (rare), hypoglycemia (rare)
Other	Drug fever, chills, periarteritis nodosa, lupus erythematosus phenomena

DRUG INTERACTIONS

Para-aminobenzoic acid	⇩ Bacteriostatic effect of sulfamethoxazole
Oral anticoagulants, oral hypoglycemics, methotrexate, phenytoin, thiopental	Effects increased or prolonged ⇧ Toxicity
Methenamine	⇧ Risk of crystalluria

ALTERED LABORATORY VALUES

Blood/serum values	⇩ PBI ⇩ ^{131}I thyroid uptake
Urinary values	⇧ Glucose (with Clinitest tablets)

Use in children

Contraindicated for use in infants under 2 mo of age except in the treatment of congenital toxoplasmosis as adjunctive therapy with pyrimethamine; maximum dose, 75 mg/kg/24 h. Prolonged or recurrent therapy in children under 6 yr of age with chronic renal diseases has been insufficiently studied.

Use in pregnancy or nursing mothers

Safe use has not been established during pregnancy; contraindicated at term and in nursing mothers. Sulfonamides cross the placental barrier, are excreted in breast milk, and may cause kernicterus.

GANTRISIN (Sulfisoxazole) Roche

Tabs: 0.5 g sulfisoxazole **Pediatric susp, pediatric syrup:** acetyl sulfisoxazole equivalent to 0.5 g sulfisoxazole/5 ml
Amps: 400 mg sulfisoxazole diolamine/ml (5 ml)

LIPO GANTRISIN (Acetyl sulfisoxazole) Roche

Susp (long-acting): acetyl sulfisoxazole equivalent to 1 g sulfisoxazole/5 ml

INDICATIONS	ORAL DOSAGE	PARENTERAL DOSAGE
Acute, recurrent, or chonic urinary-tract infections caused by susceptible strains of *Escherichia coli, Klebsiella-Enterobacter*, staphylococci, *Proteus mirabilis*, and *P vulgaris* in the absence of obstructive uropathy and foreign bodies **Meningococcal meningitis** caused by sulfonamide-sensitive strains ***Haemophilus influenzae* meningitis** (as an adjunct to parenteral streptomycin therapy) **Prophylaxis of meningococcal meningitis** caused by sulfonamide-sensitive Group A strains **Acute otitis media** caused by *Haemophilus influenzae* when used concomitantly with penicillin **Trachoma, inclusion conjunctivitis, nocardiosis, chancroid** **Toxoplasmosis** (adjunctive therapy) **Malaria** caused by chloroquine-resistant strains of *Plasmodium falciparum* (adjunctive therapy)	**Adult:** 2–4 g to start, followed by 4–8 g/24 h in 4–6 divided doses; long-acting susp: 4–5 g q12h **Infant (≥2 mo) and child:** 75 mg/kg (2 g/m²) to start, followed by 150 mg/kg/24 h (4 g/m²/24 h) in 4–6 divided doses, up to 6 g/24 h; long-acting susp: 60–75 mg/kg to start, followed by 60–75 mg/kg bid, up to 6 g/24 h	**Adult:** 50 mg/kg (1.25 g/m²) to start, followed by 100 mg/kg/24 h (2.25 g/m²/24 h) SC in 3 divided doses, IV (slowly) in 4 divided doses, or IM in 2–3 divided doses **Infant (≥2 mo) and child:** same as for adult

ADMINISTRATION/DOSAGE ADJUSTMENTS

Therapeutic blood levels	For most infections, 5–15 mg/dl; for serious infections, 12–15 mg/dl; blood levels >20 mg/dl increase the probability of adverse reactions
Dilution of parenteral form	For SC or IV administration, dilute solution supplied to 5% in sterile distilled water (use of other diluents may cause precipitation); for IM use, the solution supplied may be given undiluted. Up to 10 ml may be given IM to adults, but not more than 5 ml in any one site; children should receive correspondingly smaller volumes. Do not administer in combination with parenteral fluids. Rapid IV administration may precipitate severe systemic reactions.

CONTRAINDICATIONS

Hypersensitivity to sulfonamides

WARNINGS/PRECAUTIONS

Group A beta-hemolytic streptococcal infections	Sulfonamides have no place in the treatment of such infections, as they will neither eradicate the causative organism nor prevent complications
In vitro sulfonamide sensitivity tests	May not be reliable; coordinate test results with bacteriological and clinical response
Blood dyscrasias	May occur and can be fatal (see ADVERSE REACTIONS); obtain CBC frequently and watch for early signs (eg, sore throat, fever, pallor, purpura, jaundice) of serious blood disorders
Hypersensitivity reactions	May occur and can be fatal (see ADVERSE REACTIONS); use with caution in patients allergic to some goitrogens, diuretics, and oral hypoglycemia agents
Renal complications	May occur (see ADVERSE REACTIONS); perform a urinalysis, with microscopic examination, frequently
Crystalluria, urinary calculi	May be prevented by maintaining adequate fluid intake
Special-risk patients	Use with caution in patients with impaired renal or hepatic function, severe allergy, bronchial asthma, G6PD deficiency, or porphyria[1]

[1] *United States Pharmacopeia Dispensing Information 1980.* Rockville, Md., United States Pharmacopeial Convention, Inc., 1980

Table continued on following page

ADVERSE REACTIONS

Hematological	Agranulocytosis, aplastic anemia, thrombocytopenia, leukopenia, hemolytic anemia, purpura, hypoprothrombinemia, methemoglobinemia
Allergic	Erythema multiforme (Stevens-Johnson syndrome), generalized skin eruptions, epidermal necrolysis, urticaria, serum sickness, pruritus, exfoliative dermatitis, anaphylactoid reactions, periorbital edema, conjunctival and scleral injection, photosensitization, arthralgia, allergic myocarditis
Gastrointestinal	Nausea, vomiting, abdominal pain, hepatitis, diarrhea, anorexia, pancreatitis, stomatitis
Central nervous system	Headache, peripheral neuritis, mental depression, convulsions, ataxia, hallucinations, tinnitus, vertigo, insomnia
Renal	Toxic nephrosis with oliguria and anuria, crystalluria, urinary calculi, diuresis (rare)
Endocrinological	Goiter (rare), hypoglycemia (rare)
Other	Drug fever, chills, periarteritis nodosa, lupus erythematosus phenomena, local reactions (with IM use)

OVERDOSAGE

Signs and symptoms	See ADVERSE REACTIONS
Treatment	Discontinue use of drug; treat symptomatically

DRUG INTERACTIONS

Para-aminobenzoic acid	⇩ Bacteriostatic effect of sulfisoxazole
Oral anticoagulants, oral hypoglycemics, methotrexate, phenytoin, thiopental	Effects increased or prolonged ⇧ Toxicity
Methenamine	⇧ Risk of crystalluria

ALTERED LABORATORY VALUES

Blood/serum values	⇩ PBI ⇩ ^{131}I thyroid uptake ⇩ Glucose (rare)
Urinary values	⇧ Glucose (with Clinitest tablets) ⇧ Protein (with sulfosalicylic acid method)

Use in children

Contraindicated for use in infants under 2 mo of age except in the treatment of congenital toxoplasmosis as adjunctive therapy with pyrimethamine

Use in pregnancy or nursing mothers

Safe use has not been established during pregnancy; contraindicated at term and in nursing mothers. Sulfonamides cross the placental barrier, are excreted in breast milk, and may cause kernicterus.

HIPREX (Methenamine hippurate) Merrell-National

Tabs: 1 g

INDICATIONS	ORAL DOSAGE
Prophylaxis or suppression of frequently recurring urinary-tract infections following eradication of acute infection by other appropriate antimicrobial agents	**Adult:** 1 g bid in AM and PM **Child (6–12 yr):** 0.5–1.0 g bid in AM and PM

CONTRAINDICATIONS

Renal insufficiency ●	Severe dehydration ●
Severe hepatic insufficiency ●	Concurrent sulfonamide therapy ●

WARNINGS/PRECAUTIONS

High-dosage therapy (8 g/day for 3–4 wk)	May lead to bladder irritation, painful and frequent micturition, albuminuria, and gross hematuria
Urine acidity	Should be maintained, especially in treating infections due to urea-splitting organisms, such as *Proteus* and strains of *Pseudomonas*; restrict alkalinizing foods and medications, and provide supplemental acidifying medications, if necessary
Elevated serum transaminase levels	Perform liver-function studies periodically, especially in patients with liver dysfunction
Urine cultures	Should be obtained periodically to monitor efficacy of regimen

ADVERSE REACTIONS

Gastrointestinal	Nausea, upset stomach
Genitourinary	Dysuria
Dermatological	Rash

DRUG INTERACTIONS

Urinary alkalinizing agents, antacids, carbonic anhydrase inhibitors, thiazide diuretics	⇩ Antibacterial effectiveness
Sulfonamides	⇧ Risk of crystalluria

ALTERED LABORATORY VALUES

Blood/serum values	⇧ SGOT ⇧ SGPT (see WARNINGS/PRECAUTIONS)
Urinary values	⇧ Catecholamines (with fluorometric methods) ⇧ 17-OHCS (with Reddy method) ⇩ Estriol (with acid hydrolysis method) ⇩ 5-HIAA (with nitrosonaphthol reagent test)

Use in children

See INDICATIONS; general guidelines not established for use in children under 6 yr of age

Use in pregnancy or nursing mothers

Safe use not established in early pregnancy; appears to be safe for use during 3rd trimester. General guidelines not established for use in nursing mothers.

MACRODANTIN (Nitrofurantoin macrocrystals) Norwich-Eaton

Caps: 25, 50, 100 mg

INDICATIONS	ORAL DOSAGE
Urinary-tract infections caused by susceptible strains of *Escherichia coli*, enterococci, and *Staphylococcus aureus*,[1] and *Klebsiella, Enterobacter*, and *Proteus*	**Adult:** 50–100 mg qid **Child:** 5–7 mg/kg/24 h in 4 divided doses

ADMINISTRATION/DOSAGE ADJUSTMENTS

Cultures and susceptibility tests	Should be obtained prior to and during therapy
Gastric irritation	May be minimized by administering with food or milk
Duration of therapy	Continue treatment for a minimum of 1 wk and at least 3 days after urine becomes sterile

CONTRAINDICATIONS

Anuria or oliguria ● Significantly impaired renal function ● Hypersensitivity to nitrofurantoin ●

WARNINGS/PRECAUTIONS

Pulmonary reactions	May occur and can be fatal; discontinue drug and take appropriate measures
Long-term therapy	May lead to insidious onset of diffuse interstitial pneumonitis and/or pulmonary fibrosis;
Hemolytic anemia of the primaquine-sensitivity type	May be induced in patients with G6PD deficiency; discontinue therapy
Superinfection	May occur, caused primarily by *Pseudomonas*
Severe or irreversible peripheral neuropathy	May occur and can be fatal; administer with caution to patients with renal impairment, anemia, diabetes, electrolyte imbalance, vitamin B deficiency, or debilitating disease

ADVERSE REACTIONS

	Frequent reactions are italicized
Gastrointestinal	*Anorexia, nausea, vomiting*, abdominal pain, diarrhea
Dermatological	Maculopapular, erythematous, or eczematous eruption; pruritus, urticaria, angioedema
Hematological	Hemolytic anemia, granulocytopenia, leukopenia, eosinophilia, megaloblastic anemia
Central nervous system	Peripheral neuropathy, headache, dizziness, nystagmus, drowsiness
Acute hypersensitivity[2]	Fever, chills, cough, chest pain, dyspnea, pulmonary infiltration, eosinophilia
Chronic hypersensitivity[3]	Malaise, dyspnea on exertion, cough, altered pulmonary function, diffuse interstitial pneumonitis and/or fibrosis, fever (rarely prominent)
Other sensitivity reactions	Anaphylaxis, asthmatic attack (in patients with a history of asthma), cholestatic jaundice, drug fever, arthralgia
Other	Transient alopecia, genitourinary superinfection, hepatitis (rare)

OVERDOSAGE

Signs and symptoms	See ADVERSE REACTIONS
Treatment	Discontinue therapy; treat symptomatically

DRUG INTERACTIONS

Nalidixic acid	⇩ Effect of nitrofurantoin
Probenecid, sulfinpyrazone	⇧ Nitrofurantoin serum level and/or toxicity

ALTERED LABORATORY VALUES

Urinary values	⇧ Glucose (with Clinitest tablets)

No clinically significant alterations in blood/serum values occur at therapeutic dosages

Use in children	Use in pregnancy or nursing mothers
Contraindicated in infants under 1 mo of age because of the risk of hemolytic anemia due to glutathione instability	Contraindicated at term; safe use not established during pregnancy or in nursing mothers

[1]Not indicated for associated renal cortical or perinephric abscesses
[2]Usually occurs within the first week of treatment and is reversible with cessation of therapy; if drug is not withdrawn, symptoms may worsen
[3]Usually occurs after the first 6 mo of continuous treatment; permanent impairment of pulmonary function may remain even after drug is discontinued

Table continued on following page

MANDELAMINE (Methenamine mandelate) Parke-Davis

Tabs: 0.25, 0.5, 1.0 g **Granules:** 0.5, 1.0 g **Susp:** 250 mg/5 ml, 500 mg/5 ml (Forte)

INDICATIONS	ORAL DOSAGE
Suppression or elimination of bacteruria associated with pyelonephritis, cystitis, and other chronic urinary-tract infections **Infected residual urine** accompanying neurological disease	**Adult:** 1 g qid after each meal and at bedtime **Child (<6 yr):** 0.25 g/30 lb qid **Child (6–12 yr):** 0.5 g qid after each meal and at bedtime

CONTRAINDICATIONS

Renal insufficiency ●

When urine acidification is contraindicated or unattainable ●

WARNINGS/PRECAUTIONS

Dysuria	May occur, especially at dosages higher than those recommended above. Control by reducing dosage and acidification; restrict alkalinizing foods and medication and, if necessary, provide supplemental acidifying agents.
Elderly and/or debilitated patients	Administer suspension formulas with caution to avoid inducing lipid pneumonia

ADVERSE REACTIONS

Gastrointestinal	GI disturbance
Dermatological	Rash

OVERDOSAGE

Signs and symptoms	See ADVERSE REACTIONS
Treatment	Discontinue medication; treat symptomatically

DRUG INTERACTIONS

Urinary alkalinizing agents, antacids, carbonic anhydrase inhibitors, thiazide diuretics	⇩ Antibacterial effectiveness
Sulfonamides	⇧ Risk of crystalluria

ALTERED LABORATORY VALUES

Urinary values	⇧ Catecholamines (with fluorometric methods) ⇧ 17-OHCS (with Reddy method) ⇩ Estriol (with acid hydrolysis method) ⇩ 5-HIAA (with nitroso-naphthol reagent test)

No clinically significant alterations in blood/serum values occur at therapeutic dosages

Use in children

See INDICATIONS

Use in pregnancy or nursing mothers

General guidelines not established

NegGram (Nalidixic acid) Winthrop

Tabs: 250, 500, 1,000 mg **Susp:** 250 mg/5 ml

INDICATIONS	ORAL DOSAGE
Urinary-tract infections caused by susceptible Gram-negative microorganisms, including most *Proteus* strains, *Klebsiella*, *Enterobacter*, and *Escherichia coli*	**Adult:** 1 g qid for 1–2 wk, followed by 2 g/day for prolonged therapy **Child:** 55 mg/kg/day in 4 divided doses for 1–2 wk, followed by 33 mg/kg/day for prolonged therapy

ADMINISTRATION/DOSAGE ADJUSTMENTS

Susceptibility tests	Should be performed with 30-μg disc prior to therapy, as well as during treatment if warranted by the clinical response
Bacterial resistance	May emerge within 48 h after start of therapy; repeat cultures and sensitivity tests and institute appropriate anti-infective therapy

CONTRAINDICATIONS

Hypersensitivity to nalidixic acid ●	History of convulsive disorders ●

WARNINGS/PRECAUTIONS

Prolonged therapy	Perform blood counts and renal- and liver-function tests periodically if treatment continues for longer than 2 wk
Special-risk patients	Use with caution in patients with liver disease, epilepsy, severe cerebral arteriosclerosis, or severe renal failure
Photosensitivity	Avoid undue exposure to direct sunlight; discontinue therapy if photosensitivity occurs. Bullae may continue to appear with successive exposures to sunlight or with mild skin trauma for up to 3 mo after discontinuation of drug.
Underdosage during initial therapy	May lead to emergence of bacterial resistance
CNS toxicity (rare)	Brief convulsions, increased intracranial pressure, and toxic psychosis may occur, especially in infants, children, and elderly patients (usually from overdosage) and in patients with predisposing factors. Discontinue therapy and institute appropriate corrective measures; diagnostic procedures involving risk to the patient should be undertaken only if CNS symptoms do not rapidly disappear within 48 h.
Cross-resistance	May occur with oxolinic acid

ADVERSE REACTIONS

Central nervous system	Drowsiness, weakness, headache, dizziness, vertigo, toxic psychosis, brief convulsions, 6th cranial nerve palsy, paresthesia (rare)
Ophthalmic	Reversible visual disturbances, including overbrightness of lights, change in color perception, difficulty in focusing, decreased acuity, double vision
Gastrointestinal	Abdominal pain, nausea, vomiting, diarrhea, cholestasis (rare)
Allergic	Rash, pruritus, urticaria, angioedema, eosinophilia, arthralgia with joint stiffness and swelling, anaphylaxis, photosensitivity reactions, including erythema and bullae
Metabolic	Acidosis (rare)
Hematological	Thrombocytopenia (rare), leukopenia (rare), hemolytic anemia (rare), G6PD deficiency (rare)

OVERDOSAGE

Signs and symptoms	Toxic psychosis, convulsions, increased intracranial pressure, metabolic acidosis, vomiting, nausea, lethargy
Treatment	Drug is rapidly excreted. If overdosage is noted early, empty stomach contents by gastric lavage. Employ supportive measures, and administer IV fluids. Provide assisted ventilation, if needed. For severe toxicity, anticonvulsant therapy may be indicated.

DRUG INTERACTIONS

Oral anticoagulants	⇧ Anticoagulant effect

Table continued on following page

ALTERED LABORATORY VALUES

Urinary values ——— ⇧ Glucose (with Clinitest tablets) ⇧ 17-Ketosteroids (with Zimmerman method)

No clinically significant alterations in blood/serum values occur at therapeutic dosages

Use in children

Contraindicated in children under 3 mo of age; reversible increased intracranial pressure, with bulging anterior fontanels, papilledema, and headache, has been reported in infants and children receiving therapeutic doses

Use in pregnancy or nursing mothers

Safe use not established during 1st trimester; general guidelines not established for use in nursing mothers

PROLOPRIM (Trimethoprim) Burroughs Wellcome

Tabs: 100 mg

INDICATIONS	ORAL DOSAGE
Initial episodes of uncomplicated urinary-tract infections caused by susceptible strains of *Escherichia coli, Proteus mirabilis, Klebsiella pneumoniae,* and *Enterobacter*	**Adult:** 100 mg q12h for 10 days

ADMINISTRATION/DOSAGE ADJUSTMENTS

Cultures and susceptibility tests	Should be performed to determine bacterial susceptibility to trimethoprim, although therapy may be initiated prior to test results
Patients with renal impairment	Reduce dosage to 50 mg q12h if creatinine clearance rate (CCr)=15–30 ml/min; do not administer if CCr <15 ml/min

CONTRAINDICATIONS

Hypersensitivity to trimethoprim ●	Established megaloblastic anemia due to folate deficiency ●

WARNINGS/PRECAUTIONS

Blood dyscrasias	May occur rarely, especially with high doses and/or prolonged therapy. Obtain CBC if early signs develop (eg, sore throat, fever, pallor, or purpura). If signs of bone marrow depression (thrombocytopenia, leukopenia, and/or megaloblastic anemia) are present, discontinue therapy and administer leucovorin, 3–6 mg/day IM, for 3 days or until hematopoiesis is normal.
Suspected folate deficiency	Use with caution; concomitant administration of folates does not interfere with antibacterial action
Hepatic or renal impairment	Use with caution (see ADMINISTRATION/DOSAGE ADJUSTMENTS)

ADVERSE REACTIONS

	Frequent reactions are italicized
Dermatological	*Mild-to-moderate maculopapular, morbilliform rash (2.9%); pruritus;* exfoliative dermatitis
Gastrointestinal	Epigastric distress, nausea, vomiting, glossitis
Hematological	Thrombocytopenia, leukopenia, neutropenia, megaloblastic anemia, methemoglobinemia
Other	Fever

OVERDOSAGE

Signs and symptoms	Nausea, vomiting, dizziness, headache, mental depression, confusion, bone marrow depression (manifested as thrombocytopenia, leukopenia, megaloblastic anemia)
Treatment	Evacuate stomach by gastric lavage and institute general supportive measures. Acidify urine to increase renal elimination. Peritoneal dialysis is ineffective and hemodialysis only moderately effective.

DRUG INTERACTIONS

No clinically significant drug interactions have been observed

ALTERED LABORATORY VALUES

Blood/serum values	⇧ SGOT ⇧ SGPT ⇧ Bilirubin ⇧ BUN ⇧ Creatinine

No clinically significant alterations in urinary values occur at therapeutic dosages

Use in children

Safety in infants under 2 mo of age not established; effectiveness not established in children under 12 yr of age

Use in pregnancy or nursing mothers

Pregnancy category C. Teratogenicity has been shown in rats at doses 40 times human dose; in rabbits, doses 6 times human dose have been associated with an increase in fetal loss. Human studies have been inconclusive. Trimethoprim may interfere with folic acid metabolism and appears in breast milk. Use during pregnancy or lactation with caution, and only if potential benefit outweighs risk to fetus or nursing infant.

RENOQUID (Sulfacytine) Parke-Davis

Tabs: 250 mg

INDICATIONS	ORAL DOSAGE
Acute urinary-tract infections caused by susceptible strains	**Adult:** 500 mg to start, followed by 250 mg qid for 10 days

CONTRAINDICATIONS

Hypersensitivity to sulfonamides

WARNINGS/PRECAUTIONS

In vitro sulfonamide sensitivity tests	May not be reliable; coordinate test results with bacteriological and clinical response
Blood dyscrasias	May occur and can be fatal (see ADVERSE REACTIONS); obtain CBC frequently
Hypersensitivity reactions	May occur and can be fatal (see ADVERSE REACTIONS)
Renal complications	May occur (see ADVERSE REACTIONS); perform a urinalysis
Crystalluria, urinary calculi	May be prevented by maintaining adequate fluid intake
Special-risk patients	Use with caution in patients with impaired renal or hepatic function, severe allergy, bronchial asthma, or G6PD deficiency

ADVERSE REACTIONS[1]

Hematological	Agranulocytosis, aplastic anemia, thrombocytopenia, leukopenia, hemolytic anemia, purpura, hypoprothrombinemia, methemoglobinemia
Allergic	Erythema multiforme (including Stevens-Johnson syndrome), generalized skin eruptions, epidermal necrolysis, urticaria, serum sickness, pruritus, exfoliative dermatitis, anaphylactoid reactions, periorbital edema, conjunctival and scleral injection, photosensitization, arthralgia, allergic myocarditis
Gastrointestinal	Nausea, vomiting, abdominal pain, hepatitis, diarrhea, anorexia, pancreatitis, stomatitis
Central nervous system	Headache, peripheral neuritis, mental depression, convulsions, ataxia, hallucinations, tinnitus, vertigo, insomnia
Renal	Toxic nephrosis with oliguria and anuria, crystalluria, urinary calculi, diuresis (rare)
Endocrinological	Goiter (rare), hypoglycemia (rare)
Other	Drug fever, chills, periarteritis nodosa, lupus erythematosus phenomena

OVERDOSAGE

Signs and symptoms	See ADVERSE REACTIONS
Treatment	Discontinue use of drug; treat symptomatically

DRUG INTERACTIONS

Para-aminobenzoic acid (PABA)	⇩ Bacteriostatic effect of sulfacytine
Oral anticoagulants, oral hypoglycemics, methotrexate, phenytoin, thiopental	Effects increased or prolonged ⇧ Toxicity
Methenamine	⇧ Risk of crystalluria

ALTERED LABORATORY VALUES

Blood/serum values	⇩ PBI ⇩ ^{131}I thyroid uptake	Urinary values	⇧ Glucose

Use in children	Use in pregnancy or nursing mothers
Contraindicated for use in infants under 2 mo of age; not recommended for use in children under 14 yr of age	Safe use has not been established during pregnancy; contraindicated at term and in nursing mothers. Sulfonamides cross the placental barrier, are excreted in breast milk, and may cause kernicterus.

[1]Includes reactions common to sulfonamides in general

Table continued on following page

SEPTRA (Trimethoprim and sulfamethoxazole) Burroughs Wellcome

Tabs: 80 mg trimethoprim and 400 mg sulfamethoxazole **Susp:** 40 mg trimethoprim and 200 mg sulfamethoxazole per 5 ml

SEPTRA DS (Trimethoprim and sulfamethoxazole) Burroughs Wellcome

Tabs: 160 mg trimethoprim and 800 mg sulfamethoxazole

INDICATIONS	ORAL DOSAGE
Urinary-tract infections caused by susceptible strains of *Escherichia coli, Klebsiella-Enterobacter, Proteus mirabilis, P vulgaris,* and *P morganii*[1]	**Adult:** 2 Septra tabs, 1 Septra DS tab, or 20 ml (4 tsp) q12h for 10–14 days **Child:** 4 mg/kg trimethoprim and 20 mg/kg sulfamethoxazole q12h for 10 days, or as follows: **Child (10 kg or 22 lb):** ½ Septra tab or 5 ml (1 tsp) q12h for 10 days **Child (20 kg or 44 lb):** 1 Septra tab or 10 ml (2 tsp) q12h for 10 days **Child (30 kg or 66 lb):** 1½ Septra tabs or 15 ml (3 tsp) q12h for 10 days **Child (40 kg or 88 lb):** 2 Septra tabs, 1 Septra DS tab, or 20 ml (4 tsp) q12h for 10 days
Acute otitis media caused by susceptible strains of *Haemophilus influenzae* or *Streptococcus pneumoniae*[2]	**Child:** Same as child dosage above.
Acute exacerbations of chronic bronchitis caused by susceptible strains of *Haemophilus influenzae* or *Streptococcus pneumoniae*	**Adult:** Same as adult dosage above.
Enteritis caused by susceptible strains of *Shigella flexneri* and *S sonnei*	**Adult:** same as adult's dosage above for 5 days **Child:** same as child's dosage above for 5 days
***Pneumocystis carinii* pneumonitis**	**Adult:** 5 mg/kg trimethoprim and 25 mg/kg sulfamethoxazole q6h for 14 days **Child:** same as for adult, or as follows: **Child (8 kg or 18 lb):** ½ Septra tab or 5 ml (1 tsp) q6h for 14 days **Child (16 kg or 35 lb):** 1 Septra tab or 10 ml (2 tsp) q6h for 14 days **Child (24 kg or 53 lb):** 1½ Septra tabs or 15 ml (3 tsp) q6h for 14 days **Child (32 kg or 70 lb):** 2 Septra tabs, 1 Septra DS tab, or 20 ml (4 tsp) q6h for 14 days

ADMINISTRATION/DOSAGE ADJUSTMENTS

Patients with renal impairment	Follow the usual dosage regimen if creatinine clearance rate (CCr)>30 ml/min. Administer half the usual dosage if CCr=15-30 ml/min. Use is not recommended if CCr<15 ml/min.

CONTRAINDICATIONS

Hypersensitivity to trimethoprim or sulfonamides

WARNINGS/PRECAUTIONS

Group A beta-hemolytic streptococcal pharyngitis	Sulfonamides have no place in the treatment of such infections, as they will neither eradicate the causative organism from the tonsillopharyngeal area nor prevent complications
Blood dyscrasias	May occur and can be fatal (see ADVERSE REACTIONS); obtain CBC frequently and watch for early signs (eg, sore throat, fever, pallor, purpura, jaundice) of serious blood disorders. Discontinue treatment if count of any formed blood element falls significantly.
Hypersensitivity reactions	May occur and can be fatal (see ADVERSE REACTIONS); use with caution in patients allergic to some goitrogens, diuretics, and oral hypoglycemic agents
Renal complications	May occur (see ADVERSE REACTIONS); perform a urinalysis, with careful microscopic examination, during therapy, particularly if renal function is impaired
Crystalluria, urinary calculi	May be prevented by maintaining adequate fluid intake
Special-risk patients	Use with caution in patients with impaired renal or hepatic function, folate deficiency, severe allergy, bronchial asthma, G6PD deficiency, or porphyria[3] and in elderly patients being treated with certain diuretics, particularly thiazides

[1]Initial episodes of uncomplicated infections should be treated with a single, effective antibacterial agent, rather than a combination
[2]Not indicated for prophylaxis or prolonged administration
[3]*United States Pharmacopeia Dispensing Information 1980.* Rockville, Md., United States Pharmacopeial Convention, Inc., 1980
[4]Includes reactions common to sulfonamides in general

Table continued on following page

SEPTRA/SEPTRA DS continued

ADVERSE REACTIONS[1]

Hematological	Agranulocytosis, aplastic anemia, megaloblastic anemia, thrombopenia, leukopenia, hemolytic anemia, purpura, hypoprothrombinemia, methemoglobinemia
Allergic	Erythema multiforme (Stevens-Johnson syndrome), generalized skin eruptions, epidermal necrolysis, urticaria, serum sickness, pruritus, exfoliative dermatitis, anaphylactoid reactions, periorbital edema, conjunctival and scleral injection, photosensitization, arthralgia, allergic myocarditis
Gastrointestinal	Glossitis, stomatitis, nausea, vomiting, abdominal pain, hepatitis, diarrhea, pancreatitis
Central nervous system	Headache, peripheral neuritis, mental depression, convulsions, ataxia, hallucinations, tinnitus, vertigo, insomnia, apathy, fatigue, muscle weakness, nervousness
Renal	Toxic nephrosis with oliguria and anuria, crystalluria, urinary calculi, diuresis (rare)
Endocrinological	Goiter (rare), hypoglycemia (rare)
Other	Drug fever, chills, periarteritis nodosa, lupus erythematosus phenomena

OVERDOSAGE

Signs and symptoms	See ADVERSE REACTIONS
Treatment	Discontinue use of drug; treat symptomatically

DRUG INTERACTIONS

Diuretics (especially thiazides)	⇧ Risk of thrombopenia with purpura in elderly patients
Para-aminobenzoic acid	⇩ Bacteriostatic effect of sulfamethoxazole
Warfarin	⇧ Prothrombin time
Oral hypoglycemics, methotrexate, phenytoin, thiopental	Effects increased or prolonged ⇧ Toxicity
Methenamine	⇩ Risk of crystalluria

ALTERED LABORATORY VALUES

Blood/serum values	⇩ PBI ⇩ ^{131}I thyroid uptake

No clinically significant alterations in urinary values occur at therapeutic dosages

Use in children

See INDICATIONS. Data on the safety of repeated use in children under 2 yr of age are limited; contraindicated for infants under 2 mo of age.

Use in pregnancy or nursing mothers

Contraindicated during pregnancy and in nursing mothers

[1]Includes reactions common to sulfonamides in general

THIOSULFIL (Sulfamethizole) Ayerst

Tabs: 0.25 g

THIOSULFIL FORTE (Sulfamethizole) Ayerst

Tabs: 0.5 g

INDICATIONS	ORAL DOSAGE
Urinary-tract infections caused by susceptible strains of *Escherichia coli, Klebsiella-Enterobacter, Staphylococcus aureus, Proteus mirabilis,* and *P vulgaris* in the absence of obstructive uropathy and foreign bodies	**Adult:** 0.5–1.0 g tid or qid **Infant (>2 mo) and child:** 30–45 mg/kg/day in 4 divided doses

ADMINISTRATION/DOSAGE ADJUSTMENTS

Therapeutic blood levels	For most infections, 5–15 mg/dl; for serious infections, 12–15 mg/dl. Blood levels >20 mg/dl increase the probability of adverse reactions.

CONTRAINDICATIONS

Hypersensitivity to sulfonamides

WARNINGS/PRECAUTIONS

Group A beta-hemolytic streptococcal infections	Sulfonamides have no place in the treatment of such infections, as they will neither eradicate the causative organism nor prevent complications
In vitro sulfonamide sensitivity tests	May not be reliable; coordinate test results with bacteriological and clinical response
Blood dyscrasias	May occur and can be fatal (see ADVERSE REACTIONS); obtain frequent blood counts and watch for early signs (eg, sore throat, fever, pallor, purpura, jaundice) of serious blood disorders
Hypersensitivity reactions	May occur and can be fatal (see ADVERSE REACTIONS); use with caution in patients allergic to some goitrogens, diuretics, and oral hypoglycemic agents
Renal complications	May occur (see ADVERSE REACTIONS); obtain frequent renal-function studies and perform a weekly urinalysis, with microscopic examination, if patient is treated for longer than 2 wk
Crystalluria, urinary calculi	May be prevented by maintaining adequate fluid intake
Special-risk patients	Use with caution in patients with severe renal or hepatic impairment, severe allergy, bronchial asthma, or G6PD deficiency

ADVERSE REACTIONS

Hematological	Agranulocytosis, aplastic anemia, thrombocytopenia, leukopenia, hemolytic anemia, purpura, hypoprothrombinemia, methemoglobinemia
Allergic	Erythema multiforme (Stevens-Johnson syndrome), generalized skin eruptions, epidermal necrolysis, urticaria, serum sickness, pruritus, exfoliative dermatitis, anaphylactoid reactions, periorbital edema, conjunctival and scleral injection, photosensitization, arthralgia, allergic myocarditis
Gastrointestinal	Nausea, vomiting, abdominal pain, hepatitis, diarrhea, anorexia, pancreatitis, stomatitis
Central nervous system	Headache, peripheral neuritis, mental depression, convulsions, ataxia, hallucinations, tinnitus, vertigo, insomnia
Renal	Toxic nephrosis with oliguria and anuria, diuresis (rare)
Endocrinological	Goiter (rare), hypoglycemia (rare)
Other	Drug fever, chills, periarteritis nodosa, lupus erythematosus phenomena

OVERDOSAGE

Signs and symptoms	See ADVERSE REACTIONS
Treatment	Discontinue use of drug; treat symptomatically

Table continued on following page

THIOSULFIL/THIOSULFIL FORTE continued

DRUG INTERACTIONS

Para-aminobenzoic acid (PABA)	⇩ Bacteriostatic effect of sulfamethizole
Oral anticoagulants, oral hypoglycemics, methotrexate, phenytoin, thiopental	Effects increased or prolonged ⇧ Toxicity
Methenamine	⇧ Risk of crystalluria

ALTERED LABORATORY VALUES

Blood/serum values	⇩ PBI ⇩ ^{131}I thyroid uptake
Urinary values	⇧ Glucose (with Clinitest tablets)

Use in children

Contraindicated for use in infants under 2 mo of age

Use in pregnancy or nursing mothers

Safe use has not been established during pregnancy; contraindicated at term and in nursing mothers. Sulfonamides cross the placental barrier, are excreted in breast milk, and may cause kernicterus.

TRIMPEX (Trimethoprim) **Roche**

Tabs: 100 mg

INDICATIONS	ORAL DOSAGE
Initial episodes of uncomplicated urinary-tract infections caused by susceptible strains of *Escherichia coli, Proteus mirabilis, Klebsiella pneumoniae,* and *Enterobacter*	**Adult:** 100 mg q12h for 10 days

ADMINISTRATION/DOSAGE ADJUSTMENTS

Cultures and susceptibility tests	Should be performed to determine bacterial susceptibility to trimethoprim, although therapy may be initiated prior to test results
Patients with renal impairment	Reduce dosage to 50 mg q12h if creatinine clearance rate (CCr)=15–30 ml/min; do not administer if CCr <15 ml/min

CONTRAINDICATIONS

Hypersensitivity to trimethoprim ●	Established megaloblastic anemia due to folate deficiency ●

WARNINGS/PRECAUTIONS

Blood dyscrasias	May occur rarely, especially with high doses and/or prolonged therapy. Obtain CBC if early signs develop (eg, sore throat, fever, pallor, or purpura). If signs of bone marrow depression (thrombocytopenia, leukopenia, and/or megaloblastic anemia) are present, discontinue therapy and administer leucovorin, 3–6 mg/day IM, for 3 days or until hematopoiesis is normal.
Suspected folate deficiency	Use with caution; concomitant administration of folates does not interfere with antibacterial action
Hepatic or renal impairment	Use with caution (see ADMINISTRATION/DOSAGE ADJUSTMENTS)

ADVERSE REACTIONS

Frequent reactions are italicized

Dermatological	*Mild-to-moderate maculopapular, morbilliform rash (2.9%); pruritus;* exfoliative dermatitis
Gastrointestinal	Epigastric distress, nausea, vomiting, glossitis
Hematological	Thrombocytopenia, leukopenia, neutropenia, megaloblastic anemia, methemoglobinemia
Other	Fever

OVERDOSAGE

Signs and symptoms	Nausea, vomiting, dizziness, headache, mental depression, confusion, bone marrow depression (manifested as thrombocytopenia, leukopenia, megaloblastic anemia)
Treatment	Evacuate stomach by gastric lavage and institute general supportive measures. Acidify urine to increase renal elimination. Peritoneal dialysis is ineffective and hemodialysis only moderately effective.

DRUG INTERACTIONS

No clinically significant drug interactions have been observed

ALTERED LABORATORY VALUES

Blood/serum values	⇧ SGOT ⇧ SGPT ⇧ Bilirubin ⇧ BUN ⇧ Creatinine

No clinically significant alterations in urinary values occur at therapeutic dosages

Use in children

Safety in infants under 2 mo of age not established; effectiveness not established in children under 12 yr of age

Use in pregnancy or nursing mothers

Pregnancy category C. Teratogenicity has been shown in rats at doses 40 times human dose; in rabbits, doses 6 times human dose have been associated with an increase in fetal loss. Human studies have been inconclusive. Trimethoprim may interfere with folic acid metabolism and appears in breast milk. Use during pregnancy or lactation with caution, and only if potential benefit outweighs risk to fetus or nursing infant.

URISED (Atropine sulfate, hyoscyamine, methenamine, methylene blue, phenyl salicylate, and benzoic acid) Webcon

Tabs: 0.03 mg atropine sulfate, 0.03 mg hyoscyamine, 40.8 mg methenamine, 5.4 mg methylene blue, 18.1 mg phenyl salicylate, and 4.5 mg benzoic acid

INDICATIONS

Lower urinary-tract discomfort caused by hypermotility
Cystitis, urethritis, and trigonitis caused by organisms susceptible to formaldehyde
Prophylaxis prior to **urinary-tract instrumentation or operation**
Relief of **urinary-tract symptoms during diagnostic procedures**

ORAL DOSAGE

Adult: 2 tabs qid, followed by liberal fluid intake
Child: reduce adult dosage in proportion to age and weight

CONTRAINDICATIONS

Urinary bladder-neck or pyloric obstruction ●

Duodenal obstruction ●

Glaucoma ●

Cardiospasm ●

Hypersensitivity to any component ●

WARNINGS/PRECAUTIONS

Known idiosyncratic reaction to atropine-like compounds	Administer with caution
Urine discoloration	Urine may appear blue in color; advise patients accordingly
Acute urinary retention	May be precipitated in patients with prostatic hypertrophy

ADVERSE REACTIONS

Gastrointestinal	Dry mouth
Genitourinary	Difficult micturition, acute urinary retention
Central nervous system	Blurred vision, dizziness
Cardiovascular	Rapid pulse, flushing

OVERDOSAGE

Signs and symptoms	See ADVERSE REACTIONS
Treatment	Reduce dosage or discontinue medication; treat symptomatically

DRUG INTERACTIONS

Other antimuscarinics, amantadine, antihistamines, haloperidol, phenothiazines, MAO inhibitors, tricyclic antidepressants	⇧ Atropine-like effects
Urinary alkalinizing agents, antacids, carbonic anhydrase inhibitors, thiazide diuretics	⇩ Antibacterial effectiveness
Sulfonamides	⇧ Risk of crystalluria

ALTERED LABORATORY VALUES

Urinary values	⇧ Catecholamines (with fluorometric methods) ⇧ 17-OHCS (with Reddy method) ⇩ Estriol (with acid hydrolysis method) ⇩ 5-HIAA (with nitrosonaphthol reagent test)

No clinically significant alterations in blood/serum values occur at therapeutic dosages

Use in children

General guidelines not established for use in younger children

Use in pregnancy or nursing mothers

General guidelines not established

Product (Manufacturer)	Ingredients	Actions
Achromycin Ointment (Lederle) Ointment **Dosage** Apply to affected areas as needed	3% Tetracycline hydrochloride	Inhibits bacterial growth
Baciguent Ointment (Upjohn) Ointment **Dosage** Apply to affected areas as needed	500 units/g Bacitracin	Inhibits bacterial growth
Bacimycin (Merrell-National) Ointment **Dosage** Apply to affected areas as needed	500 units/g Bacitracin	Inhibits bacterial growth
	3.5 mg/g Neomycin	Inhibits bacterial growth
	Petrolatum	Ointment base
Bactine (Miles) Liquid **Dosage** Apply to affected areas as needed	Benzalkonium chloride	Antiseptic
	3.17% Alcohol	Astringent and antiseptic base
Betadine Solution (Purdue Frederick) Liquid **Dosage** Apply to affected areas as needed	10% Povidone-iodine	Antiseptic
Desenex Ointment (Pennwalt) Ointment **Dosage** Apply to affected areas each AM and PM	20% Zinc undecylenate	Inhibits fungal growth
	5% Undecylenic acid	Inhibits fungal growth
Isodine Antiseptic Skin Cleanser (Blair) Liquid **Dosage** Apply liberally to affected areas as needed	7.5% Povidone-iodine	Antiseptic
Isodine Antiseptic Solution (Blair) Liquid **Dosage** Apply liberally to affected areas as needed	10% Povidone-iodine	Antiseptic
Isodine Antiseptic Ointment (Blair) Ointment **Dosage** Apply liberally to affected areas as needed	10% Povidone-iodine	Antiseptic
Myciguent Cream (Upjohn) Cream **Dosage** Apply to affected areas as needed	5 mg/g Neomycin sulfate	Inhibits bacterial growth
Mycitracin Ointment (Upjohn) Ointment **Dosage** Apply to affected areas as needed	5000 units/g Polymyxin B sulfate	Inhibits bacterial growth
	500 units/g Bacitracin	Inhibits bacterial growth
	5 mg/g Neomycin sulfate	Inhibits bacterial growth

Table continued on following page

NONPRESCRIPTION TOPICAL ANTIBIOTICS

Product (Manufacturer)	Ingredients	Actions
Neo-Polycin Ointment (Dow) Ointment **Dosage** Apply to affected areas as needed	5000 units/g Polymyxin B sulfate	Inhibits bacterial growth
	400 units/g Bacitracin zinc	Inhibits bacterial growth
	3.5 mg/g Neomycin (as sulfate)	Inhibits bacterial growth
	Fuzene	Ointment base
	Polyethyene glycol dilaurate	Ointment base
	Polyethyene glycol disterate	Ointment base
	Light liquid petrolatum	Ointment base
	Synthetic glyceride wax	Hardening agent
	White petrolatum	Ointment base
Neosporin Ointment (Burroughs Wellcome) Ointment **Dosage** Apply to affected areas as needed	5000 units/g Polymyxin B sulfate	Inhibits bacterial growth
	400 units/g Bacitracin zinc	Inhibits bacterial growth
	3.5 mg/g Neomycin (as sulfate)	Inhibits bacterial growth
	White petrolatum	Ointment base
Polysporin Ointment (Burroughs Wellcome) Ointment **Dosage** Apply to affected areas as needed	10,000 units/g Polymyxin B sulfate	Inhibits bacterial growth
	500 units/g Bacitracin zinc	Inhibits bacterial growth
	White petrolatum	Ointment base
S.T. 37 (Beecham) Liquid **Dosage** Apply undiluted to affected areas; bandage lightly if desired. Use as needed.	Hexylresorcin	Antiseptic
	Glycerin	Emollient
Terramycin Ointment with Polymyxin B Sulfate (Pfipharmecs) Ointment **Dosage** Apply to affected areas as needed	30 mg/g Oxytetracycline hydrochloride	Inhibits bacterial growth
	10,000 units/g Polymyxin B sulfate	Inhibits bacterial growth
Vioform Cream (CIBA) Cream **Dosage** Apply to affected areas as needed	3% Iodochlorhydroxyquin	Antiseptic
	Water-washable base	
Zephiran Chloride Solution (Winthrop) Liquid **Dosage** Apply to affected areas as needed	0.13% Benzalkonium chloride	Antiseptic
Zephiran Chloride Spray (Winthrop) Liquid **Dosage** Apply onto affected areas as needed	0.13% Benzalkonium chloride	Antiseptic

Fungal Infections

About fifty different varieties of fungi—primitive plant-like organisms that lack chlorophyll and therefore live off other living or dead material—are capable of causing disease in human beings. Fungi exist in two interchangeable forms—a single-cell or yeast form and a multicellular mold form. Its environment at any given time determines which form the fungus will adopt. Most fungi that cause disease in human beings do so in the yeast form, but when these fungi are cultured for identification in the laboratory, they transform themselves into the mold form.

Fungal infections, also called mycotic infections, develop in three characteristic patterns. By far the most common are the superficial infections of the skin and nails, as seen in athlete's foot or ringworm. Deep, widespread systemic fungal infections of the liver, lung, kidney, and other internal organs are relatively rare. Finally, there are the fungal infections caused by opportunistic fungi that live harmlessly in the environment or are present in man as "normal flora," but are capable of causing disease in persons who have diminished immune and white-cell defenses. Persons with diabetes, leukemia and other cancers, and kidney disease are particularly susceptible. Patients on long-term steroid medication, broad-spectrum antibiotics, and anticancer chemotherapy, as well as those who have received organ transplants, all have weakened (compromised) immune defenses and therefore are even more dangerously susceptible to these opportunistic fungi. In addition, while fungal disease usually progresses very slowly, it can be explosively invasive and deadly in persons with lowered or compromised defenses. For example, fungal infections are a major problem in hospitals that treat large numbers of cancer patients.

The most common superficial fungal infections, as well as the rarer but more serious systemic infections, will be reviewed in this section.

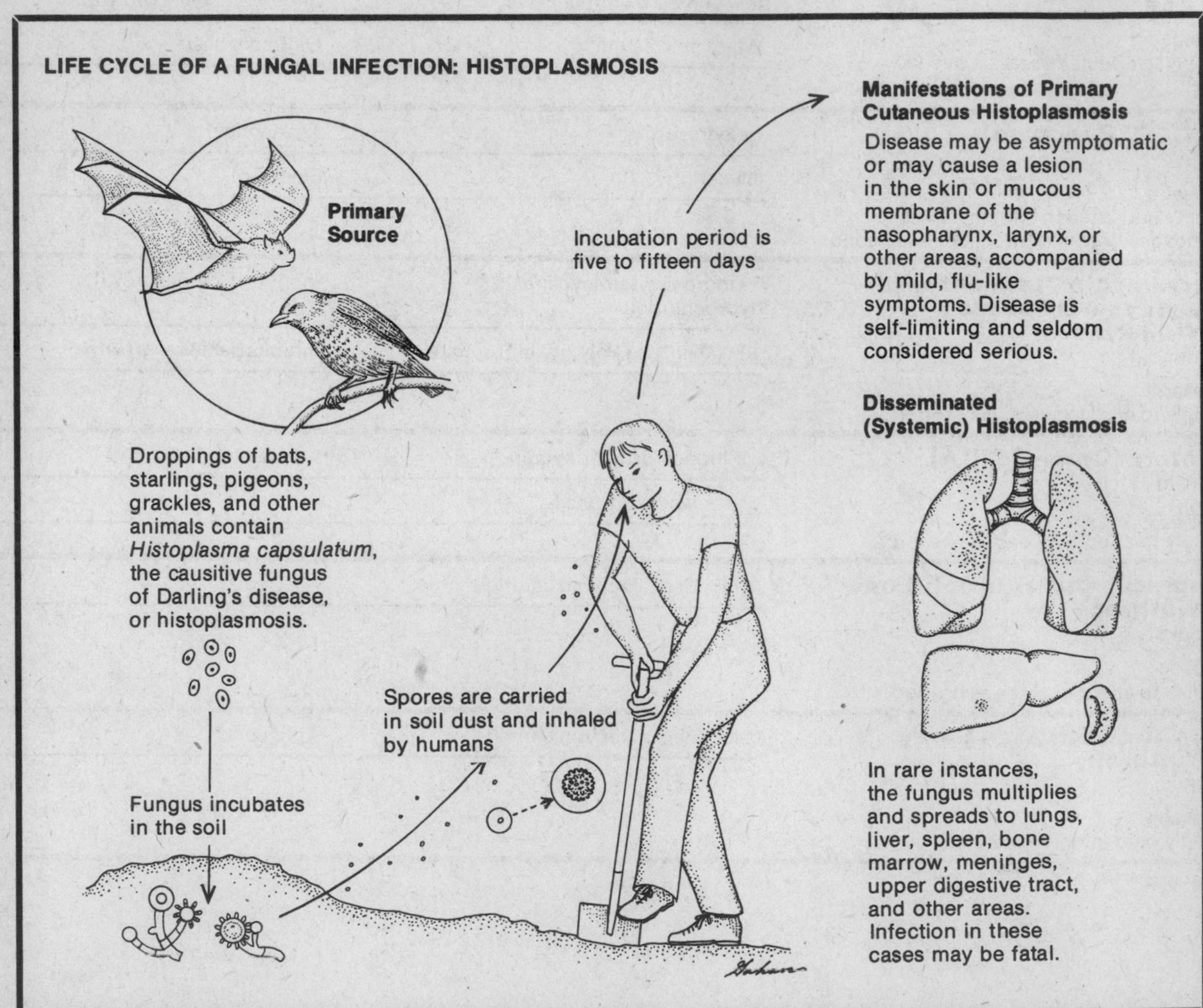

SUPERFICIAL FUNGAL INFECTIONS

Ringworm

The common forms of ringworm infections—tinea cruris (jock itch), tinea corporis (ringworm of the body), tinea pedis (athlete's foot), tinea barbae (ringworm of the beard), tinea capitis (ringworm of the scalp), and tinea unguium (ringworm of the nails)—are among the nuisance disorders of mankind. They are somewhat unpleasant to look at and usually cause mild but persistent discomfort. Most are fairly contagious and entire families are often affected, as are people who share gymnasium and bathroom facilities.

These superficial infections are caused by a group of about ten fungi, the dermatophytes (*Trichophyton, Epidermophyton,* and *Microsporum* species), that have adapted so well to their human hosts that they never kill and, until recently, were nearly impossible to treat. They cause dry, flaky rashes with mild to maddening itch. Fingernails and toenails can be thickened and disfigured. If cracking of the skin occurs, as it does in athlete's foot, pain is produced. Ringworm of the scalp can lead to hair loss, which may be permanent if scarring results. The discomfort is exacerbated in hot and moist environments, such as in the tropics, but even so, the infections will remain superficial.

These common superficial fungal infections usually can be diagnosed simply by looking at them, but occasionally laboratory tests are needed, especially if the infection is resistant to treatment. In these cases, the affected skin or nail can be gently scraped and a small sample placed on a glass slide, dissolved by a potassium hydroxide solution, and then examined under a microscope. If doubt persists, the scrapings can be cultured in a special fungal growth medium. These tests are often necessary in diagnosing nail problems because there are a number of conditions that may injure the nail beds, resulting in abnormal nail growth that resembles fungal infections. Suspected fungal infection of the scalp or hairy areas can be diagnosed by inspection under a long-wave ultraviolet light (Wood's lamp), which causes the infected area to glow or fluoresce.

Treatment of Superficial Fungal Infections

These superficial fungal disorders usually yield to modern treatment, although some resistance still occurs. For example, athlete's foot is often difficult to cure, but this can be accomplished with persistence, provided that reinfection can be avoided. Topical medications of clotrimazole (Lotrimin), haloprogin (Halotex), and tolnaftate (Tinactin) in the form of powders, creams, or fluids should be applied regularly two or three times a day for about ten to fourteen days. Infection between the toes may need a month of diligent applications. Persistence and regularity are keys to success.

Undecylenic acid (in Desenex and other products) is a useful agent to prevent or control the spread of athlete's foot. To prevent reinfection, one should avoid wearing shoes or other garments that may harbor the fungus. In general, self-medication of athlete's foot with nonprescription drugs should be avoided unless it is done under a physician's supervision. This is particularly important if the toenails appear to be involved in the infection, or if the foot is inflamed or swollen or the infection is widespread. The same is true of other ringworm infections, such as jock itch. Some of the nonprescription products can control uncomplicated infections, especially if they are not widespread. But a physician should be consulted before self-medication is attempted..

Griseofulvin (Fulvicin, Grifulvin, Grisactin, and other brands), an oral medication, is very effective in treating ringworm and other superficial fungal infections, especially those affecting the beard or scalp. Griseofulvin, taken for two to four months, is also the drug of choice for treating dry, scaly fungal diseases of the hands, and is the only agent effective in the treatment of fungal infections of the nails. In the latter case, it must be taken for six months to a year, and even then success is not guaranteed, particularly if the toenails are affected.

Although griseofulvin is a very safe drug, it may cause rashes and hypersensitivity to sunlight, and can interact with barbiturates and the coumadin anticoagulants. In some cases of extensive infection, particularly of the scalp, the body will sometimes respond with a severe allergic reaction to griseofulvin at the site of disease. A short course (one week) of concomitant treatment with corticosteroids can quiet this reaction until the antifungal medication takes control of the infection.

Tinea Versicolor

Tinea versicolor, caused by a fungus called *Malassezia furfur,* is a superficial infection that is often spread from person to person. It causes a shiny, dry, scaly rash, generally on the chest and back. White skin affected by this fungus will not tan and stands out in pale patches, while black or heavily pigmented skin is often made darker. Topical preparations of griseofulvin or a selenium sulfide shampoo (Selsun) will clear up the infection quickly, but it may take longer for normal pigmentation to return.

OPPORTUNISTIC FUNGAL INFECTIONS

Candidiasis

Candidiasis, also known as moniliasis or thrush, is caused mainly by *Candida albicans*, a fungus that can cause both oral and superficial disease in healthy persons and widespread systemic disease in patients with compromised resistance.

Candida, a normal inhabitant of the female genital tract, is a major cause of vaginitis, and active infection may be encouraged or worsened by use of antibiotics. Vaginal infection can be symptomless or can be itchy and painful with a heavy discharge. These infections are treated with a cream or suppository containing clotrimazole (Lotrimin), nystatin (Mycostatin), miconazole (MicaTin and Monistat), or a sulfa combination (Vagitrol). The sulfa combinations are particularly useful if the cause of the vaginitis is uncertain because they are usually effective against candidiasis, trichomoniasis, and nonspecific vaginitis. These various medications also can be taken as a preventive measure when vaginitis is likely to arise, such as during antibiotic therapy. Another common form of vaginitis is caused by *Trichomonas vaginalis*, which is a protozoan (single-cell primitive animal) rather than a fungus. Metronidazole (Flagyl) is the drug of choice for trichomoniasis, although specific therapy is not always required. (See *Parasitic Infections,* page 469, for a more complete discussion.)

Candidiasis of the skin occurs in warm moist areas, such as the groin, under the breasts, and in the armpits. It can be treated topically with nystatin, clotrimazole, miconazole, and if necessary, amphotericin B (Fungizone) in a cream base. Sometimes a steroid is prescribed along with an antifungal drug to quiet inflammation. Griseofulvin does not clear up *Candida* infections; in fact, it may make them worse.

Candida infection in healthy individuals is unpleasant but seldom serious. It can be life-threatening, however, in patients with cancer, nutritional and metabolic disorders, and suppression of the immune system from chronic disease, steroids, or anticancer drugs. For example, mouth thrush—white patches of *Candida*—is relatively common in both healthy adults and children, and is easily treated with nystatin drops. Patients with an impaired defense system contract thrush with great ease, but in these persons, the candidiasis is likely to spread via the bloodstream to the intestinal tract, particularly in the esophagus and stomach, the liver, eyes, heart, kidneys, and brain—a potential disaster that never happens in healthy persons.

There are five or six other opportunistic fungi like *Candida* that attack patients with weakened resistance to infection. *Aspergillus,* for example, can grow as a symptomless "fungus ball" within the lung, or more seriously, it can become invasive, attacking the brain, kidney, or heart valves. It can also cause blood clots and emboli. In contrast, in healthy persons the *Aspergillus* fungus usually causes only an allergic asthma-like reaction. Mucormycosis—an infection caused by one of the Mucorales fungi—is found in patients with kidney failure or poorly controlled diabetes. Still another opportunistic fungal infection is cryptococcosis, which causes a type of meningitis and encephalitis of slow and insidious progression.

Problems in Diagnosis

Diagnosis of the opportunistic and other systemic fungal diseases is often complicated by the fact that they may mimic other conditions, and, except for physicians in large medical centers, they are seen infrequently in most medical practices. Diagnosis often can be obtained by physical examination alone or culture of appropriate body fluids (urine, sputum, blood, spinal fluid, abscess exudate, etc.). In some cases, biopsy of tissue from the lung, liver, and brain or other affected organs may be required, particularly in cases of rapid deterioration. Skin and blood tests are available that can often indicate the presence of a fungus, although sometimes a positive result means only that the fungus was present at one time and may no longer be so.

Treatment

Treatment of the opportunistic fungi causing systemic infection is often difficult, especially in the very ill. Amphotericin B (Fungizone), which is given intravenously, is the oldest and most reliable drug in these cases. Flucytosine (Ancobon) is a newer addition, and can be used independently of or as an adjunct to amphotericin B. Flucytosine is a convenient oral medication but its usefulness when administered alone is limited because it is only fungistatic, meaning it immobilizes the fungus, but does not kill it, and resistance to it arises frequently. Miconazole (Monistat I.V.), another antifungal drug that is administered intravenously, also is used to treat systemic fungal infections either alone or in combination with other drugs. In addition, actinomycosis, another opportunistic fungal infection, can be treated with penicillin. Unfortunately, these systemic fungal infections are not always cured and the adverse reactions to the drugs used in their treatment are often serious. For example, kidney damage is common with these drugs, particularly amphotericin B, and is not always totally reversible. Bone marrow suppression occurs frequently. Amphotericin B infusions cause local phlebitis, and allergic reactions, fever, nausea, and falling blood pressures also occur. Steroids and anticoagulants are sometimes added to the infusion bottles to minimize these reactions. Despite these various problems, these drugs have greatly increased the success rate of treatment and are life-saving to many patients with systemic fungal infections.

DEEP FUNGAL INFECTIONS

The deep fungi, like the opportunistic ones, are not spread from person to person; instead, these fungal organisms are found naturally in the environment or live harmlessly in all of us. Many are found in the soil and are acquired by inhalation, especially in dry, dusty areas. One fungus, *Cryptococcus neoformans,* which can cause meningitis, can be found in pigeon droppings.

Fungi in this category cause deep systemic disease, but unlike the opportunistic fungi, their serious effect is not limited to persons with weakened resistance. Diseases in this category include coccidioidomycosis, histoplasmosis, and blastomycosis. In many instances, the fungi are harbored in the soil and may be spread by bird, bat, or rodent droppings. They enter the body by inhalation; therefore most infections from these fungi are centered in the lungs and respiratory tract, and rarely spread any further. These diseases may be totally symptomless in their primary pulmonary form or they may cause cough, fever, shortness of breath, and chest pain. San Joaquin or valley fever, which is seen in the desert regions of California and the Southwest, for example, has been recognized to be a self-limited lung infection caused by *Coccidioides immitis*. It has been estimated that thousands of cases occur each year, but most of them are mistaken for flu or colds, and go unrecognized as being of fungal origin.

Very rarely, these diseases may become progressive and widespread, even in healthy individuals. When this occurs, the liver, brain, lymph nodes, bone, or lungs may be severely or fatally affected. Amphotericin B is the drug of first choice for the systemic spread of these potentially serious deep fungal infections. For the mild pulmonary pattern of disease, supportive and symptomatic care is often all that is required.

IN CONCLUSION

In most instances, fungal infections are more bothersome than serious, but for persons who are weakened by other serious diseases or whose immune system is compromised, they may prove life-threatening. Certain types of fungi may cause systemic infections that are usually so mild that they go unnoticed or require little or no treatment.

The following charts cover the drugs most commonly prescribed to treat fungal infections. In addition, the major nonprescription athlete's foot products are listed in an overall chart on Athlete's Foot Medications, and other topical nonprescription antifungal drugs are included in the chart on Topical Antifungal Medications.

ANCOBON (Flucytosine) Roche

Caps: 250, 500 mg

INDICATIONS	ORAL DOSAGE
Serious mycotic infections caused by susceptible strains of *Candida* and *Cryptococcus*	**Adult:** 50–150 mg/kg/day div q6h

ADMINISTRATION/DOSAGE ADJUSTMENTS

Nausea or vomiting	May be reduced or avoided by administering capsules a few at a time over a 15-minute period
Renal impairment	Reduce dosage to lowest effective level

CONTRAINDICATIONS

Hypersensitivity to flucytosine

WARNINGS/PRECAUTIONS

Renal impairment	May lead to drug accumulation; use with extreme caution and monitor blood levels
Bone-marrow depression	Use with extreme caution in patients with hematological disease or history of chemotherapy or radiotherapy and in those undergoing radiotherapy; monitor hepatic function (alkaline phosphatase, SGOT, SGPT) and hematopoietic system frequently

ADVERSE REACTIONS

Gastrointestinal	Nausea, vomiting, diarrhea
Dermatological	Rash
Hematological	Anemia, leukopenia, thrombocytopenia
Central nervous system	Confusion, hallucinations, headache, sedation, vertigo

OVERDOSAGE

Signs and symptoms	See ADVERSE REACTIONS
Treatment	Discontinue medication; institute supportive measures, as required

DRUG INTERACTIONS

Amphotericin B	⇧ Antifungal activity and toxicity
Myelosuppressive agents	⇧ Potential toxicity

ALTERED LABORATORY VALUES

Blood/serum values	⇧ Alkaline phosphatase ⇧ SGOT ⇧ SGPT

No clinically significant alterations in urinary values occur at therapeutic dosages

Use in children	Use in pregnancy or nursing mothers
General guidelines not established	Safe use not established

AVC (Sulfanilamide, aminacrine hydrochloride, and allantoin) Merrell-National

Cream: 15% sulfanilamide, 0.2% aminacrine hydrochloride, and 2% allantoin (¼, 4 oz) **Supp:** 1.05 g sulfanilamide, 0.014 g aminacrine hydrochloride, and 0.14 g allantoin

INDICATIONS	INTRAVAGINAL DOSAGE
Vulvovaginitis when isolation of causative organism is not possible[1] **Trichomoniasis, vulvovaginal candidiasis, and vaginitis** due to *Haemophilus vaginalis* or other susceptible bacteria[2]	**Adult:** 1 applicatorful or supp qd or bid through 1 complete menstrual cycle, unless specific therapy is initiated

CONTRAINDICATIONS

Sensitivity to sulfonamides

WARNINGS/PRECAUTIONS

Local or systemic toxicity or sensitivity	May occur; discontinue therapy if manifestations (eg, skin rash) appear

ADVERSE REACTIONS

Mucocutaneous	Increased discomfort, burning

Use in children

General guidelines not established

Use in pregnancy or nursing mothers

General guidelines not established

[1]Probably effective
[2]Possibly effective

FULVICIN P/G (Griseofulvin ultramicrosize) Schering

Tabs: 125, 250 mg

INDICATIONS	ORAL DOSAGE
Tinea corporis, tinea pedis, tinea cruris, tinea barbae, tinea capitis, and tinea unguium (onychomycosis) caused by *Trichophyton rubrum, T tonsurans, T mentagrophytes, T interdigitalis, T verrucosum, T megninii, T gallinae, T crateriform, T sulphureum, T schoenleinii, Microsporum audouini, M canis, M gypseum,* and *Epidermophyton floccosum* unresponsive or likely to be unresponsive to topical therapy alone	**Adult:** 250 mg/day in a single dose or div until infecting organism is completely eradicated; for resistant infections, 500 mg/day div until infecting organism is completely eradicated (see ADMINISTRATION/DOSAGE ADJUSTMENTS) **Child (30-50 lb):** 62.5-125 mg/day; for tinea capitis, administer a single daily dose until infecting organism is eradicated **Child (>50 lb):** 125-250 mg/day; for tinea capitis, administer a single daily dose until infecting organism is eradicated

FULVICIN-U/F (Griseofulvin microsize) Schering

Tabs: 250, 500 mg

INDICATIONS	ORAL DOSAGE
Same as for Fulvicin P/G	**Adult:** 500 mg/day in a single dose or div until infecting organism is completely eradicated; for resistant infections, 1 g/day div until infecting organism is completely eradicated (see ADMINISTRATION/DOSAGE ADJUSTMENTS) **Child (30-50 lb):** 125-250 mg/day **Child (>50 lb):** 250-500 mg/day

ADMINISTRATION/DOSAGE ADJUSTMENTS

Pretreatment evaluation	The type of fungi responsible for the infection should be identified before initiating therapy; identification may be made by direct microscopic examination or culture
Duration of treatment	Therapy must be continued until infecting organism is completely eradicated. Representative treatment periods are for tinea corporis, 2-4 wk; tinea capitis, 4-6 wk; tinea pedis, 4-8 wk; tinea unguium, depending on rate of growth, at least 4 mo for fingernails and at least 6 mo for toenails (see WARNINGS/PRECAUTIONS)
Concomitant antifungal therapy	Concomitant use of topical agents is usually necessary, particularly in the treatment of tinea pedis (athlete's foot); general hygienic measures should be observed to control sources of infection or reinfection

CONTRAINDICATIONS

History of sensitivity to griseofulvin●	Porphyria●	Hepatocellular failure●

WARNINGS/PRECAUTIONS

Unwarranted uses	Griseofulvin should not be used for bacterial infections, candidiasis (moniliasis), histoplasmosis, actinomycosis, sporotrichosis, chromoblastomycosis, coccidioidomycosis, North American blastomycosis, cryptococcosis (torulosis), tinea versicolor, and nocardiosis, or for minor or trivial infections that will respond to topical agents alone
Antifungal prophylaxis	Safety and efficacy of griseofulvin for prophylaxis of fungal infections have not been established
Prolonged therapy	Periodically monitor organ system functions, including renal, hepatic, and hematopoietic function, of patients on long-term therapy
Penicillin-allergic patients	May be treated without difficulty, despite theoretical possibility of cross-sensitivity with penicillin
Photosensitivity	May occur, and can aggravate pre-existing lupus erythematosus; caution patients against undue exposure to artificial or natural sunlight
Hypersensitivity reactions	May occur (see ADVERSE REACTIONS); therapy may need to be withdrawn and appropriate countermeasures instituted
Granulocytopenia	May occur; discontinue medication

Table continued on following page

FULVICIN P/G/FULVICIN-U/F continued

ADVERSE REACTIONS

Hypersensitivity	Skin rash, urticaria, angioneurotic edema (rare)
Central nervous system	Paresthesias of hands and feet, headache, fatigue, dizziness, insomnia, mental confusion, impaired performance of routine activities
Gastrointestinal	Nausea, vomiting, epigastric distress, diarrhea
Hematological	Leukopenia (rare), granulocytopenia
Other	Oral thrush, photosensitivity, proteinuria (rare)

OVERDOSAGE

Signs and symptoms	See ADVERSE REACTIONS
Treatment	Discontinue medication; treat symptomatically

DRUG INTERACTIONS

Oral anticoagulants	⇩ Anticoagulant effect
Barbiturates	⇩ Antifungal effect

ALTERED LABORATORY VALUES

No clinically significant alterations in blood/serum or urinary values occur at therapeutic dosages

Use in children

See INDICATIONS; dosage has not been established for children under 2 yr of age

Use in pregnancy or nursing mothers

Safe use not established during pregnancy; embryotoxicity and teratogenic effects have been reported in the rat and dog but have not yet been confirmed in other animal species or man. General guidelines not established for use in nursing mothers.

Note: Griseofulvin ultramicrosize also marketed as **GRIS-PEG** (Dorsey); griseofulvin microsize also marketed as **GRIFULVIN V** (Ortho) and **GRISACTIN** (Ayerst)

FUNGIZONE (Amphotericin B) Squibb

Cream: 3% (20 g) **Lotion:** 3% (30 ml) **Ointment:** 3% (20 g) **Vial:** 50 mg (10 ml)

INDICATIONS	TOPICAL DOSAGE	PARENTERAL DOSAGE
Cutaneous and mucocutaneous candidiasis	**Adult:** Apply liberally to candidal lesion bid to qid	—
Cryptococcosis; North American blastomycosis; coccidioidomycosis; invasive phycomycosis (caused by *Mucor, Rhizopus, Absidia, Entomophthora,* and *Basidiobolus*) and **aspergillosis; disseminated sporotrichosis, histoplasmosis,** and **candidiasis**	—	**Adult:** 0.25 mg/kg/day IV (slowly) to start, followed by gradual increases as tolerance permits, up to 1 mg/kg/day or 1.5 mg/kg every other day, usually for several months

ADMINISTRATION/DOSAGE ADJUSTMENTS

Selection of patients for intravenous therapy	Use only in hospitalized patients, or in those under close clinical observation; use should be restricted to patients with diagnosis of progressive, potentially fatal forms of susceptible mycotic infections that have been firmly established, preferably by culture or histologically
Rate of intravenous infusion	Administer slowly over 6 h; recommended concentration, 0.1 mg/ml (1 mg/10 ml)
Supplemental medication	Adverse reactions resulting from IV therapy may be partially alleviated by giving aspirin, antihistamines, and antiemetics. Alternate-day therapy may decrease anorexia and phlebitis. IV administration of adrenal corticosteroids just prior to, or during, infusion of amphotericin B may decrease febrile reactions. (Dosage and duration of corticosteroid treatment should be kept to a minimum.) Adding small amounts of heparin to the infusion may decrease incidence of thrombophlebitis.
Interruption of intravenous therapy	If lapse is longer than 7 days, reinstitute therapy at lowest dosage level and increase dosage gradually
Clinical response of mycotic skin infections	Intertriginous lesions usually respond within a few days, and treatment may be completed within 1-3 wk. Candidiasis in other than interdigital areas usually resolves within 1-2 wk, whereas interdigital lesions and paronychias may require 2-4 wk of intensive treatment. Onychomycotic infections that respond may require several months or more of treatment.

CONTRAINDICATIONS

Hypersensitivity to amphotericin B, unless condition is life-threatening and amenable only to amphotericin B therapy

WARNINGS/PRECAUTIONS[1]

Renal impairment	Determine BUN and serum creatinine levels (or endogenous creatinine clearance) at least weekly; if BUN >40 mg/dl or serum creatinine >3.0 mg/dl, discontinue therapy or reduce dosage markedly until renal function improves. Some permanent impairment often occurs, especially with cumulative doses >5 g. Supplemental alkalinization of the urine may reduce renal tubular acidosis complications.
Hepatic impairment	Obtain weekly liver-function studies; if sulfobromophthalein retention, serum alkaline phosphatase concentration, and/or bilirubin level rise, therapy may have to be discontinued
Hematopoietic abnormalities	May occur (see ADVERSE REACTIONS); obtain weekly hemograms
Hypokalemia	Occurs frequently and may be potentiated by concomitant corticosteroid therapy; determine serum potassium level at least weekly during therapy
Hypersensitivity reactions	Discontinue therapy and institute appropriate treatment
Other nephrotoxic antibiotics	Should be used with great caution, if at all, in combination with amphotericin B; concomitant treatment with antineoplastic agents (eg, nitrogen mustard) also should be avoided, if possible
Rhinocerebral phycomycosis	Generally occurs in association with diabetic ketoacidosis; diabetic control must be restored before successful antifungal treatment can be accomplished
Oleaginous ointment	May be irritating to moist intertriginous areas

[1]The topical preparations have no evident systemic toxicity or side effects

Table continued on following page

ADVERSE REACTIONS[1]
Frequent reactions are italicized

Central nervous system	*Headache, malaise,* convulsions
Otic	Hearing loss, tinnitus, transient vertigo
Ophthalmic	Blurred vision or diplopia
Gastrointestinal	*Anorexia, nausea, vomiting, dyspepsia, diarrhea, cramping epigastric pain,* melena or hemorrhagic gastroenteritis, acute liver failure
Hematological	*Normochromic, normocytic anemia;* coagulation defects, thrombocytopenia, leukopenia, agranulocytosis, eosinophilia, leukocytosis
Renal	*Hypokalemia, azotemia, hyposthenuria, renal tubular acidosis, nephrocalcinosis,* anuria, oliguria
Cardiovascular	Arrhythmias, ventricular fibrillation, cardiac arrest, hypertension, hypotension
Dermatological	Slight sensitization (with topical preparations); erythema, pruritus, or burning sensation (with cream); pruritus, with or without other signs of local irritation (with lotion and IV form); maculopapular rash (with IV form)
Other	*Fever, sometimes with shaking chills; weight loss; generalized pain, including muscle and joint pain; pain and irritation at injection site, with phlebitis and thrombophlebitis;* peripheral neuropathy, anaphylactoid reactions, flushing

OVERDOSAGE

Signs and symptoms	See ADVERSE REACTIONS
Treatment	Discontinue medication; institute supportive measures, as required

DRUG INTERACTIONS

Digitalis	⇧ Risk of digitalis toxicity
Corticosteroids	⇧ Risk of hypokalemia
Flucytosine	⇧ Toxicity of flucytosine
Nephrotoxic antibiotics	⇧ Risk of renal toxicity

ALTERED LABORATORY VALUES

Blood/serum values	⇧ BUN ⇧ Creatinine ⇧ Sulfobromophthalein retention ⇧ Alkaline phosphatase ⇧ Bilirubin ⇩ Potassium ⇩ Magnesium ⇩ Sodium ⇩ Calcium

No clinically significant alterations in urinary values occur at therapeutic dosages

Use in children

General guidelines not established

Use in pregnancy or nursing mothers

Safe use of parenteral administration not established during pregnancy; general guidelines not established for use in nursing mothers

GYNE-LOTRIMIN (Clotrimazole) Schering

Tabs: 100 mg **Cream:** 1% (50 mg/applicatorful) (45 g)

INDICATIONS	INTRAVAGINAL DOSAGE
Vulvovaginal candidiasis	**Adult:** 1 tab or applicatorful/day, preferably at bedtime, for 7 consecutive days (tabs) or 7–14 days (cream) or, if patient is not pregnant, 2 tabs/day for 3 consecutive days

CONTRAINDICATIONS

Hypersensitivity to clotrimazole or any other component

WARNINGS/PRECAUTIONS

Lack of response	Re-evaluate diagnosis by appropriate microbiological studies before instituting another course of therapy

ADVERSE REACTIONS

Mucocutaneous	Burning; erythema and irritation (with cream)
Dermatological	Rash (with tabs)
Gastrointestinal	Lower abdominal cramps (with tabs)
Genitourinary	Slight urinary frequency (with tabs)
Other	Burning or irritation in sexual partner (with tabs), intercurrent cystitis (with cream)

Use in children

General guidelines not established

Use in pregnancy or nursing mothers

Safe use not established during pregnancy, although use during the 2nd and 3rd trimesters has not been associated with ill effects. General guidelines not established for use in nursing mothers.

HALOTEX (Haloprogin) Westwood

Cream: 1% (15, 30 g) **Sol:** 1% (10, 30 ml)

INDICATIONS	TOPICAL DOSAGE
Tinea pedis, cruris, corporis, and manuum caused by *Trichophyton rubrum, T tonsurans, T mentagrophytes, Microsporum canis,* and *Epidermophyton floccosum* **Tinea versicolor** caused by *Malassezia furfur*	**Adult:** Apply cream or solution liberally to affected area bid for 2-3 wk; interdigital lesions may require 2-4 wk of treatment

CONTRAINDICATIONS

Hypersensitivity to haloprogin or other components

WARNINGS/PRECAUTIONS

Irritation or sensitivity	Discontinue therapy and institute appropriate treatment; avoid contact with eyes
Mixed infections	May require supplementary systemic anti-infective therapy
Lack of response after 4 wk	Re-evaluate diagnosis

ADVERSE REACTIONS

Dermatological	Local irritation, burning, vesicle formation, increased maceration, pruritus, exacerbation of pre-existing lesions

Use in children	Use in pregnancy or nursing mothers
General guidelines not established	Safe use not established; general guidelines not established for use in nursing mothers

LOTRIMIN (Clotrimazole) **Schering**

Sol: 1% (10, 30 ml) **Cream:** 1% (15, 30 g)

INDICATIONS	TOPICAL DOSAGE
Tinea pedis, cruris, and corporis caused by *Trichophyton rubrum, T mentagrophytes, Epidermophyton floccosum*, and *Microsporum canis* **Candidiasis** caused by *Candida albicans* **Tinea versicolor** caused by *Malassezia furfur*	**Adult:** Gently massage solution or cream into affected and surrounding areas bid, in AM and PM

CONTRAINDICATIONS

Hypersensitivity to clotrimazole or other components

WARNINGS/PRECAUTIONS

Irritation or sensitivity	Discontinue therapy and institute appropriate treatment; avoid contact with eyes
Lack of response after 4 wk	Re-evaluate diagnosis

ADVERSE REACTIONS

Dermatological	Erythema, stinging, blistering, peeling, edema, pruritus, urticaria, irritation

Use in children	Use in pregnancy or nursing mothers
General guidelines not established	Safe use has not been established in pregnant women. During 1st trimester, use only when considered essential. General guidelines not established

Note: Clotrimazole also marketed as **MYCELEX** and **MYCELEX-G** (Dome)

MICATIN (Miconazole nitrate) Ortho

Cream: 2% (15 g; 1, 3 oz) **Lotion:** 2% (12, 30 ml)

INDICATIONS	TOPICAL DOSAGE
Tinea pedis, cruris, and corporis caused by *Trichophyton rubrum, T mentagrophytes,* and *Epidermophyton floccosum;* **cutaneous candidiasis**	**Adult:** Apply cream or lotion to affected area bid, in AM and PM, for 2 wk (for candidiasis, tinea cruris, and tinea corporis) or 1 mo (for tinea pedis)
Tinea versicolor	**Adult:** Apply cream or lotion to affected area qd

ADMINISTRATION/DOSAGE ADJUSTMENTS

Intertriginous areas	**Use lotion form; if cream is used, apply sparingly and smooth in well**

CONTRAINDICATIONS

Hypersensitivity to miconazole

WARNINGS/PRECAUTIONS

Irritation or sensitivity	**Discontinue use immediately; avoid contact with eyes**
Lack of response after 4 wk	**Re-evaluate diagnosis**

ADVERSE REACTIONS

Dermatological	**Irritation, burning, maceration**

Use in children

General guidelines not established

Use in pregnancy or nursing mothers

General guidelines not established

MONISTAT 7 (Miconazole nitrate) Ortho

Vaginal cream: 2% (47 g)

INDICATIONS	INTRAVAGINAL DOSAGE
Vulvovaginal candidiasis (moniliasis)	**Adult:** One applicatorful at bedtime for 7 days; repeat course, if necessary

CONTRAINDICATIONS

Hypersensitivity to miconazole

WARNINGS/PRECAUTIONS

Irritation or sensitivity	Discontinue use immediately
Lack of response	Perform appropriate microbiological studies to confirm diagnosis and rule out other pathogens

ADVERSE REACTIONS
Frequent reactions are italicized

Genitourinary	*Vulvovaginal burning, itching, or irritation (6.6%),* vaginal burning, pelvic cramps
Other	Hives, skin rash, headache

Use in children

General guidelines not established

Use in pregnancy or nursing mothers

Safe use not established during pregnancy; use during 1st trimester should be considered only when deemed essential to patient's welfare, since some absorption from the vagina may occur. General guidelines not established for use in nursing mothers.

MONISTAT i.v. (Miconazole) Janssen

Amps: 10 mg/ml (20 ml)

INDICATIONS	PARENTERAL DOSAGE
Coccidioidomycosis	**Adult:** 1,800-3,600 mg/day by IV infusion (30-60 min) in a single daily dose or in 3 divided doses for 3-20 wk or longer; for relapse or reinfection, repeat course **Child:** 20-40 mg/kg/day by IV infusion (30-60 min) in divided doses no greater than 15 mg/kg
Cryptococcosis	**Adult:** 1,200-2,400 mg/day by IV infusion (30-60 min) in a single daily dose or in 3 divided doses for 3-12 wk or longer; for relapse or reinfection, repeat course **Child:** 20-40 mg/kg/day by IV infusion (30-60 min) in divided doses no greater than 15 mg/kg
Candidiasis **Chronic mucocutaneous candidiasis**	**Adult:** 600-1,800 mg/day by IV infusion (30-60 min) in a single daily dose or in 3 divided doses for 1-20 wk or longer; for relapse or reinfection, repeat course **Child:** 20-40 mg/kg/day by IV infusion (30-60 min) in divided doses no greater than 15 mg/kg
Paracoccidioidomycosis	**Adult:** 200-1,200 mg/day by IV infusion (30-60 min) in a single daily dose or in 3 divided doses for 2-16 wk or longer; for relapse or reinfection, repeat course **Child:** 20-40 mg/kg/day by IV infusion (30-60 min) in divided doses no greater than 15 mg/kg
Fungal meningitis (adjunctive therapy)	**Adult:** 20 mg (undiluted) intrathecally every 3-7 days by alternate lumbar, cervical, and cisternal punctures
Urinary bladder mycoses (adjunctive therapy)	**Adult:** 200 mg by bladder instillation

ADMINISTRATION/DOSAGE ADJUSTMENTS

Preparation of IV infusion	Dilute contents of 1 amp in at least 200 ml of 0.9% sodium chloride or 5% dextrose
Initial therapy	Give 200 mg to start with the physician in attendance and under stringent hospital conditions
Nausea and vomiting	May be mitigated by giving antihistaminic or antiemetic drugs before miconazole infusion or by reducing the dose, slowing the rate of infusion, or avoiding administration at mealtime

CONTRAINDICATIONS

Hypersensitivity to miconazole

WARNINGS/PRECAUTIONS

Transient tachycardia or arrhythmia	May occur with rapid injection of undiluted miconazole
Patient monitoring	Obtain hemoglobin, hematocrit, electrolyte, and lipid determinations
Ambulatory patients	Closely monitor suitable patients
Unwarranted use	Trivial forms of fungal diseases should not be treated with IV miconazole
Systemic fungal mycoses	May be complications of chronic underlying disease; take appropriate diagnostic and therapeutic measures, if indicated
Severe pruritus and skin rashes	May occur; discontinue medication

ADVERSE REACTIONS

Frequent reactions are italicized

Dermatological	*Pruritus (21%), rash (9%)*
Gastrointestinal	*Nausea (18%), vomiting (7%)*, diarrhea, anorexia
Central nervous system	Drowsiness
Hematological	Decreased hematocrit, thrombocytopenia, RBC aggregation or rouleau formation on blood smears
Other	*Phlebitis (29%), fever and chills (10%)*, hyperlipemia (due to vehicle), flushes

Table continued on following page

MONISTAT i.v. continued

OVERDOSAGE

Signs and symptoms	See WARNINGS/PRECAUTIONS and ADVERSE REACTIONS
Treatment	Discontinue medication; treat symptomatically and institute supportive measures, as required

DRUG INTERACTIONS

Oral anticoagulants	⇧ Anticoagulant effect
Agents containing cremophor-type vehicles	Abnormal lipoprotein electrophoresis

ALTERED LABORATORY VALUES

Blood/serum values	⇩ Sodium

No clinically significant alterations in urinary values occur at therapeutic dosages

Use in children

Safe use not established in children under 1 yr of age

Use in pregnancy or nursing mothers

Safe use not established during pregnancy; general guidelines not established for use in nursing mothers

MYCELEX-G (Clotrimazole) Miles

Cream: 1% **Tabs:** 100 mg

INDICATIONS	TOPICAL DOSAGE
Vulvovaginal candidiasis (moniliasis)	**Adult:** 1 applicatorful, inserted intravaginally, qd (preferably at bedtime) for 7–14 days, or 1 vaginal tab qd (preferably at bedtime) for 7 consecutive days or, if patient is not pregnant, 2 tabs/day for 3 consecutive days

ADMINISTRATION/DOSAGE ADJUSTMENTS

Diagnostic confirmation	Obtain KOH smears and/or cultures; rule out other pathogens associated with vulvovaginitis (*Trichomonas* and *Haemophilus vaginalis*) by appropriate laboratory methods

CONTRAINDICATIONS

Hypersensitivity to any component

WARNINGS/PRECAUTIONS

Treatment failure	Repeat appropriate antimicrobial studies to confirm the diagnosis and rule out other pathogens before instituting another course of antimycotic therapy

ADVERSE REACTIONS

Local	Burning, erythema, irritation
Genitourinary	Intercurrent cystitis (with cream), slight urinary frequency (with tabs)
Gastrointestinal	Lower abdominal cramps (with tabs)
Other	Burning or irritation in sexual partner (rare; with tabs)

Use in children

General guidelines not established

Use in pregnancy or nursing mothers

Use during the second and third trimesters of pregnancy has not been associated with ill effects; general guidelines not established for use in nursing mothers

MYCOSTATIN (Nystatin) Squibb

Oral susp: 100,000 units/ml (60 ml) **Oral tabs:** 500,000 units **Vaginal tabs:** 100,000 units **Cream:** 100,000 units/g (15, 30 g) **Ointment:** 100,000 units/g (15, 30 g) **Powder:** 100,000 units in talc (15 g)

INDICATIONS	ORAL DOSAGE	TOPICAL DOSAGE
Candidiasis of the oral cavity	**Adult:** 400,000-600,000 units (2-3 ml in each side of mouth) qid **Infant:** 200,000 units (1 ml in each side of mouth) qid **Child:** same as for adult	—
Intestinal candidiasis	**Adult:** 500,000-1,000,000 units (1-2 tabs) tid	
Cutaneous or mucocutaneous candidiasis	—	**Adult:** Apply cream or ointment liberally to affected areas bid or as needed until healing is complete; if powder is used, apply to candidal lesions bid or tid until lesions have healed
Vulvovaginal candidiasis (moniliasis)	—	**Adult:** 100,000 units (1 vaginal tab) qd for 2 wk

ADMINISTRATION/DOSAGE ADJUSTMENTS

Candidal infections of the feet	Powder should be dusted freely on feet, shoes, and socks
Premature or low-birth-weight infants	For treatment of oral candidiasis, 100,000 units (1 ml) qid may be effective
Duration of therapy	Continue treatment of candidiasis of the oral cavity for at least 48 h after perioral symptoms have cleared and cultures have returned to normal; to prevent relapse, treatment of intestinal candidiasis should be continued for at least 48 h after clinical cure has been achieved

CONTRAINDICATIONS

Hypersensitivity to nystatin or other components

WARNINGS/PRECAUTIONS

Sensitivity or irritation	Discontinue therapy immediately
Tartrazine sensitivity	Presence of FD&C Yellow No. 5 (tartrazine) in oral tabs may cause allergic-type reactions, including bronchial asthma, in susceptible individuals

ADVERSE REACTIONS

Gastrointestinal	Diarrhea, distress, nausea, vomiting
Dermatological	Irritation, sensitization

Use in children and infants

See INDICATIONS and ADMINISTRATION/DOSAGE ADJUSTMENTS; general guidelines not established for other uses and appropriate dosages

Use in pregnancy or nursing mothers

Safe use has not been established during pregnancy; no adverse effects or complications have been attributed to nystatin in infants born to women treated with nystatin. General guidelines not established for use in nursing mothers.

VAGISEC PLUS (9-Aminoacridine hydrochloride, polyoxyethylene nonyl phenol, sodium edetate, and sodium dioctyl sulfosuccinate) Schmid

Supp: 6 mg 9-aminoacridine hydrochloride, 5.25 mg polyoxyethylene nonyl phenol, 0.66 mg sodium edetate, and 0.07 mg sodium dioctyl sulfosuccinate

INDICATIONS	INTRAVAGINAL DOSAGE
Vaginitis caused by *Trichomonas vaginalis,* as well as **mixed vaginal infections** complicated by a bacterial moiety	**Adult:** 1 supp in AM and at bedtime for 14 days

ADMINISTRATION/DOSAGE ADJUSTMENTS

Concomitant treatment	Vagisec liquid scrubs are advisable
Re-examination	Perform 3 days after cessation of home treatment
Chronic or stubborn cases	Therapy may be repeated with no interval between courses
Cure	Vaginal smears or cultures, taken once per month for 3 mo, should show absence of trichomonads and return to normal vaginal flora

CONTRAINDICATIONS

Conception	Product is spermicidal and should not be used on days when patient is trying to conceive

WARNINGS/PRECAUTIONS

Recurrent vaginitis	Often indicates extravaginal foci or infection in cervical, vestibular, or urethral glands, or reinfection by the sexual partner; during treatment, advise patient to refrain from sexual intercourse or have her partner wear a condom

ADVERSE REACTIONS

Mucocutaneous	Minor irritation

Use in children	Use in pregnancy or nursing mothers
General guidelines not established	General guidelines not established

VAGITROL (Sulfanilamide, allantoin, and aminacrine hydrochloride) Syntex

Cream: 15.0% sulfanilamide, 2.0% allantoin, and 0.2% aminacrine hydrochloride (4 oz) **Supp:** 1.05 g sulfanilamide, 0.14 g allantoin, and 0.014 g aminacrine hydrochloride

INDICATIONS	INTRAVAGINAL DOSAGE
Vulvovaginitis when isolation of causative organism is not possible[1] **Trichomoniasis; vulvovaginal candidiasis; vaginitis** caused by *Haemophilus vaginalis* or other susceptible bacteria[2]	**Adult:** 1 applicatorful or suppository qd or bid; continue treatment through one complete menstrual cycle, unless a definite diagnosis is made and specific therapy initiated

CONTRAINDICATIONS

Hypersensitivity to sulfonamides or other components●	Kidney disease●

WARNINGS/PRECAUTIONS

Lack of response or recurrence of symptoms	Discontinue treatment, attempt to isolate causative organism, and institute specific therapy
Blood dyscrasias	May occur and can be fatal (see ADVERSE REACTIONS); watch for early signs (eg, sore throat, fever, pallor, purpura, jaundice) of serious blood disorders, and discontinue treatment if evidence of systemic toxicity occurs
Hypersensitivity reactions	May occur and can be fatal (see ADVERSE REACTIONS); use with caution in patients allergic to some goitrogens, diuretics, and oral hypoglycemic agents
Crystalluria, urinary calculi	May be prevented by maintaining adequate fluid intake
Special-risk patients	Use with caution in patients with impaired renal or hepatic function, severe allergy, bronchial asthma, G6PD deficiency, or porphyria[3]

ADVERSE REACTIONS

Hematological	Agranulocytosis, aplastic anemia, thrombocytopenia, leukopenia, hemolytic anemia, purpura, hypoprothrombinemia, methemoglobinemia
Allergic	Erythema multiforme (Stevens-Johnson syndrome), generalized skin eruptions, epidermal necrolysis, urticaria, serum sickness, pruritus, exfoliative dermatitis, anaphylactoid reactions, periorbital edema, conjunctival and scleral injection, photosensitization, arthralgia, allergic myocarditis
Gastrointestinal	Nausea, emesis, abdominal pains, hepatitis, diarrhea, anorexia, pancreatitis, stomatitis
Central nervous system	Headache, peripheral neuritis, mental depression, convulsions, ataxia, hallucinations, tinnitus, vertigo, insomnia
Endocrinological	Goiter (rare), hypoglycemia (rare)
Other	Drug fever, chills, toxic nephrosis with oliguria and anuria, periarteritis nodosum, lupus erythematosus phenomenon, diuresis (rare)

Use in children

General guidelines not established

Use in pregnancy or nursing mothers

Safe use not established during pregnancy; general guidelines not established for use in nursing mothers

[1]Probably effective
[2]Possibly effective
[3]*United States Pharmacopeia Dispensing Information 1980.* Rockville, Md., United States Pharmacopeial Convention, Inc., 1980

VANOBID (Candicidin) **Merrell-National**

Ointment: 0.6 mg/g (75 g) **Tabs:** 3 mg

INDICATIONS	INTRAVAGINAL DOSAGE
Vaginitis caused by *Candida albicans* and other *Candida* species	**Adult:** 1 applicatorful or tab in AM and at bedtime for 14 days

CONTRAINDICATIONS

Hypersensitivity to candicidin

WARNINGS/PRECAUTIONS

Sexual intercourse during treatment	Not recommended; partner should wear a condom to avoid reinfection
Contraceptive diaphragm	May deteriorate during prolonged contact with candicidin; substitute another form of contraception during treatment
Persistent or recurrent symptoms	Repeat treatment

ADVERSE REACTIONS

Mucocutaneous	Sensitization and temporary irritation (extremely rare)

Use in children

General guidelines not established

Use in pregnancy or nursing mothers

During pregnancy, the use of an applicator may be contraindicated; manual insertion may be preferred. General guidelines not established for use in nursing mothers.

TOPICAL ANTIFUNGAL MEDICATIONS

Product (Manufacturer)	Ingredients	Actions
Cruex Medicated Cream (Pennwalt) Cream **Dosage** Apply liberally to affected areas as needed	3% Chloroxylenol	Antiseptic
	20% Zinc undecylenate	Inhibits fungal growth
Cruex Powder (Pennwalt) Powder **Dosage** Apply to affected areas 1–2 times daily	10% Calcium undecylenate	Inhibits fungal growth
Desenex Liquid (Pennwalt) Liquid **Dosage** Spray onto affected areas as needed	10% Undecylenic acid	Inhibits fungal growth
	40% Alcohol	Astringent and antiseptic
Desenex Powder (Pennwalt) Powder **Dosage** Apply to affected areas as needed	20% Zinc undecylenate	Inhibits fungal growth
	2% Undecylenic acid	Inhibits fungal growth
Desenex Ointment (Pennwalt) Ointment **Dosage** Apply to affected areas each AM and PM	20% Zinc undecylenate	Inhibits fungal growth
	5% Undecylenic acid	Inhibits fungal growth

ATHLETE'S FOOT MEDICATIONS

Product (Manufacturer)	Ingredients	Actions
Aftate (Plough) Liquid **Dosage** Spray on affected areas twice daily	1% Tolnaftate	Inhibits fungal growth
Aftate (Plough) Spray powder **Dosage** Spray on affected areas twice daily	1% Tolnaftate	Inhibits fungal growth
Aftate (Plough) Powder **Dosage** Apply to affected areas twice daily	1% Tolnaftate	Inhibits fungal growth
Aftate (Plough) Gel **Dosage** Apply to affected areas twice daily	1% Tolnaftate	Inhibits fungal growth

Table continued on following page

Product (Manufacturer)	Ingredients	Actions
Daliderm (Dalin) Powder **Dosage** Apply to affected areas several times daily	Zinc undecylenate	Inhibits fungal growth
	Sodium propionate	Inhibits fungal growth
	Salicylic acid	Peeling agent with irritant effect; aid in fungus removal
	Methylbenzethonium chloride	Antiseptic
	Corn starch	Skin protective
	Magnesium carbonate	Absorbing agent
	Boric acid	Antiseptic
	Bentonite	Emulsifier
	Zinc oxide	Astringent and antiseptic
	Talc	Skin protective
	Aromatic oils	Anesthetic
Desenex Liquid (Pharmacraft) Liquid **Dosage** Apply to affected areas several times daily	10% Undecylenic acid	Inhibits fungal growth
	40% Isopropyl alcohol	Antiseptic and astringent
	Propylene glycol	Solvent
	Triethanolamine	Buffer
Desenex Ointment (Pharmacraft) Ointment **Dosage** Apply liberally to affected areas each PM	5% Undecylenic acid	Inhibits fungal growth
	20% Zinc undecylenate	Inhibits fungal growth
Desenex Powder (Pharmacraft) Powder **Dosage** Apply to affected areas each AM and PM	20% Zinc undecylenate	Inhibits fungal growth
	2% Undecylenic acid	Inhibits fungal growth
Desenex Aerosol (Pharmacraft) Aerosol **Dosage** Spray on affected areas each AM and PM	20% Zinc undecylenate	Inhibits fungal growth
	2% Undecylenic acid	Inhibits fungal growth
Desenex Soap (Pharmacraft) Soap **Dosage** Lather into affected areas with hot water and rinse, twice daily	2% Undecylenic acid	Inhibits fungal growth
Domeboro (Dome) Liquid **Dosage** Apply to affected areas several times daily	Aluminum sulfate	Astringent
	Calcium acetate	Stabilizing agent
Enzactin (Norwich) Cream **Dosage** Massage cream into affected areas daily	250 mg/g Triacetin	Inhibits fungal growth

Table continued on following page

Product (Manufacturer)	Ingredients	Actions
NP 27 Cream (Norwich) Cream **Dosage** Massage cream into skin until cream disappears, then apply second generous coating to affected areas, each AM and PM	8-Hydroxyquinoline	Inhibits fungal growth
	Benzoic acid	Inhibits fungal growth
	Salicylic acid	Peeling agent with irritant effect; aids in fungus removal
	Propylparaben	Antifungal agent and astringent
	Methylparaben	Antifungal agent and astringent
NP 27 Liquid (Norwich) Liquid **Dosage** Spray liberally onto affected areas each AM and PM	Benzoic acid	Inhibits fungal growth
	Chlorothymol	Inhibits fungal growth
	Salicylic acid	Peeling agent with irritant effect; aids in fungus removal
	50% Isopropyl alcohol	Antiseptic and astringent
	Propylparaben	Antifungal agent and astringent
	Benzyl alcohol	Antiseptic
NP 27 Powder (Norwich) Powder **Dosage** Apply generously to affected areas once daily	Benzoic acid	Inhibits fungal growth
	Salicylic acid	Peeling agent with irritant effect; aids in fungus removal
	Eucalyptol	Astringent
	Menthol	Mild anesthetic; reduces itching
Solvex Athlete's Foot Spray (Scholl) Aerosol **Dosage** Spray on affected areas several times daily	Undecylenic acid	Inhibits fungal growth
	Chlorothymol	Inhibits fungal growth
	Triclosan	Inhibits fungal growth
	Dichlorophene	Antifungal and antiprotozoan agent
	Benzocaine	Mild anesthetic agent; reduces itching
	Propylene glycol	Solvent
	Alcohol	Antiseptic and astringent
Solvex Ointment (Scholl) Ointment **Dosage** Massage into affected areas several times daily	Benzoic acid	Inhibits fungal growth
	Salicylic acid	Peeling agent with irritant effect; aids in fungus removal
	Thymol	Mild antifungal agent
Solvex Powder (Scholl) Powder **Dosage** Apply to affected areas several times daily	8-Hydroxyquinoline sulfate	Inhibits fungal growth
	Chlorothymol	Inhibits fungal growth
	Colloidal sulfur	Peeling agent with irritant effect; aids in fungus removal

Table continued on following page

Product (Manufacturer)	Ingredients	Actions
Tinactin Cream (Schering) Cream **Dosage** Massage generous amount into affected areas twice daily	1% Tolnaftate	Inhibits fungal growth
	Polyethylene glycol 400	Cream base
	Propylene glycol	Solvent
	Butylated hydroxytoluene	Antiseptic
	Titanium dioxide	Skin protective
Tinactin Solution (Schering) Liquid **Dosage** Massage 2–3 drops into affected areas twice daily	1% Tolnaftate	Inhibits fungal growth
	Polyethylene glycol 400	Cream base
	Butylated hydroxytoluene	Antiseptic
Tinactin Powder (Schering) Powder **Dosage** Apply liberally to affected areas and into shoes and socks, as needed	1% Tolnaftate	Inhibits fungal growth
	Corn starch	Skin protective
	Talc	Skin protective
Tinactin Aerosol (Schering) Aerosol **Dosage** Spray liberally onto affected areas and into shoes and socks, as needed	1% Tolnaftate	Inhibits fungal growth
	Talc	Skin protective
	Propellants	
	Butylated hydroxytoluene	Antiseptic
Ting (Pharmacraft) Cream **Dosage** Massage into affected areas several times daily	Zinc stearate	Inhibits fungal growth
	Benzoic acid	Inhibits fungal growth
	Boric acid	Antiseptic
	Zinc oxide	Astringent and antiseptic
	16% Alcohol	Astringent and antiseptic
Ting (Pharmacraft) Powder **Dosage** Apply liberally to affected areas several times daily	Zinc stearate	Inhibits fungal growth
	Benzoic acid	Inhibits fungal growth
	Boric acid	Antiseptic
	Zinc oxide	Astringent and antiseptic

Parasitic Infections

Parasitic disease is generally regarded as a major health problem only in the tropical or developing nations, but, in truth, certain types of parasitic infections are found in both rural and urban areas in industrialized nations, including the United States. In addition, the increased ease and popularity of world travel have added to the incidence of tropical and other exotic parasites in developed countries. Certain other parasites, such as head lice, appear to be increasing in all strata of American society. This section will review the most common types of parasitic diseases seen in the United States and their treatment.

GENERAL CHARACTERISTICS

By definition, a parasite is an organism that lives off another organism. In human beings, the parasitic organisms are larger than bacteria, ranging in size from microscopic protozoans (primitive one-cell organisms) to ten-yard-long intestinal tapeworms Parasitic infections are often chronic, and the organisms are commonly spread throughout the environment—in the soil, water, or in animal reservoirs—making eradication and control difficult or impossible. The extent of disease often depends on the parasitic burden—the number of infecting organisms—with low numbers producing asymptomatic or mild disease, and greater numbers producing more serious, even life-threatening effects.

Parasites travel in varied ways. Many are spread by vectors that carry the infection from victim to victim, but are not affected themselves. Malaria, which is spread by mosquitoes, is one such disease. Other parasites exist in the soil. Hookworm, for example, enters the skin directly, making it unwise to walk barefoot in the areas in the southern United States in which it is endemic. The schistosomes, a group of tropical parasitic worms, are found in water. Trichinosis is acquired by eating infected meat. Still other parasites are transmitted by fecal contamination of food and water.

Some parasites, such as ticks, bedbugs, fleas, and lice, are relatively harmless themselves but can be vectors of such diseases as Rocky Mountain spotted fever and typhus. Plague—the "Black Death" of medieval Europe—actually is a disease of rats that is transmitted by the oriental flea, a parasite that occasionally spreads to man and carries the disease with it.

Control and Prevention

The control and prevention of parasitic disease have been a major concern of governments, military forces, and international organizations. Control

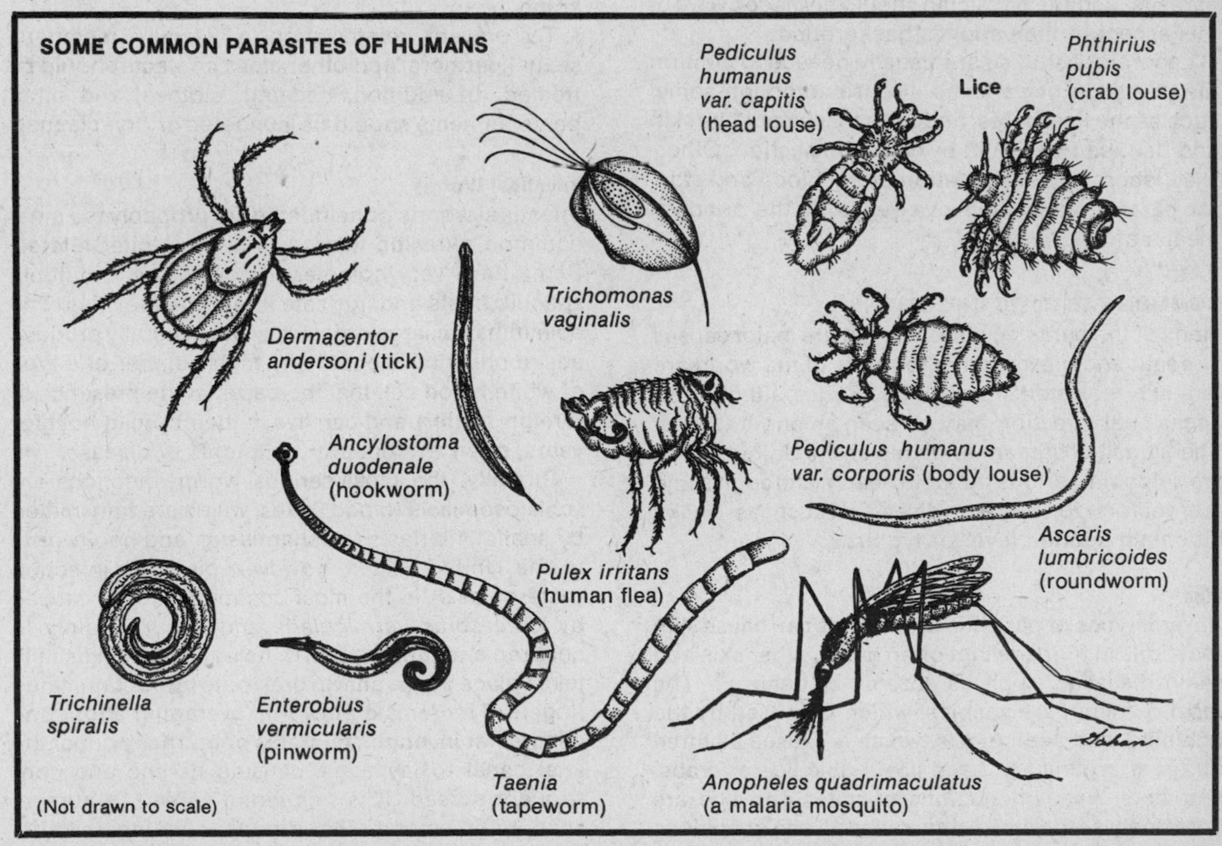

usually relies, not on direct elimination of the parasite but, rather, on altering the environment that is conducive to its continued presence, eliminating its vector, or simple avoidance. Malaria is best attacked by eliminating the mosquito. Unfortunately, mosquitoes that are resistant to insecticides have developed, and malaria is again on the increase. Therefore, travelers to areas in which malaria is endemic are advised to undergo preventive treatment. Simply avoiding contact with likely sources of intestinal parasites—e.g., not swimming, drinking unboiled water, or eating uncooked foods, especially salads and fruits, in endemic areas—is a prudent but not foolproof course. Other parasitic infections such as trichinosis and tapeworms can be totally prevented by never eating undercooked meat, particulary pork and fish.

Diagnosis

Symptoms of parasitic infection vary according to the causative organism. In many cases, it may take weeks, even years, for the disease to manifest itself. In countries where particular parasitic diseases are common, physicians are more attuned to their symptoms and manifestations than doctors in the United States. For example, the usual cause of severe heart failure in parts of Chile is Chagas' disease, which is caused by a protozoan, *Trypanosoma cruzi*. In contrast, most American physicians would assume the cause to be arteriosclerotic vascular disease, and never consider the possibility of a parasitic infection. Travel to a foreign country, even years before, suggests the possibility of a parasite, and the physician should be made aware of this aspect of the patient's background.

Laboratory studies are usually needed to confirm the presence of parasitic disease, although some, such as the lice, mites, and ticks that inhabit the skin and hair, can be found by visual inspection. Otherwise, laboratory examination of the blood and stool for parasites and their ova (eggs) is the principal means of diagnosis.

COMMON PARASITIC INFECTIONS

Many of the parasitic diseases that are major causes of death and disease in other parts of the world are rare or nonexistent in the United States, although an occasional infection may be seen among travelers. The parasites that are endemic to the United States are seldom a serious threat to health, although some are vectors for serious diseases, such as Rocky Mountain spotted fever or typhus.

Lice

Several types of parasitic arthropods can cause skin reactions in humans that often mimic other skin and scalp diseases, such as eczema or dandruff. The most common are scabies, which is caused by the itch mite, and pediculosis, which is caused by three different organisms: head lice, pubic lice or crabs, and body lice. Infestations of mites and lice are commonly associated with crowded living conditions and poor hygiene, but these are not prerequisites—scabies occurs in all social classes, and head lice are most common among middle-class white children. The crab louse is spread by sexual contact or through common use of towels and other personal items. It inhabits the pubic area, although it may also infest the beard and, more rarely, the eyebrows and eyelashes. Occasionally, crabs may spread to the trunk and legs.

Itching and inflammation of the skin are the primary symptoms of louse and mite infestations, and secondary infections at the site of itching and scratching are relatively common. The itching is caused by irritating secretions injected into the skin as the female mites burrow under the outer layer to lay their eggs. The lice in and of themselves usually are more of an irritant and psychological humiliation than a serious threat to health, although some lice are vectors for typhus.

The goals of treatment are twofold: to eliminate the parasite completely and to prevent reinfection. The main drugs used to treat scabies and louse infestations in the United States are gamma benzene hexachloride (Kwell) and crotamiton (Eurax). Two applications, in the form of a shampoo, cream, or lotion, may be needed: the first to eliminate the adult insects and a few days later to kill any that might have hatched in the interim. Since the medications may be irritating to the skin, mucous membranes, and eyes, they should be used with care and only as instructed. In treating head lice, the nits or eggs that are attached near the roots of the hair must be combed out, usually with a fine-tooth metal comb.

To prevent reinfestation, all family members, sexual partners, and other close contacts should be treated. In addition, bedding, clothes, and other personal items should be laundered or dry-cleaned.

Intestinal Worms

Intestinal worms or helminths are probably the most common parasitic infections in the United States. Some have very complex life cycles with multiple specific hosts and intricate interdependencies. The helminths are large organisms that generally produce eosinophilia (an abnormally high number of a type of white blood cell that increases in the presence of foreign matter) and can live in their human host for years, often without any symptoms of disease.

Globally, the most serious worm infections are schistosomiasis (blood flukes, which are transmitted by snails), filariasis (elephantiasis), and hookworm. In the United States, however, pinworm infection (enterobiasis) is the most common. This is caused by *Enterobius vermicularis* and occurs mainly in children and family groups. Its transmission usually takes place by the anal to oral route by contaminated fingers. The female pinworm, averaging about one centimeter in length, migrates nocturnally out of the anal canal to lay eggs, causing itching and consequent spread. It is frequently spread in nursery school and among other groups of young children.

Pinworm infection has also become one of the diseases increasingly associated with homosexual practices.

Drugs used to treat pinworm infections include single oral doses of mebendazole (Vermox), pyrantel pamoate (Antiminth), and pyrvinium pamoate (Povan). A second dose of the latter may be prescribed two weeks after the first to ensure against reinfection. Drugs used to treat roundworm and other helminthic infections, such as piperazine (Antepar) or thiabendazole (Mintezol), also may be used, although the latter is somewhat more toxic than other pinworm medications.

Roundworm infections (ascariasis) are relatively rare in the United States, but are the most common intestinal parasites in the world. The eggs hatch in the small intestine, travel to the lungs via the veins and lymph system, and up the pulmonary tree to the epiglottis, where they are swallowed and returned to the intestine to develop into adult worms. Symptoms of roundworm infection include cough, fever, and vague abdominal complaints, such as pain, nausea and vomiting, and loss of appetite. Since the worms may migrate to the liver, pancreas, and other abdominal organs, the infection should be treated, even if there are no serious symptoms. The drugs used to treat roundworms are essentially the same as those prescribed for pinworms.

Intestinal hookworms may cause anemia, iron loss, and nutritional deficiencies. This parasitic disease is seen mostly in the southern United States, where it is caused by *Necator americanus*. The parasite enters the skin, usually through the feet, migrates through the blood vessels to the lungs, is coughed up, swallowed, and takes up residence in the intestine for as long as fifteen years. The worm causes eosinophilia and its ova are readily found in stool. Mebendazole (Vermox) and pyrantel pamoate (Antiminth) are safe, effective drugs for hookworm infections and will also eliminate any coexistent *Ascaris lumbricoides*, a type of roundworm found in the United States. Wearing shoes in endemic areas protects against contracting the parasite.

Trichinosis, a self-limited infection of intestine and muscle found in the United States and Europe, is acquired by eating the encysted larvae of *Trichinella spiralis* found in raw or inadequately cooked pork. There have been reports of trichinosis in persons who have eaten rare beef or other undercooked meat, but investigation usually finds that these meats had come in contact with pork, either at the meat processors or during home preparation. The larvae are released in the human intestine by digestive enzymes. They mature to adults, mate, and produce more larvae, which then wander about the body to ultimately form cysts in muscle. Most trichinosis is symptomless because there are not enough parasites to produce noticeable discomfort. In some rare cases, however, patients may have intestinal distress, fever, myalgia (muscle pain), weakness, cardiac failure, and encephalitis, especially during the stage of larval migration. Edema, hives, and eosinophilia can occur also.

Trichinosis is diagnosed by muscle biopsy and by finding rising levels of antibodies to the foreign organism. Treatment is rarely indicated, but thiabendazole (Mintezol) is effective if treatment is necessary, and corticosteroids may be prescribed to reduce muscle pain and fever. Total prevention can be achieved by thoroughly cooking all pork products or meat that has come in contact with pork.

Infection by fish, beef, and pork tapeworms is uncommon in the United States and rarely causes the degree of malnutrition and wasting popularly imagined. The fish tapeworm is fairly harmless but, oddly, can cause a deficiency anemia by absorbing most of the vitamin B_{12} ingested by its host. The pork tapeworm can reach four yards in length and beef tapeworm up to ten yards. Larval cysts of the pork tapeworm can cause severe disease by invading the muscle and brain of their host, although the adult worm in the intestine causes little difficulty. Niclosamide (Yomesan) kills all three worms by inhibiting their oxygen uptake, and quinacrine hydrochloride (Atabrine Hydrochloride) can be used if niclosamide is ineffective. Again, prevention can be achieved by thorough cooking of all fish, beef, and pork.

Protozoan Parasites

Worldwide, amebiasis, malaria, leishmaniasis, African trypanosomiasis ("sleeping sickness"), and Chagas' disease are the most serious parasitic infections caused by protozoans. These diseases affect hundreds of millions of people, shortening their lives, and leaving many of their victims chronically weak and ill. They pose a massive public health problem and slow economic progress. In the highly developed countries of Europe and the United States, these diseases are unknown or unusual.

Throughout the world, malaria is the most common serious infectious disease, and it remains the major cause of death and disease in many developing countries of Asia and Africa. In the United States, malaria was once a major health problem in mosquito-infested areas but has been largely controlled in most areas. It re-emerged as a public health concern in the last decade when Vietnam War veterans brought back many cases.

Malaria has a complex life cycle with different stages in *Anopheles*, its mosquito vector, and in the human liver and blood. Disease severity depends on the particular malarial species. *Plasmodium vivax* malaria is relatively mild, while *Plasmodium falciparum* malaria can be fatal, causing "blackwater fever" and coma. Typically, the disease is characterized by attacks of chills, fever, and sweating that are believed to occur when the infected red blood cells rupture, releasing the malarial parasites to infect other blood cells. In some patients, however, this synchronization is not established; instead, the patient may suffer from chronic or periodic flu-like symptoms.

A number of drugs are available to both relieve the disease symptoms and to help prevent establishment of the disease in exposed persons. Travelers planning to visit areas in which malaria is endemic are advised to see their physician before leaving for guidance and possible prophylactic treatment with one of the major antimalaria drugs, chloroquine (Aralen). However, some malaria strains are resistant to this drug; therefore, information on current malaria outbreaks and resistance should be obtained from the Center for Disease Control in Atlanta, Georgia (404-329-3670 or 404-329-3644).

Malaria can be transmitted via mosquitoes or blood transfusions. Since the parasite is very difficult to eliminate totally, persons with a history of malaria generally are not acceptable blood donors.

Drugs used to treat malaria include various forms of quinine, chloroquine (Aralen), amodiaquine (Camoquine), pyrimethamine (Daraprim), and hydroxychloroquine (Plaquenil). In addition, antibiotics such as tetracycline or sulfa combined with pyrimethamine may be prescribed.

The most common protozoan infection in the United States is vaginal trichomoniasis. Most types of vaginal trichomoniasis are asymptomatic—of the three kinds of human trichomonads, only one, *Trichomonas vaginalis*, produces disease with vaginal discharge, pain, and itch in women and recurrent prostatitis in men. Trichomoniasis is transmitted sexually, and both partners must be treated, usually with metronidazole (Flagyl), to avoid recurrence.

Amebiasis, caused by *Entamoeba histolytica*, is spread by fecal contamination of food and water, with flies and food handlers being important links in the chain of transmission. It is found in about 2 percent of Americans, particularly travelers. Its incidence is also higher among homosexuals. Although some infections may be asymptomatic, amebiasis is usually characterized by colonic ulceration, cramping pain, diarrhea, bloody stools, and general weakness. Amebic liver abscess is a serious complication, and severe infection can mimic ulcerative colitis, colon cancer, and appendicitis. To effect a cure, the amebae in both the liver and the bowel must be eliminated. Metronidazole (Flagyl), emetine hydrochloride (sold under that brand name), and tetracycline are effective in symptomatic disease, while iodoquinol (Yodoxin) or metronidazole can eliminate the parasite in asymptomatic carriers. Prevention is achieved by eating properly cooked foods. A stool examination for evidence of infection is advised for travelers who have been to areas where parasitic diseases are known to exist.

Giardiasis, infestation with *Giardia lamblia*, a protozoan, produces abdominal pains, gas, and foul-smelling diarrhea. It is transmitted in contaminated food and water. Chronic giardiasis can produce a malabsorption syndrome in which food nutrients are not absorbed from the intestine, causing malnutrition. Metronidazole (Flagyl) is effective in treating giardiasis, as is quinacrine hydrochloride (Atabrine Hydrochloride), a drug once used to prevent malaria. Asymptomatic carriers should be detected and treated to prevent spread. Homosexuals have an increased incidence of giardiasis, as do patients with lymphoma and some other cancers.

IN CONCLUSION

Although parasitic disease remains the major cause of death and disease in many parts of the world, in the United States most infections do not pose a major threat to health. However, they should not be dismissed as trivial or left to self-medication. Whenever a parasitic disease is suspected, especially among persons who have traveled to areas where they are endemic, a physician should be consulted. Most of the common parasitic infections seen in the United States are readily treated. The following drug charts cover the medications prescribed for parasitic skin infections, intestinal worms, and protozoan infections. Antibiotics that may be prescribed to treat certain parasitic infections are listed in the *Bacterial Infections* section (pages 339–443).

ANTEPAR (Piperazine citrate) Burroughs Wellcome

Tabs: 550 mg (equivalent to 500 mg piperazine hexahydrate)
Syrup: 550 mg/5 ml (equivalent to 500 mg piperazine hexahydrate per 5 ml)

INDICATIONS	ORAL DOSAGE
Ascariasis (roundworm infection)	**Adult:** 3.5 g piperazine hexahydrate (7 tabs or tsp) qd for 2 consecutive days; for severe infections, repeat course after 1 wk **Child:** 75 mg/kg piperazine hexahydrate qd, up to 3.5 g/day, for 2 consecutive days; for severe infections, repeat course after 1 wk
Enterobiasis (pinworm infection)	**Adult:** 65 mg/kg piperazine hexahydrate qd, up to 2.5 g (5 tabs or tsp)/day, for 7 consecutive days; for severe infections, repeat course after 1 wk **Child:** same as adult

ADMINISTRATION/DOSAGE ADJUSTMENTS

Adjunctive measures	Dietary restriction, laxatives, and enemas are unnecessary
Mass treatment of ascariasis	As a public health measure and when repeated therapy is impractical, give a single dose of 70 mg piperazine hexahydrate per pound of body weight, up to 3 g; this dose will remove the organism in most cases but is not as effective as the recommended multiple-dose regimen

CONTRAINDICATIONS

Hypersensitivity to piperazine and its salt ●

Impaired renal or hepatic function ●

Convulsive disorders ●

WARNINGS/PRECAUTIONS

Neurotoxicity	May occur, especially in children, with prolonged or repeated treatment exceeding recommended dosages and duration
Occurrence of side effects	Discontinue therapy if CNS, significant gastrointestinal, or hypersensitivity reactions occur (see ADVERSE REACTIONS)
Special-risk patients	Use with appropriate caution in anemic or severely malnourished patients

ADVERSE REACTIONS

Gastrointestinal	Nausea, vomiting, abdominal cramps, diarrhea
Central nervous system and neuromuscular	Headache, vertigo, ataxia, tremors, choreiform movement, muscular weakness, hyporeflexia, paresthesia, blurred vision, paralytic strabismus, convulsions, EEG abnormalities, sense of detachment, memory defect
Hypersensitivity	Urticaria, erythema multiforme, purpura, fever, arthralgia

OVERDOSAGE

Signs and symptoms	See ADVERSE REACTIONS; in lethal doses, convulsions, respiratory depression
Treatment	Discontinue medication and treat symptomatically. In cases of massive overdose, empty stomach by aspiration and gastric lavage. Maintain an open airway and assist ventilation, if necessary. Convulsions may be treated with a short-acting barbiturate.

DRUG INTERACTIONS

Pyrantel pamoate	⇩ Anthelmintic effect

ALTERED LABORATORY VALUES

No clinically significant alterations in blood/serum or urinary values occur at therapeutic dosages

Use in children

See INDICATIONS

Use in pregnancy or nursing mothers

Safe use not established during pregnancy; general guidelines not established for use in nursing mothers

ANTIMINTH (Pyrantel pamoate) Roerig

Susp: 50 mg/ml

INDICATIONS	ORAL DOSAGE
Ascariasis (roundworm infection) **Enterobiasis** (pinworm infection)	**Adult:** 11 mg/kg (1 ml/10 lb), up to 1 g, in a single dose with milk or fruit juice, if desired **Child (>2 yr):** same as adult

ADMINISTRATION/DOSAGE ADJUSTMENTS

Timing of administration — May be administered without regard to meal times or time of day

Adjunctive measures — Purging is unnecessary prior to, during, or after therapy

CONTRAINDICATIONS

None

WARNINGS/PRECAUTIONS

Hepatic impairment — Use with caution; drug may cause minor transient elevations of SGOT

ADVERSE REACTIONS

Frequent reactions are italicized

Gastrointestinal — *Anorexia, nausea, vomiting, gastralgia, abdominal cramps, diarrhea, tenesmus*

Central nervous system — Headache, dizziness, drowsiness, insomnia

Dermatological — Rash

OVERDOSAGE

Signs and symptoms — See ADVERSE REACTIONS

Treatment — Discontinue medication and treat symptomatically

DRUG INTERACTIONS

Piperazine — ⇩ Anthelmintic effect

ALTERED LABORATORY VALUES

Blood/serum values — ⇧ SGOT (transient)

No clinically significant alterations in urinary values occur at therapeutic dosages

Use in children

See INDICATIONS; safety in children under 2 yr has not been established

Use in pregnancy or nursing mothers

Safe use not established during pregnancy; general guidelines not established for use in nursing mothers

EMETINE HYDROCHLORIDE (Emetine hydrochloride) Lilly

Amps: 65 mg/ml

INDICATIONS	PARENTERAL DOSAGE
Acute fulminating or acute exacerbations of chronic **amoebic dysentery**	**Adult:** 65 mg qd or 32 mg bid in AM and PM, or 1 mg/kg/day up to 65 mg/day SC (deeply) (preferred) or IM for 3-5 days **Child (<8 yr):** ≤10 mg/day **Child (>8 yr):** ≤20 mg/day
Amoebic hepatitis or abscess	**Adult:** 65 mg qd or 32 mg bid AM and PM or 1 mg/kg/day up to 65 mg/day SC (deeply) (preferred) or IM for 10 days **Child** (**<8 yr**): ≤10 mg/day **Child** (**>8 yr**): ≤20 mg/day
Balantidiasis **Fascioliasis** **Paragonimiasis**	

ADMINISTRATION/DOSAGE ADJUSTMENTS

Patient supervision	Strict medical supervision, with daily examination, is mandatory; confine patients to bed during treatment and for several days afterward. Record pulse rate and blood pressure 2-3 times daily. Take an ECG before emetine is started, after the fifth dose, upon completion of therapy, and one week later.
Lethal dose	10-25 mg/kg
Parenteral administration	IV route is contraindicated; avoid entrance into a vein by retracting the syringe plunger before injecting the material
Extraintestinal amebiasis	Institute adequate amebicidal treatment simultaneously or as immediate follow-up to ensure eradication of *Entamoeba histolytica* from primary intestinal lesions

CONTRAINDICATIONS

Organic cardiac or renal disease	Except when amoebic abscess or hepatitis is not controlled by chloroquine
Recent use of emetine (within 6 wk to 2 mo)	

WARNINGS/PRECAUTIONS

Aged or debilitated patients	Use with utmost caution
Fatalities	Have occurred with repeated doses, even when the total dose did not exceed 600 mg; do not extend the course of therapy beyond 10 days or exceed a total dose of 650 mg
Irritation	May occur; avoid contact with the cornea or mucous membranes, especially of the conjunctiva
Tachycardia	May occur; discontinue use
Precipitous fall in blood pressure	May occur; discontinue use
Neuromuscular symptoms	May occur; discontinue use
Marked gastrointestinal effects	May occur; discontinue use
ECG abnormalities	May occur; discontinue use if the significance of these changes outweighs the severity and type of disease and the need for emetine

ADVERSE REACTIONS

Local	Aching, tenderness, and muscle weakness at injection site
Dermatological	Eczematous, urticarial, or purpuric lesions
Gastrointestinal	Nausea, vomiting
Central nervous system and neuromuscular	Dizziness; headache; weakness; aching and tender muscles; skeletal-muscle stiffness
Cardiovascular	Hypotension, tachycardia, precordial pain, dyspnea, ECG abnormalities, gallop rhythm, cardiac dilatation, congestive heart failure, death

Table continued on following page

EMETINE HYDROCHLORIDE continued

OVERDOSAGE

Signs and symptoms	Muscular tremors, weakness, and pain, especially in the extremities; purpura, dermatitis, or hemoptysis; neuritis, vertigo; bloody diarrhea with prostration; arrhythmias; myocardial weakness with congestive failure; sudden cardiac failure
Treatment	Discontinue use and institute supportive measures, as required

DRUG INTERACTIONS

No clinically significant drug interactions have been reported

ALTERED LABORATORY VALUES

No clinically significant alterations in blood/serum or urinary values occur at therapeutic dosages

Use in children

Use only when severe dysentery is not counteracted by other amebicides

Use in pregnancy or nursing mothers

Contraindicated for use during pregnancy; emetine may cause harm to the fetus. Use with caution in nursing mothers.

MINTEZOL (Thiabendazole) **Merck Sharp & Dohme**

Tabs (chewable): 500 mg **Susp:** 500 mg/5 ml

INDICATIONS	ORAL DOSAGE
Enterobiasis (pinworm infection)	**Adult (<150 lb):** 25 mg/kg (1 ml/10 lb) bid, up to 3 g/day, for 2 doses, followed in 7 days by an additional 2 doses of 25 mg/kg each; if a repeated course is impractical, give 4 doses of 25 mg/kg each, up to 3 g/day, over 2 consecutive days **Child:** same as adult
Strongyloidiasis **Ascariasis** (roundworm infection) **Uncinariasis** (hookworm infection) caused by *Necator americanus* and *Ancylostoma duodenale* **Trichuriasis** (whipworm infection)[1] **Cutaneous larva migrans** (creeping eruptions)	**Adult (<150 lb):** 25 mg/kg (1 ml/10 lb) bid, up to 3 g/day, for 4 doses over 2 consecutive days; alternatively, a single daily dose of 50 mg/kg may be used at the risk of a higher incidence of side effects **Child:** same as adult
Symptomatic relief of trichinosis during invasive phase	**Adult (<150 lb):** 25 mg/kg (1 ml/10 lb) bid, up to 3 g/day, for 2–4 consecutive days (optimal dosage has not been established) **Child:** same as adult

ADMINISTRATION/DOSAGE ADJUSTMENTS

Patients weighing ≥150 lb	Give 1.5 g (15 ml, or 1 tbsp) at recommended intervals
Persistent cutaneous larva migrans	If active lesions are still present 2 days after completion of therapy, administer a second course of therapy
Adjunctive measures	Dietary restriction, complementary medication, and enemas are unnecessary

CONTRAINDICATIONS

Hypersensitivity to thiabendazole

WARNINGS/PRECAUTIONS

Hypersensitivity reactions	May occur and in severe cases may be fatal; discontinue drug immediately and do not resume therapy (see CONTRAINDICATIONS)
CNS side effects	May occur frequently (see ADVERSE REACTIONS); caution patients to avoid activities requiring mental alertness
Anemic, dehydrated, or malnourished patients	Institute supportive therapy prior to initiating anthelmintic therapy
Hepatic or renal impairment	Carefully monitor patient

ADVERSE REACTIONS

Frequent reactions are italicized

Gastrointestinal	*Anorexia, nausea, vomiting,* diarrhea, epigastric distress
Central nervous system	*Dizziness,* weariness, drowsiness, giddiness, headache; rarely, tinnitus, hyperirritability, numbness
Hypersensitivity	Fever, facial flushing, chills, conjunctival injection, angioedema, anaphylaxis, skin rash, erythema multiforme (including Stevens-Johnson syndrome), lymphadenopathy
Dermatological	Pruritus; perianal rash (rare)
Ophthalmic	Abnormal sensation in eyes, blurred vision, xanthopsia (all rare)
Cardiovascular	Hypotension, circulatory collapse (both rare)
Genitourinary	Enuresis, malodorous urine, crystalluria, hematuria (all rare)
Hepatic	Jaundice, cholestasis, parenchymal liver damage (all rare)
Metabolic	Hyperglycemia (rare)
Hematological	Transient leukopenia (rare)
Other	Appearance of live *Ascaris* in mouth and nose (rare)

OVERDOSAGE

Signs and symptoms	See ADVERSE REACTIONS
Treatment	Discontinue medication and treat symptomatically; insititute supportive measures, as required

[1] Therapeutic effect is limited

Table continued on following page

MINTEZOL continued

DRUG INTERACTIONS

No clinically significant drug interactions have been reported

ALTERED LABORATORY VALUES

Blood/serum values	⇧ Glucose ⇧ SGOT (transient) ⇧ Cephalin flocculation (transient)

No clinically significant alterations in urinary values occur at therapeutic dosages

Use in children

See INDICATIONS; clinical experience with thiabendazole for treatment of strongyloidiasis, ascariasis, uncinariasis, trichuriasis, and trichinosis in children weighing under 30 lb is limited

Use in pregnancy or nursing mothers

Safe use not established

POVAN (Pyrvinium pamoate) Parke-Davis

Tabs: 50 mg **Susp:** 10 mg/ml

INDICATIONS	ORAL DOSAGE
Enterobiasis (pinworm infection)	**Adult:** 5 mg/kg (5 ml/10 kg), up to 350 mg, in a single dose; if necessary, dose may be repeated in 2 or 3 wk **Child:** same as adult

ADMINISTRATION/DOSAGE ADJUSTMENTS

Mass treatment of enterobiasis	To ensure complete parasite eradication, consider treatment of all members of family or institution group

CONTRAINDICATIONS

None

WARNINGS/PRECAUTIONS

Red stool and vomitus	Patient (or parent) should be cautioned in advance to expect red discoloration due to pyrvinium pamoate; vomitus will stain most materials
Gastrointestinal reactions	Occur more often in older children and adults who have received large doses

ADVERSE REACTIONS

Gastrointestinal	Nausea, vomiting (especially with suspension), cramping, diarrhea
Hypersensitivity	Photosensitivity, allergic reactions

OVERDOSAGE

Signs and symptoms	See ADVERSE REACTIONS
Treatment	Discontinue medication; treat symptomatically

DRUG INTERACTIONS

No clinically significant drug interactions have been reported

ALTERED LABORATORY VALUES

No clinically significant alterations in blood/serum or urinary values occur at therapeutic dosages

Use in children

See INDICATIONS

Use in pregnancy or nursing mothers

Safety has not been established during pregnancy; general guidelines not established for use in nursing mothers

VERMOX (Mebendazole) Janssen

Tabs (chewable): 100 mg

INDICATIONS	ORAL DOSAGE
Enterobiasis (pinworm infection)	**Adult:** 100 mg in a single dose; if patient is not cured 3 wk later, repeat; tablet may be chewed, swallowed whole, or crushed and mixed with food **Child (>2 yr):** same as adult
Ascariasis (roundworm infection) **Trichuriasis** (whipworm infection) **Uncinariasis** (hookworm infection) caused by *Necator americanus* and *Ancylostoma duodenale*	**Adult:** 100 mg bid in AM and PM, for 3 consecutive days; if patient is not cured 3 wk later, repeat; tablet may be chewed, swallowed whole, or crushed and mixed with food **Child (>2 yr):** same as adult

ADMINISTRATION/DOSAGE ADJUSTMENTS

Adjunctive measures — Fasting and purging are unnecessary

CONTRAINDICATIONS

Hypersensitivity to mebendazole

WARNINGS/PRECAUTIONS

See information below on use in children and during pregnancy

ADVERSE REACTIONS

Gastrointestinal — Transient abdominal pain and diarrhea in cases of massive infection and expulsion of worms

OVERDOSAGE

Systemic toxicity has not occurred in clinical use, probably because of poor absorption

DRUG INTERACTIONS

No clinically significant drug interactions have been reported

ALTERED LABORATORY VALUES

No clinically significant alterations in blood/serum or urinary values occur at therapeutic dosages

Use in children	Use in pregnancy or nursing mothers
See INDICATIONS; safety in children under 2 yr of age has not been established	Contraindicated during pregnancy; general guidelines not established for use in nursing mothers

ARALEN PHOSPHATE (Chloroquine phosphate) Winthrop

Tabs: 500 mg (equivalent to 300 mg chloroquine base)

ARALEN HYDROCHLORIDE (Chloroquine hydrochloride) Winthrop

Amps: 50 mg (equivalent to 40 mg chloroquine base per ml) (5 ml)

INDICATIONS	ORAL DOSAGE	PARENTERAL DOSAGE
Acute malaria attacks due to *Plasmodium vivax*, *P malariae*, *P ovale*, and susceptible strains of *P falciparum*	**Adult:** 1 g to start, followed after 6–8 h by 500 mg and a single dose of 500 mg on each of two consecutive days; total dose: 2.5 g **Child:** 10 mg (base)/kg, up to 600 mg (base) to start, followed after 6 h by 5 mg (base)/kg up to 300 mg (base), followed after 18 h by 5 mg (base)/kg, followed after 24 h by 5 mg (base)/kg; total dose: 25 mg (base)/kg	**Adult:** 160–200 mg (base) IM to start, repeated in 6 h, if needed, up to 800 mg (base)/24 h **Child:** 5 mg (base)/kg IM to start, repeated in 6 h, if needed, up to 10 mg/kg/24 h
Suppression of malaria due to *P vivax* and *P malariae*	**Adult:** 500 mg/wk on exactly the same day of the week **Child:** 5 mg (base)/kg/wk, up to 300 mg (base)/wk on exactly the same day of the week	—
Extraintestinal ambiasis	**Adult:** 1 g/day for 2 days, followed by 500 mg/day for at least 2–3 wk	**Adult:** 160–200 mg (base)/day for 10–12 days

ADMINISTRATION/DOSAGE ADJUSTMENTS

IV administration	Should be replaced by oral therapy as soon as feasible
Suppressive therapy	Should begin 2 wk prior to exposure; failing this, give adults 1 g to start and children 10 mg (base)/kg in 2 divided doses 6 h apart to start. Continue suppressive therapy for 8 wk after leaving the endemic area.
Radical cure of *P vivax* and *P malariae* malaria	Necessitates concomitant therapy with an 8-aminoquinoline compound
Extraintestinal amebiasis	Treatment is usually combined with an effective intestinal amebicide

CONTRAINDICATIONS

Retinal or visual field changes	Attributable to either 4-aminoquinoline compounds or any other etiology
Hypersensitivity to 4-aminoquinoline compounds	

WARNINGS/PRECAUTIONS

Resistant *P falciparum* strains	Should be treated with quinine or other specific forms of therapy
Psoriatic patients	Severe attack may be precipitated; use chloroquine only if benefit outweighs risk
Porphyria	May be exacerbated; use chloroquine only if benefit outweighs risk
Irreversible retinal damage	May occur with long-term or high-dose therapy; if there is any indication (past or present) of abnormality in visual acuity, visual field, or retinal macular areas (ie, pigmentary changes, loss of foveal reflex) or any visual symptoms (ie, light flashes and streaks) which are not fully explainable by difficulties of accommodation or corneal opacities, discontinue use immediately and closely observe patient for possible progression. Retinal changes and visual disturbances may progress even after cessation of therapy. Initial and periodic ophthalmologic examinations (including visual acuity, expert slit-lamp, funduscopic, and visual field tests) should be performed when prolonged therapy is contemplated.
Muscular weakness	May occur with prolonged therapy; question and examine patients periodically, including testing knee and ankle reflexes. Discontinue use if weakness occurs.
Special-risk patients	Use with caution in patients with hepatic disease, alcoholism, or G6PD deficiency and in those receiving known hepatotoxic drugs
Blood dyscrasias	May occur with prolonged therapy; perform periodic CBC. Consider discontinuing use if any severe blood disorder appears which is not attributable to the disease under treatment.

Table continued on following page

ARALEN continued

ADVERSE REACTIONS

Central nervous system	Mild and transient headache, psychic stimulation, psychotic episodes and convulsions (rare), neuromyopathy
Auditory	Nerve deafness, tinnitus, reduced hearing
Dermatological	Pruritus, lichen planus-like eruptions, pigmentary changes
Gastrointestinal	Anorexia, nausea, vomiting, diarrhea, abdominal cramps
Cardiovascular	Hypotension, ECG changes
Ophthalmic	Blurred vision, difficulty in focusing or accommodation; reversible corneal changes (transient edema or opaque deposits in the epithelium) which may be asymptomatic or cause visual halos, focusing difficulties, or blurred vision; irreversible, sometimes progressive, or (rarely) delayed retinal changes, such as narrowing of the arterioles, macular lesions (loss of foveal reflex, areas of edema, atrophy, abnormal pigmentation), pallor of the optic disc, optic atrophy, and patchy retinal pigmentation; scotomatous vision with retinal change (rare)
Hematologic	Blood dyscrasias

OVERDOSAGE

Signs and symptoms	Headache, drowsiness, visual disturbances, cardiovascular collapse, convulsions, respiratory and cardiac arrest (sometimes fatal); ECG may reveal atrial standstill, nodal rhythm, prolonged intraventricular conduction time, and progressive bradycardia leading to ventricular fibrillation and/or arrest
Treatment	Following acute ingestion, empty stomach immediately by emesis or gastric lavage followed by activated charcoal in a dose at least five times the estimated dose of chloroquine ingested. Tracheal intubation or tracheostomy may be necessary. Peritoneal dialysis and exchange transfusions may be helpful. Control convulsions before attempting gastric lavage; if due to cerebral stimulation, administer an ultra-short-acting barbiturate cautiously, but if due to anoxia, correct with oxygen, artificial respiration or, in shock with hypotension, by vasopressor therapy. For patients who survive acute ingestion, observe closely, force fluids, and give 8 g ammonium chloride in divided doses (for adults) to acidify the urine; exercise caution in patients with renal impairment and/or metabolic acidosis.

DRUG INTERACTIONS

Gold salts	⇧ Risk of severe skin reaction
Phenylbutazone	⇧ Risk of severe skin reaction

ALTERED LABORATORY VALUES

No clinically significant alterations in blood/serum or urinary values occur at therapeutic dosages

Use in children

See INDICATIONS: children are especially sensitive to 4-aminoquinolines and fatalities have been reported following accidental ingestion, sometimes of small doses; sudden death has been reported following overdose of parenteral chloroquine; in no instance should single parenteral dose exceed 5 mg (base)/kg

Use in pregnancy or nursing mothers

Use during pregnancy should be avoided except in the suppression or treatment of malaria when in the judgment of the physician the benefit outweighs the possible hazard; general guidelines not established for use in nursing mothers

FLAGYL (Metronidazole) **Searle**

Tabs: 250 mg

INDICATIONS	ORAL DOSAGE
Symptomatic trichomoniasis when the presence of trichomonads has been confirmed by appropriate laboratory procedures **Asymptomatic trichomoniasis** associated with endocervicitis, cervicitis, or cervical erosion Treatment of **asymptomatic partners** of treated patients	**Adult:** 250 mg tid for 7 days or, if patient is not pregnant, 2 g in a single dose or in 2 divided doses of 1 g each for 1 day
Acute intestinal amebiasis	**Adult:** 750 mg tid for 5–10 days **Child:** 35–50 mg/kg/24 h in 3 divided doses for 10 days
Amebic liver abscess	**Adult:** 500–750 mg tid for 5–10 days **Child:** same as child dosage above

ADMINISTRATION/DOSAGE ADJUSTMENTS

Repeated therapy	Wait 4–6 wk and reconfirm diagnosis by culture before repeating course of therapy

CONTRAINDICATIONS

Past or present blood dyscrasias ●	Active organic CNS disease ●	Hypersensitivity to metronidazole ●

WARNINGS/PRECAUTIONS

Carcinogenicity	Has been reported in mice and rats; unnecessary use should be avoided
Mild leukopenia	May occur; obtain total and differential leukocyte counts before and after treatment, especially if a second course is necessary
Neurological signs	May occur (see ADVERSE REACTIONS); discontinue use immediately
Unrecognized candidiasis	Symptoms may be exacerbated; treat appropriately
Amebic liver abscess	Therapy may not obviate need to aspirate pus
Alcohol ingestion	May evoke a disulfiram-like reaction (see DRUG INTERACTIONS)

ADVERSE REACTIONS
Frequent reactions are italicized

Gastrointestinal	*Nausea, anorexia, vomiting, diarrhea, epigastric distress, abdominal cramping,* constipation, metallic sharp unpleasant taste, furry tongue, glossitis, stomatitis, dry mouth
Central nervous system and neurological	Headache, dizziness, vertigo, incoordination, ataxia, convulsive seizures, confusion, irritability, depression, weakness, insomnia, peripheral neuropathy (numbness, paresthesia of extremities)
Hematological	Leukopenia (reversible)
Dermatological	Erythematous eruption, urticaria, flushing, pruritus
Genitourinary	Dysuria, cystitis, dyspareunia, polyuria, incontinence, decreased libido, pyuria, dark urine, dryness of the vagina or vulva, pelvic pressure
Other	Joint pain (resembling serum sickness), nasal congestion, fever, proctitis, flattening of T-wave on ECG

OVERDOSAGE

Signs and symptoms	See ADVERSE REACTIONS
Treatment	Stop medication; treat symptomatically and institute supportive measures, as needed

DRUG INTERACTIONS

Alcohol	Abdominal cramps, nausea, vomiting, headache, flushing
Oral anticoagulants	⇧ Prothrombin time

Table continued on following page

ALTERED LABORATORY VALUES

Blood/serum values —— ⇧ or ⇩ SGOT (test interference)

No clinically significant alterations in urinary values occur at therapeutic dosages

Use in children

General guidelines not established

Use in pregnancy or nursing mothers

Contraindicated during 1st trimester of pregnancy; use in 2nd and 3rd trimesters and in nursing mothers is restricted to patients in whom local palliative treatment has been inadequate in controlling symptoms. Metronidazole crosses the placental barrier and enters fetal circulation rapidly. It is also excreted in breast milk; patient should stop nursing if drug is prescribed.

PLAQUENIL (Hydroxychloroquine sulfate) **Winthrop**

Tabs: 200 mg (equivalent to 155 mg hydroxychloroquine base)

INDICATIONS	ORAL DOSAGE
Acute attacks of malaria due to *Plasmodium vivax, P malariae, P ovale,* and susceptible strains of *P falciparum*	**Adult:** 800 mg to start, followed after 6-8 h by 400 mg, and 400 mg on each of two consecutive days (total dose, 2 g); alternative regimen, 800 mg as a single dose **Child:** 10 mg (base)/kg, up to 620 mg (base), to start, followed after 6 h by 5 mg (base)/kg, up to 310 mg (base), followed after 18 h by 5 mg (base)/kg, followed after 24 h by 5 mg (base)/kg (total dosage, 25 mg (base)/kg)
Suppression of malaria due to *P vivax* and *P malariae*	**Adult:** 400 mg/wk on exactly the same day of the week **Child:** 5 mg (base)/kg/wk, up to 310 mg (base), on exactly the same day of the week
Discoid and systemic lupus erythematosus in patients refractory to drugs with less potential for serious side effects	**Adult:** 400 mg qd or bid for several weeks or months; for prolonged maintenance 200-400 mg/day
Rheumatoid arthritis in patients refractory to drugs with less potential for serious side effects	**Adult:** 400-600 mg/day with food or milk, followed in 4-12 wk by a 50% reduction in dosage to 200-400 mg for maintenance

ADMINISTRATION/DOSAGE ADJUSTMENTS

Duration of therapy for rheumatoid arthritis	Discontinue use if objective improvement, such as reduced joint swelling and increased mobility, does not occur within 6 mo; should relapse occur after medication is withdrawn, therapy may be resumed or continued on an intermittent schedule, if there are no ocular contraindications
Combination therapy of rheumatoid arthritis	Corticosteroids and salicylates may be used in conjunction with hydroxychloroquine; they can generally be decreased in dosage or eliminated after hydroxychloroquine has been used for several weeks. Reduce every 4-5 days the dose of cortisone by no more than 5-15 mg; of hydrocortisone by 5-10 mg; of prednisolone and prednisone by 1-2.5 mg; of methylprednisolone and triamcinolone by 1-2 mg; and of dexamethasone by 0.25-0.5 mg.
Suppressive therapy of malaria	Should begin 2 wk prior to exposure; failing this, give adults 800 mg to start and children 10 mg (base)/kg in 2 divided doses 6 h apart to start. Continue suppressive therapy for 8 wk after leaving endemic area.
Radical cure of *P vivax* and *P malariae* malaria	Necessitates concomitant therapy with an 8-aminoquinoline compound

CONTRAINDICATIONS

Retinal or visual field changes	Attributable to 4-aminoquinoline compounds
Hypersensitivity to 4-aminoquinoline compounds	

WARNINGS/PRECAUTIONS

Resistant *P falciparum* strains	Should be treated with quinine or other specific forms of therapy
Psoriatic patients	Severe attack may be precipitated; use hydroxychloroquine only if benefit outweighs risk
Porphyria	May be exacerbated; use hydroxychloroquine only if benefits outweigh risks
Irreversible retinal damage	May occur with long-term or high-dose therapy; if there are any indications (past or present) of abnormality in visual acuity, visual field, or retinal macular areas (ie, pigmentary changes, loss of foveal reflex) or any visual symptoms (ie, light flashes and streaks) which are not fully explainable by difficulties of accommodation or corneal opacities, discontinue use immediately and closely observe patient for possible progression. Retinal changes and visual disturbances may progress even after cessation of therapy. Initial and periodic ophthalmological examinations (including visual acuity, expert slit-lamp, funduscopic, and visual field tests) should be performed when prolonged therapy is contemplated.
Muscular weakness	May occur with prolonged therapy; question and examine patients periodically, including testing knee and ankle reflexes. Discontinue use if weakness occurs.
Special-risk patients	Use with caution in patients with hepatic disease, alcoholism, or G6PD deficiency and in those receiving known hepatotoxic drugs
Blood dyscrasias	May occur with prolonged therapy; perform periodic CBC. Consider discontinuing use if any severe blood disorder appears which is not attributable to the disease under treatment.
Dermatological reactions	May occur; use with caution in patients with dermatitis

Table continued on following page

PLAQUENIL continued

ADVERSE REACTIONS[1]	
Central nervous system and neuromuscular	Mild and transient headache, dizziness, irritability, nervousness, emotional changes, nightmares, psychosis, lassitude, vertigo, tinnitus, nystagmus, nerve deafness, convulsions, ataxia, extraocular muscle palsies, skeletal muscle weakness, absent or hypoactive deep-tendon reflexes
Gastrointestinal	Diarrhea, anorexia, nausea, abdominal cramps, weight loss, vomiting (rare)
Ophthalmic	Disturbance of accommodation, blurred vision; reversible corneal changes (transient edema, punctate to lineal opacities, decreased sensitivity with or without blurred vision, visual halos, photophobia)[2]; retinal changes, such as macular lesions (edema, atrophy, abnormal pigmentation, loss of foveal reflex); increased macular recovery time following exposure to a bright light, elevated retinal threshold to red light in macular, paramacular, and peripheral retinal areas; other fundus changes, including optic disc pallor and atrophy, attenuation of retinal arterioles, fine granular pigmentary disturbance in the peripheral retina, and prominent choroidal patterns in advanced stage; visual field defects (pericentral or paracentral scotoma, central scotoma with decreased visual acuity, field constriction [rare])
Dermatological	Bleaching of hair, alopecia, pruritus, skin and mucosal pigmentation, skin eruptions (urticarial, morbilliform, lichenoid, maculopapular, purpuric, erythema annulare centrifigum and exfoliative dermatitis)
Hematological	Blood dyscrasias, including aplastic anemia, agranulocytosis, leukopenia, thrombocytopenia (hemolysis in those with G6PD deficiency)

OVERDOSAGE	
Signs and symptoms	Headache, drowsiness, visual disturbances, cardiovascular collapse, convulsions, respiratory and cardiac arrest (sometimes fatal); ECG may reveal atrial standstill, nodal rhythm, prolonged intraventricular conduction time, and progressive bradycardia leading to ventricular fibrillation and/or arrest.
Treatment	Following acute ingestion, empty stomach immediately by emesis or gastric lavage, followed by activated charcoal in a dose at least five times the estimated dose of chloroquine ingested. Tracheal intubation or tracheostomy may be necessary. Peritoneal dialysis and exchange transfusions may be helpful. Control convulsions before attempting gastric lavage; if due to cerebral stimulation, administer an ultra-short-acting barbiturate cautiously, but if due to anoxia, correct with oxygen, artificial respiration or, in shock with hypotension, by vasopressor therapy. For patients who survive acute ingestion, observe closely, force fluids, and give 8 g ammonium chloride in diluted dose (for adults) to acidify the urine; exercise caution in patients with renal impairment and/or metabolic acidosis.

DRUG INTERACTIONS	
Gold salts	⇧ Risk of severe skin reaction
Phenylbutazone	⇧ Risk of severe skin reaction

ALTERED LABORATORY VALUES

No clinically significant alterations in blood/serum or urinary values occur at therapeutic dosages

Use in children

See INDICATIONS; children are especially sensitive to 4-aminoquinolines, and fatalities have been reported following accidental ingestion, sometimes of small doses. Safe use not established in juvenile arthritis.

Use in pregnancy or nursing mothers

Use during pregnancy should be avoided except in the suppression or treatment of malaria when in the judgment of the physician the benefit outweighs the possible hazard; general guidelines not established for use in nursing mothers

[1]These adverse reactions have been observed with 4-aminoquinoline compounds, and may not necessarily occur with hydroxychloroquine

[2]Incidence of corneal changes and visual side effects is lower with hydroxychloroquine than with chloroquine

EURAX (Crotamiton) Geigy

Cream: 10% (60 g) **Lotion:** 10% (60 ml)

INDICATIONS	TOPICAL DOSAGE
Scabies *(Sarcoptes scabiei)*	**Adult:** after bathing or showering, thoroughly massage 30 g or 30 ml into the skin of the whole body from the chin down, paying particular attention to folds and creases; repeat 24 h later, and bathe 48 h after last application **Child:** same as adult
Pruritus	**Adult:** massage into affected area; repeat as needed **Child:** same as adult

ADMINISTRATION/DOSAGE ADJUSTMENTS

Contaminated clothing and linen — Should be changed the morning after application. Contaminated clothing and bed linen may be dry-cleaned or washed in the hot cycle of a washing machine.

CONTRAINDICATIONS

Allergy to any component

WARNINGS/PRECAUTIONS

Special-risk areas — Acutely inflamed skin, raw and weeping surfaces, eyes and mouth; defer use until acute inflammation subsides

Severe irritation or sensitization — May occur; discontinue use and institute appropriate therapy

ADVERSE REACTIONS

Allergic — Sensitivity

Dermatological — Irritation

OVERDOSAGE

None

Use in children

See INDICATIONS; do not use on infants

Use in pregnancy or nursing mothers

General guidelines not established

KWELL (Lindane) Reed & Carnrick

Cream: 1% (57, 454 g) **Lotion:** 1% (59, 472 ml; 3.8 liter) **Shampoo:** 1% (59, 472 ml; 3.8 liter)

INDICATIONS	TOPICAL DOSAGE
Scabies *(Sarcoptes scabiei)*	**Adult:** apply a thin layer of the cream or lotion in sufficient quantity (usually 1 oz for an adult) to cover the entire body from the neck down; thoroughly massage the preparation into all skin surfaces from the neck to the toes, leave it in place for 8–12 h, and then wash thoroughly **Child:** same as for adult
Pediculosis capitis (head lice)	**Adult:** apply a sufficient amount of shampoo to thoroughly wet the hair and skin of the infested and surrounding areas, followed by enough water to work up a lather while rubbing the shampoo into the hair and scalp; continue shampooing for 4 min, then rinse thoroughly and towel dry. When hair is dry, remove any remaining nits or nit shells with a fine-tooth comb or tweezers. Alternatively, apply a sufficient amount of cream or lotion to cover only the infested and surrounding hairy areas, rub it well into the hair and scalp, leave in place for 12 h, and then wash thoroughly. **Child:** same as for adult
Pediculosis pubis (crab lice).	**Adult:** apply a thin layer of the cream or lotion in sufficient quantity to cover only the hair and skin of the pubic area, and if infested, the thighs, trunk, and auxillary regions; rub the preparation into the hair and skin, leave it in place for 12 h, and then wash thoroughly. Alternatively, apply a sufficient amount of shampoo to thoroughly wet the hair and skin of the infested and surrounding hairy areas, followed by enough water to work up a lather while rubbing the shampoo into the hair and skin; continue shampooing for 4 min, then rinse thoroughly and towel dry. **Child:** same as for adult

ADMINISTRATION/DOSAGE ADJUSTMENTS

Crusted scabies, lesions — A warm bath preceding medication may be helpful in removing crusts or scaling

Retreatment of lice infestations — Usually unnecessary; retreat only if living lice are demonstrable after 7 days

CONTRAINDICATIONS

Sensitivity to any component

WARNINGS/PRECAUTIONS

CNS toxicity — May occur, especially in young patients

Percutaneous absorption — May be enhanced by simultaneous application of creams, ointments, or oils

Contact with eyes — If accidental contact occurs, flush with water

Irritation or sensitization — May occur; discontinue use

Pruritus — May persist after treatment due to acquired sensitivity to mites and their products

ADVERSE REACTIONS

Local — Eczematous eruptions due to irritation

Other — Seizures (causal relationship not established)

OVERDOSAGE

Signs and symptoms — Vomiting, restlessness, irritability, muscle spasms, ataxia, clonic and tonic convulsions, cardiac arrhythmias, ventricular fibrillation, pulmonary edema, bladder irritation, microscopic hematuria, hepatitis, prostration, stupor, coma, respiratory failure

Treatment — If poisoning follows accidental ingestion, empty stomach immediately by gastric lavage and administer a saline cathartic to dilute bowel contents and hasten evacuation; oil laxatives promote absorption of lindane and should be avoided. Treat CNS manifestations with IV diazepam, pentobarbital, or phenobarbital.

DRUG INTERACTIONS

Other skin preparations — ⇧ Percutaneous absorption of lindane

ALTERED LABORATORY VALUES

No clinically significant alterations in blood/serum or urinary values occur at therapeutic dosages

Use in children

See INDICATIONS

Use in pregnancy or nursing mothers

Use with caution during pregnancy (see WARNINGS/PRECAUTIONS); general guidelines not established for use in nursing mothers

Childhood and Adult Immunization

The discovery of vaccines quite literally changed the course of human history. For the first time, many of the major killers of mankind—smallpox, diphtheria, whooping cough, and many other contagious diseases—could be effectively prevented. Today, smallpox has been eliminated from the official roster of diseases as a result of an intensive, worldwide eradication campaign, and routine immunization against it is no longer recommended.

Most childhood diseases—measles, mumps, whooping cough, polio, and others—are now preventable by immunization, and a vaccine against one of the few remaining childhood diseases, chicken pox, is in the testing stage. The recent introduction of vaccines against bacterial pneumonia and influenza promises to greatly reduce the danger that these diseases continue to pose to the very young, the aged, or persons weakened by other diseases. The new vaccine against hepatitis B has been heralded as a means of preventing not only a serious liver disease but also a common form of liver cancer, and it is hoped that, one day, vaccines against at least some forms of cancer will be developed.

TYPES OF VACCINES

The common vaccines are fragile substances manufactured from weakened (attenuated) or killed forms of the causative microorganisms. For example, rubella, measles, and mumps vaccines are manufactured from attenuated live viruses, while diphtheria and tetanus vaccines are made from killed bacteria or modified bacterial toxins.

Vaccines are very sensitive to heat; therefore, they must be kept refrigerated until they are used—a factor that often makes immunization in the lesser developed tropical countries difficult.

HOW VACCINES WORK

All vaccines work by the same principle: They stimulate the individual's immune system to manufacture antibodies against the disease in question, thus building a natural immunity to it. Immunization against common childhood diseases usually begins in the first few weeks of life. In some instances, later reimmunization or "booster" shots may be required.

Other vaccines may be administered under specific circumstances. For example, if there is an outbreak of meningitis, persons at risk of developing the disease may be given one of the relatively new meningitis vaccines. Persons traveling to parts of the world where certain diseases, such as cholera or typhoid, are endemic also are advised to undergo these immunizations. In still other instances, special immunization may be recommended for persons who are considered particularly susceptible to disease—for example, a person undergoing cancer chemotherapy may be advised to undergo influenza and pneumonia immunization. Or tetanus immunization may be recommended for persons who sustain a deep cut or other wound.

The following tables outline the recommended schedules for childhood immunization. They also cover other types of vaccines that are available and indicate who should receive them. Specific information on immunization for travelers may be obtained by writing or calling the Center for Disease Control, 1600 Clifton Road, Atlanta, Ga. 30333, telephone 404-329-3671.

COMMON IMMUNIZATIONS FOR CHILDREN AND ADULTS

Disease	Vaccine	Usage	Administration
Diphtheria Tetanus Pertussis	DTP: Diphtheria, tetanus toxoids, pertussis	6 wk.–6 yr.: 3 doses intramuscularly at 4–8-wk. intervals; 4th dose 1 yr. after 3rd. Ideal immunization: 2–3 mo. of age or infant's 6-wk. checkup.	Active and passive immunization for tetanus must be considered in wound management. Decision is based on history of previous tetanus vaccinations and condition of wound.
	Tetanus and diphtheria toxoids, Adult type (Td) (diphtheria component in Td 10–25% of that in standard DTP)	School-age children and adults, 3 doses Td intramuscularly; 2nd dose 4–8 wk. after 1st; 3rd dose 6 mo.–1 yr. after 2nd.	Routine pertussis immunization is not recommended after the age of 7 yr.
	Tetanus toxoid (T)	Booster: ages 3–6 yr.	
	Tetanus immunoglobulin for passive immunization	Thereafter and for all other persons: recommended dose of Td intramuscularly every 10 yr. (If dose is given sooner for wound management, next booster not needed for 10 yr. hence.)	
Influenza: (1980-81) *A/Brazil/78 (H1N1) A/Bangkok/79 (H3N2) B/Singapore/79*	Official name: *influenza virus vaccine, trivalent.* Inactivated trivalent antigens representing A/Brazil, A/Bangkok, B/Singapore. Available as whole virus or split virus.	Annual vaccination: individuals at increased risk, e.g., acquired, congenital heart disease; chronic compromised pulmonary dysfunction; chronic renal disease; diabetes mellitus; chronic severe anemia; immunocompromised conditions; persons over 65.	28 yr. and older, whole or split virus: 0.5 ml (1 dose); 13–27 yr., whole or split virus: 0.5 ml (2 dose) 4 wk. apart unless had 1 dose in 1978 or 1979, then 1 dose. 3–12 yr., split virus: 0.5 ml (2 dose as above); 6–35 mo., split virus: 0.25 ml (2 dose as above, special care in this age group.)
Measles *(Roseola)*	Live measles virus vaccine. Monovalent form (measles only); Measles-rubella (MR); Measles-mumps-rubella (MMR)	15 months of age: MMR routine infant-child vaccination. Revaccination recommended for those vaccinated before 1 yr. of age with live measles vaccine or before 1968 with inactivated vaccine. No enhanced risk with revaccination.	Exposure to disease no contraindication to vaccination. Live vaccine up to 72 hr. after exposure. Immune serum globulin for susceptible exposed less than 6 days before: 0.25 ml/kg of body weight; live vaccine 3 mo. later.
Meningitis *Neisseria meningitidis* Types A, B, C	Monovalent A, monovalent C, and bivalent A-C consist of purified capsular polysaccharide, each inducing specific serogroup immunity (Type B under development; see Table 3).	Civilian use only to control outbreaks caused by serogroup A or C. Travelers to countries known to have epidemics. Also adjunct to chemoprophylaxis for contacts of cases caused by serogroups A or C; see Table 3.	Single dose of vaccine administered parenterally.
Mumps *Mumps virus*	Live mumps virus vaccine prepared in chicken embryo culture. Produces subclinical infection.	Susceptible children, adolescents, adults unless immunized before 1 yr. of age. Persons born before 1957 believed naturally immune. MMR for routine use in children at 15 mo. (Immune serum globulin recommended after exposure).	Single dose cutaneously

Contraindications	Adverse Effects	Incidence
Risk of allergy to equine antitoxin must be weighed against benefits of vaccine in casé of diphtheria exposure		Diphtheria: 200–300 cases annually: 10% of cases of respiratory diphtheria are fatal. Tetanus: (1975) 102 cases; more than half in persons 50 yr. or older. Pertussis: (1972) 2–3 reported deaths in infants less than 1 yr.
Allergy to egg protein.	Fever, malaise, myalgia within 6–12 hr., persists for 1–2 days. Guillian-Barré syndrome with self-limited reversible paralysis: Incidence 10 in 1,000,000.	• 1968–80: more than 150,000 deaths estimated in U.S. • Infections range in severity from mild to fatal. • Viruses A & B recognizable for only portion of respiratory disease. • Influenza-related deaths occur primarily among chronically ill or those over age 65.
Pregnancy; febrile illness; antibiotic allergies (for vaccines containing trace amounts of antibiotics); tuberculosis may be exacerbated by natural measles vaccine; immunodeficiency diseases; immune serum globulin for those for whom live vaccination is contraindicated. Immune serum globulin not to be used to control measles outbreaks.	5–15% of vaccinees may present with fever 6th day after vaccination. Some reports of subacute sclerosing panencephalitis (SSPE). Some inoculated with inactivated virus may present with atypical measles.	Since introduction of vaccine in 1963, 57,345 reported (1977): more than 60% of cases in which age was known occurred in persons 10 yr. or older; 20% in persons 15–19 yr.
Safety during pregnancy not established.	Infrequent and mild reactions; localized erythema 1 or 2 days.	• 1968–78: 3,000–6,000 cases in U.S.; 1966–68 and since 1972 serogroup B most often isolated from patients; 1969–71 serogroup C most common in civilian and military populations. • In 1971, USAF gave C vaccine to all recruits, virtually eliminating C disease from that population. • Now, sulfa-sensitive serogroup B causes majority of U.S. cases. • C strains account for one third of cases.
Pregnancy. Vaccines with trace amounts of antibiotics should be considered carefully for those allergic to antibiotics. Febrile illness; immunodeficiency diseases.	No association with pancreatic damage or diabetes mellitus. Orchitis in 20% of clinical cases in postpubertal males. Benign meningeal signs in 15% of cases. Nerve deafness a rare complication.	Fewer than 20 cases per year.

COMMON IMMUNIZATIONS FOR CHILDREN AND ADULTS (CONTINUED)

Disease	Vaccine	Usage	Administration
Pneumococcal disease *Streptococcus pneumoniae* (pneumococcus)	Polyvalent vaccine (Pneumovax-Pnu-Immune) unified polysaccharide from 14 of most common types.	Majority of adults respond with rise in antibody. Limited response in children under 2 yr. Mass immunization not recommended. Selective immunization recommended. Benefits of vaccination increase with age. Persons at high risk important candidates for vaccine.	Each dose contains 50 micrograms of each polysaccharide. Administered subcutaneously.
Poliomyelitis	Oral polio vaccine (OPV or Sabin vaccine) contains 3 strains of poliovirus and gives higher levels of gastrointestinal immunity. Some differences remain as to comparative OPV treatment of choice. Inactivated polio vaccine (IPV or Salk vaccine), given by subcutaneous injection, not used extensively in U.S. for over 10 yr., but a Canadian IPV product is now available in the U.S.	OPV: Infants to 18 yr. IPV: Infancy through preschool. Before entering school, children receiving either OPV or IPV should have additional dose. Children not adequately protected for preadolescent years should be reevaluated for dosage. Adults are usually immune except in special cases or exposure to epidemic.	OPV: 3 doses; in infancy integrated with DTP. First dose: 6–12 wk. 2nd dose: 6–8 wk. later. 3rd dose: 8–12 mo. later (most persons protected after single dose of OPV). IPV: 4 doses; integrated with DTP. Three doses 4–8-wk. intervals. 4th dose 6–12 mo. after 3rd dose.
Rubella	Live rubella virus vaccine prepared in embryo cell culture. Monovalent form or in combination with measles (MR) and measles-mumps-rubella (MMR).	Routine infant-child vaccination programs. 12 mo. of age or 15 mo.+ with combination vaccine. Because of increased risk to fetus, unimmunized prepubertal girls, adolescent and adult females in childbearing group should be vaccinated; nonpregnant females who lack proof of immunity.	One dose in volume specified by manufacturer.

GUIDE TO TETANUS PROPHYLAXIS IN WOUND MANAGEMENT

History of tetanus immunization (doses)	Clean, minor wounds		All other wounds	
	Td*	TIG†	Td*	TIG†
Uncertain	Yes	No	Yes	Yes
0–1	Yes	No	Yes	Yes
2	Yes	No	Yes	No‡
3 or more	No§	No	No‖	No

* Tetanus toxoid, adult type
† Tetanus immunoglobulin
‡ Unless wound more than 24 hours old
§ Unless more than 10 years since last dose
‖ Unless more than 5 years since last dose

Contraindications	Adverse Effects	Incidence
No specific information on safety re pregnancy.	Slight erythema and slight pain for 1 day at injection site occur in less than 5%.	• 400,000–500,000 cases projected annually with 5–10% fatality rate. • Pneumococcal meningitis 1.5–2.5 out of 100,000 cases annually. One half the cases in ages 1 mo.–4 yr.; 40% are fatal in this range.
Pregnancy; Immunodeficiency diseases: OPV-IPV not recommended in these cases.	In rare instances, OPV associated with paralysis in healthy individuals. No paralysis with IPV; however, persons can be infected with wild strains or attenuated vaccine virus strains subsequent to IPV vaccination (rare).	• Decline from more than 18,000 in 1954 to less than 20 in 1973–78. • Proportion of U.S. population immunized has declined in years. • 1978 survey shows only 60% of 1-4-year-olds had primary polio vaccination.
• Pregnancy. Immune serum globulin not recommended for postexposure prophylaxis in early pregnancy. • Febrile illness • Allergies to antibiotics may occur if vaccine contains trace amounts of antibiotics. • Immunodeficiency diseases.	• Rash, lymphadenopathy in children. • Joint pain • Transient arthritis in susceptible women.	• 1977: 80 million doses of live rubella virus vaccine distributed. 70% of cases in persons 15 yr. or older. Outbreaks continue among older persons: junior, senior high schools, colleges, military, hospital employees.

SPECIFIC-USE VACCINES

Disease	Vaccine	Usage	Adverse Effects	Incidence
Rabies	Vaccine contains fixed rabies virus grown in human diploid cells and inactivated with tributyl phosphate.	Following bites from animal suspected as rabid.	Fewer than with other rabies vaccine; preferable for post-exposure immunoprophylaxis and preexposure immunization. Additional experience with drug needed.	
Adenovirus	Live oral vaccine containing adenoviruses types 4 and 7. Contained in enteric coated capsule.	Live virus bypasses respiratory system and selectively infects gastrointestinal tract, inducing immunity.		
Vaccine under investigation				
Hepatitis B	HBs Ag vaccine prepared from antigen abundant in the plasma taken from blood of infected individuals.	Under investigation; vaccine reported to give protection from clinical and subclinical hepatitis B virus infection among hemodialysis patients.		In U.S., 1 of every 1,000 persons chronically infected; 10% of adults possess hepatitis antibody. Hepatitis B transmitted by blood transfusion, rarely by mouth.

Neoplastic Diseases

Cancer Chemotherapy

In recent decades, greatly improved methods of cancer detection and treatment have vastly increased the likelihood of survival. In the 1930s, for example, fewer than 20 percent of all cancer patients could expect to be alive five years after diagnosis. Today, more than three million living Americans have undergone cancer treatment, and more than half of these are considered cured, meaning they have survived for five or more years with no sign of recurrence. A third of the 750,000 persons who are newly diagnosed as having life-threatening cancer each year can now expect to be cured. Even so, cancer remains the second leading cause of death in the United States, claiming about 400,000 lives a year.

Although cancer is usually thought of as a single disease, it is actually a large group of a hundred or more diseases, all characterized by the uncontrolled growth and proliferation of abnormal cells. What causes a normal cell to alter its life cycle and trigger this uncontrolled growth is unknown, but if unchecked, the abnormal cancerous cells will form a mass (tumor) and will eventually spread to other parts of the body—a process known as metastasis.

Although there are a hundred or more distinctly different kinds of cancer, some are much more common than others. In the United States, lung cancer is by far the most prevalent life-threatening malignancy, accounting for more than 100,000 deaths a year. (Skin cancer is the most common form of the disease, but is almost always curable.) Men are the most frequent victims of lung cancer, but women are fast "catching up," a fact attributed to the marked increase in women smokers in recent years. Cancer of the colon and rectum—a highly curable disease if detected and treated early—is the second most common cause of cancer death, while breast cancer—the leading cause of cancer death among women—ranks third.

Although cancer can strike at any age and in all social and economic groups, its frequency increases with age—nearly two thirds of all cases develop in persons over the age of fifty-five. A recent study of cancer rates over the last twenty-five years found that blacks have a higher cancer incidence and death rate than whites. However, this is attributed to environmental and social factors rather than to racial or biological characteristics.

TREATMENT OF CANCER

Surgery remains the principal treatment of most cancers, particularly for tumors that are localized with no evidence of spread beyond the regional lymph nodes. Increasingly, however, surgery is combined with drug therapy (cancer chemotherapy) and/or radiation therapy in the hope of preventing recurrence and distant spread (metastasis). The concept is to employ local treatment (surgery and/or radiation) to treat the localized tumor and systemic treatment with drugs to eradicate the cancer cells that may have spread to other parts of the body. This discussion will concentrate primarily on the drugs now being used in treating the more common forms of cancer.

Cancer Chemotherapy

Modern cancer chemotherapy started in the 1940s with the observation that estrogens could induce remission in some cases of prostatic cancer. Since then, thirty to forty active anticancer agents have been developed for clinical use. At present, cancer chemotherapy is the primary treatment for persons with leukemia, multiple myeloma, Hodgkin's disease, certain non-Hodgkin's lymphomas, Burkitt's lymphoma, choriocarcinoma, oat-cell lung cancer, and many types of metastatic cancer.

Since anticancer drugs are cytotoxic—meaning they are toxic to normal as well as tumor cells—the goal of chemotherapy is to take advantage of differences between cancerous and normal cells, killing one and not the other. The timing of therapy is extremely important. The probability of effecting a cure is greatest when cancer is in an early, rapid-growth stage because fast-growing tumor cells are more vulnerable to drugs than slow-growing ones.

It should be stressed that most anticancer drugs are still considered experimental. Their toxic effects can be limited and, in some cases, completely eliminated by sufficient knowledge of their clinical pharmacology. Many drugs, however, have not been sufficiently studied in particular tumors, while in the treatment of some common cancers, almost no assessment of drugs has yet been done.

From the patient's viewpoint, nausea and vomiting are among the most common and unpleasant side effects of certain anticancer drugs. The severity of these side effects varies widely among patients and is still only partially controlled by drugs that reduce nausea and vomiting. Loss of hair (alopecia) occurs to a varying degree with many of the drugs, but the hair almost always grows back, often while the drugs are still being administered. Temporary sterility is another side effect of many anticancer drugs. Ovarian function is generally only temporarily suppressed, whereas the effect on spermatogenesis is more profound and long-lasting. Other commonly experienced side effects include loss of appetite, mouth and intestinal ulcers, skin eruptions, weakness, diarrhea, constipation, and various immunological deficiencies. Most of these are temporary or reversible.

CURRENT TRENDS IN THERAPY

In the 1950s and 1960s, the general approach to treatment was to administer a low dose of an anticancer drug until toxicity developed, a regimen that is still followed in the low-dose continuous use of chlorambucil in follicular lymphomas. However, continuous administration of cytotoxic drugs suppresses the patient's immune system (increasing susceptibility to other diseases) and interferes with bone marrow function. Therefore, the current trend is to administer the anticancer drugs at higher doses on an intermittent schedule. Studies indicate that the antitumor effect of most of the drugs increases with the dose. In addition, the intervals between courses of therapy give bone marrow cells and intestinal lining an opportunity to recover.

As in any form of therapy, patients undergoing cancer chemotherapy should be carefully monitored. In evaluating drug response, the most commonly accepted definitions are:

Complete response. Disappearance of tumor for a minimum period—usually a month or longer

Partial response. A greater than 50 percent reduction in measurable disease for a minimum period—usually a month or longer

Stable and progressive disease. The cancer is continuing to progress.

In general, therapy is often continued even in the absence of overt disease. Most cancer specialists recommend that chemotherapy be repeated in order to destroy cells that may have escaped earlier doses but that may now be in a more favorable state for treatment.

Adjuvant Chemotherapy

In the 1970s, it was recognized that certain multiple cancer therapies—for example, administering anticancer drugs following cancer surgery—were more effective than a single mode of treatment. By the time many cancers have grown large enough to be diagnosed, they have completed a large portion of their life cycle and may have metastasized. In these cases, strictly local treatment, such as surgical removal of the primary tumor, is bound to fail. Therefore, the approach of adjuvant chemotherapy in addition to local therapy has evolved. Recent studies have found, for example, that a significant number of patients with breast and colon cancer, osteosarcoma, and possibly melanoma, achieve longer disease-free survival if chemotherapy is administered after surgical removal of the primary tumor.

Drug Selection

A number of factors are considered in selecting a particular anticancer drug or combination of drugs. These include mechanism of action; type and stage of cancer involved; goal of treatment (i.e., remission, symptomatic relief, etc.); other concomitant treatment(s); age and condition of the patient; and history of previous cancer chemotherapy or other anticancer treatment.

Dosage is usually based upon body weight (or, in some instances, surface area). Initially, the drugs are administered in a dosage form and on a schedule considered most effective for the type of cancer involved. Since adjustments and alterations are often made depending on individual response, close patient monitoring throughout the course of cancer chemotherapy is considered essential.

Most anticancer drugs are given intravenously, although some, such as methotrexate, can be given orally.

Categories of Anticancer Drugs

Anticancer drugs fall into six general categories: alkylating agents, antimetabolites, antibiotics, steroid hormones, metaphase inhibitors (or plant alkaloids), and miscellaneous agents. The major uses and considerations for use of drugs in each of these categories will be briefly described here. More complete information is given in the following drug charts or may be obtained from any of the Comprehensive Cancer Centers, as designated by the National Cancer Institute (see Table).

Alkylating Agents Nitrogen mustard, which was originally developed as a poison for military use, is the prototype of these alkylating agents, which interfere with DNA function and can be manipulated to produce selective effects on the development and function of tumor cells. Alkylating agents include carmustine (BiCNU), busulfan (Myleran), chlorambucil (Leukeran), cyclophosphamide (Cytoxan), lomustine (CeeNU), melphalan (Alkeran), and triethylenethiophosphoramide (Thio-Tepa).

The alkylating agents are generally considered most useful in treating chronic leukemia, lymphomas, Hodgkin's disease, multiple myeloma, and breast, lung, and ovarian cancers. Common adverse reactions associated with these drugs include bone marrow depression, various gastrointestinal reactions (particularly loss of appetite, nausea, and vomiting), and various skin effects, such as pigmentation changes, hair loss, rashes, and itching.

Antimetabolites Antimetabolites act by interfering with various metabolic processes, particularly nucleic acid synthesis, thereby preventing tumor cell growth or hindering cell function. Agents in this category include cytarabine (Cytosar-U), fluorouracil (Adrucil and Fluorouracil), mercaptopurine (Purinethol), and methotrexate (Methotrexate).

The antimetabolites are used to treat a wide variety of cancers, but some are more useful than others against specific cancers. Cytarabine, mercaptopurine, and methotrexate all are effective against acute leukemias, but cytarabine is often more effective against acute myeloblastic leukemia in adults than in children, and mercaptopurine is often more effective against chronic myelocytic leukemia. Fluorouracil is one of the principal agents used to treat colon, breast, and ovarian malignancies, and, to a somewhat lesser degree, cancers of the rectum, stomach, and pancreas. Methotrexate, either alone or in combination with other anticancer agents, is particularly useful against choriocarcinoma and acute lymphoblastic leukemias. It is also effective against meningeal leukemia, sarcomas, and cancers of the colon, ovary, cervix, breast, testis, lung, head, and neck. Patients receiving antimetabolites should have frequent liver and kidney function tests, as well as a complete blood count before each drug administration.

Antibiotics Several antibiotics or antibiotic-like agents have been found to be effective in cancer chemotherapy, acting primarily by interfering with DNA and RNA synthesis. These agents include bleomycin (Blenoxane), which is effective against Hodgkin's disease, non-Hodgkin's lymphomas, and testicular and squamous cell carcinomas; actinomycin (Cosmegen), which is used primarily against Wilms' tumor, choriocarcinoma, and testicular carcinoma; and doxorubicin (Adriamycin), which is effective against a wide spectrum of neoplasms, including acute leukemias, Hodgkin's disease, non-Hodgkin's lymphomas, soft-tissue and bone sarcomas, and breast, lung, and ovarian carcinomas, among others.

Bleomycin should be used with caution in persons with impaired kidney or lung function. High doses of doxorubicin can cause irreversible heart damage in some patients.

Hormones Steroid hormones—androgens, progestogens, estrogens, and adrenal corticosteroids—have proved useful in treating a number of cancers, particularly those of the breast, endometrium, kidney, and prostate. The corticosteroids are also used alone or with other anticancer agents to treat acute leukemias, Hodgkin's disease, and some breast cancers. These agents appear to act by suppressing the growth of tumors dependent upon sex hormones.

In addition to the various hormone preparations, specific anticancer drugs in this category include megestrol (Megace), a progestational agent used in the treatment of advanced breast or endometrial carcinoma, and tamoxifen (Nolvadex), a nonsteroidal antiestrogenic agent used primarily in the treatment of breast cancer.

Common side effects with hormone anticancer therapy include salt and fluid retention, and hypertension. In addition, women may experience hirsutism (abnormal hairiness) and other symptoms of masculinization, whereas feminization and loss of sexual function may occur in men.

Metaphase Inhibitors or Plant Alkaloids Anticancer drugs in this category act by interfering with cell division (metaphase). The most commonly used anticancer drugs in this category are vincristine (Oncovin) and vinblastine (Velban), which are derived from the *Vinca rosea* plant, more commonly known as periwinkle.

Vincristine is used in acute leukemia and, in combination with other drugs, against a variety of cancers, including Hodgkin's disease, oat-cell lung cancer, Wilms' tumor, and sarcomas. Vinblastine is used primarily in the palliative (relief of symptoms) treatment of lymphomas, advanced Hodgkin's disease, and sarcomas.

Miscellaneous Anticancer Drugs This category includes a variety of compounds, such as cisplatin (Platinol)—a platinum complex—and dacarbazine (DTIC-Dome). These drugs have properties similar to the alkylating agents, but are different in their spectrum and degree of activity. Cisplatin is used primarily in treatment of localized testicular as well as palliative therapy of metastatic testicular and ovarian cancers, whereas dacarbazine is used mostly in the treatment of metastatic melanoma.

Combination Therapy

Combinations of anticancer agents are being used with increasing frequency. By the time most cancers are diagnosed, the tumors already contain many billions or trillions of cancer cells. Treatment with a single drug will kill a proportion of these cells, but very often a large reservoir of resistant cancer cells is left to multiply and spread. By using combinations of drugs with different mechanisms of action, this possibility is minimized.

Combination chemotherapy has made prolonged disease-free survival possible for patients with neoplasms that were considered untreatable only a few years ago—for example, those with oat-cell lung cancer. Combination chemotherapy is also being used with encouraging results in acute leukemias, Hodgkin's disease, osteogenic sarcoma, lymphoma, Wilms' tumor, and cancers of the breast, testis, ovary, and gastrointestinal tract.

When selecting a combination of anticancer drugs, physicians concentrate on those with different anticancer activities and mechanisms of action, and avoid using drugs that produce toxicity in the same organ system(s). The drugs are administered at specific intervals according to a regimen designed to kill as many cancer cells as possible and then allow the immune system and other body functions to recover before the next course of treatment.

IN CONCLUSION

The following drug charts outline the major considerations in prescribing the most commonly used anticancer drugs. It should be emphasized that most of these drugs are still considered experimental and should be administered under the close supervision of physicians who are experienced in cancer chemotherapy. Although many of the drugs produce unpleasant and sometimes serious side effects, in most instances the benefits to be derived in treating life-threatening cancer outweigh these risks. All side effects, however, should be discussed with the supervising physician.

COMPREHENSIVE CANCER CENTERS

The following have been designated Comprehensive Cancer Centers by the National Cancer Institute. The telephone numbers are those for public and professional information.

Alabama
Comprehensive Cancer Center
University of Alabama in Birmingham
University Station
Birmingham, Ala. 35294
Tel: 205/934-6612

California
UCLA Jonsson Comprehensive Cancer Center
924 Westwood Boulevard, Suite 650
Los Angeles, Calif. 90024
Tel: 213/825-5412 (professional)
213/824-6017 (public)

University of Southern California Comprehensive Cancer Center
2025 Zonal Avenue
Los Angeles, Calif. 90033
Tel: 213/224-7626

Colorado
Colorado Regional Cancer Center, Inc.
935 Colorado Boulevard
Denver, Colo. 80206
Tel: 303/320-5921

Connecticut
Yale University Comprehensive Cancer Center
333 Cedar Street
New Haven, Conn. 06510
Tel: 203/436-3779

District of Columbia
Georgetown University/Howard University Comprehensive Cancer Center

Composed of:

Cancer Research Center
Howard University Hospital
2400 Sixth Street, N.W.
Washington, D.C. 20059
Tel: 202/636-5700

Vincent T. Lombardi Cancer Research Center
Georgetown University Medical Center
3800 Reservoir Road, N.W.
Washington, D.C. 20007
Tel: 202/636-5640

Florida
Comprehensive Cancer Center for the State of Florida
University of Miami School of Medicine
Jackson Memorial Medical Center
1475 N.W. Twelfth Avenue
Miami, Fla. 33136
Tel: 305/547-7707 ext. 220

Illinois
Illinois Cancer Council
36 South Wabash Avenue, Suite 700
Chicago, Ill. 60603
Tel: 312-CANCER-1 (Illinois residents) or
312/346-9813 (out-of-state)

Other Institutions in Council include:
Northwestern University Cancer Center
303 East Chicago Avenue
Chicago, Ill. 60611
Tel: 312/649-8674

Rush-Presbyterian-St. Luke's Medical Center
1753 West Congress Parkway
Chicago, Ill. 60612
Tel: 312/942-6642

University of Chicago Cancer Research Center
905 East Fifty-Ninth Street
Chicago, Ill. 60637
Tel: 312/947-6386

University of Illinois
P.O. Box 6998
Chicago, Ill. 60608
Tel: 312/996-8843 or 312/996-6666

Maryland
The Johns Hopkins Oncology Center
600 Wolfe Street
Baltimore, Md. 21205
Tel: 301/955-3636

Massachusetts
Sidney Farber Cancer Institute
44 Binney Street
Boston, Mass. 02115
Tel: 617/732-3150 or 617/732-3000

Michigan
Comprehensive Cancer Center of Metropolitan Detroit
110 East Warren
Detroit, Mich. 48201
Tel: 313/833-0710 ext. 247

Minnesota
Mayo Comprehensive Cancer Center
20 First Street, S.W.
Rochester, Minn. 55901
Tel: 507/284-8285

New York
Columbia University Cancer Research Center
College of Physicians & Surgeons
701 West 168th Street
New York, N.Y. 10032
Tel: 212/694-4161

Memorial Sloan-Kettering Cancer Center
1275 York Avenue
New York, N.Y. 10021
Tel: 212/794-7984

Roswell Park Memorial Institute
666 Elm Street
Buffalo, N.Y. 14263
Tel: 716/845-4400

North Carolina
Comprehensive Cancer Center
Duke University Medical Center
Durham, N.C. 27710
Tel: 919/684-2230

Ohio
The Ohio State University Comprehensive Cancer Center
357 McCampbell Hall
1580 Cannon Drive
Columbus, Ohio 43210
Tel: 614/422-1382

Pennsylvania
Fox Chase/University of Pennsylvania Comprehensive Cancer Center
7701 Burholme Avenue
Philadelphia, Pa. 19111
Tel: 215/728-2717

Texas
The University of Texas Health System Cancer Center
M.D. Anderson Hospital & Tumor Institute
6723 Bertner Avenue
Houston, Tex. 77030
Tel: 713/792-3030

Washington
Fred Hutchinson Cancer Research Center
1124 Columbia Street
Seattle, Wash. 98104
Tel: 206/292-6301

Wisconsin
The University of Wisconsin Clinical Cancer Center
600 Highland Avenue
Madison, Wis. 53706
Tel: 608/262-0064

ADRIAMYCIN (Doxorubicin hydrochloride) Adria

Vials: 10, 50 mg (2 mg/ml after reconstitution) for IV use only

INDICATIONS	PARENTERAL DOSAGE
Disseminated neoplastic conditions, including acute lymphoblastic leukemia, acute myeloblastic leukemia, Wilms' tumor, neuroblastoma, soft tissue and bone sarcomas, breast carcinoma, ovarian carcinoma, transitional cell bladder carcinoma, thyroid carcinoma, Hodgkin's disease, non-Hodgkin's lymphomas, bronchogenic carcinoma (small cells most responsive)	**Adult:** 60–75 mg/m² IV every 21 days or 30 mg/m² for 3 consecutive days every 4 wk; the lower dose should be given to patients with inadequate marrow reserves due to old age, prior therapy, or neoplastic infiltration

ADMINISTRATION/DOSAGE ADJUSTMENTS

Intravenous administration	Reconstitute with Sodium Chloride Injection USP or Sterile Water for Injection USP, using 5 ml for the 10-mg vial or 25 ml for the 50-mg vial, and administer required dose slowly (not less than 3-5 min) into tubing of a freely running IV infusion of Sodium Chloride Injection USP or 5% Dextrose Injection USP; to avoid formation of a precipitate, do not mix with heparin or fluorouracil
Patients with elevated serum bilirubin levels	If serum bilirubin level = 1.2–3.0 mg/dl, give ½ the normal dose; if > 3 mg/dl, give ¼ the normal dose

CONTRAINDICATIONS

Marked myelosuppression induced by previous treatment with antitumor agents or radiotherapy ●	Previous treatment with complete cumulative doses of doxorubicin and/or daunorubicin ●	Preexisting heart disease ●

WARNINGS/PRECAUTIONS

Severe cellulitis, vesication, and local tissue necrosis	Can result if extravasation occurs during IV administration; terminate injection or infusion immediately and restart in another vein
Irreversible myocardial toxicity with delayed congestive failure	May be encountered as total dosage approaches 550 mg/m² and is often unresponsive to cardiac supportive therapy. Myocardial toxicity may occur at lower doses in patients with prior mediastinal irradiation or on concurrent cyclophosphamide therapy. Perform baseline ECG and repeat prior to each dose or course after a cumulative dose of 300 mg/m² has been given.
Impaired hepatic function	Enhances toxicity; prior to individual dosing, evaluate hepatic function with conventional clinical laboratory tests (eg, SGOT, SGPT, alkaline phosphatase, and bilirubin)
Bone-marrow depression (primarily leukopenia)	May occur and requires careful hematologic monitoring; hematologic toxicity may require dose reduction or suspension or delay of therapy. Severe myelosuppression may result in superinfection and hemorrhage.
Concurrent therapy	Doxorubicin may potentiate the toxic effects of other anticancer therapies (see DRUG INTERACTIONS)
Mutagenic, carcinogenic properties	Have been observed in experimental models
Initial therapy	Requires close observation of the patient and extensive laboratory monitoring; hospitalize patients during the 1st phase of treatment
Hyperuricemia	May occur, secondary to rapid lysis of neoplastic cells; monitor blood uric-acid level and be prepared to use appropriate supportive and pharmacological measures
Urine discoloration	Urine may appear red in color for 1–2 days after administration; inform patients accordingly

Table continued on following page

ADRIAMYCIN continued

ADVERSE REACTIONS

Hematological	Myelosuppression
Cardiovascular	Cardiotoxicity, arrhythmias, phlebosclerosis, facial flushing
Dermatological	Reversible complete alopecia; hyperpigmentation of nailbeds and dermal creases (primarily in children); recalled skin reaction due to prior radiotherapy; severe cellulitis, vesication, and tissue necrosis; erythematous streaking along the vein proximal to the injection site
Gastrointestinal	Acute nausea and vomiting, stomatitis, esophagitis, ulceration, anorexia, diarrhea
Hypersensitivity	Fever, chills, urticaria, anaphylaxis, cross-sensitivity to lincomycin
Other	Conjunctivitis, lacrimation (rare)

OVERDOSAGE

Signs and symptoms	Myelosuppression, cardiotoxicity
Treatment	Discontinue medication and institute general supportive measures, as needed; treat heart failure with digitalis, diuretics, low-salt diet, and bed rest

DRUG INTERACTIONS

Cyclophosphamide	⇧ Risk of hemorrhagic cystitis and cardiotoxicity
Mercaptopurine	⇧ Risk of hepatotoxicity
Radiotherapy	⇧ Risk of cardiac, mucosal, skin, and liver toxicity ⇧ Antineoplastic effect
Antigout agents	⇧ Serum uric-acid levels
Mitomycin	⇧ Risk of cardiotoxicity
Myelosuppressive agents	⇧ Antineoplastic effect
Smallpox vaccination	⇧ Risk of generalized vaccinia

ALTERED LABORATORY VALUES

Blood/serum values	⇧ Uric acid
Urinary values	⇧ Uric acid

Use in children

General guidelines not established

Use in pregnancy or nursing mothers

Safe use not established during pregnancy; doxorubicin is embryotoxic and teratogenic in rats and embryotoxic and an abortifacient in rabbits. General guidelines not established for use in nursing mothers.

ALKERAN (Melphalan) **Burroughs Wellcome**

Tabs: 2 mg

INDICATIONS	ORAL DOSAGE
Multiple myeloma	**Adult:** 6 mg/day for 2–3 wk to start, followed (after a wait of up to 4 wk) by 2 mg/day

ADMINISTRATION/DOSAGE ADJUSTMENTS

Therapeutic response	May be very gradual over many months; maximum benefit may be missed if treatment is abandoned too soon

CONTRAINDICATIONS

Recent or concurrent radiotherapy ●	Recent chemotherapy ●	Depressed neutrophil and/or platelet counts ●

WARNINGS/PRECAUTIONS

Bone-marrow depression	Can result from excessive dosage. Obtain frequent blood counts to determine optimal dosage and to avoid toxicity; discontinue therapy if leukocyte count <3,000/mm³ or platelet count <100,000/mm³.

ADVERSE REACTIONS

Gastrointestinal	Nausea, vomiting
Hematological	Anemia, neutropenia, thrombocytopenia

OVERDOSAGE

Signs and symptoms	Bone-marrow depression
Treatment	Discontinue medication; institute supportive measures, as required

DRUG INTERACTIONS

Antigout agents	⇧ Serum uric-acid level
Myelosuppressive agents, radiotherapy	⇧ Antineoplastic effect
Smallpox vaccination	⇧ Risk of generalized vaccinia

ALTERED LABORATORY VALUES

Blood/serum values	⇧ Uric acid
Urinary values	⇧ Uric acid ⇧ 5-HIAA

Use in children	Use in pregnancy or nursing mothers
General guidelines not established	Safe use not established during pregnancy; general guidelines not established for use in nursing mothers

BiCNU (Carmustine [BCNU]) **Bristol**

Vial: 100 mg (3.3 mg/ml after reconstitution) for IV use only

INDICATIONS	PARENTERAL DOSAGE
Palliative treatment of **brain tumors,** including glioblastoma, brain-stem glioma, medullablastoma, astrocytoma, ependymoma, and metastatic brain tumors, **multiple myeloma** (in combination with prednisone), **Hodgkin's disease** (secondary adjunctive therapy), and **non-Hodgkin's lymphomas** (secondary adjunctive therapy)	**Adult:** 200 mg/m² in a single IV dose or divided over several days every 6 wk

ADMINISTRATION/DOSAGE ADJUSTMENTS

Intravenous administration	Reconstitute contents of 100-mg vial with 3 ml of absolute alcohol (supplied) plus 27 ml of Sterile Water for Injection USP; if desired, may be further diluted with Sodium Chloride Injection USP or 5% Dextrose Injection USP; administer required dose by IV drip over a period of 1–2 h
Hematologic response to prior dose	If nadir of WBC count following previous dose is 2,000–2,999/mm³ and/or nadir of platelet count is 25,000–74,999/mm³, give 70% of prior dose during next course of therapy; if nadir of WBC count is <2,000/mm³ and/or nadir of platelet count is <25,000/mm³, give 50% of prior dose during next course. Concomitant use of other myelosuppressive agents may require further dosage adjustment.
Reduced bone-marrow reserve	Adjust dosage as needed to maintain adequate bone-marrow function

CONTRAINDICATIONS

Hypersensitivity to carmustine ●	Platelet, leukocyte, or erythrocyte depression ●

WARNINGS/PRECAUTIONS

Delayed bone-marrow toxicity	Obtain frequent blood counts, as well as liver-function studies, for at least 6 wk after administration. Do not repeat dose more often than once every 6 wk. Bone-marrow toxicity is cumulative; adjust dosage on the basis of lowest blood counts. Do not administer until WBC count >4,000/mm³ and platelet count >100,000/mm³
Nausea and/or vomiting	May occur within 2 h of dosing; may be minimized or sometimes prevented by prior antiemetic therapy

ADVERSE REACTIONS

Gastrointestinal	Nausea, vomiting
Hematological	Delayed thrombocytopenia, leukopenia, anemia
Hepatic	Reversible toxicity
Respiratory	Pulmonary infiltrates and/or fibrosis
Other	Burning at injection site, thrombosis (rare), intense flushing of skin and suffusion of conjunctiva with too rapid IV administration

OVERDOSAGE

Signs and symptoms	See ADVERSE REACTIONS
Treatment	Discontinue medication; institute supportive measures, as required

DRUG INTERACTIONS

Hepatotoxic agents	⇧ Hepatotoxicity
Nephrotoxic agents	⇧ Nephrotoxicity
Myelosuppressive agents, radiotherapy	⇧ Antineoplastic effect
Smallpox vaccination	⇧ Risk of generalized vaccinia

Table continued on following page

ALTERED LABORATORY VALUES

Blood/serum values—————— ⇧ Alkaline phosphatase ⇧ Bilirubin ⇧ SGOT ⇧ SGPT ⇧ BUN

No clinically significant alterations in urinary values occur at therapeutic dosages

Use in children	**Use in pregnancy or nursing mothers**
General guidelines not established	Safe use not established during pregnancy; carmustine is embryotoxic and teratogenic in rats and embryotoxic in rabbits at dose levels equivalent to human doses. General guidelines not established for use in nursing mothers.

BLENOXANE (Bleomycin sulfate) **Bristol**

Amps: 15 units

INDICATIONS	PARENTERAL DOSAGE
Palliative treatment of **squamous cell carcinoma** of the mouth, tongue, tonsil, nasopharynx, oropharynx, sinus, palate, lip, buccal mucosa, gingiva, epiglottis, skin, larynx, penis, cervix, and vulva and of **testicular carcinoma,** including embryonal cell carcinoma, choriocarcinoma, and teratocarcinoma	**Adult:** 0.25–0.50 units/kg SC, IM, or IV weekly or twice weekly
Palliative treatment of **lymphomas,** including Hodgkin's disease, reticulum cell sarcoma, and lymphosarcoma	**Adult:** 2 units or less for first 2 doses, then 0.25–0.50 units/kg SC, IM, or IV weekly or twice weekly

ADMINISTRATION/DOSAGE ADJUSTMENTS	
Subcutaneous or intramuscular administration	Dissolve contents of ampule in 1-5 ml of Sterile Water for Injection USP, Sodium Chloride for Injection USP, 5% Dextrose Injection USP, or Bacteriostatic Water for Injection USP before administration
Intravenous administration	Dissolve contents of ampule in 5 ml or more of suitable IV solution (eg, normal saline or glucose) and administer slowly over a period of 10 min
Therapeutic response	If no improvement in Hodgkin's disease or testicular tumors is seen within 2 wk, improvement is unlikely; squamous cell cancers may take as long as 3 wk to respond
Hodgkin's disease	After achieving a 50% response with regular dosage schedules, administer 1 unit/day or 5 units/wk IV or IM for maintenance

CONTRAINDICATIONS

Hypersensitivity or idiosyncratic reaction to bleomycin

WARNINGS/PRECAUTIONS	
High toxicity	Monitor patients carefully and frequently for adverse reactions
Pulmonary fibrosis	Nonspecific pneumonitis progressing to pulmonary fibrosis may lead to death, especially in elderly patients and those receiving a total dose exceeding 400 units. Roentgenograms should be taken every 1–2 wk; if pulmonary changes are noted, discontinue treatment until it can be determined if they are drug-related. Total doses over 400 units should be given with great caution.
Special-risk patients	Use with extreme caution in patients with impaired renal or pulmonary function
Renal or hepatic toxicity	Begins as a deterioration in renal or liver-function tests; occurs infrequently
Idiosyncratic reactions	A severe idiosyncratic reaction, consisting of hypotension, mental confusion, fever, chills, and wheezing, may occur in 1% of lymphoma patients after the 1st or 2nd dose; monitor patient carefully

ADVERSE REACTIONS	
Pulmonary	Pneumonitis, fibrosis leading to death
Dermatological	Erythema, rash, striae, vesiculation, hyperpigmentation, tender skin, hyperkeratosis, nail changes, alopecia, pruritus
Gastrointestinal	Stomatitis, vomiting, anorexia
Other	Fever, chills, weight loss, pain at tumor site, phlebitis

OVERDOSAGE	
Signs and symptoms	See ADVERSE REACTIONS
Treatment	Discontinue medication; institute supportive measures, as required

Table continued on following page

DRUG INTERACTIONS

Antineoplastics, radiotherapy —————— ⇧ Risk of toxicity, including bone-marrow depression

ALTERED LABORATORY VALUES

No clinically significant alterations in blood/serum or urinary values occur at therapeutic dosages

Use in children	**Use in pregnancy or nursing mothers**
General guidelines not established	Safe use not established during pregnancy; general guidelines not established for use in nursing mothers

CeeNU (Lomustine [CCNU]) Bristol

Caps: 10, 40, 100 mg

INDICATIONS	ORAL DOSAGE
Palliative treatment of **primary and metastatic brain tumors** (postoperative and/or postirradiation adjunctive therapy) and **Hodgkin's disease** (secondary adjunctive therapy)	**Adult:** 130 mg/m² every 6 wk **Child:** same as adult

ADMINISTRATION/DOSAGE ADJUSTMENTS

Hematologic response to prior dose	If nadir of WBC count following previous dose is 2,000–2,999/mm³, and/or nadir of platelet count is 25,000–74,999/mm³, give 70% of prior dose during next course of therapy; if nadir of WBC count is <2,000/mm³ and/or nadir of platelet count is <25,000/mm³, give 50% of prior dose during next course. Concomitant use of other myelosuppressive agents may require further dosage adjustment.
Compromised bone-marrow function	Reduce dosage to 100 mg/m² every 6 wk

CONTRAINDICATIONS

Hypersensitivity to lomustine

WARNINGS/PRECAUTIONS

Delayed bone-marrow toxicity	Use with caution in patients with decreased numbers of circulating platelets, leukocytes, or erythrocytes. Obtain frequent blood counts, as well as liver-function studies, for at least 6 wk after administration. Do not repeat dose more often than once every 6 wk. Bone-marrow toxicity is cumulative; adjust dosage on the basis of lowest blood counts. Do not administer until WBC count >4,000/mm³ and platelet count >100,000/mm³.

ADVERSE REACTIONS

Gastrointestinal	Nausea, vomiting, stomatitis
Hematological	Delayed thrombocytopenia, leukopenia, anemia
Hepatic	Reversible toxicity
Central nervous system and neuromuscular	Disorientation, lethargy, ataxia, dysarthria
Other	Alopecia

OVERDOSAGE

Signs and symptoms	See ADVERSE REACTIONS
Treatment	Discontinue medication; institute supportive measures, as required

DRUG INTERACTIONS

Myelosuppressive agents, radiotherapy	⇧ Antineoplastic effect
Smallpox vaccination	⇧ Risk of generalized vaccinia

ALTERED LABORATORY VALUES

Blood/serum values	⇧ Alkaline phosphatase ⇧ Bilirubin ⇧ SGOT ⇧ SGPT

No clinically significant alterations in urinary values occur at therapeutic dosages

Use in children

See INDICATIONS

Use in pregnancy or nursing mothers

Safe use not established during pregnancy; general guidelines not established for use in nursing mothers

CERUBIDINE (Daunorubicin hydrochloride) Ives

Vial: 20 mg (5 mg/ml after reconstitution) for IV use only

INDICATIONS	PARENTERAL DOSAGE
Induction of remission in **acute nonlymphocytic (myelogenic, monocytic, erythroid) leukemia**	**Adult:** 60 mg/m²/day IV for 3 consecutive days every 3–4 wk (up to three courses may be required for remission)

ADMINISTRATION/DOSAGE ADJUSTMENTS

Intravenous administration	Dilute contents of vial with 4 ml of Sterile Water for Injection USP; withdraw desired dose into a syringe containing 10–15 ml of normal saline and inject into tubing or sidearm of a rapidly flowing IV infusion of 5% dextrose or normal saline. Do not administer or mix with other drugs or heparin. Use extreme care to avoid extravasation, as severe local tissue necrosis may occur.
Patients with hepatic or renal impairment	If serum bilirubin = 1.2–3.0 mg/dl, give ¾ the normal dose; if serum bilirubin >3 mg/dl or serum creatinine >3 mg/dl, give ½ the normal dose
Combination therapy	Give 45 mg/m²/day of daunorubicin IV for 3 consecutive days during first course and for 2 consecutive days during following courses; in addition, give 100 mg/m²/day of cytosine arabinoside (Cytosar) IV daily for 7 days during first course and for 5 days during subsequent courses. Up to three courses may be needed for remission.

CONTRAINDICATIONS

See WARNINGS/PRECAUTIONS

WARNINGS/PRECAUTIONS

Myocardial toxicity	Possibly leading to fatal congestive heart failure may occur, especially when total cumulative dose exceeds 550 mg/m². Effects may occur during therapy or may be delayed for several months. Use with caution in patients with pre-existing heart disease, patients concomitantly receiving other potentially cardiotoxic agents, related antineoplastic compounds, such as doxorubicin (Adriamycin), or in patients who are undergoing (or have undergone) radiotherapy that encompasses the heart. Monitor ECG and/or determine systolic ejection fraction prior to each course of therapy. A decrease equal to or greater than 30% in limb lead QRS voltage may be indicative of a significant risk of drug-induced cardiomyopathy.
Pericarditis-myocarditis	Occurs rarely, irrespective of dosage
Severe myelosuppression	Occurs in all patients at therapeutic doses; do not use in patients with pre-existing drug-induced bone marrow suppression unless benefits outweigh risks.
Hepatic or renal impairment	Enhances toxicity; evaluation of hepatic and renal function prior to therapy, using conventional clinical laboratory tests, is recommended. Dosage should be reduced accordingly (see ADMINISTRATION/DOSAGE ADJUSTMENTS).
Hyperuricemia	May occur secondary to rapid lysis of leukemic cells; monitor blood uric acid levels and initiate appropriate therapy where needed
Urine discoloration	Urine may appear red; inform patient accordingly
Systemic infection	Must be controlled with appropriate measures prior to therapy
Drug toxicity	Because of the potential for severe, toxic reactions, therapy requires close patient observation; use only when facilities for extensive laboratory monitoring and immediate supportive resources are available for responding to severe hemorrhagic complications and/or overwhelming infection

ADVERSE REACTIONS

Hematological	Myelosuppression
Cardiovascular	Congestive heart failure, pericarditis-myocarditis
Dermatological	Reversible alopecia
Gastrointestinal	Acute nausea and vomiting (antiemetic therapy may be helpful), mucositis, diarrhea
Hypersensitivity	Fever, chills, skin rash

OVERDOSAGE

Signs and symptoms	Myelosuppression, cardiotoxicity
Treatment	Discontinue medication and institute supportive measures, as needed; treat congestive heart failure with digitalis, diuretics, sodium restriction, and bed rest

Table continued on following page

CERUBIDINE continued

DRUG INTERACTIONS

No clinically significant drug interactions have been observed

ALTERED LABORATORY VALUES

Blood/serum values	⇧ Uric acid
Urinary values	Discoloration (may interfere with certain colorimetric methods)

Use in children

Contraindicated

Use in pregnancy or nursing mothers

Pregnancy category D. May produce teratogenic effects; pregnant patients should be apprised of potential hazard to fetus. General guidelines not established for use in nursing mothers.

CYTOSAR-U (Cytarabine) Upjohn

Vials: 100 mg (20 mg/ml after reconstitution) and 500 mg (50 mg/ml after reconstitution) for SC or IV use

INDICATIONS	PARENTERAL DOSAGE
Acute myelocytic leukemia and other leukemias, including acute lymphocytic leukemia, chronic myelocytic leukemia, and erythroleukemia	**Adult:** 200 mg/m²/day by continuous IV infusion for 5 days, repeated approximately every 2 wk until remission occurs; for maintenance, use a similar dose at longer intervals **Child:** same as for adult

ADMINISTRATION/DOSAGE ADJUSTMENTS

Preparation of parenteral solutions	Reconstitute with Bacteriostatic Water for Injection with 0.9% benzyl alcohol (supplied), using 5 ml for the 100-mg vial or 10 ml for the 500-mg vial, and adjust pH, when necessary, with HCl and/or NaOH (pH of reconstituted solution is ~ 5)
Intrathecal use	For acute meningeal leukemia, administer 30 mg/m² intrathecally once every 4 days until CSF findings return to normal, followed by one additional dose;

CONTRAINDICATIONS

Hypersensitivity to cytarabine

WARNINGS/PRECAUTIONS

Severe bone-marrow depression	May occur; monitor patients carefully and frequently, including daily platelet and leukocyte counts, and have facilities available to manage secondary infection and hemorrhage. Suspend or modify use if platelet count falls below 50,000/mm³ or polymorphonuclear leukocyte (granulocyte) count falls below 1,000/mm³ and do not restart therapy until counts return to these levels and signs of marrow recovery appear.
Severe nausea and vomiting	May result from rapid administration of large IV doses; effects are less severe with infusion
Special-risk patients	Use with caution in patients with pre-existing, drug-induced, bone-marrow suppression; reduce dosage and use with caution in patients with poor liver function
Hyperuricemia	May occur; monitor blood uric-acid level and institute supportive measures, as required

ADVERSE REACTIONS

	Frequent reactions are italicized
Hematological	*Thrombophlebitis, bleeding (all sites),* anemia, leukopenia, thrombocytopenia, megaloblastosis, reduced reticulocyte count
Gastrointestinal	*Anorexia, nausea, vomiting, diarrhea, oral and anal inflammation or ulceration, hepatic dysfunction,* sore throat, esophagitis, esophageal ulceration, abdominal pain, jaundice
Genitourinary	Urinary retention, renal dysfunction
Dermatological	*Rash,* freckling, ulceration, alopecia
Other	*Fever,* sepsis, pneumonia, cellulitis at injection site, neuritis, neurotoxicity, chest pain, dizziness, conjunctivitis, anaphylaxis

OVERDOSAGE

Signs and symptoms	See ADVERSE REACTIONS
Treatment	Discontinue medication; institute supportive measures, as required

DRUG INTERACTIONS

Antigout agents	⇧ Blood uric-acid level
Myelosuppressive agents, radiotherapy	⇧ Antineoplastic effect
Methotrexate	Possible synergistic effect
Smallpox vaccination	⇧ Risk of generalized vaccinia

Table continued on following page

ALTERED LABORATORY VALUES

Blood/serum values	⇧ SGOT ⇧ Uric acid
Urinary values	⇧ Uric acid

Use in children

See INDICATIONS; numerous studies have shown that children with acute myelocytic leukemia have higher response rates than adults who have received similar treatment regimens

Use in pregnancy or nursing mothers

Safe use not established during pregnancy, particularly when therapy is initiated during the 1st trimester. Cytarabine causes abnormal cerebellar development in the neonatal hamster and is teratogenic in rats. Although normal infants have been born to women treated during the 2nd and 3rd trimesters, such infants should be followed. General guidelines not established for use in nursing mothers.

CYTOXAN (Cyclophosphamide) Mead Johnson

Tabs: 25, 50 mg **Vials:** 100, 200, 500 mg (20 mg/ml after reconstitution)

INDICATIONS	ORAL DOSAGE	PARENTERAL DOSAGE
Malignant lymphomas (stages III and IV), including Hodgkin's disease, follicular lymphoma, lymphocytic lymphosarcoma, reticulum cell sarcoma, lymphoblastic lymphosarcoma, Burkitt's lymphoma **Multiple myeloma; leukemias,** including chronic lymphocytic leukemia, chronic granulocytic leukemia, acute myelogenous and monocytic leukemia, acute lymphoblastic leukemia in children **Advanced mycosis fungoides, neuroblastoma, ovarian adenocarcinoma, retinoblastoma, breast carcinoma, malignant lung neoplasms**	**Adult:** 1–5 mg/kg/day	**Adult:** 40–50 mg/kg IV div over a period of 2–5 days to start, followed by 10–15 mg/kg IV every 7–10 days or 3–5 mg/kg IV twice weekly

ADMINISTRATION/DOSAGE ADJUSTMENTS

Parenteral administration	Reconstitute with Sterile (or Bacteriostatic) Water for Injection USP, using 5 ml for the 100-mg vial, 10 ml for the 200-mg vial, or 25 ml for the 500-mg vial. Reconstituted solution may be injected IV, IM, intraperitoneally, or intrapleurally or may be infused IV with 5% Dextrose Injection USP or Sodium Chloride Injection USP.
Compromised bone-marrow function	Due to previous treatment with x-ray or cytotoxic drugs or tumor infiltration may require reduction of the initial loading dose by ⅓ to ½
Maintenance therapy	Unless the disease is unusually sensitive to cyclophosphamide, give largest maintenance dose that is reasonably tolerated, using WBC count as a guide

CONTRAINDICATIONS

None

WARNINGS/PRECAUTIONS

Adrenalectomized patients	May require dosage adjustment of both replacement steroids and cyclophosphamide
Concurrent phenobarbital therapy	Chronic high-dose phenobarbital therapy increases the metabolic and leukopenic activity of cyclophosphamide
Normal wound healing	May be impaired
Special-risk patients	Use with caution in patients with leukopenia, thrombocytopenia, tumor cell infiltration of bone marrow, previous x-ray therapy, previous cytotoxic drug therapy, or impaired hepatic or renal function
Immunosuppression	May occur and interruption or modification of dosage should be considered in patients who develop bacterial, fungal, or viral infections, especially in those receiving, or with a recent history of, steroid therapy. Varicella-zoster infections are particularly dangerous under these circumstances and can lead to death.
Mutagenic potential	Both male and female patients should be advised to employ adequate methods of contraception
Cystitis	May be minimized by ensuring ample fluid intake and frequent voiding
Tartrazine sensitivity	Presence of FD&C Yellow No. 5 (tartrazine) in tablets may cause allergic-type reactions, including bronchial asthma, in susceptible individuals

Table continued on following page

CYTOXAN continued

ADVERSE REACTIONS

Secondary malignancies	Urinary bladder, myeloproliferative, lymphoproliferative (causative relationship unestablished)
Hematological	Leukopenia, thrombocytopenia, anemia
Gastrointestinal	Anorexia, nausea, vomiting, hemorrhagic colitis, oral mucosal ulceration, jaundice
Genitourinary	Severe or fatal hemorrhagic cystitis, nonhemorrhagic cystitis, and/or fibrosis of the bladder, nephrotoxicity (including hemorrhage and clot formation in the renal pelvis)
Endocrinological	Gonadal suppression leading to amenorrhea or azoospermia, ovarian fibrosis
Dermatological	Alopecia, hyperpigmentation of skin and fingernails, dermatitis
Pulmonary	Interstitial fibrosis

OVERDOSAGE

Signs and symptoms	See ADVERSE REACTIONS
Treatment	Discontinue medication; institute supportive measures, as required

DRUG INTERACTIONS

Phenobarbital	⇧ Cytotoxic and leukopenic activity
Doxorubicin, daunorubicin	⇧ Risk of hemorrhagic cystitis and cardiotoxicity
Allopurinol, chloramphenicol	⇧ Risk of bone-marrow toxicity
Antigout agents	⇧ Blood uric-acid levels
Myelosuppressive agents, radiotherapy	⇧ Antineoplastic effect
Smallpox vaccination	⇧ Risk of generalized vaccinia
Succinylcholine	⇧ Risk of prolonged apnea

ALTERED LABORATORY VALUES

Blood/serum values	⇧ Uric acid ⇩ Pseudocholinesterase
Urinary values	⇧ Uric acid

Use in children

General guidelines not established

Use in pregnancy or nursing mothers

Contraindicated during pregnancy, particularly early pregnancy, unless potential benefits of therapy outweigh possible risks to the fetus; cyclophosphamide causes teratogenic effects and fetal resorption in animals. Patient should stop breast feeding if drug is prescribed during nursing period.

DTIC-DOME (Dacarbazine) Dome

Vials: 100, 200 mg (10 mg/ml after reconstitution) for IV use only

INDICATIONS	PARENTERAL DOSAGE
Metastatic malignant melanoma	**Adult:** 2–4.5 mg/kg/day IV for 10 consecutive days every 4 wk or 250 mg/m²/day IV for 5 consecutive days every 3 wk

ADMINISTRATION/DOSAGE ADJUSTMENTS

Intravenous administration	Reconstitute with Sterile Water for Injection USP, using 9.9 ml for the 100-mg vial or 19.7 ml for the 200-mg vial; withdraw required dose into a syringe and inject directly into a vein or, if desired, further dilute reconstituted solution with 5% Dextrose injection USP or Sodium Chloride Injection USP and administer as an IV infusion. Use extreme care to avoid extravasation, as subcutaneous infiltration of the drug may cause tissue damage and severe pain.

CONTRAINDICATIONS

Hypersensitivity to dacarbazine

WARNINGS/PRECAUTIONS

Bone-marrow depression	May occur and can be fatal; monitor WBC, RBC, and platelet counts carefully. Hematopoietic toxicity may require suspension or cessation of therapy.
Nausea and vomiting	May be minimized by coadministering phenobarbital and/or prochlorperazine; restricting oral intake of food for 4–6 h before treatment may lessen severity

ADVERSE REACTIONS

Frequent reactions are italicized

Gastrointestinal	*Anorexia, nausea, vomiting,* diarrhea (rare), hepatotoxicity and liver necrosis (extremely rare)
Hematological	Leukopenia, thrombocytopenia, anemia
Dermatological	Alopecia, erythematous and urticarial rashes, photosensitivity (rare)
Other	Facial flushing, facial paresthesia, influenza-like syndrome (fever, myalgias, and malaise), anaphylaxis

OVERDOSAGE

Signs and symptoms	See ADVERSE REACTIONS
Treatment	Discontinue medication; institute supportive measures, as required

DRUG INTERACTIONS

Allopurinol	⇧ Effect of allopurinol
Myelosuppressive agents, radiotherapy	⇧ Antineoplastic effect
Smallpox vaccination	⇧ Risk of generalized vaccinia

ALTERED LABORATORY VALUES

Blood/serum values	⇧ Alkaline phosphatase ⇧ BUN ⇧ SGOT ⇧ SGPT

No clinically significant alteratons in urinary values occur at therapeutic dosages

Use in children

General guidelines not established

Use in pregnancy or nursing mothers

Safe use not established during pregnancy; dacarbazine is teratogenic in animals. General guidelines not established for use in nursing mothers.

EFUDEX (Fluorouracil) Roche

Cream: 5% (25 g) **Sol:** 2%, 5% (10 ml)

INDICATIONS	TOPICAL DOSAGE
Multiple actinic or solar keratoses	**Adult:** apply cream or solution in an amount sufficient to cover lesions bid for 2–4 wk until inflammatory response (characterized by erythema and vesiculation) progresses to erosion, ulceration, and necrosis
Superficial basal-cell carcinomas, when conventional methods are impractical (eg, multiple lesions or difficult treatment sites)	**Adult:** apply 5% cream or solution in an amount sufficient to cover lesions bid for at least 3–6 wk (up to 10–12 wk, if necessary) until lesions are obliterated

CONTRAINDICATIONS

Hypersensitivity to any of the components

WARNINGS/PRECAUTIONS

Application	Apply with caution near eyes, nose, and mouth; wash hands immediately afterward
Occlusive dressings	May increase incidence of inflammatory reactions in adjacent normal skin; porous gauze dressings may be applied for cosmetic reasons without increase in reaction
Ultraviolet rays	Prolonged exposure to sunlight or other UV radiation should be avoided during therapy because intensity of reaction may be increased
Unsightly appearance	Forewarn patients that treated areas may be unsightly during and, in some cases, for several weeks after therapy; healing of keratotic lesions may not be complete for 1–2 mo following cessation of therapy
Unresponsive solar keratoses	Perform biopsy to confirm diagnosis
Follow-up	Patients with superficial basal cell carcinoma should be followed and biopsies performed to determine whether cure has been achieved

ADVERSE REACTIONS	Frequent reactions are italicized
Local	*Pain, pruritus, hyperpigmentation, burning,* dermatitis, scarring, soreness, tenderness, suppuration, scaling, swelling
Hematological	Leukocytosis, thrombocytopenia, toxic granulation, eosinophilia
Other	Insomnia, stomatitis, irritability, medicinal taste, photosensitivity, lacrimation, and telangiectasia (causal relationship not established)

Use in children

General guidelines not established

Use in pregnancy or nursing mothers

Safe use not established during pregnancy; general guidelines not established for use in nursing mothers

FLUOROURACIL Roche

Amps: 500 mg/10 ml (10 ml)

INDICATIONS	PARENTERAL DOSAGE
Palliative treatment of **carcinoma of the colon, rectum, breast, stomach, and pancreas**	**Adult:** 12 mg/kg/day IV for 4 days, up to 800 mg/day, to start, followed by 6 mg/kg IV on the 6th, 8th, 10th, and 12th days, unless toxicity occurs; patient should be hospitalized during 1st course of therapy

ADMINISTRATION/DOSAGE ADJUSTMENTS

Dosage	Based on patient's actual weight; estimated lean body mass is used if the patient is obese or edematous
High-risk patients	Administer 6 mg/kg/day IV for 3 days, up to 400 mg/day, to start, followed by 3 mg/kg IV on the 5th, 7th, and 9th days unless toxicity occurs
Maintenance therapy	If toxicity does not develop, or if it subsides after treatment, repeat dosage of first course beginning 30 days after the last day of previous treatment *or* administer 10–15 mg/kg/wk; do not exceed 1 g/wk

CONTRAINDICATIONS

Poor nutritional state ● Depressed bone-marrow function ● Potentially serious infections ●

WARNINGS/PRECAUTIONS

Special-risk patients	Use with caution in patients with a history of high-dose pelvic irradiation, prior use of alkylating agents, widespread involvement of bone marrow by metastatic tumors, or impaired hepatic or renal function
Combination therapy	Increases toxicity if it causes additional stress to the patient, interferes with nutrition, or depresses bone-marrow function
High toxicity	Therapeutic response is unlikely to occur without some evidence of toxicity; inform patient of expected effects, particularly oral manifestations (see ADVERSE REACTIONS), and obtain WBC count with differential before giving each dose
Severe hematological toxicity, GI hemorrhage, death	May result despite meticulous patient selection and careful dosage adjustment
Conditions necessitating prompt withdrawal of therapy	Discontinue medication if any of the following toxic signs appear: stomatitis, esophagopharyngitis, leukopenia (WBC count <3,500/mm³), rapidly falling WBC count, intractable vomiting, diarrhea, GI ulceration and bleeding, thrombocytopenia (platelet count <100,000/mm³) hemorrhage

ADVERSE REACTIONS

Gastrointestinal	Stomatitis, esophagopharyngitis, sloughing, ulceration, diarrhea, anorexia, nausea, vomiting
Hematological	Leukopenia, thrombocytopenia
Dermatological	Alopecia, dermatitis (pruritic maculopapular rash), dry skin, fissuring, photosensitivity, nail changes (including loss)
Cardiovascular	Myocardial ischemia
Other	Photophobia, lacrimation, epistaxis, euphoria, acute cerebellar syndrome

OVERDOSAGE

Signs and symptoms	See ADVERSE REACTIONS
Treatment	Discontinue medication; institute supportive measures, as required

Table continued on following page

FLUOROURACIL continued

DRUG INTERACTIONS

Myelosuppressive agents, radiotherapy	⇧ Antineoplastic effect
Smallpox vaccination	⇧ Risk of generalized vaccinia

ALTERED LABORATORY VALUES

Blood/serum values	⇩ Albumin
Urinary values	⇧ 5-HIAA

Use in children

General guidelines not established

Use in pregnancy or nursing mothers

Safe use not established during pregnancy; general guidelines not established for use in nursing mothers

NOTE: Fluorouracil also marketed as **ADRUCIL** **(Adria)**

LEUKERAN (Chlorambucil) **Burroughs Wellcome**

Tabs: 2 mg

INDICATIONS	ORAL DOSAGE
Chronic lymphocytic leukemia; malignant lymphomas, including lymphosarcoma, giant follicular lymphoma, and Hodgkin's disease	**Adult:** 0.1–0.2 mg/kg/day for 3–6 wk to start, followed by 0.03–0.1 mg/kg/day, if needed

ADMINISTRATION/DOSAGE ADJUSTMENTS

Bone-marrow infiltration or hypoplastic bone marrow	Dosage should not exceed 0.1 mg/kg/day

CONTRAINDICATIONS

Radiotherapy or chemotherapy	Within 4 wk after a full course of treatment

WARNINGS/PRECAUTIONS

Irreversible bone-marrow damage	Can result; monitor patients carefully. Determine hemoglobin levels and total and differential leukocyte counts weekly. During the first 3–6 wk of therapy, obtain leukocyte counts 3–4 days after each weekly complete blood count.
Slowly progressive lymphopenia	Often develops during treatment but returns to normal upon completion of drug therapy
Neutropenia	Can be expected in most patients after the 3rd wk of treatment and for up to 10 days after the last dose; subsequently, the neutrophil count usually rapidly returns to normal. Do not discontinue medication at the first evidence of a fall in neutrophil count.
Hypoplastic or lymphomatous bone marrow	Do not administer full dosage (see ADMINISTRATION/DOSAGE ADJUSTMENTS)

ADVERSE REACTIONS

Hematological	Bone-marrow depression

OVERDOSAGE

Signs and symptoms	See ADVERSE REACTIONS
Treatment	Discontinue medication; institute supportive measures, as required

DRUG INTERACTIONS

Antigout agents	⇧ Serum uric-acid level
Myelosuppressive agents, radiotherapy	⇧ Antineoplastic effect
Smallpox vaccination	⇧ Risk of generalized vaccinia

ALTERED LABORATORY VALUES

Blood/serum values	⇧ Uric acid
Urinary values	⇧ Uric acid

Use in children	**Use in pregnancy or nursing mothers**
General guidelines not established	Contraindicated during 1st trimester of pregnancy; general guidelines not established for use in nursing mothers

MEGACE (Megestrol acetate) **Mead Johnson**

Tabs: 20, 40 mg

INDICATIONS	ORAL DOSAGE
Palliative treatment of **advanced breast cancer**	**Adult:** 40 mg qid
Palliative treatment of **recurrent, inoperable, or metastatic endometrial carcinoma**	**Adult:** 40–320 mg/day div

ADMINISTRATION/DOSAGE ADJUSTMENTS

Duration of therapy	At least 2 mo of continuous treatment is needed to determine efficacy

CONTRAINDICATIONS

As a diagnostic test for pregnancy

WARNINGS/PRECAUTIONS

Thromboembolic disorders	Use with caution in patients with a history of thrombophlebitis
Breast tumors	Risk may or may not be increased, based on increased incidence of benign and malignant breast tumors in female dogs treated with megestrol for up to 7 yr; relevance to humans is unknown but should be considered both before and during therapy
Tartrazine sensitivity	Presence of FD&C Yellow No. 5 (tartrazine) in tablets may cause allergic-type reactions, including bronchial asthma, in susceptible individuals

ADVERSE REACTIONS

None

OVERDOSAGE

No serious side effects have resulted with dosages as high as 800 mg/day

DRUG INTERACTIONS

No clinically significant drug interactions have been observed

ALTERED LABORATORY VALUES

No clinically significant alterations in blood/serum or urinary values occur at therapeutic dosages

Use in children

General guidelines not established

Use in pregnancy or nursing mothers

Contraindicated during 1st 4 mo of pregnancy; general guidelines not established for use in nursing mothers

METHOTREXATE Lederle

Tabs: 2.5 mg **Vials:** 2.5 mg/ml (2 ml), 25 mg/ml (2 ml), 20 mg

INDICATIONS	ORAL DOSAGE	PARENTERAL DOSAGE
Gestational choriocarcinoma, chorioadenoma destruens, hydatidiform mole	**Adult:** 15–30 mg/day for 5 days; repeat 3–5 times, at intervals of 1 or more wk, as required	**Adult:** 15–30 mg/day IM for 5 days; repeat 3–5 times, at intervals of 1 or more wk, as required
Palliative treatment of **acute lymphocytic (lymphoblastic) leukemia**	—	**Adult:** 3.3 mg/m² IM or IV with 60 mg prednisone/m²/day
Burkitt's lymphoma (stages I–II)	**Adult:** 10–25 mg/day for 4–8 days; repeat several times at 7- to 10-day intervals	—
Lymphosarcoma (stage III)	**Adult:** 0.625–2.5 mg/kg/day	—
Meningeal leukemia	—	**Adult:** 12 mg/m² or 15 mg intrathecally every 2–5 days until CSF cell count returns to normal, followed by one additional dose
Advanced mycosis fungoides	**Adult:** 2.5–10 mg/day	**Adult:** 50 mg/wk or 25 mg twice weekly IM
Breast cancer, epidermoid cancer of the head and neck **Lung cancer,** particularly squamous cell and small cell Advanced **lymphosarcoma (stage IV)**	Consult manufacturer	
Severe, recalcitrant, disabling **psoriasis**	**Adult:** 10–25 mg/wk, up to 50 mg/wk; 2.5 mg q12h for 3 doses or q8h for 4 doses each wk, up to 30 mg/wk; or 2.5 mg/day for 5 days, up to 6.25 mg/day, followed by a drug-free interval of 2 or more days until optimal clinical response is achieved	**Adult:** 10–25 mg/wk IM or IV, up to 50 mg/wk, until optimal clinical response is achieved

ADMINISTRATION/DOSAGE ADJUSTMENTS

Maintenance therapy for acute lymphocytic (lymphoblastic) leukemia — Administer 30 mg/m² orally or IM twice weekly or 2.5 mg/kg IV every 14 days

CONTRAINDICATIONS

Psoriatic patients with severe renal or hepatic disorders or pre-existing blood dyscrasias ●

Impaired renal function (see WARNINGS/PRECAUTIONS) ●

WARNINGS/PRECAUTIONS

Fatal or severe toxic reactions — May occur; inform patients of the risks involved; monitor patients carefully, including hemogram, hematocrit, urinalysis, renal-function and liver-function tests, chest x-ray and, with high-dose or long-term therapy, liver biopsy or bone-marrow aspiration study. In addition, death may result from use in the treatment of psoriasis; restrict therapy to severe, recalcitrant, disabling psoriasis which fails to respond to other treatment modalities, but only after the diagnosis is confirmed by biopsy and/or dermatological examination

Special-risk patients — Use with caution, if at all, in patients with pre-existing bone-marrow aplasia, anemia, leukopenia, thrombocytopenia, and bleeding, and in those with infection, peptic ulcer, ulcerative colitis, debility, and in the very young or elderly

Hepatotoxicity — May occur, particularly at high dosage or with prolonged therapy. Determine hepatic function prior to use and monitor regularly throughout therapy; avoid concomitant use of other hepatotoxic drugs, including alcohol.

Impaired renal function — Toxic accumulation or additional renal damage may occur. Determine patient's renal status prior to and during therapy and use with caution if significant impairment is disclosed; reduce dosage or discontinue medication until renal function improves or is restored.

Table continued on following page

METHOTREXATE continued

WARNINGS/PRECAUTIONS continued	
Intestinal perforation	May result in hemorrhagic enteritis and death; discontinue use if diarrhea and ulcerative stomatitis develop
Concurrent therapy	Toxicity may be increased by salicylates, sulfonamides, phenytoin, phenylbutazone, and some antibacterials
Bacterial infection	May follow profound drug-induced leukopenia; discontinue use and institute appropriate antimicrobial therapy; transfusion also may be necessary
Immunosuppressive action	Must be considered in evaluating use where immune reponses are important or essential
Vitamin preparations	Containing folic acid or its derivatives, may alter response to methotrexate

ADVERSE REACTIONS	
Gastrointestinal	Ulcerative stomatitis, nausea, abdominal distress, gingivitis, pharyngitis, stomatitis, anorexia, vomiting, diarrhea, hematemesis, melena, ulceration, bleeding, enteritis
Hematological	Leukopenia, bone-marrow depression, thrombocytopenia, anemia, hypogammaglobulinemia, hemorrhage, septicemia
Dermatological	Erythematous rashes, pruritus, urticaria, photosensitivity, depigmentation, alopecia, ecchymosis, telangiectasia, acne, furunculosis
Hepatic	Toxicity, acute atrophy, necrosis, fatty metamorphosis, periportal fibrosis, cirrhosis
Genitourinary	Renal failure, azotemia, cystitis, hematuria, defective oogenesis or spermatogenesis, transient oligospermia, menstrual dysfunction, infertility, abortion, fetal defects, severe nephropathy
Central nervous system	Headaches, drowsiness, blurred vision, aphasia, hemiparesis, paresis, convulsions, leukoencephalopathy (with IV use), arachnoiditis (with intrathecal use)
Other	Malaise, undue fatigue, chills, fever, dizziness, decreased resistance to infection, pneumonitis, metabolic changes precipitating diabetes, osteoporotic effects, abnormal tissue-cell changes, sudden death

OVERDOSAGE	
Signs and symptoms	See ADVERSE REACTIONS
Treatment	Discontinue medication; institute supportive measures, as required. Leucovorin (citrovorum factor) neutralizes the immediate toxic effects on the hematopoietic system. When large doses or overdoses are given, administer leucovorin by IV infusion in doses up to 75 mg within 12 h, followed by 12 mg IM q6h for 4 doses. When average doses produce adverse effects, administer 6–12 mg leucovorin IM q6h for 4 doses.

DRUG INTERACTIONS	
Alcohol, hepatotoxic agents	⇧ Risk of hepatotoxicity
Antigout agents	⇧ Blood uric-acid level
Asparaginase	⇩ Antineoplastic effect
Myelosuppressive agents, radiotherapy	⇧ Antineoplastic effect
Phenylbutazone, salicylates, sulfonamides, phenytoin, probenicid, tetracycline, chloramphenicol, pyrimethamine, para-aminobenzoic acid	⇧ Methotrexate toxicity
Smallpox vaccination	⇧ Risk of generalized vaccinia

Table continued on following page

METHOTREXATE continued

ALTERED LABORATORY VALUES

Blood/serum values	⇧ Isocitric acid dehydrogenase (ICD) ⇧ Uric acid
Urinary values	⇧ Uric acid

Use in children

General guidelines not established

Use in pregnancy or nursing mothers

Not recommended for women of childbearing potential; fetal death and congenital anomalies have occurred. Contraindicated for pregnant psoriatic patients; general guidelines not established for use in nursing mothers.

MUTAMYCIN (Mitomycin) Bristol

Vials: 5, 20 mg (0.5 mg/ml after reconstitution) for IV use only

INDICATIONS	PARENTERAL DOSAGE
Disseminated adenocarcinoma of the stomach or pancreas when used in combination with other chemotherapeutic agents and as palliative treatment when other modalities have failed	**Adult:** 20 mg/m^2 IV as a single dose via IV catheter or 2 mg/m^3/day IV in two courses of 5 days each (ie, 20 mg/m^2 over 10 days), separated by a drug-free interval of 2 days; repeat at intervals of 6–8 wk, if indicated (see WARNINGS/PRECAUTIONS)

ADMINISTRATION/DOSAGE ADJUSTMENTS

Intravenous administration	Reconstitute with Sterile Water for Injection USP, using 10 ml for the 5-mg vial or 40 ml for the 20-mg vial, and administer via a functioning IV catheter or, if desired, may be further diluted in various IV solutions to a concentration of 20–40 μg/ml (may be mixed with heparin) before administration. Use extreme care to avoid extravasation and resulting possible cellulitis, ulceration, and slough
Hematologic response to prior dose	If nadir of WBC count following previous dose is 2,000–2,999/mm^3 and/or nadir of platelet count is 25,000–74,999/mm^3, give 70% of prior dose during next course of therapy; if nadir of WBC count is $<$2,000/mm^3 and/or nadir of platelet count is $<$25,000/mm^3, give 50% of prior dose during next course. Concomitant use of other myelosuppressive agents may require further dosage adjustment.
Duration of therapy	If disease continues to progress after two courses of therapy, discontinue medication

CONTRAINDICATIONS

Hypersensitivity or idiosyncratic reaction to mitomycin ●	Thrombocytopenia ●	Coagulation disorders ●
Increased bleeding tendency ●	Serum creatinine level $>$1.7 mg/dl ●	

WARNINGS/PRECAUTIONS

Bone-marrow suppression	Occurs frequently; warn patients of potential toxicity and obtain following studies during therapy and for at least 7 wk afterward: platelet count, WBC count, differential, and hemoglobin. Interrupt therapy if platelet count falls below 150,000/mm^3 or WBC count falls below 4,000/mm^3 or either declines progressively. Do not reinstitute until WBC count returns to 3,000/mm^3 and platelet count to 75,000/mm^3.
Renal toxicity	May occur; monitor patient for rise in BUN and serum creatinine level (see CONTRAINDICATIONS)

ADVERSE REACTIONS	Frequent reactions are italicized
Hematological	*Myelosuppression, including thrombocytopenia and/or leukopenia (64%)*
Dermatological	*Mucous membrane toxicity (4%), cellulitis, stomatitis, alopecia*
Renal	*Functional impairment, characterized by an elevated serum creatinine level (2%)*
Pulmonary	Dyspnea, nonproductive cough, radiographic evidence of infiltrates
Gastrointestinal	*Anorexia, nausea, vomiting,* diarrhea and hematemesis (causal relationship not established)
Central nervous system	Headache, confusion, drowsiness, syncope, fatigue, and pain (causal relationship not established)
Other	*Fever,* blurring of vision, thrombophlebitis, and edema (causal relationship not established)

OVERDOSAGE

Signs and symptoms	See ADVERSE REACTIONS
Treatment	Reduce dosage or if necessary, discontinue therapy; steroids have been employed in treatment of pulmonary toxicity, but their therapeutic value has not been determined

DRUG INTERACTIONS

Myelosuppresive agents	⇧ Antineoplastic effect and myelosuppression
Smallpox vaccination	⇧ Risk of generalized vaccinia

Table continued on following page

MUTAMYCIN continued

ALTERED LABORATORY VALUES

Blood/serum values —————————— ⇧ BUN ⇧ Creatinine

No clinically significant alterations in urinary values occur at therapeutic dosages

Use in children

General guidelines not established

Use in pregnancy or nursing mothers

Safe use not established during pregnancy, mitomycin is teratogenic in animals. General guidelines not established for use in nursing mothers.

NOLVADEX (Tamoxifen citrate) Stuart

Tabs: 10 mg

INDICATIONS	ORAL DOSAGE
Palliative treatment of **advanced breast cancer** in postmenopausal women[1]	**Adult:** 1-2 tabs bid in AM and PM

CONTRAINDICATIONS

None

WARNINGS/PRECAUTIONS

Oncogenic activity	Has been observed in animals; the possibility of this potential in humans should be considered
Ocular pathology	Retinopathy, corneal changes, and a decrease in visual acuity have been reported in a few patients after long-term, high-dose therapy
Hypercalcemia	May occur with bone metastases within a few weeks after the start of therapy; take appropriate measures and, if severe, discontinue medication
Existing leukopenia or thrombocytopenia	Use with caution; obtain complete blood counts, including platelet counts, periodically

ADVERSE REACTIONS

Endocrinological	Hot flashes, vaginal bleeding or discharge, menstrual irregularities
Gastrointestinal	Nausea, vomiting, anorexia
Dermatological	Rash, pruritus vulvae
Central nervous system	Depression, dizziness, lightheadedness, headache
Other	Increased bone and tumor pain, local disease flare, increased size of pre-existing soft-tissue lesions accompanied by marked erythema and/or new lesions, peripheral edema, hypercalcemia

OVERDOSAGE

Signs and symptoms	Toxicity has not been reported in humans
Treatment	Reduce dosage or discontinue medication; treat symptomatically

DRUG INTERACTIONS

No clinically significant drug interactions have been observed

ALTERED LABORATORY VALUES

Blood/serum values	⇧ Calcium

No clinically significant alterations in urinary values occur at therapeutic dosages

Use in children	Use in pregnancy or nursing mothers
No appropriate indications	Safe use not established during pregnancy; general guidelines not established for use in nursing mothers

[1]Patients who have had a recent negative estrogen receptor assay are unlikely to respond to tamoxifen

ONCOVIN (Vincristine sulfate) Lilly

Amps: 1, 5 mg for IV use only

INDICATIONS	PARENTERAL DOSAGE
Acute leukemia, Hodgkin's disease, lymphosarcoma, reticulum-cell sarcoma, rhabdomyosarcoma, neuroblastoma, Wilms' tumor (combined oncolytic therapy)	**Adult:** 1.4 mg/m² IV at weekly intervals **Child:** 2 mg/m² IV at weekly intervals

ADMINISTRATION/DOSAGE ADJUSTMENTS

Dosage calculation	Extreme care must be used in calculating and administering the dose of vincristine; overdosage may have a very serious or fatal outcome
Intravenous administration	Reconstitute with Bacteriostatic Sodium Chloride Injection with 0.9% benzyl alcohol (supplied) or dilute in sterile water or physiological saline to a concentration of 0.01–1 mg/ml and inject required dose either directly into a vein or into the tubing of a freely running IV infusion
Local reactions	Extravasation should be avoided; local injection of hyaluronidase and application of moderate heat to area may minimize discomfort and reduce possibility of cellulitis

CONTRAINDICATIONS

None

WARNINGS/PRECAUTIONS

Acute uric-acid nephropathy	May occur; administration of the next dose warrants careful consideration in the presence of leukopenia or complicating infection
Central nervous system leukemia	May require additional agents and routes of administration
Neurotoxicity	Pay particular attention to dosage and neurological side effects when administering vincristine to patients with pre-existing neuromuscular disease, or before use with other neurotoxic drugs

ADVERSE REACTIONS

Dermatological	Alopecia
Central nervous system and neuromuscular	Neuritic pain, difficulty in walking, sensory loss, paresthesia, slapping gait, loss of deep-tendon reflexes, muscle wasting, convulsions, hypertension, ataxia, foot drop, cranial nerve manifestations, numbness of digits, headache
Hematological	Leukopenia
Gastrointestinal	Constipation, paralytic ileus (particularly in children), abdominal cramps, vomiting, diarrhea, oral ulceration
Genitourinary	Polyuria, dysuria
Other	Inappropriate antidiuretic hormone secretion syndrome, weight loss, fever

OVERDOSAGE

Signs and symptoms	See ADVERSE REACTIONS
Treatment	Discontinue medication; institute supportive measures, as required

DRUG INTERACTIONS

Antigout agents	⇧ Blood uric-acid level
Asparaginase, isoniazid and other neurotoxic drugs, spinal cord irradiation	⇧ Risk of neurotoxicity
Doxorubicin	⇧ Risk of myelosuppression
Myelosuppressive agents, radiotherapy	⇧ Antineoplastic effect
Smallpox vaccination	⇧ Risk of generalized vaccinia

Table continued on following page

ALTERED LABORATORY VALUES

Blood/serum values	⇧ Potassium ⇧ Uric acid
Urinary values	⇧ Uric acid

Use in children

See INDICATIONS

Use in pregnancy or nursing mothers

Safe use not established during pregnancy; general guidelines not established for use in nursing mothers

PLATINOL (Cisplatin) Bristol

Vial: 10, 50 mg (1 mg/ml after reconstitution) for IV use only

INDICATIONS	PARENTERAL DOSAGE
Palliative treatment of **metastatic testicular tumors**	**Adult:** 20 mg/m²/day IV for 5 consecutive days every 3 wk for 3 courses, in combination with bleomycin sulfate and vinblastine sulfate
Palliative treatment of **metastatic ovarian tumors**	**Adult:** 50 mg/m² IV once every 3 wk, in combination with doxorubicin hydrochloride, or 100 mg/m² IV once every 4 wk alone as secondary therapy for patients refractory to standard chemotherapy and who have not been previously treated with cisplatin

ADMINISTRATION/DOSAGE ADJUSTMENTS

Intravenous administration	Reconstitute with Sterile Water for Injection USP, using 10 ml for the 10-mg vial or 50 ml for the 50-mg vial; dilute the reconstituted solution with 2 liters of 5% Dextrose in 1/2 N or 1/3 N Saline with 37.5 mg mannitol and infuse over a period of 6–8 h
Hydration of patient	Infuse 1–2 liters of fluid for 8–12 h prior to administration of cisplatin and maintain adequate hydration and urinary output for 24 h after
Patient monitoring	Monitor renal function and perform audiometric testing before initiating therapy and prior to administering subsequent doses of cisplatin (see WARNINGS/PRECAUTIONS); blood counts should be obtained weekly and liver and neurological function tests periodically

CONTRAINDICATIONS

Pre-existing renal impairment ●

History of allergy to cisplatin or other platinum-containing compounds ●

Myelosuppression ●

Hearing impairment ●

WARNINGS/PRECAUTIONS

Cumulative nephrotoxicity	May be manifested by elevation in BUN, serum creatinine, and/or serum uric acid or by reduction in creatinine clearance, generally during the 2nd wk after dosing; toxicity is dose-related and becomes more prolonged and severe with repeated courses. Measure serum creatinine, BUN, and creatinine clearance before initiating therapy and prior to each course; do not administer if serum creatinine >1.5 mg/dl and/or BUN >25 mg/dl.
Myelosuppression	May occur in 25–30% of patients and is dose-related; obtain peripheral blood counts weekly and do not administer if platelet count <100,000/mm³ or WBC count <4,000/mm³
Ototoxicity	May be manifested by tinnitus and/or high-frequency hearing loss (4,000–8,000 Hz) in one or both ears; hearing loss tends to become more frequent and severe with repeated doses, particularly in children. Do not administer unless audiometry indicates normal auditory acuity.
Nausea and vomiting	May occur in almost all patients, usually within 1–4 h after treatment and lasting up to 24 h; symptoms may persist for up to 1 wk after dosing
Hyperuricemia	May occur at approximately the same frequency as increases in BUN and serum creatinine, generally between 3–5 days after treatment; may be controlled with allopurinol
Neurotoxicity	May occur; monitor neurological function regularly and discontinue therapy at first sign of symptoms
Anaphylactoid-like reactions	Consisting of facial edema, wheezing, tachycardia, and hypotension, may occur within a few minutes of drug administration; reactions may be controlled with IV epinephrine, corticosteroids, or antihistamines

Table continued on following page

ADVERSE REACTIONS

Gastrointestinal	Nausea, vomiting, anorexia
Renal	Nephrotoxicity, renal tubular damage
Otic	Tinnitus, high-frequency hearing loss
Hematological	Leukopenia, thrombocytopenia, anemia
Neurological	Peripheral neuropathies (possibly irreversible), loss of taste sensation, seizures
Allergic	Anaphylactoid-like reactions (see WARNINGS/PRECAUTIONS)
Other	Cardiac abnormalities

OVERDOSAGE

Signs and symptoms	See ADVERSE REACTIONS
Treatment	Discontinue medication; treat symptomatically and institute supportive measures, as required

DRUG INTERACTIONS

No clinically significant drug interactions have been observed

ALTERED LABORATORY VALUES

Blood/serum values	⇧ BUN ⇧ Creatinine ⇧ Uric acid ⇧ SGOT

No clinically significant alterations in urinary values occur at therapeutic dosages

Use in children

General guidelines not established

Use in pregnancy or nursing mothers

Safe use not established during pregnancy; general guidelines not established for use in nursing mothers

THIOTEPA (*N, N', N"*-Triethylenethiophosphoramide) **Lederle**

Vials: 15 mg (10 mg/ml after reconstitution)

INDICATIONS	PARENTERAL DOSAGE
Palliative treatment of **adenocarcinoma of the breast or ovary**	**Adult:** 0.3–0.4 mg/kg by rapid IV administration at intervals of 1–4 wk or 0.6–0.8 mg/kg, injected directly into the tumor, to start, followed by 0.07–0.8 mg/kg at intervals of 1–4 wk, depending on the patient's condition
Intracavitary effusions secondary to diffuse or localized neoplastic disease of various serosal cavities	**Adult:** 0.6–0.8 mg/kg injected directly into the cavity
Superficial papillary carcinoma of the urinary bladder	**Adult:** 60 mg in 30–60 ml distilled water instilled into the bladder by catheter and retained for 2 hr, once a week for 4 wk

ADMINISTRATION/DOSAGE ADJUSTMENTS	
Parenteral administration	Reconstitute contents of 15-mg vial with 1.5 ml of Sterile Water for Injection USP; the reconstituted solution may then be injected directly and rapidly into a suitable vein, injected directly into the tumor mass (see below), or, if desired, added to larger volumes of other diluents for intracavitary administration, continuous IV infusion, or perfusion therapy
Intratumor administration	First inject a small amount of local anesthetic through a 22-gauge needle, remove the syringe, and inject drug through the same needle
Intracavitary administration	Drug may be administered through same tubing used to remove fluid from involved cavity
Intravesical administration	Patient must be dehydrated for 8–12 h prior to treatment
Local injection	Drug may be mixed with 2% procaine hydrochloride or 1:1000 epinephrine hydrochloride, or both
Maintenance dose	Adjust weekly on the basis of pretreatment control and subsequent blood counts

CONTRAINDICATIONS	
Hepatic, renal, or bone-marrow damage[1] ●	Hypersensitivity to *N, N', N"*-triethylenethiophosphoramide ●

WARNINGS/PRECAUTIONS	
Hematopoietic toxicity	Leukopenia, thrombocytopenia, and anemia may occur, possibly leading to death from septicemia and hemorrhage. Obtain weekly blood and platelet counts during therapy and for at least 3 wk afterward; discontinue therapy if WBC count falls to 3,000/mm³ or less or if the platelet count falls to 150,000/mm³. Do not use other myelosuppressive agents concomitantly.
Mutagenicity	Chromosomal aberrations have been shown in vitro, with frequency increasing with increasing patient age
Carcinogenicity	Strong circumstantial evidence of human carcinogenicity exists
Other alkylating agents and radiotherapy	Do not use concomitantly; ensure complete hematologic recovery from first agent before instituting therapy with second agent

ADVERSE REACTIONS	Frequent reactions are italicized
Hematological	*Bone-marrow depression, including thrombocytopenia, leukopenia, and anemia*
Gastrointestinal	Nausea, vomiting, anorexia
Central nervous system	Dizziness, headache
Endocrinological	Amenorrhea, interference with spermatogenesis
Dermatological and hypersensitivity	Hives, rash, alopecia (one case), weeping from subcutaneous lesions (due to breakdown of tumor tissue)
Other	Pain at injection site, fever (due to breakdown of tumor tissue)

OVERDOSAGE	
Signs and symptoms	Bone-marrow depression, including leukopenia, thrombocytopenia, and anemia
Treatment	Discontinue therapy; administer transfusions of whole blood, platelets, or leukocytes, as needed

[1]If need for therapy outweighs risks, drug may be used in low dosage with adequate monitoring of hepatic, renal, and hematopoietic function

Table continued on following page

THIOTEPA continued

DRUG INTERACTIONS

Alkylating agents	⇧ Toxicity
Myelosuppressive agents, radiotherapy	⇧ Myelosuppression
Succinylcholine	⇧ Risk of prolonged apnea

ALTERED LABORATORY VALUES

No clinically significant alterations in blood/serum or urinary values occur at therapeutic dosages

Use in children

General guidelines not established

Use in pregnancy or nursing mothers

Not recommended for use during pregnancy, unless expected benefit outweighs teratogenic risk; general guidelines not established for use in nursing mothers

Neurological Diseases

Movement Disorders

It is the highest achievement of a dancer or athlete to make a challenging performance look simple. The true complexity of coordinated movement is only revealed by the variety of tragic disorders in which movement is severely distorted, difficult, or impossible. These conditions can arise from abnormal functioning within the brain, as in Parkinson's disease, Huntington's disease (or chorea), and tardive dyskinesia; from damaged nerve tissue outside the brain, as in multiple sclerosis; or from diseases of the muscles themselves, as in muscular dystrophy and myasthenia gravis.

MOVEMENT DISORDERS ARISING WITHIN THE BRAIN

Symptoms

Parkinsonism, Huntington's disease, and tardive dyskinesia usually begin in adulthood. Each involves progressive loss of normal movement and substitution of either muscular rigidity or abnormal involuntary movements. In the later stages of these diseases, the patient may develop mental and psychiatric problems as well.

About 200,000 persons in the United States are affected by parkinsonism. It is especially prevalent in older people, affecting about 1 percent of the population over the age of sixty years.

In parkinsonism, the basic problem is muscular rigidity. Movement gradually degenerates from slowed movements (bradykinesia) to the inability to initiate movement (akinesia). This is due to increased resistance in the muscles, a condition known as hypertonicity. Parkinsonism generally takes five to ten years to reach the stage of incapacitation, although in some persons, this may be extended to twenty years or more. Two other signs commonly found in parkinsonian patients are excessive salivation and tremor of the hands.

As the disease progresses, mental faculties may degenerate. First the cognitive and perceptual abilities are impaired, then occasional memory lapses and confusion occur. The patient may be subject to bouts of depression.

Huntington's disease is one of the more common hereditary nervous disorders, occurring in about one in every 10,000 people. It has gained more public attention in recent years because of one of its more famous victims, the folksinger Woody Guthrie. Its symptoms are the opposite of parkinsonism. The person with Huntington's disease is subject to abnormal unintended movements, due to decreased intrinsic resistance to motion in the muscles (hypotonicity). Because these undirected movements may resemble the gestures of a dancer, they have been called choreiform (from the Greek word for dance), and this disease was initially called Huntington's chorea. Early in the disease, the involuntary movements are mild and resemble the effects of clumsiness or nervousness. The disease is progressive, however, and eventually produces uncontrollable jerking and contortions of the body and finally death.

As in parkinsonism, the person with Huntington's disease often sustains loss of mental abilities. In addition, many of these patients experience delusions and hallucinations, and about 10 percent may suffer seizures and mental retardation. The disease course usually takes from ten to twenty years, during much of which the victim is an invalid.

Huntington's disease is a genetically transmitted condition that is inherited as an autosomal dominant trait, meaning that each child of a parent with Huntington's disease has a 50 percent chance of developing the condition and that men and women are at equal risk. Because symptoms of the disease often do not appear until age thirty or later, a person whose father or mother had Huntington's disease frequently does not know whether they have the disease until after they have had children. There is great interest in finding a way to detect the presence of the disease before symptoms appear, but so far, no such test is available.

Choreiform movements also characterize tardive dyskinesia. In this condition the limbs and trunk muscles may be affected, but a more characteristic pattern is bizarre, repetitive, involuntary movements of the mouth and facial muscles. The most typical are protrusion of the tongue, pursing of the mouth, and grimacing of the facial musculature. There is also a characteristic hyperextension of the fingers.

Tardive dyskinesia is predominantly an iatrogenic disease, meaning it is a result of medical treatment, most often affecting those who have undergone long-term treatment with antipsychotic medicines such as the phenothiazines (e.g. Thorazine) or the butyrophenones (e.g., Haldol). (See the section on *Anxiety, Depression,* and *Psychotic Disorders,* pages 736–807.)

Treatment

All three of these conditions are thought to be due to abnormalities in a part of the brain called the basal ganglia, which regulates movement.

The current therapy of parkinsonism is based on the fundamental understanding of how the balancing mechanism is altered in this disease. In the mid-1960s, examination of brains from deceased parkinsonian patients revealed degeneration of the basal ganglia nerve cells containing a substance called dopamine. This led to the postulation that enhancement of the dopaminergic pathway in the brain might be an effective treatment for parkinsonism. Dopamine itself does not enter the brain, but its immediate metabolic precursor, L-dihydroxyphenylalanine (L-dopa), does. It was then discovered that administration of the synthetic form of L-dopa, levodopa (Dopar and Larodopa), alleviated symptoms in most persons with parkinsonism. Unfortunately, 95 percent of the levodopa administered does not go to the brain; instead it acts on peripheral nerves or is broken down to other biologically active compounds, such as epinephrine. Therefore, levodopa given by itself produces many systemic side effects, including disturbances of heart rhythm, nausea, vomiting, depression, euphoria, or anxiety. Some of these problems are solved by adding levodopa to carbidopa, a compound that inhibits the enzymes that break down levodopa. Carbidopa is too large to enter the brain, so it does not interfere with levodopa's conversion and action in the basal ganglia. This combination of levodopa and carbidopa, called Sinemet, is effective in doses one fourth as large as levodopa given alone. Systemic toxicity is greatly reduced, although psychiatric side effects may still occur. It significantly alleviates rigidity, bradykinesia, and walking and balance difficulties in about two thirds of patients. The improvements in bradykinesia and rigidity are longest lasting.

Drugs that block the action of dopamine should not be given at the same time as levodopa. These include reserpine, commonly used to treat high blood pressure, and antipsychotic drugs, such as phenothiazines and haloperidol.

In patients with mild symptoms, anticholinergics such as benztropine (Cogentin) or biperiden (Akineton), may be used for initial treatment, with levodopa or Sinemet being added later. Further augmentation of dopaminergic activity can sometimes be obtained by adding antihistamines or the antiviral compound amantadine (Symmetrel) to either anticholinergics or levodopa. Two frequently used antihistamines are diphenhydramine (Benadryl) and chlorphenoxamine (Phenoxene). Another drug sometimes used for adjunctive therapy is the phenothiazine ethopropazine (Parsidol). Amantadine is sometimes used by itself for initial treatment in very mild cases. Its effect lasts for three to six months. In fact, some neurologists recommend beginning parkinsonism therapy with amantadine or anticholinergic drugs rather than levodopa. This is because the beneficial effects of levodopa diminish after three to five years of treatment. At some medical centers, physicians are investigating the "drug holiday" in prolonging the period of levodopa's effectiveness. Periodically the patient is taken off medication and kept in the hospital for a few days. Many patients can be effectively treated with much lower doses of levodopa after this drug-free period.

To date, there are no drugs that are effective in treating or controlling Huntington's disease, although several promising ones are in the testing stage.

A similar situation exists in the treatment of the choreiform movements of tardive dyskinesia. This disorder is thought to arise from augmentation of the dopaminergic nerve cells through increased sensitivity of the receptor sites at which dopamine exerts its action. Attempts to find effective treatment for this condition have been frustrating. One particularly deceptive aspect of tardive dyskinesia is that it apparently disappears when the dosage of a phenothiazine, such as chlorpromazine (Thorazine), is increased. However, this is merely a masking effect, and the symptoms are even more exaggerated when the antipsychotic drug is later stopped. Currently the most promising approach is to prevent the disease by altering prescribing of phenothiazine.

DISORDERS ARISING OUTSIDE THE BRAIN

Multiple Sclerosis

In this disease, the body's immune system goes awry and attacks the insulating material covering the spinal cord. The disease is characterized by destruction of the sheaths of certain nerves and portions of the brain. The symptoms vary according to the area affected, and may include partial one-sided paralysis, weakness, visual disturbances, loss of bladder control, and other neurological problems. It is a progressive disease, but there are often periods of remission. One of the symptoms, muscular spasm, is controllable by drugs such as baclofen (Lioresal) in some patients. (See the section on *Backache and Other Musculoskeletal Disorders, pages* 707–735.)

Muscular Dystrophy

Very little is known about this genetically transmitted group of diseases. They involve muscle wasting, generally of unknown origin. No effective therapy exists.

Myasthenia Gravis

This chronic neuromuscular disease can occur from adolescence on. It often affects women in their thirties. The chief manifestation is muscular weakness, with the patient becoming fatigued more easily as the disease progresses. Most often the ability to walk is impaired, as are chewing and breathing. One characteristic sign is drooping eyelids.

During the mid-1970s, research revealed that myasthenia gravis is caused by an impairment of cholinergic transmission at the neuromuscular junction. This is the very small area where the signal for muscular contraction is passed from the nerve to the muscle. As in multiple sclerosis, the defect in myasthenia is caused by an immune system disorder in which antibodies are produced against the receptor at which acetylcholine exerts its action. This antibody either blocks or destroys the receptor, reducing the effectiveness of the acetylcholine signal, which activates muscle, secretory glands, and other nerve cells.

Therapy of this condition consists of drugs that inhibit the breakdown of acetylcholine. These compounds, called acetylcholinesterases, produce improvement in many patients, although some symptoms and disabilities may persist. The drugs commonly used, such as pyridostigmine (Mestinon) and neostigmine (Prostigmin), are much longer-acting than edrophonium (Tensilon), a chemical that temporarily counters muscle weakness. Use of these drugs requires careful physician supervision. Occasionally some patients become temporarily refractory to therapy (myasthenic crisis), and mechanical respiration must be supplied.

The autoimmune basis of myasthenia partly explains the effectiveness of two other treatments that can be used when anticholinesterases do not help, namely, removal of the thymus gland, which is involved in the maturation of the cells of the immune system, or the administration of corticosteroid drugs, which are powerful suppressors of the immune response. The steroid most commonly used for this purpose is prednisone (Deltasone, Meticorten, and Orasone).

For patients who do not benefit from any of the above treatments, azathioprine (Imuran), an immunosuppressant often used in organ transplant patients, has recently been used experimentally with good success. Since it can produce severe toxic effects, it is unlikely that it will be approved for widespread, long-term use. However, plasmapheresis, a mechanical technique to remove the circulating antibodies, has been employed most recently with striking success.

IN CONCLUSION

Many movement disorders, such as parkinsonism, are progressive and difficult to treat or control. In recent years, new approaches to drug therapy of some of these disorders have succeeded in some improvement, and other regimens are under investigation. The following charts cover the drugs used most commonly in treating parkinsonism and myasthenia gravis.

AKINETON (Biperiden) Knoll

Tabs: 2 mg **Amps:** 5 mg/ml (1 ml)

INDICATIONS	ORAL DOSAGE	PARENTERAL DOSAGE
Parkinsonism, including postencephalitic, arteriosclerotic, and idiopathic forms (adjunctive therapy)	**Adult:** 2 mg tid or qid	—
Drug-induced extrapyramidal disturbances	**Adult:** 2 mg 1-3 times/day	**Adult:** 2 mg IM or IV q½h, as needed, up to 4 doses/24 h

ADMINISTRATION/DOSAGE ADJUSTMENTS

Gastric irritation	May be avoided by administering drug during or after meals
Dry mouth, blurred vision	May be decreased or eliminated by reducing oral dosage or by slow parenteral administration

CONTRAINDICATIONS

Hypersensitivity to biperiden

WARNINGS/PRECAUTIONS

Special-risk patients	Use with caution in patients with manifest glaucoma, prostatism, or cardiac arrythmias

ADVERSE REACTIONS

Central nervous system	Mental confusion, euphoria, agitation, disturbed behavior, disorientation, drowsiness
Gastrointestinal	Gastric irritation
Cardiovascular	Mild, transient postural hypotension
Other	Dry mouth, blurred vision, urinary retention

OVERDOSAGE

Signs and symptoms	Range from CNS depression to stimulation; atropine-like effects
Treatment	Generally symptomatic and supportive; if patient is neither precomatose nor convulsive, empty stomach by emesis or gastric lavage. Support respiration with artificial respiration or mechanical assistance, if needed. For CNS excitation, administer a short-acting barbiturate *carefully*, since excitation may precede depression. Treat circulatory collapse with vasopressors. Hyperthermia may be controlled with tepid bathing.

DRUG INTERACTIONS

Alcohol and other CNS depressants	⇧ Sedative effects
Amantadine, antihistamines, antimuscarinics, haloperidol, MAO inhibitors, tricyclic antidepressants, phenothiazines, procainamide, quinidine	⇧ Atropine-like effects
Antacids, antidiarrheals	⇧ Absorption of biperiden (allow 1-2 h between doses of different medications)

ALTERED LABORATORY VALUES

No clinically significant alterations in blood/serum or urinary values occur at therapeutic dosages

Use in children

General guidelines not established

Use in pregnancy or nursing mothers

Safe use during pregnancy not established; general guidelines not established for use in nursing mothers

ARTANE (Trihexyphenidyl hydrochloride) Lederle

Tabs: 2, 5 mg **Caps (sust rel):** 5 mg **Elixir:** 2 mg/5 ml

INDICATIONS	ORAL DOSAGE
Parkinsonism, including postencephalitic, arteriosclerotic, and idiopathic forms (adjunctive therapy)	**Adult:** 1 mg/day to start, followed, if needed, by increases of 2 mg/day at 3- to 5-day intervals, up to 6-10 mg/day in 3 divided doses at mealtimes
Drug-induced extrapyramidal disturbances	**Adult:** 1 mg to start, followed by increases, if needed, after several hours, up to 15 mg/day; usual dosage range: 5-15 mg/day

ADMINISTRATION/DOSAGE ADJUSTMENTS

Patients with arteriosclerosis or idiosyncratic reaction to other drugs	Initiate therapy with small doses and gradually increase to avoid untoward effects (see ADVERSE REACTIONS). Discontinue therapy for several days and resume at lower dosage if severe reactions occur.
Postencephalitic patients	May require 12-15 mg/day; excessive salivation may be reduced by administration after meals or concomitant use of small amounts of atropine
Excessive dry mouth, thirst	May be allayed by taking drug prior to meals, or by mints, chewing gum, or water
Drug-induced extrapyramidal reactions	Control may be rapidly achieved by reducing tranquilizer dosage when instituting trihexyphenidyl therapy
Combination therapy	Administer 3-6 mg/day when used with levodopa; when used with another parasympathetic agent, gradually increase trihexyphenidyl dosage while decreasing dosage of other agent
Sustained-release capsules	May be used for maintenance therapy after patient has been stabilized on conventional dosage forms; administer daily dose as a single dose after breakfast, or as 2 divided doses q12h. Do not use for initial therapy.

CONTRAINDICATIONS

None

WARNINGS/PRECAUTIONS

Increased intraocular pressure	May develop; perform gonioscope evaluation prior to therapy and closely monitor intraocular pressure at regular intervals thereafter. Incipient glaucoma may be precipitated.
Special-risk patients	Use with caution in patients with cardiac, hepatic, or renal disorders, hypertension, glaucoma, obstructive gastrointestinal or genitourinary tract disease, or in elderly males with prostatic hypertrophy
Elderly patients	Exhibit increased sensitivity to drug; strict dosage regulation is necessary
Prolonged therapy	Observe patient carefully for allergic or other untoward reactions

ADVERSE REACTIONS

Frequent reactions are italicized

Central nervous system	*Dizziness (30-50%), nervousness (30-50%),* delusions, hallucinations, paranoia, mental confusion,[1] agitation,[1] disturbed behavior,[1] euphoria, drowsiness, weakness, headache, psychiatric disturbances (with excessive use)
Gastrointestinal	*Mild nausea (30-50%),* dilation of the colon, paralytic ileus, nausea with vomiting,[1] constipation
Dermatological	Rash
Cardiovascular	Tachycardia
Ophthalmic	*Blurred vision (30-50%),* mydriasis, increased intraocular tension
Genitourinary	Urinary hesitancy, urinary retention
Other	*Dry mouth (30-50%),* suppurative parotitis

OVERDOSAGE

Signs and symptoms	May range from CNS stimulation (confusion, excitement, hyperpyrexia, agitation, disorientation, delirium, hallucinations) to CNS depression (drowsiness, sedation, coma)
Treatment	Treat symptomatically and employ supportive measures, as needed. If patient is neither precomatose nor convulsive, empty stomach by emesis or gastric lavage. Support respiration with artificial respiration or mechanical assistance, if needed. For CNS excitation, administer a short-acting barbiturate *carefully,* since excitation may precede depression. Treat circulatory collapse with vasopressors. Control hyperthermia with tepid bathing.

[1]In patients with arteriosclerosis or history of idiosyncratic reaction to other drugs

Table continued on following page

ARTANE continued

DRUG INTERACTIONS

Alcohol and other CNS depressants	⇧ Sedative effect
Amantadine, antihistamines, antimuscarinics, haloperidol, MAO inhibitors, phenothiazines, procainamide, quinidine, tricyclic antidepressants	⇧ Atropine-like effects
Antacids, antidiarrheals	⇧ Absorption of trihexyphenidyl (allow 1-2 h between doses of different medications)

ALTERED LABORATORY VALUES

No clinically significant alterations in blood/serum or urinary values occur at therapeutic dosages

Use in children	Use in pregnancy or nursing mothers
General guidelines not established	General guidelines not established

COGENTIN (Benztropine mesylate) Merck Sharp & Dohme

Tabs: 0.5, 1, 2 mg **Amps:** 1 mg/ml[1] (2 ml)

INDICATIONS	ORAL DOSAGE	PARENTERAL DOSAGE
Idiopathic parkinsonism (adjunctive therapy)	**Adult:** 0.5–1.0 mg at bedtime to start, followed by up to 4–6 mg/day, if needed; usual dosage: 1–2 mg/day	**Adult:** 0.5–1.0 mg IM at bedtime to start, followed by up to 4–6 mg/day, if needed; usual dosage: 1–2 mg/day
Postencephalitic parkinsonism (adjunctive therapy)	**Adult:** 2 mg/day to start, followed by up to 6 mg/day, if needed; usual dosage: 1–2 mg/day	**Adult:** 2 mg/day IM to start, followed by up to 6 mg/day, if needed; usual dosage: 1–2 mg/day
Drug-induced extrapyramidal disorders	**Adult:** 1–4 mg qd or bid	**Adult:** 1–4 mg IM qd or bid
Drug-induced acute dystonic reactions	—	**Adult:** 1–2 mg IV, followed by 1–2 mg orally bid to prevent recurrence
Prophylaxis of recurrent or transient drug-induced extrapyramidal disorders	**Adult:** 1–2 mg bid or tid, as needed; reassess need after 1–2 wk	—

ADMINISTRATION/DOSAGE ADJUSTMENTS

Medical supervision	Continued supervision is recommended due to cumulative action
Atropine-like effect, mydriasis	May be minimized by careful adjustment of daily dosage
Initiating therapy	Use smallest dose to start, followed by increase of 0.5 mg/day, if needed, at 5- to 6-day intervals
Intravenous use	As there is no significant difference in the onset of effect after IM or IV administration, the IV route is rarely needed
Dosage interval	Daily dose may be given as a single dose, preferably at bedtime, or divided
Combination therapy	May be used with levodopa/carbidopa or with levodopa alone
Patients receiving other antiparkinsonism agents	Reduce or discontinue dosage of other agents gradually when adding benztropine mesylate
Emergency situations	1–2 mg IM or IV may be used; repeat dose, if needed

CONTRAINDICATIONS

Hypersensitivity to benztropine mesylate or any component of injectable form

WARNINGS/PRECAUTIONS

Mental impairment, reflex-slowing	Performance of potentially hazardous tasks may be impaired; caution patients accordingly
Paralytic ileus	May occur in patients who are also receiving phenothiazines or tricylic antidepressants, and can be fatal. Advise patient to report gastrointestinal disturbances promptly.
Anhidrosis	Possibly leading to fatal hyperthermia, may occur. Use with caution during hot weather and in patients with sweating disorders. Concomitant administration of other atropine-like drugs in patients with chronic diseases, CNS disease, or alcoholism, or in patients who perform manual labor in a hot environment, increases risk. Monitor patient for early signs and reduce dosage accordingly.
Muscle weakness, inability to move particular muscle groups	May occur with excessive dosages; reduce dosage accordingly
Mental confusion, excitement	May occur with large doses or in susceptible individuals
Intensification of preexisting mental disorder	May occur during treatment of extrapyramidal disorders; toxic psychosis may be precipitated if dosage is increased. Monitor patient carefully when therapy is increased.
Unwarranted use	Antiparkinsonism agents do not alleviate and may exacerbate symptoms of phenothiazine-induced tardive dyskinesia
Glaucoma	Monitor patient for increased intraocular pressure

ADVERSE REACTIONS

Gastrointestinal	Nausea, vomiting, constipation
Central nervous system and neuromuscular	Nervousness, visual hallucinations, listlessness, depression
Hypersensitivity	Skin rash
Other	Dry mouth, dysuria, blurred vision

[1]Contains 9.0 mg sodium chloride/ml

Table continued on following page

COGENTIN continued

OVERDOSAGE

Signs and symptoms	CNS depression, preceded or followed by stimulation; confusion; nervousness; listlessness; intensification of mental symptoms; toxic psychoses; visual hallucinations; dizziness; muscle weakness; ataxia; dry mouth; mydriasis; blurred vision; palpitations; nausea; vomiting; dysuria; numbness of fingers; dysphagia; allergic reactions, including skin rash, headache; hot, dry, flushed skin; delirium; coma; shock; convulsions; respiratory arrest; anhidrosis; hyperthermia; glaucoma; constipation
Treatment	Generally symptomatic and supportive. Empty stomach by emesis or gastric lavage, except in precomatose, convulsive, or psychotic states. Maintain respiration. For anticholinergic intoxication, give 1–2 mg physostigmine SC or IV; repeat after 2 h, if needed. CNS excitement may be treated with a short-acting barbiturate. Do not use convulsant stimulants for depression. Treat mydriasis and cycloplegia with a local miotic. Use icebags or other cold applications and alcohol sponges for hyperpyrexia. Vasopressors and fluids may be required for circulatory collapse. Darken room for photophobia.

DRUG INTERACTIONS

Alcohol and other CNS depressants	⇧ Sedative effects
Amantadine, antihistamines, antimuscarinics, haloperidol, MAO inhibitors, tricyclic antidepressants, procainamide, quinidine	⇧ Atropine-like effects
Antacids, antidiarrheals	⇧ Absorption of benztropine (allow 1–2 h between doses of different medications)

ALTERED LABORATORY VALUES

No clinically significant alterations in blood/serum or urinary values occur at therapeutic dosages

Use in children

Contraindicated for use in children under 3 yr of age; use with caution in older children. General guidelines not established for child dosages.

Use in pregnancy or nursing mothers

Safe use not established during pregnancy; general guidelines not established for use in nursing mothers

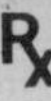

KEMADRIN (Procyclidine hydrochloride) Burroughs Wellcome

Tabs: 2, 5 mg

INDICATIONS	ORAL DOSAGE
Mild to moderate postencephalitic, arteriosclerotic, and idiopathic parkinsonism **Severe parkinsonism** (adjunctive therapy)	**Adult:** 2–2.5 mg tid after meals to start, followed by a gradual increase in dosage to 4–5 mg tid, and, if needed, 4–5 mg at bedtime
Drug-induced extrapyramidal disorders, including sialorrhea due to neuroleptic medication	**Adult:** 2–2.5 mg tid to start, followed by increases of 2–2.5 mg/day until symptoms are relieved; usual dosage range: 10–20 mg/day

ADMINISTRATION/DOSAGE ADJUSTMENTS

Bedtime dose	If dose is not well tolerated, divide total daily requirement into 3 equal daytime doses
Patients receiving other antiparkinsonism agents	Gradually substitute 2–2.5 mg procyclidine tid for all or part of original drug until optimum combination dosage or replacement with procyclidine is achieved
Elderly or arteriosclerotic patients	Lower dosage may be required
Atropine-like effects, mydriasis	May be minimized by careful dosage adjustment

CONTRAINDICATIONS

Narrow-angle glaucoma

WARNINGS/PRECAUTIONS

Special-risk patients	Use with caution in patients with hypotension or conditions in which inhibition of parasympathetic nervous system is undesirable, such as tachycardia or urinary retention
Mental confusion, disorientation	May occur, particularly in the elderly, with development of agitation, hallucinations, and psychotic-like symptoms
Psychotic episodes	May be precipitated in patients with mental disorders when dosage is increased in the treatment of drug-induced extrapyramidal disorders

ADVERSE REACTIONS

Central nervous system	Giddiness, lightheadedness
Gastrointestinal	Nausea, vomiting, epigastric distress, constipation, dry mouth, acute suppurative parotitis
Allergic	Skin rash
Musculoskeletal	Muscular weakness
Ophthalmic	Blurred vision, mydriasis

OVERDOSAGE

Signs and symptoms	May range from CNS stimulation (confusion, excitement, hyperpyrexia, agitation, disorientation, delirium, hallucinations) to depression (drowsiness, sedation, coma)
Treatment	Treat symptomatically and employ supportive measures, as needed. If patient is neither precomatose nor convulsive, empty stomach by emesis or gastric lavage. Support respiration with artificial respiration or mechanical assistance, if needed. For CNS excitation, administer a short-acting barbiturate *carefully,* since excitation may precede depression. Treat circulatory collapse with vasopressors. Control hyperthermia with tepid bathing.

DRUG INTERACTIONS

Alcohol and other CNS depressants	⇧ Sedative effect
Antihistamines, antimuscarinics, haloperidol, MAO inhibitors, tricyclic antidepressants, phenothiazines, procainamide, quinidine, amantadine	⇧ Atropine-like effects
Antacids, antidiarrheals	⇧ Absorption of procyclidine (allow 1–2 h between doses of different medications)

Table continued on following page

KEMADRIN continued

ALTERED LABORATORY VALUES

No clinically significant alterations in blood/serum or urinary values occur at therapeutic dosages

Use in children

Safety and efficacy not established

Use in pregnancy or nursing mothers

Safe use not established

LARODOPA (Levodopa) Roche

Tabs: 100, 250, 500 mg **Caps:** 100, 250, 500 mg

INDICATIONS	ORAL DOSAGE
Idiopathic Parkinson's disease (paralysis agitans) **Postencephalitic parkinsonism** **Symptomatic parkinsonism** due to carbon monoxide or manganese intoxication **Parkinsonism** in the elderly associated with cerebral arteriosclerosis	**Adult:** 0.5–1 g/day in 2 or more divided doses, with food, to start, followed by increases of up to 0.75 g/day, as tolerated, every 3–7 days, up to a total of 8 g/day, until desired therapeutic response is achieved. An exceptional patient may require higher doses; administer doses exceeding 8 g/day with caution.

ADMINISTRATION/DOSAGE ADJUSMENTS

Duration of therapy	Up to 6 mo of treatment may be required in some patients to obtain a significant therapeutic response; during prolonged therapy, perform periodic evaluations of hepatic, hematopoietic, cardiovascular, and renal function
Concomitant use with general anesthetics	Levodopa may be continued as long as the patient is able to take fluids and medication by mouth; if therapy is interrupted, give the usual daily dose as soon as the patient is able to take oral medication
Reinstitution of therapy after prolonged interruptions	Adjust dosage gradually, although in many cases the dosage can be rapidly titrated to the previous therapeutic level

CONTRAINDICATIONS

Hypersensitivity to levodopa ●	Suspicious, undiagnosed skin lesions or history of melanoma ●	Concomitant or recent use of MAO inhibitors ●
Narrow-angle glaucoma ●		

WARNINGS/PRECAUTIONS

Special-risk patients	Use with caution in patients with severe cardiovascular or pulmonary disease, bronchial asthma, or renal, hepatic, or endocrine disease
Postural hypotension	May occur; use with caution in patients receiving antihypertensive agents. Dosage adjustment of antihypertensive agents may be necessary.
MAO inhibitor therapy	Wait at least 14 days after discontinuing MAO inhibitors before initiating levodopa therapy
History of myocardial infarction with residual arrhythmias	If levodopa is essential, administer with caution in a facility with a coronary or intensive care unit
Gastrointestinal hemorrhage	May occur in patients with a history of active peptic ulcer disease
Depression with suicidal tendencies	May develop; observe patient carefully. Administer with caution to psychotics.
Patients with chronic wide-angle glaucoma	Use with caution, provided intraocular pressure is well controlled; observe for changes in intraocular pressure
Leukopenia	May occur, requiring at least temporary cessation of therapy

ADVERSE REACTIONS

Frequent reactions are italicized

Musculoskeletal	*Adventitious movements (eg, choreiform movements, dystonia), ataxia, increased hand tremor,* muscle twitching, blepharospasm, trismus
Cardiovascular	Orthostatic hypotension, cardiac irregularities, palpitations; rarely, hypertension and phlebitis
Central nervous system	*Headache, dizziness, numbness, weakness, faintness, bruxism, confusion, insomnia, nightmares, hallucinations, delusions, agitation, anxiety, malaise, fatigue, euphoria,* mental changes (eg, paranoid ideation and psychotic episodes), bradykinetic episodes, depression with or without suicidal tendencies, dementia; rarely, sense of stimulation and convulsions (causal relationship not established)
Gastrointestinal	*Anorexia, nausea, and vomiting with or without abdominal pain and distress; dry mouth, dysphagia, sialorrhea,* diarrhea, constipation, flatulence; rarely, hiccoughs, bleeding, and duodenal ulcer
Hematological	Reduced WBC count, hemoglobin, and hematocrit, leukopenia; rarely, hemolytic anemia and agranulocytosis
Dermatological	Rash, flushing; rarely, alopecia
Respiratory	Bizarre breathing patterns

Table continued on following page

LARODOPA continued

ADVERSE REACTIONS continued

Genitourinary	Urinary retention, urinary incontinence, dark urine; rarely, priapism
Ophthalmic	Diplopia, blurred vision, dilated pupils; rarely, oculogyric crises and activation of latent Horner's syndrome
Other	Burning sensation of the tongue, bitter taste, diaphoresis, hot flashes, weight gain or loss, dark sweat; rarely, edema and hoarseness

OVERDOSAGE

Signs and symptoms	See ADVERSE REACTIONS
Treatment	Empty stomach immediately by gastric lavage. Institute general supportive measures, as indicated, maintain adequate airway, and administer IV fluids. Institute ECG monitoring and observe patient carefully for possible arrhythmias; give appropriate antiarrhythmic agents, if required. Value of pyridoxine hydrochloride (vitamin B_6) in reversing the antiparkinsonism effects of levodopa has not been established. Value of dialysis is unknown. Consider the possibility of multiple-drug ingestion.

DRUG INTERACTIONS

Pyridoxine hydrochloride (vitamin B_6)	Antagonism of levodopa
Antihypertensive agents	⇧ Hypotensive effect
Methyldopa	⇩ Antiparkinsonism effect ⇧ Hypotensive effect
Butyrophenones (haloperidol), papaverine, phenothiazines, phenytoin, reserpine	⇩ Antiparkinsonism effect
MAO inhibitors	⇧ Risk of hypertensive crisis
Sympathomimetics	⇧ Risk of cardiac arrhythmias

ALTERED LABORATORY VALUES

Blood/serum levels	⇧ BUN ⇧ SGOT ⇧ SGPT ⇧ Lactic dehydrogenase ⇧ Bilirubin ⇧ Alkaline phosphatase ⇧ PBI + Coombs' test (with prolonged therapy)
Urinary values	⇧ Uric acid (with colorimetric method)

Use in children

Safe use not established in children under 12 yr of age

Use in pregnancy or nursing mothers

Safe use not established during pregnancy, or in women who may become pregnant; levodopa adversely affects fetal and postnatal growth and viability in rodents. Do not use in nursing mothers.

Note: Levodopa also marketed as **DOPAR** (Norwich-Eaton).

SINEMET (Carbidopa and levodopa) **Merck Sharp & Dohme**

Tabs: 10 mg carbidopa and 100 mg levodopa (10/100); 25 mg carbidopa and 100 mg levodopa (25/100); 25 mg carbidopa and 250 mg levodopa (25/250)

INDICATIONS	ORAL DOSAGE
Idiopathic Parkinson's disease (paralysis agitans) **Postencephalitic parkinsonism** **Symptomatic parkinsonism** due to carbon monoxide or manganese intoxication	**Adult:** one 10/100 tab or one 25/100 tab tid, followed by increases of 1 tab qd or every other day, up to 6 tabs/day; if more levodopa is required, substitute one 25/250 tab tid or qid, followed by increases of ½–1 tab/day or ½–1 tab every other day, up to 8 tabs/day, or 6 tabs/day with supplemental levodopa

ADMINISTRATION/DOSAGE ADJUSTMENTS	
Patients receiving levodopa	Discontinue levodopa before initiating therapy. Initiate therapy with a morning dose after a night (at least 8 h) when patient has not received levodopa. Suggested dose is one 25/250 tab tid or qid, or, in patients who required less than 1,500 mg levodopa/day, one 10/100 or 25/100 tab tid or qid, or a daily dose providing 25% of the previous daily levodopa dose. Adjust dosage by omitting or adding ½–1 tab/day.
Combination therapy	May be used with other antiparkinsonism agents; adjust dosages accordingly
Nausea and vomiting	Substitute one 25/100 tab for one 10/100 tab if these reactions occur with low daily dosages of the 10/100 tabs

CONTRAINDICATIONS	
Hypersensitivity to carbidopa or levodopa	
Narrow-angle glaucoma	
Suspicious, undiagnosed skin lesions or history of melanoma	
Concomitant MAO-inhibitor therapy	Discontinue MAO inhibitors at least 14 days prior to therapy

WARNINGS/PRECAUTIONS	
Depression with suicidal tendencies	May develop; observe patient carefully
Dyskinesias	May occur at lower dosages than with levodopa alone; adjust dosage accordingly. Blepharospasm is an early sign of excess dosage.
Special-risk patients	Use with caution in patients with recurrent or past psychoses, severe cardiovascular or pulmonary disease, bronchial asthma, or renal, hepatic, or endocrine disease
History of myocardial infarction with residual arrhythmias	Monitor cardiac function during initial dosage adjustment in a facility with provisions for intensive cardiac care
Gastrointestinal hemorrhage	May occur in patients with a history of peptic ulcer
Prolonged therapy	Monitor hepatic, hematopoietic, cardiovascular, and renal function periodically
Chronic wide-angle glaucoma	Use with caution, provided intraocular pressure is well controlled; observe for changes in intraocular pressure

ADVERSE REACTIONS[1]	Frequent reactions are italicized
Musculoskeletal	*Choreiform, dystonic, and other involuntary movements;* ataxia; increased hand tremor; muscle twitching; blepharospasm; trismus
Central nervous system	Mental changes (eg, paranoid ideation and psychotic episodes), bradykinetic episodes, depression with or without suicidal tendencies, dementia, dizziness, headache, numbness, weakness, faintness, confusion, bruxism, insomnia, nightmares, hallucinations, delusions, agitation, anxiety, malaise, fatigue, euphoria, sense of stimulation; convulsions (causal relationship not established)
Gastrointestinal	*Nausea,* anorexia, vomiting, abdominal pain and distress, dry mouth, dysphagia, hiccoughs, sialorrhea, diarrhea, constipation, flatulence; rarely, bleeding and duodenal ulcer
Cardiovascular	Cardiac irregularities and/or palpitations, orthostatic hypotension; rarely, hypertension and phlebitis
Hematological	Hemolytic anemia, leukopenia, and agranulocytosis (rare)
Dermatological	Flushing, rash, alopecia
Respiratory	Bizarre breathing patterns

[1]Includes reactions reported with levodopa alone

Table continued on following page

SINEMET continued

ADVERSE REACTIONS continued

Genitourinary	Urinary retention, urinary incontinence, dark urine, priapism
Ophthalmic	Diplopia, blurred vision, mydriasis, oculogyric crises, activation of latent Horner's syndrome
Other	Burning sensation of the tongue, bitter taste, diaphoresis, hot flashes, weight gain or loss, dark sweat, edema, hoarseness

OVERDOSAGE

Signs and symptoms	See ADVERSE REACTIONS
Treatment	Empty stomach immediately by gastric lavage. Institute general supportive measures, as indicated, maintain adequate airway, and administer IV fluids. Institute ECG monitoring and observe patient carefully for possible arrhythmias; give appropriate antiarrhythmic agents, if required. Value of pyridoxine hydrochloride (vitamin B_6) in reversing the antiparkinsonism effects of levodopa has not been established. Value of dialysis in unknown. Consider the possibility of multiple-drug ingestion.

DRUG INTERACTIONS

Pyridoxine hydrochloride (vitamin B_6)	Antagonism of levodopa
Antihypertensive agents	⇧ Hypotensive effect
Methyldopa	⇩ Antiparkinsonism effect ⇧ Hypotensive effect
Butyrophenones (haloperidol), papaverine, phenothiazines, phenytoin, reserpine	⇩ Antiparkinsonism effect
MAO inhibitors	⇧ Risk of hypertensive crisis
Sympathomimetics	⇧ Risk of cardiac arrhythmias

ALTERED LABORATORY VALUES

Blood/serum values	⇧ BUN ⇧ SGOT ⇧ SGPT ⇧ Lactic dehydrogenase ⇧ Bilirubin ⇧ Alkaline phosphatase ⇧ PBI + Coombs' test
Urinary values	⇧ Uric acid (with colorimetric method)

Use in children

Safe use not established in children <18 yr of age

Use in pregnancy or nursing mothers

Safe use not established during pregnancy; levodopa, alone and in combination with carbidopa, has caused skeletal and visceral malformations in rabbits. Contraindicated in nursing mothers.

SYMMETREL (Amantadine hydrochloride) Endo

Caps: 100 mg **Syrup:** 50 mg/5 ml

INDICATIONS	ORAL DOSAGE
Idiopathic and postencephalitic parkinsonism **Symptomatic parkinsonism** due to carbon monoxide intoxication **Parkinsonism** associated with cerebral arteriosclerosis in the elderly	**Adult:** 100 mg bid; increase, if necessary, up to 400 mg/day div
Drug-induced extrapyramidal reactions	**Adult:** 100 mg bid; increase, if necessary, up to 300 mg/day div
Prophylaxis and symptomatic treatment of **respiratory-tract illness** caused by influenza A virus strains	**Adult:** 200 mg/day in a single dose or 2 divided doses **Child (1–9 yr):** 2–4 mg/lb/day in 2–3 equal doses, up to 150 mg/day **Child (9–12 yr):** same as adult

ADMINISTRATION/DOSAGE ADJUSTMENTS	
Concomitant therapy	Reduce dosage of amantadine hydrochloride or concomitant anticholinergics if atropine-like effects occur. Use cautiously with CNS stimulants.
Combination therapy with levodopa	When adding levodopa, maintain constant amantadine dosage of 100 mg qd or bid, while gradually increasing levodopa dosage to optimal level
Prolonged therapy	Effectiveness may decrease after several months; increase dosage to 300 mg/day or temporarily discontinue therapy for several weeks
Seriously ill patients or those receiving other antiparkinsonism agents in high doses	Initiate therapy with 100 mg/day, followed by 100 mg bid, if necessary
CNS disturbances	May be alleviated by twice-daily administration
Duration of therapy for influenza A virus respiratory illness	For prophylaxis, continue treatment at least 10 days following known exposure. When used chemoprophylactically with inactivated influenza A virus vaccine, administer for 2–3 wk after vaccine has been given. When vaccine is unavailable or contraindicated, administer amantadine up to 90 days. Symptomatic treatment should be started as soon as possible after onset of symptoms and continued for 24–48 h after symptoms disappear.

CONTRAINDICATIONS

Hypersensitivity to amantadine

WARNINGS/PRECAUTIONS	
Seizures	May be precipitated in susceptible individuals
Congestive heart failure	May occur; use with caution and adjust dosage carefully in patients with history of congestive heart failure or peripheral edema
Mental impairment, reflex-slowing, or blurred vision	Performance of potentially hazardous tasks may be impaired; caution patients accordingly
Abrupt discontinuation of therapy	May precipitate parkinsonian crisis in patients with Parkinson's disease
Special-risk patients	Adjust dosage carefully in patients with renal impairment or orthostatic hypotension; use with caution in patients with hepatic disease, history of recurrent eczematoid rash, or with psychosis or severe psychoneurosis not controlled by chemotherapeutic agents
Renal impairment	Use with caution and monitor for signs of excessive drug accumulation

ADVERSE REACTIONS	Frequent reactions are italicized
Central nervous system	*Depression, psychosis,* hallucinations, confusion, anxiety, irritability, dizziness, lightheadedness, headache, fatigue, insomnia, weakness, slurred speech, ataxia, convulsions (rare)
Cardiovascular	*Congestive heart failure, orthostatic hypotension,* peripheral edema
Hematological	Leukopenia (rare), neutropenia (rare)
Gastrointestinal	Anorexia, nausea, constipation, vomiting, dry mouth
Dermatological	Skin rash, livedo reticularis; eczematoid dermatitis (rare)
Ophthalmic	Visual disturbances; oculogyric episodes (rare)
Other	Urinary retention, dyspnea

Table continued on following page

SYMMETREL continued

OVERDOSAGE

Signs and symptoms	Hyperactivity, convulsions, arrhythmias, hypotension
Treatment	Empty stomach by gastric lavage or emesis and institute supportive measures, including forced or IV fluids, if necessary. Acidification of urine may speed elimination of drug. Monitor vital signs, serum electrolytes, urine pH, and urinary output. Catheterization should be done if no record of recent voiding exists. Employ appropriate anticonvulsant, antiarrhythmic, or antihypotensive therapy.

DRUG INTERACTIONS

Anticholinergic agents	⇧ Atropine-like effects

ALTERED LABORATORY VALUES

No clinically significant alterations in blood/serum or urinary values occur at therapeutic dosages

Use in children

See INDICATIONS

Use in pregnancy or nursing mothers

Safe use during pregnancy not established. Embryotoxicity and teratogenicity have been observed in rats given exceedingly high doses. Do not use in nursing mothers.

MESTINON (Pyridostigmine bromide) Roche

Tabs: 60 mg **Tabs (sust rel):** 180 mg **Syrup:** 60 mg/5 ml[1] **Amps:** 5 mg/ml (2 ml)

INDICATIONS	ORAL DOSAGE	PARENTERAL DOSAGE
Symptomatic control of **myasthenia gravis**	**Adult:** 600 mg or 50 ml (10 tsp)/day, spaced to provide maximum relief; for mild cases, 60–360 mg or 5–30 ml (1–6 tsp)/day; for severe cases, up to 1,500 mg or 125 ml (25 tsp) per day; sust-rel tabs: 180–540 mg qd or bid at intervals ≥6 h **Child:** 7 mg/kg/day in 5–6 divided doses	**Adult:** 2–50 mg IM or IV (slowly) (see ADMINISTRATION/DOSAGE ADJUSTMENTS)
Transient difficulty in breathing, swallowing, and sucking in neonates of myasthenic mothers	**Neonate:** 5 mg q4–6h until symptoms are controlled, followed by gradual reduction in dosage until drug is completely withdrawn	**Neonate:** 0.05–0.15 mg/kg IM q4–6h until syrup may be taken
Antagonism of nondepolarizing muscle relaxants	—	**Adult:** 10–20 mg IV (see WARNINGS/PRECAUTIONS)

ADMINISTRATION/DOSAGE ADJUSTMENTS

Optimum control of myasthenia gravis	May require concomitant use of regular tablets or syrup and sustained-released tablets
Parenteral administration for myasthenia gravis	Indicated to supplement oral dosage, pre- and postoperatively, during myasthenic crisis, or whenever oral therapy is impractical
Antagonism of nondepolarizing muscle relaxants	Provide respiratory assistance until adequate recovery of voluntary respiration and neuromuscular transmission is obtained

CONTRAINDICATIONS

Hypersensitivity to anticholinesterase agents ●	Mechanical intestinal and urinary obstructions ●

WARNINGS/PRECAUTIONS

Excessive secretions and bradycardia	May result from large IV doses of pyridostigmine, as during antagonism of nondepolarizing muscle relaxants; to minimize these effects, give 0.6–1.2 mg atropine sulfate IV immediately before pyridostigmine
Delayed antagonism (>30 min) of nondepolarizing muscle relaxants	May occur in the presence of extreme debilitation or carcinomatosis, or with concomitant use of certain broad-spectrum antibiotics or anesthetic agents, notably ether; support ventilation until the patient resumes adequate voluntary respiration as evidenced by respiratory measurements and use of a peripheral nerve stimulator device
Extreme muscle weakness	May occur and indicate either cholinergic crisis due to overdosage or myasthenic crisis due to increasing severity of the disease; differentiate between the two types of crisis by edrophonium chloride, as well as by clinical judgment, since the treatments of the two conditions differ radically. For myasthenic crisis, provide more intensive anticholinesterase therapy. For cholinergic crisis, administer atropine sulfate (see OVERDOSAGE).
Hypersensitivity reactions	May occur, especially with parenteral use. Keep atropine and antishock medication readily available.
Gastrointestinal disturbances and other muscarinic reactions	May occur (see ADVERSE REACTIONS); relieve with atropine
Use of atropine sulfate	May mask signs of overdosage, and inadvertently lead to cholinergic crisis
Special-risk patients	Use with caution in patients with bronchial asthma or cardiac dysrhythmias
Skin rash	May occur; discontinue use

ADVERSE REACTIONS

Muscarinic	Nausea, vomiting, diarrhea, abdominal cramps, increased peristalsis, increased salivation, increased bronchial secretions, diaphoresis, miosis
Nicotinic	Muscle cramps, weakness, fasciculation
Other	Skin rash, thrombophlebitis (with IV use)

[1]Contains 5% alcohol

Table continued on following page

MESTINON continued

OVERDOSAGE

Signs and symptoms	Cholinergic crisis, characterized by nausea, vomiting, diarrhea, excessive salivation and sweating, increased bronchial secretions, miosis, lacrimation, bradycardia or tachycardia, cardiospasm, bronchospasm, hypotension, incoordination, blurred vision, muscle cramps, weakness, fasciculation, paralysis, respiratory paralysis and pulmonary edema, cardiac arrest, death
Treatment	Immediately discontinue use of pyridostigmine. Maintain adequate respiration. Give 1-4 mg atropine sulfate IV; repeat every 5-30 min, as needed, to control muscarinic symptoms. Respiratory paralysis is not alleviated by atropine.

DRUG INTERACTIONS

Depolarizing muscle relaxants (eg, succinylcholine, decamethonium)	⇧ Phase I block
Nondepolarizing muscle relaxants (eg, tubocurarine, metocurine, gallamine, pancuronium)	Antagonism of nondepolarizing muscle-relaxant effect
Atropine sulfate	⇩ Muscarinic effect

ALTERED LABORATORY VALUES

No clinically significant alterations in blood/serum or urinary values occur at therapeutic dosages

Use in children

See INDICATIONS

Use in pregnancy or nursing mothers

Safe use not established

PROSTIGMIN (Neostigmine methylsulfate) Roche

Tabs: 15 mg **Amps:** 0.25 mg/ml (1:4,000), 0.5 mg/ml (1:2,000) **Vial:** 5 mg/10 ml (1:2,000), 10 mg/10 ml (1:1,000)

INDICATIONS	ORAL DOSAGE	PARENTERAL DOSAGE
Symptomatic control of **myasthenia gravis** where no difficulty in swallowing is present	**Adult:** 15–375 mg/24 h div, as needed; usual dosage: 150 mg/24 h div, as needed	—
Acute myasthenic crisis with breathing and swallowing difficulty	—	**Adult:** 0.5 mg (1 ml of 1:2,000 sol) SC or IM; adjust subsequent doses according to patient response, switching to oral therapy as soon as possible
Prevention of postoperative distention and **urinary retention**	—	**Adult:** 0.25 mg (1 ml of 1:4,000 sol) SC or IM immediately after operation, repeated q4–6h for 2–3 days
Postoperative distention	—	**Adult:** 0.5 mg (1 ml of 1:2,000 sol) SC or IM, as needed
Postoperative urinary retention	—	**Adult:** 0.5 mg (1 ml of 1:2,000 sol) SC or IM; repeat after bladder has been emptied q3h for at least 5 injections
Delayed menstruation	—	**Adult:** 1 mg (1 ml of 1:1,000 sol)/day IM for 3 days
Antagonism of tubocurarine	—	**Adult:** 0.5–2 mg IV (slowly), repeated as needed, up to a total of 5 mg in exceptional cases

ADMINISTRATION/DOSAGE ADJUSTMENTS

Screening test for early pregnancy	Inject 1 mg (1 ml of 1:1,000 solution)/day IM for 3 days; if bleeding does not occur within 72 h of last injection, pregnancy may be assumed, providing pelvic lesions, systemic disease, menopause, and endocrine disorders have been ruled out
Antagonism of tubocurarine	Administer neostigmine while patient is being hyperventilated and carbon dioxide level is low. Do not give if high concentrations of halothane or cyclopropane are present. In small children, severely ill patients, or cardiac cases, titrate exact dosage, using peripheral nerve stimulator device. In the presence of bradycardia, increase pulse rate to 80/min with atropine before giving neostigmine. Provide respiratory assistance and closely observe the patient until adequate recovery of normal respiration is assured.
Oral regimen	Dosing intervals must be individualized for each patient. Therapy may be required day and night; larger portions may be useful during times of greatest fatigue.

CONTRAINDICATIONS

Hypersensitivity to neostigmine methylsulfate ●	Mechanical intestinal or urinary obstruction ●	Urinary tract infection (with oral form) ●
Hypersensitivity to bromides (with oral form) ●		

WARNINGS/PRECAUTIONS

Hypersensitivity reactions	May occur, especially with parenteral use; keep atropine sulfate and antishock medication readily available
Extreme muscle weakness	May occur and indicate either cholinergic crisis due to overdosage or myasthenic crisis due to increasing severity of the disease; differentiate between the two types of crisis by edrophonium chloride, as well as by clinical judgment, since the treatments of the two conditions differ radically. For myasthenic crisis, provide more intensive anticholinesterase therapy. For cholinergic crisis, administer atropine sulfate (see OVERDOSAGE).
Gastrointestinal disturbances and other muscarinic reactions	May occur (see ADVERSE REACTIONS); relieve with atropine sulfate
Use of atropine sulfate	May mask signs of overdosage, and inadvertently lead to cholinergic crisis
Use of antibiotics in the myasthenic patient	Use certain antibiotics, especially neomycin, streptomycin, and kanamycin, only where definitely indicated, as these agents have a mild but definite nondepolarizing blocking action; carefully adjust adjunctive anticholinesterase therapy
Special-risk patients	Use with caution in patients with asthma

Table continued on following page

PROSTIGMIN continued

WARNINGS/PRECAUTIONS continued

Large oral doses	Should be avoided in situations where absorption from the intestinal tract may be increased; use with caution when giving anticholinergic drugs, which may slow intestinal motility
Large parenteral doses	Should be preceded or accompanied by injection of atropine sulfate; use separate syringes

ADVERSE REACTIONS

Muscarinic	Nausea, vomiting, diarrhea, abdominal cramps, bowel cramps, increased salivation, increased bronchial secretions, diaphoresis, miosis
Nicotinic	Muscle cramps, weakness, fasciculation

OVERDOSAGE

Signs and symptoms	Cholinergic crisis, characterized by nausea, vomiting, diarrhea, excessive salivation and sweating, increased bronchial secretions, miosis, lacrimation, bradycardia or tachycardia, cardiospasm, bronchospasm, hypotension, incoordination, blurred vision, muscle cramps, weakness, fasciculation, paralysis, respiratory paralysis and pulmonary edema, cardiac arrest, death
Treatment	Immediately discontinue use of neostigmine. Maintain adequate respiration. Give 1–4 mg atropine sulfate IV; repeat every 5–30 min as needed to control muscarinic symptoms. Respiratory paralysis is not alleviated by atropine.

DRUG INTERACTIONS

Depolarizing muscle relaxants (eg, succinylcholine, decamethonium)	⇧ Phase I block
Nondepolarizing muscle relaxants (eg, tubocurarine, metocurine, gallamine, pancuronium)	Antagonism of nondepolarizing muscle-relaxant effect
Atropine sulfate	⇩ Muscarinic effect

ALTERED LABORATORY VALUES

No clinically significant alterations in blood/serum or urinary values occur at therapeutic dosages

Use in children

General guidelines not established

Use in pregnancy or nursing mothers

General guidelines not established

Seizures

During an average lifetime, one out of every ten persons can expect to experience at least one seizure, defined as a loss or alteration of consciousness, often associated with convulsive movements. Epilepsy, a condition characterized by recurring seizures, affects about 1 to 2 percent of the population, but seizures can also be due to underlying illnesses such as heart disease, low blood sugar, and drug or alcohol withdrawal. This section will concentrate on epileptic seizures and their treatment.

EPILEPSY

Classes of Epilepsy

Epilepsy, commonly referred to as "spells" or "fits," involves seizures caused by a basic defect in transmission of motor nerve impulses in the brain. In about two thirds of persons with epilepsy, the first seizure occurs before adolescence. There are many types of epileptic seizures, but only four major types are described here. Although the four categories are discussed as discrete entities, a fourth to half of all epileptics will have more than one type of seizure during their lifetime.

Petit mal Petit mal, also called absence attacks or blank spells, occurs mostly in young children. The attacks come on without warning, last a few seconds, and involve only a brief and subtle loss of consciousness. Occasionally, there is mild facial twitching or repetitive blinking. Absence attacks can occur frequently, up to one hundred each day.

Complex-partial, temporal lobe, or psychomotor These seizures are the teenage and adult counterpart of absence spells. The person loses contact with external reality for a few minutes and carries on purposeless or odd behavior, such as directionless wandering, lip-smacking, or chewing movements. A bystander may interpret this state as drunkenness or mental illness.

Both absence and complex-partial seizures may be mistaken for daydreaming or a sleep disorder. However, a person having a true seizure is not responsive to questions and cannot be "awakened."

Simple-partial or sensory motor Seizures in this category are brief disturbances of sensory perception combined with involuntary sequential contraction of muscle groups in arms and legs.

Grand mal or generalized tonic-clonic Most frightening of all seizures, grand mal attacks have two phases. They sometimes begin with a warning sensation of sinking or rising in the stomach (aura); the person's whole body then stiffens as the muscles go into spasm. Since all muscles are contracted, the person stops breathing. The seizure may be preceded by a brief cry as muscle contraction forces air out of the person's mouth. The victim may fall on the ground. After about thirty seconds of tonic

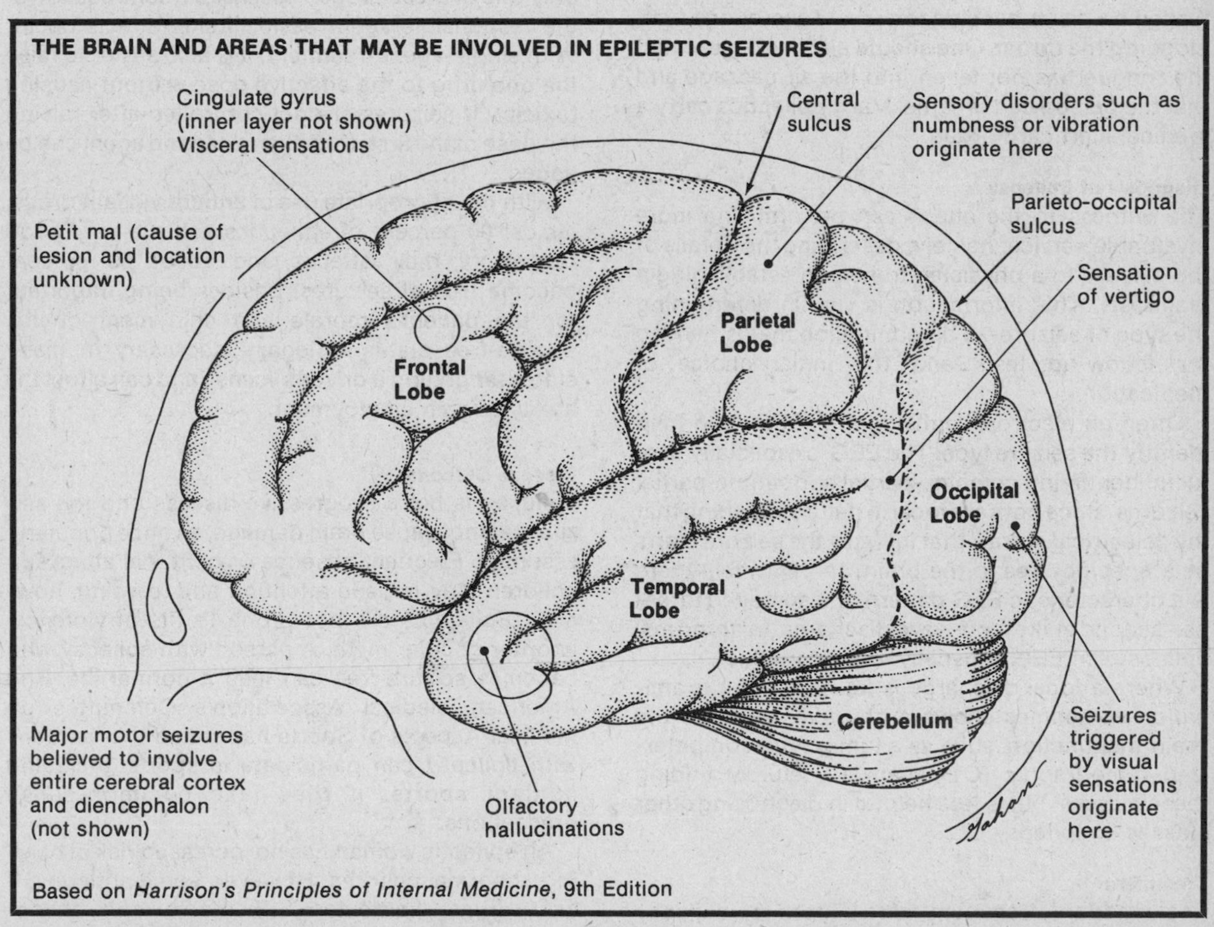

Based on *Harrison's Principles of Internal Medicine*, 9th Edition

contraction, the muscles go through a phase of rapidly alternating relaxation and contraction (clonus), which results in violent jerking, and breathing resumes irregularly. Foaming at the mouth may occur at this time. When normal consciousness returns, the person is often exhausted and may fall asleep. In some epileptics, grand mal seizures may occur infrequently, for example, once or twice a year, while others may suffer seizures once or twice each day.

A less severe form of motor seizure is bilateral massive myoclonus, in which the limbs undergo short, violent contractions. There is no loss of consciousness. This condition can progress to tonic-clonic seizures.

In those types of seizures that entail altered consciousness, the epileptic does not remember the events that occurred during the seizure. They are often preceded by the warning aura and, in some persons, they may be precipitated by lights, music, or other such stimuli, as well as alkalosis (an excess of alkali in the body, which may be caused by hyperventilation or breathing too quickly and too deeply).

First Aid

A person witnessing a seizure should take measures to keep the epileptic from injury. Furniture should be moved out of the way, clothing loosened if possible, and the person should be helped to lie down. Firm objects should not be placed in the mouth. After the tonic phase of the attack, the person should be turned on his or her side to prevent secretions from clogging the throat. One should also make sure that the tongue has not fallen into the air passage and that the person can breathe. Many epileptics carry a medical alert card or tag.

Diagnosis of Epilepsy

The witness to the attack can perform one more invaluable service; namely, describing the details of the seizure to a physician to help in establishing a diagnosis. This information is vital in determining the type of seizure—a determination that is needed for follow-up tests and the initial choice of medication.

Often an electroencephalogram (EEG) can help identify the seizure type. The EEG is especially useful in identifying complex-partial and simple-partial seizures, since both are focal in nature, meaning that the "electrical storm" that initiates the seizure starts at a specific area in the brain. In petit mal, there is a characteristic EEG pattern, the so-called three-per-second spike-and-wave discharge. In grand mal epilepsy, an EEG is usually less informative.

Where a focal discharge is found, further examination sometimes shows a physical cause for the brain malfunction, such as a tumor. The computerized tomographic (CT) scan is useful in finding these masses, but is less helpful in diagnosing other classes of epilepsy.

Treatment

The standard treatment of all types of epilepsy involves the use of anticonvulsant drugs. For the three classes of seizures known as the major triad—grand mal, complex-partial, and simple-partial—the most commonly used drugs are phenobarbital (Eskabarb and Luminal), phenytoin (Dilantin), and carbamazepine (Tegretol). Phenobarbital, the first anticonvulsant drug, was introduced in 1912 and is still considered to be very effective. Other compounds in the same chemical class as phenobarbital (barbiturates) and phenytoin (hydantoins) are sometimes useful in patients not helped by the primary drug. Another barbiturate-like drug is primidone (Mysoline).

For petit mal or absence attacks, the succinimides are the most frequently prescribed drugs, of which ethosuximide (Zarontin) is the most widely used for these patients. In 1978, the Food and Drug Administration approved valproic acid (Depakene), another anticonvulsant that is effective in controlling petit mal attacks. In refractory cases, other drugs such as trimethadione (Tridione) or clonazepam (Clonopin) may be prescribed.

Anticonvulsant drugs interact with each other and with many other medications. Phenytoin, for example, can decrease the availability of the antibiotic doxycyline, the cardiac drug digitoxin, and endogenous insulin (that manufactured by the body). Blood levels of phenytoin are decreased by antacids and alcohol.

Most experts recommend beginning therapy with only one of these drugs. This makes identification of the responsible agent easier if side effects occur. With single-agent treatment, it is also easier to raise the one drug to the effective dose without causing toxicity. If seizures are not controlled after raising the dose of the first drug, then a second agent can be added.

With the appropriate use of anticonvulsant drugs, almost 90 percent of epileptics achieve very good control of their attacks and about 50 percent become free of seizures. Besides being important for the patient's morale and enjoyment of life, seizure-free status is legally necessary in many states for getting a driver's license and can affect the ability to gain employment.

Disease Outcome

Epilepsy is not a progressive disease and the seizures do not cause brain damage, as once popularly assumed. Frequent absence or petit mal attacks in children may impede attention and learning, however. Epileptics are not prone to fits of violence, another popular myth. A person with epilepsy who becomes seizure-free can lead a normal life. The American Medical Association's Committee on Medical Aspects of Sports has stated that persons with epilepsy can participate in sports, including contact sports, if they take common-sense precautions.

An epileptic woman has no increased risk of bearing abnormal children. However, some anticonvulsant drugs, particularly phenytoin and phenobarbital, appear to increase the risk of birth defects if taken during pregnancy.

OTHER SEIZURE DISORDERS

One form of epilepsy that requires special treatment is status epilepticus, the occurrence of repeated grand mal seizures with a very brief or no interval between them. Since the patient may suffer brain damage from oxygen deprivation, immediate general anesthesia should be provided, usually with diazepam (Valium).

A particularly distressing type of non-epileptic seizure is the convulsion that can accompany high fever in children up to five years of age. In the past, some pediatricians treated children who had suffered a febrile convulsion prophylactically with phenobarbital for many years because a small fraction of them had repeated febrile seizures. At one time, it was also thought that this condition led to an increased risk of epilepsy as adults. It has now been shown that only a small fraction of children who have one seizure are prone to recurrences and that very few children with recurrent seizures go on to develop epilepsy. Because of these findings and some evidence that long-term treatment with phenobarbital may interfere with normal development, most specialists now recommend against routine prophylactic treatment of all children who have a febrile seizure. This course may still be appropriate, however, if the initial seizure lasts longer than fifteen minutes or is otherwise severe.

IN CONCLUSION

Recurrent seizures can be controlled or prevented in the large majority of patients with epilepsy through the proper use of anticonvulsant drugs. Persons who achieve seizure-free status can expect to live normal lives; others whose disease is under good control can participate in sports and other normal activities. The following charts cover the major anticonvulsant drugs prescribed to treat the various types of epilepsy.

AMYTAL SODIUM (Amobarbital sodium) Lilly

Caps: 65, 200 mg **Amps:** 125, 250, 500 mg *C-II*

INDICATIONS	ORAL DOSAGE	PARENTERAL DOSAGE
Convulsive seizures due to chorea, eclampsia, meningitis, tetanus, procaine or cocaine reactions, and strychnine or picrotoxin poisoning **Catatonic, negativistic, or manic reactions** **Epileptiform seizures**	—	**Adult:** 65–500 mg IM or IV, up to 1,000 mg/dose, as needed **Child (6–12 yr):** 65–500 mg IM or IV, as needed
Insomnia	**Adult:** 65–200 mg at bedtime	—
Preanesthetic sedation	**Adult:** 200 mg 1–2 h prior to surgery	—
Labor	**Adult:** 200–400 mg to start, followed by 200–400 mg q1–3h, if needed, up to a total of 1,000 mg	—

ADMINISTRATION/DOSAGE ADJUSTMENTS

Preparation of parenteral solutions	Dilute contents of ampul with Sterile Water for Injection; ordinarily, a 10% solution is used for IV administration and a 20% solution for IM injection
Intramuscular administration	Inject deeply into a large muscle mass, such as the gluteus maximus; to preclude irritation, give no more than 5 ml at any one site
Intravenous administration	Administer slowly (≤1 ml/min); too-rapid IV administration may result in apnea and/or hypotension

CONTRAINDICATIONS

Hypersensitivity to barbiturates ●	Manifest or latent porphyria ●	Severe hepatic impairment ●
Respiratory disease accompanied by dyspnea or obstruction ●	Previous addiction to sedative-hypnotics ●	Acute or chronic pain ●

WARNINGS/PRECAUTIONS

Hepatic impairment	Use with caution
Elderly or debilitated patients	May react with marked excitement or CNS depression; use with caution
Borderline hypoadrenal function	Effects of cortisol may be diminished; use with caution
Mental impairment, reflex-slowing	Performance of potentially hazardous tasks may be impaired; warn patient accordingly
Overdosage	Excessive doses, either alone or in combination with other CNS depressants, may cause toxic effects and death; warn patients not to exceed recommended dosage and to limit alcohol intake, and that the concomitant use of other CNS depressants can cause additional CNS depression. Use with caution in patients who have a history of emotional disturbances or suicidal ideation.
Habit-forming	Psychic and/or physical dependence and tolerance may develop, especially in addiction-prone individuals
Withdrawal symptoms	May occur after cessation of chronic use of large doses, resulting in delirium, convulsions, and death

ADVERSE REACTIONS

Central nervous system	Residual sedation (hangover), drowsiness; lethargy and headache (with oral use); idiosyncratic excitement and pain (with parenteral use)
Respiratory	Depression, apnea; laryngospasm (with parenteral use)
Cardiovascular	Circulatory collapse; vasodilation and hypotension (with rapid IV injection)
Hypersensitivity	Allergic reactions, skin eruptions
Gastrointestinal	Nausea, vomiting
Other	Postoperative atelectasis (with parenteral use)

OVERDOSAGE

Signs and symptoms	Early hypothermia followed by fever, sluggish or absent reflexes, respiratory depression, circulatory collapse, pulmonary edema, and coma
Treatment	Empty stomach by gastric lavage and institute general supportive measures, including IV fluid replacement and maintenance of blood pressure and adequate respiratory exchange. Dialysis may be helpful.

Table continued on following page

AMYTAL SODIUM continued

DRUG INTERACTIONS

Oral anticoagulants	⇩ Prothrombin time
Alcohol, tranquilizers, CNS depressants	⇧ CNS depression
Corticosteroids	⇩ Corticosteroid effects
Digitalis, digitoxin	⇩ Cardiac glycoside effects
Doxycycline	⇩ Anti-infective effect
Tricyclic antidepressants	⇩ Antidepressant effect
Griseofulvin	⇩ Griseofulvin absorption
MAO inhibitors	⇧ Antidepressant or barbiturate effects

ALTERED LABORATORY VALUES

Blood/serum values	⇩ Bilirubin

No clinically significant alterations in urinary values occur at therapeutic dosages

Use in children

Safety and efficacy not established in children under 6 yr of age

Use in pregnancy or nursing mothers

Safe use not established during pregnancy; use only when clearly indicated. Neonatal depression may occur following use during labor. Administer with caution to nursing mothers.

CELONTIN (Methsuximide) Parke-Davis

Caps: 150, 300 mg

INDICATIONS	ORAL DOSAGE
Absence (petit mal) seizures	**Adult:** 300 mg/day to start, followed by weekly increases of 300 mg/day, up to 1.2 g/day, if needed **Child:** same as adult[1]

ADMINISTRATION/DOSAGE ADJUSTMENTS

Combination therapy	May be used with other anticonvulsants when other forms of epilepsy coexist with absence (petit mal) seizures

CONTRAINDICATIONS

Hypersensitivity to succinimides

WARNINGS/PRECAUTIONS

Blood dyscrasias	May occur and may be fatal (see ADVERSE REACTIONS); obtain CBC periodically
Renal or hepatic disease	Use with caution; perform periodic urinalysis and liver-function tests in all patients taking methsuximide
Mental impairment, reflex-slowing	Performance of potentially hazardous tasks may be impaired; caution patients accordingly
Abrupt discontinuation of therapy	May precipitate absence (petit mal) status; all dosage adjustments must be gradual
Grand-mal seizures	May occur when methsuximide is used alone to treat mixed types of epilepsy
Behavioral alterations	Including unusual depression or aggressiveness may occur; withdraw drug gradually

ADVERSE REACTIONS

Frequent reactions are italicized

Gastrointestinal	*Nausea, vomiting, anorexia, diarrhea, weight loss, epigastric and abdominal pain, constipation*
Hematological	Eosinophilia, leukopenia, monocytosis, pancytopenia
Central nervous system and neuromuscular	*Drowsiness, ataxia, dizziness,* headache, irritability, nervousness, hiccoughs, insomnia, confusion, instability, mental slowness, depression, hypochondriacal behavior, aggressiveness; rarely, psychosis, suicidal behavior, and auditory hallucinations
Ophthalmic	Blurred vision, photophobia, periorbital edema
Dermatological	Urticaria; Stevens-Johnson syndrome; pruritic, erythematous rashes
Others	Hyperemia

OVERDOSAGE

Signs and symptoms	See ADVERSE REACTIONS
Treatment	Induce emesis or perform gastric lavage to empty stomach. Treat symptomatically and institute supportive measures, as required.

DRUG INTERACTIONS

Tricyclic antidepressants (high doses), antipsychotics (high doses)	Seizures

ALTERED LABORATORY VALUES

No clinically significant alterations in blood/serum or urinary values occur at therapeutic dosages

Use in children

See INDICATIONS

Use in pregnancy or nursing mothers

An increased incidence of birth defects may be associated with the use of anticonvulsants during pregnancy. However, discontinuation of therapy may be considered only if removal of the drug does not pose any serious risk, such as the precipitation of status epilepticus in patients with serious convulsive disorders. The safety of methsuximide during lactation has not been established.

[1] *United States Pharmacopeia Dispensing Information 1980.* Rockville, Md, The United States Pharmacopeial Convention, Inc, 1980

CLONOPIN (Clonazepam) Roche

Tabs: 0.5, 1, 2 mg *C-IV*

INDICATIONS	ORAL DOSAGE
Lennox-Gastaut syndrome (petit mal variant) **Akinetic and myoclonic seizures** **Absence (petit mal) seizures** in patients refractory to succinimides	**Adult:** up to 1.5 mg/day in 3 divided doses to start, followed by increases of 0.5–1.0 mg/day every 3 days until optimal clinical response is achieved, up to 20 mg/day **Infant and child (<10 yr and <30 kg):** 0.01–0.03 mg/kg/day, or up to 0.05 mg/kg/day, if necessary, in 2–3 divided doses to start, followed by increases of 0.25–0.5 mg every 3 days, up to 0.1–0.2 mg/kg/day in 3 equally divided doses, until optimal clinical response is achieved

ADMINISTRATION/DOSAGE ADJUSTMENTS

Unequally divided doses	Give largest dose before bedtime

CONTRAINDICATIONS

Hypersensitivity to benzodiazepines ●
Acute narrow-angle glaucoma ●
Significant hepatic disease ●
Open-angle glaucoma (unless patient is receiving appropriate therapy) ●

WARNINGS/PRECAUTIONS

Habit-forming	Psychic and/or physical dependence and tolerance may develop, especially in addiction-prone individuals
Mental impairment, reflex-slowing	Performance of potentially hazardous tasks may be impaired; caution patients accordingly and about additive effects of alcohol and other CNS depressants
Abrupt discontinuation of therapy	May precipitate barbiturate-like withdrawal symptoms or status epilepticus, especially with prolonged high-dose therapy; always withdraw drug gradually and, if necessary, administer another anticonvulsant concomitantly
Impaired renal function	Use with caution to avoid excessive accumulation of metabolites
Respiratory depression	May occur; use with caution in patients with chronic respiratory disease
Generalized tonic-clonic (grand mal) seizures	May be precipitated in patients with mixed-type seizures; if needed, administer additional appropriate anticonvulsants or increase anticonvulsant dosage
Increased salivation	May occur; use with caution in patients who have difficulty handling secretions
Long-term therapy	Perform a CBC and liver-function tests periodically

ADVERSE REACTIONS

Frequent reactions are italicized

Central nervous system and neuromuscular	*Drowsiness (50%), ataxia (30%), behavioral problems (25%),* aphonia, choreiform movements, coma, dysarthria, dysdiadochokinesis, headache, hemiparesis, hypotonia, slurred speech, tremor, vertigo, confusion, depression, forgetfulness, hallucinations, hysteria, increased libido, insomnia, psychosis, muscle weakness, pain
Ophthalmic	Abnormal eye movements, diplopia, "glassy-eyed" appearance, nystagmus
Respiratory	Depression, chest congestion, rhinorrhea, shortness of breath, hypersecretion in upper respiratory passages
Cardiovascular	Palpitations
Dermatological	Alopecia, hirsutism, rash, ankle and facial edema
Gastrointestinal	Anorexia or increased appetite, coated tongue, constipation, diarrhea, dry mouth, encopresis, gastritis, hepatomegaly, nausea, sore gums
Genitourinary	Dysuria, enuresis, nocturia, urinary retention
Hematological	Anemia, leukopenia, thrombocytopenia, eosinophilia
Other	Dehydration, general deterioration, lymphadenopathy, fever

OVERDOSAGE

Signs and symptoms	Somnolence, confusion, coma, diminished reflexes
Treatment	Empty stomach immediately by gastric lavage. Institute general supportive measures, including IV fluids and airway maintenance, and monitor vital signs. Treat hypotension with levarterenol or metaraminol. The value of dialysis is unknown.

Table continued on following page

CLONOPIN continued

DRUG INTERACTIONS

Valproic acid	Absence (petit mal) status
Alcohol, narcotic analgesics, barbiturates, sedative-hypnotics, anxiolytics, phenothiazine, thioxanthene and butyrophenone antipsychotics, MAO inhibitors, tricyclic antidepressants, other anticonvulsants	⇧ CNS depression

ALTERED LABORATORY VALUES

Blood/serum values	⇧ SGOT ⇧ SGPT ⇧ Alkaline phosphatase

No clinically significant alterations in urinary values occur at therapeutic dosages

Use in children

See INDICATIONS. Effects of long-term use are unknown; use for prolonged periods only if expected benefit outweighs risks

Use in pregnancy or nursing mothers

An increased incidence of birth defects may be associated with the use of anticonvulsants during pregnancy. However, discontinuation of therapy may be considered only if removal of the drug does not pose any serious risk, such as the precipitation of status epilepticus with hypoxia in patients with serious convulsive disorders. Patient should stop nursing if drug is essential.

DEPAKENE (Valproic acid) Abbott

Caps: 250 mg **Syrup:** 50 mg/ml

INDICATIONS	ORAL DOSAGE
Simple and complex absence seizures, including petit mal **Multiple seizure types** which include absence seizures (adjunctive therapy)	**Adult:** 15 mg/kg/day to start, followed by weekly increases of 5–10 mg/kg/day until optimal clinical response is achieved, up to 60 mg/kg/day; doses above 250 mg/day should be divided **Child:** same as adult

ADMINISTRATION/DOSAGE ADJUSTMENTS

Gastrointestinal irritation	May be avoided by administering drug with meals or by initiating therapy gradually
Combination therapy	Serum levels of phenytoin and phenobarbital may be affected by valproic acid (see DRUG INTERACTIONS); periodic serum determinations are recommended

CONTRAINDICATIONS

Hypersensitivity to valproic acid

WARNINGS/PRECAUTIONS

Hepatic failure	May occur, usually within first 6 mo of therapy, and may be fatal. Use with caution in patients with preexisting hepatic disease. In all patients, monitor liver function prior to initiating therapy and at frequent intervals thereafter; discontinue use of the drug in the presence of suspected or apparent significant hepatic dysfunction.
Thrombocytopenia, platelet aggregation dysfunction	May occur; perform platelet counts and bleeding-time determinations before initiating therapy and at periodic intervals thereafter, especially prior to planned surgery. Reduce dosage or withdraw drug pending investigation if hemorrhage, bruising, or a hemostasis/coagulation disorder develops.
Mental impairment, reflex-slowing	Performance of potentially hazardous tasks may be impaired; caution patients accordingly

ADVERSE REACTIONS

	Frequent reactions are italicized
Gastrointestinal	*Nausea, vomiting, indigestion,* diarrhea, abdominal cramps, constipation, anorexia with weight loss, increased appetite with weight gain
Central nervous system and neuromuscular	Sedation (usually with combination therapy), emotional upset, depression, psychosis, aggression, hyperactivity, behavioral deterioration; rarely, ataxia, headache, asterixis, tremor, dysarthria, dizziness, incoordination, weakness, coma (in patients also receiving phenobarbital)
Dermatological	Alopecia, rash, and petechiae (rare)
Ophthalmic	Nystagmus, diplopia, "spots before eyes" (rare)
Hematological	Thrombocytopenia, inhibition of platelet aggregation, lymphocytosis, hypofibrinogenemia, leukopenia, eosinophilia, bruising, hematoma formation, frank hemorrhage
Other	Severe hepatotoxicity

OVERDOSAGE

Signs and symptoms	Deep coma, diffuse EEG slowing[1]
Treatment	Employ general supportive measures. Maintain adequate urinary output. Gastric lavage is of limited value since drug is rapidly absorbed.

DRUG INTERACTIONS

Alcohol, CNS depressants	⇧ CNS depression
Phenobarbital, barbiturates	⇧ Risk of neurotoxicity
Primidone	⇧ Serum levels of barbiturate metabolite of primidone
Phenytoin	⇧ Serum phenytoin levels (possible)
Clonazepam	Absence (petit mal) status
Aspirin, warfarin, dipyridamole, sulfinpyrazone	⇧ Bleeding time

[1]Single reported case of valproic acid overdosage in combination with phenobarbital and phenytoin *Table continued on following page*

DEPAKENE continued

ALTERED LABORATORY VALUES

Blood/serum values	⇧ Alkaline phosphatase ⇧ SGOT ⇧ SGPT ⇧ Lactate dehydrogenase
Urinary values	False-positive ketone tests

Use in children

See INDICATIONS

Use in pregnancy or nursing mothers

Increased incidence of birth defects may be associated with the use of anticonvulsants during pregnancy. Teratogenicity, including skeletal and soft-tissue abnormalities, fetal resorptions, delayed parturition, and adversely affected postnatal growth and survival have been observed in animal studies. However, discontinuation of therapy may be considered only if removal of the drug does not pose any serious risk, such as the precipitation of status epilepticus with hypoxia in patients with serious convulsive disorders. Valproic acid is excreted in breast milk; patient should stop nursing if drug is prescribed.

DILANTIN (Phenytoin) Parke-Davis

Tabs: 50 mg **Susp:** 30 mg/5 ml (Dilantin-30 Pediatric Suspension), 125 mg/5 ml (Dilantin-125 Suspension)

DILANTIN (Phenytoin sodium) Parke-Davis

Caps: 30, 100 mg **Powder:** 1 oz

INDICATIONS	ORAL DOSAGE
Grand mal and psychomotor seizures	**Adult:** 100 mg tid to start, followed by up to 600 mg/day; usual maintenance dosage: 100 mg tid or qid **Child:** 5 mg/kg/day in 2–3 equally divided doses, followed by up to 300 mg/day; usual maintenance dosage: 4–8 mg/kg/day

ADMINISTRATION/DOSAGE ADJUSTMENTS	
Timing of administration	Gastrointestinal disturbances may be alleviated by giving drug with or immediately after meals
Serum level monitoring	May be useful for optimal dosage adjustments; therapeutic range of 10–20 μg/ml should be achieved in 7–10 days
Alternative regimen for adults	If seizures can be controlled with 100 mg tid, frequency of adminstration may be reduced by giving 300 mg qd
Combination therapy	Combination anticonvulsant therapy is indicated if both petit mal and grand mal seizures are present
Dosage adjustment or drug withdrawal	Must be gradual

CONTRAINDICATIONS

Hypersensitivity to hydantoins

WARNINGS/PRECAUTIONS	
Unwarranted uses	Do not use for seizures due to hypoglycemia or other identifiable and correctable causes
Abrupt discontinuation of therapy	May precipitate status epilepticus; if abrupt withdrawal is required (eg, due to an allergic or hypersensitivity reaction), substitute a non-hydantoin anticonvulsant
Hepatic impairment	Use with caution and monitor for signs of excessive drug accumulation and early toxicity
Slow phenytoin metabolism	May occur in a small percentage of patients due to genetically determined limited enzyme availability and lack of induction
Elderly and/or severely ill patients	Use with caution and monitor for signs of excessive drug accumulation and early toxicity
Reversible lymph-node hyperplasia	May occur; substitute another anticonvulsant agent or combination after ruling out other lymph-gland pathology
Skin rash	May occur; discontinue therapy and do not resume if rash is exfoliative, purpuric, or bullous. Therapy may be resumed only if rash is mild (measles-like or scarlatiniform) and has completely cleared; if rash recurs, withdraw drug permanently.

ADVERSE REACTIONS	Frequent reactions are italicized
Central nervous system	*Ataxia, slurred speech, confusion,* dizziness, insomnia, transient nervousness, motor twitching, headache
Ophthalmic	*Nystagmus*
Gastrointestinal	Nausea, vomiting, constipation
Dermatological	Scarlatiniform or morbilliform (measles-like) rash, sometimes accompanied by fever; bullous, exfoliative or purpuric dermatitis; lupus erythematosus; Stevens-Johnson syndrome
Hematological	Thrombocytopenia, leukopenia, granulocytopenia, agranulocytosis, pancytopenia, macrocytosis, megaloblastic anemia
Other	Gingival hyperplasia, polyarthropathy, hirsutism, toxic hepatitis, liver damage, periarteritis, osteomalacia

Table continued on following page

OVERDOSAGE

Signs and symptoms	Nystagmus, ataxia, and dysarthria, progressing to comatose state, fixed pupils, hypotension, respiratory depression, apnea, and death
Treatment	Induce emesis or perform gastric lavage to empty stomach. Treat symptomatically. Support airway, administer oxygen and vasopressors, and assist ventilation. Hemodialysis may be useful. Total exchange transfusion has been employed in cases of severe intoxication in children.

DRUG INTERACTIONS

Barbiturates	⇧ Phenytoin metabolism (effect varies and is unpredictable)
Oral anticoagulants, disulfiram, phenylbutazone, oxyphenbutazone, chloramphenicol, sulfaphenazole	⇧ Phenytoin toxicity
Isoniazid	⇧ Phenytoin toxicity in patients who are slow acetylators
Tricyclic antidepressants (high doses), antipsychotics (high doses)	⇧ Risk of seizures
Alcohol, folic acid	⇩ Anticonvulsant effect
Dexamethasone	⇩ Corticosteroid effects
Doxycycline	⇩ Anti-infective effect
Levodopa	⇩ Antiparkinson effect
Sympathomimetics	Hypotension, bradycardia (effect is dependent on dose and rate of administration of phenytoin)
Valproic acid	⇧ or ⇩ Serum phenytoin level

ALTERED LABORATORY VALUES

Blood/serum values	⇧ Glucose ⇧ Alkaline phosphatase ⇩ PBI

No clinically significant alterations in urinary values occur at therapeutic dosages

Use in children

See INDICATIONS

Use in pregnancy or nursing mothers

An increased incidence of birth defects may be associated with the use of anticonvulsants during pregnancy. However, discontinuation of therapy may be considered only if removal of the drug does not pose any serious risk, such as the precipitation of status epilepticus with hypoxia in patients with serious convulsive disorders. The safety of phenytoin during lactation has not been established.

DILANTIN Parenteral (Phenytoin sodium) Parke-Davis

Amps: 50 mg/ml (2, 5 ml) **Syringe:** 50 mg/ml (2 ml)

INDICATIONS	PARENTERAL DOSAGE
Grand mal status epilepticus	**Adult:** 150–250 mg IV (slowly) to start, followed by 100–150 mg after 30 min, if needed; higher doses may be required to control seizures **Child:** 250 mg/m^2 body surface, administered as for adults
Seizures associated with neurosurgery	**Adult:** 100–200 mg IM q4h during and after surgery

ADMINISTRATION/DOSAGE ADJUSTMENTS

Preparation of solution	Use only clear solutions; a faint yellow color may develop, but has no effect on potency. Do not add to IV infusion since precipitation may occur.
Intravenous administration	Administer slowly (≤50 mg/min), followed by an injection of sterile saline through the same needle or IV catheter to avoid local venous irritation stemming from alkalinity of solution. Do not give by continuous infusion.
Intramuscular administration	May be used if immobilization of extremity is impossible due to convulsions, if veins are inaccessible, in postoperative patients, in comatose patients, or in patients with GI upsets; do not use for status epilepticus due to slow absorption. When transferring a patient previously stabilized on oral phenytoin for surgical prophylaxis, IM dose should be 50% greater than oral dose; when returning to oral therapy, reduce dose to 50% of original oral dosage for 1 wk.
Combination therapy	Combination anticonvulsant therapy is indicated if phenytoin does not control seizure or if both petit mal and grand mal seizures are present

CONTRAINDICATIONS

Hypersensitivity to hydantoins ●	Sino-atrial block ●	Second- and third-degree AV block ●
Sinus bradycardia ●	Adams-Stokes syndrome ●	

WARNINGS/PRECAUTIONS

Unwarranted uses	Do not use for seizures due to hypoglycemia or other identifiable and correctable causes
Impaired liver function	Use with caution and monitor for signs of excessive drug accumulation and early toxicity
Slow phenytoin metabolism	May occur in a small percentage of patients due to a genetically determined limited enzyme availability and lack of induction
Elderly or severely ill patients	Use with caution and monitor for signs of excessive drug accumulation and early toxicity
Special-risk patients	Use with caution in patients with hypotension and severe myocardial toxicity

ADVERSE REACTIONS

Central nervous system	Drowsiness, vertigo, CNS depression
Cardiovascular[1]	Hypotension, circulatory collapse, atrial and ventricular conduction depression, ventricular fibrillation
Gastrointestinal	Nausea, vomiting (rare)
Other	Nystagmus, circumoral tingling

OVERDOSAGE

Signs and symptoms	Nystagmus, ataxia, dysarthria, progressing to comatose state, fixed pupils, hypotension, respiratory depression, apnea, and death
Treatment	Treat symptomatically. Support airway, administer oxygen and vasopressors, and assist ventilation. Hemodialysis may be useful. Total exchange transfusion has been employed in cases of severe intoxication in children.

[1]Elderly or gravely ill patients are particularly susceptible

Table continued on following page

DILANTIN Parenteral continued

DRUG INTERACTIONS

Barbiturates	⇧ Phenytoin metabolism (effect varies and is unpredictable)
Oral anticoagulants, disulfiram, phenylbutazone, oxyphenbutazone, chloramphenicol, sulfaphenazole	⇧ Phenytoin toxicity
Isoniazid	⇧ Phenytoin toxicity in patients who are slow acetylators
Tricyclic antidepressants, antipsychotics	⇧ Risk of seizures
Lidocaine, propranolol	⇧ Cardiac depression with IV use of phenytoin
Alcohol, folic acid	⇩ Anticonvulsant effect
Dexamethasone	⇩ Corticosteroid effects
Doxycycline	⇩ Anti-infective effect
Levodopa	⇩ Antiparkinson effect
Sympathomimetics	Hypotension, bradycardia (effect is dependent on dose and rate of administration of phenytoin)
Valproic acid	⇧ or ⇩ Serum phenytoin level

ALTERED LABORATORY VALUES

Blood/serum values	⇧ Glucose ⇧ Alkaline phosphatase ⇩ PBI

No clinically significant alterations in urinary values occur at therapeutic dosages

Use in children

See INDICATIONS

Use in pregnancy or nursing mothers

An increased incidence of birth defects may be associated with the use of anticonvulsants during pregnancy. However, discontinuation of therapy may be considered only if removal of the drug does not pose any serious risk, such as the precipitation of status epilepticus with hypoxia in patients with serious convulsive disorders. The safety of phenytoin during lactation has not been established.

DILANTIN with PHENOBARBITAL (Phenytoin and phenobarbital) Parke-Davis

Caps: 100 mg phenytoin and 16 mg phenobarbital; 100 mg phenytoin and 32 mg phenobarbital

INDICATIONS	ORAL DOSAGE
Grand mal and psychomotor seizures in patients requiring both drugs for seizure control	**Adult:** 3–4 caps/day, or up to 6 caps/day, if needed, as determined by titration of individual components (see ADMINISTRATION/DOSAGE ADJUSTMENTS) **Child:** up to 300 mg phenytoin/day, as determined by titration of individual components (see ADMINISTRATION/DOSAGE ADJUSTMENTS)

ADMINISTRATION/DOSAGE ADJUSTMENTS

Initiating anticonvulsant therapy	Determine daily anticonvulsant requirements by administering the two drugs separately; if total daily doses of the two drugs used separately are within recommended doses for combination form, combination may be substituted. Children should generally be started on 5 mg/kg/day of phenytoin and 2–3 mg/kg/day phenobarbital, both drugs being given in 2 or 3 equally divided doses.
Dosage adjustments	Should be accomplished by switching patient to separate phenytoin and phenobarbital dosage forms
Serum level monitoring	May be useful for optimal dosage adjustment; therapeutic range (adults) for phenytoin, 10–20 μg/ml; for phenobarbital, 10–30 μg/ml
Timing of administration	Gastrointestinal disturbances may be alleviated by giving drug with or immediately after meals
Combination therapy	Addition of an anticonvulsant effective against absence (petit mal) epilepsy is necessary if both grand mal and petit mal seizures are present

CONTRAINDICATIONS

History of confusion or restlessness from hypnotics ●	Hypersensitivity to hydantoins ●	Renal impairment ●
History of abnormal reactions or hypersensitivity to barbiturates ●	Latent or manifest porphyria ●	Hepatic impairment ●
Previous addiction to sedative/hypnotics ●	Familial history of intermittent porphyria ●	Severe pulmonary insufficiency ●

WARNINGS/PRECAUTIONS

Unwarranted uses	Phenytoin should not be used for seizures due to hypoglycemia or other identifiable and correctable causes
Habit-forming	Psychic and/or physical dependence and tolerance may develop, especially in addiction-prone individuals, due to phenobarbital component
Abrupt discontinuation of therapy	May precipitate status epilepticus; if abrupt withdrawal is required (eg, due to allergic or hypersensitivity reaction), substitute a non-hydantoin anticonvulsant. Withdrawal symptoms, including convulsions and delirium, may occur upon discontinuation of phenobarbital in patients who are chronically intoxicated.
Hepatic impairment	Use with caution and monitor for signs of excessive drug accumulation and early toxicity
Elderly and/or severely ill patients	Use with caution and monitor for signs of excessive drug accumulation and early toxicity; marked excitement, rather than depression, may occur, particularly in those patients with cerebral arteriosclerosis
Reversible lymph-node hyperplasia	May occur due to phenytoin component; substitute another anticonvulsant agent or combination after ruling out other lymph-gland pathology
Slow phenytoin metabolism	May occur in small percentage of patients due to genetically determined limited enzyme availability and lack of induction
Skin rash	May occur due to phenytoin component; discontinue therapy and do not resume if rash is exfoliative, purpuric, or bullous. Therapy may be resumed only if rash is mild (measles-like or scarlatiniform) and has completely cleared; if rash recurs, withdraw drug permanently.
Special-risk patients	Use with caution in patients with pulmonary disease, respiratory depression, severe anemia, congestive heart failure, fever, hyperthyroidism, or diabetes mellitus, due to phenobarbital component
Psychiatric disorders	Use with caution in patients with suicidal tendencies, predilection to barbiturate or alcohol abuse, or neuroses; symptoms in mentally ill, phobic, or emotionally disturbed patients may be accentuated by phenobarbital component
Mental impairment, reflex-slowing	Performance of potentially hazardous activities may be impaired due to phenobarbital component; caution patient accordingly and about additive effects of alcohol and other CNS depressants

Table continued on following page

DILANTIN with PHENOBARBITAL continued

ADVERSE REACTIONS	Frequent reactions are italicized
Central nervous system	*Nystagmus, ataxia, slurred speech, mental confusion,* dizziness, insomnia, transient nervousness, motor twitchings, headache, euphoria, drowsiness, vertigo, hebetude, delirium, stupor
Gastrointestinal	Nausea, vomiting, constipation, discomfort
Dermatological	Scarlatiniform, morbilliform, or other rashes sometimes accompanied by fever; bullous, exfoliative, or purpuric dermatitis; lupus erythematosus; Stevens-Johnson syndrome
Hypersensitivity (to phenobarbital)	Stevens-Johnson syndrome, erythematous rash, high fever, jaundice, mental confusion, toxic damage to parenchymatous organs
Hematological	Thrombocytopenia, leukopenia, granulocytopenia, agranulocytosis, pancytopenia, macrocytosis, megaloblastic anemia, lymphadenopathy
Other	Gingival hyperplasia, polyarthropathy, hirsutism, toxic hepatitis, liver damage, periarteritis nodosa, osteomalacia

OVERDOSAGE	
Signs and symptoms	*Toxic effects primarily attributable to phenytoin:* nystagmus, ataxia, dysarthria, progressing to comatose state, fixed pupils, hypotension, respiratory depression, apnea, and death; *phenobarbital-related effects:* rapid weak pulse, reduced vital signs, depressed cardiac contractility, hypotension, hypoxia, respiratory arrest and death; late complications include hypostatic pneumonia, bronchopneumonia, lung abscess, pulmonary edema, cerebral edema, circulatory collapse, irreversible renal shutdown
Treatment	Induce emesis or perform gastric lavage to empty stomach. Treat symptomatically. Support airway, administer oxygen and vasopressors, and assist ventilation. Hemodialysis may be useful. Total exchange transfusion has been employed in severe cases of phenytoin intoxication in children.

DRUG INTERACTIONS	
Oral anticoagulants	⇧ Phenytoin toxicity ⇩ Prothrombin time
Isoniazid, disulfiram, phenylbutazone, oxyphenbutazone, chloramphenicol, sulfaphenazole	⇧ Phenytoin toxicity in patients who are slow acetylators
Tricyclic antidepressants (high doses)	⇧ Risk of seizures ⇩ Antidepressant effect
Antipsychotics (high doses)	⇧ Risk of seizures
MAO inhibitors	⇧ CNS depression ⇧ MAO inhibitor effects
General anesthetics, CNS depressants	⇧ CNS depression
Alcohol	⇧ CNS depression ⇩ Anticonvulsant effect
Folic acid	⇩ Anticonvulsant effect
Corticosteroids	⇩ Corticosteroid effects
Doxycycline	⇩ Anti-infective effect
Levodopa	⇩ Antiparkinson effect
Sympathomimetics	Hypotension, bradycardia (effect is dependent on dose and rate of administration of phenytoin)
Valproic acid	⇧ or ⇧ Serum phenytoin level
Digitalis, digitoxin	⇩ Cardiac glycoside effects
Griseofulvin	⇩ Griseofulvin absorption

ALTERED LABORATORY VALUES	
Blood/serum values	⇧ Glucose ⇧ Alkaline phosphatase ⇩ Bilirubin ⇩ PBI

No clinically significant alterations in urinary values occur at therapeutic dosages

Use in children

See INDICATIONS

Use in pregnancy or nursing mothers

An increased incidence of birth defects may be associated with the use of anticonvulsants during pregnancy. However, discontinuation of therapy may be considered only if removal of the drug does not pose any serious risk, such as the precipitation of status epilepticus with hypoxia in patients with serious convulsive disorders. Patient should stop nursing if drug is prescribed.

GEMONIL (Metharbital) Abbott

Tabs: 100 mg *C-III*

INDICATIONS	ORAL DOSAGE
Grand mal, petit mal, myoclonic, and mixed-type seizures	**Adult:** 100 mg 1–3 times/day, to start, followed by gradual increases in dosage up to 600–800 mg/day, until optimal clinical response is achieved **Child:** 5–15 mg/kg/day or 50 mg 1–3 times/day, to start, followed by gradual increases in dosage until optimal clinical response is achieved

ADMINISTRATION/DOSAGE ADJUSTMENTS

Combination therapy	May be used concomitantly with trimethadione, paramethadione, phenacemide, ethotoin, phenytoin, or mephenytoin; when adding metharbital to established regimen, gradually increase the dosage of metharbital while decreasing the dosage of other agent

CONTRAINDICATIONS

Hypersensitivity to barbiturates ●	Manifest or latent porphyria ●

WARNINGS/PRECAUTIONS

Habit-forming	Psychic and/or physical dependence and tolerance may develop, especially in addiction-prone individuals
Hepatic impairment	Use with caution and observe for signs of excessive drug accumulation
Renal impairment	Use with caution; metharbital is converted in the liver to barbital (a long-acting barbiturate), which is excreted unchanged in urine[1]
Abrupt discontinuation of therapy	May precipitate status epilepticus

ADVERSE REACTIONS

Gastrointestinal	Gastric distress
Central nervous system	Irritability, dizziness, drowsiness
Dermatological	Rash

OVERDOSAGE

Signs and symptoms	Drowsiness, irritability, dizziness, and gastric distress, followed in cases of very large ingestions by loss of consciousness and coma
Treatment	Maintain and assist respiration and support circulation with vasopressors and IV fluids, as indicated. Evacuate stomach by gastric lavage, taking care to avoid pulmonary aspiration. Administer an osmotic diuretic and measure intake and output of fluids. Perform dialysis, if indicated. Administer antibiotics to control pulmonary complications, when necessary.

DRUG INTERACTIONS

Oral anticoagulants	⇩ Prothrombin time
Alcohol, general anesthetics, CNS depressants, MAO inhibitors	⇧ CNS depression
Corticosteroids	⇩ Corticosteroid effects
Digitalis, digitoxin	⇩ Cardiac glycoside effects
Tricyclic antidepressants	⇩ Antidepressant effect
Doxycycline	⇩ Anti-infective effect
Griseofulvin	⇩ Griseofulvin absorption
Phenytoin	⇧ or ⇩ Phenytoin effects, depending on dosage of metharbital

[1]Gilman AG et al (eds): *The Pharmacological Basis of Therapeutics*, ed 6. New York, Macmillan, 1980, p 458

Table continued on following page

GEMONIL continued

ALTERED LABORATORY VALUES

Blood/serum values ———————— ⇩ Bilirubin

No clinically significant alterations in urinary values occur at therapeutic dosages

Use in children

See INDICATIONS

Use in pregnancy or nursing mothers

An increased incidence of birth defects may be associated with the use of anticonvulsants during pregnancy. However, discontinuation of therapy may be considered only if removal of the drug does not pose any serious risk, such as the precipitation of status epilepticus with hypoxia in patients with serious convulsive disorders. Maternal ingestion of anticonvulsants may cause neonatal hemorrhage due to a coagulation defect. Administer prophylactic vitamin K_1 to mother 1 mo prior to and during delivery, and to infant intravenously immediately after birth. The safety of metharbital during lactation has not been established.

MEBARAL (Mephobarbital) Breon

Tabs: 32, 50, 100, 200 mg *C-IV*

INDICATIONS	ORAL DOSAGE
Grand mal and petit mal seizures	**Adult:** 400–600 mg/day **Child (<5 yr):** 16–32 mg tid or qid **Child (>5 yr):** 32–64 mg tid or qid
Sedation for the relief of anxiety, tension, and apprehension	**Adult:** 32–100 mg tid or qid; usual dose: 50 mg tid or qid **Child:** 16–32 mg tid or qid

ADMINISTRATION/DOSAGE ADJUSTMENTS

Initiating anticonvulsant therapy	Start with small doses, and gradually titrate dosage upward over 4–5 days until optimal dosage level is obtained (see ORAL DOSAGE). In patients receiving other anticonvulsants, gradually increase mephobarbital dosage while tapering dosage of other agents.
Maintenance anticonvulsant therapy	Gradually reduce dosage over 4–5 days to lowest effective level
Combination anticonvulsant therapy	Mephobarbital may be alternated with phenobarbital or given concurrently (for adults, give 200–300 mg/day of mephobarbital combined with 50–100 mg/day of phenobarbital); when used in combination with phenytoin in adults, give 600 mg/day of mephobarbital and reduce dosage of phenytoin to 230 mg/day
Timing of administration	For nocturnal epilepsy, dosage should be taken at night; for diurnal epilepsy, dosage should be taken during day

CONTRAINDICATIONS

Hypersensitivity to any barbiturate ●	Porphyria ●

WARNINGS/PRECAUTIONS

Habit-forming	Psychic and/or physical dependence and tolerance may develop, especially in addiction-prone individuals
Abrupt discontinuation of therapy	May produce withdrawal symptoms after chronic use of high doses, resulting in tremors, weakness, insomnia, convulsions, and delirium. In epileptic patients, abrupt cessation of therapeutic doses may precipitate status epilepticus. Dosage should be gradually discontinued over 4–5 days.
Mental impairment, reflex-slowing	Performance of potentially hazardous tasks may be impaired; caution patients accordingly and about additive effects of alcohol and other CNS depressants
Vitamin D deficiency	Vitamin D requirements may be increased; rickets and osteomalacia have occurred rarely following prolonged use of barbiturates
Special-risk patients	Use with caution in patients with impaired hepatic, renal, cardiac, or respiratory function, and in patients with myasthenia gravis and myxedema
Elderly or debilitated patients	Reduce dosage to avoid oversedation; confusion may occur in the elderly

ADVERSE REACTIONS

Central nervous system	Dizziness, headache, "hangover," confusion, paradoxical excitation, exacerbation of preexisting pain
Gastrointestinal	Nausea, vomiting, epigastric pain
Cardiovascular	Hypotension
Hypersensitivity	Facial edema, skin rash, bullae and vesicles, purpura, erythema multiforme, exfoliative dermatitis (rare), degeneration of liver (in severe cases)
Hematological	Megaloblastic anemia, agranulocytosis, thrombocytopenia

OVERDOSAGE

Signs and symptoms	Mild cases resemble alcohol intoxication; severe overdosage results in shock, coma, and death; respiratory depression and renal failure may occur
Treatment	Maintain patent airway and assist respiration, as needed. Gastric lavage, with endotracheal intubation, if needed, may be used if patient is seen within a few hours of ingestion. Forced diuresis and alkalinization of urine are indicated if renal failure has not occurred. Hemodialysis is effective, especially in renal failure; peritoneal dialysis is less effective. Use of analeptic agents is controversial.

Table continued on following page

MEBARAL continued

DRUG INTERACTIONS

Alcohol, CNS depressants	⇧ CNS depression
Oral anticoagulants	⇩ Prothrombin time
Antihistamines	⇩ Antihistamine effect
Corticosteroids	⇩ Corticosteroid effects
Digitalis, digitoxin	⇩ Cardiac glycoside effects
Tricyclic antidepressants	⇩ Antidepressant effect
Doxycycline	⇩ Anti-infective effect
Griseofulvin	⇩ Griseofulvin absorption
Phenytoin	⇧ or ⇩ Serum phenytoin level, depending on dose of mephobarbital

ALTERED LABORATORY VALUES

Blood/serum values	⇩ Bilirubin

No clinically significant alterations in urinary values occur at therapeutic dosages

Use in children

See INDICATIONS

Use in pregnancy or nursing mothers

An increased incidence of birth defects may be associated with the use of anticonvulsants during pregnancy. Barbiturates cross the placental barrier and may have depressant effects on the fetus when administered during labor. Neonatal withdrawal symptoms have been reported following use of barbiturates during pregnancy. Exposure to anticonvulsants in utero may cause neonatal bleeding defects; administer prophylactic vitamin K_1 to mother prior to delivery or to infant at birth. Barbiturates appear in breast milk and may have adverse effects on nursing infants.

MESANTOIN (Mephenytoin) Sandoz

Tabs: 100 mg

INDICATIONS	ORAL DOSAGE
Grand mal, focal, Jacksonian, and psychomotor seizures in patients refractory to less toxic anticonvulsants	**Adult:** 50–100 mg/day to start, followed by weekly increases of 50–100 mg/day, up to 800 mg/day, if needed; usual maintenance dosage: 200–600 mg/day **Child:** 50–100 mg/day to start, followed by weekly increases of 50–100 mg/day; usual maintenance dosage: 100–400 mg/day

ADMINISTRATION/DOSAGE ADJUSTMENTS

Patients receiving other anticonvulsants	Gradually add mephenytoin (see ORAL DOSAGE) while tapering dose of anticonvulsant to be discontinued, over a period of 3–6 wk; thereafter, dosage may be increased by 100 mg/day at weekly intervals, if needed. Phenobarbital may be continued until optimal mephenytoin dosage is achieved, and then gradually withdrawn.
Dosage reduction	Must be gradual to minimize risk of precipitating seizures

CONTRAINDICATIONS

Hypersensitivity to hydantoins

WARNINGS/PRECAUTIONS

Medical supervision	Patient must be kept under close supervision at all times due to possibility of serious adverse effects (see ADVERSE REACTIONS)
Hepatic impairment	Use with caution and observe for signs of excessive drug accumulation; pretreatment liver-function tests are recommended
Blood dyscrasias	May occur (see ADVERSE REACTIONS). Instruct patient to discontinue drug and report for examination if sore throat, fever, mucous-membrane bleeding, glandular swelling, or cutaneous reactions develop. Obtain total WBC and differential before starting treatment, 2 wk after starting therapy, 2 wk after optimal dosage is reached, monthly thereafter for 1 yr, and every 3 mo subsequently. If neutrophil count drops to between 1,600 and 2,500/mm³, obtain counts every 2 wk. If neutrophil count falls below 1,600/mm³, discontinue therapy.

ADVERSE REACTIONS

Hematological	Leukopenia, neutropenia, agranulocytosis, thrombocytopenia, pancytopenia, eosinophilia, monocytosis, leukocytosis, simple anemia, hemolytic anemia, megaloblastic anemia, aplastic anemia (rare)
Dermatological	Maculopapular, morbilliform, scarlatiniform, urticarial, purpuric, and nonspecific skin rashes; exfoliative dermatitis; erythema multiforme (Stevens-Johnson syndrome); toxic epidermal necrolysis; fatal dermatitides; skin pigmentation and rashes associated with lupus erythematosus syndrome; alopecia
Central nervous system	Drowsiness (dose-related), ataxia, fatigue, irritability, choreiform movements, depression, tremor, nervousness, sleeplessness, dizziness; mental confusion, psychotic disturbances, and increased seizures (causal relationship not established)
Neuromuscular	Dysarthria, polyarthropathy
Ophthalmic	Diplopia, nystagmus, photophobia, conjunctivitis
Gastrointestinal	Nausea, vomiting, weight gain, gum hyperplasia
Hepatic	Hepatitis and jaundice (causal relationship not established)
Other	Edema, pulmonary fibrosis, lymphadenopathy resembling Hodgkin's disease; nephrosis (causal relationship not established)

OVERDOSAGE

Signs and symptoms	See ADVERSE REACTIONS
Treatment	Induce emesis or perform gastric lavage to empty stomach. Treat symptomatically and institute supportive measures, as required.

DRUG INTERACTIONS[1]

Tricyclic antidepressants (high doses), antipsychotics (high doses)	Seizures
Oral hypoglycemics	⇩ Hypoglycemic effect

[1]Other interactions have been reported with hydantoins, but not with mephenytoin

Table continued on following page

ALTERED LABORATORY VALUES

Blood/serum values ———— ⇧ Glucose ⇧ Alkaline phosphatase ⇩ PBI

No clinically significant alterations in urinary values occur at therapeutic dosages

Use in children	**Use in pregnancy or nursing mothers**
See INDICATIONS	An increased incidence of birth defects may be associated with the use of anticonvulsants during pregnancy. However, discontinuation of therapy may be considered only if removal of the drug does not pose any serious risk, such as the precipitation of status epilepticus with hypoxia in patients with serious convulsive disorders. The safety of mephenytoin during lactation has not been established.

MILONTIN (Phensuximide) **Parke-Davis**

Caps: 500 mg **Susp:** 60 mg/ml

INDICATIONS	ORAL DOSAGE
Absence (petit mal) seizures	**Adult:** 500–1,000 mg bid or tid; usual maintenance dosage: 1,500 mg/day **Child:** 10–20 ml (2–4 tsp) bid or tid

ADMINISTRATION/DOSAGE ADJUSTMENTS

Combination therapy — May be used with other anticonvulsants when other forms of epilepsy coexist with absence (petit mal) seizures

CONTRAINDICATIONS

Hypersensitivity to succinimides

WARNINGS/PRECAUTIONS

Blood dyscrasias — May occur and may be fatal (see ADVERSE REACTIONS); obtain CBC periodically

Renal or hepatic disease — Use with caution; perform a urinalysis and liver-function tests periodically in all patients. Succinimides have produced morphological and functional changes in animal livers.

Mental impairment, reflex-slowing — Performance of potentially hazardous tasks may be impaired; caution patients accordingly

Grand mal seizures — May occur when phensuximide is used alone in mixed types of epilepsy

Abrupt discontinuation of therapy — May precipitate absence (petit mal) status; all dosage adjustments must be gradual

ADVERSE REACTIONS Frequent reactions are italicized

Gastrointestinal — *Nausea, vomiting, anorexia*

Central nervous system and neuromuscular — Drowsiness, dizziness, ataxia, headache, dream-like state, lethargy, muscle weakness

Dermatological — Pruritus, skin eruptions, erythema multiforme, erythematous rashes, alopecia

Genitourinary — Urinary frequency, renal damage, hematuria

Hematological — Granulocytopenia, transient leukopenia, pancytopenia

Other — Lupus erythematosus-like syndrome

OVERDOSAGE

Signs and symptoms — See ADVERSE REACTIONS

Treatment — Induce emesis or perform gastric lavage to empty stomach. Treat symptomatically and institute supportive measures, as required.

DRUG INTERACTIONS

Tricyclic antidepressants (high doses), antipsychotics (high doses) — Seizures

ALTERED LABORATORY VALUES

No clinically significant alterations in blood/serum or urinary values occur at therapeutic dosages

Use in children

See INDICATIONS

Use in pregnancy or nursing mothers

An increased incidence of birth defects may be associated with the use of anticonvulsants during pregnancy. However, discontinuation of therapy may be considered only if removal of the drug does not pose any serious risk, such as the precipitation of status epilepticus in patients with serious convulsive disorders. The safety of phensuximide during lactation has not been established.

MYSOLINE (Primidone) **Ayerst**

Tabs: 50, 250 mg **Susp:** 50 mg/ml

INDICATIONS	ORAL DOSAGE
Grand mal, psychomotor, and focal epileptic seizures	**Adult:** 250 mg/day to start, followed by weekly increases of 250 mg/day, up to 2 g/day div; usual maintenance dosage: 750–1,500 mg/day **Child (<8 yr):** 125 mg/day to start, followed by weekly increases of 125 mg/day; usual maintenance dosage: 500–750 mg/day div **Child (>8 yr):** same as adult

ADMINISTRATION/DOSAGE ADJUSTMENTS	
Patients receiving other anticonvulsants	Gradually increase primidone dosage while decreasing dosage of other agent until optimal combination dosage is achieved. If other medication is to be completely withdrawn, transition should not be completed for at least 2 wk.
Small fractional adjustments	May be required for initiation of combination therapy, during transfer from other anticonvulsants, and during stressful situations likely to precipitate seizures (eg, menstruation, allergic episodes, holidays); use 50-mg tabs

CONTRAINDICATIONS	
Hypersensitivity to phenobarbital●	Porphyria●

WARNINGS/PRECAUTIONS	
Abrupt discontinuation of therapy	May precipitate status epilepticus
Prolonged therapy	Perform a CBC and sequential multiple analysis-12 (SMA-12) every 6 mo
Megaloblastic anemia	Occurs rarely; may be treated with folic acid without interruption of anticonvulsant therapy

ADVERSE REACTIONS	Frequent reactions are italicized
Central nervous system	*Ataxia, vertigo,* fatigue, hyperirritability, emotional disturbances, drowsiness
Gastrointestinal	Nausea, anorexia, vomiting
Ophthalmic	Diplopia, nystagmus
Hematological	Megaloblastic anemia (see WARNINGS/PRECAUTIONS)
Dermatological	Morbilliform skin eruptions
Genitourinary	Impotence

OVERDOSAGE	
Signs and symptoms	See ADVERSE REACTIONS
Treatment	Treat symptomatically. Institute supportive measures, as required.

DRUG INTERACTIONS	
Alcohol, general anesthetics, CNS depressants, MAO inhibitors	⇧ Drug effects and/or anticonvulsant toxicity
Oral anticoagulants	⇩ Prothrombin time
Corticosteroids	⇩ Corticosteroid effects
Digitalis, digitoxin	⇩ Cardiac glycoside effects
Doxycycline	⇩ Anti-infective effect
Tricyclic antidepressants	⇩ Antidepressant effect
Griseofulvin	⇩ Griseofulvin absorption
Phenytoin, other anticonvulsants	Change in pattern of epileptiform seizures

Table continued on following page

MYSOLINE continued

ALTERED LABORATORY VALUES

Blood/serum values ———————— ⇩ Bilirubin

No clinically significant alterations in urinary values occur at therapeutic dosages

Use in children

See INDICATIONS

Use in pregnancy or nursing mothers

An increased incidence of birth defects may be associated with the use of anticonvulsants during pregnancy. However, discontinuation of therapy may be considered only if removal of the drug does not pose any serious risk, such as the precipitation of status epilepticus with hypoxia in patients with serious convulsive disorders. Neonatal hemorrhage due to a coagulation deficiency resembling vitamin K deficiency may occur. Administer prophylactic vitamin K_1 to pregnant women 1 mo prior to and during delivery. Primidone appears in breast milk in substantial quantities; patient should stop nursing if undue somnolence and drowsiness occur in nursing infants.

PARADIONE (Paramethadione) **Abbott**

Caps: 150, 300 mg **Sol:** 300 mg/ml[1]

INDICATIONS	ORAL DOSAGE
Absence (petit mal) seizures in patients refractory to less toxic anticonvulsants	**Adult:** 900 mg/day to start, followed by weekly increases of 300 mg/day, if needed, until optimal clinical response is achieved; usual maintenance dosage: 300–600 mg tid or qid **Child:** 300–900 mg/day in 3–4 equally divided doses; solution may be diluted with water, if desired

CONTRAINDICATIONS

Hypersensitivity to paramethadione

WARNINGS/PRECAUTIONS	
Medical supervision	Patient must be carefully supervised, especially during 1st year of therapy, because of the possibility of serious adverse effects (see ADVERSE REACTIONS)
Exfoliative dermatitis, severe erythema multiforme	May develop; discontinue therapy at first sign of even a mild skin rash; reinstitute therapy cautiously and only after rash has cleared completely
Blood dyscrasias	May occur and may be fatal (see ADVERSE REACTIONS); obtain baseline and monthly CBC and instruct patient to report early signs (eg, sore throat, fever, malaise, bruises, petechiae, epistaxis) of serious blood disorders. Obtain more frequent counts if neutrophil count drops to $<3,000/mm^3$. Discontinue therapy if blood count is markedly depressed or neutrophil count is $2,500/mm^3$ or less. Do not use ordinarily in patients with severe blood dyscrasias.
Hepatic impairment	May occur; perform baseline and monthly liver-function tests and discontinue if jaundice or other signs of hepatic dysfunction occur. Do not use ordinarily in patients with severe hepatic impairment.
Nephrosis	May occur and may be fatal; perform urinalysis prior to initiating therapy and at monthly intervals thereafter. Withdraw drug if persistent or increasing albuminuria or other significant renal abnormalities occur. Do not use ordinarily in patients with severe renal dysfunction.
Visual disturbances	May occur; use with caution in patients with diseases of the retina or optic nerve. Hemeralopia may be reversed by dosage reduction. Discontinue drug if scotomata occur.
Systemic lupus erythematosus	May occur; discontinue therapy if lupus-like manifestations occur
Lymphadenopathies	May occur, simulating malignant lymphoma; discontinue therapy if lymph-node enlargement occurs
Myasthenia gravis-like syndrome	May occur with chronic use; discontinue therapy if suggestive symptoms occur
Drugs with similar side effects	Should be avoided or used with extreme caution during therapy
Abrupt discontinuation of therapy	May precipitate petit mal status; if abrupt withdrawal is required (eg, because of serious adverse effects), substitute another anticonvulsant
Drowsiness	May occur but usually subsides with continued therapy; if drowsiness persists, reduce dosage
Tartrazine sensitivity	Presence of FD&C Yellow No. 5 (tartrazine) in 300-mg capsules may cause allergic-type reactions, including bronchial asthma, in susceptible individuals

ADVERSE REACTIONS	
Gastrointestinal	Nausea, vomiting, abdominal pain, gastric distress, anorexia, weight loss (rare)
Central nervous system	Drowsiness, fatigue, malaise, insomnia, vertigo, headache, paresthesias, grand mal seizures, increased irritability, personality changes
Hematological	Neutropenia, leukopenia, eosinophilia, thrombocytopenia, pancytopenia, agranulocytosis, hypoplastic anemia, fatal aplastic anemia, bleeding gums, epistaxis, petechial hemorrhage, vaginal bleeding
Dermatological	Acneform or morbilliform rash, progressing to exfoliative dermatitis or severe erythema multiforme; alopecia
Ophthalmic	Hemeralopia, photophobia, diplopia, retinal hemorrhage
Hypersensitivity	Pruritus associated with lymphadenopathy and hepatosplenomegaly
Other	Hiccoughs, blood-pressure changes, fatal nephrosis, hepatitis (rare), lupus erythematosus, lymphadenopathies simulating malignant lymphoma, myasthenia gravis-like syndrome

[1]Contains 65% alcohol

Table continued on following page

PARADIONE continued

OVERDOSAGE

Signs and symptoms	Drowsiness, nausea, dizziness, ataxia, and visual disturbances, followed by coma in cases of massive ingestions
Treatment	Induce emesis or perform gastric lavage to empty stomach. Institute general supportive measures and monitor vital signs. Alkalinization of the urine may increase metabolite excretion. Following recovery, obtain a CBC and evaluate hepatic and renal function.

DRUG INTERACTIONS

Mephenytoin, phenacemide	⇧ Risk of toxicity

ALTERED LABORATORY VALUES

Urinary values	⇧ Albumin

No clinically significant alterations in blood/serum values occur at therapeutic dosages

Use in children

See INDICATIONS

Use in pregnancy or nursing mothers

An increased incidence of birth defects may be associated with the use of paramethadione during pregnancy. Administer to women of childbearing potential only if essential to management of seizures; effective contraception should be used and, if patient becomes pregnant, termination of pregnancy should be considered. Maternal ingestion of anticonvulsants may cause neonatal hemorrhage (usually within 24 h of birth) due to a coagulation defect. Administer prophylactic vitamin K_1 to mother 1 mo prior to and during delivery, and to infant IV immediately after birth. The safety of paramethadione during lactation has not been established.

PEGANONE (Ethotoin) Abbott

Tabs: 250 mg

INDICATIONS	ORAL DOSAGE
Grand mal and psychomotor seizures	**Adult:** up to 1,000 mg/day in 4-6 divided doses to start, followed by gradual increases over several days; usual maintenance dosage: 2,000-3,000 mg/day in 4-6 divided doses **Child:** up to 750 mg/day in 4-6 divided doses to start, depending on age and weight, followed by gradual increases, as needed, up to 3,000 mg/day; usual maintenance dosage: 500-1,000 mg/day in 4-6 divided doses

ADMINISTRATION/DOSAGE ADJUSTMENTS

Timing of administration	Nausea and vomiting may be minimized by taking after meals
Patients receiving other anticonvulsants	Gradually increase ethotoin dosage while tapering dosage of other agent
Combination therapy	Ethotoin may be used with metharbital in grand mal seizures, or with trimethadione or paramethadione. Use with phenacemide is not recommended.

CONTRAINDICATIONS

Hepatic abnormalities ●	Hematological disorders ●

WARNINGS/PRECAUTIONS

Blood dyscrasias	May occur; obtain baseline and monthly CBC and instruct patient to report early signs (eg, sore throat, general malaise) of serious blood disorders. Discontinue if blood count is markedly depressed. Avoid other drugs with adverse hematological effects.
Hepatic impairment	Observe for clinical signs; if liver-function tests indicate hepatic dysfunction, discontinue therapy
Monitoring of renal function	Perform a urinalysis when therapy is begun and monthly for several months thereafter
Megaloblastic anemia	May occur due to interference with folic acid metabolism
Lymphoma-like syndrome	May occur; discontinue therapy until signs and symptoms remit

ADVERSE REACTIONS

Gastrointestinal	Nausea, vomiting, diarrhea, gum hypertrophy (rare)[1]
CNS and neuromuscular	Fatigue, insomnia, dizziness, headache, numbness, fever, ataxia (rare)[1]
Ophthalmic	Diplopia, nystagmus
Dermatological	Rash
Other	Chest pain, lymphadenopathy, systemic lupus erythematosus

OVERDOSAGE

Signs and symptoms	Drowsiness, visual disturbance, nausea, and ataxia, followed by coma massive ingestion
Treatment	Induce emesis or perform gastric lavage. Institute general supportive measures.

DRUG INTERACTIONS[2]

Phenacemide	Paranoid symptoms
Oral anticoagulants (high doses)	⇧ Anticonvulsant toxicity
Antipsychotics (high doses)	Seizures
Oral hypoglycemics	⇩ Hypoglycemic effect

ALTERED LABORATORY VALUES

Blood/serum values	⇧ Glucose

No clinically significant alterations in urinary values occur at therapeutic dosages

Use in children

See INDICATIONS

Use in pregnancy or nursing mothers

An increased incidence of birth defects may be associated with the use of anticonvulsants during pregnancy. However, discontinuation of therapy may be considered only if removal of the drug does not pose any serious risk. Administer prophylactic vitamin K[1], to pregnant women 1 mo prior to and during delivery, and to infant IV immediately after birth. If megaloblastic anemia occurs during gestation, folic acid therapy should be considered. The safety of ethotoin during lactation has not been established.

[1]Usually occurs only in patients receiving an additional hydantoin derivative
[2]Other interactions have been reported with other hydantoins, but not with ethotoin

Table continued on following page

PHENOBARBITAL various manufacturers

Tabs: 8, 15, 16, 30, 32, 60, 65, 100 mg **Caps:** 16 mg **Drops:** 16 mg/ml **Elixir:** 20 mg/5 ml *C-IV*

PHENOBARBITAL SODIUM various manufacturers

Amps: 65 mg/ml (2 ml), 130 mg/ml (1 ml), 163 mg/ml (2 ml) **Vials:** 65, 120, 130, 325 mg **Syringes:** 65 mg/ml (1 ml), 130 mg/ml (1 ml)
Cartridge-needle units: 30 mg/ml (1 ml) *C-IV*

INDICATIONS	ORAL DOSAGE	PARENTERAL DOSAGE
Grand mal and partial seizures	**Adult:** 50–100 mg bid or tid or 100–200 mg/day at bedtime **Child:** 3–6 mg/kg/day div	—
Status epilepticus	—	**Adult:** 200–325 mg IM or IV (slowly), repeated after 6 h, if necessary **Child:** 3–5 mg IM or IV (slowly)
Daytime and postoperative sedation	**Adult:** 30–120 mg/day in 2–3 divided doses **Child:** 6 mg/kg/day in 3 divided doses	**Adult:** 32–100 mg IM **Child:** 8–30 mg IM
Preoperative sedation	—	**Adult:** 100–200 mg IM 60–90 min before surgery **Child:** 16–100 mg IM 60–90 min before surgery
Hypnosis	**Adult:** 100–320 mg at bedtime **Child:** adjust according to age and weight	**Adult:** 100–320 mg IM or IV (slowly) **Child:** 3–6 mg/kg IM or IV (slowly)

ADMINISTRATION/DOSAGE ADJUSTMENTS

Intramuscular use	Inject deeply into large muscle mass; to minimize risk of tissue irritation, inject not more than 5 ml into any one site
Intravenous use	Patient should be hospitalized and closely supervised; when relatively large doses are indicated, inject slowly at a rate not greater than 60 mg/min
Discontinuing therapy	Reduce dosage gradually after prolonged use of high doses to avoid withdrawal symptoms

CONTRAINDICATIONS

Sensitivity to barbiturates●	Uncontrolled pain●	Marked hepatic impairment●
Respiratory or cardiac disease (if more than minimal)●	History of porphyria●	

WARNINGS/PRECAUTIONS

Habit-forming	Psychic and/or physical dependence and tolerance may develop, especially in addiction-prone individuals
Mental impairment, reflex-slowing	Performance of potentially hazardous activities may be impaired; caution patients accordingly and about possible additive effect of alcohol and other CNS depressants
Hepatic or renal impairment	Use with extreme caution and observe for signs of excessive drug accumulation (see OVERDOSAGE)
Withdrawal symptoms	May occur after chronic use of large doses, resulting in delirium, convulsions, or death
Excessive narcosis	May follow IM injection of large hypnotic doses; observe patients for 20–30 min after administration
Overly rapid IV administration	May cause respiratory depression or apnea, laryngospasm, or vasodilatation with hypotension (see ADMINISTRATION/DOSAGE ADJUSTMENTS)
Hypersensitivity reactions	May occur, especially in patients with asthma, urticaria, or angioneurotic edema

ADVERSE REACTIONS

Central nervous system	Residual sedation ("hangover"), drowsiness, lethargy, vertigo, ataxia, paradoxical excitation
Respiratory	Depression, apnea
Gastrointestinal	Nausea, vomiting, anorexia
Cardiovascular	Vasodilatation and hypotension (with IV use), circulatory collapse
Hypersensitivity	Urticaria, angioneurotic edema, rash, drug fever, serum sickness, erythema multiforme (Stevens-Johnson syndrome)

Table continued on following page

PHENOBARBITAL/PHENOBARBITAL SODIUM continued

OVERDOSAGE

Signs and symptoms	Respiratory depression, depressed superficial and deep reflexes, miosis or mydriasis, decreased urine formation, hypothermia, coma
Treatment	Following acute ingestion, empty stomach immediately by gastric lavage, taking care to prevent pulmonary aspiration. Maintain patent airway, assist ventilation, and administer oxygen, as needed. Monitor vital signs and fluid balance. Treat shock with fluids and other standard measures. If renal function is normal, force diuresis and alkalinize urine to help eliminate drug. Dialysis may be helpful. Antibiotics may be needed to control pulmonary complications.

DRUG INTERACTIONS

Alcohol, tranquilizers, and other CNS depressants	⇧ CNS depression
Coumarin anticoagulants	⇩ Prothrombin time
Digitalis, digitoxin	⇩ Cardiac glycoside plasma levels
Doxycycline	⇩ Doxycycline half-life
Griseofulvin	⇩ Griseofulvin absorption
Corticosteroids	⇩ Corticosteroid effects

ALTERED LABORATORY VALUES

Blood/serum values	⇧ Sulfobromophthalein (BSP) retention ⇩ Bilirubin

No clinically significant alterations in urinary values occur at therapeutic dosages

Use in children

See INDICATIONS; phenobarbital may produce paradoxical excitement or hyperactivity in children or exacerbate existing hyperkinetic behavior

Use in pregnancy or nursing mothers

Safe use has not been established during pregnancy. Phenobarbital is excreted in breast milk; patient should stop nursing if drug is prescribed and infant shows signs of barbiturate toxicity.

PHENURONE (Phenacemide) Abbott

Tabs: 500 mg

INDICATIONS	ORAL DOSAGE
Severe epilepsy, especially mixed forms of psychomotor seizures refractory to other anticonvulsants	**Adult:** 500 mg tid, followed by weekly increases of 500 mg/day, if needed, administered in additional doses, up to 5 g/day; usual maintenance dosage: 2–3 g/day **Child (5–10 yr):** ½ the adult dose at same time intervals

ADMINISTRATION/DOSAGE ADJUSTMENTS

Combination therapy	May be used with other anticonvulsants; use with extreme caution if toxic effects are similar
Patients receiving other anticonvulsants	Gradually increase phenacemide dosage while tapering dosage of anticonvulsant to be discontinued to maintain seizure control

CONTRAINDICATIONS

None

WARNINGS/PRECAUTIONS

Personality disorders, including severe psychoses and suicide attempts	May occur; use with extreme caution in patients with history of personality disorders and observe for behavioral changes (eg, apathy, depression, aggressiveness). Hospitalization during 1st wk of therapy may be advisable. Withdraw drug if severe or exacerbated personality changes occur.
Severe hepatic impairment	May occur and may be fatal; use with caution in patients with hepatic dysfunction. Perform baseline and periodic liver-function tests and discontinue therapy if jaundice or other signs of hepatitis appear.
Blood dyscrasias	May occur and may be fatal (see ADVERSE REACTIONS); obtain baseline and monthly CBC and instruct patient to report early signs (sore throat, malaise, fever) of serious blood disorders. Discontinue therapy if blood count is markedly depressed.
Nephritis	May occur; perform periodic urinalysis and discontinue therapy if abnormalities occur
Hypersensitivity reactions	Use with caution in patients with a history of allergy, especially to other convulsants, and discontinue therapy at the first sign of skin rash or other allergic manifestations

ADVERSE REACTIONS

Frequent reactions are italicized

Gastrointestinal	Disturbances, anorexia
Central nervous system and neuromuscular	Headache, drowsiness, dizziness, insomnia, paresthesias psychic changes
Dermatological	Rash
Hematological	*Leukopenia,* aplastic anemia, other blood dyscrasias
Renal	Nephritis
Hepatic	Hepatitis, jaundice

OVERDOSAGE

Signs and symptoms	Excitement and mania, followed by drowsiness, dizziness, ataxia, and coma
Treatment	Induce emesis or perform gastric lavage to empty stomach. Institute general supportive measures. Following recovery, carefully evaluate hepatic and renal function, mental state, and blood-forming organs.

DRUG INTERACTIONS

Ethotoin	Paranoid symptoms

ALTERED LABORATORY VALUES

No clinically significant alterations in blood/serum or urinary values occur at therapeutic dosages

Use in children

See INDICATIONS; general guidelines not established for use in children < 5 yr of age

Use in pregnancy or nursing mothers

An increased incidence of birth defects may be associated with the use of anticonvulsants during pregnancy. However, discontinuation of therapy may be considered only if removal of the drug does not pose any serious risk, such as the precipitation of status epilepticus with hypoxia in patients with serious convulsive disorders. Maternal ingestion of anticonvulsants may cause neonatal hemorrhage (usually within 24 h of birth) due to a coagulation defect. Administer prophylactic vitamin K_1 to mother 1 mo prior to and during delivery, and to infant IV immediately after birth. The safety of phenacemide during lactation has not been established.

TEGRETOL (Carbamazepine) Geigy

Tabs: 200 mg

INDICATIONS	ORAL DOSAGE
Epilepsy, including partial seizures with complex symptomatology (eg, psychomotor, temporal lobe), generalized tonic-clonic (grand mal) seizures, and mixed seizure patterns, in patients refractory to other anticonvulsants	**Adult:** 200 mg bid to start, followed by gradual increases of 200 mg/day up to 1,600 mg/day, if needed, in 3–4 divided doses until optimal clinical response is obtained; usual maintenance dosage: 800–1,200 mg/day **Child (6–12 yr):** 100 mg bid to start, followed by gradual increases of 100 mg/day up to 1,000 mg/day, if needed, in 3–4 divided doses until optimal clinical response is obtained; usual maintenance dosage: 400–800 mg/day **Child (12–15 yr):** same as adult, up to 1,000 mg/day, if needed **Child (>15 yr):** same as adult, up to 1,200 mg/day, if needed
Pain associated with **trigeminal neuralgia**	**Adult:** 100 mg bid, followed by increases of 100 mg q12h, up to 1,200 mg/day, if needed; usual maintenance dosage: 400–800 mg/day

ADMINISTRATION/DOSAGE ADJUSTMENTS

Combination therapy	Carbamazepine may be added to an existing anticonvulsant regimen while the dosage of other anticonvulsants is maintained or gradually reduced
Maintenance therapy	Adjust dosage gradually to minimum effective level; for trigeminal neuralgia, reassess dosage at least every 3 mo and discontinue therapy, if possible

CONTRAINDICATIONS

Previous bone-marrow depression	
Hypersensitivity	To carbamazepine or any tricyclic compounds
Concomitant MAO-inhibitor therapy	Wait at least 14 days after discontinuing MAO inhibitors before initiating carbamazepine therapy

WARNINGS/PRECAUTIONS

Unwarranted uses	Carbamazepine should not be used for absence (petit mal) seizures or seizures that are responsive to other anticonvulsants (eg, phenytoin, phenobarbital, or primidone)
Blood dyscrasias	May occur and may be fatal (see ADVERSE REACTIONS). Obtain a CBC prior to treatment, at weekly intervals for first 3 mo of therapy, and monthly thereafter. Instruct patient to discontinue drug and report for examination if early signs (eg, sore throat, fever, purpura) of serious blood disorders develop. Discontinue treatment if evidence of bone-marrow depression (erythrocytes $<4.0 \times 10^6/mm^3$, hematocrit <32%, hemoglobin <11 g/dl, leukocytes $<4{,}000/mm^3$, platelets $<100{,}000/mm^3$, reticulocytes <0.3% [$20{,}000/mm^3$], serum iron >150 μg/dl) develops. Perform a bone marrow aspiration and trephine biopsy if necessary.
Mental impairment, reflex-slowing	Performance of potentially hazardous tasks may be impaired; caution patients accordingly
Latent psychoses	May be activated
Elderly patients	May become agitated or confused
Eye changes	May occur; perform baseline and periodic eye examinations, including slit-lamp examination, funduscopy, and tonometry
Hepatic dysfunction	May occur; perform baseline and periodic liver-function tests, especially in patients with hepatic disease. Discontinue therapy if hepatic disease is activated or aggravated.
Renal dysfunction	May occur; baseline and periodic complete urinalyses and BUN determinations are recommended
Special-risk patients	Use with caution in patients with cardiac, hepatic, or renal damage, increased intraocular pressure, or a history of drug-induced hematological reactions, and in those who have had interrupted courses of carbamazepine therapy
Abrupt discontinuation of therapy	May precipitate seizures of status epilepticus

Table continued on following page

TEGRETOL continued

ADVERSE REACTIONS	Frequent reactions are italicized
Central nervous system and neuromuscular	*Dizziness, drowsiness, unsteadiness,* incoordination, confusion, headache, fatigue, speech disturbances, abnormal involuntary movements, peripheral neuritis, paresthesias, depression with agitation, talkativeness, tinnitus, hyperacusis, aching joints and muscles, leg cramps
Gastrointestinal	*Nausea, vomiting,* gastric distress, abdominal pain, diarrhea, constipation, anorexia, dry mouth and pharynx, glossitis, stomatitis
Hematological	Aplastic anemia, leukopenia, agranulocytosis, eosinophilia, leukocytosis, thrombocytopenia, purpura
Genitourinary	Urinary frequency, acute urinary retention, oliguria with hypertenion, renal failure, azotemia, impotence
Ophthalmic	Blurred vision, visual hallucinations, transient diplopia, oculomotor disturbances, nystagmus; scattered, punctate cortical lens opacities and conjunctivitis (causal relationship not established)
Dermatological	Pruritic and erythematous rashes, urticaria, Stevens-Johnson syndrome, photosensitivity, altered pigmentation, exfoliative dermatitis, alopecia, erythema multiforme and nodosum, aggravation of disseminated lupus erythematosus
Cardiovascular	Congestive heart failure, aggravation of hypertension, hypotension, syncope and collapse, edema, primary thrombophlebitis, recurrence of thrombophlebitis, aggravation of coronary-artery disease, adenopathy or lymphadenopathy, arrhythmias, AV block, myocardial infarction; cerebral arterial insufficiency with paralysis (causal relationship not established)
Other	Diaphoresis, fever, chills, inappropriate secretion of antidiuretic hormone syndrome, altered thyroid function,[1] cholestatic and hepatocellular jaundice

OVERDOSAGE	
Signs and symptoms	Dizziness, ataxia, drowsiness, stupor, nausea, vomiting, restlessness, agitation, disorientation, tremor, involuntary movements, opisthotonus, slowed or hyperactive abnormal reflexes, mydriasis, nystagmus, flushing, cyanosis, urinary retention, hypotension or hypertension, coma, leukocytosis, reduced leukocyte count, glycosuria, acetonuria, dysrhythmias
Treatment	Empty stomach by induction of emesis or gastric lavage. Treat symptomatically and monitor vital signs and ECG. Treat hyperirritability with parenteral barbiturates, unless MAO inhibitors have been taken in overdosage or within 1 wk, and have equipment available for artificial ventilation and resuscitation. Muscular hypertonus in children may be treated with paraldehyde. Treat shock with IV fluids, oxygen, corticosteroids, and other supportive measures.

DRUG INTERACTIONS	
Oral contraceptives	⇧ Risk of pregnancy and breakthrough bleeding
MAO inhibitors	Hyperpyrexia, excitability, seizures

ALTERED LABORATORY VALUES	
Blood/serum values	⇧ BUN ⇩ Thyroid-function values Abnormal liver-function tests
Urinary values	⇧ Albumin ⇧ Glucose

Use in children

See INDICATIONS; general guidelines not established for use in children < 6 yr of age

Use in pregnancy or nursing mothers

An increased incidence of birth defects may be associated with the use of anticonvulsants during pregnancy. Teratogenicity, including kinked ribs, cleft palate, and other anomalies, has been demonstrated in rats. However, discontinuation of therapy may be considered only if removal of the drug does not pose any serious risk, such as the precipitation of status epilepticus with hypoxia in patients with serious convulsive disorders. Patient should stop nursing if drug is prescribed.

[1]Combination therapy

TRIDIONE (Trimethadione) Abbott

Caps: 300 mg **Tabs (chewable):** 150 mg **Sol:** 40 mg/ml (1.2 g/fl oz)

INDICATIONS	ORAL DOSAGE
Absence (petit mal) seizures in patients refractory to less toxic anticonvulsants	**Adult:** 900 mg to start, followed by weekly increases of 300 mg/day, if needed, until optimal clinical response is achieved; usual maintenance dosage: 300–600 mg tid or qid **Child:** 300–900 mg/day in 3–4 equally divided doses

CONTRAINDICATIONS

Hypersensitivity to trimethadione

WARNINGS/PRECAUTIONS

Medical supervision	Patient must be carefully supervised, especially during 1st yr of therapy, because of possibility of serious side effects
Exfoliative dermatitis, severe erythema multiforme	May develop; discontinue therapy at first sign of even mild skin rash and reinstitute therapy (cautiously) only after rash has cleared completely
Blood dyscrasias	May occur and may be fatal (see ADVERSE REACTIONS); obtain baseline and monthly CBC and instruct patient to report early signs (eg, sore throat, fever, malaise, bruises, petechiae, epistaxis) of infection or bleeding tendency. Discontinue therapy if blood count is markedly depressed or neutrophil count drops to 2,500/mm³ or less. Do not use ordinarily in patients with severe blood dyscrasias.
Hepatic impairment	May occur; perform baseline and liver function tests and discontinue if jaundice or other signs of hepatic dysfunction occur. Do not use ordinarily in patients with severe hepatic impairment.
Nephrosis	May occur and may be fatal; perform urinalysis prior to initiating therapy and at monthly intervals thereafter. Withdraw drug if persistent or increasing albuminuria or other significant renal abnormality occurs. Do not use ordinarily in patients with severe renal dysfunction.
Visual disturbances	May occur; use with caution in patients with diseases of the retina or optic nerve. Hemeralopia may be reversed by dosage reduction. Discontinue drug if scotomata occur.
Systemic lupus erythematosus	May occur; discontinue therapy if lupus-like manifestations occur
Lymphadenopathies	May occur, simulating malignant lymphoma; discontinue therapy if lymph-node enlargement occurs
Myasthenia gravis-like syndrome	May occur with chronic use; discontinue therapy if suggestive symptoms occur
Drugs with similar side effects	Should be avoided or used with extreme caution during therapy
Abrupt discontinuation of therapy	May precipitate petit mal status; if abrupt withdrawal is required (eg, because of serious effects), substitute another anticonvulsant

ADVERSE REACTIONS

Gastrointestinal	Nausea, vomiting, abdominal pain, gastric distress, anorexia, weight loss
Central nervous system and neuromuscular	Drowsiness, fatigue, malaise, insomnia, vertigo, headache, paresthesias, grand mal seizures, increased irritability, personality changes
Hematological	Neutropenia, leukopenia, eosinophilia, thrombocytopenia, pancytopenia, agranulocytosis, hypoplastic anemia, fatal aplastic anemia, bleeding gums, epistaxis, petechial hemorrhage, vaginal bleeding
Dermatological	Acneform or morbilliform rash progressing to exfoliative dermatitis or severe erythema multiforme; alopecia
Ophthalmic	Hemeralopia, photophobia, diplopia, retinal hemorrhage
Hypersensitivity	Pruritus associated with lymphadenopathy and hepatosplenomegaly
Other	Hiccoughs, blood-pressure changes, fatal nephrosis, hepatitis (rare), lupus erythematosus, lymphadenopathies simulating malignant lymphoma, myasthenia gravis-like syndrome

OVERDOSAGE

Signs and symptoms	Drowsiness, nausea, dizziness, ataxia, and visual disturbances, followed by coma in cases of massive ingestion
Treatment	Induce emesis or perform gastric lavage to empty stomach. Institute general supportive measures and monitor vital signs. Alkalinization of the urine may increase metabolite excretion. Following recovery, obtain a CBC and evaluate hepatic and renal function.

Table continued on following page

TRIDONE continued

DRUG INTERACTIONS

Tricyclic antidepressants (high doses), antipsychotics (high doses)	Seizures
Mephenytoin	Aplastic anemia

ALTERED LABORATORY VALUES

Urinary values	⇧ Albumin

No clinically significant alterations in blood/serum values occur at therapeutic dosages

Use in children

See INDICATIONS

Use in pregnancy or nursing mothers

An increased incidence of birth defects may be associated with the use of trimethadione during pregnancy. Administer to women of childbearing potential only if essential to management of seizures; effective contraception should be used and, if patient becomes pregnant, termination of pregnancy should be considered. Maternal ingestion of anticonvulsants may cause neonatal hemorrhage (usually within 24 h of birth) due to a coagulation defect. Administer prophylactic vitamin K to mother 1 mo prior to and during delivery, and to infant IV immediately after birth. The safety of trimethadione during lactation has not been established.

ZARONTIN (Ethosuximide) Parke-Davis

Caps: 250 mg **Syrup:** 50 mg/ml

INDICATIONS	ORAL DOSAGE
Absence (petit mal) seizures	**Adult:** 500 mg/day to start, followed by increases of 250 mg/day every 4–7 days until optimal clinical response is achieved, up to 1.5 g/day div **Child (3–6 yr):** 250 mg/day to start, followed by increases of 250 mg/day every 4–7 days until optimal clinical response is achieved, up to 1.5 g/day div; normal optimal dosage: 20 mg/kg/day **Child (>6 yr):** same as adult

ADMINISTRATION/DOSAGE ADJUSTMENTS

Combination therapy	Ethosuximide may be combined with other anticonvulsants when other forms of epilepsy coexist with the absence (petit mal) form; titrate dosages gradually
Dosages exceeding 1.5 g/day	Should be administered only under the strictest medical supervision

CONTRAINDICATIONS

Hypersensitivity to succinimides

WARNINGS/PRECAUTIONS

Blood dyscrasias	May occur and may be fatal; obtain blood counts periodically
Hepatic or renal impairment	May occur; administer with extreme caution to patients with known hepatic or renal disease. Perform a urinalysis and obtain liver-function studies periodically in all patients.
Mental impairment, reflex-slowing	Performance of potentially hazardous tasks may be impaired; caution patients accordingly
Grand mal seizures	May be precipitated when ethosuximide is used alone in patients with mixed types of epilepsy
Abrupt discontinuation of therapy	May precipitate absence (petit mal) status

ADVERSE REACTIONS

	Frequent reactions are italicized
Gastrointestinal	*Anorexia, vague gastric upset, nausea, vomiting, cramps, epigastric and abdominal pain, diarrhea,* swelling of the tongue, hypertrophy
Hematological	Leukopenia, agranulocytosis, pancytopenia, aplastic anemia, eosinophilia
Central nervous system	Drowsiness, headache, dizziness, euphoria, hiccoughs, irritability, hyperactivity, lethargy, fatigue, ataxia, sleep disturbances, night terrors, poor concentration, aggressiveness; paranoid psychosis and depression with overt suicidal tendencies (rare)
Dermatological	Urticaria, Stevens-Johnson syndrome, pruritic erythematous rash, hirsutism
Other	Myopia, vaginal bleeding, systemic lupus erythematosus

OVERDOSAGE

Signs and symptoms	See ADVERSE REACTIONS
Treatment	Induce emesis or perform gastric lavage to empty stomach. Treat symptomatically and institute supportive measures, as required.

DRUG INTERACTIONS

Tricyclic antidepressants (high doses), antipsychotics (high doses)	Seizures

ALTERED LABORATORY VALUES

No clinically significant alterations in blood/serum or urinary values occur at therapeutic dosages

Use in children

See INDICATIONS; general guidelines not established for use in children under 5 yr of age

Use in pregnancy or nursing mothers

An increased incidence of birth defects may be associated with the use of anticonvulsants during pregnancy. However, discontinuation of therapy may be considered only if removal of the drug does not pose any serious risk, such as the precipitation of status epilepticus with hypoxia in patients with serious convulsive disorders. The safety of ethosuximide during lactation has not been established.

Vitamin and Mineral Supplements

More than any other aspect of human health, the area of nutrition is clouded by misconceptions, myths, fads, and incomplete knowledge. Although deficiency diseases such as pellagra and scurvy have all but disappeared from the United States, and Americans enjoy unparalleled variety and abundance of foods, millions remain convinced that somehow their diets are faulty or inadequate. As a result, they spend more than $350 million a year on a variety of vitamin, mineral, and other nutritional supplements, and an additional $500 million on so-called health foods.

In prehistoric times, when early man spent most of his time in quest of food, food magic flourished. He understood that to live, he must eat, but he did not understand how the roots, berries, meat and other substances he consumed imparted strength and essential energy. Today, although we know a good deal about the roles of various nutrients in human health, large numbers of Americans are still convinced that certain foods are almost magical.

Through the ages, certain foods have been regarded as possessing extraordinary qualities. Garlic, for example, has been credited with everything from giving extra strength (for this purpose, the Egyptians fed large quantities of it to the slaves building the pyramids) to warding off the plague and evil spirits. It is still regarded by many as capable of controlling high blood pressure and preventing or curing other disease—all suppositions that defy scientific proof. For centuries, yogurt has been considered capable of imparting health and longevity—again, a belief that still persists among many Americans despite a lack of supporting evidence. While food is essential to maintain health and life itself, it is important to remember that no single food or nutrient has extraordinary medicinal qualities.

RECOMMENDED DIETARY ALLOWANCES

In all, more than fifty different nutrients, in addition to water, have been identified. These various nutrients fall into five general catagories: proteins, carbohydrates, fats, vitamins, and minerals. The Food and Nutrition Board of the National Research Council has established Recommended Dietary Allowances (RDAs) for at least sixteen of these (Table 1). These RDAs are calculated for healthy persons of different ages; individual needs may vary, however, especially among persons with certain diseases, such as cancer or diabetes. Even so, the RDAs are a good guide as to how much of the various nutrients should be consumed daily.

Unfortunately, many persons believe that when it comes to vitamins and minerals, the more the better. Megavitamin therapy—the consumption of therapeutic pharmacological doses of nutrients that far exceed the RDAs—has become increasingly popular in recent years. There is no evidence that megavitamins are beneficial for a healthy person; indeed, they may be harmful in some circumstances. In many instances, the body will simply excrete the excess nutrient in the urine, as is the case with megadoses of vitamin C. (Even so, there is some evidence that large amounts of vitamin C may harm the kidneys.) Other nutrients, such as the fat-soluble vitamins A and D, and minerals such as iron and calcium, are stored in the body, presenting a danger of a toxic accumulation. Therefore, megadoses of vitamins should be treated like any other drugs, and used only under the supervision of a physician.

WHO NEEDS NUTRITIONAL SUPPLEMENTS?

For most healthy persons, a normal diet that includes a variety of foods will provide adequate nutrition without additional supplements. Of course, many considerations other than nutritional value go into individual food choices. Taste, the eating habits of family and friends, cost, and convenience are a few factors affecting food selection.

To help persons achieve a balanced diet and yet allow for personal food choices, the Harvard University Department of Nutrition devised the Basic Four Food Groups in the mid-1960s. These classifications are still considered valid, even though some convenience and processed foods are difficult to classify, or may fall into several groups. The Basic Four, with recommended numbers of servings per day, are:

- Meat, poultry, fish, dried peas, legumes, and other high-protein foods: two servings.
- Milk, cheese, and other dairy foods: two servings.
- Fruits and vegetables: four servings.
- Cereals and breads: four servings.

To ensure maximum nutrient content, foods

Table 1: RECOMMENDED DIETARY ALLOWANCES, REVISED 1980

	Age years	Weight kg	Weight lbs	Vitamin A IU	Vitamin D IU	Vitamin E IU	Ascorbic Acid (C) mg	Folacin µg	Niacin (B_3) mg	Riboflavin (B_2) mg	Thiamine (B_1) mg	Pyridoxine HCl (B_6) mg	Cyanocobalamin (B_{12}) µg	Calcium mg	Phosphorus mg	Iodine µg	Iron mg	Magnesium mg	Zinc mg
Infants	0.0–0.5	6	13	2,100	400	4	35	30	6	0.4	0.3	0.3	0.5	360	240	40	10	50	3
	0.5–1.0	9	20	2,000	400	6	35	45	8	0.6	0.5	0.6	1.5	540	360	50	15	70	5
Children	1–3	13	29	2,000	400	7	45	100	9	0.8	0.7	0.9	2.0	800	800	70	15	150	10
	4–6	20	44	2,500	400	9	45	200	11	1.0	0.9	1.3	2.5	800	800	90	10	200	10
	7–10	28	62	3,500	400	10	45	300	16	1.4	1.2	1.6	3.0	800	800	120	10	250	10
Males	11–14	45	99	5,000	400	12	50	400	18	1.6	1.4	1.8	3.0	1,200	1,200	150	18	350	15
	15–18	66	145	5,000	400	15	60	400	18	1.7	1.4	2.0	3.0	1,200	1,200	150	18	400	15
	19–22	70	154	5,000	300	15	60	400	19	1.7	1.5	2.2	3.0	800	800	150	10	350	15
	23–50	70	154	5,000	200	15	60	400	18	1.6	1.4	2.2	3.0	800	800	150	10	350	15
	51+	70	154	5,000	200	15	60	400	16	1.4	1.2	2.2	3.0	800	800	150	10	350	15
Females	11–14	46	101	4,000	400	12	50	400	15	1.3	1.1	1.8	3.0	1,200	1,200	150	18	300	15
	15–18	55	120	4,000	400	12	60	400	14	1.3	1.1	2.0	3.0	1,200	1,200	150	18	300	15
	19–22	55	120	4,000	300	12	60	400	14	1.3	1.1	2.0	3.0	800	800	150	18	300	15
	23–50	55	120	4,000	200	12	60	400	13	1.2	1.0	2.0	3.0	800	800	150	18	300	15
	51+	55	120	4,000	200	12	60	400	13	1.2	1.0	2.0	3.0	800	800	150	10	300	15
Pregnancy				+1,000	+200	+3	+20	+400	+2	+0.3	+0.4	+0.6	+1.0	+400	+400	+25	†	+150	+5
Lactation				+2,000	+200	+4	+40	+100	+5	+0.5	+0.5	+0.5	+1.0	+400	+400	+50	‡	+150	+10

† This increased requirement cannot be met by ordinary diets; therefore, the use of 30 to 60 mg of supplemental iron is recommended.
‡ Same requirement as for nonpregnant women, but continue supplementation for 2 to 3 months after parturition.
Reproduced from *Recommended Dietary Allowances*, 9th ed., with the permission of the National Academy of Sciences, Washington, D.C., 1980.

should be fresh or lightly processed, whenever possible. For example, whole-grain cereals and breads contain a greater number of different nutrients than enriched white bread; an orange or orange juice will have more nutrients than an orange-flavored drink that is high only in vitamin C.

ESSENTIAL NUTRIENTS AND THEIR FUNCTION

Certain vitamins and minerals are essential for specific body functions. A vitamin is defined as a chemical derived from foods (although some can now be synthesized artificially) that is necessary for normal growth, development, or body function, as well as for prevention of deficiency diseases. Minerals are inorganic chemicals, such as iron, sodium, and calcium, that also are essential to maintaining certain body functions. Table 2 lists the major vitamins and minerals with their functions, signs of deficiency, and sources.

For persons who feel that their diets may not provide adequate amounts of the various essential vitamins and minerals, or who would like extra nutritional insurance, there are a number of multiple vitamin and mineral preparations. These are generally regarded as safe for most people, and carry few if any adverse reactions. In addition, special supplements may be recommended for infants, whose diets may be low in certain nutrients; older persons, whose food intake may be limited to only a few foods; rapidly growing adolescents; and persons with certain diseases. Women who have heavy menstrual periods may require extra iron supplements, and women who are pregnant or nursing also may need nutritional supplements. Extra calcium is sometimes recommended for women approaching menopause, especially if their intake of milk and other calcium-rich dairy products is limited.

A number of drugs may alter the body's utilization of certain vitamins and minerals. By the same token, some nutrients interfere with the action of certain drugs. Examples include the potassium depletion sometimes seen in persons using thiazide diuretics to treat hypertension; the increased need for B vitamins among women using certain oral contraceptives; and the interference of calcium with the action of tetracyclines. Problems can often be avoided by informing one's physican of any vitamin supplements one may be taking whenever a drug is prescribed.

IN CONCLUSION

The vast majority of Americans can easily obtain adequate nutrients by eating a varied diet that includes the recommended number of daily servings from the Basic Four Food Groups. In some instances, additional nutritional supplements may be indicated, but a physician should be consulted before taking large therapeutic doses of any vitamin or mineral.

Several hundred nonprescription vitamin and mineral supplements are available. The following charts cover representative products. Those that are available only by prescription, such as the potassium supplements, are listed separately. Other prescription multipurpose supplements are included in the overall chart, but are indicated by the Rx (prescription) symbol.

Table 2: MAJOR ESSENTIAL NUTRIENTS, THEIR FUNCTIONS, AND SOURCES

Nutrient	Functions and Precautions	Sources
Vitamin A (Retinol)	Needed to maintain eye, skin, and nerve function. Deficiency manifested by night blindness, corneal lesions, skin, and nerve disorders. Toxic in high doses.	Liver, egg yolk, butter, fortified margarine, whole milk, dark green leafy vegetables, deep yellow vegetables and fruits, tomatoes.
Vitamin D	Needed to metabolize and retain calcium and phosphorus. Deficiency manifested by rickets and other bone disorders. Toxic in large amounts.	Liver, oily saltwater fish, fortified milk, exposure to sunlight.
Vitamin E	Believed essential for normal reproduction.	Whole-grain cereals (particularly the oils), eggs, fish, meats, and liver.
Vitamin K	Needed to regulate clotting of blood.	Green leafy vegetables, pork, liver, eggs.
Vitamin C (Ascorbic acid)	Needed in metabolism of proteins; enhances iron absorption; essential for healthy skin, blood vessels, connective tissues, gums, and other body structures.	Citrus fruits, strawberries, melons, minimally cooked vegetables, especially broccoli, peppers, brussels sprouts, cabbage, tomatoes, potatoes, and other greens.
Vitamin B_1 (Thiamin)	Needed for carbohydrate metabolism. Deficiency manifested by beriberi.	**Pork, organ meats, yeast, eggs, green leafy vegetables, whole or enriched cereals and breads, berries, nuts, and legumes.**
Vitamin B_2 (Riboflavin)	Essential for electron transport and cell growth. Deficiency is rare, and manifested by dermatitis and other skin disorders.	Organ meats, milk, cheese, meats, eggs, green leafy vegetables, whole grains, legumes.
Niacin (Nicotinic acid)	Essential for utilization of major nutrients, electrolyte transport, enzyme production and function. Deficiency manifested by pellagra.	Liver, meats, fish, whole-grain and enriched cereals and breads, nuts, peanut butter, dried peas and beans.
Vitamin B_6 (Pyridoxine hydrochloride)	Needed for protein metabolism, enzymatic reactions, fat and carbohydrate metabolism.	Liver, meats, whole-grain cereals, soybeans, peanuts, corn, bananas, avocados, potatoes.
Vitamin B_{12} (Cyanocobalamin)	**Acts with folic acid in various cellular activities; involved in fat and carbohydrate metabolism, nucleic acid synthesis, and enzyme function. Deficiency manifested by pernicious anemia.**	Organ meats, meat, fish, whole milk.
Folic acid	Needed for metabolism, nucleic acid synthesis, production of red blood cells. Deficiency manifested by anemia.	Liver, dark grean leafy vegetables, asparagus, lima beans, kidney, nuts, whole-grain cereals, lentils, and oranges.
Pantothenic acid	Needed for enzyme function and metabolism, antibody production; also has possible role in brain function. Deficiency characterized by torpor, depression, cardiovascular instability, muscle weakness, abdominal pain, movement disorder, increased susceptibility to infections.	Organ meats, egg yolk, peanuts, cabbage, broccoli, cauliflower, whole grains, cereal brans, and many other plant and animal sources.
Biotin	Acts as coenzyme in metabolic functions. Deficiency manifested by dermatitis, loss of appetite, muscle pain, insomnia, slight anemia.	Organ meats, peanuts, egg yolk, cauliflower, mushrooms, chocolate. Also produced by intestinal flora.
Calcium	**Essential for building and maintaining bones and teeth, blood clotting, maintaining cellular integrity, heart and muscle function. Dietary deficiency unknown; stores may be depleted by kidney and other diseases. Excessive calcium intake can be toxic.**	Milk and other dairy products, egg yolk, shellfish, canned sardines and salmon (with bones), soybeans, dark green vegetables such as broccoli, kale, and mustard greens.
Phosphorus	**Acts with calcium to harden bones and teeth, essential for most metabolic processes, maintenance of blood chemistry, transport of fatty acids, normal growth and development, and other functions.**	Meats, fish, poultry, eggs, milk, cheese, legumes, and other high-protein foods.

Table 2: MAJOR ESSENTIAL NUTRIENTS, THEIR FUNCTIONS, AND SOURCES continued

Nutrient	Functions and Precautions	Sources
Iron	Component of hemoglobin and myoglobin (blood cells); essential in oxygen transport function of blood. Deficiency manifested by anemia. Iron overload may lead to liver failure, heart attack, and death.	Liver, kidney, heart, lean meats, shellfish, egg yolk, dried beans and other legumes, dried fruits, nuts, green leafy vegetables, dark molasses, whole-grain and enriched cereals and breads.
Potassium	Essential for muscle function and excitability of nerve tissue. Deficiency manifested by nervous irritability, mental disorientation, irregular heart beat. Potassium overload can be life-threatening.	Oranges, tomatoes, bananas, peanuts, legumes, dried apricots, peaches, and other dried fruits.
Zinc	Needed for normal growth of children, wound healing, taste, smell, and appetite function.	Eggs, herring, liver, meats, fish, nuts, legumes, whole-grain breads and cereals, yeast, oysters, and peanut butter.

Note: Other trace elements considered essential to human health include copper, selenium, iodine, fluorine, chromium, manganese, magnesium, molybdenum, and cobalt. All are widely distributed in the diet, and deficiency states are rare. Sodium (salt) is also an essential mineral, but is found in many foods, and deficiency is not a problem in the United States.

KAOCHLOR 10% LIQUID (Potassium chloride) **Warren-Teed**

Liq: 1.5 g (20 mEq)/15 ml (15 ml, 4 fl oz, 1 pt, 1 gal)

KAOCHLOR-EFF (Potassium chloride, potassium citrate, potassium bicarbonate, and betaine hydrochloride) **Warren-Teed**

Effervescent tabs: 0.60 g potassium chloride, 0.20 g potassium citrate, 1.00 g potassium bicarbonate, and 1.84 g betaine hydrochloride (20 mEq each of potassium and chloride) *sugar-free*

KAOCHLOR S-F 10% LIQUID (Potassium chloride) **Warren-Teed**

Liq: 1.5 g (20 mEq)/15 ml (15 ml, 4 fl oz, 1 pt, 1 gal) *sugar-free*

INDICATIONS	ORAL DOSAGE
Hypokalemia and metabolic acidosis; digitalis intoxication	**Adult:** 15 ml (1 tbsp) or 1 tab diluted or dissolved in 3 oz or more of water or other liquid 2–5 times/day (40–100 mEq/day)
Prevention of potassium depletion when dietary potassium intake is inadequate in patients receiving digitalis and diuretics for congestive heart failure, diuretics for hypertension or hepatic cirrhosis with ascites, or corticosteroids, and in patients with hyperaldosteronism and normal renal function, the nephrotic syndrome, and certain diarrheal states	**Adult:** 15 ml (1 tbsp) or 1 tab diluted or dissolved in 3 oz or more of water or other liquid qd (20 mEq/day)

CONTRAINDICATIONS

Hyperkalemia	Further elevation of serum potassium level may produce cardiac arrest

WARNINGS/PRECAUTIONS

Chronic renal disease or impaired potassium excretion	Asymptomatic hyperkalemia may rapidly develop, leading to cardiac arrest and death; carefully monitor serum potassium level and adjust dosage as needed
Concomitant metabolic acidosis	Should be treated with an alkalizing potassium salt, such as potassium bicarbonate, citrate, acetate, or gluconate
Total body potassium stores	May not be accurately reflected by serum potassium levels; monitor acid-base status, serum electrolytes, ECG, and clinical status, particularly in patients with cardiac or renal disease or in the presence of acidosis

ADVERSE REACTIONS — Frequent reactions are italicized

Gastrointestinal	*Nausea, vomiting, diarrhea, abdominal discomfort,* obstruction, bleeding, perforation
Other	Hyperkalemia

OVERDOSAGE

Signs and symptoms	Hyperkalemia, ECG changes (peaked T waves, ST-segment depression, loss of P wave, prolongation of Q-T interval, widening and slurring of QRS complex), paresthesias of the extremities, muscle weakness, heaviness, flaccid paralysis, listlessness, mental confusion, peripheral vascular collapse with fall in blood pressure, cardiac arrhythmias, and heart block
Treatment	Discontinue medication and eliminate potassium-rich foods and drugs and use of potassium-sparing diuretics. Administer over a period of 1 h 300–500 ml of 10% dextrose containing 10–20 units of insulin per liter of solution. Correct acidosis, if present, with IV sodium bicarbonate. Use of sodium or ammonium cation exchange resins, hemodialysis, and/or peritoneal dialysis may be needed (ammonium compounds should not be used in patients with hepatic cirrhosis). If patient is receiving digitalis, too rapid lowering of the serum potassium level may result in digitalis toxicity.

DRUG INTERACTIONS

Blood from blood bank, potassium-sparing diuretics, low-salt milk, potassium-containing medications, salt substitutes	⇧ Serum potassium level
Sodium cycle exchange resins, glucose-insulin infusions, sodium bicarbonate, laxatives	⇩ Serum potassium level

Table continued on following page

KAOCHLOR continued

ALTERED LABORATORY VALUES

Blood/serum values	⇧ Potassium
Urinary values	⇧ Potassium

Use in children
General guidelines not established

Use in pregnancy or nursing mothers
General guidelines not established

KAON-CL TABS/KAON-CL 20% (Potassium chloride) Warren-Teed

Tabs (slow rel): 500 mg (6.67 mEq) **Liq:** 3 g (40 mEq)/15 ml(15 ml, 4 fl oz, 1 pt, 1 gal) *sugar-free*

INDICATIONS	ORAL DOSAGE
Hypokalemia with or without metabolic acidosis; **digitalis intoxication; hypokalemic familial periodic paralysis; hypokalemia secondary to diuretic therapy** of essential hypertension when dietary supplementation alone is inadequate	**Adult:** 2–5 tabs tid or 15–37.5 ml (1–2½ tbsp) in 6 oz or more of water per tbsp qd (40–100 mEq/day); some patients may require higher doses
Prevention of potassium depletion when dietary potassium intake is inadequate in patients receiving digitalis and diuretics for congestive heart failure or diuretics for hepatic cirrhosis with ascites, and in patients with hyperaldosteronism and normal renal function, potassium-wasting nephropathies, and certain diarrheal states	**Adult:** 1 tab tid or 7.5 ml (½ tbsp) in 6 oz or more of water qd (20 mEq/day)

ADMINISTRATION/DOSAGE ADJUSTMENTS

GI irritation	Nausea, vomiting, abdominal discomfort, and diarrhea may ocur; do not administer Kaon-CL 20% full strength

CONTRAINDICATIONS

Hyperkalemia	Further elevation of serum potassium level may produce cardiac arrest
Esophageal compression due to left-atrial enlargement	Esophageal ulceration may occur
GI motility problems or obstruction	Use a liquid preparation for potassium supplementation if tablet passage through the GI tract is likely to be delayed or arrested

WARNINGS/PRECAUTIONS

Chronic renal disease or impaired potassium excretion	Asymptomatic hyperkalemia may develop, leading to cardiac arrest and death; carefully monitor serum potassium level and adjust dosage as needed
GI obstruction, hemorrhage, or perforation	Stenotic and/or ulcerative small-bowel lesions and death may occur with tablets because of a high local concentration of potassium ion near the bowel wall; discontinue medication immediately if severe vomiting, abdominal pain, distention, or GI bleeding occurs. Use of slow-release tablets should be reserved for patients who cannot tolerate or refuse to take liquid or effervescent preparations or when a compliance problem exists.
Concomitant metabolic acidosis	Should be treated with an alkalizing potassium salt, such as potassium bicarbonate, citrate, acetate, or gluconate
Total body potassium stores	May not be accurately reflected by serum potassium levels; monitor acid-base status, serum electrolytes, ECG, and clinical status, particularly in patients with cardiac or renal disease or in the presence of acidosis

ADVERSE REACTIONS

Frequent reactions are italicized

Gastrointestinal	*Nausea, vomiting, abdominal discomfort, diarrhea,* obstruction, bleeding, perforation
Other	Hyperkalemia

OVERDOSAGE

Signs and symptoms	Hyperkalemia, ECG changes (peaked T waves, ST-segment depression, loss of P wave, prolongation of Q-T interval, widening and slurring of QRS complex), paresthesias of the extremities, muscle weakness, heaviness, flaccid paralysis, listlessness, mental confusion, peripheral vascular collapse with fall in blood pressure, cardiac arrhythmias, and heart block
Treatment	Discontinue medication and eliminate potassium-rich foods and drugs and use of potassium-sparing diuretics. Administer over a period of 1 h 300–500 ml of 10% dextrose containing 10–20 units of insulin per liter of solution. Correct acidosis, if present, with IV sodium bicarbonate. Use of sodium or ammonium cation exchange resins, hemodialysis, and/or peritoneal dialysis may be needed (ammonium compounds should not be used in patients with hepatic cirrhosis). If patient is receiving digitalis, too rapid lowering of the serum potassium level may result in digitalis toxicity.

Table continued on following page

DRUG INTERACTIONS

Blood from blood bank, potassium-sparing diuretics, low-salt milk, potassium-containing medications, salt substitutes	⇧ Serum potassium level
Sodium cycle exchange resins, glucose-insulin infusions, sodium bicarbonate, laxatives	⇩ Serum potassium level

ALTERED LABORATORY VALUES

Blood/serum values	⇧ Potassium
Urinary values	⇧ Potassium

Use in children

General guidelines not established

Use in pregnancy or nursing mothers

General guidelines not established

KAON ELIXIR (Potassium gluconate) Warren-Teed

Elixir: 4.68 g (20 mEq)/15 ml (15 ml, 4 fl oz, 1 pt, 1 gal) *sugar-free*

INDICATIONS	ORAL DOSAGE
Hypokalemia and metabolic acidosis; digitalis intoxication	**Adult:** 15 ml (1 tbsp) in 1 oz or more of water or other liquid 2-5 times/day (40-100 mEq/day)
Prevention of potassium depletion when dietary potassium intake is inadequate in patients receiving digitalis and diuretics for congestive heart failure, diuretics for hypertension or hepatic cirrhosis with ascites, or corticosteroids, and in patients with hyperaldosteronism and normal renal function, the nephrotic syndrome, and certain diarrheal states	**Adult:** 15 ml (1 tbsp) in 1 oz or more of water or other liquid qd (20 mEq/day)

KAON TABLETS (Potassium gluconate) Warren-Teed

Tabs: 1.17 g (5 mEq)

INDICATIONS	ORAL DOSAGE
Prevention and treatment of **hypokalemia** secondary to diuretic or corticosteroid therapy **Cardiac arrhythmias** caused by digitalis intoxication	**Adult:** 2 tabs qid after meals and at bedtime (40 mEq/day)

CONTRAINDICATIONS

Severe renal impairment with oliguria or azotemia ●

Untreated Addison's disease ●

Adynamia episodica hereditaria ●

Acute dehydration ●

Heat cramps ●

Hyperkalemia ●

WARNINGS/PRECAUTIONS

Monitoring of therapy	Since the amount of potassium deficiency or daily dosage needed for replacement is not accurately known, frequently check patient's clinical status and periodically monitor ECG and/or serum potassium level, especially in the presence of cardiac or renal disease or acidosis
Chronic renal disease or impaired potassium excretion	Asymptomatic hyperkalemia may rapidly develop, leading to cardiac arrest and death; carefully monitor serum potassium level and adjust dosage as needed
GI obstruction, hemorrhage, or perforation	Stenotic and/or ulcerative small-bowel lesions and death may occur with tablets because of a high local concentration of potassium ion near the bowel wall; discontinue medication immediately if abdominal pain, distention, nausea, vomiting, or GI bleeding occurs. Coated potassium tablets should be used only when adequate dietary supplementation is impractical.
Hypochloremic alkalosis	May occur, especially in hypokalemic patients on salt-free diets, requiring chloride, as well as potassium, supplementation

ADVERSE REACTIONS

Gastrointestinal	Nausea, vomiting, abdominal discomfort, diarrhea

OVERDOSAGE

Signs and symptoms	Hyperkalmeia, ECG changes (peaked T waves, ST-segment depression, loss of P wave, prolongation of Q-T interval, widening and slurring of QRS complex), paresthesias of the extremities, muscle weakness, heaviness, flaccid paralysis, listlessness, mental confusion, peripheral vascular collapse with fall in blood pressure, cardiac arrhythmias, and heart block
Treatment	Discontinue medication and eliminate potassium-rich foods and drugs and use of potassium-sparing diuretics. Administer over a period of 1 h 300-500 ml of 10% dextrose containing 10-20 units of insulin per liter of solution. Correct acidosis, if present, with IV sodium bicarbonate. Use of sodium or ammonium cation exchange resins, hemodialysis, and/or peritoneal dialysis may be needed (ammonium compounds should not be used in patients with hepatic cirrhosis). If patient is receiving digitalis, too rapid lowering of the serum potassium level may result in digitalis toxicity.

Table continued on following page

KAON ELIXIR/KAON TABLETS continued

DRUG INTERACTIONS

Blood from blood bank, potassium-sparing diuretics, low-salt milk, potassium-containing medications, salt substitutes	⇧ Serum potassium level
Sodium cycle exchange resins, glucose-insulin infusions, sodium bicarbonate, laxatives	⇩ Serum potassium level

ALTERED LABORATORY VALUES

Blood/serum values	⇧ Potassium
Urinary values	⇧ Potassium

Use in children

General guidelines not established

Use in pregnancy or nursing mothers

General guidelines not established

KAY CIEL (Potassium chloride) Berlex

Elixir: 1.5 g (20 mEq)/15 ml (118, 473, 3,785 ml)[1] **Powder:** 1.5 g (20 mEq) per packet *sugar-free*

INDICATIONS

Prevention and treatment of **potassium deficiency** caused by thiazide diuretic or corticosteroid therapy, digitalis intoxication, low dietary intake of potassium, or as a result of vomiting or diarrhea, or for correction of associated hypochloremic alkalosis

ORAL DOSAGE

Adult: 15 ml (1 tbsp) or 1.5 g (1 packet) in 4 oz of cold water or fruit juice bid, preferably after meals (40 mEq/day)

CONTRAINDICATIONS

- Impaired renal function ●
- Untreated Addison's disease ●
- Dehydration ●
- Heat cramps ●
- Hyperkalemia ●

WARNINGS/PRECAUTIONS

Monitoring of therapy	Potassium supplementation should be done with caution, with dosage adjusted to meet individual requirements; frequently check patient's clinical status and periodically monitor ECG and/or serum potassium level, especially in the presence of cardiac disease
Hypokalemia	Frequently associated hypochloremic alkalosis should be corrected
GI injury	Caution patients to adhere to dilution instructions to avoid injury

ADVERSE REACTIONS

Gastrointestinal	Nausea, vomiting, abdominal discomfort, diarrhea

OVERDOSAGE

Signs and symptoms	Hyperkalemia, ECG changes (peaked T waves, ST-segment depression, loss of P wave, prolongation of Q-T interval, widening and slurring of QRS complex), paresthesias of the extremities, muscle weakness, heaviness, flaccid paralysis, listlessness, mental confusion, peripheral vascular collapse with fall in blood pressure, cardiac arrhythmias, and heart block
Treatment	Discontinue medication and eliminate potassium-rich foods and drugs and use of potassium-sparing diuretics. Administer over a period of 1 h 300-500 ml of 10% dextrose containing 10-20 units of insulin per liter of solution. Correct acidosis, if present, with IV sodium bicarbonate. Use of sodium or ammonium cation exchange resins, hemodialysis, and/or peritoneal dialysis may be needed (ammonium compounds should not be used in patients with hepatic cirrhosis). If patient is receiving digitalis, too rapid lowering of the serum potassium level may result in digitalis toxicity.

DRUG INTERACTIONS

Blood from blood bank, potassium-sparing diuretics, low-salt milk, potassium-containing medications, salt substitutes	⇧ Serum potassium level
Sodium cycle exchange resins, glucose-insulin infusions, sodium bicarbonate, laxatives	⇩ Serum potassium level

ALTERED LABORATORY VALUES

Blood/serum values	⇧ Potassium
Urinary values	⇧ Potassium

Use in children

General guidelines not established

Use in pregnancy or nursing mothers

General guidelines not established

[1]Contains 4% alcohol

K-LOR (Potassium chloride) Abbott

Powder: 1.125 g (15 mEq), 1.5 g (20 mEq) per packet

INDICATIONS

Prevention and treatment of **hypochloremic alkalosis** and **hypokalemia** caused by diarrhea, vomiting, decreased potassium intake, increased renal excretion of potassium (eg, due to acidosis, diuresis, or adrenocortical hyperactivity), administration of exogenous adrenocortical steroids, injection of potassium-free fluids, and increased glucose uptake

ORAL DOSAGE

Adult: 1 K-Lor 15-mEq packet dissolved in 3 oz or more of cold water or juice 2–5 times/day after meals (30–75 mEq/day) or 1 K-Lor 20-mEq packet dissolved in 4 oz or more of cold water or juice 1–4 times/day after meals (20–80 mEq/day)

CONTRAINDICATIONS

Severe renal impairment with oliguria or azotemia ●

Acute dehydration ●

Patients receiving potassium-sparing agents ●

Untreated Addison's disease ●

Heat cramps ●

Adynamia episodica hereditaria ●

Hyperkalemia ●

WARNINGS/PRECAUTIONS

Special-risk patients	Use with caution in the presence of cardiac disease and systemic acidosis
Monitoring of therapy	Since dietary or daily amount of potassium-supplement need is not accurately known, check patient's clinical status frequently, and monitor ECG and/or serum potassium levels periodically

ADVERSE REACTIONS

Gastrointestinal	Abdominal discomfort, nausea, vomiting, diarrhea

OVERDOSAGE

Signs and symptoms	Hyperkalemia, ECG changes (peaked T waves, ST-segment depression, loss of P wave, prolongation of Q-T interval, widening and slurring of QRS complex), paresthesias of the extremities, muscle weakness, heaviness, flaccid paralysis, listlessness, mental confusion, peripheral vascular collapse with fall in blood pressure, cardiac arrhythmias, and heart block
Treatment	Discontinue medication and eliminate potassium-rich foods and drugs and use of potassium-sparing diuretics. Administer over a period of 1 h 300-500 ml of 10% dextrose containing 10–20 units of insulin per liter of solution. Correct acidosis, if present, with IV sodium bicarbonate. Use of sodium or ammonium cation exchange resins, hemodialysis, and/or peritoneal dialysis may be needed (ammonium compounds should not be used in patients with hepatic cirrhosis). If patient is receiving digitalis, too rapid lowering of the serum potassium level may result in digitalis toxicity.

DRUG INTERACTIONS

Blood from blood bank, potassium-sparing diuretics, low-salt milk, potassium-containing medications, salt substitutes	⇧ Serum potassium level
Sodium cycle exchange resins, glucose-insulin infusions, sodium bicarbonate, laxatives	⇩ Serum potassium level

ALTERED LABORATORY VALUES

Blood/serum values	⇧ Potassium
Urinary values	⇧ Potassium

Use in children

General guidelines not established

Use in pregnancy or nursing mothers

General guidelines not established

KLORVESS 10% LIQUID (Potassium chloride) Dorsey

Liq: 1.5 g (20 mEq)/15 ml (15 ml, 4 fl oz, 1 pt, 1 gal)

KLORVESS EFFERVESCENT TABLETS, GRANULES (Potassium chloride, potassium bicarbonate, and L-lysine monohydrochloride) Dorsey

Effervescent tabs, granules (per packet): 1.125 g potassium chloride, 0.5 g potassium bicarbonate, and 0.913 g L-lysine monohydrochloride (20 mEq each of potassium and chloride) *sugar-free*

INDICATIONS	ORAL DOSAGE
Prevention and treatment of **potassium depletion and hypokalemic-hypochloremic alkalosis**	**Adult:** 15 ml (1 tbsp) or 1 tab or packet completely diluted or dissolved in 3–4 oz of water bid to qid, ingested slowly with or immediately after meals (40–80 mEq/day)

CONTRAINDICATIONS

Severe renal impairment with azotemia or oliguria ●

Untreated Addison's disease ●

Familial periodic paralysis ●

Acute dehydration ●

Heat cramps ●

Hyperkalemia ●

Concomitant use of aldosterone-inhibiting or potassium-sparing diuretics ●

WARNINGS/PRECAUTIONS

GI irritation	Caution patient to adhere to dilution instructions to avoid injury
Monitoring of therapy	Since the extent of potassium deficiency cannot be determined accurately, use with caution and periodically monitor patient's clincial status, serum electrolytes, and ECG, particularly if the patient has cardiac disease or is receiving digitalis

ADVERSE REACTIONS

Gastrointestinal	Nausea, vomiting, abdominal discomfort, diarrhea

OVERDOSAGE

Signs and symptoms	Hyperkalemia, ECG changes (peaked T waves, ST-segment depression, loss of P wave, prolongation of Q-T interval, widening and slurring of QRS complex), paresthesias of the extremities, muscle weakness, heaviness, flaccid paralysis, listlessness, mental confusion, peripheral vascular collapse with fall in blood pressure, cardiac arrhythmias, and heart block
Treatment	Discontinue medication and eliminate potassium-rich foods and drugs and use of potassium-sparing diuretics. Administer over a period of 1 h 300–500 ml of 10% dextrose containing 10–20 units of insulin per liter of solution. Correct acidosis, if present, with IV sodium bicarbonate. Use of sodium or ammonium cation exchange resins, hemodialysis, and/or peritoneal dialysis may be needed (ammonium compounds should not be used in patients with hepatic cirrhosis). If patient is receiving digitalis, too rapid lowering of the serum potassium level may result in digitalis toxicity.

DRUG INTERACTIONS

Blood from blood bank, potassium-sparing diuretics, low-salt milk, potassium-containing medications, salt substitutes	⇧ Serum potassium level
Sodium cycle exchange resins, glucose-insulin infusions, sodium bicarbonate, laxatives	⇩ Serum potassium level

ALTERED LABORATORY VALUES

Blood/serum values	⇧ Potassium
Urinary values	⇧ Potassium

Use in children

General guidelines not established

Use in pregnancy or nursing mothers

General guidelines not established

KLOTRIX (Potassium chloride) Mead Johnson

Tabs (slow rel): 750 mg (10 mEq)

INDICATIONS	ORAL DOSAGE
Hypokalemia with or without metabolic acidosis; **digitalis intoxication; hypokalemic familial periodic paralysis; hypokalemia secondary to diuretic therapy** of essential hypertension when dietary supplementation alone is inadequate	**Adult:** 4–8 tabs (40–80 mEq)/day; tablets must be swallowed whole and never crushed or chewed
Prevention of potassium depletion when dietary potassium intake is inadequate in patients receiving digitalis and diuretics for congestive heart failure or diuretics for hepatic cirrhosis with ascites, and in patients with hyperaldosteronism and normal renal function, potassium-wasting nephropathies, and certain diarrheal states	**Adult:** 2 tabs (20 mEq)/day; tablets must be swallowed whole and never crushed or chewed

ADMINISTRATION/DOSAGE ADJUSTMENTS

GI irritation	Nausea, vomiting, abdominal discomfort, and diarrhea may occur; reduce dose or instruct patient to take dose with meals

CONTRAINDICATIONS

Hyperkalemia	Further elevation of serum potassium level may produce cardiac arrest
Esophageal compression due to left-atrial enlargement	Esophageal ulceration may occur
GI motility problems or obstruction	Use a liquid preparation for potassium supplementation if tablet passage through the GI tract is likely to be delayed or arrested

WARNINGS/PRECAUTIONS

Chronic renal or impaired potassium excretion	Asymptomatic hyperkalemia may develop, leading to cardiac arrest and death; carefully monitor serum potassium level and adjust dosage as needed
GI obstruction, hemorrhage, or perforation	Stenotic and/or ulcerative small-bowel lesions and death may occur because of a high local concentration of potassium ion near the bowel wall; discontinue medication immediately if severe vomiting, abdominal pain, distention, or GI bleeding occurs. Use of slow-release tablets should be reserved for patients who cannot tolerate or refuse to take liquid or effervescent preparations or when some other compliance problem exists.
Concomitant metabolic acidosis	Should be treated with an alkalizing potassium salt, such as potassium bicarbonate, citrate, acetate, or gluconate
Total body potassium stores	May not be accurately reflected by serum potassium levels; monitor acid-base status, serum electrolytes, ECG, and clinical status, particularly in patients with cardiac or renal disease or in the presence of acidosis

ADVERSE REACTIONS

Frequent reactions are italicized

Gastrointestinal	*Nausea, vomiting, abdominal discomfort, diarrhea,* obstruction, bleeding, ulceration, perforation (see WARNINGS/PRECAUTIONS)
Other	Hyperkalemia, skin rash (rare)

OVERDOSAGE

Signs and symptoms	Hyperkalemia, ECG changes (peaked T waves, ST-segment depression, loss of P wave, prolongation of Q-T interval, widening and slurring of QRS complex), paresthesias of the extremities, muscle weakness, heaviness, flaccid paralysis, listlessness, mental confusion, peripheral vascular collapse with fall in blood pressure, cardiac arrhythmias, and heart block
Treatment	Discontinue medication and eliminate potassium-rich foods and drugs and use of potassium-sparing diuretics. Administer over a period of 1 h 300–500 ml of 10% dextrose containing 10–20 units of insulin per liter of solution. Correct acidosis, if present, with IV sodium bicarbonate. Use of sodium or ammonium cation exchange resins, hemodialysis, and/or peritoneal dialysis may be needed (ammonium compounds should not be used in patients with hepatic cirrhosis). If patient is receiving digitalis, too rapid lowering of the serum potassium level may result in digitalis toxicity.

Table continued on following page

DRUG INTERACTIONS

Blood from blood bank, potassium-sparing diuretics, low-salt milk, potassium-containing medications, salt substitutes	⇧ Serum potassium level
Sodium cycle exchange resins, glucose-insulin infusions, sodium bicarbonate, laxatives	⇩ Serum potassium level

ALTERED LABORATORY VALUES

Blood/serum values	⇧ Potassium
Urinary values	⇧ Potassium

Use in children	**Use in pregnancy or nursing mothers**
General guidelines not established	General guidelines not established

K-LYTE/K-LYTE DS (Potassium bicarbonate and potassium citrate) Mead Johnson

Effervescent tabs: 25 mEq (K-Lyte); 50 mEq (K-Lyte DS)

INDICATIONS	ORAL DOSAGE
Prevention and treatment of **potassium deficiency** caused by thiazide diuretics, corticosteroids, severe vomiting, diarrhea, low dietary intake of potassium, and digitalis intoxication	**Adult:** 1 K-Lyte tab completely dissolved in 3–4 oz of cold or ice water bid to qid or 1 K-Lyte DS tab completely dissolved in 6–8 oz of cold or ice water qd or bid, sipped slowly with meals (50–100 mEq/day)

K-LYTE/CL/K-LYTE/CL 50 (Potassium chloride) Mead Johnson

Effervescent tabs: 1.875 mg (25 mEq), 3.75 mg (50 mEq) | **Powder:** 1.875 mg (25 mEq)/scoop

INDICATIONS	ORAL DOSAGE
Same as K-Lyte	**Adult:** 1 K-Lyte/CL tab completely dissolved in 3–4 oz of cold or ice water or 25 mEq powder (1 scoop) completely dissolved in 6 oz of cold or ice water bid to quid, sipped slowly (5–10 min) with meals (500–100 mEq/day); K-Lyte/CL 50 tabs: 1 tab completely dissolved in 6–8 oz of cold or ice water qd or bid

CONTRAINDICATIONS

Impaired renal function with oliguria or azotemia ●	Hyperkalemia from any cause ●	Addison's disease ●

WARNINGS/PRECAUTIONS

Monitoring of therapy	Since the degree of potassium deficiency may be difficult to determine accurately, use with caution, adjust dosage to individual requirements, and frequently monitor patient's clinical status, ECG and serum potassium level, particularly if the patient is taking digitalis
GI irritation	Caution patients to dissolve each dose completely, as indicated (see ORAL DOSAGE)
Established hypokalemia	Attention should also be paid to other potential electrolyte disturbances

ADVERSE REACTIONS

Gastrointestinal	Nausea, vomiting, diarrhea, abdominal discomfort

OVERDOSAGE

Signs and symptoms	Hyperkalemia, ECG changes (peaked T waves, ST-segment depression, loss of P wave, prolongation of Q-T interval, widening and slurring of QRS complex), paresthesias of the extremities, muscle weakness, heaviness, flaccid paralysis, listlessness, mental confusion, peripheral vascular collapse with fall in blood pressure, cardiac arrhythmias, and heart block
Treatment	Discontinue medication and eliminate potassium-rich foods and drugs and use of potassium-sparing diuretics. Administer over a period of 1 h 300–500 ml of 10% dextrose containing 10-20 units of insulin per liter of solution. Correct acidosis, if present, with IV sodium bicarbonate. Use of sodium or ammonium cation exchange resins, hemodialysis, and/or peritoneal dialysis may be needed (ammonium compounds should not be used in patients with hepatic cirrhosis). If patient is receiving digitalis, too rapid lowering of the serum potassium level may result in digitalis toxicity.

DRUG INTERACTIONS

Blood from blood bank, potassium-sparing diuretics, low-salt milk, potassium-containing medications, salt substitutes	⇧ Serum potassium level
Sodium cycle exchange resins, glucose-insulin infusions, sodium bicarbonate, laxatives	⇩ Serum potassium level

Table continued on following page

ALTERED LABORATORY VALUES

Blood/serum values	⇧ Potassium
Urinary values	⇧ Potassium

Use in children	Use in pregnancy or nursing mothers
General guidelines not established	General guidelines not established

SLOW-K (Potassium chloride) Ciba

Tabs (slow rel): 600 mg (8 mEq)

INDICATIONS	ORAL DOSAGE
Hypokalemia with or without metabolic acidosis; **digitalis intoxication; hypokalemic familial periodic paralysis; hypokalemia secondary to diuretic therapy** of essential hypertension when dietary supplementation alone is inadequate	**Adult:** approximately 5-12 tabs (approximately 40-100 mEq)/day; tablets must be swallowed whole and never crushed or chewed
Prevention of potassium depletion when dietary potassium intake is inadequate in patients receiving digitalis and diuretics for congestive heart failure or diuretics for hepatic cirrhosis with ascites, and in patients with hyperaldosteronism and normal renal function, potassium-wasting nephropathies, and certain diarrheal states	**Adult:** approximately 2-3 tabs (about 20 mEq)/day; tablets must be swallowed whole and never crushed or chewed

ADMINISTRATION/DOSAGE ADJUSTMENTS

GI irritation	Nausea, vomiting, abdominal discomfort, and diarrhea may occur; reduce dose or instruct patient to take dose with meals

CONTRAINDICATIONS

Hyperkalemia	Further elevation of serum potassium may produce cardiac arrest
Esophageal compression due to an enlarged left atrium	Esophageal ulceration may occur
GI motility problems or obstruction	Use liquid preparation for potassium supplementation if tablet passage through the GI tract is likely to be delayed or arrested

WARNINGS/PRECAUTIONS

Chronic renal disease or impaired potassium excretion	Asymptomatic hyperkalemia may develop, leading to cardiac arrest and death; carefully monitor serum potassium level and adjust dosage as needed
GI obstruction, hemorrhage, or perforation	Stenotic and/or ulcerative lesions of the small bowel and death can occur because of the high localized concentration of potassium ion; discontinue medication if severe vomiting, abdominal pain, distention, or gastrointestinal bleeding occurs. Use of slow-release tablets should be reserved for patients who cannot tolerate or refuse to take liquid or effervescent preparations or when some other compliance problem exists.
Concomitant metabolic acidosis	Should be treated with an alkalizing potassium salt, such as potassium bicarbonate, citrate, acetate, or gluconate
Total body potassium stores	May not be accurately reflected by serum potassium levels; monitor acid-base status, serum electrolytes, ECG, and clinical status, particularly in patients with cardiac or renal disease or in the presence of acidosis

ADVERSE REACTIONS

Frequent reactions are italicized

Gastrointestinal	*Nausea, vomiting, abdominal discomfort, diarrhea,* obstruction, bleeding, ulceration, perforation (see WARNINGS/PRECAUTIONS)
Other	Hyperkalemia, skin rash (rare)

OVERDOSAGE

Signs and symptoms	Hyperkalemia, ECG changes (peaked T waves, ST-segment depression, loss of P wave, prolongation of Q-T interval, widening and slurring of QRS complex), paresthesias of the extremities, muscle weakness, heaviness, flaccid paralysis, listlessness, mental confusion, peripheral vascular collapse with fall in blood pressure, cardiac arrhythmias, and heart block
Treatment	Discontinue medication and eliminate potassium-rich foods and drugs and use of potassium-sparing diuretics. Administer over a period of 1 h 300-500 ml of 10% dextrose containing 10-20 units of insulin per liter of solution. Correct acidosis, if present, with IV sodium bicarbonate. Use of sodium or ammonium cation exchange resins, hemodialysis, and/or peritoneal dialysis may be needed (ammonium compounds should not be used in patients with hepatic cirrhosis). If patient is receiving digitalis, too rapid lowering of the serum potassium level may result in digitalis toxicity.

Table continued on following page

SLOW-K continued

DRUG INTERACTIONS

Blood from blood bank, potassium-sparing diuretics, low-salt milk, potassium-containing medications, salt substitutes	⇧ Serum potassium level
Sodium cycle exchange resins, glucose-insulin infusions, sodium bicarbonate, laxatives	⇩ Serum potassium level

ALTERED LABORATORY VALUES

Blood/serum values	⇧ Potassium
Urinary values	⇧ Potassium

Use in children

General guidelines not established

Use in pregnancy or nursing mothers

General guidelines not established

Product (Manufacturer)	Vitamin A (IU)	Vitamin D (IU)	Vitamin C (mg)	Thiamine or B_1 (mg)	Riboflavin or B_2 (mg)	Niacin (mg)
ABDEC BABY DROPS (Parke-Davis)	5,000	400	50	1	1.2	10
ABDEC KAPSEAL (Parke-Davis)	10,000	400	75	5	3.0	25
ABDOL $\overline{c}$ MINERALS (Parke-Davis)	5,000	400	50	2.5	2.5	20
ALLBEE C-800 (Robins)	-	-	800	15	17	100
ALLBEE C-800 PLUS IRON (Robins)	-	-	800	15	17	100
ALLBEE-T (Robins)	-	-	500	15.5	10	100
ALLBEE WITH C (Robins)	-	-	300	15	10.2	50
B COMPLEX TABLETS (Squibb)	-	-	-	7	0.7	9
BECOTIN (Dista)	-	-	-	10	10	50
BECOTIN-T (Dista)	-	-	300	15	10	100
BECOTIN WITH VITAMIN C (Dista)	-	-	150	10	10	50
Rx BEROCCA (Roche)	-	-	500	15	15	100
Rx BEROCCA-C (Roche)	-	-	100	10	10	80
Rx BEROCCA-C 500 (Roche)	-	-	500	10	10	80
CENTRUM (Lederle)	5,000	400	90	2.25	2.6	20
CHOCKS/ CHOCKS-BUGS BUNNY (Miles)	2,500	400	60	1.05	1.2	13.5
CHOCKS PLUS IRON/ CHOCKS-BUGS BUNNY PLUS IRON (Miles)	2,500	400	60	1.05	1.2	13.5
COD LIVER OIL CONCENTRATE CAPSULES (Schering)	10,000	400	-	-	-	-
COD LIVER OIL CONCENTRATE TABLETS (Schering)	4,000	200	-	-	-	-
COD LIVER OIL CONCENTRATE TABLETS WITH VITAMIN C (Schering)	4,000	200	50	-	-	-

[1]Dexpanthenol [2]Dexpanthenol (equivalent to 23.2 mg calcium panthothenate)

	Pyridoxine or B_6 (mg)	Cyanocobalamin or B_{12} (μg)	Folic Acid (μg)	Pantothenic Acid (mg)	Vitamin E (IU)	Calcium (mg)	Iron (mg)	Magnesium (mg)	Potassium (mg)	Zinc (mg)
	1	-	-	5	-	-	-	-	-	-
	1.5	2	-	10	5	-	-	-	-	-
	.5	1	100	2.5	-	44	15	1	5	5
	25	12	-	25	45	-	-	-	-	-
	25	12	400	25	45	-	27	-	-	-
	8.2	5	-	23	-	-	-	-	-	-
	5	-	-	10	-	-	-	-	-	-
	9	2	-	-	-	-	-	-	-	-
	4.1	1	-	25	-	-	-	-	-	-
	5	4	-	20	-	-	-	-	-	-
	4.1	1	-	26	-	-	-	-	-	-
	5	5	500	20	-	-	-	-	-	-
	20	-	-	20[1]	-	-	-	-	-	-
	20	-	-	23.2[2]	-	-	-	-	-	-
	3	9	400	10	30	162	27	100	7.5	22.5
	1.05	4.5	300	-	15	-	-	-	-	-
	1.05	4.5	300	-	15	-	15	-	-	-
	-	-	-	-	-	-	-	-	-	-
	-	-	-	-	-	-	-	-	-	-
	-	-	-	-	-	-	-	-	-	-

Product (Manufacturer)	Vitamin A (IU)	Vitamin D (IU)	Vitamin C (mg)	Thiamine or B_1 (mg)	Riboflavin or B_2 (mg)	Niacin (mg)
EN-CEBRIN (Lilly)	4,000	400	50	3	2	10
Rx EN-CEBRIN F (Lilly)	4,000	400	50	3	2	10
FEMININS (Mead Johnson)	5,000	400	200	1.5	3	15
FEMIRON (J.B. Williams)	-	-	-	-	-	-
FEMIRON WITH VITAMINS (J.B. Williams)	5,000	400	60	1.5	1.7	20
FEOSOL CAPSULES (Menley & James)	-	-	-	-	-	-
FEOSOL ELIXIR (Menley & James)	-	-	-	-	-	-
Rx FEOSOL PLUS (Smith Kline & French)	-	-	50	2	2	20
FEOSOL TABLETS (Menley & James)	-	-	-	-	-	-
FERGON TABLETS (Breon)	-	-	-	-	-	-
FERGON CAPSULES (Breon)	-	-	-	-	-	-
FERGON ELIXIR (Breon)	-	-	-	-	-	-
FERGON PLUS (Breon)	-	-	75	-	-	-
FER-IN-SOL DROPS (Mead Johnson)	-	-	-	-	-	-
FER-IN-SOL SYRUP (Mead Johnson)	-	-	-	-	-	-
FER-IN-SOL CAPSULES (Mead Johnson))	-	-	-	-	-	-
Rx FERO-FOLIC-500 (Abbott)	-	-	500	-	-	-
FERO-GRAD-500 (Abbott)	-	-	500	-	-	-
FERO-GRADUMET (Abbott)	-	-	-	-	-	-
FERRO-SEQUELS (Lederle)	-	-	-	-	-	-
FLINTSTONES (Miles)	2,500	400	60	1.05	1.2	13.5

	Pyridoxine or B_6 (mg)	Cyanocobalamin or B_{12} (μg)	Folic Acid (μg)	Pantothenic Acid (mg)	Vitamin E (IU)	Calcium (mg)	Iron (mg)	Magnesium (mg)	Potassium (mg)	Zinc (mg)
	1.7	5	-	5	-	250	30	5	-	1.5
	2	5	1,000	5	-	250	30	5	-	1.5
	25	10	100	10	10	-	18	-	-	10
	-	-	-	-	-	-	20	-	-	-
	2	6	400	10	15	-	20	-	-	-
	-		-	-	-	-	50	-	-	-
	-	-	-	-	-	-	44	-	-	-
	2	5	400	-	-	-	65	-	-	-
	-	-	-	-	-	-	65	-	-	-
	-	-	-	-	-	-	37	-	-	-
	-	-	-	-	-	-	50	-	-	-
	-	-	-	-	-	-	35	-	-	-
	-	.5	-	-	-	-	58	-	-	-
	-	-	-	-	-	-	15	-	-	-
	-	-	-	-	-	-	18	-	-	-
	-	-	-	-	-	-	60	-	-	-
	-	-	800	-	-	-	105	-	-	-
	-	-	-	-	-	-	105	-	-	-
	-	-	-	-	-	-	105	-	-	-
	-	-	-	-	-	-	50	-	-	-
	1.05	4.5	300	-	15	-	-	-	-	-

Product (Manufacturer)	Vitamin A (IU)	Vitamin D (IU)	Vitamin C (mg)	Thiamine or B_1 (mg)	Riboflavin or B_2 (mg)	Niacin (mg)
FLINTSTONES WITH IRON (Miles)	2,500	400	60	1.05	1.2	13.5
GANATREX (Merrell-National)	5,000	400	60	1.5	1.7	20
GERILETS (Abbott)	5,000	400	90	2.25	2.6	30
GEVRABON (Lederle)	-	-	-	5	2.5	50
GERITOL LIQUID (J.B. Williams)	-	-	-	5	5	100
GERITOL TABLETS (J.B. Williams)	-	-	75	5	5	30
GOLDEN BOUNTY B COMPLEX WITH VITAMIN C (Squibb)	-	-	100	4	4.8	4.7
GOLDEN BOUNTY MULTIVITAMIN SUPPLEMENT WITH IRON (Squibb)	5,000	400	60	1.5	1.7	20
IBERET (Abbott)	-	-	150	6	6	30
IBERET-500 (Abbott)	-	-	500	6	6	30
Rx IBERET-FOLIC-500 (Abbott)	-	-	500	6	6	30
IBERET-LIQUID (Abbott)	-	-	37.5	1.5	1.5	7.5
IBERET-500 LIQUID (Abbott)	-	-	125	1.5	1.5	7.5
INCREMIN (Lederle)	-	-	-	10	-	-
Rx MATERNA 1.60 (Lederle)	8,000	400	120	3	3.4	20
MI-CEBRIN (Dista)	10,000	400	100	10	5	30
MI-CEBRIN-T (Dista)	10,000	400	150	15	10	100
MOL-IRON CAPSULES (Schering)	-	-	-	-	-	-
MOL-IRON TABLETS & LIQUID (Schering)	-	-	-	-	-	-
MOL-IRON WITH VITAMIN C TABLETS (Schering)	-	-	75	-	-	-

	Pyridoxine or B_6 (mg)	Cyanocobalamin or B_{12} (μg)	Folic Acid (μg)	Pantothenic Acid (mg)	Vitamin E (IU)	Calcium (mg)	Iron (mg)	Magnesium (mg)	Potassium (mg)	Zinc (mg)
	1.05	4.5	300	-	15	-	15	-	-	-
	2	6	-	-	30	-	-	-	-	-
	3	9	400	15	45	-	27	-	-	-
	1	1	-	10	-	-	15	2	-	2
	1	1.5	-	4	-	-	100	-	-	-
	.5	3	-	2	-	-	50	-	-	-
	-	25	-	-	-	-	-	-	-	-
	2	6	400	-	30	-	18	-	-	-
	5	25	-	10	-	-	105	-	-	-
	5	25	-	10	-	-	105	-	-	-
	5	25	800	10	-	-	105	-	-	-
	1.25	6.25	-	2.5[2]	-	-	26.25	-	-	-
	1.25	6.25	-	2.5[2]	-	-	26.25	-	-	-
	5	25	-	-	-	-	30	-	-	-
	4	12	1,000	-	30	350	60	100	-	15
	1.7	3	-	10	5.5	-	15	5	-	1.5
	2	7.5	-	10	5.5	-	15	5	-	1.5
	-	-	-	-	-	-	78	-	-	-
	-	-	-	-	-	-	39	-	-	-
	-	-	-	-	-	-	39	-	-	-

Product (Manufacturer)	Vitamin A (IU)	Vitamin D (IU)	Vitamin C (mg)	Thiamine or B_1 (mg)	Riboflavin or B_2 (mg)	Niacin (mg)
MOL-IRON WITH VITAMIN C CAPSULES (Schering)	-	-	150	-	-	-
MYADEC (Parke-Davis)	10,000	400	250	10	10	100
NATABEC KAPSEALS (Parke-Davis)	4,000	400	50	3	2	20
Rx NATABEC KAPSEALS Rx (Parke-Davis)	4,000	400	50	3	2	10
Rx NATAFORT FILMSEAL (Parke-Davis)	6,000	400	120	3	2	20
NATALINS (Mead Johnson)	8,000	400	90	1.7	2	20
Rx NATALINS Rx (Mead Johnson)	8,000	400	90	2.55	3	20
ONE-A-DAY BRAND VITAMINS (Miles)	5,000	400	60	1.5	1.7	20
ONE-A-DAY BRAND VITAMINS PLUS IRON (Miles)	5,000	400	60	1.5	1.7	20
ONE-A-DAY BRAND VITAMINS PLUS MINERALS (Miles)	5,000	400	60	1.5	1.7	20
OPTILETS-500 (Abbott)	10,000	400	500	15	10	100
OPTILETS-M-500 (Abbott)	10,000	400	500	15	10	100
PALS (Bristol-Myers)	3,500	400	60	.8	1.3	14
PALS WITH IRON (Bristol-Myers)	3,500	400	60	.8	1.3	14
Rx POLY-VI-FLOR WITH IRON CHEWABLE TABLETS (Mead Johnson)	2,500	400	60	1.05	1.2	13.5
Rx POLY-VI-FLOR WITH IRON DROPS (Mead Johnson)	1,500	400	35	.5	.6	8
Rx POLY-VI-SOL CHEWABLE TABLETS (Mead Johnson)	2,500	400	60	1.05	1.2	13.5
Rx POLY-VI-SOL WITH IRON CHEWABLE TABLETS (Mead Johnson)	2,500	400	60	1.05	1.2	13.5

Pyridoxine or B_6 (mg)	Cyanocobalamin or B_{12} (μg)	Folic Acid (μg)	Pantothenic Acid (mg)	Vitamin E (IU)	Calcium (mg)	Iron (mg)	Magnesium (mg)	Potassium (mg)	Zinc (mg)
-	-	-	-	-	-	78	-	-	-
5	6	400	20	30	-	20	100	-	20
3	5	-	-	-	600	30	-	-	-
3	5	1,000	-	-	600	30	-	-	-
15	6	1,000	-	30	350	65	100	-	25
4	8	800	-	30	200	45	100	-	-
10	8	1,000	15	30	200	60	100	-	15
2	6	400	-	15	-	-	-	-	-
2	6	400	-	15	-	18	-	-	-
2	6	400	10	15	100	18	100	-	15
5	12	-	20	30	-	-	-	-	-
5	12	-	20	30	-	20	80	-	1.5
1	2.5	50	5	-	-	-	-	-	-
1	2.5	50	5	-	-	12	-	-	-
1.05	4.5	300	-	5	-	12	-	-	-
.4	-	-	-	5	-	10	-	-	-
1.05	4.5	300	-	15	-	-	-	-	-
1.05	4.5	300	-	15	-	12	-	-	-

Product (Manufacturer)	Vitamin A (IU)	Vitamin D (IU)	Vitamin C (mg)	Thiamine or B_1 (mg)	Riboflavin or B_2 (mg)	Niacin (mg)
PRAMET FA (Ross)	4,000	400	100	3	2	10
STRESSCAPS (Lederle)	-	-	300	10	10	100
STRESSTABS 600 (Lederle)	-	-	600	15	15	100
STRESSTABS 600 WITH IRON (Lederle)	-	-	600	15	15	100
STRESSTABS 600 WITH ZINC (Lederle)	-	-	600	20	10	100
STUARTINIC (Stuart)	-	-	500	6	6	20
Rx STUART NATAL 1+1 (Stuart)	8,000	400	90	2.55	3	20
STUART PRENATAL (Stuart)	8,000	400	60	1.7	2	20
SURBEX (Abbott)	-	-	-	6	6	30
SURBEX WITH C (Abbott)	-	-	250	6	6	30
SURBEX-750 WITH IRON (Abbott)	-	-	750	15	15	100
SURBEX-750 WITH ZINC (Abbott)	-	-	750	15	15	100
SURBEX-T (Abbott)	-	-	500	15	10	100
Rx TABRON (Parke-Davis)	-	-	500	6	6	30
THERA-COMBEX H-P (Parke-Davis)	-	-	500	25	15	100
THERAGRAN TABLETS (Squibb)	10,000	400	200	10.3	10	100
THERAGRAN LIQUID (Squibb)	10,000	400	200	10	10	100
Rx THERAGRAN HEMATINIC (Squibb)	8,333	133	100	3.3	3.3	33.3
THERAGRAN-M (Squibb)	10,000	400	200	10.3	10	100
THERAGRAN-2[3] (Squibb)	10,000	400	200	10.3	10	100
Rx TRIHEMIC 600 (Lederle)	-	-	600	-	-	-

[3]Theragran-2 also contains 1.5 mg iodine, 2 mg copper, and 1 mg manganese

Pyridoxine or B_6 (mg)	Cyanocobalamin or B_{12} (μg)	Folic Acid (μg)	Pantothenic Acid (mg)	Vitamin E (IU)	Calcium (mg)	Iron (mg)	Magnesium (mg)	Potassium (mg)	Zinc (mg)
5	3	1,000	92	-	250	60	-	-	-
2	6	-	20	-	-	-	-	-	-
5	12	-	20	30	-	-	-	-	-
25	12	400	20	30	-	27	-	-	-
10	25	400	25	45	-	-	-	-	23.9
1	25	-	10	-	-	100	-	-	-
10	12	1,000	-	30	200	65	100	-	-
4	8	800	-	30	200	60	100	-	-
2.5	5	-	10	-	-	-	-	-	-
2.5	5	-	10	-	-	-	-	-	-
25	12	400	20	30	-	27	-	-	-
20	12	400	20	30	-	-	-	-	22.5
5	10	-	20	-	-	-	-	-	-
5	25	1,000	10	30	-	100	-	-	-
10	5	-	20	-	-	-	-	-	-
4.1	5	-	18.4	15	-	-	-	-	-
4.1	5	-	21.4	-	-	-	-	-	-
3.3	50	330	11.7	5	-	66.7	11.7	-	-
4.1	5	-	18.4	15	-	12	65	-	1.5
4.1	5	-	18.4	15	-	12	-	-	22.5
-	25	1,000	-	30	-	115	-	-	-

Product (Manufacturer)	Vitamin A (IU)	Vitamin D (IU)	Vitamin C (mg)	Thiamine or B_1 (mg)	Riboflavin or B_2 (mg)	Niacin (mg)
Rx **TRINSICON** (Dista)	-	-	75	-	-	-
Rx **TRINSICON M** (Dista)	-	-	75	-	-	-
TRI-VI-SOL DROPS (Mead Johnson)	1,500	400	35	-	-	-
TRI-VI-SOL Tablets (Mead Johnson)	2,500	400	60	-	-	-
TRI-VI-SOL WITH IRON (Mead Johnson)	1,500	400	35	-	-	-
UNICAP (Upjohn)	5,000	400	60	1.5	1.7	20
UNICAP M (Upjohn)	5,000	400	60	1.5	1.7	20
UNICAP PLUS IRON (Upjohn)	5,000	400	60	1.5	1.7	20
UNICAP SENIOR (Upjohn)	5,000	400	60	1.2	1.7	14
UNICAP T (Upjohn)	5,000	400	300	10	10	100
VICON-C (Glaxo)	-	-	300	20	10	100
Rx **VICON FORTE** (Glaxo)	8,000	-	150	10	5	25
VICON PLUS (Glaxo)	4,000	-	150	10	5	25
VI-DAYLIN ADC DROPS (Ross)	1,500	400	35	-	-	-
VI-DAYLIN CHEWABLE (Ross)	2,500	400	60	1.05	1.2	13.5
VI-DAYLIN DROPS (Ross)	1,500	400	35	.5	.6	8
VI-DAYLIN LIQUID (Ross)	2,500	400	60	1.05	1.2	13.5
VI-DAYLIN + IRON ADC DROPS (Ross)	1,500	400	35	-	-	-
VI-DAYLIN + IRON CHEWABLE (Ross)	2,500	400	60	1.05	1.2	13.5
VI-DAYLIN + IRON DROPS (Ross)	1,500	400	35	.5	.6	8
VI-DAYLIN + IRON LIQUID (Ross)	2,500	400	60	1.05	1.2	13.5

	Pyridoxine or B_6 (mg)	Cyanocobalamin or B_{12} (μg)	Folic Acid (μg)	Pantothenic Acid (mg)	Vitamin E (IU)	Calcium (mg)	Iron (mg)	Magnesium (mg)	Potassium (mg)	Zinc (mg)
	-	15	500	-	-	-	110	-	-	-
	-	15	-	-	-	-	110	-	-	-
	-	-	-	-	-	-	-	-	-	-
	-		-	-	-	-	-	-	-	-
	-	-	-	-	-	-	10	-	-	-
	2	6	400	-	15	-	-		-	
	2	6	400	10	15	-	18	-	5	15
	2	6	400	10	15	-	18	-	-	-
	2	6	400	10	15	-	10	-	5	15
	6	18	400	10	15	-	18	-	5	15
	5	-	-	20	-	-	-	70	-	80
	-	10	1,000	10	50	-	-	70	-	80
	2	-	-	10	50	-	-	70	-	80
	-	-	-	-	-	-	-	-	-	-
	1.05	4.5	300	-	15	-	-	-	-	-
	.4	1.5	-	-	5	-	-	-	-	-
	1.05	4.5	-	-	15	-	-	-	-	-
	-	-	-	-	-	-	10	-	-	-
	1.05	4.5	300	-	15	-	-	-	-	-
	.4	1.5	-	-	5	-	10	-	-	-
	1.05	4.5	-	-	15	-	10	-	-	-

Product (Manufacturer)	Vitamin A (IU)	Vitamin D (IU)	Vitamin C (mg)	Thiamine or B_1 (mg)	Riboflavin or B_2 (mg)	Niacin (mg)
Rx VI-DAYLIN W/FLUORIDE CHEWABLE (Ross)	2,500	400	60	1.02	1.2	13.4
VI-DAYLIN/F ADC DROPS (Ross)	1,500	400	35	-	-	-
VI-DAYLIN/F ADC + IRON DROPS (Ross)	1,500	400	35	-	-	-
VI-DAYLIN/F DROPS (Ross)	1,500	400	35	.5	.6	8
Rx VI-DAYLIN/F + IRON CHEWABLE (Ross)	2,500	400	60	1.05	1.2	13.5
Rx VI-DAYLIN/F + IRON DROPS (Ross)	1,500	400	35	.5	.6	8
Z-BEC (Robins)	-	-	600	15	10.2	100

Calcium Supplements

Product (Manufacturer)	Calcium (mg)
Rx Calcium Gluconate (Lilly)	45
Rx Calcium Lactate (Lilly)	42.25
Dibasic calcium phosphate (Lilly)	145
Os-Cal 500	500

	Pyridoxine or B_6 (mg)	Cyanocobalamin or B_{12} (μg)	Folic Acid (μg)	Pantothenic Acid (mg)	Vitamin E (IU)	Calcium (mg)	Iron (mg)	Magnesium (mg)	Potassium (mg)	Zinc (mg)
	1.28	4.5	200	-	15	-	-	-	-	-
	-	-	-	-	-	-	-	-	-	-
	-	-	-	-	-	-	10	-	-	-
	.4	-	-	-	5	-	-	-	-	-
	1.05	4.5	300	-	15	-	12	-	-	-
	.4	1.5	-	-	5	-	10	-	-	-
	10	6	-	25	45	-	-	-	-	22.5

Weight Control

Overweight is by far the most common nutritional disorder in the United States today. About forty million Americans are overweight, and twenty-five million of those are obese, a condition defined as being 20 percent or more above optimum weight, as calculated on standard insurance tables, for a given height, age, sex, and body frame.

CONTRIBUTING FACTORS

In some societies, obesity is a desired state, since it is considered a sign of prosperity and leadership—"if you are fat, you obviously have enough to eat and are in a position where you don't have to work it all off." In most western industrialized societies, however, the opposite ideal prevails, as summed up by the socialite who once quipped: "You can't be too rich or too thin." Why, then, are so many people markedly overweight?

Weight gain is the direct result of consuming more energy (calories) than one expends. Although Americans today eat less than they did in 1900, the more sedentary life-style made possible by modern technology has greatly reduced the amount of caloric energy expended in work and recreation. Despite the current popularity of activities like running and jogging, studies have found that the average American still spends many more hours watching television than engaged in physical activity. As a result, even moderate food consumption can result in an energy imbalance, with the excess calories being stored as adipose or fat tissue.

Although the cause-and-effect aspect of obesity is relatively simple, it is actually a complex, poorly understood phenomenon. Why do some people overeat and become fat while others with a similar background and life-style automatically adjust their food intake appropriately and remain slim? In addition, recent studies have documented a fact that many obese persons have long maintained: Some people can simply consume more food than others without excessive weight gain.

Appetite and satiety are poorly understood mechanisms. Some studies suggest that the appetite center in the hypothalamus, which regulates hunger and satiety, does not function properly at very low levels of activity, implying that persons who are inactive may have difficulty in regulating their food intake. In addition, some persons appear to be more susceptible to food stimuli than others, which may explain why certain persons chronically overeat. Social and economic status also appears to be a factor; in the United States, obesity is more common among the economically and socially disadvantaged.

Heredity and early food conditioning are other factors that may affect weight. Obesity tends to run in families, but this is generally attributed to family eating habits rather than genetic factors. Still, inherited body type does play a role in weight gain—endomorphs, who have a soft, round body type tend to be overweight, while the taller, finer-boned ectomorphs are frequently thin.

Eating habits established in childhood are considered important in determining whether a person will develop later weight problems. Babies who are offered food as a pacifier, even when they may not be hungry, are likely to turn to food throughout their lives whenever they are under stress. Also, research suggests that fat babies produce an abnormal number of fat cells, which remain with them through life. While these fat cells can be "starved" during a period of dieting, their very presence appears to make future weight gain easier than for persons with a normal number of fat cells.

HEALTH RISKS OF OBESITY

Obesity is associated with an increased mortality rate as well as a number of serious health risks, including a higher incidence of diabetes, hypertension, heart attacks, and gallbladder and kidney diseases. Premature death is more common among the obese. The excess weight also contributes to various musculoskeletal disorders, such as arthritis, gout, and back problems. In some diseases, such as adult diabetes or mild hypertension, weight loss is often the only treatment required.

TREATMENT

Dieting has been called the great American obsession; every few months, yet another dieting scheme is introduced. These diets are usually touted as being "painless," and are built around a gimmick, such as rigidity or limitation in food choices (e.g., the grapefruit, Pritikin, or Scarsdale diets); low carbohydrate, high protein intake (e.g., the Stillman or Scarsdale diets); fasting (usually with liquid protein supplements); and a variety of faddist approaches. Although the gimmicks vary, virtually all of these diets embody reduced energy consumption, and if followed, will help most people reduce. The problem, however, is maintaining the weight loss once the diet is stopped and former eating habits are resumed. In addition, some of the dieting schemes may be hazardous to health unless carried out under the supervision of a physician, dietitian, nutritionist, or other trained health professional.

In general, diets that provide fewer than 1,000 calories a day should be supervised by a physician. It also should be emphasized that more lasting results are likely to be obtained from a nutritionally balanced diet that provides for a gradual weight loss of two to three pounds a week, and one that is combined with an attempt to change eating behavior. Regardless of the dieting regimen, to lose a pound of excess weight, caloric intake must be reduced to a level that is less than the amount required to maintain basic body functions added to those expended in physical activity. A pound equals 3,500 calories; to lose a pound a week, daily intake has to be reduced by at least 500 calories below the number needed for normal function. If 1,700 calories are normally required per day, a diet that provides 1,200 should result in a weight loss of a pound a week.

Behavior Modification

Altering one's eating behavior is considered the most difficult part of weight control. Hypnosis, biofeedback, meditation, psychoanalysis, peer support groups, and exercise and health clubs are but a few of the supportive techniques employed by persons who want to succeed in losing weight. More extreme approaches, which are usually reserved for the morbidly obese whose overweight is considered life-threatening, include intestinal bypass surgery and wiring the jaw to prevent chewing.

In general, the best results are achieved by careful self-examination of present eating patterns, and modification of those that contribute to overeating. While this may sound simple, in practice it is often very difficult, because it often means changing long-established habits. Turning to food during periods of stress is an example of an eating pattern established early in life. Many overweight persons share common eating patterns. Many tend to eat very fast, literally gulping down large quantities of food before the appetite center in the hypothalamus has an opportunity to signal satiety. Others feel compelled to eat everything on their plates, and then help themselves to seconds. Frequent snacking on high-calorie, low-nutrition foods, consuming a diet high in fats and sweets, eating all the leftovers to avoid waste, and constant nibbling while watching television or performing routine tasks are still other common eating habits that contribute to weight gain.

Many overweight persons are truly unaware of just how much food they consume in the course of a normal day. Keeping a faithful and accurate food diary is one way of determining just how much food is being consumed, as well as times of day or situations that trigger snacking. Learning portion size and how to calculate calories is another important aspect of dieting. Foods vary tremendously in size—apples, for example, may range from 80 calories for one an average of two inches in diameter to almost 150 for the premium oversized ones. A serving of meat may vary from three or four ounces of lean roast beef to nearly a pound of marbled (high-fat) steak. Most calorie charts specify serving size; using precise measures and a scale will help ensure proper calorie count.

Recognizing hidden sources of calories is also important. Many people, for example, overlook beverages when calculating what they eat. But a twelve-ounce bottle of beer contains 185 calories, an eight-ounce soft drink 105 calories, a scotch and soda 150. Adding cream and two teaspoons of sugar to coffee raises its calorie content from zero to ninety-five. Using artificial sweeteners and low-calorie diet foods is one way to reduce energy consumption.

Drastic change is seldom recommended in framing a weight-control program—once the novelty wears off, it is too easy to revert to old habits and patterns. Instead, commonsense and moderation are more likely to bring success. Examples of commonsense modifications in diet and eating habits include the following:

- Don't eat between meals and don't skip meals.
- Don't "taste" while cooking.
- Don't have tempting high-calorie snack foods handy; instead, keep a supply of raw vegetables and fruits for those times when you feel compelled to eat something.
- Scale down portion size and learn to calculate calories.
- Eat slowly, taking time to chew and savor each bite.
- When eating out, avoid eating the bread and butter, ask for salad dressings to be served on the side, order a baked potato instead of french fries, and have fruit instead of pastry for dessert. Fish or poultry are not as high in calories as the high-fat red meats, unless fried. Order the smaller meat portions; if they are unavailable, ask that half be packed in a carry-home bag.
- Don't feel compelled to eat everything, including the leftovers.
- When possible, turn to low-calorie substitutes, such as skim milk, low-calorie cheeses and spreads, herbs instead of butter for flavoring vegetables, etc.
- Increase your physical activity.
- Drink lots of water.
- Weigh yourself daily and keep a record of gains and losses.
- Avoid eating alone and engage in conversation during meals.

APPETITE-SUPPRESSING DRUGS

Amphetamines and Amphetamine Derivatives

Drugs to suppress the appetite (anorexigenics) are usually reserved for those persons unable to lose weight by dieting alone. A number of prescription and nonprescription agents, as well as low-calorie dietary substitutes, are available. Most of the prescription drugs contain amphetamines, which are derivatives of phentylamine and suppress the appetite by acting as central nervous system stimulants. Routine use of amphetamines, commonly called "uppers," has fallen into disfavor in recent years because of the high potential for drug abuse. Amphetamines also can be habit-forming. Appetite-suppressing drugs that are derived from amphetamines or substances with similar actions include methamphetamine (Desoxyn), benzphetamine (Didrex), dextroamphetamine (Dexedrine), phentermine (Fastin and Ionamin), phenmetrazine (Preludin), diethylpropion (Tenuate and Tepanil), and mazindol (Sanorex). Some drugs are combinations of amphetamines, such as amphetamine and dextroamphetamine (Biphetamine) or dextroamphetamine and amobarbital (Dexamyl).

Other Weight-Loss Drugs

Hormones Another pharmacological approach to weight loss entails giving certain hormones, such as thyroid hormone, to alter metabolism and thereby consume more energy. While this approach may effect weight loss, there is also a very high risk of adverse effects. Therefore, the use of thyroid and other hormones as diet aids is considered medically unsound. In addition, some hormones such as human chorionic growth hormone (HCG), a placental hormone that helps supply energy to the growing fetus, have been promoted as weight-loss drugs, but studies have disproved their value.

Diuretics These agents, which promote weight loss by removing fluids from the body, are sometimes used to achieve dramatic, short-term reduction. However, these effects are temporary and the potential adverse effects of diuretics used for this purpose outweigh their usefulness. Caution should be exercised in taking nonprescription diuretic or "water pills," especially by persons with high blood pressure and heart or kidney diseases.

Laxatives or cathartics Theoretically, certain types of laxatives may promote weight loss by speeding food through the digestive tract and thereby preventing normal absorption. The bulking laxatives, such as bran or Metamucil, are preferable to the laxatives that stimulate the bowel nerves.

Taste alteration Some diet products contain a mild anesthetic such as benzocaine, which temporarily "deadens" the taste buds. The theory is that if taste is altered, people will not be tempted to overeat.

Low-Calorie Substitutes

In addition to appetite suppressants, there are a number of foods and food substitutes that are intended to meet nutritional needs and satisfy hunger, but with fewer calories than regular foods. These range from sugar substitutes and low-calorie meals to the protein supplements that are used in many fasting programs. The latter were introduced in the late 1970s, and although they were originally intended for use in a controlled medical setting, they almost immediately became the newest diet fad. Fasting diets do enable people to lose large amounts of weight in a relatively short time, but if unsupervised, they can lead to very serious medical problems. Several deaths, for example, have been attributed to heart attacks that were a direct result of protein-sparing fasting diets. In some areas, nonprescription liquid protein supplements are still available, but they should not be used in a fasting regimen except under the direct supervision of a physician.

IN CONCLUSION

Weight loss and control is an often frustrating seesaw process for millions of Americans. Although overeating is the major cause of obesity, the reasons why the natural satiety mechanism does not prevent this from happening are, in many cases, unknown. In others, a complex interplay of social, psychological, and physiological factors are involved.

The preferred approach to weight loss is dietary modification coupled with changes in eating behavior to prevent weight regain. In patients unable to lose weight through this method or for the morbidly obese, drugs that suppress the appetite may be recommended. The following drug charts cover the major prescription appetite suppressants as well as nonprescription diet aids, artificial sweeteners, and low-calorie and dietary supplements. Bulk-producing laxatives are included in the section on *Constipation* (pages 264–274).

BIPHETAMINE (Amphetamine and dextroamphetamine) Pennwalt

Caps: 12.5, 20 mg *C-II*

INDICATIONS	ORAL DOSAGE
Exogenous obesity, as a short-term adjunct to caloric restriction	**Adult:** 7.5–20 mg qd 10–14 h before bedtime

CONTRAINDICATIONS

Hypersensitivity or idiosyncratic reaction to sympathomimetic amines ●

Concomitant or recent MAO-inhibitor therapy ●

History of drug abuse ●

Advanced arteriosclerosis ●

Symptomatic cardiovascular disease ●

Moderate to severe hypertension ●

Hyperthyroidism ●

Glaucoma ●

Agitated states ●

WARNINGS/PRECAUTIONS

Habit-forming	Psychic and/or physical dependence and tolerance may develop, especially in addiction-prone individuals; if tolerance develops, discontinue drug rather than increase recommended dosage
Mental impairment	Performance of potentially hazardous activities may be impaired; caution patients accordingly
Abrupt discontinuation of therapy	May result in extreme fatigue and mental depression after prolonged use of high doses; changes in sleep EEG may also occur
Hypertension	May worsen; use with caution in patients with even mild hypertension
Insulin requirements	May be altered by drug directly and by reduction in caloric intake
MAO-inhibitor therapy	Wait at least 14 days after discontinuing amphetamine and dextroamphetamine before instituting MAO inhibitors (see DRUG INTERACTIONS)

ADVERSE REACTIONS

Cardiovascular	Palpitations, tachycardia, increase in blood pressure
Central nervous system	Overstimulation, restlessness, dizziness, insomnia, euphoria, dysphoria, tremor, headache, psychotic episodes (rare)
Gastrointestinal	Dry mouth, unpleasant taste, diarrhea, constipation, other disturbances
Allergic	Urticaria
Endocrinological	Impotence, altered libido

OVERDOSAGE

Signs and symptoms	Restlessness, tremor, hyperreflexia, tachypnea, confusion, assaultiveness, hallucinations, panic states, fatigue, depression, arrhythmias, hypertension, hypotension, circulatory collapse, nausea, vomiting, diarrhea, abdominal cramps, convulsions, coma
Treatment	Treat symptomatically. Use gastric lavage to empty stomach; administer barbiturates, as required; for acute, severe hypertension, administer IV phentolamine; acidify urine to increase drug excretion.

DRUG INTERACTIONS

MAO inhibitors	Hypertensive crisis
Urinary alkalizers	⇧ Sympathomimetic effect
Phenothiazines, tricyclic antidepressants	⇩ Sympathomimetic effect
Guanethidine	⇩ Antihypertensive effect

ALTERED LABORATORY VALUES

No clinically significant alterations in blood/serum or urinary values occur at therapeutic dosages

Use in children

Not recommended for children less than 12 yr of age

Use in pregnancy or nursing mothers

Safe use not established during pregnancy; general guidelines not established for use in nursing mothers

DESOXYN (Methamphetamine hydrochloride) Abbott

Tabs: 2.5, 5 mg **Tabs (sust rel):** 5, 10, 15 mg *C-II*

INDICATIONS	ORAL DOSAGE
Exogenous obesity, as a short-term adjunct to caloric restriction	**Adult:** 2.5–5 mg tid, 30 min before each meal; sust-rel tabs: 10–15 mg qd in AM
Attention deficit disorder	**Child (>6 yr):** 2.5–5 mg qd or bid to start, followed by weekly increments of 5 mg/day until optimal response is achieved; usual maintenance dosage: 20–25 mg/day

ADMINISTRATION/DOSAGE ADJUSTMENTS

Initial therapy	Initiate therapy for behavioral syndrome only after a complete, thorough history and an appropriate evaluation of the child have been compiled; sustained-release tablets should not be used to initiate therapy or for maintenance until conventionally titrated daily dose equals or exceeds dose provided by sustained-release tablet
Duration of therapy for behavioral syndrome in children	Interrupt therapy occasionally to determine whether symptoms recur, warranting continued administration

CONTRAINDICATIONS

Hypersensitivity or idiosyncratic reaction to sympathomimetic amines ●	Advanced arteriosclerosis ●	Glaucoma ●
Concomitant or recent MAO-inhibitor therapy ●	Hyperthyroidism ●	Symptomatic cardiovascular disease ●
History of drug abuse ●	Moderate to severe hypertension ●	Agitated states ●

WARNINGS/PRECAUTIONS

Habit-forming	Psychic and/or physical dependence and tolerance may develop, especially in addiction-prone individuals; if tolerance develops, discontinue drug rather than increase recommended dosage
Mental impairment	Performance of potentially hazardous activities may be impaired; caution patients accordingly
Abrupt discontinuation of therapy	May result in extreme fatigue and mental depression after prolonged use of high doses
Hypertension	May worsen; use with caution in patients with even mild hypertension
Insulin requirements	May be altered by drug directly and by reduction in caloric intake
MAO-inhibitor therapy	Wait at least 14 days after discontinuing methamphetamine before instituting MAO inhibitors (see DRUG INTERACTIONS)
Inappropriate use	Methamphetamine should not be used to combat fatigue or to replace rest in normal individuals
Tartrazine sensitivity	Presence of FD&C Yellow No. 5 (tartrazine) in 15-mg sustained-release tablets may cause allergic-type reactions, including bronchial asthma, in susceptible individuals

ADVERSE REACTIONS

Cardiovascular	Palpitations, tachycardia, hypertension
Central nervous system	Overstimulation, restlessness, dizziness, insomnia, euphoria, dysphoria, tremor, headache, psychotic episodes (rare)
Gastrointestinal	Dry mouth, unpleasant taste, diarrhea, constipation, other disturbances
Dermatological	Urticaria
Endocrinological	Impotence, altered libido

Table continued on following page

DESOXYN continued

OVERDOSAGE

Signs and symptoms	Restlessness, tremor, hyperreflexia, tachypnea, confusion, assaultiveness, hallucinations, panic states, fatigue, depression, arrhythmias, hypertension, hypotension, circulatory collapse, nausea, vomiting, diarrhea, abdominal cramps, convulsions, coma
Treatment	Treat symptomatically. Use gastric lavage to empty stomach; administer barbiturates, as required; for acute, severe hypertension, administer IV phentolamine; acidify urine to increase drug excretion.

DRUG INTERACTIONS

MAO inhibitors	Hypertensive crisis
Urinary alkalizers	⇧ Sympathomimetic effect
Guanethidine	⇩ Antihypertensive effect
Phenothiazines; tricyclic antidepressants	⇩ Sympathomimetic effect

ALTERED LABORATORY VALUES

No clinically significant alterations in blood/serum or urinary values occur at therapeutic dosages

Use in children

See INDICATIONS; prescription of this drug for attention deficit disorder should take into account the chronicity and severity of the child's symptoms and their appropriateness for his or her age. Methamphetamine should not be used in children under 6 yr of age or, in most cases, for symptoms associated with acute stress reactions. The drug is also not recommended as an anorectic agent for use in children less than 12 yr of age; in psychotic children, use of methamphetamine may exacerbate symptoms of behavior disturbance and thought disorder. Growth should be monitored during treatment. Long-term effects in children are unknown.

Use in pregnancy or nursing mothers

Safe use not established during pregnancy; general guidelines not established for use in nursing mothers

DEXEDRINE (Dextroamphetamine sulfate) **Smith Kline & French**

Tabs: 5 mg **Caps (sust rel):** 5, 10, 15 mg **Elixir:** 5 mg/5 ml *C-II*

INDICATIONS	ORAL DOSAGE
Exogenous obesity, as a short-term adjunct to caloric restriction	**Adult:** 30 mg/day in divided doses of 5–10 mg 30–60 min before meals; sust-rel caps: 10–15 mg qd in AM
Narcolepsy	**Adult:** 5–60 mg/day div **Child (6–12 yr):** 5 mg/day to start, followed by weekly increments of 5 mg/day until optimal response is obtained; sust-rel caps: 5 mg qd, followed by weekly increments of 5 mg/day, where appropriate **Child (>12 yr):** 10 mg/day to start, followed by weekly increments of 10 mg/day until optimal response is obtained; sust-rel caps: 10 mg qd, followed by weekly increments of 10 mg/day, where appropriate
Behavioral syndrome in children	**Child (3–5 yr):** 2.5 mg/day to start, followed by weekly increments of 2.5 mg/day until optimal response is obtained **Child (6–12 yr):** 5 mg qd or bid to start, followed by weekly increments of 5 mg/day until optimal response is obtained; sust-rel caps: 5 mg qd to start, followed by weekly increments of 5 mg/day, where appropriate

ADMINISTRATION/DOSAGE ADJUSTMENTS

Insomnia or anorexia	Dosage should be reduced if bothersome adverse reactions appear; late-evening doses tend to cause insomnia, particularly with sust-rel caps, and should be avoided
Child dosage intervals	With tablets or elixir, give 1st dose on awakening and 1–2 additional doses at intervals of 4–6 h
Duration of therapy for behavioral syndrome in children	Interrupt therapy occasionally to determine whether symptoms recur, warranting continued administration

CONTRAINDICATIONS

Hypersensitivity or idiosyncratic reaction to sympathomimetic amines •	Advanced arteriosclerosis •	Hyperthyroidism •
Concomitant or recent MAO-inhibitor therapy •	Symptomatic cardiovascular disease •	Glaucoma •
History of drug abuse •	Moderate to severe hypertension •	Agitated states •

WARNINGS/PRECAUTIONS

Habit-forming	Psychic and/or physical dependence and tolerance may develop, especially in addiction-prone individuals; if tolerance develops, discontinue drug rather than increase recommended dosage
Mental impairment	Performance of potentially hazardous activities may be impaired; caution patients accordingly
Abrupt discontinuation of therapy	May result in extreme fatigue and mental depression after prolonged use of high doses; changes in sleep EEG may also occur
Hypertension	May worsen; use with caution in patients with even mild hypertension
Insulin requirements	May be altered by drug directly and by reduction in caloric intake
MAO-inhibitor therapy	Wait at least 14 days after discontinuing dextroamphetamine before instituting MAO inhibitors (see DRUG INTERACTIONS)

ADVERSE REACTIONS

Cardiovascular	Palpitations, tachycardia, hypertension
Central nervous system	Overstimulation, restlessness, dizziness, insomnia, euphoria, dyskinesia, dysphoria, tremor, headache, psychotic disturbances (rare)
Gastrointestinal	Dry mouth, unpleasant taste, diarrhea, constipation, anorexia, other disturbances
Dermatological	Urticaria
Endocrinological	Impotence, altered libido, weight loss

Table continued on following page

OVERDOSAGE

Signs and symptoms	Restlessness, tremor, hyperreflexia, rapid respiration, confusion, assaultiveness, hallucinations, panic, fatigue, depression, arrhythmias, hypertension, hypotension, circulatory collapse, nausea, vomiting, diarrhea, abdominal cramps, convulsions, coma, death
Treatment	Empty stomach by gastric lavage. Use saline cathartics to hasten evacuation of sustained-release caps. Administer a barbiturate to provide sedation. Acidify the urine to promote dextroamphetamine sulfate excretion. For acute, severe hypertension, administer IV phentolamine.

DRUG INTERACTIONS

MAO inhibitors	Hypertensive crisis
Urinary alkalizers	⇧ Sympathomimetic effect
Phenothiazines, tricyclic antidepressants	⇩ Sympathomimetic effect
Guanethidine	⇩ Antihypertensive effect

ALTERED LABORATORY VALUES

No clinically significant alterations in blood/serum or urinary values occur at therapeutic dosages

Use in children

See INDICATIONS; prescription of this drug for behavioral syndrome in children should take into account the chronicity and severity of the child's symptoms and their appropriateness for his or her age. Dextroamphetamine should not be used in children under 3 yr of age or, in most cases, for symptoms associated with acute stress reactions. The drug is also not recommended for use as an anorectic in children under 12 yr of age. In psychotic children, use of amphetamines may exacerbate behavior disturbances and thought disorder. Growth should be monitored during treatment. Long-term effects in children are unknown.

Use in pregnancy or nursing mothers

Safe use has not been established. Animal reproductive studies have suggested embryotoxicity and teratogenicity. Drug should not be used by women who are or may become pregnant, especially during 1st trimester, unless potential benefit clearly outweighs possible risk to fetus. General guidelines not established for use in nursing mothers.

DIDREX (Benzphetamine hydrochloride) Upjohn

Tabs: 25, 50 mg *C-III*

INDICATIONS

Exogenous obesity, as a short-term adjunct to caloric restriction

ORAL DOSAGE

Adult: 25–50 mg qd, bid, or tid

ADMINISTRATION/DOSAGE ADJUSTMENTS

Initial therapy	Begin with 25–50 mg qd in AM; adjust dosage in accordance with patient response

CONTRAINDICATIONS

Hypersensitivity or idiosyncratic reaction to sympathomimetic amines ●

Concomitant or recent MAO-inhibitor therapy ●

Concomitant use of other CNS stimulants ●

Advanced arteriosclerosis ●

Symptomatic cardiovascular disease ●

Moderate to severe hypertension ●

Hyperthyroidism ●

Agitated states ●

History of drug abuse ●

WARNINGS/PRECAUTIONS

Drug dependence	Psychic and/or physical dependence may develop, especially in addiction-prone individuals
Abrupt discontinuation of therapy	May result in extreme fatigue and mental depression after prolonged use of high doses; changes in sleep EEG may also occur
Insulin requirements	May be altered by drug directly and by reduction in caloric intake
MAO-inhibitor therapy	Wait at least 14 days after discontinuing benzphetamine before instituting MAO inhibitors (see DRUG INTERACTIONS)
Psychological disturbances	May result from concurrent use of an anorectic agent and restrictive dietary regimen

ADVERSE REACTIONS

Central nervous system	Overstimulation, restlessness, dizziness, insomnia, tremor, headache, psychotic episodes (rare), depression
Gastrointestinal	Various disturbances, nausea, diarrhea, dry mouth, unpleasant taste
Cardiovascular	Palpitations, tachycardia, elevation of blood pressure
Hypersensitivity	Urticaria, other skin reactions
Other	Diaphoresis, altered libido

OVERDOSAGE

Signs and symptoms	See ADVERSE REACTIONS
Treatment	Treat symptomatically. Administer barbiturates, as required. For hypertension, consider a nitrite or a rapidly acting alpha-adrenergic-blocking agent. The value of hemodialysis or peritoneal dialysis is currently unknown.

DRUG INTERACTIONS

General anesthetics	Cardiac arrhythmias
Other CNS stimulants	⇧ CNS stimulation
Guanethidine	⇩ Antihypertensive effect
Hypoglycemics	Altered blood glucose level
MAO inhibitors	Hypertensive crisis
Phenothiazines	⇩ Sympathomimetic effect

ALTERED LABORATORY VALUES

No clinically significant alterations in blood/serum or urinary values occur at therapeutic dosages

Use in children

Not recommended for use in children under 12 yr of age

Use in pregnancy or nursing mothers

Safe use has not been established during pregnancy. Animal reproductive studies have suggested embryotoxicity and teratogenicity. Drug should not be used by women who are or who may become pregnant, especially during 1st trimester, unless potential benefit clearly outweighs possible risk to fetus. General guidelines not established for use in nursing mothers.

ESKATROL (Dextroamphetamine sulfate and prochlorperazine maleate) Smith Kline & French

Caps: (sust rel): 15 mg dextroamphetamine sulfate and 7.5 mg prochlorperazine maleate *C-II*

INDICATIONS	ORAL DOSAGE
Exogenous obesity, as a short-term adjunct to caloric restriction[1]	**Adult:** 1 cap/day in the AM; for appetite control through evening hours, shift dose to midmorning

ADMINISTRATION/DOSAGE ADJUSTMENTS

Tolerance	Anorectics are usually most effective for a period of 4–8 wk; if a longer period of therapy is indicated, discontinue medication for 2–4 wk before reinstituting the regimen

CONTRAINDICATIONS

- Hypersensitivity or idiosyncratic reaction to sympathomimetic amines ●
- History of phenothiazine-induced jaundice or blood dyscrasias ●
- History of drug abuse ●
- Nausea and vomiting associated with intestinal obstruction or brain tumor ●
- Advanced arteriosclerosis ●
- Symptomatic cardiovascular disease ●
- Moderate to severe hypertension ●
- Hyperthyroidism ●
- Agitated states ●
- Bone-marrow depression ●
- Concomitant or recent MAO-inhibitor therapy ●

WARNINGS/PRECAUTIONS

Habit-forming	Psychic and/or physical dependence and tolerance may develop, especially in addiction-prone individuals; if tolerance develops, discontinue drug rather than increase recommended dosage
Mental impairment	Performance of potentially hazardous activities may be impaired; caution patients accordingly
Abrupt discontinuation of therapy	May result in extreme fatigue and mental depression after prolonged use of high doses; changes in sleep EEG may also occur
Hypertension	May worsen; use with caution in patients with even mild hypertension
Insulin requirements	May be altered by drug directly and by reduction in caloric intake
MAO-inhibitor therapy	Wait at least 14 days after discontinuing MAO inhibitors before instituting Eskatrol therapy (see DRUG INTERACTIONS)
Insomnia	May result from late afternoon or evening medication

ADVERSE REACTIONS[2]

Cardiovascular	Palpitations, tachycardia, elevation of blood pressure, hypotension
Central nervous system	Overstimulation, restlessness, dizziness, insomnia, euphoria, dyskinesia, dysphoria, tremor, headache, psychotic disturbances (rare), sedation, tinnitus, vertigo, miosis, lethargy, extrapyramidal or parkinsonian-like symptoms, convulsions, catatonic-like reactions
Gastrointestinal	Dry mouth, unpleasant taste, diarrhea, other disturbances, cholestatic jaundice
Dermatological	Urticaria, rash
Endocrinological	Impotence, altered libido
Hematological	Leukopenia, agranulocytosis
Other	Nasal congestion

[1]Possibly effective
[2]Other adverse reactions have been observed with one or more phenothiazines, including prochlorperazine, and should be considered when phenothiazine compounds are administered (cf Compazine)

Table continued on following page

ESKATROL continued

OVERDOSAGE

Signs and symptoms	*Dextroamphetamine-related effects:* restlessness, dizziness, hyperreflexia, tremor, insomnia, tenseness, irritability, confusion, assaultiveness, hallucinations, panic states, fatigue, depression, chills, pallor, flushing, diaphoresis, palpitations, hypertension, hypotension, headache, extrasystoles and other arrhythmias, anginal pain, circulatory collapse, syncope, nausea, vomiting, diarrhea, abdominal cramps, convulsions, coma; *prochlorperazine-related effects:* extrapyramidal reactions, CNS depression, somnolence, coma, agitation, restlessness, convulsions, fever, hypotension, dry mouth, ileus
Treatment	Empty stomach by gastric lavage. *Do not induce emesis.* Maintain open airway. Administer oral or parenteral barbiturates, as required. To provide a basal level of sedation, administer one or more doses of sodium amobarbital orally or IM. Treat extrapyramidal symptoms with antiparkinsonism drugs, barbiturates, or diphenhydramine. Avoid convulsion-inducing stimulants (eg, pecrotoxin or pentylenetetrazol). For severe hypotension, administer levarterenol or phenylephrine; *do not administer epinephrine.* Provide saline cathartics to hasten evacuation of sustained-released pellets. Dialysis is not helpful in phenothiazine overdosage; the value of hemodialysis and peritoneal dialysis in amphetamine overdosage is currently unknown.

DRUG INTERACTIONS

General anesthetics	⇧ Risk of cardiac arrhythmias
MAO inhibitors	Hypertensive crisis
Other CNS stimulants	⇧ CNS stimulation
Alcohol, anesthetics, narcotics, and other CNS depressants	⇧ CNS depression
Phenothiazines, tricyclic antidepressants	⇩ Sympathomimetic effect
Guanethidine	⇩ Antihypertensive effect
Epinephrine	Severe hypotension
Antacids, antidiarrheal suspensions	⇩ Absorption of prochlorperazine component
Urinary alkalizers	⇩ Excretion of dextroamphetamine component
Anticonvulsants	⇩ Convulsion threshold
Antimuscarinics	⇧ Atropine-like effect
Levodopa	⇩ Antiparkinsonian effect

ALTERED LABORATORY VALUES

Urinary values	⇧ Bilirubin (methodological interference) False-positive or false-negative pregnancy tests

No clinically significant alterations in blood/serum values occur at therapeutic dosages

Use in children	Use in pregnancy or nursing mothers
Not recommended for use in children under 12 yr of age	Safe use has not been established. Animal reproductive studies have suggested embryotoxicity and teratogenicity. Drug should not be used by women who are or may become pregnant, especially during 1st trimester, unless potential benefit clearly outweighs possible risk to fetus. Use in nursing mothers is contraindicated.

FASTIN (Phentermine hydrochloride) Beecham

Caps (sust rel): 30 mg *C-IV*

INDICATIONS

Exogenous obesity, as a short-term adjunct to caloric restriction

ORAL DOSAGE

Adult: 30 mg 2 h after morning meal

CONTRAINDICATIONS

Hypersensitivity or idiosyncratic reaction to sympathomimetic amines ●

Concomitant or recent MAO-inhibitor therapy ●

History of drug abuse ●

Advanced arteriosclerosis ●

Symptomatic cardiovascular disease ●

Moderate to severe hypertension ●

Glaucoma ●

Hyperthyroidism ●

Agitated states ●

WARNINGS/PRECAUTIONS

Habit-forming	Psychic and/or physical dependence and tolerance may develop, especially in addiction-prone individuals; if tolerance develops, discontinue drug rather than increase recommended dosage
Mental impairment	Performance of potentially hazardous activities may be impaired; caution patients accordingly
Abrupt discontinuation of therapy	May result in extreme fatigue and mental depression after prolonged use of high doses; changes in sleep EEG may also occur
Hypertension	May worsen; use with caution in patients with even mild hypertension
Insulin requirements	May be altered by drug directly and by reduction in caloric intake
MAO-inhibitor therapy	Wait at least 14 days after discontinuing phentermine before instituting MAO inhibitors (see DRUG INTERACTIONS)

ADVERSE REACTIONS

Cardiovascular	Palpitations, tachycardia, hypertension
Central nervous system	Overstimulation, restlessness, dizziness, insomnia, euphoria, dysphoria, tremor, headache, psychotic episodes (rare)
Gastrointestinal	Dry mouth, unpleasant taste, diarrhea, constipation, other disturbances
Dermatological	Urticaria
Endocrinological	Impotence, altered libido

OVERDOSAGE

Signs and symptoms	Restlessness, tremor, hyperreflexia, tachypnea, confusion, assaultiveness, hallucinations, panic states, fatigue, depression, arrhythmias, hypertension, hypotension, circulatory collapse, nausea, vomiting, diarrhea, abdominal cramps, convulsions, coma
Treatment	Treat symptomatically; use gastric lavage to empty stomach; administer barbiturates, as required. For acute, severe hypertension, administer IV phentolamine; acidify urine to increase drug excretion.

DRUG INTERACTIONS

MAO inhibitors	Hypertensive crisis
Other CNS stimulants	⇧ CNS stimulation
Phenothiazines	⇩ Sympathomimetic effect
Guanethidine	⇩ Antihypertensive effect

ALTERED LABORATORY VALUES

No clinically significant alterations in blood/serum or urinary values occur at therapeutic dosages

Use in children

Not recommended for use in children under 12 yr of age

Use in pregnancy or nursing mothers

Safe use not established during pregnancy; general guidelines not established for use in nursing mothers

IONAMIN (Phentermine resin) Pennwalt

Caps: 15, 30 mg *C-IV*

INDICATIONS

Exogenous obesity, as a short-term adjunct to caloric restriction

ORAL DOSAGE

Adult: 15–30 mg qd before breakfast or 10–14 h before bedtime

CONTRAINDICATIONS

- Hypersensitivity or idiosyncratic reaction to sympathomimetic amines ●
- Concomitant or recent MAO-inhibitor therapy ●
- History of drug abuse ●
- Advanced arteriosclerosis ●
- Symptomatic cardiovascular disease ●
- Moderate to severe hypotension ●
- Glaucoma ●
- Hyperthyroidism ●
- Agitated states ●

WARNINGS/PRECAUTIONS

Habit-forming	Psychic and/or physical dependence and tolerance may develop, especially in addiction-prone individuals; if tolerance develops, discontinue drug rather than increase recommended dosage
Mental impairment	Performance of potentially hazardous activities may be impaired; caution patients accordingly
Abrupt discontinuation of therapy	May result in extreme fatigue and mental depression after prolonged use of high doses; changes in sleep EEG may also occur
Hypertension	May worsen; use with caution in patients with even mild hypertension
Insulin requirements	May be altered by drug directly and by reduction in caloric intake
MAO-inhibitor therapy	Wait at least 14 days after discontinuing phentermine before instituting MAO inhibitors (see DRUG INTERACTIONS)

ADVERSE REACTIONS

Cardiovascular	Palpitations, tachycardia, hypertension
Central nervous system	Overstimulation, restlessness, dizziness, insomnia, euphoria, dysphoria, tremor, headache, psychotic episodes (rare)
Gastrointestinal	Dry mouth, unpleasant taste, diarrhea, constipation, other disturbances
Dermatological	Urticaria
Endocrinological	Impotence, altered libido

OVERDOSAGE

Signs and symptoms	Restlessness, tremor, hyperreflexia, tachypnea, confusion, assaultiveness, hallucinations, panic states, fatigue, depression, arrhythmias, hypertension, hypotension, circulatory collapse, nausea, vomiting, diarrhea, abdominal cramps, convulsions, coma
Treatment	Treat symptomatically; use gastric lavage to empty stomach; administer barbiturates, as required; for acute, severe hypertension, administer IV phentolamine; acidify urine to increase drug excretion

DRUG INTERACTIONS

MAO inhibitors	Hypertensive crisis
Other CNS stimulants	⇧ CNS stimulation
Phenothiazines	⇩ Sympathomimetic effect
Guanethidine	⇩ Antihypertensive effect

ALTERED LABORATORY VALUES

No clinically significant alterations in blood/serum or urinary values occur at therapeutic dosages

Use in children

Not recommended for use in children under 12 yr of age

Use in pregnancy or nursing mothers

Safe use not established during pregnancy; general guidelines not established for use in nursing mothers

PRELUDIN (Phenmetrazine hydrochloride) **Boehringer Ingelheim**

Tabs: 25 mg **Tabs (sust rel):** 50, 75 mg *C-II*

INDICATIONS	ORAL DOSAGE
Exogenous obesity, as a short-term adjunct to caloric restriction	**Adult:** 25 mg bid or tid 1 h before meals; sust-rel tabs: 50–75 mg qd

ADMINISTRATION/DOSAGE ADJUSTMENTS

Timing of administration	Since sustained-release tabs suppress appetite for approximately 12 h, time of administration should be determined by period of day over which anorectic effect is desired

CONTRAINDICATIONS

Hypersensitivity or idiosyncratic reaction to sympathomimetic amines ●	Advanced arteriosclerosis ●	Hyperthyroidism ●
Concomitant use of CNS stimulants or MAO inhibitors ●	Symptomatic cardiovascular disease ●	Glaucoma ●
History of drug abuse ●	Moderate to severe hypertension ●	Agitated states ●

WARNINGS/PRECAUTIONS

Habit-forming	Psychic and/or physical dependence and tolerance may develop, especially in addiction-prone individuals; if tolerance develops, discontinue drug rather than increase recommended dosage
Mental impairment	Performance of potentially hazardous activities may be impaired; caution patients accordingly
Abrupt discontinuation of therapy	May result in extreme fatigue and mental depression after prolonged use of high doses; changes in sleep EEG may also occur
Hypertension	May worsen; use with caution in patients with even mild hypertension
Insulin requirements	May be altered by drug directly and by reduction in caloric intake
MAO-inhibitor therapy	Wait at least 14 days after discontinuing phenmetrazine before instituting MAO inhibitors (see DRUG INTERACTIONS)
Tartrazine sensitivity	Presence of FD&C Yellow No. 5 (tartrazine) in 75-mg sustained-release tablets may cause allergic-type reactions, including bronchial asthma, in susceptible individuals

ADVERSE REACTIONS

Cardiovascular	Palpitations, tachycardia, increase in blood pressure
Central nervous system	Overstimulation, restlessness, dizziness, insomnia, euphoria, dysphoria, tremor, headache, psychotic disturbances (rare)
Gastrointestinal	Dry mouth, unpleasant taste, diarrhea, constipation, other disturbances
Allergic	Urticaria
Endocrinological	Impotence, altered libido

OVERDOSAGE

Signs and symptoms	Restlessness, tremor, hyperreflexia, rapid respiration, confusion, assaultiveness, hallucinations, panic, fatigue, depression, arrhythmias, hypertension, hypotension, circulatory collapse, nausea, vomiting, diarrhea, abdominal cramps, convulsions, coma, death
Treatment	Empty stomach by gastric lavage. Administer a barbiturate to provide sedation. Acidify the urine to promote phenmetrazine excretion. For acute, severe hypertension, administer IV phentolamine.

Table continued on following page

PRELUDIN continued

DRUG INTERACTIONS

MAO inhibitors	Hypertensive crisis
Other CNS stimulants	⇧ CNS stimulation
Phenothiazines	⇩ Anorectic effect
Guanethidine	⇩ Antihypertensive effect

ALTERED LABORATORY VALUES

Urinary values	⇧ 5-HIAA

No clinically significant alterations in blood/serum values occur at therapeutic dosages

Use in children

Not recommended for use in children under 12 yr of age

Use in pregnancy or nursing mothers

Safe use not established during pregnancy. Animal reproductive studies have demonstrated no teratogenicity; however, fertility, survival of offspring, and body weight of pups at weaning have been adversely affected. Congenital malformations have been reported in clinical studies, but causal relationship has not been proved. Drug should not be used by women who are or may become pregnant, especially during 1st trimester, unless potential benefit clearly outweighs possible risk to fetus. General guidelines not established for use in nursing mothers.

SANOREX (Mazindol) Sandoz

Tabs: 1, 2 mg *C-III*

INDICATIONS	ORAL DOSAGE
Exogenous obesity, as a short-term adjunct to caloric restriction	**Adult:** 1 mg tid 1 h before meals or 2 mg qd 1 h before lunch; take with meals if GI discomfort occurs

CONTRAINDICATIONS

Hypersensitivity or idiosyncratic reaction to mazindol ●

Concurrent or recent MAO-inhibitor therapy ●

History of drug abuse ●

Symptomatic cardiovascular disease ●

Severe hypertension ●

Glaucoma ●

Agitated states ●

WARNINGS/PRECAUTIONS

Habit-forming	Psychic and/or physical dependence and tolerance may develop, especially in addiction-prone individuals; if tolerance develops, discontinue drug rather than increase recommended dosage
Mental impairment	Performance of potentially hazardous activities may be impaired; caution patients accordingly
Insulin requirements	May be altered by drug directly and by reduction in caloric intake
Hypertension	May worsen; use with caution in patients with hypertension
MAO-inhibitor therapy	Wait at least 14 days after discontinuing mazindol before instituting MAO inhibitors
Pressor therapy	If it should be necessary to give a pressor amine agent to a patient in shock who has recently been taking mazindol, monitor blood pressure with extreme care at frequent intervals and initiate pressor therapy with a low dose

ADVERSE REACTIONS

Frequent reactions are italicized

Cardiovascular	*Tachycardia,* palpitations
Central nervous system	*Nervousness, insomnia,* overstimulation, restlessness, dizziness, dysphoria, tremor, headache, depression, drowsiness, weakness
Gastrointestinal	*Dry mouth, constipation,* unpleasant taste, diarrhea, nausea, other disturbances
Other	Rash, hyperhidrosis, clamminess, impotence (rare), altered libido (rare)

OVERDOSAGE

Signs and symptoms	Restlessness, tremor, tachypnea, dizziness, fatigue, depression, tachycardia, hypertension, circulatory collapse, nausea, vomiting, abdominal cramps
Treatment	Treat symptomatically

DRUG INTERACTIONS

MAO inhibitors	⇧ Risk of hypertensive crisis
Other CNS stimulants	⇧ CNS stimulation
Phenothiazines	⇩ Anorectic effect
Guanethidine	⇩ Antihypertensive effect
Vasopressors	⇧ Pressor effect

ALTERED LABORATORY VALUES

No clinically significant alterations in blood/serum or urinary values occur at therapeutic dosages

Use in children

Not recommended for children under 12 yr of age

Use in pregnancy or nursing mothers

Safe use not established during pregnancy; general guidelines not established for use in nursing mothers

TENUATE (Diethylpropion hydrochloride) Merrell-National

Tabs: 25 mg **Tabs (sust rel):** 75 mg *C-IV*

INDICATIONS	ORAL DOSAGE
Exogenous obesity, as a short-term adjunct to caloric restriction	**Adult:** 25 mg tid, 1 h before meals and in mid-evening, if desired; sust-rel tabs: 75 mg qd in midmorning

CONTRAINDICATIONS

Hypersensitivity or idiosyncratic reaction to sympathomimetic amines ●

Concomitant or recent MAO-inhibitor therapy ●

History of drug abuse ●

Advanced arteriosclerosis ●

Hyperthyroidism ●

Severe hypertension ●

Glaucoma ●

Agitated states ●

WARNINGS/PRECAUTIONS

Habit-forming	Psychic and/or physical dependence and tolerance may develop, especially in addiction-prone individuals; if tolerance develops, discontinue drug rather than increase recommended dosage
Mental impairment	Performance of potentially hazardous activities may be impaired; caution patients accordingly
Abrupt discontinuation of therapy	May result in extreme fatigue and mental depression after prolonged use of high doses; changes in sleep EEG may also occur
Hypertension	May worsen; use with caution in patients with hypertension or symptomatic cardiovascular disease, including arrhythmias
Insulin requirements	May be altered by drug directly and by reduction in caloric intake
MAO-inhibitor therapy	Wait at least 14 days after discontinuing diethylpropion before instituting MAO inhibitors (see DRUG INTERACTIONS)
Convulsions	May occur in some epileptics; monitor patients carefully and, if necessary, titrate dose or discontinue use

ADVERSE REACTIONS

Cardiovascular	Palpitations, tachycardia, hypertension, precordial pain, arrhythmias, T-wave changes in ECG
Central nervous system and neuromuscular	Overstimulation, nervousness, restlessness, dizziness, jitteriness, insomnia, anxiety, euphoria, depression, dysphoria, tremor, dyskinesia, drowsiness, headache, psychotic episodes (rare), convulsions, muscle pain
Gastrointestinal	Dry mouth, unpleasant taste, nausea, vomiting, abdominal discomfort, diarrhea, constipation, other disturbances
Genitourinary	Dysuria, polyuria
Dermatological	Urticaria, rash, ecchymoses, erythema, alopecia
Endocrinological	Impotence, altered libido, gynecomastia, menstrual upset
Hematological	Bone-marrow depression, agranulocytosis, leukopenia
Other	Dyspnea, mydriasis, malaise, diaphoresis

OVERDOSAGE

Signs and symptoms	Restlessness, tremor, hyperreflexia, tachypnea, confusion, assaultiveness, hallucinations, panic states, fatigue, depression, arrhythmias, hypertension, hypotension, circulatory collapse, nausea, vomiting, diarrhea, abdominal cramps, convulsions, coma
Treatment	Treat symptomatically; use gastric lavage to empty stomach. Administer barbiturates, as required. For acute, severe hypertension, use IV phentolamine.

Table continued on following page

TENUATE continued

DRUG INTERACTIONS

MAO inhibitors	Hypertensive crisis
Other CNS stimulants	⇧ CNS stimulation
Phenothiazines	⇩ Anorectic effect
Guanethidine	⇩ Antihypertensive effect

ALTERED LABORATORY VALUES

No clinically significant alterations in blood/serum or urinary values occur at therapeutic dosages

Use in children	Use in pregnancy or nursing mothers
Not recommended for use in children under 12 yr of age	Safe use not established during pregnancy; general guidelines not established for use in nursing mothers

Note: Diethylpropion hydrochloride also marketed as **TEPANIL** (Riker).

Product (Manufacturer)	Ingredients	Actions
Appedrine Tablets (Thompson) Tablets **Dosage** 1 tab at midmorning and midafternoon	25 mg Phenylpropanolamine hydrochloride	Stimulant that suppresses appetite
	50 mg Carboxymethylcellulose sodium	Laxative
	100 mg Caffeine	Stimulant that suppresses appetite
	1667 IU Vitamin A	Dietary supplement
	133 IU Vitamin D	Dietary supplement
	1 mg Thiamine	Dietary supplement
	1 mg Riboflavin	Dietary supplement
	0.33 mg Pyridoxine hydrochloride	Dietary supplement
	0.33 g Cyanocobalamin	Dietary supplement
	20 mg Ascorbic acid	Dietary supplement
	7 mg Niacinamide	Dietary supplement
	0.33 mg Calcium pantothenate	Dietary supplement
Dexatrim Capsules (Thompson) **Dosage** One cap with full glass of water each morning	50 mg Phenylpropanolamine hydrochloride	Stimulant that suppresses appetite
	200 mg Caffeine	Stimulant that suppresses appetite
Dexatrim Extra Strength Capsules (Thompson) **Dosage** One cap with full glass of water each morning	75 mg Phenylpropanolamine hydrochloride	Stimulant that suppresses appetite
	200 mg Caffeine	Stimulant that suppresses appetite
Dietac 12-Hour Diet Aid Tablets (Menley & James) Tablets **Dosage** One tab each morning	50 mg Phenylpropanolamine hydrochloride	Stimulant that suppresses appetite
	200 mg Caffeine	Stimulant that suppresses appetite
Dietac Pre-Meal Diet Aids (Menley & James) Tablets **Dosage** One tab 30 min before meals 3 times a day Liquid **Dosage** 5 drops in hot or cold beverage 30 min before meals 3 times a day	25 mg Phenylpropanolamine hydrochloride	Stimulant that suppresses appetite
Diet-Trim Tablets (Pharmex) Tablets **Dosage** 1 tab at midmorning and midafternoon	Carboxymethylcellulose	Laxative
	Benzocaine	Mild anesthetic that reduces taste sensitivity

Table continued on following page

Product (Manufacturer)	Ingredients	Actions
Prolamine Capsules (Thompson) Capsules **Dosage** 1 tab at midmorning and midafternoon	35 mg Phenylpropanolamine hydrochloride	Stimulant that suppresses appetite
	140 mg Caffeine	Stimulant that suppresses appetite
Slim-Line Candy (Thompson) Solid drops **Dosage** Before meals, in place of snacks and in place of dessert. Use whenever sweet food is craved.	6 mg Benzocaine	Mild anesthetic that reduces taste sensitivity
	Sucrose	Sweetener

ARTIFICIAL SWEETENERS

Product (Manufacturer)	Ingredients	Actions
Sucaryl Sodium (Abbott) Tablet **Dosage** 1 tab dissolved into beverage. Use in place of sugar.	16 mg Saccharin sodium	Noncaloric sweetener
Sucaryl Sodium (Abbott) Liquid **Dosage** 1–2 drops mixed into beverage. Use in place of sugar.	1.21% Saccharin sodium	Noncaloric sweetener
Sweeta (Squibb) Tablet **Dosage** 1 tab dissolved into beverage. Use in place of sugar.	15 mg Saccharin sodium	Noncaloric sweetener
Sweeta (Squibb) Liquid **Dosage** 1–2 drops mixed into beverage. Use in place of sugar.	7 mg/drop Saccharin sodium	Noncaloric sweetener
Sweet 'N Low (Cumberland) Powder **Dosage** Use 1 packet for sweetness of 2 tsp sugar in beverages and cooking	40 mg/packet Saccharin sodium	Noncaloric sweetener
	Dextrose	Sweetener
	Cream of tartar	Vehicle
	Drying agent	

Product (Manufacturer)	Ingredients	Actions
Metrecal (Drackett) Cookie (25 calories) **Dosage** Use as low-calorie snack or dessert	Flour	Baking ingredient
	Sugars	Sweeteners
	Milk protein concentrate	Protein and dietary supplement
	Vegetable shortening	Baking ingredient
	Yeast	Baking ingredient
	Vitamins	Dietary supplements
	Minerals	Dietary supplements
Slender (Carnation) Liquid (225 calories/10 fl oz) **Dosage** 1 serving up to 4 times daily	Nonfat dry milk	Protein and dietary supplement
	Sucrose	Sweetener
	Vegetable oil	Cooking ingredient
	Artificial flavors	Taste
	Vitamins	Dietary supplements
	Minerals	Dietary supplements
Slender (Carnation) Powder (170 calories mixed with 6 oz skim, and 225 calories mixed with 6 oz whole milk) **Dosage** Dissolve contents of 1 packet into 6 oz milk. Use up to 4 times daily.	Nonfat dry milk	Protein supplement
	Sucrose	Sweetener
	Vegetable oil	Cooking ingredient
	Artificial flavors	Taste
	Vitamins	Dietary supplements
	Minerals	Dietary supplements
Slender (Carnation) Bar (275 calories/2 bars) **Dosage** Two-bar servings, up to 4 times daily	Nonfat dry milk	Protein supplement
	Sucrose	Sweetener
	Vegetable oil	Cooking ingredient
	Artificial flavors	Taste
	Vitamins	Dietary supplements
	Minerals	Dietary supplements

Pain Relief

Pain

Although pain in and of itself is not a disease, it is by far mankind's most common medical complaint. It is considered the earliest symptom of most illnesses, and almost all maladies have a component of pain. Perception and tolerance of pain, however, are highly individualized and are influenced by many factors, including anxiety, fatigue, fear, cultural background, and personality type.

While pain is generally regarded as an unpleasant experience to be avoided as much as possible, it serves an essential purpose in human development and survival, warning of actual or threatened damage to body tissue from disease or external factors. A classic example is the pain experienced from a burn: a young child quickly learns not to touch a hot stove or other objects that can burn. Other common examples include chest pain, which may warn of an impending heart attack; a painful shoulder or elbow, which may indicate a faulty tennis swing or other pattern of misuse; and frequent headaches, which may be a symptom of a serious illness or an indication of undue stress.

TYPES OF PAIN

Pain may be organic or psychogenic, or a combination of the two. Although the perception of pain is frequently altered by psychological factors, this discussion will be devoted primarily to the causes and treatments of organic pain, which is caused by a demonstrable injury to the body's pain detection system.

There are three major categories of organic pain: superficial or cutaneous pain, which arises from the skin; deep pain, which originates in the muscles, tendons, joints, and bones; and visceral pain, which originates in the various internal organs such as the heart or kidneys. Cutaneous pain is characterized by a short-lived burning or prickling sensation. It is perceived almost immediately, and its location is easily identifiable and the causes quickly discriminated. In contrast, deep or visceral pain tends to be a more vague, persistent, dull, aching sensation, whose precise location is not always apparent—at times it may be felt in a place some distance from the source, a phenomenon known as "referred pain." Although a tiny pinprick in the skin will produce a sensation of pain, extensive damage to an internal organ may produce little or no pain.

Regardless of the source, the sensation of pain is transmitted through specific pain sensors and pathways throughout the body. A network of pain receptors in the form of minute, branching nerve endings is found in most parts of the body, but is most highly developed in the skin. There are two sizes of pain sensory nerve fibers: the thicker "A" fibers, which transmit the "fast pain," perceived as sharp, stabbing, or prickling sensations; and the thinner "C" fibers, which transmit "slow pain," perceived as a burning or aching sensation.

The pain receptors may be stimulated by chemical substances or tissue injury. The precise mechanism is still unclear, but it is believed that the pain receptor nerve endings are stimulated by a polypeptide, a substance produced by the release of an enzyme at the site of tissue injury. The resulting pain impulse travels along pain fibers in the nerve cells to the spinal cord, then to pain centers in the thalamus, where it is perceived, and ultimately to the cortex of the brain, where it is interpreted.

COMMON CAUSES OF PAIN

Headache

In any given week, about 15 percent of the population suffers from headache. There are many types of headache, both serious and benign. One of the most common is the so-called "tension headache," which is caused by muscular spasms in the neck or scalp. The pain is often localized at the base of the skull or forehead, and there is usually a feeling of pressure or "tightness" in the back of the neck where it meets the skull. Areas surrounding the sinus cavities, which are situated near the nose and eyes, are another common source of headache. A dull pain behind or around the eyes, or in the frontal area of the scalp or forehead, characterizes the so-called "sinus headache," which is often accompanied by nasal congestion, and a feeling of pressure around the nose and eyes.

The throbbing or pulsating headaches of vascular origin, such as migraine and cluster headaches, afflict large segments of the population. (These are discussed in detail in the section on *Migraine and Other Headaches,* page 696.) Uncorrected visual problems are still another common cause of headache, especially persistent or recurring pain around or behind the eyes.

Pain originating *inside* the skull itself (intracranial) is usually a more serious warning sign and warrants prompt medical attention. Causes of intracranial headache include tumors, injury, ruptured blood vessels, abscesses, and infection. These headaches are usually described as deep, aching, steady, and dull, and are seldom throbbing or pulsating. The pain is usually continuous and is often more intense in the morning. A headache accompanied by dizziness, blurred vision, loss of hearing or memory, nausea, personality changes, or loss of consciousness is a common warning sign of intracranial injury or disease, and is cause for seeing a physician as soon as possible.

Joint and Muscle Pain
Arthritis, an inflammation of the connective tissue surrounding the joint and tendons, is the most common source of joint pain. (See the section on *Arthritis and Gout,* page 996, for a more detailed discussion.)

Myalgia, pain arising in skeletal muscles, is usually caused by overexertion or straining of muscles that are not accustomed to the demands being placed on them. For example, undertaking jogging or some other form of vigorous exercise without proper conditioning usually results in sore, aching muscles. Tension or maintaining a certain position for a prolonged period are other common causes of myalgia.

Nerve Pain
Neuralgia, defined as pain arising in the sensory nerves, usually manifests itself as sharp, stabbing pain in the afflicted area. The trigeminal nerve, which is located in the facial area, is commonly afflicted, resulting in the severe, often excruciating pain in the jaw and face known as *tic douloureux*. The cause of most neuralgia is unknown, since it does not appear to be related to organic damage to the nerves themselves.

Pain Associated with Disease
Many diseases have pain as a major symptom, primarily because they cause inflammation or swelling in organs or body parts that are pain sensitive. For example, angina pectoris—the chest pain caused by insufficient circulation to the heart muscle—is a hallmark of coronary heart disease; epigastric pain may indicate an ulcer; abdominal pain may be a symptom of gallbladder disease or any number of other disorders involving the abdominal organs; and pain frequently accompanies many types of cancer.

TREATMENT OF PAIN

Ideally, the best and most effective treatment of pain is identification and elimination of its cause. Obviously, this is not always possible; besides, the diagnosis and treatment may require varying

PATHWAY OF PAIN FROM SKIN TO THE BRAIN

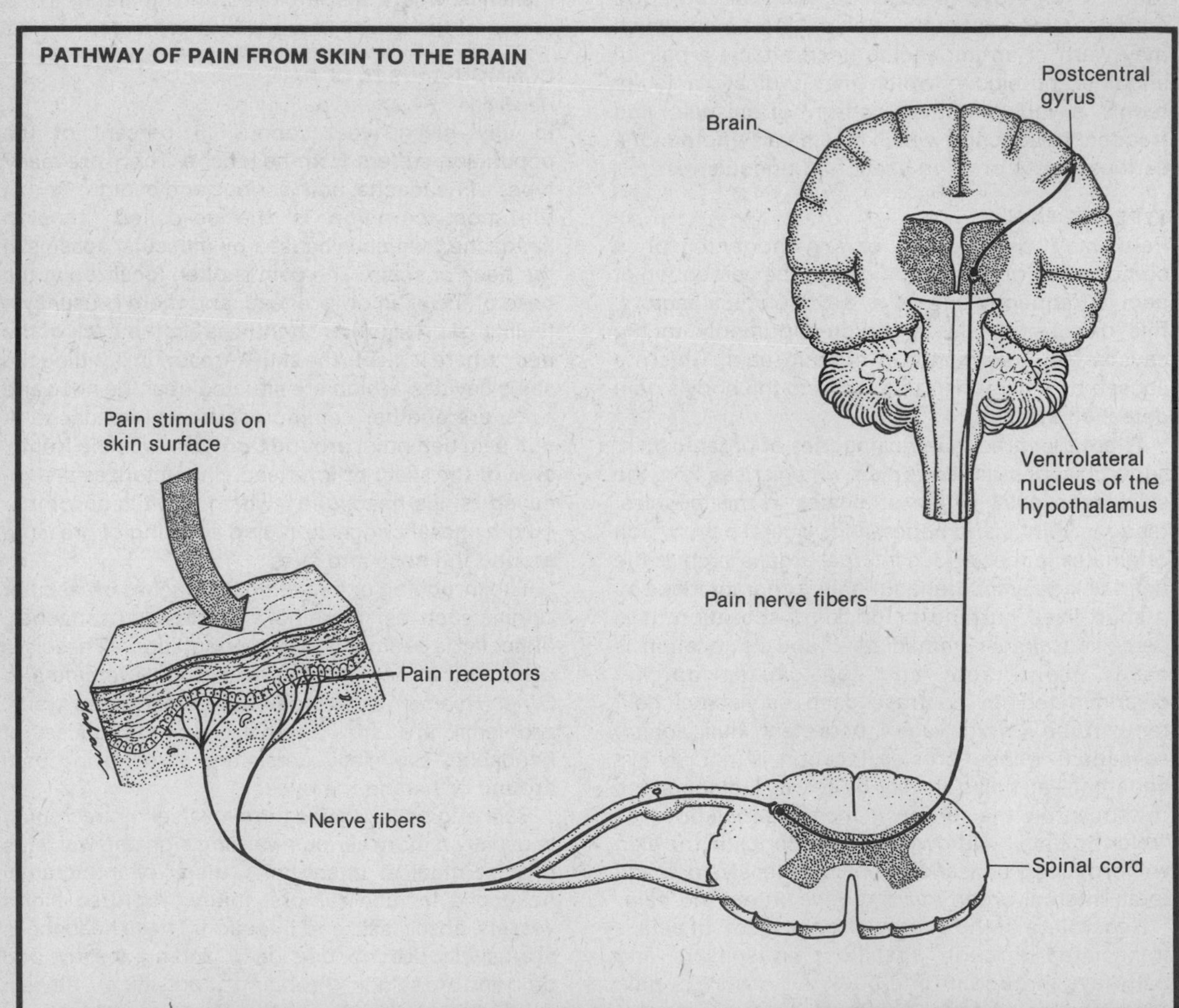

amounts of time. In either instance, analgesics, commonly referred to as "painkillers," are often needed to relieve the pain.

TYPES OF ANALGESICS

In this book, painkillers are divided into two broad categories: strong analgesics and mild-to-moderate analgesics. As might be expected, the strong analgesics are used to relieve moderate-to-severe and very severe pain, while the mild ones are used for mild-to-moderate pain. Some mild-to-moderate analgesics are chemically related to strong analgesics, and there are some instances in which the milder painkillers are sufficient to control moderately severe pain. The following discussion will give a brief overview of the various classes of analgesics, while the charts at the end of this section list specific indications and other prescribing considerations.

The Strong Analgesics

Strong analgesics are further divided into two categories: narcotics, such as morphine and other derivatives of opium, and non-narcotic medications, which often produce morphine-like effects, but are not as likely to be habit forming.

To many physicians and patients alike, the specter of drug dependence is a major objection to the use of strong narcotic analgesics. As a result, many persons who suffer from a temporary painful condition, such as a broken leg or post-surgical pain, are denied adequate relief because of the fear of addiction. Most experts in pain control agree that the administration of morphine or a morphine-like drug to a person who is hospitalized with a short-term painful condition is not likely to cause addiction. However, in treating a chronic painful condition, such as rheumatoid arthritis, caution must be exercised in using these strong analgesics, as well as habit-forming mild analgesics that are chemically related to morphine and other narcotics, because dependence can develop within a few weeks. In addition, patients develop "tolerance" to many of these drugs, meaning that ever-increasing doses are needed to produce the same degree of pain relief. Although tolerance to the beneficial effects may develop, unfortunately, the same is not true of the adverse effects. Thus, the danger of respiratory arrest, reduced blood pressure, and other potential adverse effects increases along with the increasing doses.

How Strong Analgesics Work

Most strong analgesics appear to work through the opiate receptors in the central nervous system to alter the sensation of pain, suppress anxiety, and produce sedation. In contrast, the mild painkillers seem to reduce the sensitivity of the pain receptors in the nerve endings, rather than to affect the central nervous system.

Most strong analgesics are given by injection, and virtually all are effective against moderate to moderately severe pain. However, some, such as morphine, hydromorphone, oxymorphone, levorphanol, methadone, and methotrimeprazine, seem to be more effective against severe and very severe pain than others, such as meperidine, alphaprodine, anileridine and pentazocine. Morphine, which is derived from the most active alkaloid in opium, is the most frequently used strong analgesic, and the actions of the others are similar to that of morphine.

Precautions and Adverse Reactions

As noted earlier, most of the strong analgesics are narcotics and thus are potentially habit forming. However, addiction to morphine and other strong painkillers rarely occurs if the drugs are used in a hospital setting, as needed, for short periods of time, such as after surgery or an accident. There is now little controversy over the use of morphine or similar narcotics in these patients; in contrast, there is considerable controversy over the use of narcotics to relieve pain in end-stage cancer, with some doctors arguing that the relief of pain in these patients is more important than concern over possible addiction, and others contending that alternative means of pain relief should be found.

The most common adverse effects of strong analgesics are nausea and vomiting, which can usually be managed by staying in bed or using an antinauseant medication; respiratory depression, which can be life-threatening in elderly or debilitated patients, especially those with chronic lung disease; constipation, which can be controlled with diet and/or laxatives; orthostatic hypotension, which is a sudden drop in blood pressure upon standing up that can be controlled by staying in bed or getting up slowly; and drowsiness, which is often considered an advantage in strong analgesics should be used cautiously in persons with liver disease, asthma and other lung disorders, head injuries, and reduced blood volume due to severe bleeding.

The Mild Analgesics

Many mild analgesics are related both chemically and by mechanism of action to strong analgesics, while others are markedly different. In some instances, such as following surgery or an accident, a mild analgesic may be sufficient to control even moderately severe pain. There are also some analgesics, such as those containing oxycodone (Percodan and Tylox) that may be classified as either strong or mild because, in some conditions, they are effective against moderately severe pain. Whenever mild analgesics provide satisfactory pain relief, they are preferable to the strong ones because they entail less danger of adverse effects.

In general, mild analgesics are divided into two groups: those that are chemically related to the strong analgesics (codeine, ethoheptazine, oxycodone, and propoxyphene) and those painkillers with an added antipyretic effect, meaning that they also reduce fever. This group includes the salicylates (aspirin), acetaminophen (Tylenol), and combinations of mild painkillers.

Derivatives of Strong Analgesics

This group of drugs includes codeine, a derivative of morphine; propoxyphene (Darvon), which is related to methadone; ethoheptazine (Zactane), which is related to meperidine; and oxycodone, which is derived from opium and, when combined with other painkillers, is sold as Percodan, Tylox, and Percocet. All of these drugs are classified as narcotics, and while they are generally not as potent in relieving severe pain as the strong analgesics, they are often prescribed for moderate-to-severe pain. All are habit forming and should be used with caution, especially when prescribed for chronic conditions outside a hospital setting.

The Salicylates

Aspirin is the major salicylate sold in the United States. Of all the painkillers, it is the most widely used and one of the safest and most effective of all analgesics. It is also one of the least expensive.

In addition to its ability to relieve pain, aspirin has powerful anti-inflammatory and antipyretic effects. It remains the drug of first choice in treating headache, rheumatoid arthritis and other types of musculoskeletal pain, and neuralgia. It is less effective against visceral pain, but is still often the only painkiller needed by many surgery, trauma, and even cancer patients.

As with all drugs, aspirin does have the potential for adverse reactions and toxicity; overdoses of aspirin, for example, remain a leading cause of accidental poisoning death in young children. Gastrointestinal problems, such as heartburn, nausea, cramps, and intestinal bleeding abnormalities, are the most common adverse effects of aspirin. When taken in high doses, aspirin may cause ringing in the ears (tinnitus), deafness, dizziness, and headache. These adverse effects usually can be reversed by lowering the dosage, or, if necessary, stopping the drug. Because of the possibility of hemorrhage, aspirin probably should be avoided by persons who have peptic ulcer, although there are buffered and coated aspirin preparations that may help minimize this danger.

Allergic reactions to aspirin are relatively rare and occur most often in persons who suffer from asthma. In fact, 3 to 5 percent of all asthma patients will show an allergic response (wheezing, itching, runny nose, etc.) to aspirin and should avoid this drug.

Acetaminophen

Acetaminophen, which is sold as Tylenol and under a number of other brand names, is an alternative to aspirin in most non-inflammatory conditions. It is often recommended in treating moderately severe pain such as that of cancer, surgery, and postpartum trauma, as well as the milder pain associated with tension and other mild headaches, menstrual discomfort, and other such disorders. It also will lower a fever, but since it does not have an anti-inflammatory effect, it is not as effective a pain reliever as aspirin for persons with rheumatoid arthritis or other conditions in which inflammation is a cause of the pain. However, acetaminophen is recommended instead of aspirin for gout patients or others taking drugs to lower elevated uric acid.

Damage to the liver is the major potential danger of acetaminophen, although this usually occurs only when large doses (more than 13 to 15 grams or 40 to 46 tablets) are taken. However, there have been reports of serious, even fatal, liver damage among alcoholics who have taken only the recommended dosages of acetaminophen. It does not have the high potential for gastrointestinal disturbances commonly associated with aspirin and is therefore a popular alternative to aspirin in persons predisposed to intestinal problems.

Mixtures of Mild Analgesics

Combinations of various mild analgesics are widely promoted as painkillers, but their use is debated by many experts. Some contend that the combinations of painkillers increase effectiveness, while others maintain that they offer few, if any, advantages over aspirin or acetaminophen. A combination of aspirin, phenacetin, and caffeine (A.P.C.) is one of the most common drugs in this category, although a number of studies have failed to demonstrate that it is any more effective than plain aspirin. Since phenacetin has little or no action against inflammation, it is less effective than plain aspirin against rheumatoid arthritis and other inflammatory conditions.

Other common combinations include aspirin and codeine; Empirin with codeine; Darvon and acetaminophen; Darvon and A.P.C.; Darvon and aspirin; and Tylenol with codeine.

Several mixtures of analgesics are sold as pain relievers for specific types of pain. For example, there are a number of drugs exclusively for the relief of menstrual pain. In general, these work either by including a diuretic to remove the excess body fluid that sometimes accumulates at certain times during the menstrual cycle; or by addition of aspirin, acetaminophen, or other analgesics. Examples of diuretic-based menstrual products include Aqua-Ban and Fluidex, while those that are primarily analgesics include Midol and Pamprin.

More recently, researchers ascertained that an excessive release of prostaglandins is the major cause of menstrual cramps—a disorder that afflicts 30 to 50 percent of all menstruating women. Since a number of the anti-inflammatory drugs used to treat arthritis are prostaglandin inhibitors, some of these drugs are now being used to prevent menstrual pain. Drugs in this category with a specific indication for dysmenorrhea include naproxen sodium (Anaprox) and naproxen (Naprosyn). The other prostaglandin inhibitors that may be recommended for menstrual cramps have a more general indication for mild-to-moderate pain. Examples include ibuprofen (Motrin) and mefenamic acid (Ponstel).

Topical Analgesics

Another large category of nonprescription pain relievers is the topical analgesics (i.e., Absorbine Jr. or Ben Gay), which are used primarily to treat muscular pain, such as that occurring in bursitis, sprains, arthritis, athletic injuries, and other such causes.

Most of these products act as counterirritants, meaning that when they are applied to the skin, a perception of pain occurs that acts to block or reduce the perception of the underlying pain. Ingredients used in topical analgesics include methyl salicylate, menthol, turpentine oil, clove oil, and thymol, among others. These pain relievers may be applied as liniments, gels, lotions, or ointments. They are relatively safe, the major hazard being a hypersensitive or allergic reaction. They also may be very toxic if swallowed; therefore, they should be used only externally, and as with all medications, kept out of the reach of children and others who may try to ingest them.

More detailed information on both strong and mild analgesics, as well as combination drugs, may be found in the following drug charts. In addition, specific types of pain are discussed in the sections on *Migraine and Other Headaches* (page 696); *Arthritis and Gout* (page 996); *Coronary Artery Disease* (page 7); *Heartburn, Indigestion, and Ulcers* (page 199); and *Backache and other Musculoskeletal Disorders* (page 707).

ANAPROX (Naproxen sodium) Syntex

Tabs: 275 mg

INDICATIONS	ORAL DOSAGE
Mild-to-moderate pain; dysmenorrhea	**Adult:** 550 mg to start, followed by 275 mg q6-8h, as needed, up to 1,375 mg/day
Rheumatoid arthritis; osteoarthritis	**Adult:** 275 mg bid (AM and PM) or 275 mg in AM and 550 mg in PM

ADMINISTRATION/DOSAGE ADJUSTMENTS	
Therapeutic response in arthritis	Should be observed within 2 wk; in some patients, symptomatic improvement may not be seen for up to 4 wk
Combination therapy	Added benefits in arthritis have not been demonstrated with corticosteroids; however, use with gold salts has resulted in greater improvement. Use with salicylates is not recommended. Use with related drug naproxen is not recommended.
Adrenal function tests	Discontinue naproxen sodium therapy 72 h prior to testing

CONTRAINDICATIONS	
Hypersensitivity	To naproxen sodium or aspirin and other nonsteroidal, anti-inflammatory drugs when manifested by asthma, rhinitis, or urticaria

WARNINGS/PRECAUTIONS	
Peptic ulcer, perforation, GI bleeding	May occur and can be severe or even fatal; use with caution in patients with a history of peptic ulcer disease or active gastric or duodenal ulcers
Renal damage	Chronic therapy has caused nephritis in animal studies; use with great caution in patients with significant renal functional impairment, and monitor serum creatinine and/or creatinine clearance periodically
Corticosteroid therapy	If discontinued, reduce dosage gradually to avoid complications of sudden steroid withdrawal
Impaired vision	May occur with some nonsteroidal anti-inflammatory drugs; perform ophthalmologic studies periodically
Drowsiness, dizziness, vertigo, depression	Performance of potentially hazardous activities may be impaired; caution patients accordingly
Peripheral edema	May occur, especially in patients with questionable or compromised cardiac function
Prolonged bleeding time	May occur due to inhibition of platelet aggregation; use with caution in patients with coagulation defects or in those on anticoagulant therapy
Initial low hemoglobin values (≤10 g)	Obtain periodic hemoglobin determinations during long-term therapy

ADVERSE REACTIONS[1]	Frequent reactions are italicized
Gastrointestinal	*Constipation (3-9%), heartburn (3-9%), abdominal pain (3-9%), nausea (3-9%), dyspepsia (1-3%), diarrhea (1-3%), stomatitis (1-3%),* bleeding, peptic ulcer with bleeding and/or perforation, vomiting, melena, hematemesis
Central nervous system and neuromuscular	*Headache (3-9%), dizziness (3-9%), drowsiness (3-9%), lightheadedness (1-3%), vertigo (1-3%),* myalgia, muscle weakness, inability to concentrate, depression, malaise, dream abnormalities
Dermatological	*Pruritus (3-9%), eruption (3-9%), ecchymoses (3-9%), sweating (1-3%), purpura (1-3%),* rash, alopecia; urticaria (causal relationship not established)
Cardiovascular	*Edema (3-9%), dyspnea (3-9%), palpitations (1-3%),* congestive heart failure
Hepatic	Abnormal liver function tests, jaundice
Renal	Glomerular nephritis, interstitial nephritis, nephrotic syndrome, hematuria
Hematological	Thrombocytopenia, leukopenia, granulocytopenia, eosinophilia; agranulocytosis, aplastic anemia, and hemolytic anemia (causal relationship not established)
Other	*Tinnitus (3-9%), thirst (1-3%),* menstrual disorders, chills, fever; angioneurotic edema, hypoglycemia, and hyperglycemia (causal relationship not established)

OVERDOSAGE	
Signs and symptoms	Drowsiness, heartburn, indigestion, nausea, vomiting
Treatment	Induce emesis or use gastric lavage to empty stomach, and institute supportive measures. Activated charcoal may be helpful.

[1]Adverse reactions occurring in patients treated for rheumatoid arthritis or osteoarthritis are listed; in general, these reactions were reported 2–10 times more frequently than they were in patients treated for mild-to-moderate pain or dysmenorrhea

Table continued on following page

DRUG INTERACTIONS

Albumin-bound drugs	Displacement of either drug
Coumarin anticoagulants	⇧ Prothrombin time
Hydantoins	⇧ Hydantoin plasma level
Sulfonylureas	⇧ Sulfonylurea plasma level
Sulfonamides	⇧ Sulfonamide plasma level
Aspirin	⇧ Excretion of naproxen sodium
Probenecid	⇧ Naproxen sodium plasma half-life

ALTERED LABORATORY VALUES

Blood/serum values	⇧ BUN	
Urinary values	⇧ 17-Ketogenic steroids	Interference with 5-HIAA determinations

Use in children	Use in pregnancy or nursing mothers
Safety and effectiveness have not been established	Not recommended; naproxen anion appears in breast milk at a concentration of 1% of that in the maternal plasma

CODEINE PHOSPHATE Lilly

Soluble (hypodermic) tabs: 15, 30, 60 mg *C-II*

CODEINE SULFATE Lilly

Tabs: 15, 30, 60 mg **Soluble (hypodermic) tabs:** 15, 30, 60 mg *C-II*

INDICATIONS	ORAL DOSAGE	PARENTERAL DOSAGE
Mild to moderate pain	**Adult:** 15–60 mg q4h **Child:** 0.5 mg/kg q4h	**Adult:** 15–60 mg IM or SC q4h

CONTRAINDICATIONS

Hypersensitivity to codeine

WARNINGS/PRECAUTIONS

Habit-forming	Psychic and/or physical dependence and tolerance may develop, especially in addiction-prone individuals
Head injury, increased intracranial pressure	Respiratory depression and elevation of CSF pressure may be exaggerated; clinical course may be masked
Mental impairment, reflex-slowing	Performance of potentially hazardous activities may be impaired; caution patients accordingly
Acute abdominal conditions	Diagnosis or clinical course may be masked
Special-risk patients	Use with caution in the elderly or debilitated and in patients with severe hepatic or renal impairment, hypothyroidism, Addison's disease, prostatic hypertrophy, or urethral stricture

ADVERSE REACTIONS Frequent reactions are italicized

Central nervous system	*Light-headedness, dizziness, sedation,* euphoria, dysphoria
Gastrointestinal	*Nausea, vomiting,* constipation
Dermatological	Pruritus

OVERDOSAGE

Signs and symptoms	Respiratory depression, miosis, extreme somnolence progressing to stupor or coma, skeletal-muscle flaccidity, cold and clammy skin, hypotension, bradycardia, and, in severe cases, apnea, circulatory collapse, and cardiac arrest
Treatment	Give primary attention to re-establishing adequate respiratory exchange through provision of an adequate airway and assisted or controlled ventilation; positive-pressure respiration may be desirable if pulmonary edema is present. If respiratory depression is significant, promptly administer naloxone (adult, 0.4 mg; child, 0.01 mg/kg), preferably IV, and repeat at 2- to 3-min intervals until satisfactory breathing is restored. *Do not use analeptic agents.* Oxygen, IV fluids, vasopressors, and other supportive measures should be employed, as needed. Gastric lavage, followed by instillation of activated charcoal, may be useful; dialysis is of little value unless other, dialyzable substances (such as barbiturates) have been simultaneously ingested.

DRUG INTERACTIONS

Other narcotic analgesics; sedative-hypnotics, antianxiety agents, phenothiazines, general anesthetics, and other CNS depressants (including alcohol); MAO inhibitors; tricyclic antidepressants	⇧ CNS depression; reduce dose of one or both agents if used concomitantly or in close succession
Anticholinergic agents	⇧ Risk of paralytic ileus

ALTERED LABORATORY VALUES

Blood/serum values	⇧ Amylase ⇧ Lipase

No clinically significant alterations in urinary values occur at therapeutic dosages

Use in children

See INDICATIONS

Use in pregnancy or nursing mothers

Safe use not established during pregnancy; general guidelines not established for use in nursing mothers

DARVOCET-N 50 (Propoxyphene napsylate and acetaminophen) **Lilly**

Tabs: 50 mg propoxyphene napsylate and 325 mg acetaminophen *C-IV*

DARVOCET-N 100 (Propoxyphene napsylate and acetaminophen) **Lilly**

Tabs: 100 mg propoxyphene napsylate and 650 mg acetaminophen *C-IV*

INDICATIONS	ORAL DOSAGE
Mild to moderate pain alone or accompanied by fever	**Adult:** 2 Darvocet-N 50 tabs or 1 Darvocet-N 100 tab q4h, as needed

CONTRAINDICATIONS

Suicidal or addiction-prone individuals ●	Hypersensitivity to propoxyphene or acetaminophen ●

WARNINGS/PRECAUTIONS

Habit-forming	Psychic dependence and, less often, physical dependence and tolerance may develop when taken in higher-than-recommended doses for prolonged periods, especially in addiction-prone individuals
Overdosage	Excessive doses of propoxyphene, either alone or in combination with other CNS depressants, including alcohol (see DRUG INTERACTIONS), are a major cause of drug-related deaths; caution patients not to exceed recommended dosage and to limit their alcohol intake, and that the concomitant use of other CNS depressants can cause additional CNS depression
Mental impairment, reflex-slowing	Performance of potentially hazardous activities may be impaired; caution patients accordingly and about additive effect of alcohol and other CNS depressants (see DRUG INTERACTIONS)

ADVERSE REACTIONS[1]

Central nervous system	Dizziness, sedation, light-headedness, euphoria, dysphoria, minor visual disturbances, weakness, headache
Gastrointestinal	Nausea, vomiting, constipation, abdominal pain, liver dysfunction
Dermatological	Rash

OVERDOSAGE

Signs and symptoms	*Propoxyphene-related effects:* CNS depression, ranging from somnolence (usually) to stupor and coma; respiratory depression, progressing to Cheyne-Stokes respiration, cyanosis, hypoxia, and apnea; pinpoint pupils, becoming dilated as hypoxia increases, fall in blood pressure and deterioration in cardiac performance, culminating in pulmonary edema and circulatory collapse; respiratory and metabolic acidosis; cardiac conduction delay and arrhythmias; convulsions; *acetaminophen-related effects*: nausea, vomiting, diaphoresis, and general malaise; clinical and laboratory evidence of hepatotoxicity (vomiting, right upper quadrant tenderness, increased SGOT, SGPT, serum bilirubin, and prothrombin time, and possible hypoglycemia) may not be apparent until 48–72 h after ingestion
Treatment	Give primary attention to re-establishing adequate respiratory exchange through provision of adequate airway and assisted or controlled ventilation; positive-pressure respiration may be desirable if pulmonary edema is present. If respiratory depression is significant, promptly administer naloxone (adult, 0.4 mg; child, 0.01 mg/kg), preferably IV, and repeat at 2- to 3-min intervals until satisfactory breathing is restored. *Do not use analeptic agents.* Monitor blood gases, pH, and electrolytes and promptly correct any acid-base or electrolyte abnormalities present (lactic acidosis may require IV sodium bicarbonate for prompt correction). Administer an anticonvulsant in carefully titrated doses if seizures occur. Oxygen, IV fluids, vasopressors, and other supportive measures should be employed, as needed. ECG monitoring is essential. Gastric lavage, followed by instillation of activated charcoal, may be useful; the charcoal must be lavaged out after 1 h and before instilling acetylcysteine as an antidote. (Call the Rocky Mountain Poison Center, [800] 525-6115, for assistance in diagnosing acetaminophen overdosage and for directions for administering acetylcysteine as an antidote [currently investigational].) Determine serum acetaminophen level as soon as possible, but not earlier than 4 h after suspected ingestion. Liver function studies should be obtained initially and repeated at 24-h intervals. Acetylcysteine can be given up to 24 h postingestion, but should be administered as early as possible, within 16 h of suspected ingestion for optimal results.

[1]For other possible adverse reactions, see acetaminophen

Table continued on following page

DARVOCET-N continued

DRUG INTERACTIONS

Other narcotic analgesics; sedative-hypnotics, antianxiety agents, phenothiazines, general anesthetics, muscle relaxants, and other CNS depressants; MAO inhibitors; tricyclic antidepressants	⇧ CNS depression; use with caution in patients who require concomitant administration of other CNS depressants
Alcohol	⇧ CNS depression; use with caution in patients who consume excessive amounts of alcohol
Warfarin	⇧ Hypoprothrombinemia (slight)

ALTERED LABORATORY VALUES

Blood/serum values	⇧ Prothrombin time ⇧ Uric acid (with phosphotungstate method)
Urinary values	⇧ 5-HIAA (with nitrosonaphthol reagent test)

Use in children

Not recommended

Use in pregnancy or nursing mothers

Safe use during pregnancy not established relative to fetal development; however, neonatal withdrawal symptoms have been reported following propoxyphene usage during pregnancy. Although low levels of propoxyphene have been found in human milk, no adverse effects have been noted in nursing infants.

DARVON (Propoxyphene hydrochloride) Lilly

Caps: 32, 65 mg *C-IV*

INDICATIONS	ORAL DOSAGE
Mild to moderate pain	**Adult:** 65 mg q4h, as needed

CONTRAINDICATIONS

Suicidal or addiction-prone individuals ● Hypersensitivity to propoxyphene ●

WARNINGS/PRECAUTIONS

Habit-forming	Psychic dependence and, less often, physical dependence and tolerance may develop when taken in higher-than-recommended doses for prolonged periods, especially in addiction-prone individuals
Overdosage	Excessive doses of propoxyphene, either alone or in combination with other CNS depressants, including alcohol (see DRUG INTERACTIONS), are a major cause of drug-related deaths; caution patients not to exceed recommended dosage, to limit their alcohol intake, and that the concomitant use of other CNS depressants can cause additional CNS depression
Mental impairment, reflex-slowing	Performance of potentially hazardous activities may be impaired; caution patients accordingly and about additive effect of alcohol and other CNS depressants (see DRUG INTERACTIONS)

ADVERSE REACTIONS	Frequent reactions are italicized
Central nervous system	*Dizziness, sedation,* light-headedness, headache, weakness, euphoria, dysphoria, minor visual disturbances
Gastrointestinal	*Nausea, vomiting,* constipation, abdominal pain, liver dysfunction
Dermatological	Rash

OVERDOSAGE

Signs and symptoms	CNS depression, ranging from somnolence (usually) to stupor and coma; respiratory depression, progressing to Cheyne-Stokes respiration, cyanosis, hypoxia, and apnea; pinpoint pupils, becoming dilated as hypoxia increases; fall in blood pressure and deterioration in cardiac performance, culminating in pulmonary edema and circulatory collapse; respiratory and metabolic acidosis; cardiac conduction delay and arrhythmias; convulsions
Treatment	Give primary attention to re-establishing adequate respiratory exchange through provision of an adequate airway and assisted or controlled ventilation; positive-pressure respiration may be desirable if pulmonary edema is present. If respiratory depression is significant, promptly administer naloxone (adult, 0.4 mg; child, 0.01 mg/kg), preferably IV, and repeat at 2- to 3-min intervals until satisfactory breathing is restored. *Do not use analeptic agents.* Oxygen, IV fluids, vasopressors, and other supportive measures should be employed, as needed. Gastric lavage, followed by instillation of activated charcoal, may be useful; dialysis is of little value unless other, dialyzable substances (such as barbiturates) have been simultaneously ingested.

DRUG INTERACTIONS

Other narcotic analgesics; sedative-hypnotics, antianxiety agents, phenothiazines, general anesthetics, muscle relaxants, and other CNS depressants; MAO inhibitors; tricyclic antidepressants	⇧ CNS depression; use with caution in patients who require concomitant administration of other CNS depressants
Alcohol	⇧ CNS depression; use with caution in patients who consume excessive amounts of alcohol

ALTERED LABORATORY VALUES

No clinically significant alterations in blood/serum or urinary values occur at therapeutic dosages

Use in children

Not recommended

Use in pregnancy or nursing mothers

Safe use in pregnancy has not been established relative to fetal development; however, neonatal withdrawal symptoms have been reported following propoxyphene usage during pregnancy. Although low levels of propoxyphene have been found in human milk, no adverse effects have been noted in nursing infants.

DARVON COMPOUND/DARVON COMPOUND-65 (Propoxyphene hydrochloride, aspirin, phenacetin, and caffeine) Lilly

Caps: 32 mg (Darvon Compound) or 65 mg (Darvon Compound-65) propoxyphene hydrochloride, 227 mg aspirin, 162 mg phenacetin, and 32.4 mg caffeine *C-IV*

INDICATIONS	ORAL DOSAGE
Mild to moderate pain alone or accompanied by fever	**Adult:** 1 cap q4h, as needed

CONTRAINDICATIONS[1]	
Suicidal or addiction-prone individuals ●	Hypersensitivity to propoxyphene, aspirin, phenacetin, or caffeine ●

WARNINGS/PRECAUTIONS[1]	
Habit-forming	Psychic dependence and, less often, physical dependence and tolerance may develop when taken in higher-than-recommended doses for prolonged periods, especially in addiction-prone individuals
Overdosage	Excessive doses of propoxyphene, either alone or in combination with other CNS depressants, including alcohol (see DRUG INTERACTIONS), are a major cause of drug-related deaths; caution patients not to exceed recommended dosage, to limit their alcohol intake, and that the concomitant use of other CNS depressants can cause additional CNS depression
Mental impairment, reflex-slowing	Performance of potentially hazardous activities may be impaired; caution patients accordingly and about additive effect of alcohol and other CNS depressants (see DRUG INTERACTIONS)
Severe kidney disease, cancer of the kidney	May occur with prolonged (1-3 yr) use of phenacetin in high doses (1 g/day or more) in combination with other anti-inflammatory analgesics or with total ingestions of 2 kg of phenacetin or more
Special-risk patients	Use with extreme caution in patients with peptic ulcer or coagulation abnormalities

ADVERSE REACTIONS[1]	Frequent reactions are italicized
Central nervous system	*Dizziness, sedation,* light-headedness, euphoria, dysphoria, headache, weakness, minor visual disturbances
Gastrointestinal	*Nausea, vomiting,* constipation, abdominal pain, liver dysfunction
Dermatological	Rash

OVERDOSAGE	
Signs and symptoms	*Propoxyphene-related effects:* CNS depression, ranging from somnolence (usually) to stupor and coma; respiratory depression, progressing to Cheyne-Stokes respiration, cyanosis, hypoxia, and apnea; pinpoint pupils, becoming dilated as hypoxia increases; fall in blood pressure and deterioration in cardiac performance, culminating in pulmonary edema and circulatory collapse; respiratory and metabolic acidosis; cardiac conduction delay and arrhythmias; convulsions; *aspirin-related effects:* hyperpnea, nausea, vomiting, vertigo, tinnitus, flushing, sweating, thirst, headache, drowsiness, diarrhea, and tachycardia, progressing to hyperthermia, hemorrhage, acid-base disturbances, restlessness, confusion, convulsions, vasomotor depression, coma, and respiratory failure; *phenacetin-related effects:* nausea, vomiting, abdominal pain, chills, excitement, delirium, cyanosis due to methemoglobinemia, respiratory depression, cardiac arrest; *caffeine-related effects:* insomnia, restlessness, and excitement progressing to mild delirium, dehydration, fever, tachycardia, extrasystoles, tremor, and convulsions

[1] For other possible contraindications, warnings and precautions, and adverse reactions, see aspirin

Table continued on following page

OVERDOSAGE continued

Treatment	Give primary attention to re-establishing adequate respiratory exchange through provision of an adequate airway and assisted or controlled ventilation; positive-pressure respiration may be desirable if pulmonary edema is present. If respiratory depression is significant, promptly administer naloxone (adult, 0.4 mg; child, 0.01 mg/kg), preferably IV, and repeat at 2- to 3-min intervals until satisfactory breathing is restored. *Do not use analeptic agents.* Monitor blood gases, pH, and electrolytes and promptly correct any acid-base or electrolyte abnormalities present (lactic acidosis may require IV sodium bicarbonate for prompt correction). Administer an anticonvulsant in carefully titrated doses if seizures occur. Oxygen, IV fluids, vasopressors, and other supportive measures should be employed, as needed. ECG monitoring is essential. Gastric lavage, followed by instillation of activated charcoal, may be useful if performed within 4 h of ingestion. In moderately severe cases of salicylate poisoning, cautiously administer sodium bicarbonate IV in sufficient quantity, if possible, to maintain an alkaline diuresis; intermittent peritoneal dialysis may also be helpful. In severe cases, hemodialysis should be seriously considered. Hyperthermia, particularly in children, and dehydration require prompt correction. Hemorrhagic phenomena may necessitate whole-blood transfusions and phytonadione (vitamin K_1). Severe cyanosis resulting from phenacetin-induced methemoglobinemia can be corrected with 1% methylene blue (1–2 mg/kg IV). Do not administer barbiturates to treat excitement or convulsions.

DRUG INTERACTIONS

Other narcotic analgesics; sedative-hypnotics, antianxiety agents, phenothiazines, general anesthetics, muscle relaxants, and other CNS depressants; MAO inhibitors; tricyclic antidepressants	⇧ CNS depression; use with caution in patients who require concomitant administration of other CNS depressants
Anticoagulants	⇧ Risk of bleeding
Alcohol	⇧ Risk of GI ulceration and CNS depression; use with caution in patients who consume excessive amounts of alcohol
Corticosteroids, phenylbutazone, oxyphenbutazone	⇧ Risk of GI ulceration
Probenecid, sulfinpyrazone	⇩ Uricosuric effect
Spironolactone	⇩ Diuretic effect
Methotrexate	⇧ Methotrexate plasma level and risk of toxicity

ALTERED LABORATORY VALUES

Blood/serum values	⇧ Prothrombin time ⇧ Uric acid (with low doses) ⇩ Uric acid (with high doses) ⇩ Thyroxine (T_4) ⇩ Thyroid-stimulating hormone ⇧ Glucose ⇩ Bilirubin
Urinary values	⇧ Glucose (with Clinitest tablets) ⇧ 5-HIAA (with nitrosonaphthol reagent test)

Use in children

Not recommended

Use in pregnancy or nursing mothers

Safe use not established relative to fetal development; however, neonatal withdrawal symptoms have been reported following propoxyphene usage during pregnancy. Although low levels of propoxyphene have been found in human milk, no adverse effects have been noted in nursing infants.

DARVON-N (Propoxyphene napsylate) Lilly

Tabs: 100 mg **Susp:** 50 mg/5 ml (16 oz) *C-IV*

INDICATIONS	**ORAL DOSAGE**
Mild to moderate pain	**Adult:** 100 mg or 10 ml (2 tsp) q4h, as needed

CONTRAINDICATIONS

Suicidal or addiction-prone individuals ● Hypersensitivity to propoxyphene ●

WARNINGS/PRECAUTIONS

Habit-forming	Psychic dependence and, less often, physical dependence and tolerance may develop when taken in higher-than-recommended doses for prolonged periods, especially in addiction-prone individuals
Overdosage	Excessive doses of propoxyphene, either alone or in combination with other CNS depressants, including alcohol (see DRUG INTERACTIONS) are a major cause of drug-related deaths; caution patients not to exceed recommended dosage, to limit their alcohol intake, and that concomitant use of other CNS depressants can cause additional CNS depression
Mental impairment, reflex-slowing	Performance of potentially hazardous activities may be impaired; caution patients accordingly and about additive effect of alcohol and other CNS depressants (see DRUG INTERACTIONS)

ADVERSE REACTIONS	Frequent reactions are italicized
Central nervous system	*Dizziness, sedation,* light-headedness, weakness, euphoria, dysphoria, minor visual disturbances
Gastrointestinal	*Nausea, vomiting,* constipation, abdominal pain, liver dysfunction
Dermatological	Rash

OVERDOSAGE

Signs and symptoms	CNS depression, ranging from somnolence (usually) to stupor and coma; respiratory depression, progressing to Cheyne-Stokes respiration, cyanosis, hypoxia, and apnea; pinpoint pupils, becoming dilated as hypoxia increases; fall in blood pressure and deterioration in cardiac performance, culminating in pulmonary edema and circulatory collapse; respiratory and metabolic acidosis; cardiac conduction delay and arrhythmias; convulsions
Treatment	Give primary attention to re-establishing adequate respiratory exchange through provision of an adequate airway and assisted or controlled ventilation; positive-pressure respiration may be desirable if pulmonary edema is present. If respiratory depression is significant, promptly administer naloxone (adult, 0.4 mg; child, 0.01 mg/kg), preferably IV, and repeat at 2- to 3-min intervals until satisfactory breathing is restored. *Do not use analeptic agents.* Oxygen, IV fluids, vasopressors, and other supportive measures should be employed, as needed. Gastric lavage, followed by instillation of activated charcoal, may be useful; dialysis is of little value unless other, dialyzable substances (such as barbiturates) have been simultaneously ingested.

DRUG INTERACTIONS

Other narcotic analgesics; sedative-hypnotics, antianxiety agents, phenothiazines, general anesthetics, muscle relaxants, and other CNS depressants; MAO inhibitors; tricyclic antidepressants	⇧ CNS depression; use with caution in patients who require concomitant administration of other CNS depressants
Alcohol	⇧ CNS depression; use with caution in patients who consume excessive amounts of alcohol

ALTERED LABORATORY VALUES

No clinically significant alterations in blood/serum or urinary values occur at therapeutic dosages

Use in children	**Use in pregnancy or nursing mothers**
Not recommended	Safe use during pregnancy not established relative to fetal development; however, neonatal withdrawal symptoms have been reported following propoxyphene usage during pregnancy. Although low levels of propoxyphene have been found in human milk, no adverse effects have been noted in nursing infants.

EMPIRIN with CODEINE (Aspirin and codeine phosphate) Burroughs Wellcome

Tabs: 325 mg aspirin with 15 (#2), 30 (#3), or 60 (#4) mg codeine phosphate *C-III*

INDICATIONS	ORAL DOSAGE
Mild, moderate, and moderate to severe pain	**Adult:** 1-2 #2 or #3 tabs q4h, as needed, or 1 #4 tab q4h, as needed

CONTRAINDICATIONS[1]

Hypersensitivity to aspirin or codeine

WARNINGS/PRECAUTIONS[1]	
Habit-forming	Psychic and/or physical dependence and tolerance may develop, especially in addiction-prone individuals
Nasal polyps, asthma, hay fever	May predispose to salicylate hypersensitivity
Mental impairment, reflex-slowing	Performance of potentially hazardous activities may be impaired; caution patients accordingly
Head injury, increased intracranial pressure	Respiratory depression and elevation of CSF pressure may be exaggerated; clinical course may be masked
Acute abdominal conditions	Diagnosis or clinical course may be obscured
Special-risk patients	Use with caution in the elderly or debilitated and in patients with severe hepatic or renal impairment, hypothyroidism, Addison's disease, prostatic hypertrophy, urethral stricture, peptic ulcer, or coagulation abnormalities

ADVERSE REACTIONS[1]	Frequent reactions are italicized
Gastrointestinal	*Nausea, vomiting,* constipation, gastric irritation and bleeding
Central nervous system	*Dizziness, light-headedness, sedation,* drowsiness, euphoria, dysphoria, headache, tinnitus, mental confusion, vertigo
Dermatological	Rash, pruritus
Hypersensitivity	Anaphylaxis
Other	Thirst, diaphoresis

OVERDOSAGE	
Signs and symptoms	*Toxic effects primarily attributable to codeine:* respiratory depression, miosis, extreme somnolence progressing to stupor or coma, skeletal-muscle flaccidity, cold and clammy skin, bradycardia, hypotension, and, in severe cases, apnea, circulatory collapse, and cardiac arrest: *aspirin-related effects:* hyperpnea, nausea, vomiting, vertigo, tinnitus, flushing, sweating, thirst, headache, drowsiness, diarrhea, and tachycardia, progressing to hyperthermia, hemorrhage, acid-base disturbances, restlessness, confusion, convulsions, vasomotor depression, coma, and respiratory failure
Treatment	Give primary attention to re-establishing adequate respiratory exchange through provision of an adequate airway and assisted or controlled ventilation; positive-pressure respiration may be desirable if pulmonary edema is present. If respiratory depression is significant, promptly administer naloxone (adult, 0.4 mg; child, 0.01 mg/kg), preferably IV, and repeat at 2- to 3-min intervals until satisfactory breathing is restored. *Do not use analeptic agents.* Oxygen, IV fluids, vasopressors, and other supportive measures should be employed, as needed. Gastric lavage, followed by instillation of activated charcoal, may be used if performed within 4 h of ingestion. In moderately severe cases of salicylate poisoning, cautiously administer sodium bicarbonate IV in sufficient quantity, if possible, to maintain an alkaline diuresis; intermittent peritoneal dialysis may also be helpful. In severe cases, hemodialysis should be seriously considered. Hyperthermia, particularly in children, and dehydration require prompt correction. Hemorrhagic phenomena may necessitate whole-blood transfusions and phytonadione (vitamin K_1).

DRUG INTERACTIONS	
Other narcotic analgesics; sedative-hypnotics, antianxiety agents, phenothiazines, general anesthetics, and other CNS depressants (including alcohol); MAO inhibitors; tricyclic antidepressants	⇧ CNS depression; reduce dose of one or both agents if used concomitantly or in close succession
Anticholinergic agents	⇧ Risk of paralytic ileus
Methotrexate	⇧ Methotrexate plasma level and risk of toxicity

[1]For other possible contraindications, warnings and precautions, and adverse reactions, see aspirin

Table continued on following page

DRUG INTERACTIONS continued

Anticoagulants	⇧ Risk of bleeding
Alcohol, corticosteroids, phenylbutazone, oxyphenbutazone	⇧ Risk of GI ulceration
Probenecid, sulfinpyrazone	⇩ Uricosuria
Spironolactone	⇩ Diuretic effect

ALTERED LABORATORY VALUES

Blood/serum values	⇧ Amylase ⇧ Lipase ⇧ Prothrombin time ⇧ Uric acid (with low doses) ⇩ Uric acid (with high doses) ⇩ Thyroxine (T_4) ⇩ Thyroid-stimulating hormone
Urinary values	⇧ Glucose (with Clinitest tablets)

Use in children

General guidelines not established

Use in pregnancy or nursing mothers

Safe use not established during pregnancy; general guidelines not established for use in nursing mothers

FIORINAL with CODEINE (Butalbital, aspirin, phenacetin, caffeine, and codeine phosphate) Sandoz

Caps: 50 mg butalbital, 200 mg aspirin, 130 mg phenacetin, 40 mg caffeine, and 7.5 (#1), 15 (#2), or 30 (#3) mg codeine phosphate *C-III*

INDICATIONS	ORAL DOSAGE
Mild to moderate pain	**Adult:** 1-2 caps to start, up to 6 caps/day, as needed

CONTRAINDICATIONS[1]

Hypersensitivity to aspirin, phenacetin, caffeine, or butalbital

WARNINGS/PRECAUTIONS[1]

Habit-forming	Psychic and/or physical dependence and tolerance may develop, especially in addiction-prone individuals

ADVERSE REACTIONS[1]

Central nervous system	Dizziness, drowsiness
Gastrointestinal	Nausea, vomiting, constipation
Dermatological	Rash
Other	Miosis

OVERDOSAGE

Signs and symptoms	*Toxic effects primarily attributable to butalbital:* drowsiness, confusion, coma, respiratory depression, hypotension, shock; *aspirin-related effects:* hyperpnea, nausea, vomiting, vertigo, tinnitus, flushing, sweating, thirst, headache, drowsiness, diarrhea, and tachycardia, progressing to hyperthermia, hemorrhage, acid-base disturbances, restlessness, confusion, convulsions, vasomotor depression, coma, and respiratory failure; *phenacetin-related effects:* nausea, vomiting, abdominal pain, chills, excitement, delirium, cyanosis due to methemoglobinemia, respiratory depression, cardiac arrest; *caffeine-related effects:* insomnia, restlessness, and excitement progressing to mild delirium, dehydration, fever, tachycardia, extrasystoles, tremor, and convulsions
Treatment	Induce emesis if patient is conscious. Gastric lavage may be used if pharyngeal and laryngeal reflexes are intact and less than 4 h have elapsed since ingestion; a cuffed endotracheal tube should be inserted before performing lavage on an unconscious patient or when necessary to provide assisted respiration. Meticulous attention should be given to maintaining adequate pulmonary ventilation. Severe hypotension may require IV use of levarterenol or phenylephrine for correction. If respiratory depression is significant, promptly administer naloxone (adult, 0.4 mg; child, 0.01 mg/kg), preferably IV, and repeat at 2- to 3-min intervals until satisfactory breathing is restored. *Do not use analeptic agents.* In moderately severe cases of salicylate poisoning, cautiously administer sodium bicarbonate in sufficient quantity, if possible, to maintain an alkaline diuresis; intermittent peritoneal dialysis may also be helpful. In severe cases, hemodialysis should be seriously considered. Hyperthermia, particularly in children, and dehydration require prompt correction. Hemorrhagic phenomena may necessitate whole-blood transfusions and phytonadione (vitamin K_1). Severe cyanosis resulting from phenacetin-induced methemoglobinemia can be corrected with 1% methylene blue (1-2 mg/kg IV). Do not administer barbiturates to treat excitement or convulsions.

DRUG INTERACTIONS

Other sedative-hypnotics; narcotic analgesics, antianxiety agents, phenothiazines, general anesthetics, and other CNS depressants (including alcohol); MAO inhibitors	⇧ CNS depression; reduce dose of one or both agents if used concomitantly or in close succession
Anticholinergic agents	⇧ Risk of paralytic ileus
Alcohol, corticosteroids, phenylbutazone, oxyphenbutazone	⇧ Risk of GI ulceration
Probenecid, sulfinpyrazone	⇩ Uricosuric effect
Spironolactone	⇩ Diuretic effect
Methotrexate	⇧ Methotrexate plasma level and risk of toxicity
Corticosteroids, digitalis, digitoxin, doxycycline, tricyclic antidepressants	⇩ Serum half-life and drug effect
Griseofulvin	⇩ Absorption of griseofulvin

[1]For other possible contraindications, warnings and precautions, and adverse reactions, see Fiorinal

Table continued on following page

ALTERED LABORATORY VALUES

Blood/serum values	⇧ Amylase ⇧ Lipase ⇧ Prothrombin time ⇧ Uric acid (with low doses) ⇩ Uric acid (with high doses) ⇩ Thyroxine (T_4) ⇩ Thyroid-stimulating hormone ⇧ Glucose ⇩ Bilirubin
Urinary values	⇧ Glucose (with Clinitest tablets) ⇧ 5-HIAA (with nitrosonaphthol reagent test)

Use in children

General guidelines not established

Use in pregnancy or nursing mothers

General guidelines not established

MICRAININ (Meprobamate and aspirin) Wallace

Tabs: 200 mg meprobamate and 325 mg aspirin *C-IV*

INDICATIONS	ORAL DOSAGE
Pain accompanied by tension and/or anxiety in patients with musculoskeletal disease (adjunctive therapy)	**Adult:** 1-2 tabs tid or qid, as needed, up to 2,400 mg meprobamate/day

ADMINISTRATION/DOSAGE ADJUSTMENTS

Discontinuation of therapy after prolonged and excessive use	Gradually reduce dosage over a period of 1-2 wk, or substitute (and then gradually withdraw) a short-acting barbiturate to minimize withdrawal symptoms

CONTRAINDICATIONS

Acute intermittent porphyria ●	Hypersensitivity or severe intolerance to aspirin, meprobamate, or related compounds ●

WARNINGS/PRECAUTIONS

Habit-forming	Psychic and/or physical dependence and tolerance may develop; use with caution in addiction-prone individuals and watch for signs of chronic intoxication, such as ataxia, slurred speech, and vertigo
Abrupt discontinuation of therapy after prolonged or excessive use	May precipitate recurrence of pre-existing symptoms, such as anxiety, anorexia, or insomnia, or withdrawal symptoms, such as vomiting, ataxia, tremors, muscle twitching, confusion, hallucinations, and rarely, convulsive seizures, especially in patients with CNS damage or pre-existing or latent convulsive disorders (see ADMINISTRATION/DOSAGE ADJUSTMENTS)
Mental impairment, reflex-slowing	Performance of potentially hazardous activities may be impaired; caution patient accordingly
Hepatic or renal impairment	Use with caution and monitor for signs of excess drug accumulation (see OVERDOSAGE)
Seizures	May be precipitated occasionally in epileptic patients
Allergic or idiosyncratic reactions	May occur due to meprobamate component (see ADVERSE REACTIONS); cross-sensitivity with metabumate and carbromal may exist. Institute appropriate symptomatic therapy, including, where appropriate, antihistamines, epinephrine, and, in severe cases, corticosteroids. Rarely, use of aspirin in persons allergic to salicylates can result in life-threatening allergic episodes.
Special-risk patients	Use with extreme caution in patients with peptic ulcer or coagulation abnormalities due to presence of aspirin

ADVERSE REACTIONS

Central nervous system	Drowsiness, ataxia, dizziness, slurred speech, headache, vertigo, weakness, paresthesias, impairment of visual accommodation, euphoria, overstimulation, paradoxical excitement, fast EEG activity
Gastrointestinal	Nausea, vomiting, diarrhea
Cardiovascular	Palpitations, tachycardia, arrhythmias, transient ECG changes, syncope, hypotensive crisis (one fatal case)
Hypersensitivity	Itchy, urticarial, or erythematous maculopapular rash (either generalized or confined to groin); leukopenia; acute nonthrombocytopenic purpura; petechiae, ecchymoses; eosinophilia; peripheral edema; adenopathy; fever; fixed drug eruption; rarely, hyperpyrexia, chills, angioneurotic edema, bronchospasm, oliguria, anuria, anaphylaxis, erythema multiforme, exfoliative dermatitis, stomatitis, proctitis, Stevens-Johnson syndrome, and bullous dermatitis (one fatal case)
Hematological	Agranulocytosis and aplastic anemia (causal relationship not established); thrombocytopenic purpura (rare)
Other	Exacerbation of porphyric symptoms

OVERDOSAGE

Signs and symptoms	*Toxic effects primarily attributable to meprobamate:* drowsiness, lethargy, stupor, ataxia, coma, shock, vasomotor and respiratory collapse; *aspirin-related effects:* hyperpnea, nausea, vomiting, vertigo, tinnitus, flushing, sweating, thirst, headache, drowsiness, diarrhea, and tachycardia progressing to hyperthermia, hemorrhage, acid-base disturbances, restlessness, confusion, convulsions, vasomotor depression, coma, and respiratory failure

Table continued on following page

MICRAININ continued

OVERDOSAGE continued

Treatment	Induce emesis or perform gastric lavage, followed by activated charcoal, to remove any remaining drug from stomach. (Incomplete gastric emptying and delayed absorption may lead to fatal relapse.) Institute appropriate supportive measures, including respiratory assistance, and cautious use of pressor agents, as indicated. In moderately severe cases of salicylate poisoning, cautiously administer sodium bicarbonate IV in sufficient quantity, if possible, to maintain an alkaline diuresis; intermittent peritoneal dialysis may also be helpful. In severe cases, hemodialysis should be seriously considered. Hyperthermia, particularly in children, and dehydration require prompt correction. Hemorrhagic phenomena may necessitate whole-blood transfusions and phytonadione (vitamin K_1).

DRUG INTERACTIONS

Other narcotic analgesics and sedative-hypnotics; antianxiety agents, phenothiazines, general anesthetics, and other CNS depressants (including alcohol); MAO inhibitors; tricyclic antidepressants	⇧ CNS depression; reduce dose of one or both agents if used concomitantly or in close succession
Alcohol, corticosteroids phenylbutazone, oxyphenbutazone	⇧ Risk of GI ulceration
Probenecid, sulfinpyrazone	⇩ Uricosuric effect
Spironolactone	⇩ Diuretic effect
Methotrexate	⇧ Methotrexate plasma level and/or toxicity

ALTERED LABORATORY VALUES

Blood/serum values	⇧ Prothrombin time ⇧ Uric acid (with low doses) ⇩ Uric acid (with high doses) ⇩ Thyroxine (T_4) ⇩ Thyroid-stimulating hormone
Urinary values	⇧ Glucose (with Clinitest tablets)

Use in children

Not recommended for use in children under 12 yr of age

Use in pregnancy or nursing mothers

Drug should almost always be avoided during pregnancy. An increased risk of congenital malformations during the 1st trimester has been associated with minor tranquilizers, including meprobamate. Aspirin may also have teratogenic effects. Both meprobamate and aspirin cross the placental barrier and have been detected in human milk. Meprobamate appears in breast milk in concentrations 2–4 times that of maternal plasma.

MOTRIN (Ibuprofen) **Upjohn**

Tabs: 300, 400, 600 mg

INDICATIONS	ORAL DOSAGE
Mild to moderate pain	**Adult:** 400 mg q4-6h, as needed, up to 2,400 mg/day
Rheumatoid arthritis, osteoarthritis	**Adult:** 300-600 mg tid or qid

CONTRAINDICATIONS	
Hypersensitivity	To ibuprofen or to aspirin and other nonsteroidal, anti-inflammatory drugs when manifested by nasal polyps, angioedema, or bronchospasm

NOTE: Full chart appears on page 1012.

NALFON 200 (Fenoprofen calcium) Dista

Caps: 200 mg

INDICATIONS	ORAL DOSAGE
Mild to moderate pain	**Adult:** 200 mg q4–6h, as needed

ADMINISTRATION/DOSAGE ADJUSTMENTS

Timing of administration	Since food decreases fenoprofen blood levels, administer 30 min before or 2 h after meals; if gastrointestinal complaints occur, administer with meals or milk
Combination therapy	Neither benefits nor harmful interactions have been demonstrated with gold salts or corticosteroids. Concomitant therapy with salicylates is not recommended; aspirin may increase excretion rate of fenoprofen, and no additional benefit is obtained beyond the effect of aspirin alone.

CONTRAINDICATIONS

Hypersensitivity	To fenoprofen or to aspirin and other nonsteroidal, anti-inflammatory drugs when manifested by asthma, rhinitis, or urticaria
Significantly impaired renal function	Drug may accumulate, since it is eliminated primarily by the kidneys

WARNINGS/PRECAUTIONS

Peptic ulcer, perforation, GI bleeding	May occur and can be severe; use with extreme caution in patients with a history of upper-GI-tract disease or with active peptic ulcer
Genitourinary tract problems	Have been reported (see ADVERSE REACTIONS); do not use in patients who have had such reactions with other nonsteroidal anti-inflammatory drugs. In patients with possibly compromised renal function, examine renal function periodically.
Liver function	Test periodically for alterations (see ALTERED LABORATORY VALUES); discontinue therapy if significant abnormalities appear
Corticosteroid therapy	If discontinued, reduce dosage gradually to avoid complications of sudden steroid withdrawal
Initial low hemoglobin values	Obtain periodic hemoglobin determinations during long-term therapy
Peripheral edema	May occur; use with caution in patients with compromised cardiac function or hypertension
Prolonged bleeding time	May occur due to inhibition of platelet aggregation
Impaired hearing	Monitor auditory function periodically
Mental impairment	Performance of potentially hazardous activities may be impaired; caution patients accordingly
Visual impairment	May occur with some nonsteroidal anti-inflammatory drugs; perform ophthalmologic studies periodically

ADVERSE REACTIONS[1]	Frequent reactions are italicized
Gastrointestinal	*Dyspepsia (3–9%), constipation (3–9%), nausea (3–9%), vomiting (3–9%), abdominal pain (1–2%), anorexia (1–2%), occult blood loss (1–2%), diarrhea (1–2%), flatulence (1–2%), dry mouth (1–2%),* gastritis, peptic ulcer with or without perforation and/or GI hemorrhage; aphthous ulcerations or the buccal mucosa, metallic taste, and pancreatitis (causal relationship not established)
Hepatic	Jaundice, cholestatic hepatitis
Central nervous system	*Headache (15%), somnolence (15%), dizziness (3–9%), nervousness (3–9%), asthenia (3–9%), tremor (1–2%), confusion (1–2%), insomnia (1–2%), fatigue (1–2%), malaise (1–2%);* depression, disorientation, seizures, trigeminal neuralgia, and personality change (causal relationship not established)
Dermatological	*Pruritus (3–9%), rash (1–2%), increased sweating (1–2%), urticaria (1–2%);* Stevens-Johnson syndrome, angioneurotic edema, exfoliative dermatitis, and alopecia (causal relationship not established)
Cardiovascular	*Palpitations (3–9%), tachycardia (1–2%);* atrial fibrillation, pulmonary edema, ECG changes, and supraventricular tachycardia (causal relationship not established)

[1]Reactions observed during clinical trials of fenoprofen in the treatment of rheumatoid arthritis and osteoarthritis; when fenoprofen was used for analgesia in short-term studies, the incidence of adverse reactions was markedly lower than that observed during long-term trials

Table continued on following page

NALFON 200 continued

ADVERSE REACTIONS continued

Ophthalmic	*Blurred vision (1-2%);* diplopia and optic neuritis (causal relationship not established)
Otic	*Tinnitus (1-2%), decreased hearing (1-2%)*
Genitourinary	Dysuria, cystitis, hematuria, oliguria, azotemia, anuria, allergic nephritis, nephrosis, papillary necrosis
Hematological	Purpura, bruising, hemorrhage, thrombocytopenia, hemolytic anemia, agranulocytosis, pancytopenia; aplastic anemia (causal relationship not established)
Other	*Dyspnea (1-2%),* peripheral edema, anaphylaxis; lymphadenopathy, mastodynia, burning tongue, and fever (causal relationship not established)

OVERDOSAGE

Signs and symptoms	See ADVERSE REACTIONS
Treatment	Induce emesis or use gastric lavage to empty stomach, followed by activated charcoal. Employ supportive measures, as indicated. Urinary alkalinization and forced diuresis may be helpful. Furosemide does *not* lower blood levels of fenoprofen.

DRUG INTERACTIONS

Albumin-bound drugs	Displacement of either drug
Hydantoins	⇧ Hydantoin plasma level; observe for signs of toxicity
Sulfonamides	⇧ Sulfonamide plasma level; observe for signs of toxicity
Sulfonylureas	⇧ Sulfonylurea plasma level; observe for signs of toxicity
Coumarin anticoagulants	⇧ Prothrombin time; observe patient carefully
Aspirin	⇩ Plasma half-life of fenoprofen; do not use concomitantly
Phenobarbital	⇩ Plasma half-life of fenoprofen; if necessary, adjust fenoprofen dosage

ALTERED LABORATORY VALUES

Blood/serum values	⇧ Alkaline phosphatase ⇧ SGOT ⇧ Lactate dehydrogenase ⇧ BUN

No clinically significant alterations in urinary values occur at therapeutic dosages

Use in children

Safety and effectiveness have not been established

Use in pregnancy or nursing mothers

Not recommended due to lack of proof that use is safe in pregnant patients and nursing mothers

NAPROSYN (Naproxen) **Syntex**

Tabs: 250, 375 mg

INDICATIONS	ORAL DOSAGE
Mild to moderate pain, dysmenorrhea	**Adult:** 500 mg to start, followed by 250 mg q6–8h, as needed; maximum daily dose: 1250 mg
Rhematoid arthritis,[1] osteoarthritis	**Adult:** 250–375 mg bid (in AM and PM)

CONTRAINDICATIONS	
Hypersensitivity	To naproxen or aspirin and other nonsteroidal, anti-inflammatory drugs when manifested by asthma, rhinitis, or urticaria

NOTE: Full chart appears on page 1018.

PONSTEL (Mefenamic acid) **Parke-Davis**

Caps: 250 mg

INDICATIONS	ORAL DOSAGE
Mild to moderate pain	**Adult:** 500 mg to start, with food, followed by 250 mg q6h, as needed, for no longer than 1 wk

CONTRAINDICATIONS

Gastrointestinal ulceration ●	Chronic gastrointestinal inflammation ●	Hypersensitivity to mefenamic acid ●

WARNINGS/PRECAUTIONS

Diarrhea	May occur; discontinue therapy promptly
Renal or hepatic disease	Use with caution
Gastrointestinal inflammation	Use with caution
Rash	May occur; discontinue therapy promptly
Concomitant anticoagulant therapy	Prothrombin time may be prolonged; monitor frequently
Asthma	May be acutely exacerbated

ADVERSE REACTIONS

Gastrointestinal	Nausea, discomfort, vomiting, gas, diarrhea, bowel inflammation or hemorrhage, mild hepatic toxicity
Hematological	Severe autoimmune hemolytic anemia (with prolonged use), leukopenia, eosinophilia, thrombocytopenic purpura, agranulocytosis, pancytopenia, bone-marrow hypoplasia
Central nervous system	Drowsiness, dizziness, nervousness, headache, blurred vision, insomnia
Dermatological	Urticaria, rash, facial edema
Renal	Mild toxicity dysuria, hematuria
Ophthalmic	Irritation, reversible loss of color vision (rare)
Cardiovascular	Palpitations (rare), dyspnea (rare)
Other	Ear pain, diaphoresis, increased insulin requirements in diabetics (one case)

OVERDOSAGE

Signs and symptoms	Drowsiness, dizziness, nausea, vomiting, diarrhea, rash, various blood dyscrasias
Treatment	Empty stomach by inducing emesis or gastric lavage, followed by activated charcoal. Treat symptomatically and institute supportive measures, as indicated.

DRUG INTERACTIONS

Oral anticoagulants	⇧ Risk of bleeding
Insulin	⇩ Hypoglycemic effect
Aspirin and other salicylates, corticosteroids, indomethacin, phenylbutazone, oxyphenbutazone	⇧ Risk of GI ulceration

ALTERED LABORATORY VALUES

Blood/serum values	⇧ BUN ⇧ Prothrombin time + Coombs' test
Urinary values	+ Bile (with diazo tablet test)

Use in children

Contraindicated for use in children under 14 yr of age

Use in pregnancy or nursing mothers

Safe use during pregnancy not established. Animal studies have shown a decreased rate of survival to weaning, delayed parturition, decreased fertility, and an increased number of resorptions, but no fetal anomalies. General guidelines not established

TYLENOL with CODEINE (Acetaminophen and codeine phosphate) **McNeil Pharmaceutical**

Tabs: 300 mg acetaminophen and 7.5 (#1), 15 (#2), 30 (#3), or 60 (#4) mg codeine phosphate *C-III* **Elixir:** 120 mg acetaminophen and 12 mg codeine phosphate per 5 ml *C-V*

INDICATIONS	ORAL DOSAGE
Mild to moderate pain	**Adult:** 1–2 #1, #2, or #3 tabs or 15 ml (1 tbsp) q4h, as needed **Child (3–6 yr):** 5 ml (1 tsp) tid or qid **Child (7–12 yr):** 10 ml (2 tsp) tid or qid
Moderate to severe pain	**Adult:** 1 #4 tab q4h, as needed

CONTRAINDICATIONS

Hypersensitivity to acetaminophen or codeine

WARNINGS/PRECAUTIONS

Habit-forming	Psychic and/or physical dependence and tolerance may develop, especially in addiction-prone individuals
Mental impairment, reflex-slowing	Performance of potentially hazardous activities may be impaired; caution patients accordingly
Head injury, increased intracranial pressure	Respiratory depression and elevation of CSF pressure may be impaired; clinical course may be masked
Acute abdominal conditions	Diagnosis and clinical course may be masked
Special-risk patients	Use with caution in the elderly and debilitated and in patients with severe renal or hepatic impairment, hypothyroidism, Addison's disease, prostatic hypertrophy, or urethral stricture

ADVERSE REACTIONS[1]	Frequent reactions are italicized
Central nervous system	*Light-headedness, dizziness, sedation,* euphoria, dysphoria
Gastrointestinal	*Nausea, vomiting,* constipation
Dermatological	Pruritus

OVERDOSAGE

Signs and symptoms	*Toxic effects primarily attributable to codeine:* respiratory depression, miosis, extreme somnolence progressing to stupor or coma, skeletal-muscle flaccidity, cold and clammy skin, bradycardia, hypotension, and, in severe cases, apnea, circulatory collapse, and cardiac arrest; *acetaminophen-related effects:* nausea vomiting, diaphoresis, and general malaise; clinical and laboratory evidence of hepatotoxicity (vomiting, right upper quadrant tenderness, increased SGOT, SGPT, serum bilirubin, and prothrombin time, and possible hypoglycemia) may not be apparent until 48–72 h after ingestion
Treatment	Give primary attention to re-establishing adequate respiratory exchange through provision of an adequate airway and assisted or controlled ventilation; positive-pressure respiration may be desirable if pulmonary edema is present. If respiratory depression is significant, promptly administer naloxone (adult, 0.4 mg; child, 0.01 mg/kg), preferably IV, and repeat at 2- to 3-min intervals until satisfactory breathing is restored. *Do not use analeptic agents.* Oxygen, IV fluids, vasopressors, and other supportive measures should be employed, as needed. Gastric lavage, followed by instillation of activated charcoal, may be useful; the charcoal *must* be lavaged out after 1 h and before instilling acetylcysteine as an antidote. (Call the Rocky Mountain Poison Center, [800] 525-6115, for assistance in diagnosing acetaminophen overdosage and for directions for administering acetylcysteine as an antidote [currently investigational].) Determine serum acetaminophen level as soon as possible, but not earlier than 4 h after suspected ingestion. Liver function studies should be obtained initially and repeated at 24-h intervals. Acetylcysteine can be given up to 24 h postingestion, but should be administered as early as possible, within 16 h of suspected ingestion for optimal results.

DRUG INTERACTIONS

Other narcotic analgesics; sedative-hypnotics, antianxiety agents, phenothiazines, general anesthetics, and other CNS depressants (including alcohol); MAO inhibitors; tricyclic antidepressants	⇧ CNS depression; reduce dose of one or both agents if used concomitantly or in close succession

[1]For other possible adverse reactions, see acetaminophen

Table continued on following page

DRUG INTERACTIONS continued

Anticholinergic agents	⇧ Risk of paralytic ileus
Warfarin	⇧ Hypoprothrombinemia (slight)

ALTERED LABORATORY VALUES

Blood/serum values	⇧ Amylase ⇧ Lipase ⇧ Prothrombin time ⇧ Uric acid (with phosphotungstate method)
Urinary values	⇧ 5-HIAA (with nitrosonaphthol reagent test)

Use in children

See INDICATIONS; safe dosage in children under 3 yr of age has not been established

Use in pregnancy or nursing mothers

Safe use not established during pregnancy; general guidelines not established for use in nursing mothers

Note: Acetaminophen with codeine also marketed as **EMPRACET with CODEINE** (Burroughs Wellcome); **PHENAPHEN with CODEINE** and **PHENAPHEN-650 with CODEINE** (Robins)

WYGESIC (Propoxyphene hydrochloride and acetaminophen) Wyeth

Tabs: 65 mg propoxyphene and 650 mg acetaminophen *C-IV*

INDICATIONS	ORAL DOSAGE
Mild to moderate pain	**Adult:** 1 tab q4h, as needed

CONTRAINDICATIONS

Hypersensitivity to propoxyphene or acetaminophen

WARNINGS/PRECAUTIONS

Habit-forming	Psychic and, less often, physical dependence and tolerance may develop.
Overdosage	Excessive doses of propoxyphene, either alone or in combination with other CNS depressants, including alcohol (see DRUG INTERACTIONS), have resulted in toxic effects and fatalities.

ADVERSE REACTIONS[1] Frequent reactions are italicized

Central nervous system	*Dizziness, sedation,* light-headedness, headache, weakness, euphoria, dysphoria, minor visual disturbances
Gastrointestinal	*Nausea, vomiting,* constipation, abdominal pain, liver dysfunction
Dermatological	*Rash*

OVERDOSAGE

Signs and symptoms	*Propoxyphene-related effects:* CNS depression, ranging from somnolence (usually) to stupor and coma; respiratory depression, progressing to Cheyne-Stokes respiration, cyanosis, hypoxia, and apnea; pinpoint pupils, becoming dilated as hypoxia increases; fall in blood pressure and deterioration in cardiac performance, culminating in pulmonary edema and circulatory collapse; respiratory and metabolic acidosis; cardiac conduction delay and arrhythmias; convulsions; *acetaminophen-related effects:* nausea, vomiting, diaphoresis, and general malaise; clinical and laboratory evidence of hepatotoxicity may not be apparent until 48-72 h after ingestion
Treatment	Give primary attention to re-establishing adequate respiratory exchange through provision of an adequate airway and assisted or controlled ventilation; positive-pressure respiration may be desirable if pulmonary edema is present. If respiratory depression is significant, promptly administer naloxone (adult, 0.4 mg; child, 0.01 mg/kg), preferably IV, and repeat at 2- to 3-min intervals until satisfactory breathing is restored. *Do not use analeptic agents.* Monitor blood gases, pH, and electrolytes, and promptly correct any acid-base or electrolyte abnormalities present (lactic acidosis may require IV sodium bicarbonate for prompt correction). Administer an anticonvulsant in carefully titrated doses if seizures occur. Oxygen, IV fluids, vasopressors, and other supportive measures should be employed, as needed. ECG monitoring is essential. Gastric lavage, followed by instillation of activated charcoal, may be useful; the charcoal *must* be lavaged out after 1 h and before instilling acetylcysteine as an antidote. Determine serum acetaminophen level as soon as possible, but not earlier than 4 h after suspected ingestion. Liver function studies should be obtained initially and repeated at 24-h intervals.

DRUG INTERACTIONS

Other narcotic analgesics; sedative-hypnotics, antianxiety agents, phenothiazines, general anesthetics, and other CNS depressants (including alcohol); MAO inhibitors; tricyclic antidepressants	⇧ CNS depression
Warfarin	⇧ Hypoprothrombinemia (slight)

ALTERED LABORATORY VALUES

Blood/serum values	⇧ Prothrombin time ⇧ Uric acid (with phosphotungstate method)
Urinary values	⇧ 5-HIAA (with nitrosonaphthol reagent test)

Use in children	Use in pregnancy or nursing mothers
Not recommended for use in children	Safe use during pregnancy not established relative to fetal development; however, neonatal withdrawal symptoms have been reported following propoxyphene usage during pregnancy. General guidelines not established for use in nursing mothers.

[1]For other possible adverse reactions, see acetaminophen

ZOMAX (Zomepirac sodium) McNeil Pharmaceutical

Tabs: 100 mg

INDICATIONS	ORAL DOSAGE
Mild to moderately severe pain	**Adult:** 100 mg q4-6h, as needed; for mild pain, 50 mg q4-6h may be adequate

CONTRAINDICATIONS

Intolerance to zomepirac	Hypersensitivity to aspirin and other nonsteroidal anti-inflammatory drugs manifested by bronchospasm, rhinitis, urticaria, or other sensitivity reactions

WARNINGS/PRECAUTIONS

Peptic ulcer, GI bleeding	May occur; use with caution in patients with a history of upper GI disease
Prolonged use	May result in adverse effects on the urinary tract (see ADVERSE REACTIONS) and tumorigenicity, based on studies in rats; use with caution in patients treated for longer than 6 mo and perform periodic renal function tests
Patients with renal impairment	Reduce dosage and monitor closely for signs of excessive drug accumulation
Peripheral edema	May occur with prolonged therapy; use with caution in patients with fluid retention, hypertension, or heart failure
Inhibited platelet function and prolonged bleeding time	Use with caution in patients with coagulation disorders
Ocular changes	Have been reported in animals exposed to other nonsteroidal anti-inflammatory drugs; if visual symptoms develop, perform an ophthalmic examination
Fever and inflammation	May be reduced, masking complications of presumed noninfectious, noninflammatory, painful conditions
Concurrent use of aspirin	Not recommended, as there have been no controlled clinical trials demonstrating whether the interaction of zomepirac and aspirin is beneficial or harmful

ADVERSE REACTIONS

	Frequent reactions are italicized
Gastrointestinal	*Nausea (12%), distress (3-9%), diarrhea (3-9%), abdominal pain (3-9%), dyspepsia (3-9%), constipation (3-9%), flatulence (3-9%), vomiting (3-9%), gastritis (1-2%), anorexia (1-2%), taste change (1-2%),* peptic ulcer, GI bleeding; liver function abnormalities (causal relationship not established)
Central nervous system	*Dizziness (3-9%), insomnia (3-9%), drowsiness (1-2%), paresthesia (1-2%), tinnitus (1-2%), nervousness (1-2%), anxiety (1-2%), depression (1-2%)*
Cardiovascular	*Edema (3-9%), elevated blood pressure (3-9%); cardiac irregularity (1-2%), palpitations (1-2%)*
Dermatological	*Rash (3-9%); pruritus (1-2%), skin irritation (1-2%), sweating (1-2%),* urticaria
Genitourinary	*Urinary tract infection (3-9%), urinary frequency (1-2%), vaginitis (1-2%),* hematuria
Other	*Asthenia (3-9%),* periorbital edema; chills (causal relationship not established)

OVERDOSAGE

Toxicity has not been reported in clinical use[1]

DRUG INTERACTIONS

No clinically significant drug interactions have been observed

ALTERED LABORATORY VALUES

Blood/serum values	⇧ BUN ⇧ Creatinine

No clinically significant alterations in urinary values occur at therapeutic dosages

Use in children

Not recommended

Use in pregnancy or nursing mothers

Not recommended during pregnancy or in nursing mothers

[1]Although there has been no experience with acute overdose ingestions of zomepirac, standard measures, including gastric evacuation, instillation of activated charcoal, and general supportive therapy, would presumably apply; animal studies indicate that alkalinization of the urine by administration of bicarbonate enhances zomepirac elimination and may be beneficial in a clinical overdosage situation.

ASPIRIN (Various manufacturers)

Tabs: mg/gr per tab varies by manufacturer; see table on page 675.

INDICATIONS	ORAL DOSAGE
Pain, including headache, muscular aches and pains, minor arthritis pains, rheumatism, bursitis, lumbago, sciatica, toothache, teething pains, pain following dental procedures, neuralgia, neuritis, and dysmenorrhea; **sleeplessness** due to minor painful discomfort **Fever and discomfort** of colds and "flu" or accompanying immunizations	**Adult:** 325–650 mg q4h, up to 3,900 mg/day; sust-rel tabs: 1,300 mg q8h, up to 3,900 mg/day **Child (2–4 yr):** 162 mg/2.5 gr q4h, up to 5 doses/day **Child (4–6 yr):** 243 mg/3.75 gr q4h, up to 5 doses/day **Child (6–9 yr):** 325 mg/5 gr q4h, up to 5 doses/day **Child (9–11 yr):** 407 mg/6.25 gr q4h, up to 5 doses/day **Child (11–12 yr):** 488 mg/7.5 gr q4h, up to 5 doses/day
Reducing the risk of **recurrent transient ischemic attacks or stroke** in men who have had transient ischemia of the brain due to fibrin platelet emboli[1]	**Adult:** 325 mg qid or 650 mg bid

CONTRAINDICATIONS[2]

Bleeding ulcer ●	Hemorrhagic states ●
Hemophilia ●	Hypersensitivity to salicylates ●

WARNINGS/PRECAUTIONS[2]

Gastric irritation	Especially in patients with gastric ulcers, erosive gastritis, or bleeding tendencies; use with caution
Blood coagulation abnormalities	Including pre-existing hypoprothrombinemia and vitamin K deficiency; use with caution
Nasal polyps, asthma, hay fever	May predispose to salicylate hypersensitivity; use with caution
Before surgery	Drug interferes with platelet aggregation

ADVERSE REACTIONS[2,3]

Gastrointestinal	Nausea, dyspepsia, heartburn, epigastric discomfort, anorexia, diarrhea, occult blood loss, hemorrhage
Central nervous system	Dizziness, tinnitus, headache, deafness
Respiratory	Hyperventilation
Cardiovascular	Increased pulse rate
Dermatological	Skin eruptions
Other	Sweating, thirst, electrolyte and acid-base imbalance

OVERDOSAGE

Signs and symptoms	*Early*: rapid and deep breathing, hyperventilation, nausea, vomiting, vertigo, tinnitus, flushing, sweating, thirst, headache, drowsiness, diarrhea, tachycardia; *late*: fever, hemorrhage, excitement, confusion, convulsions, vasomotor depression, coma, respiratory failure, and respiratory alkalosis followed by respiratory and metabolic acidosis (primarily in children)

[1]*FDA Drug Bulletin* 10(1):2 1980. Applies to Ascriptin, Bayer, and Bufferin.
[2]Miller RL et al, in Melmon KL, Morelli HF (eds): *Clinical Pharmacology.* New York, Macmillan, 1978, pp 657–708 Moertel CG et al: *N Eng J Med 286:813-815, 1972; Tainter ML, Ferus AJ: Aspirin in Modern Therapy: A Review.* New York, Bayer Company Division of Sterling Drug, Inc, 1969, pp 1–128; *United States Pharmacopeia Dispensing Information 1980.* Rockville, Md, United States Pharmacopeial Convention, Inc, 1980
[3]Adverse reactions are dose related. Most reactions associated with intoxication resulting from continued usage of large doses

Table continued on following page

OVERDOSAGE continued

Treatment	If less than 4 h have elapsed since ingestion, induce emesis or perform gastric lavage, followed by activated charcoal, to remove any remaining drug from the stomach. Initial therapy should be directed at reducing hyperthermia by external sponging with tepid water, correcting dehydration by appropriate IV fluid replacement, and maintaining adequate cardiorespiratory and renal function. In moderately severe cases of salicylate poisoning, cautiously administer sodium bicarbonate IV in sufficient quantity, if possible, to maintain an alkaline diuresis; intermittent peritoneal dialysis may also be helpful. In severe cases, hemodialysis should be seriously considered. Potassium should be added to the repair solution to compensate for potassium losses once urine formation is deemed adequate. Glucose may be provided to correct ketosis and hypoglycemia. Plasma transfusion may be beneficial if shock intervenes. Hemorrhagic phenomena may necessitate whole-blood transfusions and phytonadione (vitamin K_1). Do not administer barbiturates to treat excitement or convulsions.

DRUG INTERACTIONS

Anticoagulants	⇧ Risk of bleeding
Alcohol	⇧ Risk of GI ulceration
Corticosteroids	⇧ Risk of GI ulceration
Pheynylbutazone, oxyphenbutazone	⇧ Risk of GI ulceration
Probenecid, sulfinpyrazone	⇩ Uricosuria
Spironolactone	⇩ Diuretic effect
Methotrexate	⇧ Methotrexate plasma level and risk of toxicity

ALTERED LABORATORY VALUES

Blood/ serum values	⇧ Prothrombin time ⇧ Uric acid (with low doses) ⇩ Uric acid (with high doses) ⇩ Thyroxine (T_4) ⇩ Thyroid-stimulating hormone
Urinary values	⇧ Glucose (with Clinitest tablets)

Use in children

See INDICATIONS

Use in pregnancy or nursing mothers

High doses are not recommended . General guidelines not established for use during pregnancy and in nursing mothers.

Note: Other nonprescription analgesics containing aspirin are listed in the table on page 675.

EXCEDRIN (Aspirin, acetaminophen, salicylamide, and caffeine) Bristol-Myers

Tabs: 3 gr (194.4 mg) aspirin, 1.5 gr (97.2 mg) acetaminophen, 2 gr (129.6 mg) salicylamide, and 1 gr (64.8 mg) caffeine

INDICATIONS	ORAL DOSAGE
Pain, including headache, sinusitis, muscular ache, menstrual discomfort, toothache, and minor arthritic pain **Discomfort** of colds and flu	**Adult:** 2 tab q4h, as needed, up to 8 tabs/24 h **Child (6–10 yr):** 1 tab q4h, as needed, up to 4 tabs/24 h

CONTRAINDICATIONS

Hypersensitivity to salicylates or acetaminophen ●	Also see CONTRAINDICATIONS for both aspirin and acetaminophen ●

WARNINGS/PRECAUTIONS

Patient self-medication	Patient should not use product if pain persists for more than 10 days, if sinus or arthritic pain persists, if skin redness is present, or in arthritic conditions affecting children under 12 yr of age without advice and supervision of physician

Also see WARNINGS/PRECAUTIONS for both aspirin and acetaminophen

ADVERSE REACTIONS

See ADVERSE REACTIONS for both aspirin and acetaminophen

OVERDOSAGE

Signs and symptoms In all cases of suspected overdose, immediately call the Rocky Mountain Poison Center (800) 525-6115, for assistance in diagnosis and for directions in administering N-acetylcysteine as an antidote (currently investigational)	*Aspirin-related effects:* rapid and deep breathing, hyperventilation, nausea, vomiting, vertigo, tinnitus, flushing, sweating, thirst, headache, drowsiness, diarrhea, tachycardia, fever, hemorrhage, excitement, confusion, convulsions, vasomotor depression, coma, respiratory failure, and respiratory alkalosis followed by respiratory and metabolic acidosis (primarily in children). *Acetaminophen-related effects:* nausea, vomiting, diaphoresis, and general malaise (some patients may be asymptomatic); clinical and laboratory evidence of hepatotoxicity (vomiting; right upper quadrant tenderness; increased SGOT, SGPT, serum bilirubin, and prothrombin time; and possible hypoglycemia) may not be apparent until 48–72 h after ingestion; *Caffeine-related effects:* insomnia, restlessness, tremors, delirium, tachycardia, extrasystoles, tinnitus, urinary frequency.
Treatment	If less than 4 h have elapsed since ingestion, induce emesis or perform gastric lavage, followed by activated charcoal, to remove any remaining drug from the stomach; the charcoal *must* be lavaged out after 1 h and before instilling acetylcysteine as an antidote for acetaminophen overdosage. Initial therapy should be directed at reducing hyperthermia by external sponging with tepid water, correcting dehydration by appropriate IV fluid replacement, and maintaining adequate cardiorespiratory and renal function. Determine serum acetaminophen level as soon as possible, but not earlier than 4 h after suspected ingestion. Liver function studies should be obtained initially and repeated at 24-h intervals. Acetylcysteine can be given up to 24 h postingestion, but should be administered as early as possible, within 16 h of suspected overdose ingestion for optimal results. In moderately severe cases of salicylate poisoning, cautiously administer sodium bicarbonate IV in sufficient quantity, if possible, to maintain an alkaline diuresis; intermittent peritoneal dialysis may also be helpful. In severe cases, hemodialysis should be seriously considered. Potassium should be added to the repair solution to compensate for potassium losses once urine formation is deemed adequate. Glucose may be provided to correct ketosis and hypoglycemia. Plasma transfusion may be beneficial if shock intervenes. Hemorrhagic phenomena may necessitate whole-blood transfusions and phytonadione (vitamin K). Do not administer barbiturates to treat excitement or convulsions.

DRUG INTERACTIONS

Anticoagulants	⇧ Risk of bleeding
Alcohol, corticosteroids, phenylbutazone, oxyphenbutazone	⇧ Risk of GI ulceration
Probenecid, sulfinpyrazone	⇩ Uricosuric effect
Spironolactone	⇩ Diuretic effect
Methotrexate	⇧ Methotrexate plasma level and risk of toxicity

Table continued on following page

ALTERED LABORATORY VALUES

Blood/serum values	⇧ Prothrombin time ⇧ Uric acid (with low doses and phosphotungstate method) ⇩ Uric acid (with high doses) ⇩ Thyroxine (T_4)
Urinary values	⇩ Thyroid-stimulating hormone ⇧ Glucose (with Clinitest tablets) ⇧ 5-HIAA (with nitrosonaphthol reagent test)

Use in children

See INDICATIONS; contraindicated for use in children under 6 yr of age

Use in pregnancy or nursing mothers

High doses are not recommended during pregnancy; general guidelines not established for use during pregnancy and in nursing mothers

Note: Aspirin and acetaminophen are also the principal analgesics in **VANQUISH** (Glenbrook).

TYLENOL, REGULAR-STRENGTH (Acetaminophen) McNeil Consumer Products

Tabs: 325 mg

INDICATIONS	ORAL DOSAGE
Mild to moderate pain **Fever and discomfort** associated with bacterial and viral infections	**Adult:** 325–650 mg q4–6h, up to 3,900 mg/day **Child (6–12 yr):** 160–325 mg (½–1 tab) tid or qid

TYLENOL, EXTRA-STRENGTH (Acetaminophen) McNeil Consumer Products

Tabs: 500 mg **Caps:** 500 mg **Liq:** 1 g/30 ml

INDICATIONS	ORAL DOSAGE
Same as for Regular-Strength Tylenol	**Adult:** 1 g or 1 fl oz tid or qid, up to 4 doses/day

TYLENOL (Acetaminophen) DROPS, ELIXIR, and CHEWABLE TABLETS McNeil Consumer Products

Drops: 60 mg/0.6 ml (one dropperful) **Elixir:** 120 mg/5 ml **Tabs:** 80 mg

INDICATIONS	ORAL DOSAGE
Mild to moderate pain, including headache, myalgias, post-immunization reactions, and post-tonsillectomy pain **Fever and discomfort** associated with bacterial and viral infections	**Infant (<1 yr):** ½ tsp or 1 dropperful tid or qid **Child (1–3 yr):** 1 tab, ½–1 tsp, or 1–2 droppersful tid or qid **Child (3 yr):** 1½ tabs, 1 tsp, or 2 droppersful tid or qid **Child (4–5 yr):** 2½ tabs, 1½ tsp, or 3 droppersful tid or qid **Child (6–8 yr):** 3 tabs or 2 tsp tid or qid **Child (9–12 yr):** 4 tabs or 3 tsp tid or qid

CONTRAINDICATIONS

None

WARNINGS/PRECAUTIONS

Patient self-medication — Patient should not exceed maximum recommended dosage or use product for more than 10 days without advice and supervision of physician

ADVERSE REACTIONS[1]

Hematological (rare) — Anemia, neutropenia, leukopenia, thrombocytopenia, pancytopenia

Hypersensitivity (rare) — Erythematous or urticarial skin rashes, mucosal lesions, laryngeal edema, drug fever

OVERDOSAGE

In all cases of suspected overdose, immediately call the Rocky Mountain Poison Center, (800) 525-6115, for assistance in diagnosis and for directions in administering *N*-acetylcysteine as an antidote (currently investigational)

Signs and symptoms — *Early*: nausea, vomiting, diaphoresis, and general malaise (some patients may be asymptomatic); *late*: clinical and laboratory evidence of hepatotoxicity (vomiting; right upper quadrant tenderness; increased SGOT, SGPT, serum bilirubin, and prothrombin time; and possible hypoglycemia) may not be apparent until 48–72 h.

Treatment — Remove stomach contents promptly by inducing emesis or by gastric lavage; *do not use activated charcoal.* Determine serum acetaminophen level as soon as possible, but not earlier than 4 h after ingestion. Liver function studies should be obtained initially and repeated at 24-h intervals. Acetylcysteine should be administered as early as possible.

DRUG INTERACTIONS

Warfarin — ⇧ Hypoprothrombinemia (slight)

ALTERED LABORATORY VALUES

Blood/serum values — ⇧ Prothrombin time ⇧ Uric acid (with phosphotungstate method)

Urinary values — ⇧ 5-HIAA (with nitrosonaphthol reagent test)

Use in children	Use in pregnancy or nursing mothers
See INDICATIONS. Extra-Strength Adult Liquid is contraindicated for use in children under 12 yr of age.	General guidelines not established

Note: Other nonprescription analgesics containing acetaminophen are listed in the table on page 675.

[1]Koch-Weser J; *N Engl J Med* 295:1297, 1976; *United States Pharmacopeia Dispensing Information 1980,* Rockville, Md, United States Pharmacopeial Convention, Inc. 1980

Composition of Nonprescription Analgesics

Product (Manufacturer)	Acetaminophen (mg)	Aspirin (mg)	Other analgesic (mg)	Caffeine (mg)	Buffered
Alka-Seltzer Effervescent Pain Reliever (Miles)	—	324	—	—	Yes
Anacin (Whitehall)	—	400	—	32	No
Anacin Maximum Strength	—	500	—	32	No
A.P.C. (various mfgrs)	—	227	162 Phen	32	No
Arthritis Pain Formula (Whitehall)	—	486	—	—	Yes
Arthritis Strength Bufferin (Bristol-Myers)	—	486	—	—	Yes
Ascriptin (Rorer)	—	325	—	—	Yes
Aspergum (Plough)	—	228	—	—	No
Bayer Aspirin (Glenbrook)	—	325	—	—	No
Bayer Children's Chewable Aspirin (Glenbrook)	—	81	—	—	No
Bayer Timed-Release Aspirin (Glenbrook)	—	650	—	—	No
Bufferin (Bristol-Meyers)	—	324.15	—	—	Yes
Cope (Glenbrook)	—	421.2	—	32	Yes
Datril (Bristol-Meyers)	325	—	—	—	No
Datril 500 (Bristol-Meyers)	500	—	—	—	No
Ecotrin (Menley & James)	—	300	—	—	No[1]
Empirin (Burroughs Wellcome)	—	227	—	32	No
Excedrin (Bristol-Meyers)	97.2	194.4	129.6 Sal	64.8	No
Femcaps (Buffington)	—	162	65 Phen 8 Ephd	32	No
Measurin (Breon) (time-release)	—	660	—	—	No
Midol (Glenbrook)[2]	—	454	—	32.4	No
Percogesic (Endo)[3]	325	—	—	—	No
St. Joseph Aspirin (Plough)	—	325	—	—	No
St. Joseph Aspirin for Children (Plough)	—	81	—	—	No
Tylenol, Regular Strength (McNeil)	325	—	—	—	No
Tylenol, Extra Strength (McNeil)	—	500	—	—	No
Vanquish (Glenbrook)	—	324	—	—	Yes

[1]Enteric coating
[2]Also contains 14.9 mg cinnamedrine
[3]Also contains 30 mg phenyltoloxamine citrate

Abbreviations

A.P.C.—Aspirin, phenacetin, and caffeine
Ephd—Epinephrine sulfate
Phen—Phenacetin
Sal—Salicylamide

DEMEROL (Meperidine hydrochloride) **Winthrop**

Tabs: 50, 100 mg **Syrup:** 50 mg/5 ml (16 oz) **Amps:** 50 mg/ml (0.5, 1.0, 1.5, 2.0 ml), 100 mg/ml (1 ml)
Vials: 50 mg/ml (30 ml), 100 mg/ml (20 ml) **Syringe:** 25, 75, 100 mg/ml (1 ml) *C-II.*

INDICATIONS	ORAL DOSAGE	PARENTERAL DOSAGE
Moderate to severe pain	**Adult:** 50–150 mg q3–4h, as needed **Child:** 0.5–0.8 mg/lb q3–4h, up to 150 mg, as needed	**Adult:** 50–150 mg SC or IM q3–4h, as needed **Child:** 0.5–0.8 mg/lb SC or IM q3–4h, up to 150 mg, as needed
Preoperative medication	—	**Adult:** 50–100 mg SC or IM, 30–90 min before onset of anesthesia **Child:** 0.5–1.0 mg/lb SC or IM, up to 100 mg, 30–90 min before onset of anesthesia
Anesthesia support	—	**Adult:** repeated slow IV injections of fractional doses (eg, 10 mg/ml) or continuous IV infusion of a more dilute solution (eg, 1 mg/ml); titrate dose to individual needs, based on patient response, premedication, type of anesthesia, and nature and duration of operation **Child:** same as adult
Obstetrical analgesia	—	**Adult:** 50–100 mg SC or IM q1–3h, as needed, when pain is regular; repeat q1–3h, as needed

ADMINISTRATION/DOSAGE ADJUSTMENTS

Intravenous administration	Rapid IV injection increases risk of adverse reactions, including severe respiratory depression, apnea, hypotension, peripheral circulatory collapse, and cardiac arrest. If IV route is necessary, inject very slowly, preferably in dilute form, and have a narcotic antagonist and facilities for assisted or controlled respiration on hand. Patient should be lying down. Do not mix with barbiturates; solutions are incompatible.
Combination therapy	Use with caution and reduce dosage in patients who are concurrently receiving other CNS depressants. Respiratory depression, hypotension, and profound sedation or coma may result.

CONTRAINDICATIONS

Hypersensitivity to meperidine	
MAO-inhibitor therapy	Therapeutic doses of meperidine have precipitated unpredictable, severe, and occasionally fatal reactions in patients who have received MAO inhibitors within 14 days of treatment with meperidine

WARNINGS/PRECAUTIONS

Habit-forming	Psychic and/or physical dependence and tolerance may develop, especially in addiction-prone individuals
Mental impairment, reflex-slowing	Performance of potentially hazardous activities may be impaired; caution patients accordingly
Head injury, increased intracranial pressure	Respiratory depression and elevation of CSF pressure may be exaggerated; clinical course may be masked
Asthma and other respiratory conditions	Therapeutic doses may decrease respiratory drive while increasing airway resistance to the point of apnea; use with extreme caution during an acute asthmatic attack and in the presence of chronic obstructive pulmonary disease, cor pulmonale, substantially decreased respiratory reserve, respiratory depression, hypoxia, or hypercapnea
Increased ventricular response rate	May occur due to potential vagolytic action of meperidine; use with caution in patients with atrial flutter and other supraventricular tachycardias
Convulsive disorders	May be aggravated; convulsions may occur in patients with no prior history of seizures if tolerance develops and doses substantially exceeding recommended levels are taken
Special-risk patients	Reduce initial dosage and use with caution in the elderly or debilitated and patients with hepatic or renal impairment, hypothyroidism, Addison's disease, prostatic hypertrophy, or urethral stricture

Table continued on following page

DEMEROL continued

ADVERSE REACTIONS[1]	Frequent reactions are italicized
Central nervous system and neuromuscular	*Light-headedness, dizziness, sedation,* euphoria, dysphoria, weakness, agitation, tremor, transient hallucinations, disorientation, visual disturbances, headache, sensory motor paralysis caused by inadvertent injection too near a nerve trunk, uncoordinated muscle movements
Gastrointestinal	*Nausea, vomiting,* dry mouth, constipation, biliary tract spasm
Dermatological	Pruritus, urticaria, rash, wheal and flare over vein at IV site
Respiratory	Depression, arrest
Cardiovascular	Flushed face, tachycardia, bradycardia, palpitations, hypotension, shock, syncope, phlebitis with IV use, cardiac arrest
Genitourinary	Urinary retention
Other	*Sweating,* pain at injection site, local induration and irritation after SC injection, edema

OVERDOSAGE	
Signs and symptoms	Respiratory depression, miosis, extreme somnolence progressing to stupor or coma, skeletal-muscle flaccidity, cold and clammy skin, hypotension, bradycardia, and, in severe cases, apnea, circulatory collapse, and cardiac arrest
Treatment	Give primary attention to re-establishing adequate respiratory exchange through provision of an adequate airway and assisted or controlled ventilation; positive-pressure respiration may be desirable if pulmonary edema is present. If respiratory depression is significant, promptly administer naloxone (adult, 0.4 mg; child, 0.01 mg/kg), preferably IV, and repeat at 2- to 3-min intervals until satisfactory breathing is restored. *Do not use analeptic agents.* Oxygen, IV fluids, vasopressors, and other supportive measures should be employed, as needed. Gastric lavage, followed by instillation of activated charcoal, may be useful; dialysis is of little value unless other, dialyzable substances (such as barbiturates) have been simultaneously ingested.

DRUG INTERACTIONS	
Other narcotic analgesics; sedative-hypnotics, antianxiety agents, phenothiazines, general anesthetics, and other CNS depressants (including alcohol); MAO inhibitors; tricyclic antidepressants	⇧ CNS depression; reduce dose of one or both agents if used concomitantly or in close succession
Anticholinergic agents	⇧ Risk of paralytic ileus

ALTERED LABORATORY VALUES	
Blood/serum values	⇧ Amylase ⇧ Lipase

No clinically significant alterations in urinary values occur at therapeutic dosages

Use in children

See INDICATIONS

Use in pregnancy or nursing mothers

Safe use not established in pregnancy, except during labor. Neonatal respiratory depression, possibly requiring resuscitation, may occur.

[1]Some adverse reactions in ambulatory patients may be alleviated if the patient lies down

DILAUDID (Hydromorphone hydrochloride) Knoll

Tabs: 1, 2, 3, 4 mg **Vials:** 2 mg/ml (10, 20 ml) **Amps:** 1, 2, 3, 4 mg/ml (1 ml) **Supp:** 3 mg
Powder: 15 gr (for prescription compounding) *C-II*

INDICATIONS	ORAL DOSAGE	PARENTERAL DOSAGE
Moderate to severe pain	**Adult:** 2 mg q4–6h, as needed; for more severe pain, 4 mg or more q4–6h	**Adult:** 2 mg SC or IM (preferred) q4–6h, as needed (IV route is hazardous); see ADMINISTRATION/DOSAGE ADJUSTMENTS

ADMINISTRATION/DOSAGE ADJUSTMENTS

Rectal use	Suppositories provide long-lasting relief and are particularly useful at night; usual adult dosage: 1 supp q6–8h
Intravenous administration	Rapid IV injection increases risk of hypotension and respiratory depression; if IV route must be used, inject very slowly, taking at least 2–3 min to administer, and monitor patient closely

CONTRAINDICATIONS

Intracranial lesion associated with increased intracranial pressure ●	Depressed ventilatory function ●	Hypersensitivity to hydromorphone ●

WARNINGS/PRECAUTIONS

Habit-forming	Psychic and/or physical dependence and tolerance may develop with prolonged use, especially in addiction-prone patients
Respiratory depression	Characterized by an increase in respiratory rate and/or tidal volume, Cheyne-Stokes respiration, and cyanosis, as well as irregular and periodic breathing, may occur, depending on dose (see OVERDOSAGE)
Head injury, increased intracranial pressure	Respiratory depression and elevation of CSF pressure may be exaggerated; clinical course may be masked
Acute abdominal conditions	Diagnosis or clinical course may be obscured
Mental impairment, reflex-slowing	Performance of potentially hazardous activities may be impaired; caution patients accordingly
Cough suppression	May occur; use with caution postoperatively and in patients with pulmonary disease
Special-risk patients	Use with caution in elderly or debilitated patients and in the presence of hepatic or renal impairment, hypothyroidism, Addison's disease, prostatic hypertrophy, and urethral stricture
Tartrazine sensitivity	Presence of FD&C Yellow No. 5 (tartrazine) in 1-, 2-, and 4-mg tablets may cause allergic-type reactions, including bronchial asthma, in susceptible individuals

ADVERSE REACTIONS

Central nervous system	Sedation, drowsiness, mental clouding, lethargy, impairment of mental and physical performance, anxiety, fear, dysphoria, dizziness, psychic dependence, mood changes
Gastrointestinal	Nausea, vomiting; constipation (with prolonged use)
Cardiovascular	Circulatory depression, peripheral circulatory collapse, and cardiac arrest following rapid IV injection; orthostatic hypotension and fainting upon sudden standing after injection
Genitourinary	Ureteral spasm, vesical sphincter spasm, urinary retention
Respiratory	Depression, irregularities

OVERDOSAGE

Signs and symptoms	Respiratory depression, miosis, extreme somnolence progressing to stupor or coma, skeletal-muscle flaccidity, cold and clammy skin, hypotension, bradycardia, and, in severe cases, apnea, circulatory collapse, and cardiac arrest
Treatment	Maintain patient airway and institute assisted or controlled ventilation, if needed. If drug is not completely absorbed and patient is conscious, induce emesis or use gastric lavage to empty stomach. For significant respiratory depression, administer naloxone (0.005 mg/kg IV) simultaneously with ventilatory assistance. Administer oxygen, IV fluids, vasopressors, and other supportive measures, as needed.

Table continued on following page

DILAUDID continued

DRUG INTERACTIONS

Other narcotic analgesics; sedative-hypnotics, antianxiety agents, phenothiazines, general anesthetics, and other CNS depressants (including alcohol); MAO inhibitors; tricyclic antidepressants	⇧ CNS depression; reduce dose of one or both agents if used concomitantly or in close succession
Anticholinergic agents	⇧ Risk of paralytic ileus

ALTERED LABORATORY VALUES

No clinically significant alterations in blood/serum or urinary values occur at therapeutic dosages

Use in children

Safety and effectiveness not established

Use in pregnancy or nursing mothers

Safe use not established during pregnancy. Teratogenicity has been reported in animals at doses 600 times the normal human dose. Infants born to mothers taking opioids regularly prior to delivery will be physically dependent; those born to mothers taking opioids shortly before delivery may have respiratory depression. Because of the potential for serious adverse effects in nursing infants, patients who are breast-feeding should either discontinue nursing or not receive the drug.

MEPERGAN (Meperidine hydrochloride and promethazine hydrochloride) Wyeth

Cartridge-needle unit: 25 mg meperidine hydrochloride and 25 mg promethazine hydrochloride per ml (2 ml)
Vial: 25 mg meperidine hydrochloride and 25 mg promethazine hydrochloride per ml (10 ml) *C-II*

INDICATIONS	PARENTERAL DOSAGE
Preanesthetic medication, when both analgesia and sedation are desired **As an adjunct to local or general anesthesia**	**Adult:** 1-2 ml (25-50 mg of each component) IM, repeated q3-4h, as needed **Child:** 0.02 ml (0.5 mg of each component)/lb IM, repeated q3-4h, as needed

MEPERGAN FORTIS (Meperidine hydrochloride and promethazine hydrochloride) Wyeth

Caps: 50 mg meperidine hydrochloride and 25 mg promethazine hydrochloride *C-II*

INDICATIONS	ORAL DOSAGE
Moderate pain, when both analgesia and sedation are desired	**Adult:** 1 cap q4-6h, as needed

ADMINISTRATION/DOSAGE ADJUSTMENTS

Intravenous administration	Rapid IV injection increases risk of adverse reactions, including severe respiratory depression, apnea, hypotension, peripheral circulatory collapse, and cardiac arrest. If IV administration is necessary, inject very slowly (≤1 ml/min), preferably through the tubing of an IV infusion set that is functioning satisfactorily. Patient should be lying down, and a narcotic antagonist and facilities for assisted or controlled respiration should be on hand. If patient complains of pain, perivascular extravasation or inadvertent intra-arterial injection, which can result in gangrene of the affected extremity, may have occurred; stop injection immediately and evaluate cause of pain. Injection into or near peripheral nerves may result in permanent neurological deficit.
Concomitant use of other CNS depressants	Use with great caution and at reduced dosage in patients who are concurrently receiving other CNS depressants (see DRUG INTERACTIONS); respiratory depression, hypotension, and profound sedation or coma may result. Reduce dosage of barbiturates by at least ½ and of other analgesic CNS depressants by ¼ to ½. Do not mix barbiturates with Mepergan in the same syringe; solutions are chemically incompatible.
Concomitant use of anticholinergic agents for preoperative medication	If desired, Mepergan may be mixed in the same syringe with 0.3-0.4 mg atropine sulfate, 0.25-0.4 mg scopolamine hydrobromide, or other appropriate atropine-like drugs

CONTRAINDICATIONS

Hypersensitivity	To meperidine or promethazine
MAO-inhibitor therapy	Therapeutic doses of meperidine have precipitated unpredictable, severe, and occasionally fatal reactions in patients who have received MAO inhibitors within 14 days of treatment with meperidine
Subcutaneous injection	Chemical irritation and, rarely, necrotic lesions, may occur
Intra-arterial injection	Severe arteriospasm and resultant gangrene may occur

WARNINGS/PRECAUTIONS

Habit-forming	Psychic and/or physical dependence and tolerance may develop, especially in addiction-prone individuals
Head injury, increased intracranial pressure	Respiratory depression and elevation of CSF pressure may be exaggerated; clinical course may be masked
Asthma and other respiratory conditions	Therapeutic doses may decrease respiratory drive while increasing airway resistance to the point of apnea; use with extreme caution during an acute asthmatic attack and in the presence of chronic obstructive pulmonary disease, cor pulmonale, substantially decreased respiratory reserve, respiratory depression, hypoxia, or hypercapnea
Severe hypotension	May occur in postoperative patients or in any patient whose ability to maintain blood pressure is lowered by depleted blood volume or by administration of phenothiazines or certain anesthetics; ambulatory patients may experience orthostatic hypotension
Mental impairment, reflex-slowing	Performance of potentially hazardous tasks may be impaired; caution patients accordingly
Increased ventricular response rate	May occur due to potential vagolytic action of meperidine; use with caution in patients with atrial flutter and other supraventricular tachycardias
Convulsive disorders	May be aggravated; convulsions may occur in patients with no prior history of seizures if tolerance develops and doses substantially exceeding recommended levels are taken
Acute abdominal conditions	Diagnosis and/or clinical course may be obscured
Antiemetic effect	May mask symptoms of unrecognized disease and interfere with diagnosis

Table continued on following page

ADVERSE REACTIONS[1]	Frequent reactions are italicized
Central nervous system and neuromuscular	*Light-headedness, dizziness, sedation,* euphoria, dysphoria, weakness, headache, agitation, tremor, uncoordinated muscle movements, transient hallucinations, disorientation, visual disturbances, extrapyramidal reactions (rare)
Respiratory	Depression, arrest
Gastrointestinal	*Nausea, vomiting,* dry mouth, constipation, biliary tract spasm
Cardiovascular	Flushing of the face, tachycardia, bradycardia, palpitations, faintness, syncope, mild hypotension or hypertension, venous thrombosis (at injection site), circulatory depression, shock, cardiac arrest
Genitourinary	Urinary retention, antidiuretic effect
Hypersensitivity	Pruritus, urticaria, rash, wheal and flare over vein at IV site; photosensitivity (rare)
Hematological	Leukopenia (rare), agranulocytosis (one case)
Other	*Sweating,* pain at injection site, local induration and irritation following SC injection

OVERDOSAGE	
Signs and symptoms	*Toxic effects primarily attributable to meperidine:* respiratory depression, miosis, extreme somnolence progressing to stupor or coma, skeletal-muscle flaccidity, cold and clammy skin, bradycardia, hypotension, and, in severe cases, apnea, circulatory collapse, and cardiac arrest; *promethazine-related effects:* deep sedation, coma, and (rarely) convulsions and cardiorespiratory symptoms compatible with the depth of sedation present; extrapyramidal reactions
Treatment	Give primary attention to re-establishing adequate respiratory exchange through provision of an adequate airway and assisted or controlled ventilation; positive-pressure respiration may be desirable if pulmonary edema is present. If respiratory depression is significant, promptly administer naloxone (adult, 0.4 mg; child, 0.01 mg/kg), preferably IV, and repeat at 2- to 3-min intervals until satisfactory breathing is restored. *Do not use analeptic agents.* Oxygen, IV fluids, vasopressors, and other supportive measures should be employed, as needed. Treat extrapyramidal reactions with anticholinergic antiparkinson agents or diphenhydramine. Severe hypotension may be treated with levarterenol or phenylephrine; do not use epinephrine. Gastric lavage, followed by instillation of activated charcoal, may be useful in cases of acute overdose ingestion; dialysis is of little value unless other, dialyzable substances (such as barbiturates) have been simultaneously ingested.

DRUG INTERACTIONS	
Other narcotic analgesics and phenothiazines; sedative-hypnotics, antianxiety agents, general anesthetics, and other CNS depressants (including alcohol); MAO inhibitors; tricyclic antidepressants	⇧ CNS depression; reduce dose of one or both agents if used concomitantly or in close succession
Anticholinergic agents	⇧ Risk of paralytic ileus
Anticonvulsants	⇩ Convulsive threshold; anticonvulsant dosage may need upward adjustment
Epinephrine	Severe hypotension

ALTERED LABORATORY VALUES	
Blood/serum values	⇧ Amylase ⇧ Lipase
Urinary values	False-positive or false-negative pregnancy tests

Use in children

See INDICATIONS

Use in pregnancy or nursing mothers

Safe use not established during pregnancy, except during labor. Neonatal respiratory depression, possibly requiring resuscitation, may occur. Meperidine is excreted in breast milk.

[1]Some adverse reactions in ambulatory patients may be alleviated if the patient lies down

MORPHINE SULFATE Wyeth

Cartridge-needle units: 2, 4 mg (1 ml); 8, 10, 15 mg (1, 2 ml) *C-II*

INDICATIONS	PARENTERAL DOSAGE
Severe pain **Preoperative medication**	**Adult:** 5–20 mg SC or IM q4h, as needed **Child:** 0.1–0.2 mg/kg SC or IM, up to 15 mg/dose, q4h, as needed

CONTRAINDICATIONS

Hypersensitivity to morphine ● Bronchial asthma ● Respiratory depression ●

WARNINGS/PRECAUTIONS

Habit-forming	Psychic and/or physical dependence and tolerance may develop, especially in addiction-prone individuals
Special-risk patients	Use with caution in the elderly, infants, or debilitated, or in those with toxic psychoses, myxedema, or prostatic hypertrophy
Head injury, increased intracranial pressure	Respiratory depression and elevation of CSF pressure may be exaggerated; clinical course may be masked
Mental impairment, reflex-slowing	Performance of potentially hazardous activities may be impaired; caution patients accordingly
Acute abdominal conditions	Clinical course or diagnosis may be masked
Convulsive disorders	May aggravate pre-existing conditions
Supraventricular tachycardias	Vagolytic action may increase ventricular response rate
Hepatic impairment	Administer with caution and monitor for signs of excessive drug accumulation[1]

ADVERSE REACTIONS

Central nervous system	Light-headedness, dizziness, sedation, euphoria, dysphoria, weakness, headache, transient hallucinations, disorientation, visual disturbances, uncoordinated muscle movements; injection near a nerve trunk may result in sensory-motor paralysis
Gastrointestinal	Nausea, vomiting, dry mouth, anorexia, constipation, biliary-tract spasm
Cardiovascular	Flushing, tachycardia, bradycardia, palpitations, hypotension, faintness, syncope, phlebitis
Genitourinary	Urinary retention or hesitancy, antidiuretic effect, reduced libido and/or potency
Dermatological	Pruritus, urticaria, rash
Other	Diaphoresis, pain at injection site, irritation and induration at SC site, wheal and flare over IV site

OVERDOSAGE

Signs and symptoms	Respiratory depression, miosis, extreme somnolence progressing to stupor or coma, skeletal-muscle flaccidity, cold and clammy skin, bradycardia, hypotension, and, in severe cases, apnea, circulatory collapse, and cardiac arrest
Treatment	Give primary attention to re-establishing adequate respiratory exchange through provision of an adequate airway and assisted or controlled ventilation; positive-pressure respiration may be desirable if pulmonary edema is present. If respiratory depression is significant, promptly administer naloxone (adult, 0.4 mg; child, 0.01 mg/kg), preferably IV, and repeat at 2- to 3-min intervals until satisfactory breathing is restored. *Do not use analeptic agents.* Oxygen, IV fluids, vasopressors, and other supportive measures should be employed, as needed. Gastric lavage, followed by instillation of activated charcoal, may be useful; dialysis is of little value unless other, dialyzable substances (such as barbiturates) have been simultaneously ingested.

DRUG INTERACTIONS

Other narcotic analgesics; sedative-hyponotics, antianxiety agents, phenothiazines, general anesthetics, and other CNS depressants (including alcohol); MAO inhibitors; tricyclic antidepressants	⇧ CNS depression; reduce dose of one or both agents if used concomitantly or in close succession
Anticholingeric agents	⇧ Risk of paralytic ileus

[1]Blaschke TF: Protein binding and kinetics of drugs in liver diseases. *Clinical Pharmacokinetics* 2:32–44, 1977

Table continued on following page

ALTERED LABORATORY VALUES

Blood/serum values —————— ⇧ Amylase ⇧ Lipase ⇩ Lactate

No clinically significant alterations in urinary values occur at therapeutic dosages

Use in children

See INDICATIONS

Use in pregnancy or nursing mothers

Safe use during pregnancy not established; morphine crosses the placental barrier and can produce respiratory depression in the newborn. Not recommended for use in nursing mothers; drug appears in breast milk.

PERCOCET-5 (Oxycodone hydrochloride and acetaminophen) Endo

Tabs: 5 mg oxycodone hydrochloride and 325 mg acetaminophen *C-II*

INDICATIONS	ORAL DOSAGE
Moderate to moderately severe pain	**Adult:** 1 tab q6h, as needed; dosage may need to be increased in cases of more severe pain or if tolerance to narcotic analgesics has developed

CONTRAINDICATIONS

Hypersensitivity to oxycodone or acetaminophen

WARNINGS/PRECAUTIONS	
Habit-forming	Psychic and/or physical dependence and tolerance may develop, especially in addiction-prone individuals
Mental impairment, reflex-slowing	Performance of potentially hazardous activities may be impaired; caution patients accordingly
Head injury, increased intracranial pressure	Respiratory depression and elevation of CSF may be exaggerated; clinical course may be masked
Acute abdominal conditions	Diagnosis and/or clinical course may be obscured
Special-risk patients	Use with caution in the elderly or debilitated and in patients with severe hepatic or renal impairment, hypothyroidism, Addison's disease, prostatic hypertrophy, or urethral stricture

ADVERSE REACTIONS[1]	Frequent reactions are italicized
Central nervous system	*Light-headedness, dizziness, sedation,* euphoria, dysphoria
Gastrointestinal	*Nausea, vomiting,* constipation
Dermatological	Rash, pruritus

OVERDOSAGE	
Signs and symptoms	*Toxic effects primarily attributable to oxycodone:* respiratory depression, miosis, extreme somnolence progressing to stupor or coma, skeletal-muscle flaccidity, cold and clammy skin, bradycardia, hypotension, and, in severe cases, apnea, circulatory collapse, and cardiac arrest; *acetaminophen-related effects:* nausea, vomiting, diaphoresis, and general malaise; clinical and laboratory evidence of hepatotoxicity (vomiting, right upper quadrant tenderness, increased SGOT, SGPT, serum bilirubin, and prothrombin time, and possible hypoglycemia) may not be apparent until 48–72 h after ingestion
Treatment	Give primary attention to re-establishing adequate respiratory exchange through provision of an adequate airway and assisted or controlled ventilation; positive-pressure respiration may be desirable if pulmonay edema is present. If respiratory depression is significant, promptly administer naloxone (adult, 0.4 mg; child, 0.01 mg/kg), preferably IV, and repeat at 2- to 3-min intervals until satisfactory breathing is restored. *Do not use analeptic agents.* Oxygen, IV fluids, vasopressors, and other supportive measures should be employed, as needed. Gastric lavage, followed by instillation of activated charcoal, may be useful in removing unabsorbed drug; the charcoal must be lavaged out after 1 h and before instilling acetylcysteine as an antidote (call the Rocky Mountain Poison Center, [800] 525-6115, for assistance in diagnosing acetaminophen overdosage and for directions for administering acetylcysteine as an antidote [currently investigational]). Determine serum acetaminophen level as soon as possible, but not earlier than 4 h after suspected ingestion. Liver function studies should be obtained initially and repeated at 24-h intervals. Acetylcysteine can be given up to 24 h postingestion, but should be administered as early as possible, within 16 h of suspected overdose ingestion for optimal results.

DRUG INTERACTIONS	
Other narcotic analgesics; sedative-hypnotics, antianxiety agents, phenothiazines, general anesthetics, and other CNS depressants (including alcohol); MAO inhibitors; tricyclic antidepressants	⇧ CNS depression; reduce dose of one or both agents if used concomitantly or in close succession
Anticholinergic agents	⇧ Risk of paralytic ileus
Warfarin	⇧ Hypoprothrombinemia (slight)

[1]Some frequent reactions may be alleviated if the patient lies down; for other possible side effects, see acetaminophen

Table continued on following page

ALTERED LABORATORY VALUES

Blood/serum values	⇧ Amylase ⇧ Lipase ⇧ Prothrombin time ⇧ Uric acid (with phosphotungstate method)
Urinary values	⇧ 5-HIAA (with nitrosonaphthol reagent test)

Use in children

Contraindicated for use in children

Use in pregnancy or nursing mothers

Safe use not established during pregnancy; general guidelines not established for use in nursing mothers

PERCODAN (Oxycodone hydrochloride, oxycodone terephthalate, and aspirin) **Endo**

Tabs: 4.5 mg oxycodone hydrochloride, 0.38 mg oxycodone terephthalate, and 325 mg aspirin *C-II*

PERCODAN-DEMI (Oxycodone hydrochloride, oxycodone terephthalate, and aspirin) **Endo**

Tabs: 2.25 mg oxycodone hydrochloride, 0.19 mg oxycodone terephthalate, and 325 mg aspirin *C-II*

INDICATIONS	ORAL DOSAGE
Moderate to moderately severe pain	**Adult:** 1 Percodan tab or 1-2 Percodan-Demi tabs q6h **Child (6-12 yr):** ¼ Percodan-Demi tab q6h **Child (>12 yr):** ½ Percodan-Demi tab q6h

CONTRAINDICATIONS[1]

Hypersensitivity to oxycodone or aspirin

WARNINGS/PRECAUTIONS[1]

Habit-forming	Psychic and/or physical dependence and tolerance may develop, especially in addiction-prone individuals
Mental impairment, reflex-slowing	Performance of potentially hazardous activities may be impaired; caution patients accordingly
Head injury, increased intracranial pressure	Respiratory depression and elevation of CSF pressure may be exaggerated; clinical course may be masked
Acute abdominal conditions	Diagnosis or clinical course may be obscured
Special-risk patients	Use with caution in the elderly or debilitated and in patients with severe hepatic or renal impairment, hypothyroidism, Addison's disease, prostatic hypertrophy, urethral stricture, peptic ulcer, or coagulation abnormalities

ADVERSE REACTIONS[1]

	Frequent reactions are italicized
Central nervous system	*Light-headedness, dizziness, sedation,* euphoria, dysphoria
Gastrointestinal	*Nausea, vomiting,* constipation
Dermatological	Pruritus

OVERDOSAGE

Signs and symptoms	*Toxic effects primarily attributable to oxycodone:* respiratory depression, extreme somnolence progressing to stupor or coma, skeletal-muscle flaccidity, cold and clammy skin, bradycardia, hypotension, and, in severe cases, apnea, circulatory collapse, and cardiac arrest; *aspirin-related effects:* hyperpnea, nausea, vomiting, vertigo, tinnitus, flushing, sweating, thirst, headache, drowsiness, diarrhea, and tachycardia progressing to hyperthermia, hemorrhage, acid-base disturbances, restlessness, confusion, convulsions, vasomotor depression, coma, and respiratory failure
Treatment	Give primary attention to re-establishing adequate respiratory exchange through provision of an adequate airway and assisted or controlled ventilation; positive-pressure respiration may be desirable if pulmonary edema is present. If respiratory depression is significant, promptly administer naloxone (adult, 0.4 mg; child, 0.01 mg/kg), preferably IV, and repeat at 2- to 3-min intervals until satisfactory breathing is restored. *Do not use analeptic agents.* Oxygen, IV fluids, vasopressors, and other supportive measures should be employed, as needed. Gastric lavage, followed by instillation of activated charcoal, may be useful if performed within 4 h of ingestion. In moderately severe cases of salicylate poisoning, cautiously administer sodium bicarbonate IV in sufficient quantity, if possible, to maintain an alkaline diuresis; intermittent peritoneal dialysis may also be helpful. In severe cases, hemodialysis should be seriously considered. Hyperthermia, particularly in children, and dehydration require prompt correction. Hemorrhagic phenomena may necessitate whole-blood transfusions and phytonadione (vitamin K_1).

DRUG INTERACTIONS

Other narcotic analgesics; sedative-hypnotics, antianxiety agents, phenothiazines, general anesthetics, and other CNS depressants (including alcohol); MAO inhibitors; tricyclic antidepressants	⇧ CNS depression; reduce dose of one or both agents if used concomitantly or in close succession
Anticholinergic agents	⇧ Risk of paralytic ileus

[1]For other possible contraindications, warnings and precautions, and adverse reactions, see aspirin

Table continued on following page

DRUG INTERACTIONS continued

Anticoagulants	⇧ Risk of bleeding
Alcohol, corticosteroids, phenylbutazone, oxyphenbutazone	⇧ Risk of GI ulceration
Probenecid, sulfinpyrazone	⇩ Uricosuric effect
Spironolactone	⇩ Diuretic effect
Methotrexate	⇧ Methotrexate plasma level and risk of toxicity

ALTERED LABORATORY VALUES

Blood/serum values	⇧ Amylase ⇧ Lipase ⇧ Prothrombin time ⇧ Uric acid (with low doses) ⇩ Uric acid (with high doses) ⇩ Thyroxine (T_4) ⇩ Thyroid-stimulating hormone
Urinary values	⇧ Glucose (with Clinitest tablets)

Use in children

Percodan is not recommended. For use of Percodan-Demi, see INDICATIONS. Both forms are contraindicated in children under 6 yr of age.

Use in pregnancy or nursing mothers

Safe use not established during pregnancy; general guidelines not established for use in nursing mothers

SYNALGOS-DC (Dihydrocodeine bitartrate, promethazine hydrochloride, aspirin, phenacetin, and caffeine) **Ives**

Caps: 16 mg dihydrocodeine bitartrate, 6.25 mg promethazine hydrochloride, 194.4 mg aspirin, 162 mg phenacetin, and 30 mg caffeine *C-III*

INDICATIONS	ORAL DOSAGE
Moderate to moderately severe pain when mild sedative effect is also desired[1]	**Adult:** 2 caps q4h, as needed

CONTRAINDICATIONS[2]

Hypersensitivity to dihydrocodeine, promethazine, aspirin, or phenacetin

WARNINGS/PRECAUTIONS[2]

Habit-forming	Psychic and/or physical dependence and tolerance may develop, especially in addiction-prone individuals
Mental impairment, reflex-slowing	Performance of potentially hazardous activities may be impaired; caution patients accordingly
Renal damage	May occur with prolonged use of phenacetin in high doses
Phenothiazine hypersensitivity	Use with caution, if at all, and only in those patients for whom the potential benefits of treatment outweigh the risks of re-exposure to phenothiazine
Special-risk patients	Use with caution in the elderly or debilitated and in patients with cardiovascular or liver disease, hypothyroidism, Addison's disease, prostatic hypertrophy, or urethral stricture; use with extreme caution in the presence of peptic ulcer or coagulation abnormalities

ADVERSE REACTIONS[2]

Central nervous system	Light-headedness, dizziness, drowsiness, sedation
Gastrointestinal	Nausea, vomiting, constipation
Dermatological	Pruritus, skin reactions
Cardiovascular	Hypotension (rare)

OVERDOSAGE

Signs and symptoms	*Toxic effects primarily attributable to dihydrocodeine:* respiratory depression, miosis, extreme somnolence progressing to stupor or coma, skeletal-muscle flaccidity, cold and clammy skin, bradycardia, hypotension, and, in severe cases, apnea, circulatory collapse, and cardiac arrest; *promethazine-related effects:* deep sedation, coma, and (rarely) convulsions and cardiorespiratory symptoms compatible with the depth of sedation present; extrapyramidal symptoms; *aspirin-related effects:* hyperpnea, nausea, vomiting, vertigo, tinnitus, flushing, sweating, thirst, headache, drowsiness, diarrhea, and tachycardia, progressing to hyperthermia, hemorrhage, acid-base disturbances, restlessness, confusion, convulsions, vasomotor depression, coma, and respiratory failure; *phenacetin-related effects:* nausea, vomiting, abdominal pain, chills, excitement, delirium, cyanosis due to methemoglobinemia, respiratory depression, cardiac arrest; *caffeine-related effects:* insomnia, restlessness, and excitement progressing to mild delirium, dehydration, fever, tachycardia, extrasystoles, tremor, convulsions
Treatment	Give primary attention to re-establishing adequate respiratory exchange through provision of an adequate airway and assisted or controlled ventilation; positive-pressure respiration may be desirable if pulmonary edema is present. If respiratory depression is significant, promptly administer naloxone (adult, 0.4 mg; child, 0.01 mg/kg), preferably IV, and repeat at 2- to 3-min intervals until satisfactory breathing is restored. *Do not use analeptic agents.* Oxygen, IV fluids, vasopressors, and other supportive measures should be employed, as needed. Gastric lavage, followed by instillation of activated charcoal, may be useful if performed within 4 h of ingestion. In moderately severe cases of salicylate poisoning, cautiously administer sodium bicarbonate IV in sufficient quantity, if possible, to maintain an alkaline diuresis; intermittent peritoneal dialysis may also be helpful. In severe cases, hemodialysis should be seriously considered. Hyperthermia, particularly in children, and dehydration require prompt correction. Hemorrhagic phenomena may necessitate whole-blood transfusions and phytonadione (vitamin K_1). Severe cyanosis resulting from phenacetin-induced methemoglobinemia can be corrected with 1% methylene blue (1–2 mg/kg IV). Do not administer barbiturates to treat excitement or convulsions.

[1]Possibly effective
[2]For other possible contraindications, warnings and precautions, and adverse reactions, see aspirin

Table continued on following page

DRUG INTERACTIONS

Other narcotic analgesics and phenothiazines; sedative-hypnotics, antianxiety agents, general anesthetics, and other CNS depressants (including alcohol); MAO inhibitors; tricyclic antidepressants	⇧ CNS depression; reduce dose of one or both agents if used concomitantly or in close succession
Anticholinergic agents	⇧ Risk of paralytic ileus
Tranquilizers, sedative-hypnotics, and other CNS depressants	⇧ CNS depression
Alcohol, corticosteroids, phenylbutazone, oxyphenbutazone	⇧ Risk of GI ulceration
Probenecid, sulfinpyrazone	⇩ Uricosuric effect
Spironolactone	⇩ Diuretic effect
Methotrexate	⇧ Methotrexate plasma level and risk of toxicity
Anticonvulsants	⇩ Convulsive threshold; anticonvulsant dosage may need upward adjustment
Epinephrine	Severe hypotension

ALTERED LABORATORY VALUES

Values	Alteration
Blood/serum values	⇧ Amylase ⇧ Lipase ⇧ Prothrombin time ⇧ Uric acid (with low doses) ⇩ Uric acid (with high doses) ⇩ Thyroxine (T_4) ⇩ Thyroid-stimulating hormone
Urinary values	⇧ Glucose (with Clinitest tablets) ⇩ Bilirubin ⇧ 5-HIAA (with nitrosonaphthol reagent test) False-positive or false-negative pregnancy tests

Use in children

Safety and efficacy not established

Use in pregnancy or nursing mothers

Safe use not established during pregnancy; general guidelines not established for use in nursing mothers

TALWIN 50 (Pentazocine hydrochloride) **Winthrop**

Tabs: 50 mg *C-IV*

INDICATIONS	ORAL DOSAGE
Moderate to severe pain	**Adult:** 50 mg q3–4h to start, or, when needed, 100 mg q3–4h, up to 600 mg/day

CONTRAINDICATIONS

Hypersensitivity to pentazocine

WARNINGS/PRECAUTIONS

Habit-forming	Psychic and/or physical dependence may develop, especially in addiction-prone individuals; abrupt discontinuation may precipitate withdrawal symptoms
Established narcotic dependence	Administration of pentazocine may precipitate withdrawal symptoms
Mental impairment, reflex-slowing	Performance of potentially hazardous activities may be impaired; caution patients accordingly
Head injury, increased intracranial pressure	Respiratory depression and elevation of CSF pressure may be exaggerated; clinical course may be masked. Use with extreme caution and only if pentazocine is essential.
Respiratory depression	May result or worsen; use cautiously and lower dosage in patients with bronchial asthma, severely limited respiratory reserve, respiratory obstruction, or cyanosis
Impaired renal or hepatic function	Use with caution; extensive hepatic disease may predispose to increased side effects
Myocardial infarction with nausea, vomiting	Use with caution
Seizures	May occur in predisposed patients
Biliary surgery	Spasm of the sphincter of Oddi may occur
Acute CNS reactions (rare)	Transient hallucinations, disorientation, and confusion have occurred and cleared spontaneously after several hours. Vital signs should be checked. Exercise caution if drug is reinstated.

ADVERSE REACTIONS	Frequent reactions are italicized
Gastrointestinal	*Nausea, vomiting,* constipation; abdominal distress, anorexia, and diarrhea (rare)
Central nervous system and neuromuscular	*Dizziness, light-headedness, sedation, euphoria, headache,* weakness, disturbed dreams, insomnia, syncope, visual blurring and focusing difficulty, hallucinations; confusion, tremor, irritability, excitement, paresthesia, and tinnitus (rare)
Allergic	Rash; urticaria and facial edema (rare)
Cardiovascular	Hypotension, tachycardia
Hematological	Depression of WBC count (usually reversible) and moderate transient eosinophilia (rare)
Other	*Sweating,* flushing; chills, urinary retention, respiratory depression, and toxic epidermal necrolysis (rare)

OVERDOSAGE

Signs and symptoms	See ADVERSE REACTIONS
Treatment	Employ IV fluids, oxygen, vasopressors, and other supportive measures. For respiratory depression, administer naloxone (usual adult dose: 0.4 mg, preferably IV), simultaneously with respiratory resuscitation. Assisted or controlled ventilation may be indicated.

DRUG INTERACTIONS

Other narcotic analgesics; sedative-hypnotics, antianxiety agents, phenothiazines, general anesthetics, and other CNS depressants (including alcohol); MAO inhibitors; tricyclic antidepressants	⇧ CNS depression; reduce dose of one or both agents if used concomitantly or in close succession
Anticholinergic agents	⇧ Risk of paralytic ileus
Morphine, meperidine	⇩ Analgesic effect of morphine or meperidine

Table continued on following page

ALTERED LABORATORY VALUES

Blood/serum values—————— ⇧ Amylase ⇧ Lipase

No clinically significant alterations in urinary values occur at therapeutic dosages

Use in children

Not recommended for use in children under 12 yr of age

Use in pregnancy or nursing mothers

Safe use in pregnancy (other than during labor) has not been established; use with caution if infant is premature. There are rare reports of a possible abstinence syndrome in newborns following prolonged use of pentazocine during pregnancy. Pentazocine is excreted in human milk.[1]

[1] *United State Pharmacopeia Dispensing Information 1980.* Rockville, Md, United States Pharmacopeial Convention, Inc, 1980

TYLOX (Oxycodone hydrochloride, oxycodone terephthalate, and acetaminophen) **McNeil Pharmaceutical**

Caps: 4.5 mg oxycodone hydrochloride, 0.38 mg oxycodone terephthalate, and 500 mg acetaminophen *C-II*

INDICATIONS	ORAL DOSAGE
Moderate to moderately severe pain	**Adult:** 1 cap q6h, as needed

CONTRAINDICATIONS

Hypersensitivity to oxycodone or acetaminophen

WARNINGS/PRECAUTIONS

Habit-forming	Psychic and/or physical dependence and tolerance may develop, especially in addiction-prone individuals
Mental impairment	Performance of potentially hazardous activities may be impaired; caution patients accordingly
Head injury, increased intracranial pressure	Respiratory depression and elevation of CSF pressure may be exaggerated; clinical course may be masked
Acute abdominal conditions	Diagnosis and clinical course may be masked
Special-risk patients	Use with caution in the elderly or debilitated and in patients with severe hypothyroidism, Addison's disease, prostatic hypertrophy, or urethral stricture

ADVERSE REACTIONS[1]	Frequent reactions are italicized
Central nervous system	*Light-headedness, dizziness, sedation,* euphoria, dysphoria
Gastrointestinal	*Nausea, vomiting,* constipation
Dermatological	Pruritus, rash

OVERDOSAGE

Signs and symptoms	*Toxic effects primarily attributable to oxycodone:* respiratory depression, miosis, extreme somnolence progressing to stupor or coma, skeletal-muscle flaccidity, cold and clammy skin, bradycardia, hypotension, and, in severe cases, apnea, circulatory collapse, and cardiac arrest; *acetaminophen-related effects:* nausea, vomiting, diaphoresis, and general malaise; clinical and laboratory evidence of hepatotoxicity (vomiting, right upper quadrant tenderness, increased SGOT, SGPT, serum bilirubin, and prothrombin time, and possible hypoglycemia) may not be apparent until 48–72 h after ingestion
Treatment	Give primary attention to re-establishing adequate respiratory exchange through provision of an adequate airway and assisted or controlled ventilation; positive-pressure respiration may be desirable if pulmonary edema is present. If respiratory depression is significant, promptly administer naloxone (adult, 0.4 mg; child, 0.01 mg/kg), preferably IV, and repeat at 2- to 3-min intervals until satisfactory breathing is restored. *Do not use analeptic agents.* Oxygen, IV fluids, vasopressors, and other supportive measures should be employed, as needed. Gastric lavage, followed by instillation of activated charcoal, may be useful; the charcoal *must* be lavaged out after 1 h and before instilling acetylcysteine as an antidote. (Call the Rocky Mountain Poison Center, [800] 525-6115, for assistance in diagnosing acetaminophen overdosage and for directions for administering acetylcysteine as an antidote [currently investigational].) Determine serum acetaminophen level as soon as possible, but not earlier than 4 h after suspected ingestion. Liver function studies should be obtained initially and repeated at 24-h intervals. Acetylcysteine can be given up to 24 h postingestion, but should be administered as early as possible, within 16 h of suspected overdose ingestion for optimal results.

DRUG INTERACTIONS

Other narcotic analgesics; sedative-hypnotics, antianxiety agents, phenothiazines, general anesthetics, and other CNS depressants (including alcohol); MAO inhibitors; tricyclic antidepressants	⇧ CNS depression; reduce dose of one or both agents if used concomitantly or in close succession
Anticholinergic agents	⇧ Risk of paralytic ileus
Warfarin	⇧ Hypoprothrombinemia (slight)

[1]For other possible adverse reactions, see acetaminophen

Table continued on following page

ALTERED LABORATORY VALUES

Blood/serum values	⇧ Amylase ⇧ Lipase ⇧ Prothrombin time ⇧ Uric acid (with phosphotungstate method)
Urinary values	⇧ 5-HIAA (with nitrosonaphthol reagent test)

Use in children

Not recommended for use in children

Use in pregnancy or nursing mothers

Safe use not established during pregnancy; general guidelines not established for use in nursing mothers

VICODIN (Hydrocodone bitartrate and acetaminophen) Knoll

Tabs: 5 mg hydrocodone bitartrate and 500 mg acetaminophen *C-III*

INDICATIONS	ORAL DOSAGE
Moderate to moderately severe pain	**Adult:** 1 tab q6h, as needed; for more severe pain, 2 tabs q6h or 1 tab at more frequent intervals

CONTRAINDICATIONS

Hypersensitivity to hydrocodone or acetaminophen

WARNINGS/PRECAUTIONS	
Habit-forming	Psychic and/or physical dependence and tolerance may develop, especially in addiction-prone individuals
Mental impairment, reflex-slowing	Performance of potentially hazardous activities may be impaired; caution patients accordingly
Head injury, increased intracranial pressure	Respiratory depression and elevation of CSF pressure may be exaggerated; clinical course may be masked
Acute abdominal conditions	Diagnosis and clinical course may be obscured
Special-risk patients	Use with caution in the elderly and debilitated and in patients with severe hepatic or renal impairment, hypothyroidism, Addison's disease, prostatic hypertrophy, or urethral stricture

ADVERSE REACTIONS[1]	Frequent reactions are italicized
Central nervous system	*Light-headedness, dizziness, sedation,* euphoria, dysphoria
Gastrointestinal	*Nausea, vomiting,* constipation
Dermatological	Rash, pruritus

OVERDOSAGE	
Signs and symptoms	*Toxic effects primarily attributable to hydrocodone:* respiratory depression, miosis, extreme somnolence progressing to stupor or coma, skeletal-muscle flaccidity, cold and clammy skin, bradycardia, hypotension, and, in severe cases, apnea, circulatory collapse, and cardiac arrest; *acetaminophen-related effects:* nausea vomiting, diaphoresis, and general malaise; clinical and laboratory evidence of hepatotoxicity (vomiting, right upper quadrant tenderness, increased SGOT, SGPT, serum bilirubin, and prothrombin time, and possible hypoglycemia) may not be apparent until 48–72 h after ingestion
Treatment	Give primary attention to re-establishing adequate respiratory exchange through provision of an adequate airway and assisted or controlled ventilation; positive-pressure respiration may be desirable if pulmonary edema is present. If respiratory depression is significant, promptly administer naloxone (adult, 0.4 mg; child, 0.01 mg/kg), preferably IV, and repeat at 2- to 3-min intervals until satisfactory breathing is restored. *Do not use analeptic agents.* Oxygen, IV fluids, vasopressors, and other supportive measures should be employed, as needed. Gastric lavage, followed by instillation of activated charcoal, may be useful; the charcoal *must* be lavaged out after 1 h and before instilling acetylcysteine as an antidote. (Call the Rocky Mountain Poison Center, [800] 525-6115, for assistance in diagnosing acetaminophen overdosage and for directions for administering acetylcysteine as an antidote [currently investigational].) Determine serum acetaminophen level as soon as possible, but not earlier than 4 h after suspected ingestion. Liver function studies should be obtained initially and repeated at 24-h intervals. Acetylcysteine can be given up to 24 h postingestion, but should be administered as early as possible, within 16 h of suspected overdose ingestion for optimal results.

DRUG INTERACTIONS	
Other narcotic analgesics; sedative-hypnotics, antianxiety agents, phenothiazines, general anesthetics, and other CNS depressants (including alcohol); MAO inhibitors; tricyclic antidepressants	⇧ CNS depression; reduce dose of one or both agents if used concomitantly or in close succession
Anticholinergic agents	⇧ Risk of paralytic ileus
Warfarin	⇧ Hypoprothrombinemia (slight)

[1]Some frequent reactions may be alleviated if the patient lies down; for other possible side effects, see acetaminophen

Table continued on following page

VICODIN continued

ALTERED LABORATORY VALUES

Blood/serum values	⇧ Amylase ⇧ Lipase ⇧ Prothrombin time ⇧ Uric acid (with phosphotungstate method)
Urinary values	⇧ 5-HIAA (with nitrosonaphthol reagent test)

Use in children

Contraindicated for use in children under 12 yr of age

Use in pregnancy or nursing mothers

Safe use not established during pregnancy.

Migraine and Other Headaches

Through the ages, headache has persisted as one of mankind's most common afflictions. Babylonian poets of some 6,000 years ago eloquently described the miseries of headache, while the Egyptian medical papyruses contain accounts of "a sickness of half the head." By the start of the Christian era, the Greeks had named this sickness "hemicrania"—an illness in half the skull. Time corrupted the term to "migraine," which is characteristically a one-sided headache.

Mankind's first documented surgical procedure was trephining, which involved cutting out round plugs of bone from the skull to relieve head pain. In fact, Stone Age medicine men cut as many as five holes—some several inches in diameter—in a single skull. Despite their crude instruments, unsterile conditions, and lack of anesthesia, many of these first surgical patients survived, as evidenced by the new bone that formed about these holes.

Today, it is estimated that nearly 90 percent of the population suffers from at least an occasional headache and about 15 percent of these episodes are severe enough to prompt the sufferer to see a physician. Of these headaches, migraine commands

BLOOD VESSELS OF THE HEAD AND SITES OF MIGRAINE HEADACHES

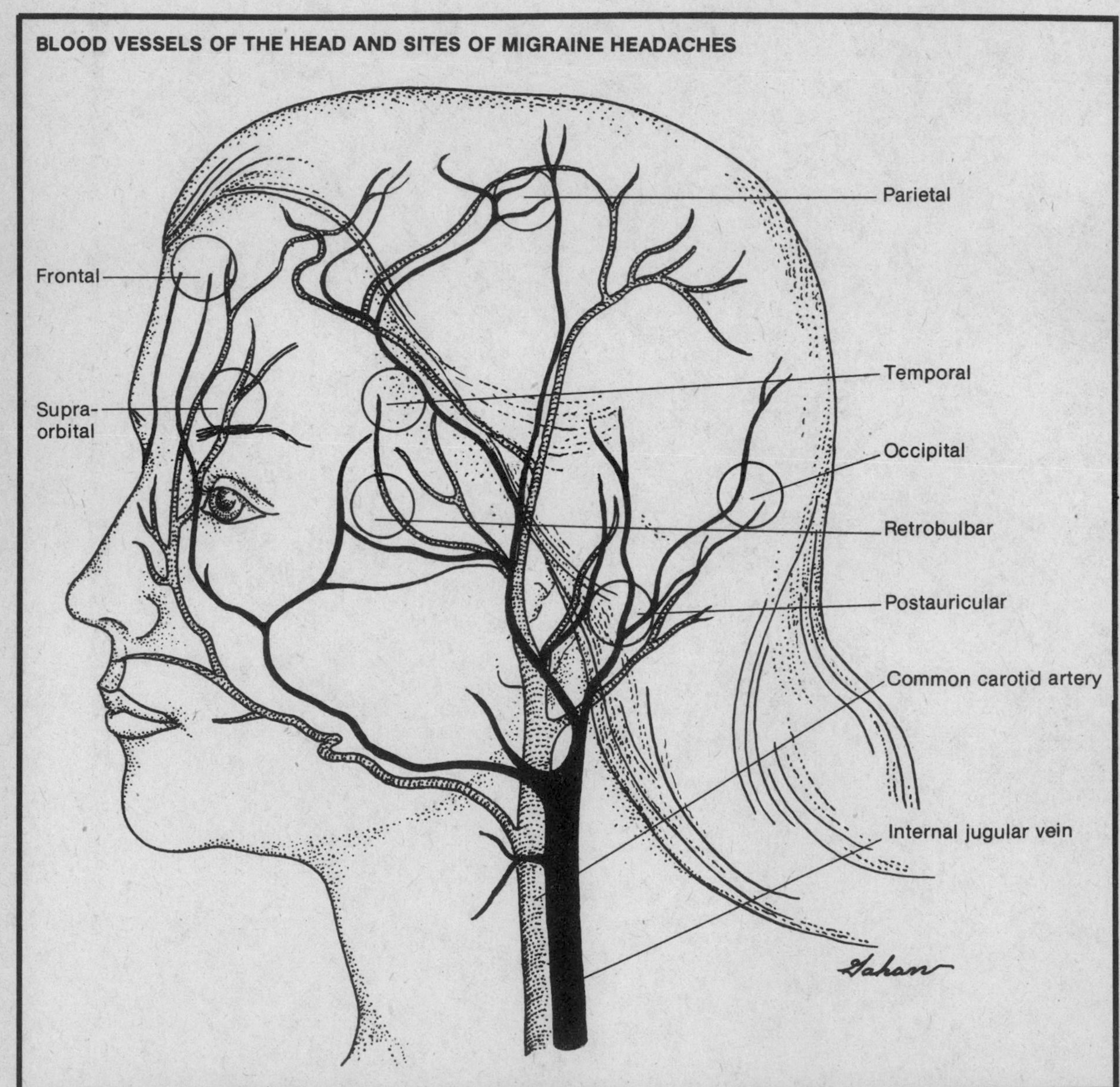

the most attention, and this discussion will focus primarily upon this type of headache and its treatment.

MIGRAINE

Although migraine is not the most common type of headache, it stands out for a variety of reasons: It affects a broad range of bodily systems, causing bizarre physical and cerebral (brain) manifestations that are uniquely individual; in some persons, its intensity can prostrate the sufferer for days; in others, it may cause little or no pain, yet produce other symptoms, such as distorted vision and hearing; and finally, its control remains a difficult medical problem.

It has been estimated that migraine afflicts one out of every eight Americans. About three fourths of adult migraineurs (those who suffer from migraine) are women, while among children it is more common in boys. Cluster headaches, a variant of migraine, are the most common in young adult men. Migraine appears to run in families; about 80 percent of migraineurs have relatives who also suffer from this disorder. It is found in all age groups—migraine has been reported in children as young as four months of age and in adults in their eighties. However, it usually first appears in young adulthood. Pregnant women are usually free from attacks and migraine often disappears with age, particularly after menopause.

More than any other headache, migraine is uniquely individual in its symptoms and manifestations, but is relatively easy to diagnose. Most commonly, it is a throbbing, recurrent headache that is usually felt on one side of the forehead or about one eye. It may start on one side of the upper neck, forehead, or temple and spread to one half or even the entire head. A variation is the so-called "facial migraine," which usually starts around one eye and spreads downward to the jaw.

A classic migraine attack may last for hours or days, although eight to twenty-four hours is most common. Many patients experience a warning of an impending attack, often in the form of visual or perceptual distortions. Indeed, migraine is sometimes referred to as the Alice-in-Wonderland syndrome; Lewis Carroll was a migraineur, and the bizarre distortions of size, position, time, and place experienced by Alice are frequent characteristics of migraine attacks. Glittering and scintillating visual patterns, often in weird geometric design, may precede the headache as well as other sensory disturbances, such as strange hearing and taste sensations. Many patients will experience emotional and intellectual disturbances, such as excitement, fear, or feelings of foreboding. Nausea, vomiting, and sensitivity to light (photophobia) commonly accompany migraine headaches. There may be chills, fever, dizziness, diarrhea, and excessive urination, as well as arm, leg, or abdominal pain.

The precise mechanism of migraine is still unclear, although it is known to be vascular (related to the blood vessels) in origin. It is thought that migraine has three phases: The blood vessels (particularly the arteries, but the veins also may be involved) of the scalp, as well as those supplying the brain, constrict to cause the sensory disturbances and other painless symptoms of migraine. These same blood vessels then dilate, releasing chemicals that result in the throbbing headache of migraine. The third and final phase of migraine is due to the inflammation and increased fluid (edema) of the tissues surrounding the blood vessels. At this point, the pain is dull and steady, and there may be nausea, vomiting, and various other symptoms.

Although the cause of migraine is unknown, there are triggering factors that may set off an attack. Migraine sufferers are likely to be sensitive, rigid, and compulsively perfectionist, proud of their accomplishments and demanding in personal standards of behavior. Migraineurs usually suppress both their anger and any resentment felt against parents or other authority figures. Emotional reactions, nervous tension, stress, and fatigue may precipitate attacks, as can relaxation after intense striving. Some migraine sufferers have attacks only on weekends or during vacations.

Hormones also may be involved. Many women, for example, experience migraine attacks preceding their menstrual periods. Alcohol and certain food substances, such as monosodium glutamate or tyramine (a chemical found in cheese, yogurt, red wine, and other foods), may trigger attacks in susceptible individuals. Some doctors believe that some migraines (as well as other headaches) may be caused by an allergic reaction to foods. Corn products, food additives, and chocolate are among the substances that have been implicated.

Treatment of Migraine

There is no sure cure for migraine, but most sufferers can obtain relief through the use of drugs and other therapies. The British have long advocated aspirin and a cup of tea supplied by a sympathetic nurse, who then puts the victim to bed in a dark, quiet room. Recent research in the United States indicates that one or two aspirin taken daily may indeed help prevent migraine, but more study is needed to confirm this. Analgesics, such as aspirin, are generally not effective in treating most adult migraineurs, but one or two aspirin may well control the attack in children. The generally preferred approach is to administer drugs that will prevent or abort an attack. These drugs must be used before the attack becomes full-blown; otherwise they have little or no effect.

The most widely used drug is ergotamine (Cafergot, Gynergen), an ergot derivative. This drug acts by constricting the arteries in the scalp. Sometimes caffeine, belladonna, and pentobarbital are added (as in Cafergot P-B) to increase blood vessel constriction, control nausea and vomiting, and relax or sedate the sufferer.

Another drug that constricts the cranial blood

vessels is isometheptene. This agent is combined with dichloralphenazone, a sedative, and the analgesic, acetaminophen (a combination marketed as Midrin).

Methysergide (Sansert) is used to prevent migraine. This drug, which is chemically related to the ergot derivatives, also constricts the cranial blood vessels.

One of the newest drugs used to prevent migraine is propranolol (Inderal), a beta-adrenergic blocker commonly used in treating cardiovascular disease. Propranolol prevents dilation of the cerebral arteries and thus helps prevent migraine attacks.

Cluster Headaches

Cluster headaches—a variant migraine—are also vascular in nature and are among the most painful of all headaches. The headaches come in clusters or bunches, and may strike several times a day for a week or more, with each headache lasting ten minutes to two hours. They usually appear at times of relaxation, sleep, a work break, the start of a vacation, etc., and often at the same time each day.

Nearly nine out of ten victims are men, usually in the twenty-to-forty age bracket. In a cluster period, an attack may be triggered by an alcoholic drink or a chemical that dilates blood vessels. The pain is usually excruciating and may be burning, throbbing, or steady. In most victims, the headaches occur on one side of the face and head, although the pain may change sides with different clusters. One eye may tear and become reddened. The nose on that side will be "stuffy" and the face swollen, especially around the eye. During an attack, the sufferer often strikes or clutches his head, digs at his eyes, and goes through other violent motions.

The condition is commonly treated with any of the drugs used for migraine, with ergotamine considered the most effective. Propranolol may be prescribed in an attempt to prevent cluster headaches. However, the medication must be used fairly early in the attack, before the blood vessels dilate, if the pain is to be successfully aborted. Therefore, drugs often are administered by injection or suppository to speed their entry into the bloodstream.

OTHER HEADACHES

Tension Headaches

By far the most common headache is the simple tension or muscle-contraction headache, which—as its name implies—is related to stress. The pain associated with this type of headache is steady rather than throbbing—many victims describe it as a "tightness," a "drawing," or "soreness," rather than outright pain. Nausea and vomiting only rarely accompany tension headaches, although dizziness and an anxious feeling may be present. These headaches occur with equal frequency in children and adults of both sexes.

Relief for tension headaches may come from relaxation techniques, massage, or heat applied to the muscles involved. Aspirin or acetaminophen are the principal drugs used to treat tension headaches, although butalbital (Fiorinal) may be prescribed for patients who do not receive adequate relief from nonprescription products.

Sinus Headaches

The cause of the so-called sinus headache is usually related to an infection or swelling of the mucous membranes that line the sinuses connecting with the nasal passages. The pain, which may be severe, is usually dull and aching, and may increase with movement or on bending over. There may also be tenderness of the cheekbones. Treatment is aimed at clearing up the sinusitis, which may be accomplished with decongestants or, in some cases, antibiotics. Simple analgesics—aspirin or acetaminophen—help relieve the pain.

THE DANGER SIGNALS OF HEADACHES

Very few headaches are symptoms of serious or life-threatening conditions. However, it is important to recognize these headaches and seek prompt medical attention. Headaches in children are more likely to represent a serious illness than in adults; therefore, a child's headache should not be neglected. Warning signs that call for prompt medical consultation and diagnosis include:

- Any severe headache that strikes suddenly without apparent cause or warning.
- Headaches accompanied by fever.
- Headaches accompanied by convulsions.
- Headaches in persons who are confused or have reduced levels of consciousness.
- Headaches following a blow on the head.
- Headaches accompanied by localized pain (i.e., in the eye, ear, etc.).
- Recurring headaches in children.
- Headaches that interfere with normal living patterns.
- Headaches that become daily or frequent.
- Headaches aggravated by coughing, sneezing, straining, or stooping.
- Headaches that awaken the person in the night.
- Any sudden change in the character or pattern of headaches.

IN CONCLUSION

Although headaches are our most common medical problem, most do not represent serious or life-threatening conditions and can be controlled through medication or certain life-style changes. The following charts cover the drugs intended specifically for migraine and other vascular headaches, as well as for severe tension headaches. Charts on aspirin and acetaminophen—the drugs most commonly used to relieve ordinary headaches—as well as other analgesics that may be recommended for headache are included in the section on *Pain* (pages 641-695).

CAFERGOT (Ergotamine tartrate and caffeine) Sandoz

Tabs: 1 mg ergotamine tartrate and 100 mg caffeine **Supp:** 2 mg ergotamine tartrate and 100 mg caffeine

INDICATIONS	ORAL DOSAGE	RECTAL DOSAGE
Vascular headache, to prevent or abort migraine, migraine variants, "histaminic cephalalgia"	**Adult:** 2 tabs at once, followed by 1 tab q½h, if needed, up to 6 tabs/attack or 10 tabs/wk	**Adult:** 1 supp at once, followed by 1 supp 1 h later, if needed, up to 2 supp/attack or 5 supp/wk

ADMINISTRATION/DOSAGE ADJUSTMENTS

Excessive nausea, vomiting — Use suppositories

Short-term prevention — Give at bedtime, within recommended dosage limits; only for carefully selected patients

CONTRAINDICATIONS

Peripheral vascular disease●

Coronary heart disease●

Hypertension●

Impaired hepatic or renal function●

Sepsis●

Hypersensitivity to ergotamine tartrate or caffeine●

WARNINGS/PRECAUTIONS

Ergotism — Although rare, may develop with high dosages or long-term use

ADVERSE REACTIONS

Cardiovascular — Precordial distress and pain, transient tachycardia and bradycardia

Gastrointestinal — Nausea, vomiting

Dermatological — Pruritus

Other — Numbness and tingling of fingers and toes, muscle pains in extremities, leg weakness, localized edema

OVERDOSAGE

Signs and symptoms — Toxic effects primarily attributable to ergotamine: vomiting, numbness, tingling, pain and cyanosis of extremities with diminished or absent peripheral pulses, hypertension or hypotension, drowsiness, stupor, coma, convulsions, shock; *caffeine-related effects:* insomnia, restlessness, tremors, delirium, tachycardia, extrasystoles

Treatment — Remove drug by induced emesis, gastric lavage, and catharsis. Maintain adequate pulmonary ventilation, correct hypotension, and control convulsions. Treat peripheral vasospasm with warmth *(not heat)* and protect ischemic limbs from cold. Use vasodilators cautiously.

DRUG INTERACTIONS

No clinically significant drug interactions have been observed

ALTERED LABORATORY VALUES

No clinically significant alterations in blood/serum or urinary values occur at therapeutic dosages

Use in children

General guidelines not established

Use in pregnancy or nursing mothers

Contraindicated during pregnancy. Not recommended for use in nursing mothers; ergotamine tartrate may cause adverse reactions in infants, including vomiting, diarrhea, weak pulse, and unstable blood pressure[1]

[1] Arena JM: *Clin Pediatr* 5:472, 1966; Katz CS, Giacoia GP: *Symp Pediatr Pharmacol* 19:151, 1972; Illingworth RS: *Practitioner* 171:533, 1953; Knowles JA: *J Pediatr* 66:1068, 1965

Note: Ergotamine tartrate also marketed as **ERGOSTAT** (Parke-Davis) and **GYNERGEN** (Sandoz).

CAFERGOT P-B (Ergotamine tartrate, caffeine, belladonna alkaloids, and pentobarbital) Sandoz

Tabs: 1 mg ergotamine tartrate, 100 mg caffeine, 0.125 mg belladonna alkaloids, and 30 mg sodium pentobarbital
Supp: 2 mg ergotamine tartrate, 100 mg caffeine, 0.25 mg belladonna alkaloids, and 60 mg pentobarbital

INDICATIONS	ORAL DOSAGE	RECTAL DOSAGE
Vascular headache complicated by tension and GI disturbances	**Adult:** 2 tabs at once, followed by 1 tab q½h, if needed, up to 6 tabs/attack or 10 tabs/wk	**Adult:** 1 supp at once, followed by 1 supp 1 h later, if needed, up to 2 supp/attack or 5 supp/wk

ADMINISTRATION/DOSAGE ADJUSTMENTS

Excessive nausea, vomiting — Use suppositories

Short-term prevention — Give at bedtime, within recommended dosage limits; only for carefully selected patients

CONTRAINDICATIONS

Peripheral vascular disease ●
Coronary heart disease ●
Hypertension ●
Impaired hepatic or renal function ●
Sepsis ●
Hypersensitivity to ergotamine, caffeine, belladonna alkaloids, or pentobarbital ●

WARNINGS/PRECAUTIONS

Habit-forming — Psychic and/or physical dependence and tolerance may develop, especially in addiction-prone individuals

Ergotism — Although rare, may develop with high dosages or long-term use

Drowsiness — Performance of potentially hazardous tasks may be impaired; caution patients accordingly

ADVERSE REACTIONS

Central nervous system — Drowsiness

Cardiovascular — Precordial distress and pain, transient tachycardia and bradycardia

Gastrointestinal — Nausea, vomiting

Dermatological — Pruritus

Other — Numbness and tingling of fingers and toes, muscle pains in extremities, leg weakness, localized edema

OVERDOSAGE

Signs and symptoms — *Toxic effects primarily attributable to ergotamine:* vomiting, numbness, tingling, pain and cyanosis of extremities with diminished or absent peripheral pulses, hypertension or hypotension, drowsiness, stupor, coma, convulsions, shock; *caffeine-related effects:* insomnia, restlessness, tremors, delirium, tachycardia, extrasystoles; *pentobarbital-related effects:* drowsiness, confusion, coma, respiratory depression, hypotension, shock; *belladonna alkaloid-related effects:* dry mouth and throat, blurred vision, urinary retention, CNS excitation, restlessness, confusion, delirium, convulsions, stupor, and coma, leading to death

Treatment — Remove drug by induced emesis, gastric lavage, and catharsis. Maintain adequate pulmonary ventilation, correct hypotension, and control convulsions. Treat peripheral vasospasm with warmth *(not heat)* and protect ischemic limbs from cold. Use vasodilators cautiously.

DRUG INTERACTIONS

Alcohol, tranquilizers, sedative-hypnotics, and other CNS depressants — ⇧ CNS depression

ALTERED LABORATORY VALUES

No clinically significant alterations in blood/serum or urinary values occur at therapeutic dosages

Use in children

General guidelines not established

Use in pregnancy or nursing mothers

Contraindicated during pregnancy; not recommended for use in nursing mothers; ergotamine tartrate may cause adverse reactions in infants, including vomiting, diarrhea, weak pulse, and unstable blood pressure[1]

[1]Arena JM: *Clin Pediatr* 5:472, 1966; Katz CS, Giacoia GP: *Symp Pediatr Pharmacol* 19:151, 1972; Illingworth RS: *Practitioner* 171:533, 1953; Knowles JA: *J Pediatr* 66:1068, 1965

Note: Ergotamine tartrate, caffeine, belladonna alkaloids, and phenacetin combination marketed as **WIGRAINE** (Organon). Ergotamine tartrate, cyclizine hydrochloride, and caffeine combination marketed as **MIGRAL** (Burroughs Wellcome).

FIORINAL (Butalbital, aspirin, phenacetin, and caffeine) Sandoz

Tabs, caps: 50 mg butalbital, 200 mg aspirin, 130 mg phenacetin, and 40 mg caffeine *C-III*

INDICATIONS	ORAL DOSAGE
Tension (muscle contraction) headache	**Adult:** 1-2 tabs or caps q4h, up to 6 tabs or caps per day
CONTRAINDICATIONS[1]	
Porphyria	Hypersensitivity to aspirin, phenacetin, caffeine, or barbiturates
WARNINGS/PRECAUTIONS[1]	
Habit-forming	Psychic and/or physical dependence and tolerance may develop, especially in addiction-prone individuals
Mental impairment, reflex-slowing	Performance of potentially hazardous activities may be impaired; caution patients accordingly
Renal damage	May occur with prolonged use of phenacetin in high doses; use with caution in patients with renal disease
ADVERSE REACTIONS[1]	Frequent reactions are italicized
Central nervous system	*Drowsiness, dizziness,* light-headedness
Gastrointestinal	Nausea, vomiting, flatulence
OVERDOSAGE	
Signs and symptoms	*Toxic effects primarily attributable to butalbital:* drowsiness, confusion, coma, respiratory depression, hypotension, shock; *aspirin-related effects:* hyperpnea, nausea, vomiting, vertigo, tinnitus, flushing, sweating, thirst, headache, drowsiness, diarrhea, and tachycardia, progressing to hyperthermia, hemorrhage, acid-base disturbances, restlessness, confusion, convulsions, vasomotor depression, coma, and respiratory failure; *phenacetin-related effects:* nausea, vomiting, abdominal pain, chills, excitement; delirium, cyanosis due to methemoglobinemia, respiratory depression, cardiac arrest; *caffeine-related effects:* insomnia, restlessness, and excitement progressing to mild delirium, dehydration, fever, tachycardia, extrasystoles, tremor, and convulsions
Treatment	Induce emesis if patient is conscious. Gastric lavage may be used if pharyngeal and laryngeal reflexes are intact and less thant 4 h have elapsed since ingestion; a cuffed endotracheal tube should be inserted before performing lavage on an unconscious patient or when necessary to provide assisted respiration. Meticulous attention should be given to maintaining adequate pulmonary ventilation. Severe hypotension may require IV use of levarterenol or phenylephrine for correction. In moderately severe cases of salicylate poisoning, cautiously administer sodium bicarbonate in sufficient quantity, if possible, to maintain an alkaline diuresis; intermittent peritoneal dialysis may also be helpful. In severe cases, hemodialysis should be seriously considered. Hyperthermia, particularly in children, and dehydration require prompt correction. Hemorrhagic phenomena may necessitate whole-blood transfusions and phytonadione (vitamin K). Severe cyanosis resulting from phenacetin-induced methemoglobinemia can be corrected with 1% methylene blue (1-2 mg/kg IV). Do not administer barbiturates to treat excitement or convulsions.
DRUG INTERACTIONS	
Other sedative-hypnotics; narcotic analgesics, antianxiety agents, phenothiazines, general anesthetics, and other CNS depressants (including alcohol); MAO inhibitors	⇧ CNS depression; reduce dose of one or both agents if used concomitantly or in close succession
Alcohol, corticosteroids, phenylbutazone, oxyphenbutazone	⇧ Risk of GI ulceration
Probenecid, sulfinpyrazone	⇩ Uricosuric effect
Spironolactone	⇩ Diuretic effect
Methotrexate	⇧ Methotrexate plasma level and risk of toxicity
Corticosteroids, digitalis, digitoxin, doxycycline, tricyclic antidepressants	⇩ Serum half-life and drug effect
Griseofulvin	⇩ Absorption of griseofulvin

[1]For other possible contraindications, warnings and precautions, and adverse reactions, see aspirin

Table continued on following page

FIORINAL continued

ALTERED LABORATORY VALUES

Blood/serum values	⇧ Prothrombin time ⇧ Uric acid (with low doses) ⇩ Uric acid (with high doses) ⇩ Thyroxine (T_4) ⇩ Thyroid-stimulating hormone ⇧ Glucose ⇩ Bilirubin
Urinary values	⇧ Glucose (with Clinitest tablets) ⇧ 5-HIAA (with nitrosonaphthol reagent test)

Use in children

Safety and effectiveness have not been established in children under 12 yr of age

Use in pregnancy or nursing mothers

Safe use not established during pregnancy; use in pregnant women only when clearly indicated. Aspirin and barbiturates appear in breast milk. Effects on infants are unknown, although serum levels are considered insignificant with therapeutic doses.

INDERAL (Propranolol hydrochloride) **Ayerst**

Tabs: 10, 20, 40, 80 mg **Amps:** 1 mg/ml (1 ml)

INDICATIONS	ORAL DOSAGE	PARENTERAL DOSAGE
Migraine prophylaxis	**Adult:** 80 mg/day div to start, followed by gradual increments until optimal response is achieved; usual maintenance dosage: 160-240 mg/day	—
Prophylaxis of moderate to severe **angina pectoris**	**Adult:** 10-20 mg/day tid or qid, before meals and at bedtime, to start, followed by gradual increments every 3-7 days until optimal response is achieved, up to 320 mg/day; usual maintenance dosage: 160 mg/day	—
Hypertension	**Adult:** 40 mg bid (alone or with a diuretic) to start, followed by gradual increases until optimal response is achieved, up to 640 mg/day; usual maintenance dosage: 160-480 mg/day	—
Cardiac arrhythmias, including supraventricular arrhythmias, ventricular tachycardias, digitalis-induced tachyarrhythmias, and resistant tachyarrhythmias due to excessive catecholamine activity during anesthesia	**Adult:** 10-30 mg tid or qid, before meals and at bedtime	**Adult:** 1-3 mg IV, slowly (see ADMINISTRATION/DOSAGE ADJUSTMENTS)
Hypertrophic subaortic stenosis	**Adult:** 20-40 mg tid or qid, before meals and at bedtime	—
As an adjunct to alpha-adrenergic blocking agents in the management of **pheochromocytoma**	**Adult:** 60 mg/day div for 3 days prior to surgery, concomitantly with an alpha-adrenergic blocking agent, or 30 mg/day div for inoperable tumors	—

Note: Full chart appears on page 15.

MIDRIN (Isometheptene mucate, dichloralphenazone, and acetaminophen) **Carnrick**

Caps: 65 mg isometheptene mucate, 100 mg dichloralphenazone, and 325 mg acetaminophen

INDICATIONS	ORAL DOSAGE
Migraine headache[1]	**Adult:** 2 caps at once, followed by 1 cap qh, up to 5 caps/12 h, as needed
Tension headache	**Adult:** 1-2 caps q4h, up to 8 caps/day

CONTRAINDICATIONS

Glaucoma●	Organic heart disease●	Hepatic disease●
Severe renal disease●	Severe hypertension●	MAO-inhibitor therapy●

WARNINGS/PRECAUTIONS[2]

Hypertension ●	Peripheral vascular disease ●	Recent cardiovascular attacks ●

ADVERSE REACTIONS[2]

Central nervous system	Dizziness
Dermatological	Rash

OVERDOSAGE

Signs and symptoms	Human experience with gross overdosage is limited
Treatment	Induce emesis or use gastric lavage, followed by activated charcoal, to empty stomach. Administer supportive measures, as needed.

DRUG INTERACTIONS

Warfarin	⇧ Hypoprothrombinemia (slight)

ALTERED LABORATORY VALUES

Blood/serum values	⇧ Prothrombin time ⇧ Uric acid (with phosphotungstate method)

Use in children	**Use in pregnancy or nursing mothers**
General guidelines not established	General guidelines not established

[1]Possibly effective
[2]For other possible warnings/precautions, as well as adverse reactions, see acetaminophen

SANSERT (Methysergide maleate) Sandoz

Tabs: 2 mg

INDICATIONS	ORAL DOSAGE
Prophylaxis of frequent[1] and/or severe and uncontrollable **vascular headaches**	**Adult:** 4–8 mg/day with meals

ADMINISTRATION/DOSAGE ADJUSTMENTS

Treatment course	Discontinue medication for 3–4 wk after each 6-mo course of treatment (see WARNINGS/PRECAUTIONS)
Trial period	If after 3-wk trial period efficacy has not been demonstrated, methysergide maleate is unlikely to be of benefit

CONTRAINDICATIONS

Peripheral vascular disease●	Severe arteriosclerosis●	Severe hypertension●
Coronary-artery disease●	Phlebitis or cellulitis of the lower limbs●	Pulmonary disease●
Collagen diseases or fibrotic processes●	Impaired liver or renal function●	Valvular heart disease●
Debilitated states●	Serious infections●	

WARNINGS/PRECAUTIONS

Retroperitoneal fibrosis, pleuropulmonary fibrosis, and fibrotic thickening of cardiac valves	May occur with long-term, uninterrupted use; caution patients to report immediately the following symptoms: cold, numb, and painful hands and feet; leg cramps on walking; girdle, flank, or chest pain; or any associated symptomatology. Discontinue use if any of these symptoms develops (see ADMINISTRATION/DOSAGE ADJUSTMENTS).
Rebound headache	May occur with abrupt discontinuation of therapy; reduce dosage gradually during the last 2–3 wk of each treatment course (see ADMINISTRATION/DOSAGE ADJUSTMENTS)

ADVERSE REACTIONS

Fibrotic	Retroperitoneal fibrosis accompanied by general malaise, fatigue, weight loss, backache, low grade fever, urinary obstruction (girdle or flank pain, dysuria, polyuria, oliguria, elevated BUN), and/or vascular insufficiency of lower limbs (leg pain, Leriche syndrome, edema of the legs, thrombophlebitis); pleuropulmonary complications with dyspnea, tightness and pain in the chest, pleural friction rubs, and pleural effusion; *cardiac complications*: nonrheumatic fibrotic thickening of the aortic root and of the aortic and mitral valves with cardiac murmurs and dyspnea, fibrotic plaques simulating Peyronie's disease
Cardiovascular	Vascular insufficiency of lower limbs, intrinsic vasoconstriction of large and small arteries (involving one or more vessels or a segment of a vessel) presenting as chest pain, abdominal pain, or cold, numb, painful extremities with or without paresthesias and diminished or absent pulses; ischemic tissue damage (rare); postural hypotension; tachycardia
Gastrointestinal	Nausea, vomiting, diarrhea, heartburn, abdominal pain, constipation
Central nervous system[2]	Insomnia, drowsiness, mild euphoria, dizziness, ataxia, light-headedness, hyperesthesia, hallucinatory experiences
Dermatological	Facial flush, telangiectasia, rash (all rare), increased hair loss
Hematological	Neutropenia, eosinophilia
Other	Peripheral edema, localized brawny edema, weight gain, weakness, arthralgia, myalgia

OVERDOSAGE

Signs and symptoms	See ADVERSE REACTIONS
Treatment	Treat symptomatically. Institute supportive measures, as required.

DRUG INTERACTIONS

No clinically significant drug interactions have been reported

[1] One or more severe vascular headaches per week
[2] May be associated with vascular headaches, and therefore may be unrelated to methysergide maleate

Table continued on following page

SANSERT continued

ALTERED LABORATORY VALUES

Blood/serum values ———— ⇩ Insulin-induced (hypoglycemia) growth hormone secretion

No clinically significant alterations in urinary values occur at therapeutic dosages

Use in children	**Use in pregnancy or nursing mothers**
Not recommended for use in children; no pediatric dosage has been established	Contraindicated during pregnancy; general guidelines not established for use in nursing mothers

Backache and Other Musculoskeletal Problems

Backache is second only to headache as man's most common source of pain. Indeed, although the human back is extremely pliable, it is by its very structure vulnerable to injury.

The spinal column, the central structure of the skeletal system, consists of thirty-three vertebrae, nine of which are fused at the base to form the sacrum and coccyx. The other twenty-four are separated by round discs that are pads of fibrous protein with jelly-like nuclei as cushions. The spinal column, held firmly, yet flexibly, by a complex maze of tendons, ligaments, and muscles, supports the head, shoulder bones, and pelvis. Running through it is a channel that houses the spinal cord—the mass of nerves that controls motor function and transmits messages to and from the brain.

It is generally assumed that man's problems with his back started when he first rose from all fours to stand and walk on his hind legs. Certainly the spine undergoes far less pressure when a person is lying down than when one is sitting or standing. The pressure increases many times over when a person lifts a heavy object or even bends forward or to either side. Obesity further adds to the spinal strain.

Back pain has many causes, the most common being muscle strain or disc problems. Other causes include tumors of the spine or any of several types of curvature, such as scoliosis, in which the spine tilts to one side, or lordosis, where the normal hollow of the back is greatly increased. Osteoporosis, a thinning out or rarefaction of the bones that is frequently seen in postmenopausal women or in

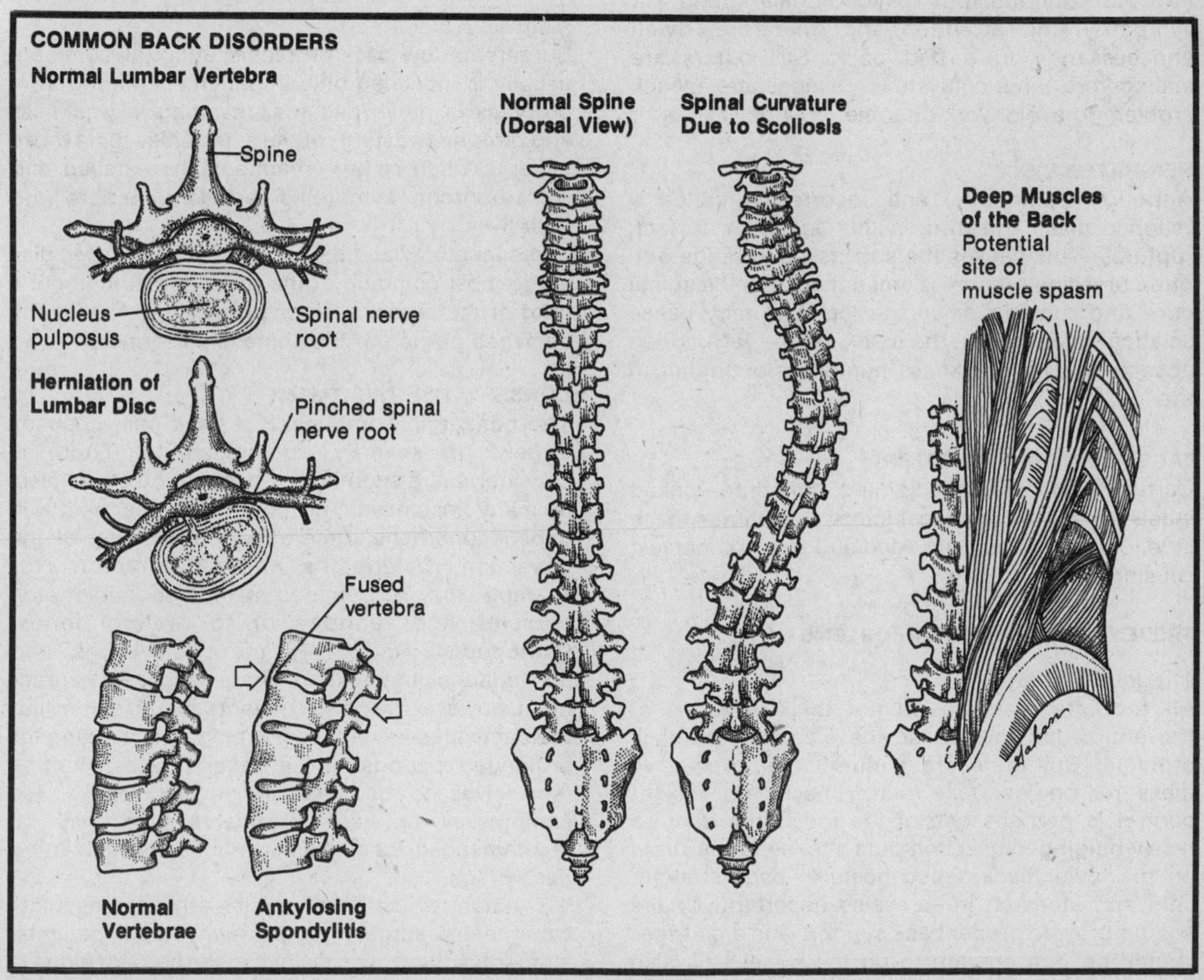

older men, leads to a collapse of the discs, resulting in pain. Still another cause of back pain is ankylosing spondylitis, an arthritis of the spine. (See *Arthritis and Gout,* pages 996-1037.)

Pain may occur at any point along the back and may radiate into adjacent areas, such as the neck or leg. The lumbosacral region—the lower back—is, however, the most common site of back pain because it bears the most weight. Most cases of low-back pain will have one of three causes: (1) muscle strain, (2) a herniated disc, or (3) facet-joint dysfunction.

MUSCLE STRAIN

Muscles contract and relax during the body's normal movements, but overstressed or overworked muscles often go into spasm, causing them to knot hard. Usually, as in the case of a sedentary person who suddenly takes up calisthenics or vigorous exercise, this results in minor aches and pains that disappear in a few days. But if the muscle remains in spasm, any movement, including walking or even standing erect, will be painful and difficult. Many persons make the mistake of trying to "work it off," which only aggravates the problem.

Psychological factors such as tension, depression, or anxiety can play a role in triggering muscle spasm. Worry or depression about an existing back problem can exacerbate it, while some persons may have an unconscious psychological need for sympathy and attention and, therefore, dwell unnecessarily on a bad back. Still others are malingerers who cultivate or exaggerate a back problem to avoid work or some other obligation.

HERNIATED DISC

Although commonly, and incorrectly, called a "slipped disc," the disc, in this condition, in fact, ruptures. This causes the soft tissue to bulge out, often pressing on nerves emanating from the spinal cord and running down the leg. This may cause sciatica (pain down the back of the leg), often accompanied by weakness, numbness, or tingling in the leg.

FACET-JOINT DYSFUNCTION

Certain surfaces of adjoining vertebrae—called facets—meet to form facet joints. Sometimes these little joints become dislocated and press on nerves, causing severe pain.

PREVENTING LOW-BACK PROBLEMS

Change of Life-Style

All too often, people do not think in terms of prevention until they already have developed a back problem. But there are a number of preventive measures one can take to avert back pain. Weight control is perhaps one of the most important—a heavy bulging midsection puts a tremendous strain on the lower back. Good posture—back straight, chin and stomach in—are also important. Chairs should provide proper back support, and a mattress should be firm enough to do the same. It is also important to lift things—no matter how light—in the correct way. If the object is below waist level, bend the knees, and then—keeping the object close to the body—rise up with the back straight and the stomach pressed in. In this way, the legs and not the back are doing the lifting.

Exercise, of course, is important in maintaining general health and well-being; but there are certain types of exercise that are especially helpful in preventing back problems. These are aimed at strengthening the abdominal muscles and increasing the elasticity of the lumbar and hamstring muscles.

DIAGNOSIS OF BACK PROBLEMS

In diagnosing a back problem, the possibility of tumors or other possible organic causes should be eliminated. Reflexes should be tested and, where indicated, a neurological examination may be undertaken to assess possible nerve involvement. X-rays of the spine are also indicated.

In some patients, a myelogram, lumbar venogram, or discogram (x-ray studies in which a dye is injected into the spinal canal) may be conducted. Computerized tomography—a computerized method using multiple x-ray images to study a cross section of the body—is sometimes useful in studying the spine.

TREATMENT

Surgery

Surgery for low-back problems, although common, usually is indicated only in patients suffering from progressive nerve damage, resulting in weakness and atrophy (wasting) of the extremities, or in those patients where other treatments have failed and whose chronic symptoms seriously interfere with their lives.

Laminectomy and the removal of a herniated disc is the most common of the procedures. In about a third of the cases, a second procedure to fuse the damaged portion of the spine is performed.

CONSERVATIVE TREATMENT

The nonsurgical treatment of back pain depends largely on severity and disability. There is considerable disagreement over various therapies; in many instances, the course of treatment will depend upon the preference and training of the physician. Osteopaths and chiropractors, for example, may recommend manipulation to stretch muscles and tendons or to realign bones. Orthopedists may rely more on drugs and conventional modalities. There is general agreement, however, that back patients should either limit their activities—avoiding stooping and standing for prolonged periods or, in severe cases, confine themselves to bed rest for a few weeks. Ice compresses or heat treatments also may be recommended, as well as wearing a specially fitted back brace.

Traction, which is sometimes regarded as a last step before surgery, helps many back patients, although some critics claim that the bed rest alone is responsible for the improvement. Several different techniques are used, including pelvic traction, in which a canvas girdle over the pelvis and hips is attached to weights overhanging the end of the bed. Gravity traction, a more recent technique, involves strapping the patient to a bed that is then tilted upward until he or she is almost upright.

DRUGS USED TO TREAT BACK PAIN

A wide variety of drugs is used to treat low-back pain. These include local anesthetics, analgesics, anti-inflammatory drugs, and muscle relaxants that may be used singly or in combination, depending upon the problem being treated.

Local Anesthetics

Many persons with chronic muscle pain develop trigger points, which are tender areas or nodules in the affected muscles. Injecting the trigger points with a local anesthetic, such as lidocaine hydrochloride (Xylocaine), often brings instant relief. Some physicians also use this approach in treating facet-joint dysfunction.

Analgesics

Because of the fear of addiction or dependence, many physicians are reluctant to give patients with low-back pain strong analgesics—particularly the narcotics—even for a short period during the acute stage. Others disagree, asserting that one or two adequate doses of morphine or meperidine (Demerol) may disrupt the cycle of muscle spasm and pain, after which the patient can be maintained on milder nonaddictive drugs.

Aspirin is the most commonly recommended analgesic for low-back pain. If a stronger pain-killer is needed, an aspirin-codeine combination, or codeine alone, may be recommended. (See the drug charts in the *Pain* section, page 641, for data on specific analgesics that may be prescribed for back pain.)

Various nonprescription analgesics, in the form of liniments, oils, lotions, and gels, are also described in this section.

Anti-Inflammatory Drugs

Aspirin, in higher dosages than when used as an analgesic, is among the anti-inflammatory agents often recommended to alleviate back pain due to any cause. But if this does not help, drugs such as phenylbutazone (Butazolidin), its derivative oxyphenbutazone (Tandearil), indomethacin (Indocin), or a corticosteroid may be prescribed. (See the section on *Arthritis and Gout,* page 996.)

Muscle Relaxants

Certain of these drugs can play an important role in the treatment of low-back pain problems involving muscle spasticity. They act by reducing muscle activity without affecting function. The drugs generally are used as adjuncts to treatments such as bed rest, cold or hot applications, and physical therapy. Muscle relaxants are often prescribed to take with painkillers.

Although the mechanical action of muscle relaxants is unclear in most instances, they generally work in one of two ways. Drugs such as cyclobenzaprine (Flexeril), baclofen (Lioresal), chlorphenesin (Maolate), orphenadrine (Norflex), carisoprodol (Soma), and diazepam (Valium) act indirectly on the muscles, in some cases by affecting the transmission of impulses from the spine to the skeletal muscles, in other cases by acting, for example, on the brain stem. Dantrolene (Dantrium) and quinine with aminophylline (Quinamm) are the relaxants that act directly on the muscles.

Dantrium and Lioresal are recommended for the syptomatic treatment of the muscular symptoms of spinal cord injuries and serious diseases such as multiple sclerosis—but not for rheumatoid-type disorders and the more routine types of low-back pains. Quinamm is indicated for the treatment of various types of leg muscle cramps. The others are indicated for acute low-back pain and other musculoskeletal disorders. Diazepam (Valium), which is best known as an antianxiety agent, is often used in connection with other types of muscle spasm, such as that from cerebral palsy or tetanus.

Most muscle relaxants can only be taken orally, but methocarbamol (Robaxin) and Valium come in injectable forms as well. Most muscle relaxants do not have analgesic properties, but an exception is Norflex. Some drugs combine analgesics with muscle relaxants. Examples include Norgesic, which contains aspirin, phenacetin, and caffeine in addition to orphenadrine citrate; Norgesic Forte, which is the same composition as Norgesic, but twice the strength; Parafon Forte, which is made up of chlorzoxazone and acetaminophen; Robaxisal, made up of methocarbamol and aspirin, and two combination forms of Soma—Soma Compound, which contains carbisoprodol, phenacetin, and caffeine, and Soma Compound with Codeine.

As is true of all drugs that act on the central nervous system, the most common side effects of muscle relaxants include drowsiness, lightheadedness, fatigue, depression, and insomnia. The drugs should be used with caution by persons who must stay alert, such as machine operators, and by persons who have liver or kidney disease.

OTHER TREATMENTS

There are a certain number of patients who try various conventional treatments and still suffer from back pain. Some are helped by other approaches, such as hypnosis, biofeedback, and acupuncture. Special pain centers or clinics are also helping growing numbers of persons who suffer from chronic pain. These centers use a multidisciplinary approach, which includes exercise, medication, and social factors.

IN CONCLUSION

Back pain is a common problem that often requires a multifaceted approach. The drug charts that follow cover the muscle relaxants that are most commonly prescribed for back pain. Other drugs used to treat back problems are included in sections on *Pain* (page 641) and *Arthritis and Gout* (page 996).

DANTRIUM (Dantrolene sodium) Norwich-Eaton

Caps: 25, 50, 100 mg

INDICATIONS	ORAL DOSAGE
Spasticity resulting from upper motor neuron disorders (eg, spinal-cord injury, stroke, cerebral palsy, multiple sclerosis)	**Adult:** 25 mg qd to start; increase to 25 mg bid to qid, followed by 25-mg increments at 4- to 7-day intervals, up to 100 mg bid to qid, as needed **Child (5-12 yr):** 0.5 mg/kg bid to start; increase to 0.5 mg/kg tid or qid, followed by increments of 0.5 mg/kg at 4- to 7-day intervals, up to 3 mg/kg bid to qid, as needed, but not more than 100 mg qid

ADMINISTRATION/DOSAGE ADJUSTMENTS	
Titration of dosage	Dosage must be individually titrated; use lowest dose compatible with optimal response. Maintain each dosage level for 4 to 7 days to determine response. Do not increase dosage beyond level at which patient received maximal benefit without adverse effects (dose may have to be reduced to this level). If benefits are not evident within 45 days, stop therapy because of potential for liver damage (see WARNINGS/PRECAUTIONS).

CONTRAINDICATIONS	
Active hepatic disease	Including hepatitis and cirrhosis
Spasticity	When utilized to maintain upright posture and balance in locomotion or to obtain or maintain increased function

WARNINGS/PRECAUTIONS	
Hepatic dysfunction or injury	May occur, sometimes fatally. Overt hepatitis can occur at any time during therapy but is most frequently observed between 3rd and 12th months. If clinical signs of hepatitis appear, accompanied by abnormal liver function tests or jaundice, treatment should be discontinued. Risk of liver damage is greater in females and in patients over 35 yr of age (see also DRUG INTERACTIONS). Liver function studies should be performed at appropriate intervals. If results are abnormal, therapy should be re-evaluated and the possibility of discontinuing therapy considered. If therapy is stopped, reinstitution should be attempted only after clinical and laboratory abnormalities have returned to normal. The patient should be hospitalized and closely monitored.
Drowsiness, dizziness	Performance of potentially hazardous activities may be impaired; caution patients accordingly
Photosensitivity	May occur; caution patients about exposure to sunlight
Diarrhea	May be severe and necessitate temporary withdrawal of therapy; if diarrhea recurs upon reinstitution of therapy, discontinue use of dantrolene permanently
Special-risk patients	Use with caution in patients with pre-existing liver disease or dysfunction, pulmonary function impairment (particularly obstructive pulmonary disease), or with severely impaired cardiac function owing to myocardial disease

ADVERSE REACTIONS	Frequent reactions are italicized
Central nervous system and neuromuscular	*Drowsiness, dizziness, weakness, malaise, fatigue*, speech disturbances, seizures, headache, lightheadedness, taste alterations, insomnia, mental depression, confusion, increased nervousness, myalgia, backache
Ophthalmic	Visual disturbances, diplopia
Cardiovascular	Tachycardia, erratic blood pressure, phlebitis
Respiratory	Feeling of suffocation
Gastrointestinal	*Diarrhea*, constipation, GI bleeding, anorexia, difficulty in swallowing, gastric irritation, abdominal cramps
Hepatic	Hepatitis
Genitourinary	Increased urinary frequency, crystalluria, hematuria, difficult erection, urinary incontinence and/or nocturia, difficult urination and/or urinary retention

Table continued on following page

DANTRIUM continued

ADVERSE REACTIONS continued

Dermatological	Abnormal hair growth, acne-like rash, pruritus, urticaria, eczematoid eruption, sweating, photosensitivity
Hypersensitivity	Pleural effusion with pericarditis
Other	Chills, fever

OVERDOSAGE

Signs and symptoms	See ADVERSE REACTIONS
Treatment	Generally supportive; immediately empty stomach by gastric lavage. Maintain adequate airway; resuscitation equipment should be readily available. Administer IV fluids to maintain adequate urine output and to prevent crystalluria. Monitor ECG and observe patient closely. Value of dialysis is unknown.

DRUG INTERACTIONS

Estrogens	⇧ Hepatotoxicity, especially in women over 35 yr of age
Alcohol, sedative-hypnotics, tranquilizers, and other CNS depressants	⇧ CNS depression

ALTERED LABORATORY VALUES

Blood/serum values	⇧ Alkaline phosphatase ⇧ SGOT ⇧ SGPT ⇧ Bilirubin (total)

No clinically significant alterations in urinary values occur at therapeutic dosages

Use in children

See INDICATIONS. Long-term safety of drug in children under 5 yr of age is not established. Benefit-risk considerations of long-term use of drug are particularly important.

Use in pregnancy or nursing mothers

Safe use has not been established in pregnancy. Contraindicated for use in nursing mothers; patient should stop nursing if drug is prescribed.

EQUAGESIC (Meprobamate, ethoheptazine citrate, and aspirin) Wyeth

Tabs: 150 mg meprobamate, 75 mg ethoheptazine citrate, and 250 mg aspirin *C-IV*

INDICATIONS	ORAL DOSAGE
Pain accompanied by tension and/or anxiety associated with musculoskeletal disease or tension headache	**Adult:** 1–2 tabs tid or qid, as needed

ADMINISTRATION/DOSAGE ADJUSTMENTS	
Long-term use (>4 mo)	Effectiveness for prolonged use has not been tested in systematic clinical studies; reassess need for continued therapy periodically
Discontinuation of therapy	Withdrawal reactions may occur with prolonged, excessive use. Reduce dosage gradually; abrupt withdrawal of doses exceeding recommended amounts has caused epileptiform seizures.

CONTRAINDICATIONS

Sensitivity or severe intolerance to meprobamate, ethoheptazine citrate, or aspirin

WARNINGS/PRECAUTIONS	
Habit-forming	Psychic and/or physical dependence and tolerance may develop, especially in addiction-prone individuals
Alcohol tolerance	May be lowered, with resultant slowing of reaction time and impairment of judgment and coordination; caution patients accordingly
Drowsiness, ataxia, visual disturbances	May occur and can usually be controlled by reduction of dosage; if symptoms continue, advise patient not to operate a motor vehicle or any dangerous machinery
Potentially suicidal patients	Should not have access to large quantities of the drug; prescribe smallest amount feasible
Allergic or idiosyncratic reactions	May occur, in rare instances, due to meprobamate component (see ADVERSE REACTIONS); treatment is symptomatic, including epinephrine, antihistamines, and, when appropriate, hydrocortisone. Discontinue use of Equagesic and do not reinstitute therapy.

ADVERSE REACTIONS	
Central nervous system	Dizziness, drowsiness, ataxia; impairment of accommodation and visual acutiy (rare)
Gastrointestinal	Nausea, vomiting, epigastric distress
Hematological	Aplastic anemia (one fatal case reported), thrombocytopenic purpura, agranulocytosis, hemolytic anemia, leukopenia (usually transient)
Allergic	Itchy, urticarial, or erythematous maculopapular rash (generalized or confined to groin); cytopenic purpura with cutaneous petechiae, ecchymoses, peripheral edema, and fever; in more severe cases (very rarely), fever, fainting spells, angioneurotic edema, bronchial spasm, hypotensive crisis (one fatal case reported), anaphylaxis, stomatitis, proctitis (one case), and hypothermia

OVERDOSAGE	
Signs and symptoms	*Meprobamate-related effects:* hyperventilation, drowsiness, lethargy, stupor, ataxia, coma, shock, vasomotor and respiratory collapse; *ethoheptazine-related effects:* CNS stimulation or depression, including drowsiness and light-headedness; nausea; vomiting; *aspirin-related effects:* hyperpnea, nausea, vomiting, vertigo, tinnitus, flushing, sweating, thirst, headache, drowsiness, diarrhea, and tachycardia progressing to hyperthermia, hemorrhage, acid-base disturbances, restlessness, confusion, convulsions, vasomotor depression, coma, and respiratory failure
Treatment	Induce emesis or perform gastric lavage, followed by activated charcoal, to remove any remaining drug from the stomach. Institute appropriate supportive measures, including respiratory assistance and parenteral use of pressor amines if severe hypotension develops. In moderately severe cases of salicylate poisoning, cautiously administer sodium bicarbonate IV in sufficient quantity, if possible, to maintain an alkaline diuresis; intermittent peritoneal dialysis may also be helpful. In severe cases, hemodialysis should be seriously considered. Hyperthermia, particularly in children, and dehydration require prompt correction. Hemorrhagic phenomena may necessitate whole-blood transfusions and phytonadione (vitamin K_1).

Table continued on following page

EQUAGESIC continued

DRUG INTERACTIONS

Other narcotic analgesics and anti-anxiety agents; sedative-hypnotics, phenothiazines, general anesthetics, and other CNS depressants (including alcohol); MAO inhibitors; tricyclic antidepressants	⇧ CNS depression; reduce dose of one or both agents if used concomitantly or in close succession
Anticoagulants	⇧ Risk of bleeding
Alcohol, corticosteroids, phenylbutazone, oxyphenbutazone	⇧ Risk of GI ulceration
Probenecid, sulfinpyrazone	⇩ Uricosuria
Spironolactone	⇩ Diuretic effect
Methotrexate	⇧ Methotrexate plasma level and risk of toxicity

ALTERED LABORATORY VALUES

Blood/serum values	⇧ Prothrombin time ⇧ Uric acid (with low doses) ⇩ Uric acid (with high doses) ⇩ Thyroxine (T_4) ⇩ Thyroid-stimulating hormone
Urinary values	⇧ Glucose (with Clinitest tablets)

Use in children

Not recommended for use in children 12 yr of age and under

Use in pregnancy or nursing mothers

Drug should almost always be avoided during pregnancy. An increased risk of congenital malformations during the 1st trimester has been associated with minor tranquilizers, including meprobamate. Meprobamate appears in breast milk in concentrations 2-4 times that of maternal plasma.

FLEXERIL (Cyclobenzaprine hydrochloride) **Merck Sharp & Dohme**

Tabs: 10 mg

INDICATIONS	ORAL DOSAGE
Muscle spasm associated with acute, painful musculoskeletal conditions (adjunctive therapy)	**Adult:** 20–60 mg/day div for no more than 2–3 wk; usual therapeutic dosage: 10 mg tid

CONTRAINDICATIONS

Hyperthyroidism	
Cardiovascular conditions	Arrhythmias, heart block, conduction disturbances, congestive heart failure, and during acute recovery phase of myocardial infarction
MAO-inhibitor therapy	Should not be used concomitantly or within 14 days of discontinuation of cyclobenzaprine therapy
Hypersensitivity	To cyclobenzaprine

WARNINGS/PRECAUTIONS

Mental impairment, reflex-slowing	Performance of potentially hazardous activities may be impaired; caution patients accordingly
Atropine-like, anticholinergic activity	Use with caution in patients with narrow-angle glaucoma, increased intraocular pressure, urinary retention, or those taking anticholinergic medication
Abrupt termination of therapy	May produce nausea, headache, and malaise after prolonged administration
Potentially suicidal patients	Deaths by deliberate or accidental overdosage have occurred with this class of drug

ADVERSE REACTIONS[1]
Frequent reactions are italicized

Central nervous system	*Drowsiness (40%), dizziness (11%),* paresthesias, insomnia, weakness, fatigue, dysarthria (rare), headache (rare), tremors (rare), hallucinations (rare), ataxia (rare)
Cardiovascular	Increased heart rate (including several cases of tachycardia), dyspnea (rare)
Gastrointestinal	*Dry mouth (28%),* dyspepsia, nausea, abdominal pain (rare), constipation (rare)
Genitourinary	Urinary retention (rare), decreased bladder tone (rare)
Musculoskeletal	Myalgia (rare)
Psychiatric	Euphoria, nervousness, disorientation, confusion, depressed mood (all rare)
Ophthalmic	Blurred vision
Allergic	Skin rash, urticaria, edema of the face and tongue (all rare)
Other	Unpleasant taste, coated tongue (rare), sweating (rare)

OVERDOSAGE

Signs and symptoms	Temporary confusion, disturbed concentration, transient visual hallucinations, agitation, hyperactive reflexes, muscle rigidity, and vomiting or hyperpyrexia, in addition to any of the previously noted ADVERSE REACTIONS. Overdosage may also cause drowsiness. hypothermia, tachycardia, and other cardiac-rhythm abnormalities, such as bundle-branch block, ECG evidence of impaired conduction, and congestive heart failure, as well as dilated pupils, convulsions, severe hypotension, stupor, and coma.

[1]Various other side effects common to tricyclic compounds in general may occur but have not been observed with cyclobenzaprine

Table continued on following page

OVERDOSAGE continued

Treatment	Institute symptomatic and supportive therapy. Empty stomach quickly by emesis and then use gastric lavage; may be followed by administration of 20–30 g activated charcoal q4–6h for first 24–48 h. Monitor ECG and cardiac function closely. Maintain open airway, adequate fluid intake, and body temperature. Physostigmine (1–3 mg IV) may be helpful. Use standard measures to manage circulatory shock and metabolic acidosis. Treat arrhythmias with neostigmine, pyridostigmine, or propranolol. Consider use of short-acting digitalis when there are signs of cardiac failure; monitor cardiac function closely for at least 5 days. Use anticonvulsants to control seizures. Dialysis is probably not helpful.

DRUG INTERACTIONS

MAO inhibitors	Hyperpyretic crisis, severe convulsions, and death have occurred
Anticholinergic medication	⇧ Anticholinergic effect
Alcohol, tranquilizers, sedative-hypnotics, and other CNS depressants	⇧ CNS depression
Guanethidine, clonidine	⇩ Antihypertensive effect

ALTERED LABORATORY VALUES

No clinically significant alterations in blood/serum or urinary values occur at therapeutic dosages

Use in children

Safety and effectiveness have not been established in children under 15 yr of age

Use in pregnancy or nursing mothers

Safe use has not been established during pregnancy or in nursing mothers. Drug probably appears in breast milk; patient should stop nursing if therapy is essential.

LIORESAL (Baclofen) **Geigy**

Tabs: 10 mg

INDICATIONS	ORAL DOSAGE
Spasticity associated with multiple sclerosis **Spinal cord injuries and diseases**	**Adult:** 5 mg tid for 3 days to start, then 10 mg tid for 3 days, 15 mg tid for 3 days, 20 mg tid for 3 days, and gradual increases thereafter, as necessary, up to 80 mg/day (20 mg qid); usual therapeutic dosage: 40–80 mg/day

CONTRAINDICATIONS

Hypersensitivity to baclofen

WARNINGS/PRECAUTIONS	
Abrupt withdrawal	Has precipitated hallucinations; reduce dose slowly when discontinuing drug, except when adverse reactions are serious
Impaired renal function	Drug is primarily excreted unchanged through the kidneys, so caution should be exercised; dosage reduction may be necessary
Stroke patients	Have shown poor tolerance to the drug and do not appear to benefit from its use
Sedation	Performance of potentially hazardous activities may be impaired; caution patients accordingly
Epilepsy	Deterioration in seizure control and EEG patterns has been reported; patients with epilepsy should be monitored clinically and electroencephalographically at regular intervals
Spasticity	Use with caution in patients in whom spasticity is utilized to sustain upright posture and balance in locomotion or to obtain increased function
Ovarian cysts	Animal studies have shown a dose-related increase
Adrenal gland enlargement or hemorrhage	Has been observed in animal studies

ADVERSE REACTIONS	Frequent reactions are italicized
Central nervous system	*Transient drowsiness (10–63%), dizziness (5–15%), weakness (5–15%), confusion (1–11%), headache (4–8%), fatigue (2–4%), insomnia (2–7%),* euphoria, excitement, depression, hallucinations, paresthesias, tinnitus, slurred speech, ataxia, epileptic seizures, syncope, dysarthria
Cardiovascular	*Hypotension (0–9%),* dyspnea, palpitations, chest pain
Ophthalmic	Blurred vision, nystagmus, strabismus, miosis, mydriasis, diplopia
Gastrointestinal	*Nausea (4–12%), constipation (2–6%),* dry mouth, taste disorders, anorexia, abdominal pain, vomiting, diarrhea, positive test for occult blood in stool
Genitourinary	*Urinary frequency (2–6%),* enuresis, urinary retention, dysuria, nocturia, hematuria, ejaculatory inhibition, impotence
Musculoskeletal	Muscle pain, coordination disorders, rigidity, tremor, dystonia
Dermatological	Rash, pruritus
Respiratory	Nasal congestion
Other	Ankle edema, excessive perspiration, weight gain

OVERDOSAGE	
Signs and symptoms	Vomiting, muscular hypotonia, drowsiness, accommodation disorders, coma, respiratory depression, seizures
Treatment	*Alert patient:* Empty stomach promptly by induced emesis, followed by gastric lavage. *Obtunded patient:* Do not induce emesis. Secure airway with a curved endotracheal tube before beginning lavage. Maintain adequate respiratory exchange. *Do not use respiratory stimulants.*

DRUG INTERACTIONS	
Alcohol, tranquilizers, sedative-hypnotics, and other CNS depressants	⇧ CNS depression

Table continued on following page

LIORESAL continued

ALTERED LABORATORY VALUES

Blood/serum values ———— ⇧ Alkaline phosphatase ⇧ SGOT ⇧ Glucose

No clinically significant alterations in urinary values occur at therapeutic dosages

Use in children	**Use in pregnancy or nursing mothers**
Not recommended for use in children under 12 yr of age	Safe use has not been established in pregnancy. Excretion of drug into breast milk is unknown; general guidelines not established for use in nursing mothers.

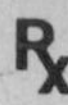

MAOLATE (Chlorphenesin carbamate) Upjohn

Tabs: 400 mg

INDICATIONS	ORAL DOSAGE
Acute, painful musculoskeletal conditions (adjunctive therapy)	**Adult:** 800 mg tid until desired effect has been achieved, then 400 mg qid or less, as needed

CONTRAINDICATIONS

Hypersensitivity to chlorphenesin

WARNINGS/PRECAUTIONS

Mental impairment, reflex-slowing	Performance of potentially hazardous activities may be impaired; caution patients accordingly
Pre-existing liver disease or impaired hepatic function	Use with caution
Hypersensitivity reactions	Anaphylaxis, drug fever, skin rash, or other allergic phenomena may occur; discontinue medication
Tartrazine sensitivity	Presence of FD&C Yellow No. 5 (tartrazine) in tablets may cause allergic-type reactions, including bronchial asthma, in susceptible individuals
Long-term safety	Safety of administration for more than 8 wk has not been established

ADVERSE REACTIONS

Central nervous system and neuromuscular	Drowsiness, dizziness, confusion, paradoxical stimulation (including insomnia, increased nervousness, and headache)[1]
Gastrointestinal	Nausea, epigastric distress, GI bleeding (two cases; causal relationship not established)
Hematological	Leukopenia, thrombocytopenia, agranulocytosis, pancytopenia
Allergic	Anaphylactoid reactions, drug fever, possibly other allergic phenomena

OVERDOSAGE

Signs and symptoms	Nausea, drowsiness
Treatment	Induce emesis or use gastric lavage and/or saline cathartics to empty stomach. Remainder of therapy is mostly supportive.

DRUG INTERACTIONS

No clinically significant drug interactions have been observed

ALTERED LABORATORY VALUES

No clinically significant alterations in blood/serum or urinary values occur at therapeutic dosages

Use in children	Use in pregnancy or nursing mothers
Not recommended for children under 12 yr of age	Safe use not established

[1]Can usually be controlled by dose reduction

NORFLEX (Orphenadrine citrate) Riker

Tabs: 100 mg **Amps:** 30 mg/ml (2 ml)

INDICATIONS	ORAL DOSAGE	PARENTERAL DOSAGE
Acute, painful musculoskeletal conditions (adjunctive therapy)	**Adult:** 100 mg bid in AM and PM	**Adult:** 60 mg IM or IV q12h, as needed

CONTRAINDICATIONS

Glaucoma ●	Prostatic hypertrophy ●	Myasthenia gravis ●
Pyloric or duodenal obstruction ●	Bladder-neck obstruction ●	Hypersensitivity to orphenadrine ●
Stenosing peptic ulcer ●	Cardiospasm (megaesophagus) ●	

WARNINGS/PRECAUTIONS

Lightheadedness, dizziness, syncope	Performance of potentially hazardous activities may be impaired; caution patients accordingly
Special-risk patients	Use with caution in patients with tachycardia, cardiac decompensation, coronary insufficiency, or cardiac arrhythmias
Long-term safety	Not established; monitor blood, urine, and liver function periodically if therapy is prolonged
Concomitant use of propoxyphene	May have additive effect; if confusion, anxiety, or tremors occur, reduce dosage and/or discontinue one or both agents

ADVERSE REACTIONS

Central nervous system and neuromuscular	Weakness, headache, dizziness, drowsiness, hallucinations, agitation, tremor, mental confusion (in the elderly)
Cardiovascular	Tachycardia, palpitations
Genitourinary	Urinary hesitancy or retention
Gastrointestinal	Dry mouth, nausea, vomiting, constipation, gastric irritation
Hematological	Aplastic anemia (very rare; causal relationship not established)
Ophthalmic	Blurred vision, pupillary dilation, increased ocular tension
Hypersensitivity	Allergic reactions, pruritus, urticaria, other dermatoses, anaphylactic reactions (following IM injection)

OVERDOSAGE

Signs and symptoms	CNS depression, nystagmus (horizontal and vertical), blurred vision, dry mouth, muscular incoordination, hypertension, convulsions
Treatment	Institute supportive therapy and maintain patent airway. Induce emesis or use gastric lavage, followed by activated charcoal, to empty stomach. Monitor vital signs and fluid and electrolyte balance.

DRUG INTERACTIONS

Tolbutamide, chlorpropamide	⇧ Hypoglycemic effect
Anticholinergic agents	⇧ Anticholinergic effect
Alcohol, general anesthetics, and other CNS depressants	⇧ CNS depression
MAO inhibitors, tricyclic antidepressants	⇧ CNS depression ⇧ Antidepressant effect

ALTERED LABORATORY VALUES

No clinically significant alterations in blood/serum or urinary values occur at therapeutic dosages

Use in children

Not recommended for use in children under 12 yr of age

Use in pregnancy or nursing mothers

Safe use not established during pregnancy; general guidelines not established for use in nursing mothers

NORGESIC (Orphenadrine citrate, aspirin, phenacetin, and caffeine) **Riker**

Tabs: 25 mg orphenadrine citrate, 225 mg aspirin, 160 mg phenacetin, and 30 mg caffeine

INDICATIONS	ORAL DOSAGE
Mild to moderate pain of acute musculoskeletal disorders (adjunctive therapy)	**Adult:** 1–2 tabs tid or qid

NORGESIC FORTE (Orphenadrine citrate, aspirin, phenacetin, and caffeine) **Riker**

Tabs: 50 mg orphenadrine citrate, 450 mg aspirin, 320 mg phenacetin, and 60 mg caffeine

INDICATIONS	ORAL DOSAGE
Same as for NORGESIC	**Adult:** ½–1 tab tid or qid

CONTRAINDICATIONS

Glaucoma ●	Prostatic hypertrophy ●	Hypersensitivity to orphenadrine, aspirin, phenacetin, or caffeine ●
Pyloric or duodenal obstruction ●	Bladder-neck obstruction ●	
Achalasia ●	Myasthenia gravis ●	

WARNINGS/PRECAUTIONS[1]

Renal disorders	Use with caution; prolonged or excessive use may result in GI disturbances, anemia, methemoglobinemia, and renal damage
Drowsiness	Performance of potentially hazardous activities may be impaired; caution patients accordingly
Special-risk patients	Use with caution in patients with tachycardia, peptic ulcers, or coagulation abnormalities
Long-term safety	Not established; monitor blood, urine, and liver function values if therapy is prolonged
Concomitant use of propoxyphene	May have additive effects; if confusion, anxiety, or tremors occur, reduce dosage and/or discontinue one or both agents

ADVERSE REACTIONS

Cardiovascular	Tachycardia, palpitations
Central nervous system	Weakness, headache, dizziness, drowsiness, confusion (in the elderly), mild excitation (occasionally), hallucinations, lightheadedness, syncope
Ophthalmic	Blurred vision, pupillary dilatation, increased intraocular tension
Genitourinary	Urinary hesitancy or retention
Gastrointestinal	Dry mouth, nausea, vomiting, constipation, hemorrhage (rare)
Dermatological	Urticaria (rare), other dermatoses (rare)
Hematological	Aplastic anemia (one case; causal relationship not established)

OVERDOSAGE

Signs and symptoms	*Aspirin-related effects:* hyperpnea, acid-base disturbances, vomiting, abdominal pain, tinnitus, hyperthermia, hypoprothrombinemia, restlessness, delirium, convulsions; *phenacetin-related effects:* vomiting, chills, hypotension, cyanosis, convulsions; *caffeine-related effects:* insomnia, restlessness, tremor, delirium, tachycardia, extrasystoles; *orphenadrine-related effects:* dry mouth, blurred vision, urinary retention, tachycardia, confusion, paralytic ileus
Treatment	Treat symptomatically and supportively. Induce emesis or use gastric lavage to empty stomach. Force diuresis, alkalinize urine, and correct electrolyte disturbances with IV fluids. Maintain adequate pulmonary ventilation. Correct hypotension with levarterenol or phenylephrine. For severe toxicity, peritoneal dialysis, hemodialysis, or exchange transfusion may be life-saving.

[1]For other possible warnings/precautions, see aspirin

Table continued on following page

DRUG INTERACTIONS

Anticoagulants	⇧ Risk of bleeding
Alcohol, corticosteroids, phenylbutazone, oxyphenbutazone	⇧ Risk of GI ulceration
Probenecid, sulfinpyrazone	⇩ Uricosuria
Spironolactone	⇩ Diuretic effect
Methotrexate	⇧ Methotrexate plasma level and risk of toxicity
Tolbutamide, chlorpropamide	⇧ Hypoglycemic effect
Anticholinergic agents	⇧ Anticholinergic effect

ALTERED LABORATORY VALUES

Blood/serum values	⇧ Prothrombin time ⇧ Uric acid (with low doses) ⇩ Uric acid (with high doses) ⇩ Thyroxine (T_4) ⇩ Thyroid-stimulating hormone
Urinary values	⇧ Glucose (with Clinitest tablets)

Use in children

Safety and effectiveness not established; not recommended for use in children under 12 yr of age

Use in pregnancy or nursing mothers

Safe use not established; high doses are not recommended

PARAFLEX (Chlorzoxazone) McNeil Pharmaceutical

Tabs: 250 mg

INDICATIONS	ORAL DOSAGE
Acute, painful musculoskeletal conditions (adjunctive therapy)	**Adult:** 500 mg tid or qid to start, followed by an increase in dosage to 750 mg tid or qid, if necessary; usual maintenance dosage: 250 mg tid or qid **Child:** 125-500 mg tid or qid, according to age and weight

CONTRAINDICATIONS

Hypersensitivity to chlorzoxazone

WARNINGS/PRECAUTIONS

Allergies	Use with caution in patients with allergies or a history of drug allergy; discontinue use if urticaria, redness, itching, or other sensitivity reactions occur
Liver dysfunction	Discontinue use if any suggestive signs or symptoms develop

ADVERSE REACTIONS

Gastrointestinal	Occasional disturbances, bleeding (rare)
Central nervous system	Drowsiness, dizziness, lightheadedness, malaise
Allergic	Skin rashes, petechiae, ecchymoses (all rare), angioneurotic edema (very rare), anaphylactic reactions (very rare)
Hepatic	Liver damage (about 27 cases)

OVERDOSAGE

Signs and symptoms	See ADVERSE REACTIONS
Treatment	Treatment is symptomatic. Institute supportive measures, as indicated.

DRUG INTERACTIONS

Alcohol, general anesthetics, other CNS depressants	⇧ CNS depression
MAO inhibitors, tricyclic antidepressants	⇧ CNS depression ⇧ Antidepressant effect

ALTERED LABORATORY VALUES

Urinary values	Discoloration (orange, purple-red)

No clinically significant alterations in blood/serum values occur at therapeutic dosages

Use in children

See INDICATIONS; tablets may be crushed and mixed with food or a suitable vehicle for administration

Use in pregnancy or nursing mothers

Safe use not established during pregnancy; general guidelines not established for use in nursing mothers

PARAFON FORTE (Chlorzoxazone and acetaminophen) McNeil Pharmaceutical

Tabs: 250 mg chlorzoxazone and 300 mg acetaminophen

INDICATIONS	ORAL DOSAGE
Acute, painful musculoskeletal conditions (adjunctive therapy)[1]	**Adult:** 2 tabs qid

CONTRAINDICATIONS

Hypersensitivity to chlorzoxazone or acetaminophen

WARNINGS/PRECAUTIONS

Liver dysfunction — Discontinue use if signs or symptoms occur

Allergies — Use with caution in patients with allergies or history of drug allergy; discontinue use if urticaria, redness, or itching occurs

ADVERSE REACTIONS[2]

Gastrointestinal — Disturbances, bleeding

Hepatic — Liver damage

Central nervous system — Drowsiness, dizziness, lightheadedness, malaise, overstimulation

Dermatological — Rash, petechiae, ecchymoses

Hypersensitivity — Angioneurotic edema, anaphylactic reactions

OVERDOSAGE

In all cases of suspected acetaminophen overdosage, immediately call the Rocky Mountain Poison Center, (800) 525-6115, for assistance in diagnosis and directions for administering *N*-acetylcysteine as an antidote (currently investigational)

Signs and symptoms — *Toxic effects primarily attributable to acetaminophen:* nausea, vomiting, diaphoresis, and general malaise; clinical and laboratory evidence of hepatotoxicity (vomiting, right upper quadrant tenderness; increased SGOT, SGPT, serum bilirubin, and prothrombin time; and possible hypoglycemia) may not be apparent until 48-72 h after ingestion

Treatment — Remove stomach contents promptly by inducing emesis or by gastric lavage; *do not use activated charcoal.* Determine serum acetaminophen level as soon as possible, but not earlier than 4 h after ingestion. Liver function studies should be obtained initially and repeated at 24-h intervals. Acetylcysteine should be administered as early as possible, within 16 h of suspected overdose ingestion for optimal results.

DRUG INTERACTIONS

Warfarin — ⇧ Hypoprothrombinemia (slight)

ALTERED LABORATORY VALUES

Blood/serum values — ⇧ Prothrombin ⇧ Uric acid (with phosphotungstate method)

Urinary values — Discoloration of urine

Use in children

General guidelines not established

Use in pregnancy or nursing mothers

Safe use not established during pregnancy; general guidelines not established for use in nursing mothers

[1]Probably effective
[2]For other possible adverse reactions, see acetaminophen

ROBAXIN (Methocarbamol) Robins

Tabs: 500, 750 mg **Vial:** 100 mg/ml (10 ml)

INDICATIONS	ORAL DOSAGE	PARENTERAL DOSAGE
Acute, painful musculoskeletal conditions (adjunctive therapy)	**Adult:** 1.5 g qid for initial 48–72 h, followed by 1 g qid or 4.5 g/day (750 mg q4h or 1.5 g tid)	**Adult:** 100–300 mg/day IM or IV, up to 3 consecutive days; 3-day course may be repeated after a lapse of 48 h if condition persists
Tetanus (adjunctive therapy)	—	**Adult:** 100–300 mg IV q6h until an NG tube can be inserted (see ADMINISTRATION/DOSAGE ADJUSTMENTS) **Child:** 15 mg/kg or more IV q6h, as needed (tetanus only)

ADMINISTRATION/DOSAGE ADJUSTMENTS

Severe musculoskeletal pain	Begin with 8 g/day orally and reduce the dosage to approximately 4 g/day after 48–72 h, or start with 200–300 mg/day IM or IV and switch to the oral form as soon as possible
Intramuscular use	Inject not more than 5 ml into each buttock; repeat, if necessary, q8h
Intravenous use	Administer directly into vein at a rate not exceeding 3 ml/min, or dilute one 10-ml vial in not more than 250 ml of isotonic sodium chloride or 5% dextrose-in-water, and give by infusion, with care taken to avoid extravasation; patient should be recumbent during delivery and for at least 10–15 min afterward to minimize risk of side effects
Tetanus	Inject 100–200 mg (10–20 ml) directly into the IV tubing; if desired, an additional 100–200 mg (10–20 ml) may be added to the infusion bottle so that a total of 300 mg is given. Repeat q6h until an NG tube can be inserted. Continue treatment orally with crushed methocarbamol tablets suspended in water or saline and delivered through the NG tube. Up to 24 g/day may be given in this manner, as needed.

CONTRAINDICATIONS

Hypersensitivity to methocarbamol ●	Known or suspected renal pathology (injectable form only) ●

WARNINGS/PRECAUTIONS

Epileptic patients	Use injectable form with caution in suspected or known epileptic subjects; convulsive seizures have occurred during IV administration
Extravasation	Must be avoided since injectable form is hypertonic; thrombophlebitis and sloughing at injection site have been reported

ADVERSE REACTIONS

Central nervous system and neuromuscular	Dizziness, lightheadedness, drowsiness, vertigo (injectable form only), fainting (injectable form only), mild muscular incoordination (injectable form only), headache, convulsions (injectable form only)
Gastrointestinal	Nausea, GI upset (injectable form only), metallic taste (injectable form only)
Cardiovascular	Syncope (injectable form only), hypotension (injectable form only), bradycardia (injectable form only)
Ophthalmic	Nystagmus (injectable form only), diplopia (injectable form only), blurred vision
Hypersensitivity	Urticaria, pruritus, rash, conjunctivitis with nasal congestion, anaphylactic reaction (injectable form only)
Other	Thrombophlebitis (injectable form only), pain and sloughing at injection site, flushing (injectable form only), fever

OVERDOSAGE

Signs and symptoms	See ADVERSE REACTIONS
Treatment	Methocarbamol is excreted via the kidney within 24 h; therapy is largely supportive during this time period

DRUG INTERACTIONS

No clinically significant drug interactions have been observed

Table continued on following page

ALTERED LABORATORY VALUES

Urinary values ———— ⇧ 5-HIAA (color interference) ⇧ VMA (color interference)

No clinically significant alterations in blood/serum values occur at therapeutic dosages

Use in children	**Use in pregnancy or nursing mothers**
Safety and effectiveness have not been established in children under 12 yr of age (except for tetanus)	Safe use has not been established during pregnancy or in nursing mothers. Methocarbamol may or may not be excreted in breast milk; patient probably should stop nursing if drug is prescribed.

QUINAMM (Quinine sulfate and aminophylline) Merrell-National

Tabs: 260 mg quinine sulfate and 195 mg aminophylline

INDICATIONS	ORAL DOSAGE
Nocturnal recumbency leg cramps, including those associated with arthritis, diabetes, varicose veins, thrombophlebitis, arteriosclerosis, and static foot deformities	**Adult:** 1 tab at bedtime; may be increased to 1 tab after dinner and at bedtime, if needed

CONTRAINDICATIONS

Hypersensitivity to quinine

G6PD deficiency

WARNINGS/PRECAUTIONS

Thrombocytopenic purpura	May occur after administration to highly sensitive patients; recovery follows withdrawal of medication
Tinnitus, deafness, skin rash, or visual disturbances	May occur; discontinue use

ADVERSE REACTIONS

Gastrointestinal	Cramps, GI disturbances
Central nervous system	Tinnitus, dizziness, deafness
Dermatological	Rash
Ophthalmic	Visual disturbances

OVERDOSAGE

Signs and symptoms	See ADVERSE REACTIONS
Treatment	Induce emesis or use gastric lavage, followed by activated charcoal, to empty stomach. Careful observation and symptomatic treatment are advisable. Convulsions may be controlled by IV-administered diazepam. Employ supportive measures, as needed.

DRUG INTERACTIONS

Coumarin anticoagulants	⇧ Hypoprothrombinemic effect

ALTERED LABORATORY VALUES

No clinically significant alterations in blood/serum or urinary values occur at therapeutic dosages

Use in children	Use in pregnancy or nursing mothers
General guidelines not established	Contraindicated during pregnancy; general guidelines not established for use in nursing mothers

ROBAXISAL (Methocarbamol and aspirin) **Robins**

Tabs: 400 mg methocarbamol and 325 mg aspirin

INDICATIONS	ORAL DOSAGE
Acute painful musculoskeletal conditions (adjunctive therapy)	**Adult:** 2 tabs qid

ADMINISTRATION/DOSAGE ADJUSTMENTS	
Severe conditions	Dosage may be increased to 3 tabs qid for 1-3 days in patients able to tolerate salicylates

CONTRAINDICATIONS[1]

Hypersensitivity to methocarbamol or aspirin

WARNINGS/PRECAUTIONS	
Gastritis, peptic ulcer	May be exacerbated by aspirin component
Drowsiness	Performance of potentially hazardous activities may be impaired; caution patients accordingly

ADVERSE REACTIONS	Frequent reactions are italicized
Gastrointestinal[2]	*Nausea (4-5%)*, gastritis, gastric erosion, vomiting, constipation, diarrhea
Central nervous system	*Dizziness or lightheadedness (4-5%)*, drowsiness, headache
Ophthalmic	Blurred vision
Hypersensitivity	Angioedema, asthma, rash, pruritus, urticaria
Other	Fever

OVERDOSAGE	
Signs and symptoms	*Toxic effects primarily attributable to aspirin:* rapid and deep breathing, hyperventilation, nausea, vomiting, vertigo, tinnitus, flushing, sweating, thirst, headache, drowsiness, diarrhea, tachycardia; *late symptoms:* fever, hemorrhage, excitement, confusion, convulsions, vasomotor depression, coma, respiratory failure, and respiratory alkalosis followed by respiratory and metabolic acidosis (primarily in children)
Treatment	If less than 4 h have elapsed since ingestion, induce emesis or perform gastric lavage, followed by activated characoal, to remove any remaining drug from the stomach. Initial therapy should be directed a reducing hyperthermia by external sponging with tepid water, correcting dehydration by appropriate IV fluid replacement, and maintaining adequate cardiorespiratory and renal function. In moderately severe cases of salicylate poisoning, cautiously administer sodium bicarbonate IV in sufficient quantity, if possible, to maintain an adequate diuresis; intermittent peritoneal dialysis may also be helpful. In severe cases, hemodialysis should be seriuosly considered. Potassium should be added to the repair solution to compensate for potassium losses once urine formation is deemed adequate. Glucose may be provided to correct ketosis and hypoglcemia. Plasma transfusion may be beneficial if shock intervenes. Hemorrhagic phenomena may necessitate whole-blood transfusions and phytonadione (vitamin K). Do not administer barbituates to treat excitement or convulsions.

DRUG INTERACTIONS	
Anticoagulants	⇧ Risk of bleeding
Alcohol, corticosteroids, phenylbutazone, oxyphenbutazone	⇧ Risk of GI ulceration
Probenecid, sulfinpyrazone	⇩ Uricosuria
Spironolactone	⇩ Diuretic effect
Methotrexate	⇧ Methotrexate plasma level and risk of toxicity

[1]For other possible contraindications, see aspirin
[2]May be minimized by taking drug with meals

Table continued on following page

ROBAXISAL continued

ALTERED LABORATORY VALUES

Blood/serum values	⇧ Prothrombin time ⇧ Uric acid (with low doses) ⇩ Uric acid (with high doses) ⇩ Thyroxine (T_4) ⇩ Thyroid-stimulating hormone
Urinary values	⇧ Glucose (with Clinitest tablets) ⇧ 5-HIAA (color interference) ⇧ VMA (color interference)

Use in children

Safety and effectiveness have not been established

Use in pregnancy or nursing mothers

Safe use not established during pregnancy. Moderate amounts of aspirin are excreted in human milk and may interfere with platelet function or decrease prothrombin levels in the infant, resulting in an increased risk of bleeding. Risk appears to be minimal if drug is taken by the mother just after nursing and if the infant has adequate stores of vitamin K. Whether methocarbamol is also excreted in human milk is unknown.

SKELAXIN (Metaxalone) Robins

Tabs: 400 mg

INDICATIONS	ORAL DOSAGE
Acute, painful musculoskeletal conditions (adjunctive therapy)	**Adult:** 800 mg tid or qid

CONTRAINDICATIONS

Hypersensitivity to metaxalone ●	Known tendency to drug-induced hemolytic or other anemias ●	Significantly impaired renal or hepatic function ●

WARNINGS/PRECAUTIONS

Elevations in cephalin flocculation tests	May occur without concurrent changes in other liver-function parameters. Use with extreme caution in patients with preexisting liver damage; perform serial liver function studies, as required.

ADVERSE REACTIONS

Gastrointestinal	Nausea, vomiting, upset
Central nervous system	Drowsiness, dizziness, nervousness, headache, irritability
Dermatological	Light rash with or without pruritus
Hematological	Leukopenia, hemolytic anemia
Hepatic	Jaundice

OVERDOSAGE

Signs and symptoms	No documented case of major toxicity has been reported. In rats and mice, progressive sedation, hypnosis, and respiratory failure were noted as the dosage increased. In dogs, higher doses produced an emetic action.
Treatment	Employ gastric lavage and supportive therapy, as required

DRUG INTERACTIONS

Alcohol	⇧ Sedative effect

ALTERED LABORATORY VALUES

Urinary values	⇧ Glucose (with Benedict's solution)

No clinically significant alterations in blood/serum values occur at therapeutic dosages

Use in children

Safety and efficacy not established

Use in pregnancy or nursing mothers

Use during pregnancy only when clearly needed; patient should stop nursing if drug is prescribed

SOMA (Carisoprodol) Wallace

Tabs: 350 mg

INDICATIONS	ORAL DOSAGE
Acute, painful musculoskeletal conditions (adjunctive therapy)	**Adult:** 350 mg tid and at bedtime

CONTRAINDICATIONS

Acute intermittent porphyria	Allergic or idiosyncratic reactions to carisoprodol or related compounds, such as meprobamate, mebutamate, or tybamate

WARNINGS/PRECAUTIONS

Idiosyncratic reactions	On very rare occasions such reactions have been reported within minutes or hours of the first dose, including extreme weakness, transient quadriplegia, dizziness, ataxia, temporary loss of vision, diplopia, mydriasis, dysarthria, agitation, euphoria, confusion, and disorientation. Symptoms usually subside over the course of the next several hours. Supportive and symptomatic therapy, including hospitalization, may be necessary (see ADVERSE REACTIONS).
Dependence	**Mild withdrawal symptoms (abdominal cramps, insomnia, chills, headache, and nausea) have followed abrupt cessation of therapy with doses of 100 mg/kg/day; use with caution in addiction-prone individuals**
Mental impairment, reflex-slowing	Performance of potentially hazardous activities may be impaired; caution patients accordingly
Compromised hepatic or renal function	Carisoprodol is metabolized by the liver and excreted by the kidney; watch for signs of excessive drug accumulation (see OVERDOSAGE)

ADVERSE REACTIONS

Central nervous system and neuromuscular	Drowsiness, dizziness, vertigo, ataxia, tremor, agitation, irritability, headache, depression, syncope, insomnia
Allergic or idiosyncratic[1]	Skin rash, erythema multiforme, pruritus, eosinophilia, fixed-drug eruption, asthmatic episodes, fever, weakness, dizziness, angioneurotic edema, smarting eyes, hypotension, anaphylactic shock
Cardiovascular	Tachycardia, postural hypotension, facial flushing
Gastrointestinal	Nausea, vomiting, hiccoughs, epigastric distress
Hematological	Leukopenia (cause not firmly established), pancytopenia (probably unrelated)

OVERDOSAGE

Signs and symptoms	Stupor, coma, shock, respiratory depression, and (very rarely) death
Treatment	Induce emesis or use gastric lavage, followed by activated charcoal. Should respiration or blood pressure become compromised, administer respiratory assistance and pressor agents cautiously, as indicated. Careful monitoring of urinary output is necessary, and caution should be taken to avoid overhydration. Observe for possible relapse due to incomplete gastric emptying and delayed absorption.

DRUG INTERACTIONS

Alcohol, tranquilizers, sedative-hypnotics, and other CNS depressants	⇧ CNS depression

ALTERED LABORATORY VALUES

No clinically significant alterations in blood/serum or urinary values occur at therapeutic dosages

Use in children	Use in pregnancy or nursing mothers
Not recommended for children under 12 yr of age	Safe use not established; carisoprodol levels in breast milk are 2 to 4 times maternal plasma concentrations

[1]Discontinue drug and institute symptomatic therapy, including use of epinephrine, antihistamines, and, in severe cases, corticosteroids; consider allergic reactions to excipients in all cases

SOMA COMPOUND (Carisoprodol, phenacetin, and caffeine) **Wallace**

Tabs: 200 mg carisoprodol, 160 mg phenacetin, and 32 mg caffeine

INDICATIONS	ORAL DOSAGE
Acute, painful musculoskeletal conditions (adjunctive therapy)	**Adult:** 1–2 tabs tid and at bedtime

CONTRAINDICATIONS	
Hypersensitivity to carisoprodol, phenacetin, caffeine, meprobamate, mebutamate, or tybamate ●	Acute intermittent porphyria ●

WARNINGS/PRECAUTIONS	
Idiosyncratic reactions	On very rare occasions such reactions have been reported within minutes or hours of the first dose, including extreme weakness, transient quadriplegia, dizziness, ataxia, temporary loss of vision, diplopia, mydriasis, dysarthria, agitation, euphoria, confusion, and disorientation. Symptoms usually subside over the course of the next several hours. Supportive and symptomatic therapy, including hospitalization, may be necessary (see ADVERSE REACTIONS).
Dependence	Mild withdrawal symptoms (abdominal cramps, insomnia, chills, headache, and nausea) have followed abrupt cessation of therapy with carisoprodol doses of 100 mg/kg/day; use with caution in addiction-prone individuals
Mental impairment, reflex-slowing	Performance of potentially hazardous activities may be impaired; caution patients accordingly
Compromised hepatic or renal function	Carisoprodol is metabolized by the liver and excreted by the kidney; watch for signs of excessive drug accumulation (see OVERDOSAGE)
Kidney disease	May occur following prolonged use (1–3 yr) of high doses of phenacetin
Special-risk patients	Use with caution in patients with anemia or cardiac, pulmonary, renal, or hepatic disease or in persons extremely sensitive to the CNS-stimulating activity of caffeine

ADVERSE REACTIONS	
Central nervous system and neuromuscular	Drowsiness, lightheadedness, dizziness, vertigo, ataxia, tremor, agitation, irritability, headache, depression, syncope, insomnia, nervousness
Allergic or idiosyncratic[1]	Skin rash, erythema multiforme, pruritus, eosinophilia, fixed-drug eruption, asthmatic episodes, fever, weakness, dizziness, angioneurotic edema, smarting eyes, hypotension, anaphylactic shock
Cardiovascular	Tachycardia, postural hypotension, facial flushing, palpitations
Gastrointestinal	Nausea, vomiting, hiccoughs, epigastric distress
Hematological	Leukopenia (causative role not firmly established), pancytopenia (probably unrelated), anemia, methemoglobinemia
Genitourinary	Diuresis

OVERDOSAGE	
Signs and symptoms	*Phenacetin-related effects:* dyspnea, cyanosis, hemolytic anemia, skin reactions with or without fever, anorexia, hypothermia, insomnia, stupor, coma, and vascular collapse, leading to death; *caffeine-related effects:* restlessness, nervousness, tolerance, delirium, tinnitus, tremors, tachycardia, scintillating scotomata, diuresis, cardiac arrhythmias; *carisoprodol-related effects:* stupor, coma, shock, respiratory depression, and (very rarely) death
Treatment	Induce emesis or use gastric lavage, followed by activated charcoal. Should respiration or blood pressure become compromised, administer respiratory assistance and pressor agents cautiously, as indicated. Careful monitoring of urinary output is necessary, and caution should be taken to avoid overhydration. For cyanosis due to methemoglobinemia, give 1% aqueous solution of methylene blue, 1–2 mg/kg body weight IV at hourly intervals up to 7 mg/kg. Observe for relapse due to incomplete gastric emptying and delayed absorption.

DRUG INTERACTIONS	
Alcohol, tranquilizers, sedative-hypnotics, and other CNS depressants	⇧ CNS depression

[1]Discontinue drug and institute symptomatic therapy, including use of epinephrine, antihistamines, and, in severe cases, corticosteroids; consider allergic reactions to excipients in all cases

Table continued on following page

ALTERED LABORATORY VALUES

No clinically significant alterations in blood/serum or urinary values occur at therapeutic dosages

Use in children

Not recommended for children under 5 yr of age. General guidelines not established for use in older children.

Use in pregnancy or nursing mothers

Safe use not established; carisoprodol levels in breast milk are 2 to 4 times maternal plasma concentrations

SOMA COMPOUND with CODEINE (Carisoprodol, phenacetin, caffeine, and codeine phosphate)

Wallace

Tabs: 200 mg carisoprodol, 160 mg phenacetin, 32 mg caffeine, and 16 mg codeine phosphate *C-III*

INDICATIONS	ORAL DOSAGE
Acute, painful musculoskeletal conditions (adjunctive therapy)	**Adult:** 1–2 tabs tid and at bedtime

CONTRAINDICATIONS

Acute intermittent porphyria ●	Allergic or idiosyncratic reactions to components and related compounds, such as meprobamate, mebutamate, or tybamate ●

WARNINGS/PRECAUTIONS

Idiosyncratic reactions	On very rare occasions such reactions have been reported within minutes or hours of the first dose, including extreme weakness, transient quadriplegia, dizziness, ataxia, temporary loss of vision, diplopia, mydriasis, dysarthria, agitation, euphoria, confusion, and disorientation. Symptoms usually subside over the course of the next several hours. Supportive and symptomatic therapy, including hospitalization, may be necessary (see ADVERSE REACTIONS).
Dependence	Mild withdrawal symptoms (abdominal cramps, insomnia, chills, headache, and nausea) have followed abrupt cessation of therapy with carisoprodol doses of 100 mg/kg/day; in addition, morphine-type drug dependence may result, owing to the presence of codeine. Use with caution in addiction-prone individuals.
Mental impairment, reflex-slowing	Performance of potentially hazardous activities may be impaired; caution patients accordingly
Compromised hepatic or renal function	Carisoprodol is metabolized by the liver and excreted by the kidney; watch for signs of excessive drug accumulation (see OVERDOSAGE)
Kidney disease	May occur following prolonged use (1–3 yr) of high doses of phenacetin
Special-risk patients	Use with caution in patients with anemia or cardiac, pulmonary, renal, or hepatic disease or in persons extremely sensitive to the CNS-stimulating activity of caffeine

ADVERSE REACTIONS

Central nervous system and neuromuscular	Drowsiness, sedation, dizziness, vertigo, ataxia, tremors, agitation, irritability, headache, depression, syncope, insomnia, nervousness
Ophthalmic	Miosis
Allergic or idiosyncratic[1]	Skin rash, erythema multiforme, pruritus, eosinophilia, fixed-drug eruption, asthmatic episodes, fever, weakness, dizziness, angioneurotic edema, smarting eyes, hypotension, anaphylactic shock
Cardiovascular	Tachycardia, postural hypotension, facial flushing
Gastrointestinal	Nausea, vomiting, constipation, hiccoughs, epigastric distress
Hematological	Leukopenia (causative role not firmly established), pancytopenia (probably unrelated), anemia, methemoglobinemia
Genitourinary	Diuresis

OVERDOSAGE

Signs and symptoms	*Phenacetin-related effects:* dyspnea, cyanosis, hemolytic anemia, skin reactions with or without fever, anorexia, hypothermia, insomnia, stupor, coma, and vascular collapse, leading to death; *caffeine-related effects:* restlessness, nervousness, tolerance, delirium, tinnitus, tremor, tachycardia, scintillating scotomata, diuresis, cardiac arrhythmias; *codeine-related effects:* coma, pinpoint pupils, respiratory depression, and shock; *carisoprodol-related effects:* stupor, coma, shock, respiratory derpession, and (very rarely) death
Treatment	Induce emesis or use gastric lavage, followed by activated charcoal. Should respiration or blood pressure become compromised, administer respiratory assistance and pressor agents cautiously, as indicated. For severe respiratory depression, administer a narcotic antagonist (eg, nalorphine or levallorphan), along with attempts at resuscitation. Careful monitoring of urinary output is necessary, and caution should be taken to avoid overhydration. For cyanosis due to methemoglobinemia, give 1% aqueous solution of methylene blue, 1–2 mg/kg body weight IV at hourly intervals up to 7 mg/kg. Observe for relapse due to incomplete gastric emptying and delayed absorption.

[1]Discontinue drug and institute symptomatic therapy, including use of epinephrine, antihistamines, and, in severe cases, corticosteroids; consider allergic reactions to excipients in all cases

Table continued on following page

SOMA COMPOUND with CODEINE continued

DRUG INTERACTIONS

Alcohol, tranquilizers, sedative-hypnotics, and other CNS depressants	⇧ CNS depression

ALTERED LABORATORY VALUES

No clinically significant alterations in blood/serum or urinary values occur at therapeutic dosages

Use in children

Not recommended for children under 5 yr of age. General guidelines not established for use in older children.

Use in pregnancy or nursing mothers

Safe use not established; carisoprodol levels in breast milk are 2 to 4 times maternal plasma concentrations

VALIUM (Diazepam) **Roche**

Tabs: 2, 5, 10 mg **Amps:** 10 mg/2 ml (2 ml) **Vial:** 50 mg/10 ml (10 ml) **Syringe:** 10 mg/2 ml (2 ml) *C-IV*

INDICATIONS	ORAL DOSAGE	PARENTERAL DOSAGE
Skeletal-muscle spasm (adjunctive therapy)	**Adult:** 2-10 mg tid or qid **Child (>6 mo):** 1-2.5 mg tid or qid to start; increase gradually, as needed	**Adult:** 5-10 mg IM or IV to start; repeat 3-4 h later, if needed
Tension and anxiety; moderate to severe psychoneurotic states	**Adult:** 2-10 mg bid to qid	**Adult:** 2-10 mg IM or IV to start; repeat 3-4 h later, if needed
Acute alcohol withdrawal syndrome	**Adult:** 10 mg tid or qid over initial 24 h; then 5 mg tid or qid, as needed	**Adult:** 10 mg IM or IV to start; then 5-10 mg 3-4 h later, if needed
Preoperative medication	—	**Adult:** 10 mg IM (preferred) before surgery
Tetanus (adjunctive therapy)	—	**Adult:** same as for muscle spasm, except that larger doses may be needed **Child (1 mo to 5 yr):** 1-2 mg IM or IV (slowly); repeat q3-4h, as needed **Child (>5 yr):** 5-10 mg IM or IV (slowly); repeat q3-4h, as needed
Convulsive disorders (adjunctive therapy)	**Adult:** 2-10 mg bid to qid **Child (>6 mo):** 1-2.5 mg tid or qid to start; increase gradually, as needed	—
Status epilepticus; severe recurrent convulsive seizures	—	**Adult:** 5-10 mg IM or IV (preferred), slowly, q10-15 min, up to 30 mg; repeat 2-4 h later, if needed **Child (1 mo to 5 yr):** 0.2-0.5 mg IM or IV (preferred), slowly, q2-5 min, up to 5 mg; repeat 2-4 h later, if needed **Child (>5 yr):** 1 mg IM or IV (preferred), slowly, q2-5 min, up to 10 mg; repeat 2-4 h later, if needed
Endoscopic procedures (adjunctive therapy)	—	**Adult:** 5-10 mg IM 30 min prior to procedure or 10-20 mg, or less, IV (preferred), slowly, just prior to procedure
Cardioversion (adjunctive therapy)	—	**Adult:** 5-15 mg IV within 5-10 min before procedure

Note: Full chart appears on page 748.

Psychological Problems

Anxiety, Depression, and Psychotic Disorders

Mood-altering drugs—tranquilizers, antianxiety agents, stimulants, sedatives, and others—are among the most commonly prescribed medications in the United States, accounting for about 20 percent of all prescriptions. Although these drugs have revolutionized the treatment of psychiatric disorders, most do not solve the underlying causes of emotional and mental problems. In addition, individual responses to mood-altering medications vary greatly. The extent and frequency of adverse reactions depend on the type of drug, dosage, method of administration (i.e., intravenous, intramuscular, or oral), and various physical and psychological characteristics of individual patients, such as age, weight, sex, genetic factors, emotional status, life-style, and past drug experience. This section will cover the three major classes of mental and emotional illness—anxiety, depression, and psychotic disorders (primarily schizophrenia)—and the drugs most commonly used in their treatment.

BEFORE STARTING THERAPY

Several initial determinations should be made before embarking on psychotropic drug therapy: Can the symptoms be attributed to an organic disease? Is the condition acute, a crisis situation, cyclic or chronic? Is it caused by internal or external stresses or a combination of factors? What are the possibilities for addiction to the medication? What therapeutic approaches (e.g., individual or group psychotherapy, biofeedback, relaxation techniques, meditation, etc.) other than drugs should be considered? What related areas of the patient's life (nutrition, exercise, sleep, work, social and love relationships, sex, etc.) should be evaluated?

ANXIETY

Anxiety is defined as varying degrees of heightened apprehension, worry, or dread of impending disaster without apparent cause. Everyone on occasion experiences feelings of anxiety and fear. Indeed, these are characteristic responses to any threat and act as protective mechanisms against danger. The psychological feelings are usually accompanied by physical reactions, such as breathing irregularities, muscle tension, especially in the chest area, excessive sweating, increased pulse rate, stomach upset, and other gastrointestinal problems, such as indigestion.

When the apprehension and fear result from real danger or impending conflict, the response is appropriate. But when there is no external threat or conflict and the feelings are attributed to unresolved internal conflicts, the reaction is considered pathological (abnormal) anxiety. In other words, does the response help or hinder in dealing with the situation at hand? If the answer is to hinder, the anxiety is likely to be abnormal, and if it persists and continues to interfere with ability to function or feelings of well-being, medical help should be sought.

Not all persons suffering from anxiety have feelings of fear or dread; instead, the disorder may manifest itself in a variety of physical symptoms, often related to either the cardiovascular or pulmonary systems. For example, the patient may complain of vague chest pains, irregular heart beats, fatigue, or breathlessness. Gastrointestinal complaints such as indigestion, constipation, diarrhea, frequent belching, or "gas" are also common. When no physical cause for these symptoms can be found, the answer is often anxiety.

Treatment of Anxiety

The traditional approach to the treatment of anxiety is to delve into the patient's past and try to pinpoint unresolved conflicts or associations that may be producing the symptoms. The symptoms may be associated with ongoing problems over which the person feels he has no control. Very often, the patient has sought other "escapes," such as the use of alcohol and other drugs. While these may temporarily ease the feelings of anxiety, they are unlikely to solve the underlying problem(s). Therefore, while many physicians and/or psychiatrists prescribe antianxiety drugs to help their patients cope and function, they also try to help them understand the basis of their anxiety and help them deal with the problem itself.

Antianxiety Drugs

Since the 1950s, the number and types of mood-altering drugs to ease the symptoms of anxiety have proliferated. These drugs include antianxiety drugs (anxiolytics), certain antihistamines, and, experimentally, beta-adrenergic blocking agents.

Anxiolytics The anxiolytic agents, often referred to as tranquilizers, are used most frequently in treating anxiety. In general, these drugs have sedative/hypnotic properties. Other drugs may have sedating effects; these agents include the potent antipsychotic drugs used to treat schizophrenia, as well as some of the antidepressants (neuroleptics).

The most frequently prescribed anxiolytics are the benzodiazepines, which include diazepam (Valium), chlordiazepoxide (Librium), prazepam (Centrax and Verstran), clorazepate (Tranxene), oxazepam (Serax), and lorazepam (Ativan). Benzodiazepines are generally considered safer and more effective in treating anxiety than the older antianxiety drugs, such as meprobamate (Equanil and Miltown), or the barbiturates, which include phenobarbitol and butabarbital. These other agents also produce stronger adverse effects on psychomotor functions, such as incoordination, mental confusion, and drowsiness, than do the benzodiazepines.

Although the benzodiazepines are remarkably effective and relatively safe antianxiety agents, they should not be taken as a matter of course to ease the stresses of everyday life. When taken over a long period of time, these drugs may become habit forming; therefore, they generally should not be used for more than two weeks at a time except under the close supervision of a physician. Certain adverse reactions to benzodiazepines, such as fatigue, headache, dizziness, and incoordination, which make it dangerous to drive a car or operate machinery, often can be avoided by taking the drug at bedtime. Alcohol, antihistamines, barbiturates, narcotics, and other antianxiety agents should not be taken concurrently with benzodiazepines, since they add to the depression of the central nervous system.

Since the liver is the main organ that removes these drugs from the body, they may be contraindicated in persons with severe liver disease. Although not specifically contraindicated, they should be used cautiously in a person with any serious medical problem. On occasion, the benzodiazepines release feelings of hostility, rage, or excitement, disturb sleep, or cause nightmares. During the use of a drug, any unusual symptom, such as a fever, eye pain, unusual bleeding, bruising, or sore throat unrelated to a cold or other illness, should be reported to the prescribing physician. Abruptly stopping the use of any sedative drug may cause delirium and convulsions if the doses have been high and used for a prolonged period; therefore, the drug should be tapered off over a period of time. An overdosage can cause coma, shock, and death.

Other drugs used to treat anxiety Barbiturates, such as amobarbital, phenobarbital, and butabarbital, have long been used to treat anxiety. These drugs depress the central nervous system, causing drowsiness, impaired mental function, and other undesired effects. Overdose is a major danger with these agents, and a major reason that their use is rather limited.

The propanediols, which include Equanil and Miltown, were once considered preferable to barbiturates in treating anxiety, especially when they were first introduced in the mid-1950s. This view has changed, however, and it is now felt that their spectrum of adverse reactions, as well as their positive effects, is comparable to those of the barbiturates.

Antihistamines, such as Atarax and Vistaril, have a sedative effect, and are therefore sometimes used in treating anxiety. Again, depression of the central nervous system is a major adverse reaction of these agents. Overdoses may be life-threatening.

Nonprescription drugs Most over-the-counter or nonprescription psychotropic drugs have been withdrawn from the market or switched to prescription use. The preparations that remain, such as Cope, are mild analgesics and are not likely to be effective against clinical anxiety.

DEPRESSION

Feelings of grief, sadness, and depression are part of normal, everyday life. At times, everyone experiences sadness, demoralization, and the grief of personal loss. But when these feelings lead to a decreased ability to function and cope with normal life, or when they have no identifiable cause, they may be symptoms of pathological depression. Since depression may mimic a number of other diseases, and very often goes undiagnosed, the American Psychiatric Association has established the following criteria for diagnosing depression:

- *Dysphoric mood* Persistent and overriding feelings of depression, hopelessness, emptiness, and other such feelings
- *Cluster of symptoms* The presence of at least five of the following: appetite disturbance and weight change (unusual increase or decrease); marked change in sleep (insomnia or increased sleep need); loss of energy; slowed thinking; decreased ability to concentrate or remember; psychomotor agitation or retardation; loss of interest in usually pleasurable activities, such as sex, social events, etc.; inappropriate feelings of guilt and self-blame; and recurrent thoughts of death or suicide
- *General impaired ability to function*

If the above have been present for two weeks, a diagnosis of depression is likely.

It also should be noted that many disease states have a component of depression. This is particularly common after a heart attack or the diagnosis of a chronic or life-threatening disease such as cancer.

Types of Depression

About 40 million Americans—two thirds of them women—suffer from depression. There are different types of depression; for example, one kind is characterized by great swings in mood, from elation or mania to the depths of depression. Or the depression may be recurrent without the intervening periods of elation. Manic depression usually manifests itself early in life and often seems to run in families. Suicide is relatively common among manic-depressives, as are accidents from reckless acts during manic phases.

The most common recurrent depression is often found in persons plagued by feelings of inadequacy. They often have trouble establishing friendships or holding a job. Even a minor disappointment or setback can trigger a state of depression.

Treatment of Depression

In most cases of depression, attempts to alter lifestyle or attitudes are ineffective. Instead, medical treatment is usually necessary, and in many persons, especially manic-depressives, this need is lifelong.

Electroconvulsive therapy For persons suffering from recurrent depression, electroconvulsive (shock) therapy is often more effective than drugs in producing a cure. Controversy surrounds this approach to depression, and unless suicide is an imminent risk, it is generally not the initial treatment of choice. However, when drugs and other therapies fail, it is considered the best alternative. Unfortunately, many persons have been unnecessarily frightened by the prospect of shock therapy through sensationalized reports of "brain damage" and other adverse effects. When properly administered, electroconvulsive therapy is relatively safe, although its risks and expense are greater than those of antidepressant drugs.

Antidepressant drugs The most widely used antidepressant agents are the tricyclic antidepressants, which work through the central nervous system.

About two thirds of patients taking tricyclic antidepressants experience decreased or total disappearance of the depression within one month, and the figure rises when the dosage is increased to the maximum for four to six weeks. Tricyclic antidepressants include amoxapine (Asendin), doxepin (Adapin and Sinequan), amitriptyline (Elavil and Endep), desipramine (Norpramin), nortriptyline (Pamelor), trimipramine (Surmontil), and imipramine (Tofranil). Some antidepressants, such as Etrafon and Triavil (perphenazine with amitriptyline), and Limbitrol (chlordiazepoxide with amitriptyline), offer combinations of antidepressant and antianxiety agents.

Since these drugs may impair the mental and/or physical abilities required for driving a car or operating machinery, they should be used with caution in these circumstances, if at all.

Monoamine oxidase inhibitors Another class of drugs, the monoamine oxidase (MAO) inhibitors, may be recommended to treat depression when antidepressant agents fail or cannot be tolerated. These drugs, which include isocarboxazid (Marplan) and phenelzine (Nardil), block the action of an enzyme and usually work rapidly, within twenty-four hours. Persons taking these drugs should not eat foods containing tyramine, such as certain types of ripe cheeses and wine, because this may precipitate a hypertensive crisis. The combination of MAO inhibitors and certain drugs, such as nasal decongestants found in cold remedies, may produce a similar response.

Lithium salts Lithium carbonate is a crystalline salt used to treat manic depression. The drug may be used with an antipsychotic or antidepressant during an acute manic or depressive phase, and alone for long-term maintenance. Since the dose of lithium must be carefully adjusted, it is important to take it exactly as prescribed and under the close supervision of a physician. Even a slight overdose can have toxic effects. Use with a thiazide diuretic lowers the amount of lithium needed, and may result in an overdose, even when only a usual amount is consumed.

PSYCHOSIS

Schizophrenia in its various manifestations is the most common form of psychosis in the United States. The term schizophrenia actually refers to a group of mental diseases characterized by impaired thinking, inappropriate behavior, hallucinations, delusions, and emotional changes. Some patients become withdrawn; others may be violent. Movement disturbances, such as agitation, bizarre positions, strange motions, or even stupor, are also common. Until the 1950s, little could be done to help these patients, who were generally institutionalized. Now many schizophrenics can lead reasonably normal lives by using antipsychotic agents.

More than twenty antipsychotic drugs are now in use in this country and the choice of a specific agent depends upon individual circumstances and physician preference.

Although antipsychotic drugs differ in mechanism of action, potency, and types of side effects, all are powerful agents capable of controlling treatable schizophrenia. They also affect many organ systems and must be carefully administered. They are generally given in three phases: an initial or loading dose, usually given during the acute stage in a hospital setting; the second or early therapeutic phase, in which the dose is adjusted to control symptoms and is then gradually lowered; and the third, or maintenance phase, in which the patient receives the lowest possible dose to prevent recurrence of the psychotic symptoms. In addition, some physicians use drug-free periods of a few weeks or even months to avoid some of the serious long-term side effects, such as movement disorders (tardive dyskinesia).

IN CONCLUSION

The introduction of various mood-altering and antipsychotic drugs has made it possible to treat a wide range of emotional and mental illnesses. It must be remembered, however, that these drugs all have the potential for serious side effects, and should not be used except under close supervision of a physician. They also should not be taken routinely to cope with the everyday stress and anxiety that is a normal part of life.

The following drug charts cover the major drugs prescribed to treat anxiety, depression, and psychotic (schizophrenic) disorders. The barbiturates and nonprescription agents sometimes promoted for anxiety may be found in the section on *Sleep Disorders* (pages 808–824).

ATIVAN (Lorazepam) Wyeth

Tabs: 0.5, 1, 2 mg *C-IV*

INDICATIONS	ORAL DOSAGE
Anxiety, tension, agitation, irritability, and insomnia associated with anxiety neuroses and transient situational disturbances **Anxiety** associated with **depression** **Anxiety in functional or organic disorders,** particularly GI or cardiovascular disease	**Adult:** 2–3 mg bid or tid to start, followed by 1–10 mg/day, as needed, in divided doses, with the largest being taken before bedtime; usual maintenance dosage: 2–6 mg/day div

ADMINISTRATION/DOSAGE ADJUSTMENTS

Insomnia	Administer 2–4 mg in a single daily dose at bedtime
Elderly and debilitated patients	Initiate therapy with 1–2 mg/day div; adjust dosage as needed
Long-term use (>4 mo)	Effectiveness for prolonged use as an antianxiety agent has not been tested in systematic clinical studies; reassess need for continued therapy periodically

CONTRAINDICATIONS

Hypersensitivity to benzodiazepines • Psychotic reactions • Primary depressive disorder •

Acute narrow-angle glaucoma •

WARNINGS/PRECAUTIONS

Habit-forming	Psychic and/or physical dependence may develop, especially in addiction-prone individuals
Mental impairment, reflex-slowing	Performance of potentially hazardous activities may be impaired; caution patients accordingly, as well as about the additive effects of alcohol and other CNS depressants
Potentially suicidal patients	Should not have access to large quantities of lorazepam; prescribe smallest amount feasible
Abrupt discontinuation of therapy	May produce barbiturate-like withdrawal symptoms or precipitate recurrence of pre-existing symptoms, including anxiety, agitation, irritability, tension, insomnia, and convulsions
Prolonged therapy	Blood counts and liver-function tests should be performed periodically; use with caution in the elderly and monitor frequently for symptoms of upper GI disease
Hepatic or renal impairment	May lead to excessive drug accumulation; monitor patient closely
Ataxia or oversedation	May develop in elderly and/or debilitated patients (see ADMINISTRATION/DOSAGE ADJUSTMENTS)
GI or cardiovascular disorders associated with anxiety	Lorazepam has not been shown to be of significant benefit in treating GI or cardiovascular symptoms

ADVERSE REACTIONS
Frequent reactions are italicized

Central nervous system	*Sedation (16%), dizziness (6.9%), weakness (4.2%), unsteadiness (3.4%),* disorientation, depression, headache, sleep disturbance, agitation
Cardiovascular	Slight hypotension
Gastrointestinal	Nausea, altered appetite, various disturbances
Other	Dermatological symptoms, visual disturbances, autonomic manifestations

OVERDOSAGE

Signs and symptoms	Somnolence, confusion, coma
Treatment	Empty stomach immediately by inducing emesis or by gastric lavage. Employ general supportive measures, as needed, and monitor vital signs. Combat hypotension with levarterenol. For CNS-depressive effects, administer caffeine and sodium benzoate. The benefit of dialysis is unknown.

Table continued on following page

ATIVAN continued

DRUG INTERACTIONS

Alcohol, tricyclic antidepressants, sedative-hypnotics, MAO inhibitors, and other CNS depressants	⇧ CNS depression

ALTERED LABORATORY VALUES

Blood/serum values	⇧ Lactate dehydrogenase

No clinically significant alterations in urinary values occur at therapeutic dosages

Use in children

Safety and effectiveness have not been established in children under 12 yr of age

Use in pregnancy or nursing mothers

Drug should almost always be avoided during early pregnancy. Although lorazepam has not been sufficiently studied to determine conclusively its effects during pregnancy, an increased risk of congenital malformations during the 1st trimester has been associated with minor tranquilizers (chlordiazepoxide, diazepam, meprobamate). Patient should stop nursing if drug is prescribed.

CENTRAX (Prazepam) Parke-Davis

Tabs: 5, 10 mg *C-IV*

INDICATIONS	ORAL DOSAGE
Anxiety and tension associated with anxiety disorders, transient situational disturbances, and functional or organic disorders	**Adult:** 30 mg/day div to start, followed by 20–60 mg/day div, as needed; alternative regimen: 20 mg at bedtime, followed several days later by 20–40 mg/day div, as needed

ADMINISTRATION/DOSAGE ADJUSTMENTS

Elderly or debilitated patients	Reduce initial dosage to 10–15 mg/day div
Long-term use (>4 mo)	Effectiveness for prolonged use as an antianxiety agent has not been tested in systematic clinical studies; reassess need for continued therapy periodically

CONTRAINDICATIONS

Hypersensitivity to prazepam ●

Acute narrow-angle glaucoma ●

Psychiatric disorders in which anxiety is not prominent ●

Psychotic reactions ●

WARNINGS/PRECAUTIONS

Habit-forming	Psychic and/or physical dependence may develop, especially in one addiction-prone
Mental impairment, reflex-slowing	Performance of potentially hazardous activities may be impaired; caution patients accordingly, as well as about the additive effect of alcohol and other CNS depressants
Potentially suicidal patients	Should not have access to large quantities; prescribe smallest amount feasible
Barbiturate-like withdrawal symptoms	May result when drug is discontinued abruptly
Prolonged therapy	Blood counts and liver-function tests should be performed periodically
Hepatic or renal impairment	May lead to excessive drug accumulation; monitor patient closely
Ataxia or oversedation	May develop in elderly or debilitated patients

ADVERSE REACTIONS

Frequent reactions are italicized

Central nervous system	*Fatigue (12%), dizziness (8.7%), weakness (7.7%), drowsiness (6.8%), lightheadedness (6.8%), ataxia (5.0%),* headache, confusion, tremor, vivid dreams, slurred speech, stimulation, blurred vision, paradoxical excitement[1]
Cardiovascular	Palpitations, syncope, slight hypotension
Gastrointestinal	Dry mouth, various other complaints
Dermatological	Diaphoresis, pruritus, skin rash
Hepatic	Altered liver-function tests
Genitourinary	Various complaints
Other	Swelling of feet, joint pains, slight weight gain

OVERDOSAGE

Signs and symptoms	See ADVERSE REACTIONS
Treatment	Induce emesis if vomiting has not occurred spontaneously and use gastric lavage immediately to empty stomach. Monitor vital signs frequently and employ general supportive measures, as needed. Combat hypotension with levarterenol or metaraminol.

DRUG INTERACTIONS

Alcohol, tricyclic antidepressants, sedative-hypnotics, MAO inhibitors, and other CNS depressants	⇧ CNS depression

ALTERED LABORATORY VALUES

No clinically significant alterations in blood/serum or urinary values occur at therapeutic dosages

Use in children

Safety and effectiveness in patients under 18 yr of age have not been established

Use in pregnancy or nursing mothers

Drug should almost always be avoided during early pregnancy. Although prazepam has not been sufficiently studied to determine conclusively its effects during pregnancy, an increased risk of congenital malformations during the 1st trimester has been associated with minor tranquilizers (chlordiazepoxide, diazepam, meprobamate). Patient should stop nursing if drug is prescribed.

[1]Greenblatt DJ, Shader RI: *Benzodiazepines in Clinical Practice.* New York, Raven Press, 1974

Note: Prazepam also marketed as **VERSTRAN** (Parke-Davis).

LIBRIUM (Chlordiazepoxide hydrochloride) Roche

Caps: 5, 10, 25 mg **Amps:** 100 mg (5 ml) *C-IV*

LIBRITABS (Chlordiazepoxide hydrochloride) Roche

Tabs: 5, 10, 25 mg *C-IV*

INDICATIONS	ORAL DOSAGE	PARENTERAL DOSAGE
Mild to moderate anxiety and tension	**Adult:** 5–10 mg tid or qid **Child (> 6 yr):** 5 mg bid to qid, up to 10 mg bid or tid, if needed	—
Severe anxiety and tension, acute anxiety	**Adult:** 20–25 mg tid or qid **Child:** same as above	**Adult:** 50–100 mg IM (preferred) or IV to start, followed by 25–50 mg tid or qid, if needed
Preoperative apprehension and anxiety	**Adult:** 5–10 mg tid or qid on days before surgery **Child:** same as above	**Adult:** 50–100 mg IM 1 h before surgery
Withdrawal symptoms of acute alcoholism	**Adult:** 50–100 mg, repeated as needed, up to 300 mg/day, until agitation is controlled	**Adult:** 50–100 mg IM (preferred) or IV, repeated in 2–4 h, if needed

ADMINISTRATION/DOSAGE ADJUSTMENTS

Intramuscular administration	Immediately before use, prepare solution by adding 2 ml of special IM diluent (supplied) to contents of 5-ml amber ampul; agitate gently until powder is completely dissolved. Inject slowly and deeply into upper outer quadrant of gluteus muscle. Patient should be kept under observation, preferably in bed, for up to 3 h after injection.
Intravenous administration	Immediately before use, prepare solution by adding 5 ml of physiologic saline or sterile water for injection to contents of 5-ml amber ampul; agitate gently until powder is completely dissolved. Inject slowly over a period of 1 min. Patient should be kept under observation, preferably in bed, for up to 3 h after injection.
Maximum parenteral dosage	Up to 300 mg may be given IM or IV during a 6-h period, but no more than this amount in any 24-h period
Elderly or debilitated patients	Reduce dosage to 5 mg bid to qid orally or 25–50 mg IM or IV
Long-term use (>4 mo)	Effectiveness for prolonged use as an antianxiety agent has not been tested in systematic clinical studies; reassess need for continued therapy periodically

CONTRAINDICATIONS

Hypersensitivity to chlordiazepoxide ● Shock ● Comatose states ●

WARNINGS/PRECAUTIONS

Habit-forming	Psychic and/or physical dependence may develop, especially in addiction-prone individuals
Mental impairment, reflex slowing	Performance of potentially hazardous activities may be impaired; caution patients accordingly, as well as about the additive effects of alcohol and other CNS depressants; ambulatory patients should not be permitted to drive after receiving an injection
Barbiturate-like withdrawal symptoms	May result when drug is discontinued
Prolonged therapy	Blood counts and liver-function tests should be performed periodically
Hepatic or renal impairment	May lead to excessive drug accumulation; monitor patient closely
Concomitant psychotropic therapy	Use with extreme caution, if at all, particularly when use of known potentiating compounds (see DRUG INTERACTIONS) is contemplated
Paradoxical reactions	Excitement, stimulation, and acute rage may occur in psychiatric patients and in hyperactive children; monitor such patients closely during therapy
Ataxia or oversedation	May develop in elderly and/or debilitated patients (see ADMINISTRATION/DOSAGE ADJUSTMENTS)

Table continued on following page

LIBRIUM/LIBRITABS continued

ADVERSE REACTIONS

Central nervous system	Drowsiness, ataxia, confusion, EEG pattern changes, extrapyramidal symptoms, blurred vision (with parenteral use)
Cardiovascular	Syncope, hypotension (with parenteral use), tachycardia (with parenteral use)
Gastrointestinal	Nausea, constipation
Dermatological	Skin eruptions, edema
Hematological	Blood dyscrasias, including agranulocytosis
Hepatic	Jaundice, dysfunction
Genitourinary	Menstrual irregularities, altered libido

OVERDOSAGE

Signs and symptoms	Somnolence, confusion, coma, diminished reflexes, excitation, hypotension
Treatment	Empty stomach immediately by gastric lavage. Employ general supportive measures, as needed. Administer IV fluids and maintain adequate airway. Combat hypotension with levarterenol or metaraminol. For CNS-depressive effects, administer methylphenidate or caffeine and sodium benzoate. If excitation occurs, do not give barbiturates. Dialysis is of limited value.

DRUG INTERACTIONS

Alcohol, tricyclic antidepressants, sedative-hypnotics, MAO inhibitors, and other CNS depressants	⇧ CNS depression
Oral anticoagulants	⇧ or ⇩ Anticoagulant effect

ALTERED LABORATORY VALUES

No clinically significant alterations in blood/serum or urinary values occur at therapeutic dosages

Use in children

See INDICATIONS. Oral form is not recommended for children under 6 yr of age; parenteral form is not recommended for children under 12 yr of age.

Use in pregnancy or nursing mothers

Drug should almost always be avoided during early pregnancy. Although chlordiazepoxide has not been sufficiently studied to determine conclusively its effects during pregnancy, an increased risk of congenital malformations during the 1st trimester has been associated with minor tranquilizers, including chlordiazepoxide. General guidelines not established for use in nursing mothers.

MILTOWN (Meprobamate) Wallace

Tabs: 200, 400 mg *C-IV*

MILTOWN 600 (Meprobamate) Wallace

Tabs: 600 mg *C-IV*

INDICATIONS	ORAL DOSAGE
Anxiety and tension and as an adjunct in the treatment of various disease states in which anxiety and tension are manifest **Sedation** of anxious, tense patients	**Adult:** 1,200–1,600 mg/day in 3–4 divided doses or 1 Miltown 600 tab bid, or up to 2,400 mg/day, if needed **Child (6–12 yr):** 100–200 mg bid or tid

ADMINISTRATION/DOSAGE ADJUSTMENTS

Long-term use (>4 mo)	Effectiveness for prolonged use as an antianxiety agent has not been tested in systematic clinical studies; reassess need for continued therapy periodically

CONTRAINDICATIONS

Hypersensitivity or idiosyncratic reaction to meprobamate and related compounds ●	Acute intermittent porphyria ●

WARNINGS/PRECAUTIONS

Habit-forming	Psychic and/or physical dependence may develop, especially in addiction-prone individuals
Mental impairment, reflex-slowing	Performance of potentially hazardous activities may be impaired; caution patients accordingly, as well as about the additive effects of alcohol and other CNS depressants
Potentially suicidal patients	Should not have access to large quantities of meprobamate; prescribe smallest amount feasible
Abrupt discontinuation of therapy	May precipitate recurrence of pre-existing symptoms, including anxiety, anorexia, or insomnia, or withdrawal reactions, including vomiting, ataxia, tremors, muscle twitching, confusion, hallucinosis, and convulsive seizures (rare). Seizures are more likely to occur in patients with CNS damage or pre-existing or latent convulsive disorders. After prolonged high-dose therapy, reduce dosage gradually over a period of 1–2 wk or substitute a short-acting barbiturate.
Hepatic or renal impairment	May lead to excessive drug accumulation (see OVERDOSAGE); monitor patient closely
Ataxia or oversedation	May develop in elderly and/or debilitated patients; administer the lowest effective dose
Seizures	May develop in epileptic patients

ADVERSE REACTIONS

Central nervous system	Drowsiness, ataxia, dizziness, slurred speech, headache, vertigo, weakness, paresthesias, impairment of visual accommodation, euphoria, overstimulation, paradoxical excitement, fast EEG activity
Gastrointestinal	Nausea, vomiting, diarrhea
Cardiovascular	Palpitations, tachycardia, arrhythmias, transient ECG changes, syncope, hypotensive crisis
Allergic or idiosyncratic	Pruritic, urticarial, or erythematous maculopapular rash in groin area or generalized; leukopenia, acute nonthrombocytopenic purpura, petechiae, ecchymoses, eosinophilia, peripheral edema, adenopathy, fever, fixed drug eruption with cross-reaction to carisoprodol, cross-sensitivity between meprobamate/mebutamate and meprobamate/carbromal; in severe cases (rare): hyperpyrexia, chills, angioneurotic edema, bronchospasm, oliguria, anuria, anaphylaxis, erythema multiforme, exfoliative dermatitis, Stevens-Johnson syndrome, bullous dermatitis
Hematological	Agranulocytosis and aplastic anemia (causal relationship not established), thrombocytopenic purpura (rare)
Other	Exacerbation of porphyric symptoms

Table continued on following page

OVERDOSAGE

Signs and symptoms	Drowsiness, lethargy, stupor, ataxia, coma, shock, vasomotor and respiratory collapse
Treatment	Empty stomach immediately by gastric lavage. Treat symptomatically. Provide respiratory assistance, CNS stimulants, and pressor agents cautiously, as needed. Diuretics, osmotic (mannitol) diuresis, peritoneal dialysis, and hemodialysis may be helpful. Monitor urinary output and avoid overhydration.

DRUG INTERACTIONS

Alcohol, tricyclic antidepressants, sedative-hypnotics, MAO inhibitors, and other CNS depressants	⇧ CNS depression

ALTERED LABORATORY VALUES

No clinically significant alterations in blood/serum or urinary values occur at therapeutic dosages

Use in children

Safety and effectiveness have not been established for children under 6 yr of age. The 600-mg tablet is not intended for use in children.

Use in pregnancy or nursing mothers

Drug should almost always be avoided during early pregnancy. Although meprobamate has not been sufficiently studied to determine conclusively its effects during pregnancy, an increased risk of congenital malformations during the 1st trimester has been associated with minor tranquilizers, including meprobamate. Patient should stop nursing if drug is prescribed.

Note: Meprobamate also marketed as **EQUANIL** (Wyeth).

SERAX (Oxazepam) Wyeth

Tabs: 15 mg **Caps:** 10, 15, 30 mg *C-IV*

INDICATIONS	ORAL DOSAGE
Mild to moderate anxiety associated with tension, irritability, agitation, or related symptoms of functional origin or secondary to organic disease	**Adult:** 10–15 mg tid or qid
Severe anxiety syndromes, agitation, or **anxiety** associated with depression	**Adult:** 15–30 mg tid or qid
Alcoholics with **acute inebriation, tremulousness,** or withdrawal **anxiety**	**Adult:** 15–30 mg tid or qid

ADMINISTRATION/DOSAGE ADJUSTMENTS

Elderly patients with anxiety, tension, irritability, and agitation	Initiate therapy with 10 mg tid; if necessary, increase dosage gradually to 15 mg tid or qid
Long-term use (>4 mo)	Effectiveness for prolonged use as an antianxiety agent has not been tested in systematic clinical studies; reassess need for continued therapy periodically

CONTRAINDICATIONS

Hypersensitivity to oxazepam ● Psychoses ●

WARNINGS/PRECAUTIONS

Habit-forming	Psychic and/or physical dependence may develop, especially in the addiction-prone
Drowsiness, dizziness	Performance of potentially hazardous activities may be impaired; caution patients accordingly, as well as about the additive effects of alcohol and other CNS depressants
Abrupt discontinuation of therapy	May cause epileptiform seizures or barbiturate-like withdrawal symptoms; reduce dosage gradually after prolonged therapy
Special-risk patients	Use with caution in patients in whom a drop in blood pressure could lead to cardiac complications, especially the elderly
Potentially suicidal patients	Should not have access to large quantities; prescribe smallest amount feasible
Prolonged therapy	Blood counts and liver-function tests should be performed periodically

ADVERSE REACTIONS[1]

Central nervous system	Transient mild drowsiness, dizziness, vertigo, headache, syncope (rare), paradoxical excitement or stimulation of affect, lethargy, slurred speech, tremor, ataxia (rare)
Gastrointestinal	Nausea
Dermatological	Morbilliform, urticarial, or maculopapular rash
Hematological	Leukopenia (rare)
Hepatic	Dysfunction, including jaundice (rare)
Other	Altered libido, edema

OVERDOSAGE

Signs and symptoms	Somnolence, confusion, coma, diminished reflexes, excitation, hypotension
Treatment	Empty stomach immediately by gastric lavage. Employ general supportive measures, as needed. Administer IV fluids and maintain adequate airway. Combat hypotension with levarterenol or metaraminol. For CNS-depressive effects, administer caffeine and sodium benzoate.

DRUG INTERACTIONS

Alcohol, tricyclic antidepressants, sedative-hypnotics, MAO inhibitors, and other CNS depressants	⇧ CNS depression

ALTERED LABORATORY VALUES

No clinically significant alterations in blood/serum or urinary values occur at therapeutic dosages

Use in children

Contraindicated for children under 6 yr of age; absolute dosage for children 6–12 yr of age has not been established

Use in pregnancy or nursing mothers

Drug should almost always be avoided during early pregnancy. Although oxazepam has not been sufficiently studied to determine conclusively its effects during pregnancy, an increased risk of congenital malformations during the 1st trimester has been associated with minor tranquilizers. General guidelines not established for use in nursing mothers.

TRANXENE (Clorazepate dipotassium) **Abbott**

Tabs: 3.75, 7.5, 15 mg **Caps:** 3.75, 7.5, 15 mg *C-IV*

TRANXENE-SD (Clorazepate dipotassium) **Abbott**

Tabs: 11.25 mg (Tranxene-SD Half Strength), 22.5 mg (Tranxene-SD) *C-IV*

INDICATIONS	ORAL DOSAGE
Anxiety disorders **Short-term symptomatic relief of anxiety**	**Adult:** 15 mg/day to start, followed by 15–60 mg/day in a single daily dose at bedtime or div, or 1 Tranxene-SD Half Strength or Tranxene-SD tab q24h (should not be used to initiate therapy)
Acute alcohol withdrawal symptoms	**Adult:** day 1, 30 mg to start, followed by 30–60 mg div; day 2, 45–90 mg div; day 3, 22.5–45 mg div; day 4, 15–30 mg div; thereafter, gradually reduce dosage to 7.5–15 mg/day and discontinue as soon as patient's condition stabilizes

ADMINISTRATION/DOSAGE ADJUSTMENTS

Elderly or debilitated patients — Initiate treatment with 7.5-15 mg/day; increase dosage gradually, as needed

Long-term use (>4 mo) — Effectiveness for prolonged use as an antianxiety agent has not been tested in systematic clinical studies; reassess need for continued therapy periodically

CONTRAINDICATIONS

Hypersensitivity to clorazepate ● Psychotic reactions ● Depressive neuroses ● Acute glaucoma ●

WARNINGS/PRECAUTIONS

Habit-forming — Psychic and/or physical dependence may develop, especially in the addiction-prone

Mental impairment, reflex-slowing — Performance of potentially hazardous activities may be impaired; caution patients accordingly, as well as about the additive effects of alcohol and other CNS depressants

Potentially suicidal patients — Should not have access to large quantities; prescribe smallest amount feasible

Barbiturate-like withdrawal symptoms — May result when drug is discontinued abruptly; withdrawal symptoms have also been reported following abrupt discontinuation of benzodiazepines taken continuously at therapeutic levels for several months

Prolonged therapy — Blood counts and liver-function tests should be performed periodically

Hepatic or renal impairment — May lead to excessive drug accumulation (see OVERDOSAGE); monitor patient closely

Ataxia or oversedation — May develop in elderly and/or debilitated patients

ADVERSE REACTIONS

Central nervous system — Drowsiness, dizziness, nervousness, headache, fatigue, ataxia, confusion, insomnia, blurred vision, irritability, diplopia, depression, slurred speech

Cardiovascular — Decreased systolic blood pressure

Gastrointestinal — Various complaints, dry mouth

Dermatological — Skin rash, edema

Other — Altered renal and hepatic function tests, decreased hematocrit, genitourinary complaints

OVERDOSAGE

Signs and symptoms — Somnolence, confusion, coma, diminished reflexes, excitation, hypotension

Treatment — Empty stomach immediately by induction of emesis and/or gastric lavage. Employ general supportive measures, as needed. Monitor vital signs frequently and keep patient under close observation. For hypotension, use levarterenol or metaraminol.

DRUG INTERACTIONS

Alcohol, tricyclic antidepressants, sedative-hypnotics, MAO inhibitors, and other CNS depressants — ⇧ CNS depression

ALTERED LABORATORY VALUES

No clinically significant alterations in blood/serum or urinary values occur at therapeutic dosages

Use in children

Not recommended for use in patients less than 18 yr of age

Use in pregnancy or nursing mothers

Drug should almost always be avoided during early pregnancy. Although clorazepate has not been sufficiently studied to determine conclusively its effects during pregnancy, an increased risk of congenital malformations during the 1st trimester has been associated with minor tranquilizers (chlordiazepoxide, diazepam, meprobamate). Patient should stop nursing if drug is prescribed.

VALIUM (Diazepam) Roche

Tabs: 2, 5, 10 mg **Amps:** 10 mg/2 ml (2 ml) **Vial:** 50 mg/10 ml (10 ml) **Syringe:** 10 mg/2 ml (2 ml) *C-IV*

INDICATIONS	ORAL DOSAGE	PARENTERAL DOSAGE
Tension and anxiety; moderate to severe psychoneurotic states	**Adult:** 2–10 mg bid to qid	**Adult:** 2–10 mg IM or IV to start; repeat 3–4 h later, if needed
Acute alcohol withdrawal syndrome	**Adult:** 10 mg tid or qid over initial 24 h; then 5 mg tid or qid, as needed	**Adult:** 10 mg IM or IV to start; then 5–10 mg 3–4 h later, if needed
Preoperative medication	—	**Adult:** 10 mg IM (preferred) before surgery
Skeletal-muscle spasm (adjunctive therapy)	**Adult:** 2–10 mg tid or qid **Child (>6 mo):** 1–2.5 mg tid or qid to start; increase gradually, as needed	**Adult:** 5–10 mg IM or IV to start; repeat 3–4 h later, if needed
Tetanus (adjunctive therapy)	—	**Adult:** same as for muscle spasm, except that larger doses may be needed **Child (1 mo to 5 yr):** 1–2 mg IM or IV (slowly); repeat q3–4h, as needed **Child (>5 yr):** 5–10 mg IM or IV (slowly); repeat q3–4h, as needed
Convulsive disorders (adjunctive therapy)	**Adult:** 2–10 mg bid to qid **Child (>6 mo):** 1–2.5 mg tid or qid to start; increase gradually, as needed	—
Status epilepticus; severe recurrent convulsive seizures	—	**Adult:** 5–10 mg IM or IV (preferred), slowly, q10–15 min, up to 30 mg; repeat 2–4 h later, if needed **Child (1 mo to 5 yr):** 0.2–0.5 mg IM or IV (preferred), slowly, q2–5 min, up to 5 mg; repeat 2–4 h later, if needed **Child (>5 yr):** 1 mg IM or IV (preferred), slowly, q2–5 min, up to 10 mg; repeat 2–4 h later, if needed
Endoscopic procedures (adjunctive therapy)	—	**Adult:** 5–10 mg IM 30 min prior to procedure or 10–20 mg, or less, IV (preferred), slowly, just prior to procedure
Cardioversion (adjunctive therapy)	—	**Adult:** 5–15 mg IV within 5–10 min before procedure

ADMINISTRATION/DOSAGE ADJUSTMENTS

Elderly and/or debilitated patients	To preclude ataxia or oversedation, start with 2–2.5 mg qd or bid orally and increase dosage gradually; when using the injectable form, reduce dosage to 2–5 mg to start and then increase gradually (see WARNINGS/PRECAUTIONS)
Concomitant therapy with narcotic analgesics	Reduce narcotic dosage by at least ⅓ and administer in small increments
Long-term use (>4 mo)	Effectiveness for prolonged use as an antianxiety agent has not been tested in systematic clinical studies; reassess need for continued therapy periodically

CONTRAINDICATIONS

Hypersensitivity to diazepam	
Acute narrow-angle glaucoma	
Open-angle glaucoma	Unless patient is receiving appropriate antiglaucoma therapy
Psychosis	Diazepam is of no value in psychotic patients
Shock, coma	
Acute alcohol intoxication	With depression of vital signs

WARNINGS/PRECAUTIONS

Habit-forming	Psychic and/or physical dependence may develop, especially in addiction-prone individuals
Mental impairment, reflex-slowing	Performance of potentially hazardous activities may be impaired; caution patients accordingly, as well as about the additive effects of alcohol and other CNS depressants
Abrupt discontinuation of therapy	May precipitate barbiturate-like withdrawal symptoms, including convulsions, tremor, abdominal and muscle cramps, vomiting, and sweating; taper dosage gradually after extended treatment
Potentially suicidal patients	Should not have access to large quantities of diazepam; prescribe smallest amount feasible

Table continued on following page

VALIUM continued

WARNINGS/PRECAUTIONS continued

Intravenous use	May result in venous thrombosis, phlebitis, local irritation, swelling, and (rarely) vascular impairment. Administer solution slowly, no faster than 5 mg (1 ml)/min, *into large veins only;* carefully avoid intra-arterial administration or extravasation. Do not mix or dilute with other drugs or solutions. If direct IV administration is not possible, slow injection through infusion tubing as close as possible to vein insertion (since diazepam is sparingly soluble) may be substituted.
Apnea and/or cardiac arrest	May occur in the elderly or gravely ill or in patients with limited pulmonary reserve when parenteral route (particularly IV) is used; risk of apnea is increased by concomitant use of CNS depressants (see DRUG INTERACTIONS)
Convulsive disorders	May increase frequency and/or severity of grand mal seizures. Dosages of standard anticonvulsants may have to be increased. Abrupt withdrawal may also be associated temporarily with increased seizure activity. The parenteral form should be used with extreme care in patients with chronic lung disease or unstable cardiovascular status.
Hepatic or renal impairment	Monitor patient closely to avoid excessive drug accumulation (see OVERDOSAGE)
Prolonged therapy	Blood counts and liver-function tests should be performed periodically

ADVERSE REACTIONS Frequent reactions are italicized

Central nervous system and neuromuscular	*Drowsiness, fatigue ataxia,* confusion, depression, dysarthria, headache, hypoactivity, slurred speech, syncope, tremor, vertigo, acute hyperexcitability, anxiety, hallucinations, increased muscle spasticity, insomnia, rage, sleep disturbances, stimulation, EEG changes, muscular weakness (with parenteral use)
Cardiovascular	Bradycardia, cardiovascular collapse, hypotension, cardiac arrest
Gastrointestinal	Constipation, nausea, hiccoughs, salivary changes
Hepatic	Jaundice
Genitourinary	Incontinence, urinary retention
Ophthalmic	Blurred vision, diplopia, nystagmus
Respiratory	Coughing, depressed respiration, dyspnea, hyperventilation, laryngospasm, throat or chest pain (during peroral endoscopy)
Dermatological	Urticaria, skin rash
Hematological	Neutropenia
Other	*Venous thrombosis and phlebitis at injection site,* changes in libido

OVERDOSAGE

Signs and symptoms	Somnolence, confusion, coma, diminished reflexes, hypotension
Treatment	Empty stomach immediately by gastric lavage. Monitor respiration, pulse, and blood pressure. Employ general supportive measures, as needed. Administer IV fluids and maintain adequate airway. Hypotension may be treated with levarterenol or metaraminol. Dialysis is of limited value.

DRUG INTERACTIONS

Alcohol, narcotic analgesics, sedative-hypnotics, and other CNS depressants	⇧ CNS depression ⇧ Hypotension (with parenteral use) ⇧ Muscular weakness (with parenteral use)
MAO inhibitors and other antidepressants	⇧ CNS effects

ALTERED LABORATORY VALUES

No clinically significant alterations in blood/serum or urinary values occur at therapeutic dosages

Use in children

When using the injectable form, give no more than 0.25 mg/kg over a 3-min period; the initial dose may be safely repeated after 15–30 min. Oral diazepam is not indicated for use in infants under 6 mo of age. General guidelines not established for use of the injectable form in newborns (≤ 30 days of age); prolonged CNS depression has been observed in neonates.

Use in pregnancy or nursing mothers

Drug should almost always be avoided during early pregnancy. Although diazepam has not been sufficiently studied to determine conclusively its effects during pregnancy, an increased risk of congenital malformations during the 1st trimester has been associated with minor tranquilizers (meprobamate, diazepam, and chlordiazepoxide). Patient should stop breast-feeding if drug is prescribed; lethargy, weight loss, and hyperbilirubinemia in nursing infants have been reported.[1]

[1]Erkkola R, Kanto J: *Lancet* 1:542, 1972; Patrick MJ, Tilstone WJ: *Lancet* 1:542, 1972; Takyi BE: *J Hosp Pharm* 28:317, 1970

VISTARIL (Hydroxyzine pamoate) Pfizer

Caps: 25, 50, 100 mg **Susp:** 25 mg/5 ml

INDICATIONS	ORAL DOSAGE
Anxiety and tension associated with psychoneurosis **Anxiety** associated with organic disease (adjunctive therapy)	**Adult:** 50–100 mg qid **Child (< 6 yr):** 50 mg/day div **Child (>6 yr):** 50–100 mg/day div
Pruritus due to allergic conditions, including chronic urticaria and atopic and contact dermatoses **Histamine-mediated pruritus**	**Adult:** 25 mg tid or qid **Child (<6 yr):** 50 mg/day div **Child (>6 yr):** 50–100 mg/day div
Preoperative sedation and following general anesthesia	**Adult:** 50–100 mg **Child:** 0.6 mg/kg

ADMINISTRATION/DOSAGE ADJUSTMENTS

Long-term use (>4 mo) — Effectiveness for prolonged use as an antianxiety agent has not been tested in systematic clinical studies; reassess need for continued therapy periodically

CONTRAINDICATIONS

Hypersensitivity to hydroxyzine

WARNINGS/PRECAUTIONS

Drowsiness — Performance of potentially hazardous activities may be impaired; caution patients accordingly

Concomitant use of CNS depressants — May potentiate hydroxyzine's effect; reduce dosage of these agents accordingly and caution patients about simultaneous use of other CNS depressants, as well as about the increased effect of alcohol

ADVERSE REACTIONS

Central nervous system — Drowsiness (transitory), involuntary motor activity, including tremor and convulsions (rare)

Gastrointestinal — Dry mouth

OVERDOSAGE

Signs and symptoms — Excessive sedation, hypotension, CNS depression

Treatment — Induce emesis or use gastric lavage immediately to empty stomach. Monitor respiration, pulse, and blood pressure. Employ general supportive measures, as needed. Hypotension may be combatted with IV fluids and levarterenol or metaraminol. Do not use epinephrine, since hydroxyzine counteracts its pressor action. Caffeine and sodium benzoate may be used to counteract CNS depression. Dialysis is of limited value, unless other agents such as barbiturates have been ingested concomitantly.

DRUG INTERACTIONS

Alcohol, narcotic analgesics, sedative-hypnotics, and other CNS depressants — ⇧ CNS depression

Tricyclic antidepressants — ⇧ CNS depression

ALTERED LABORATORY VALUES

Urinary values — ⇧ 17-Hydroxycorticosteroids

No clinically significant alterations in blood/serum values occur at therapeutic dosages

Use in children

See INDICATIONS

Use in pregnancy or nursing mothers

Contraindicated during early pregnancy; fetal abnormalities have been reported in mice, rats, and rabbits. Clinical data are inadequate in humans to establish safety in early pregnancy. Patient should stop nursing if drug is prescribed.

NOTE: Hydroxyzine hydrochloride also marketed as **ATARAX** (Roerig).

ASENDIN (Amoxapine) **Lederle**

Tabs: 50, 100, 150 mg

INDICATIONS	ORAL DOSAGE
Neurotic or reactive depression, endogenous depression, psychotic depression, depression with anxiety or agitation	**Adult:** 50 mg tid to start, followed by an increase in dosage on 3rd day to 100 mg tid, if tolerated; usual maintenance dosage: 200–300 mg/day in a single bedtime dose

ADMINISTRATION/DOSAGE ADJUSTMENTS	
Initiation of therapy	If no response is seen at 300 mg/day during a trial period of at least 2 wk, dosage may be increased, if tolerated, up to 400 mg/day div
Refractory patients	Hospitalized patients with no history of convulsive seizures may be given up to 600 mg/day div, with caution
Elderly patients	Give 25 mg tid to start, followed by an increase in dosage on the 3rd day to 50 mg tid, if tolerated; if necessary, dosage may be carefully increased up to 300 mg/day
Maintenance therapy	Use lowest dose that will control symptoms; if symptoms reappear, increase dosage to earlier level until controlled

CONTRAINDICATIONS	
Hypersensitivity to dibenzoxapines	
MAO-inhibitor therapy	Wait at least 14 days after discontinuing MAO inhibitor before giving amoxapine
Myocardial infarction	During acute recovery phase

WARNINGS/PRECAUTIONS	
Atropine-like action	Use with caution in patients with a history of urinary retention, narrow-angle glaucoma, or increased intraocular pressure; even average doses may precipitate an attack in patients with narrow-angle glaucoma
Cardiovascular disease	Use with caution and keep patient under close supervision. Tricyclic antidepressants, especially in high doses, may produce arrhythmias, sinus tachycardia, and prolongation of conduction time; myocardial infarction and stroke have followed use of these agents.
Mental and/or physical impairment	Performance of potentially hazardous activities may be impaired; caution patients accordingly and about potentiating effects of alcohol and other CNS depressants
Psychotic symptoms	May increase in schizophrenic patients; paranoia may worsen, and manic-depressive patients may shift to manic phase. Reduce dosage of amoxapine or add a major tranquilizing agent, as indicated.
Potentially suicidal patients	Should not have access to large quantities of amoxapine; prescribe smallest amount feasible
Electroconvulsive therapy	Hazard may be increased
Grand mal seizures	May occur (rarely) at dosages above recommended limits
Pancreatic islet cell hyperplasia	Has occurred in rats at doses 5–10 times the human dose
Impairment of fertility	Male rats treated with 5–10 times the human dose showed a slight decrease in fertile matings; female rats treated with therapeutic doses displayed a reversible increase in estrous cycle length

ADVERSE REACTIONS[1]	Frequent reactions are italicized
Central nervous system and neuromuscular	*Drowsiness (14%)*, anxiety, insomnia, restlessness, nervousness, tremors, confusion, excitement, nightmares, ataxia, EEG changes, tingling, paresthesias of extremities, tinnitus, disorientation, extrapyramidal symptoms, seizures, hypomania, numbness, dizziness, headache, fatigue, weakness
Anticholinergic	*Dry mouth (14%), constipation (12%), blurred vision (7%),* disturbances of accommodation, mydriasis, delayed micturition, nasal stuffiness
Cardiovascular	Palpitations, hypotension, hypertension, syncope, tachycardia, stroke (causal relationship not established)
Allergic	Skin rash, edema, drug fever, photosensitization, pruritus

[1]Various other side effects common to tricyclic antidepressants may occur but have not been observed with amoxapine

Table continued on following page

ADVERSE REACTIONS continued

Gastrointestinal	Nausea, excessive appetite, epigastric distress, vomiting, flatulence, abdominal pain, peculiar taste, weight gain or loss, diarrhea, anorexia (causal relationship not established)
Hematological	Leukopenia
Endocrinological	Increased or decreased libido, impotence, menstrual irregularity, breast enlargement and galactorrhea (in females)
Other	Increased perspiration, lacrimation, altered liver function, urinary frequency, testicular swelling (causal relationship not established for last two reactions)

OVERDOSAGE

Signs and symptoms	Experience with amoxapine overdosage has been limited; signs and symptoms reported with other tricyclic antidepressants include drowsiness, tachycardia and other arrhythmias, ECG evidence of impaired conduction, congestive heart failure, mydriasis, convulsions, severe hypotension, stupor, coma, agitation, hyperactive reflexes, muscle rigidity, vomiting, hyperpyrexia, ataxia, restlessness, athetoid and choreiform movements, respiratory depression, cyanosis, shock, diaphoresis (see also ADVERSE REACTIONS)
Treatment	Admit patient to hospital. Empty stomach by inducing emesis, followed by gastric lavage and activated charcoal. Obtain ECG and begin close monitoring of cardiac function if abnormalities appear. Maintain an open airway and adequate fluid intake. Regulate body temperature. Administer 1–3 mg physostigmine salicylate IV and repeat as needed, especially if life-threatening signs recur or persist. For circulatory shock and metabolic acidosis, institute standard supportive measures. If cardiac failure occurs, consider digitalization. (Cardiac function should be closely monitored for at least 5 days under these circumstances or if QRS interval exceeds 100 ms at any time within 24 h of overdosage.) To control convulsions, use diazepam, paraldehyde, or methocarbamol; *do not use barbiturates.* Dialysis is of no value because of low plasma drug concentrations and because of extensive tissue distribution of drug.

DRUG INTERACTIONS

Alcohol, sedative-hypnotics, and other CNS depressants	⇧ CNS depression
MAO inhibitors	Hyperpyrexia, excitability, severe convulsions, coma, death
Anticholinergic agents	Acute glaucoma, urinary retention, paralytic ileus
Epinephrine	⇧ Pressor response, arrhythmias
Ethchlorvynol	Transient delirium
Guanethidine	⇩ Antihypertensive effect
Sympathomimetic agents	Severe hypertension, hyperpyrexia
Thyroid preparations	⇧ Antidepressant effect and possible risk of arrhythmias

ALTERED LABORATORY VALUES

Blood/serum values	⇧ or ⇩ Glucose

No clinically significant alterations in urinary values occur at therapeutic dosages

Use in children

Safety and effectiveness not established in children under 16 yr of age

Use in pregnancy or nursing mothers

Animal studies show embryotoxic and fetotoxic effects as well as decreased postnatal survival. Use during pregnancy only if potential benefit to mother justifies potential risk to the fetus. Amoxapine and/or its metabolites are excreted in animal milk.

ELAVIL (Amitriptyline hydrochloride) **Merck Sharp & Dohme**

Tabs: 10, 25, 50, 75, 100, 150 mg **Vial:** 10 mg/ml (10 ml)

INDICATIONS	ORAL DOSAGE	PARENTERAL DOSAGE
Depression, especially endogenous depression	**Adult:** 75 mg/day div to start, followed by increases in late-afternoon or bedtime dose, up to a total of 150 mg/day div, if needed; alternative regimen: 50-100 mg at bedtime to start, followed by increases of 25-50 mg in bedtime dose, up to a total of 150 mg/day, if needed	**Adult:** 20-30 mg IM qid to start; replace with oral therapy as soon as possible

ADMINISTRATION/DOSAGE ADJUSTMENTS

Hospitalized patients	May require 100 mg/day to start, followed by gradual increases up to a total of 200 or, occasionally, 300 mg/day, if necessary
Adolescent and elderly patients	Reduce dosage to 10 mg tid with 20 mg at bedtime if higher dosages are not tolerated
Maintenance regimen	Usually, 50-100 mg/day, given in a single dose preferably at bedtime; some patients may require only 40 mg/day. To lessen the possibility of relapse, maintenance therapy should be continued for 3 mo or longer.

CONTRAINDICATIONS

Hypersensitivity	To amitriptyline
Concomitant MAO-inhibitor therapy	Wait at least 14 days after discontinuing MAO inhibitors before initiating amitriptyline therapy; start with low doses and increase dosage gradually with caution
Myocardial infarction	During acute recovery phase

WARNINGS/PRECAUTIONS

Atropine-like action	Use with caution in patients with a history of urinary retention, narrow-angle glaucoma, or increased intraocular pressure; even average doses may precipitate an attack in patients with narrow-angle glaucoma
Cardiovascular disease	May worsen; use with caution and keep patient under close supervision. Tricyclic antidepressants, especially in high doses, may produce arrhythmias, sinus tachycardia, and prolongation of conduction time; myocardial Infarction and stroke have followed use of these agents.
Mental and/or physical impairment	Performance of potentially hazardous activities may be impaired; caution patients accordingly and about potentiating effect on alcohol
Psychotic symptoms	May increase in schizophrenic patients; paranoia may worsen and manic-depressive patients may shift to manic phase. Reduce dosage of amitriptyline or add an antipsychotic agent, such as perphenazine.
Potentially suicidal patients	Should not have access to large quantities of amitriptyline; prescribe smallest amount feasible
Abrupt discontinuation of therapy	May produce nausea, headache, and malaise after prolonged administration; symptoms are not indicative of addiction
Elective surgery	If possible, discontinue medication several days prior to surgery
Electroconvulsive therapy (ECT)	Hazard may be increased; use ECT only when essential
Special-risk patients	Use with caution in patients with hepatic impairment, hyperthyroidism, or a history of seizures and in those taking thyroid medication, anticholinergic agents, or sympathomimetics (see DRUG INTERACTIONS)

ADVERSE REACTIONS[1]

Cardiovascular	Hypotension, hypertension, tachycardia, palpitations, myocardial infarction, arrhythmias, heart block, stroke
Central nervous system and neuromuscular	Confusion, disturbed concentration, disorientation, delusions, hallucinations, excitement, anxiety, restlessness, insomnia, nightmares, numbness, tingling, and paresthesias of the extremities; peripheral neuropathy, incoordination, ataxia, tremors, seizures, alteration in EEG patterns, extrapyramidal symptoms, tinnitus, inappropriate antidiuretic hormone (ADH) secretion syndrome, dizziness, weakness, fatigue, headache
Autonomic nervous system	Dry mouth, blurred vision, disturbance of accommodation, increased intraocular pressure, constipation, paralytic ileus, urinary retention, dilatation of urinary tract
Hematological	Bone-marrow depression, including agranulocytosis, leukopenia, eosinophilia, purpura, and thrombocytopenia

[1]Included are some tricyclic antidepressant adverse reactions not reported with this drug, but which must be considered before and during therapy

Table continued on following page

ADVERSE REACTIONS continued

Gastrointestinal	Nausea, epigastric distress, vomiting, anorexia, stomatitis, peculiar taste, diarrhea, parotid swelling, black tongue, and hepatitis, including altered liver function and jaundice (rare)
Endocrinological	Testicular swelling and gynecomastia (in males), breast enlargement and galactorrhea (in females), increased or decreased libido
Allergic	Skin rash, urticaria, photosensitization, edema of face and tongue
Other	Weight gain or loss, diaphoresis, urinary frequency, mydriasis, drowsiness, alopecia

OVERDOSAGE

Signs and symptoms	Drowsiness, hypothermia, tachycardia and other arrhythmias, ECG evidence of impaired conduction, congestive heart failure, mydriasis, convulsions, severe hypotension, stupor, coma, agitation, hyperactive reflexes, muscle rigidity, vomiting, hyperpyrexia (see also ADVERSE REACTIONS)
Treatment	Admit patient to hospital. Empty stomach by inducing emesis, followed by gastric lavage and activated charcoal (20–30 g q4–6h during initial 24–48 h). Obtain ECG and begin close monitoring of cardiac function if abnormalities appear. Maintain an open airway and adequate fluid intake. Regulate body temperature. For circulatory shock and metabolic acidosis, institute standard supportive measures. Treat cardiac arrhythmias with neostigmine, pyridostigmine, or propranolol. If cardiac failure occurs, consider digitalization. (Cardiac function should be closely monitored for at least 5 days under these circumstances.) To control convulsions, use diazepam, paraldehyde, or an inhalation anesthetic; *do not use barbiturates.* Dialysis is of no value because of low plasma drug concentrations and because of extensive tissue distribution of drug.

DRUG INTERACTIONS

Alcohol, sedative-hypnotics, and other CNS depressants	⇧ CNS depression
MAO inhibitors	Hyperpyrexia, excitability, severe convulsions, coma, death
Anticholinergic agents	Acute glaucoma, urinary retention, paralytic ileus
Epinephrine	⇧ Pressor response, arrhythmias
Ethchlorvynol	Transient delirium
Guanethidine	⇩ Antihypertensive effect
Sympathomimetic agents	Severe hypertension, hyperpyrexia
Thyroid preparations	⇧ Antidepressant effect and possible risk of arrhythmias

ALTERED LABORATORY VALUES

Blood/serum values	⇧ or ⇩ Glucose

No clinically significant alterations in urinary values occur at therapeutic dosages

Use in children	**Use in pregnancy or nursing mothers**
Not recommended for use in children under 12 yr of age	Safe use not established

Note: Amitriptyline hydrochloride also marketed as **ENDEP** (Roche).

ETRAFON (Perphenazine and amitriptyline hydrochloride) Schering

Tabs: 2 mg perphenazine and 10 mg amitriptyline hydrochloride (Etrafon 2-10); 2 mg perphenazine and 25 mg amitriptyline hydrochloride (Etrafon 2-25); 4 mg perphenazine and 10 mg amitriptyline hydrochloride (Etrafon 4-10); 4 mg perphenazine and 25 mg amitriptyline (Etrafon 4-25)

INDICATIONS	ORAL DOSAGE
Moderate to severe anxiety and/or agitation and depression or depressed mood **Anxiety and depression** associated with **chronic physical disease** Those cases in which **depression and anxiety** cannot be clearly differentiated **Depressive symptoms in schizophrenic patients**	**Adult:** 1 Etrafon 2-25 or 4-25 tab tid or qid to start, followed by decreases in dosage to the smallest amount necessary for symptom relief; usual maintenance dosage: 1 Etrafon 2-25 or 4-25 tab bid to qid

ADMINISTRATION/DOSAGE ADJUSTMENTS	
Schizophrenic patients	Give 2 Etrafon 4-25 tabs tid or qid to start, followed by up to 9 tabs/day, if necessary
Adolescent, elderly, or debilitated patients	Give 1 Etrafon 4-10 tab tid or qid to start; adjust dosage, as necessary, to achieve desired response

CONTRAINDICATIONS	
Blood dyscrasias	
Bone-marrow depression	
Hepatic impairment	
Hypersensitivity	To phenothiazines or amitriptyline
CNS depression	Caused by barbiturates, alcohol, narcotics, analgesics, or antihistamines
Concomitant MAO-inhibitor therapy	Wait at least 14 days after discontinuing MAO inhibitors before initiating therapy; start with low doses and increase dosage gradually with caution
Myocardial infarction	During acute recovery phase

WARNINGS/PRECAUTIONS	
Atropine-like action	Use with caution in patients with a history of urinary retention, narrow-angle glaucoma, or increased intraocular pressure; even average doses may precipitate an attack in patients with narrow-angle glaucoma
Cardiovascular disease	May worsen; use with caution and keep patient under close supervision. Tricyclic antidepressants, especially in high doses, may produce arrhythmias, sinus tachycardia, and prolongation of conduction time; myocardial infarction and stroke have followed use of these agents.
Mental and/or physical impairment	Performance of potentially hazardous activities may be impaired; caution patients accordingly and about potentiating effect on alcohol
Psychotic symptoms	Paranoia may worsen, and manic-depressive patients may shift to manic phase; perphenazine component minimizes the occurrence of these effects
Potentially suicidal patients	Should not have access to large quantities of this drug; prescribe smallest amount feasible
Abrupt discontinuation of therapy	May produce nausea, headache, and malaise after prolonged administration; symptoms are not indicative of addiction
Elective surgery	If possible, discontinue medication several days prior to surgery
Electroconvulsive therapy (ECT)	May increase hazard; use ECT only when essential
Antiemetic effect	May mask signs of toxicity due to overdosage of other drugs or render more difficult the diagnosis of such disorders as brain tumors or intestinal obstruction
Unexplained rise in temperature	May suggest intolerance to perphenazine component; discontinue use if a significant rise occurs
Special-risk patients	Use with caution in patients with convulsive disorders, hyperthyroidism, mitral insufficiency, pheochromocytoma, or a history of adverse reactions to phenothiazines or to imipramine, and in those exposed to heat or phosphorus insecticides or taking thyroid medication, anticholinergic agents, or sympathomimetics (see DRUG INTERACTIONS)

ADVERSE REACTIONS[1]	
Cardiovascular	Hypotension, hypertension, tachycardia, palpitations, myocardial infarction, arrhythmias, heart block, stroke, ECG abnormalities

[1]Included are some phenothiazine and tricyclic antidepressant adverse reactions not reported with this drug, but which must be considered before and during therapy

Table continued on following page

ETRAFON continued

ADVERSE REACTIONS[1] continued	
Central nervous system and neuromuscular	Confusion, disturbed concentration, disorientation, delusions, hallucinations, excitement, anxiety, restlessness, insomnia, nightmares, numbness, tingling, paresthesias of the extremities; peripheral neuropathy, incoordination, ataxia, tremors, seizures, alteration in EEG patterns, extrapyramidal reactions, tinnitus, inappropriate antidiuretic hormone (ADH) secretion syndrome, dizziness, weakness, fatigue, headache, tardive dyskinesia, reactivated psychotic symptoms, paranoia, catatonia, lassitude, photophobia, grand mal seizures (rare)
Autonomic nervous system	Dry mouth, blurred vision, disturbance of accommodation, increased intraocular pressure, constipation, paralytic ileus, urinary retention or frequency, incontinence, dilatation of urinary tract, salivation, nasal congestion, altered pulse rate
Hematological	Bone-marrow depression, including agranulocytosis, leukopenia, eosinophilia, purpura, and thrombocytopenia; pancytopenia
Gastrointestinal	Nausea, epigastric distress, heartburn, vomiting, anorexia, stomatitis, peculiar taste, diarrhea, parotid swelling, black tongue, biliary stasis, hepatitis (including altered liver function and, rarely, jaundice), polyphagia, obstipation
Endocrinological	Testicular swelling and gynecomastia (in males), breast enlargement and galactorrhea (in females), increased or decreased libido, menstrual irregularities, failure of ejaculation (rare), hyperglycemia, lactation
Allergic	Skin rash, urticaria, photosensitization, pruritus, edema of face, tongue, and larynx, eczema, erythema, exfoliative dermatitis, asthma, anaphylaxis, angioneurotic edema, cerebral edema leading to circulatory collapse and death (rare), hyperpigmentation (rare)
Other	Weight gain or loss, diaphoresis, urinary frequency, mydriasis, drowsiness, alopecia, LE-like syndrome, pigmentary retinopathy, pigmentation of cornea and lens
OVERDOSAGE	
Signs and symptoms	Drowsiness, hypothermia, tachycardia and other arrhythmias, ECG evidence of impaired conduction, congestive heart failure, mydriasis, convulsions, severe hypotension, stupor, coma, agitation, hyperactive reflexes, muscle rigidity, vomiting, hyperpyrexia (see also ADVERSE REACTIONS)
Treatment	Admit patient to hospital. Empty stomach by inducing emesis, followed by gastric lavage and activated charcoal (20–30 g q4–6h during initial 24–48h); do not use saline emetics. Obtain ECG and begin close monitoring of cardiac function for at least 5 days if abnormalities appear. Maintain an open airway and adequate fluid intake. Regulate body temperature. For circulatory shock and metabolic acidosis, institute standard supportive measures. Treat cardiac arrhythmias with neostigmine, pyridostigmine, or propranolol. If cardiac failure occurs, consider digitalization. (Cardiac function should be closely monitored for at least 5 days under these circumstances.) To control convulsions, use diazepam, paraldehyde, or an inhalation anesthetic; *do not use barbiturates.* Treat hypotension with levarterenol, not epinephrine. Administer benztropine mesylate or diphenhydramine for acute parkinsonian symptoms. Dialysis is of no value because of low plasma drug concentrations. Continue treatment for at least 48 h in patients who do not respond earlier.
DRUG INTERACTIONS	
Alcohol, sedative-hypnotics, and other CNS depressants	⇧ CNS depression
MAO inhibitors	Hyperpyrexia, excitability, severe convulsions, coma, death
Anticholinergic agents	Acute glaucoma, urinary retention, paralytic ileus
Epinephrine	Severe hypotension
Ethchlorvynol	Transient delirium
Guanethidine	⇩ Antihypertensive effect
Sympathomimetic agents	Severe hypertension, hyperpyrexia
Thyroid preparations	⇧ Antidepressant effect and possible risk of arrhythmias
Anticonvulsants	⇩ Convulsion threshold ⇧ CNS depression

Table continued on following page

ETRAFON continued

ALTERED LABORATORY VALUES

Blood/serum values———————— ⇧ or ⇩ Glucose ⇧ PBI

No clinically significant alterations in urinary values occur at therapeutic dosages

Use in children	**Use in pregnancy or nursing mothers**
Not recommended for use in children	Safe use not established

LIMBITROL (Chlordiazepoxide and amitriptyline hydrochloride) **Roche**

Tabs: 5 mg chlordiazepoxide and 12.5 mg amitriptyline hydrochloride (Limbitrol 5–12.5); 10 mg chlordiazepoxide and 25 mg amitriptyline hydrochloride (Limbitrol 10–25) *C-IV*

INDICATIONS	**ORAL DOSAGE**
Moderate to severe depression associated with **moderate to severe anxiety**	**Adult:** 3–4 Limbitrol 10–25 tabs/day div to start, or up to 6 tabs/day, if needed; some patients may require only 2 tabs/day

ADMINISTRATION/DOSAGE ADJUSTMENTS	
Elderly, debilitated, or sensitive patients	Administer 3–4 Limbitrol 5–12.5 tabs/day div to start; reduce dosage to the smallest amount needed to maintain remission

CONTRAINDICATIONS	
Hypersensitivity	To benzodiazepines or tricyclic antidepressants
Concomitant MAO-inhibitor therapy	Wait at least 14 days after discontinuing MAO inhibitors before initiating therapy; start with low doses and increase dosage gradually with caution
Myocardial infarction	During acute recovery phase

WARNINGS/PRECAUTIONS	
Atropine-like action	Use with great caution in patients with a history of urinary retention or narrow-angle glaucoma; even average doses may precipitate an attack in patients with narrow-angle glaucoma
Cardiovascular disease	May worsen; use with caution and keep patient under close supervision. Tricyclic antidepressants, especially in high doses, may produce arrhythmias, sinus tachycardia, and prolongation of conduction time; myocardial infarction and stroke have followed use of these agents.
Habit-forming	Psychic and/or physical dependence may develop, especially in addiction-prone individuals
Mental impairment, reflex-slowing	Performance of potentially hazardous activities may be impaired; caution patients accordingly, as well as about the additive effects of alcohol and other CNS depressants
Potentially suicidal patients	Should not have access to large quantities; prescribe smallest amount feasible
Concomitant psychotropic therapy	Use with extreme caution, if at all, particularly when use of known potentiating compounds is contemplated (see DRUG INTERACTIONS)
Prolonged therapy	Blood counts and liver-function tests should be performed periodically
Ataxia or oversedation	May develop in elderly and/or debilitated patients (see ADMINISTRATION/DOSAGE ADJUSTMENTS)
Abrupt discontinuation of therapy	May produce nausea, headache, malaise, and barbiturate-like withdrawal symptoms after prolonged administration
Elective surgery	If possible, discontinue medication several days prior to surgery
Electroconvulsive therapy (ECT)	Hazard may be increased; use ECT only when essential
Special-risk patients	Use with caution in patients with renal or hepatic impairment, hyperthyroidism, or a history of seizures and in those taking thyroid medication, anticholinergic agents, or sympathomimetics (see DRUG INTERACTIONS)

ADVERSE REACTIONS[1]	Frequent reactions are italicized
Cardiovascular	Hypotension, hypertension, tachycardia, palpitations, myocardial infarction, arrhythmias, heart block, stroke
Central nervous system and neuromuscular	*Drowsiness, dizziness,* vivid dreams, tremor, confusion, euphoria, apprehension, poor concentration, delusions, hallucinations, hypomania, excitement, numbness, tingling, and paresthesias of the extremities; incoordination, ataxia, alteration in EEG patterns, extrapyramidal symptoms, syncope, headache, fatigue, weakness, restlessness, lethargy

[1]Included are some phenothiazine and tricyclic antidepressant adverse reactions not reported with this drug, but which must be considered before and during therapy

Table continued on following page

ADVERSE REACTIONS continued

Autonomic nervous system	*Dry mouth, blurred vision, constipation,* nasal congestion, disturbance of accommodation, paralytic ileus, urinary retention, dilatation of urinary tract
Hematological	Bone-marrow depression (including agranulocytosis), eosinophilia, purpura, thrombocytopenia, granulocytopenia (rare)
Gastrointestinal	*Bloated feeling,* nausea, epigastric distress, vomiting, anorexia, stomatitis, peculiar taste, parotid swelling, diarrhea, black tongue, jaundice (rare), hepatic dysfunction (rare)
Endocrinological	Impotence, testicular swelling and gynecomastia (in males), breast enlargement, galactorrhea, menstrual irregularities (in females), increased or decreased libido
Allergic	Skin rash, urticaria, photosensitization, edema of face and tongue, pruritus
Other	Headache, weight gain or loss, diaphoresis, urinary frequency, mydriasis, alopecia

OVERDOSAGE

Signs and symptoms	*Toxicity primarily attributable to amitriptyline component:* hypothermia, tachycardia and other arrhythmias, ECG evidence of impaired conduction, congestive heart failure, mydriasis, convulsions, severe hypotension, stupor, coma, agitation, hyperactive reflexes, muscle rigidity, vomiting, hyperpyrexia (see also ADVERSE REACTIONS)
Treatment	Admit patient to hospital. Empty stomach by inducing emesis or by gastric lavage, followed by activated charcoal. (If patient is comatose, secure airway with a cuffed endotracheal tube before beginning lavage.) Obtain ECG and begin close monitoring of cardiac function if abnormalities appear. Maintain an open airway and adequate fluid intake. Regulate body temperature. For circulatory shock, institute standard supportive measures. If cardiac failure occurs, consider digitalization. (Cardiac function should be closely monitored for at least 5 days under these circumstances.) Treat arrhythmias with appropriate antiarrhythmic agents. To control convulsions, use an inhalation anesthetic; *do not use barbiturates.* Dialysis is of no value because of low plasma drug concentrations, but may be useful in cases of multiple drug ingestions.

DRUG INTERACTIONS

Alcohol, sedative-hypnotics, and other CNS depressants	⇧ CNS depression
MAO inhibitors	Hyperpyrexia, excitability, severe convulsions, coma, death
Anticholinergic agents	Acute glaucoma, urinary retention, severe constipation, paralytic ileus
Epinephrine	⇧ Pressor response, arrhythmias
Ethchlorvynol	Transient delirium
Guanethidine	⇩ Antihypertensive effect
Sympathomimetic agents	Severe hypertension, hyperpyrexia
Thyroid preparations	⇧ Antidepressant effect and possible risk of arrhythmias
Oral anticoagulants	⇧ or ⇩ Anticoagulant effect

ALTERED LABORATORY VALUES

Blood/serum values	⇧ or ⇩ Glucose

No clinically significant alterations in urinary values occur at therapeutic dosages

Use in children

Safety and effectiveness have not been established in children under 12 yr of age

Use in pregnancy or nursing mothers

Drug should almost always be avoided during pregnancy. Although chlordiazepoxide has not been sufficiently studied to determine conclusively its effects during pregnancy, an increased risk of congenital malformations during the 1st trimester has been associated with minor tranquilizers. Patient should stop nursing if drug is prescribed.

LITHIUM CARBONATE Philips Roxane

Tabs: 300 mg **Caps:** 300 mg

LITHIUM CITRATE Philips Roxane

Syrup: equivalent to 300 mg lithium carbonate per 5 ml (480 ml)

INDICATIONS	ORAL DOSAGE
Manic episodes of manic-depressive illness	**Adult:** for acute episodes, 600 mg or 10 ml (2 tsp) tid; for maintenance, 300 mg or 5 ml (1 tsp) tid or qid

ADMINISTRATION/DOSAGE ADJUSTMENTS

Elderly patients	May exhibit signs of toxicity at serum levels ordinarily tolerated by other patients; reduce dosage appropriately
Serum lithium levels	Should be maintained at 1.0–1.5 mEq/l during acute phase and 0.6–1.2 mEq/l during maintenance therapy; blood samples for serum lithium determinations should be drawn 8–12 h after the previous dose

CONTRAINDICATIONS

None

WARNINGS/PRECAUTIONS

Special-risk patients	In patients with significant renal or cardiovascular disease, severe debilitation or dehydration, or sodium depletion, and in those receiving diuretics, use only if the psychiatric indication is life-threatening and if the patient fails to respond to other measures; in such instances, hospitalize patient and use with extreme caution (including daily serum lithium determinations)
Morphological changes in the kidneys	Have been reported with lithium; the relationship between these changes and renal function has not been established
Concomitant use of haloperidol or other antipsychotics	May be associated with an encephalopathic syndrome characterized by weakness, lethargy, fever, tremulousness, confusion, extrapyramidal symptoms, leukocytosis, and elevated serum enzymes, BUN, and FBS, followed by irreversible brain damage. Discontinue use if signs of neurological toxicity appear. (Causal relationship not established.)
Lithium toxicity	May occur at doses close to therapeutic levels; instruct outpatients and their families to report symptoms of diarrhea, vomiting, tremors, mild ataxia, drowsiness, or muscular weakness, and to discontinue use if they occur
Serum lithium determinations	Should be obtained twice weekly during the acute phase and at least every 2 mo in uncomplicated cases receiving maintenance therapy during remission (see ADMINISTRATION/DOSAGE ADJUSTMENTS)
Neuromuscular blocking agents	Should be used with caution in patients receiving lithium (see DRUG INTERACTIONS)
Mental impairment, reflex-slowing	Performance of potentially hazardous activities may be impaired; caution patients accordingly
Sodium depletion	May occur; patient must maintain a normal diet, including salt, and an adequate fluid intake (2,500–3,000 ml/day), at least during initial stabilization period. Supplemental fluid and salt should be given if protracted sweating or diarrhea occurs.
Concomitant infection with elevated temperatures	May necessitate temporary dosage reduction or suspending of medication
Hypothyroidism	Monitor thyroid function and administer supplemental thyroid therapy, if necessary
Lithium tolerance	May decrease when manic symptoms subside

ADVERSE REACTIONS

Central nervous system and neuromuscular	Fine hand tremor, drowsiness, muscular weakness, incoordination, tremor, muscle hyperirritability (fasciculations, twitching, clonic movements of whole limbs), ataxia, choreoathetotic movements, hyperactive deep-tendon reflex, blackout spells, epileptiform seizures, slurred speech, dizziness, vertigo, somnolence, psychomotor retardation, restlessness, confusion, stupor, coma, EEG changes, fatigue, lethargy, headache, tendency to sleep, worsening of organic brain syndromes, tinnitus, giddiness
Genitourinary	Polyuria, incontinence, albuminuria, oliguria, glycosuria
Cardiovascular	Arrhythmia, hypotension, peripheral circulatory collapse, ECG changes

Table continued on following page

LITHIUM continued

ADVERSE REACTIONS continued

Autonomic nervous system	Blurred vision, dry mouth
Gastrointestinal	Nausea, diarrhea, vomiting, fecal incontinence, anorexia, metallic taste, weight changes
Thyroid	Euthyroid goiter, hypothyroidism (including myxedema), hyperthyroidism (rare), diffuse nontoxic goiter with or without hypothyroidism
Dermatological	Drying and thinning of hair, alopecia, anesthesia of skin, chronic folliculitis, exacerbation of psoriasis, xerosis cutis, pruritus with or without rash, ulcers
Other	Transient scotomata, dehydration, thirst, leukocytosis, hyperglycemia, edematous swelling of ankles or wrists, painful discoloration of fingers and toes, coldness of the extremities (1 case)

OVERDOSAGE

Signs and symptoms	Diarrhea, vomiting, drowsiness, muscular weakness, lack of coordination, ataxia, giddiness, tinnitus (see ADVERSE REACTIONS); serum lithium levels above 3.0 mEq/l may produce a complex clinical picture, involving multiple organs and organ systems
Treatment	In mild cases, reduce dosage or discontinue therapy and resume in 24–48 h at lower dosage. In severe cases, empty stomach by gastric lavage. Correct fluid and electrolyte imbalance. Regulate kidney function. Increase lithium excretion with urea, mannitol, or aminophylline. For severe toxicity, employ hemodialysis. Maintain adequate respiration. Infection prophylaxis and regular chest x-rays are essential.

DRUG INTERACTIONS

Neuromuscular blocking agents	⇧ Neuromuscular blocking effect
Methylxanthines	⇧ Lithium clearance
Sodium bicarbonate	⇧ Lithium clearance
Chlorpromazine	⇩ Serum chlorpromazine levels
Diuretics (especially thiazides)	⇩ Lithium clearance
Iodide	Hypothyroidism
Norepinephrine	⇩ Pressor effects
Haloperidol	Neurotoxicity (causal relationship not established)

ALTERED LABORATORY VALUES

Blood/serum values	⇧ ^{131}I uptake ⇩ Triiodothyronine (T_3) uptake ⇩ Thyroxine (T_4) uptake
Urinary values	⇧ Glucose ⇧ Albumin ⇧ VMA

Use in children

Not recommended

Use in pregnancy or nursing mothers

Not recommended for use during pregnancy, especially during the first trimester. Lithium is excreted in breast milk; nursing should not be undertaken during lithium therapy except in rare circumstances.

Note: Lithium carbonate also marketed as **ESKALITH** (Smith Kline & French).

MARPLAN (Isocarboxazid) **Roche**

Tabs: 10 mg

INDICATIONS	ORAL DOSAGE
Depression in patients who are refractory to tricyclic antidepressants or electroconvulsive therapy, or in whom tricyclic antidepressants are contraindicated[1]	**Adult:** 30 mg/day in single or divided doses to start, followed by reduction in dosage to 10–20 mg/day or less, for maintenance

ADMINISTRATION/DOSAGE ADJUSTMENTS

Favorable response	If not achieved within 3–4 wk, discontinue therapy

CONTRAINDICATIONS

Hypersensitivity to isocarboxazid	
Severe renal impairment	
Severe hepatic impairment	
Concomitant use of sympathomimetic drugs	Including amphetamines, methyldopa, levodopa, dopamine, tryptophan, epinephrine, and norepinephrine, may result in potentially fatal hypertensive crisis
Concomitant ingestion of food and beverages containing high amounts of pressor amines (eg, tryptophan, tyramine)	Including aged cheese (cheddar, Camembert, Stilton), processed cheese, beer, and wine (especially Chianti); also chocolate, yeast extract, avocados, pickled herring, broad-bean pods, ripe bananas, papaya products (including meat tenderizers), chicken livers, and sour cream
Concomitant or recent therapy with other MAO inhibitors or dibenzazepines	Can produce hypertensive crisis, fever, marked sweating, excitation, delirium, tremor, twitching, convulsions, coma, and circulatory collapse; wait at least 10 days after discontinuing isocarboxazid before giving another antidepressant, or after discontinuing another MAO inhibitor before giving isocarboxazid
Elective surgery requiring general anesthesia	Discontinue at least 10 days before surgery
Concomitant use of CNS depressants	Such as narcotics and alcohol (see WARNINGS/PRECAUTIONS for barbiturates); circulatory collapse and death have been reported with concomitant use of meperidine
Special-risk patients	Including the elderly or debilitated and those with hypertension, cardiovascular or cerebrovascular disease, or severe or frequent headaches
Pheochromocytoma	
Congestive heart failure	

WARNINGS/PRECAUTIONS

Hypertensive crisis	May occur within hours of ingestion of contraindicated substances; crises are characterized by headache, palpitation, neck stiffness or soreness, nausea, vomiting, sweating (sometimes with fever or cold, clammy skin), photophobia, tachycardia or bradycardia, chest pain, and dilated pupils, and may lead to potentially fatal intracranial bleeding. Monitor blood pressure frequently and discontinue use if palpitations or frequent headaches occur.
Emergency surgery	If spinal anesthesia is essential, consider possible combined hypotensive effect of isocarboxazid and the blocking agent; do not use cocaine or local anesthetic solutions containing sympathomimetic vasoconstrictors
Concomitant use of antihypertensive agents	Including thiazide diuretics, may cause hypotension; use with caution
Suicidal patients	Use only under strict medical supervision, preferably when patient is hospitalized
Patient instructions	Caution patients to avoid certain foods and proprietary cold, hay fever, or weight-reducing preparations (see CONTRAINDICATIONS), to reduce intake of alcohol and caffeine, and to report occurrence of headache or unusual symptoms
Concomitant use of other psychotropics	May have potentiating effect; wait at least 10 days after discontinuing isocarboxazid before giving another agent
Manic-depressive states	If a swing from a depressive to a manic phase occurs, discontinue use briefly and resume therapy at a lower dosage
Epileptic patients	May experience a decrease or increase in seizures
Concomitant use of *Rauwolfia* alkaloids	Use with caution

[1]Probably effective

Table continued on following page

WARNINGS/PRECAUTIONS continued	
Concomitant use of barbiturates	Reduce barbiturate dosage
Hepatic damage	Has occurred with other MAO inhibitors. Obtain liver-function studies periodically; discontinue use at the first sign of hepatic dysfunction or jaundice.
Orthostatic hypotension	May occur, manifested by dizziness, weakness, palpitations, or fainting; if severe or persistent, reduce dosage or, if necessary, discontinue therapy
Renal impairment	Use with caution and monitor for signs of excessive drug accumulation (see OVERDOSAGE)
Diabetic patients	There is conflicting evidence as to whether MAO inhibitors affect glucose metabolism or potentiate hypoglycemic agents
ADVERSE REACTIONS	
Cardiovascular	Orthostatic hypotension, disturbances in cardiac rate and rhythm
Central nervous system	Dizziness, vertigo, headache, overactivity, hyperreflexia, tremors, muscle twitching, mania, hypomania, jitteriness, confusion, memory impairment, insomnia, fatigue, weakness, akathisia,[2] ataxia,[2] coma,[2] neuritis,[2] hallucinations (rare)
Genitourinary	Dysuria,[2] incontinence,[2] urinary retention[2]
Gastrointestinal	Constipation, dry mouth, anorexia, other disturbances
Dermatological	Rash, spider telangiectases[2]
Ophthalmic	Blurred vision, amblyopia (causal relationship not established), photosensitivity[2]
Other	Peripheral edema, hyperhidrosis, black tongue,[2] hematological changes,[2] sexual disturbances[2]
OVERDOSAGE	
Signs and symptoms	Tachycardia, hypotension, coma, convulsions, respiratory depression, sluggish reflexes, pyrexia, diaphoresis
Treatment	Empty stomach by gastric lavage or emesis. Maintain an open airway and supply oxygen, if necessary. Employ general supportive measures. For hypotension, plasma may be of value; pressor amines such as levarterenol may be of limited value. For hypertensive crisis, administer phentolamine, 5 mg IV slowly, or pentolinium, 3 mg SC slowly. Perform liver-function tests and follow liver function for 4–6 wk after recovery. For hyperpyrexia, provide external cooling.
DRUG INTERACTIONS	
Alcohol, anesthetics, general narcotics (especially meperidine), other CNS depressants	Severe hypertension and hyperpyrexia; or severe hypotension
Anticonvulsants	Change in pattern of epileptiform seizures
Tricyclic antidepressants, MAO inhibitors	Hyperpyretic crisis, severe convulsions, death
Antihistamines, antimuscarinics, antiparkinsonism agents	⇧ Antimuscarinic effects
Antihypertensives, especially thiazide diuretics	Severe hypotension
Caffeine	Cardiac arrhythmias, hypotension
Dopamine, guanethidine, levodopa, methyldopa, reserpine	Severe hypertension and hyperpyrexia, leading to crisis
Insulin, oral hypoglycemics	Hypoglycemia
Indirect-acting sympathomimetics (amphetamines, ephedrine, methylphenidate, phenylpropanolamine, pseudoephedrine, tyramine, metaraminol, phenylephrine)	Severe hypotension and hyperpyrexia, leading to crisis
Direct-acting amines (epinephrine, isoproterenol, norepinephrine)	Hypertension, headache
Tyramine-containing foods and beverages	Hypertensive crisis

[2]Isolated cases

Table continued on following page

MARPLAN continued

ALTERED LABORATORY VALUES

Blood/serum values	⇩ Glucose
Urinary values	⇩ 5-HIAA ⇩ VMA

Use in children

Not recommended for use in children <16 yr of age

Use in pregnancy or nursing mothers

Safe use not established

NARDIL (Phenelzine sulfate) Parke-Davis

Tabs: 15 mg

INDICATIONS	ORAL DOSAGE
Atypical, nonendogenous, or neurotic depression, generally in patients who fail to respond to the drugs more commonly used for these conditions	**Adult:** 15 mg tid to start, followed by rapid increase in dosage to 60–90 mg/day until maximum benefit is achieved; thereafter, reduce dosage slowly over several weeks to as low as 15 mg/day or 15 mg every other day

ADMINISTRATION/DOSAGE ADJUSTMENTS

Favorable response	May not be achieved until 60-mg dosage has been continued for 4 wk

CONTRAINDICATIONS

Hypersensitivity to phenelzine sulfate	
History of liver disease or abnormal liver-function tests	
Concomitant use of sympathomimetic drugs	Including amphetamines, methyldopa, levodopa, dopamine, tryptophan, and epinephrine, may result in potentially fatal hypertensive crisis
Concomitant ingestion of food and beverages containing high amounts of pressor amines (eg, tryptophan, tyramine)	Including aged cheese (cheddar, Camembert, Stilton), processed cheese, beer, and wine (especially Chianti); also chocolate, yeast extract, avocados, pickled herring, broad-bean pods, ripe bananas, papaya products (including meat tenderizers), chicken livers, and sour cream
Concomitant or recent therapy with other MAO inhibitors	Can produce hypertensive crisis, fever, marked sweating, excitation, delirium, tremor, twitching, convulsions, coma, and circulatory collapse; wait at least 10 days after discontinuing phenelzine before giving another antidepressant, or after discontinuing another MAO inhibitor before giving phenelzine
Elective surgery requiring general anesthesia	Discontinue use at least 10 days before surgery
Concomitant use of CNS depressants	Such as narcotics and alcohol (see WARNINGS/PRECAUTIONS for barbiturates); circulatory collapse and death have been reported with concomitant use of meperidine
Concomitant use of guanethidine	
Pheochromocytoma	
Congestive heart failure	

WARNINGS/PRECAUTIONS

Hypertensive crisis	May occur within hours of ingestion of contraindicated substances; crises are characterized by headache, palpitation, neck stiffness or soreness, nausea, vomiting, sweating (sometimes with fever or cold, clammy skin), photophobia, tachycardia or bradycardia, chest pain, and dilated pupils, and may lead to potentially fatal intracranial bleeding. Monitor blood pressure frequently and discontinue use if frequent headaches or palpitations occur.
Emergency surgery	If spinal anesthesia is essential, consider possible combined hypotensive effect of phenelzine and the blocking agent; do not use cocaine or local anesthetic solutions containing sympathomimetic vasoconstrictors
Concomitant use of antihypertensive agents	Including thiazide diuretics, may cause hypotension; use with caution
Suicidal patients	Use only under strict medical supervision, preferably when patient is hospitalized
Patient instructions	Caution patients to avoid certain foods and proprietary cold, hay fever, or weight-reducing preparations and caffeine, and to report occurrence of headache or unusual symptoms
Concomitant use of tricyclic antidepressants	Has potentiating effect; if possible, wait at least 10 days after discontinuing phenelzine before giving a dibenzazepine; otherwise, use with caution and warn patients about possible adverse drug interaction
Manic-depressive states	Swing from depressive to manic phase may occur
Epileptic patients	May experience decrease or increase in seizures
Concomitant use of barbiturates	Reduce barbiturate dosage
Concomitant use of *Rauwolfia* alkaloids	Use with caution

Table continued on following page

NARDIL continued

WARNINGS/PRECAUTIONS continued	
Orthostatic hypotension	May occur, manifested by dizziness, weakness, palpitations, or fainting; if severe or persistent, reduce dosage or, if necessary, discontinue therapy
Diabetic patients	There is conflicting evidence as to whether MAO inhibitors affect glucose metabolism or potentiate hypoglycemic agents
Hypomania	May occur in hyperactive or agitated patients
Excessive stimulation	May occur in schizophrenic patients
ADVERSE REACTIONS	
Cardiovascular	Orthostatic hypotension, transient depression following electroconvulsive therapy (ECT)
Hepatic	Jaundice, fatal progressive necrotizing hepatocellular damage (rare)
Respiratory	Transient depression following ECT
Central nervous system	Dizziness, drowsiness, vertigo, overactivity, hyperreflexia, tremors, muscle twitching, mania, hypomania, jitteriness, fatigue, weakness, ataxia, coma, toxic delirium, convulsions, acute anxiety, psychosis, euphoria, palilalia
Genitourinary	Urinary retention
Gastrointestinal	Constipation, dry mouth, other disturbances
Dermatological	Rash, diaphoresis
Ophthalmic	Blurred vision, glaucoma, nystagmus
Hematological	Leukopenia, other changes
Other	Edema, sexual disturbances, hypernatremia, glottal edema
OVERDOSAGE	
Signs and symptoms	*Mild:* Drowsiness, dizziness, ataxia, irritability. *Severe:* faintness, headache, hyperactivity, marked agitation, hypotension, coma, convulsions, diaphoresis, peripheral vascular collapse.
Treatment	Maintain an open airway and supply oxygen, if necessary. Employ general supportive measures. Maintain hydration and electrolyte balance. Avoid CNS stimulants; if necessary, administer a phenothiazine IV. If vasopressors are required for hypotension, use with caution. For hypertensive crisis, administer phentolamine, 5 mg IV slowly. For hyperpyrexia, provide external cooling.
DRUG INTERACTIONS	
Alcohol, anesthetics, general narcotics (especially meperidine), other CNS depressants	Severe hypertension and hyperpyrexia; or severe hypotension
Anticonvulsants	Change in pattern of epileptiform seizures
Tricyclic antidepressants, MAO inhibitors	Hyperpyretic crises, severe convulsions, death
Antihistamines, antimuscarinics, antiparkinsonism agents	⇧ Antimuscarinic effects
Antihypertensives, especially thiazide diuretics	Severe hypotension
Caffeine	Cardiac arrhythmias, hypotension
Dopamine, guanethidine, levodopa, methyldopa, reserpine	Severe hypertension and hyperpyrexia, leading to crisis
Insulin, oral hypoglycemics	Hypoglycemia
Indirect-acting sympathomimetics (amphetamines, ephedrine, methylphenidate, phenylpropanolamine, pseudoephedrine, tyramine, metaraminol, phenylephrine)	Severe hypertension and hyperpyrexia, leading to crisis
Direct-acting amines (epinephrine, isoproterenol, norepinephrine)	Hypertension, headache
Tyramine-containing foods and beverages	Hypertensive crisis

Table continued on following page

ALTERED LABORATORY VALUES

Blood/serum values	⇩ Glucose
Urinary values	⇩ 5-HIAA ⇩ VMA

Use in children

Not recommended for use in children <16 yr of age

Use in pregnancy or nursing mothers

Safe use not established

NORPRAMIN (Desipramine hydrochloride) **Merrell-National**

Tabs: 25, 50, 75, 100, 150 mg

INDICATIONS	ORAL DOSAGE
Depression, especially endogenous depression	**Adult:** initiate at low level and increase dosage, according to clinical response and tolerance, up to 300 mg/day, if needed; usual maintenance dosage: 100–200 mg/day in a single daily dose or div

ADMINISTRATION/DOSAGE ADJUSTMENTS

Adolescent, elderly, or debilitated patients	**Administer 25–100 mg/day, or for severely ill patients, up to 150 mg/day in a single daily dose or div**
High-dose therapy	Patients requiring doses approaching 300 mg should be treated in the hospital

CONTRAINDICATIONS

Hypersensitivity	**To desipramine or other dibenzazepines**
Concomitant MAO-inhibitor therapy	Wait at least 14 days after discontinuing MAO inhibitors before initiating desipramine therapy; start with low doses and increase dosage gradually with caution
Myocardial infarction	During acute recovery phase

WARNINGS/PRECAUTIONS

Atropine-like action	**Use with extreme caution in patients with a history of urinary retention or narrow-angle glaucoma**
Cardiovascular disease	**Use with extreme caution; conduction defects, arrhythmias, tachycardias, stroke, and acute myocardial infarction may occur**
Mental and/or physical impairment	Performance of potentially hazardous activities may be impaired; caution patients accordingly and about potentiating effect on alcohol
Psychotic symptoms	May increase in schizophrenic patients; paranoia may worsen and manic-depressive patients may shift to manic phase; reduce dosage of desipramine or add an antipsychotic agent
Potentially suicidal patients	Should not have access to large quantities of desipramine; prescribe smallest amount feasible
Abrupt discontinuation of therapy	May produce nausea, headache, and malaise after prolonged administration; symptoms are not indicative of addiction
Elective surgery	If possible, discontinue medication several days prior to surgery
Electroconvulsive therapy (ECT)	Hazard may be increased; use ECT only when essential
Special-risk patients	Use with extreme caution in patients with thyroid disease or a history of seizures, and in those taking thyroid medication, anticholinergic agents, or sympathomimetics (see DRUG INTERACTIONS)
Fever and sore throat developing during therapy	Discontinue therapy if leukocyte count and differential show evidence of pathologic neutrophil depression
Tartrazine sensitivity	Presence of FD&C Yellow No. 5 (tartrazine) in all tablets except 150-mg strength may cause allergic-type reactions, including bronchial asthma, in susceptible individuals

ADVERSE REACTIONS[1]

Cardiovascular	Hypotension, hypertension, tachycardia, palpitations, myocardial infarction, arrhythmias, heart block, stroke
Central nervous system and neuromuscular	Confusion, hallucinations, disorientation, delusions, anxiety, restlessness, agitation, insomnia, nightmares, hypomania, exacerbated psychosis, numbness, tingling, paresthesias of the extremities, incoordination, ataxia, tremors, peripheral neuropathy, extrapyramidal symptoms, seizures, alteration in EEG patterns, tinnitus, drowsiness, dizziness, weakness, fatigue, headache

[1]Included are some tricyclic antidepressant adverse reactions not reported with this drug, but which must be considered before and during therapy

Table continued on following page

ADVERSE REACTIONS continued

Autonomic nervous system	Dry mouth, blurred vision, disturbance of accommodation, increased intraocular pressure, mydriasis, constipation, paralytic ileus, urinary retention, dilatation of urinary tract, sublingual adenitis (rare)
Hematological	Bone-marrow depression, including agranulocytosis, eosinophilia, purpura, and thrombocytopenia
Gastrointestinal	Anorexia, nausea, vomiting, epigastric distress, stomatitis, peculiar taste, abdominal cramps, diarrhea, parotid swelling, black tongue, altered liver function, jaundice
Endocrinological	Testicular swelling and gynecomastia (in males), breast enlargement and galactorrhea (in females), increased or decreased libido, impotence
Allergic	Skin rash, petechiae, urticaria, itching, photosensitization, edema of face and tongue or generalized, drug fever
Other	Weight gain or loss, diaphoresis, flushing, urinary frequency, nocturia, alopecia

OVERDOSAGE

Signs and symptoms	Tachycardia and other arrhythmias, cardiac output disturbances, ECG evidence of impaired conduction, congestive heart failure, mydriasis, grand mal seizures, severe hypotension, stupor, coma, agitation, hyperactive reflexes, muscle rigidity, vomiting, hyperpyrexia, shock, renal shutdown (see also ADVERSE REACTIONS)
Treatment	Admit patient to hospital. Empty stomach by gastric lavage. Obtain ECG and begin close monitoring of cardiac function for at least 72 h if abnormalities appear. Maintain an open airway and adequate fluid intake. Regulate body temperature. For cardiac arrhythmias, circulatory shock, and metabolic acidosis, institute standard supportive measures. If cardiac failure occurs, consider digitalization. (Cardiac function should be closely monitored for at least 5 days under these circumstances.) Dialysis is of no value because of low plasma drug concentrations and because of extensive tissue distribution of drug.

DRUG INTERACTIONS

Alcohol, sedative-hypnotics, and other CNS depressants	⇧ CNS depression
MAO inhibitors	Hyperpyrexia, excitability, severe convulsions, coma, death
Anticholinergic agents	Acute glaucoma, urinary retention, paralytic ileus
Ethchlorvynol	Transient delirium
Clonidine, guanethidine	⇩ Antihypertensive effect
Sympathomimetic agents	Severe hypertension, hyperpyrexia
Thyroid preparations	⇧ Antidepressant effect and possible risk of arrhythmias

ALTERED LABORATORY VALUES

Blood/serum values	⇧ or ⇩ Glucose

No clinically significant alterations in urinary values occur at therapeutic dosages

Use in children	Use in pregnancy or nursing mothers
Not recommended for use in children	Safe use not established

Note: Desipramine hydrochloride also marketed as **PERTOFRANE** (USV).

PAMELOR (Nortriptyline hydrochloride) **Sandoz**

Caps: 10, 25, 75 mg **Sol:** 10 mg/5 ml

INDICATIONS	ORAL DOSAGE
Depression, especially endogenous depression	**Adult:** 25 mg tid or qid, up to 100 mg/day, as needed; alternative regimen: give total daily dose once a day

ADMINISTRATION/DOSAGE ADJUSTMENTS

Adolescent or elderly patients	Administer 30–50 mg/day in a single daily dose or div

CONTRAINDICATIONS

Hypersensitivity	To nortriptyline or other dibenzazepines
Concomitant MAO-inhibitor therapy	Wait at least 14 days after discontinuing MAO inhibitors before initiating nortriptyline therapy; start with low doses and increase dosage gradually with caution
Myocardial infarction	During acute recovery phase

WARNINGS/PRECAUTIONS

Atropine-like action	Use with great caution in patients with a history of urinary retention or narrow-angle glaucoma
Cardiovascular disease	May worsen; use with caution, keep patient under close supervision. Tricyclic antidepressants, especially in high doses, may produce arrhythmias, sinus tachycardia, and prolongation of conduction time; myocardial infarction and stroke have followed use of these agents.
Mental and/or physical impairment	Performance of potentially hazardous activities may be impaired; caution patients accordingly and about potentiating effect on alcohol
Psychotic symptoms	May increase in schizophrenic patients; hostility may be aroused, latent symptoms may be unmasked, and manic-depressive patients may shift to manic phase
Potentially suicidal patients	Should not have access to large quantities of nortriptyline; prescribe smallest amount feasible
Abrupt discontinuation of therapy	May produce nausea, headache, and malaise after prolonged administration; symptoms are not indicative of addiction
Elective surgery	If possible, discontinue medication several days prior to surgery
Electroconvulsive therapy (ECT)	May increase hazard; use ECT only when essential
Special-risk patients	Use with caution in patients with hyperthyroidism or a history of seizures and in those taking thyroid medications, anticholinergic agents, or sympathomimetics (see DRUG INTERACTIONS)

ADVERSE REACTIONS[1]

Cardiovascular	Hypotension, hypertension, tachycardia, palpitations, myocardial infarction, arrhythmias, heart block, stroke
Central nervous system and neuromuscular	Confusion, disorientation, delusions, hallucinations, excitement, anxiety, restlessness, agitation, insomnia, panic, nightmares, hypomania, exacerbation of psychosis, numbness, tingling, paresthesias of the extremities, peripheral neuropathy, incoordination, ataxia, tremors, seizures, alteration in EEG patterns, extrapyramidal symptoms, tinnitus, drowsiness, dizziness, weakness, fatigue, headache
Autonomic nervous system	Dry mouth, blurred vision, disturbance of accommodation, increased intraocular pressure, mydriasis, constipation, paralytic ileus, urinary retention, dilatation of urinary tract, delayed micturition, sublingual adenitis (rare)
Hematological	Bone-marrow depression, including agranulocytosis, eosinophilia, purpura, and thrombocytopenia

[1]Included are some tricyclic antidepressant adverse reactions not reported with this drug, but which must be considered before and during therapy

Table continued on following page

ADVERSE REACTIONS continued

Gastrointestinal	Nausea, epigastric distress, vomiting, anorexia, stomatitis, peculiar taste, abdominal cramps, diarrhea, parotid swelling, black tongue, altered liver function, jaundice
Endocrinological	Testicular swelling, gynecomastia, and impotence (in males), breast enlargement and galactorrhea (in females), increased or decreased libido
Allergic	Skin rash, urticaria, photosensitization, edema of face and tongue or generalized, petechiae, itching, drug fever
Other	Weight gain or loss, diaphoresis, flushing, urinary frequency, nocturia, alopecia

OVERDOSAGE

Signs and symptoms	Confusion, restlessness, agitation, vomiting, hyperpyrexia, muscle rigidity, hyperactive reflexes, tachycardia, ECG evidence of impaired conduction, shock, congestive heart failure, convulsions, stupor, coma, respiratory depression, death (see also ADVERSE REACTIONS)
Treatment	Admit patient to hospital. Empty stomach by gastric lavage. Employ general supportive measures. Maintain an open airway and adequate fluid intake. To control convulsions, use diazepam or paraldehyde; *do not use barbiturates*. The value of dialysis has not been established.

DRUG INTERACTIONS

Alcohol, sedative-hypnotics, and other CNS depressants	⇧ CNS depression
MAO inhibitors	Hyperpyrexia, excitability, severe convulsions, coma, death
Anticholinergic agents	Acute glaucoma, urinary retention, paralytic ileus
Ethchlorvynol	Transient delirium
Reserpine	Stimulation ⇩ Antihypertensive effect
Guanethidine	⇩ Antihypertensive effect
Sympathomimetic agents	Severe hypertension, hyperpyrexia
Thyroid preparations	⇧ Antidepressant effect and possible risk of arrhythmias

ALTERED LABORATORY VALUES

Blood/serum values	⇧ or ⇩ Glucose

No clinically significant alterations in urinary values occur at therapeutic dosages

Use in children

Not recommended for use in children

Use in pregnancy or nursing mothers

Safe use not established

PARNATE (Tranylcypromine sulfate) Smith Kline & French

Tabs: 10 mg

INDICATIONS	ORAL DOSAGE
Severe reactive or endogenous depression in hospitalized or closely supervised patients who have not responded to other antidepressant therapy[1]	**Adult:** 10 mg in AM and 10 mg in afternoon for 2 wk, followed, if necessary, by increase in dosage to 20 mg in AM and 10 mg in afternoon for 1 wk; for maintenance, reduce dosage to 10–20 mg/day, as required

ADMINISTRATION/DOSAGE ADJUSTMENTS	
Favorable response	If not achieved within 48 h to 3 wk, discontinue therapy
Concurrent use of electroconvulsive therapy (ECT)	Give 10 mg bid to start; reduce dosage to 10 mg/day for maintenance
Dosage increases	Should be made in increments of 10 mg/day at intervals of 1–3 wk
Discontinuation of therapy	Reduce dosage from peak to maintenance levels before withdrawing medication to avoid recurrence of original symptoms
Switching from another MAO inhibitor or dibenzazepine	Wait 1 wk before initiating tranylcypromine; use ½ the normal starting dosage for at least 1 wk (see CONTRAINDICATIONS)

CONTRAINDICATIONS	
Hypersensitivity to tranylcypromine	
History of hepatic disease or abnormal liver-function tests	
Concomitant use of sympathomimetic drugs	Including amphetamines; methyldopa; levodopa; dopamine; OTC vasoconstrictor-containing cold, hay fever, or weight-reducing preparations; tryptophan; epinephrine; and norepinephrine; may result in hypertension, headache, and related symptoms
Concomitant ingestion of food and beverages containing high amounts of pressor amines (eg, tryptophan, tyramine)	Including aged cheese (cheddar, Camembert, Stilton), processed cheese, beer, and wine (especially Chianti); also chocolate, yeast extract, avocados, pickled herring, broad-bean pods, ripe bananas, papaya products (including meat tenderizers), chicken livers, and sour cream
Concomitant or recent therapy with other MAO inhibitors or dibenzazepines	Can produce hypertensive crisis, fever, marked sweating, excitation, delirium, tremor, twitching, convulsions, coma, and circulatory collapse; wait at least 1 wk after discontinuing tranylcypromine before giving another antidepressant, or after discontinuing another MAO inhibitor before giving tranylcypromine
Concomitant use of CNS depressants	Such as narcotics and alcohol
Excessive use of caffeine	
Special-risk patients	Including the elderly (>60 yr of age) or debilitated, and those with hypertension, cardiovascular or cerebrovascular disease, or history of headaches
Concomitant antiparkinsonism therapy	
Pheochromocytoma	
Concomitant use of antihypertensive agents	Including diuretics

WARNINGS/PRECAUTIONS	
Hypertensive crisis	May occur within hours of ingestion of contraindicated substance; crises are characterized by headache, palpitation, neck stiffness or soreness, nausea, vomiting, sweating, fever or cold, clammy skin, photophobia, tachycardia or bradycardia, chest pain, and dilated pupils, and may lead to potentially fatal intracranial bleeding. Monitor blood pressure frequently and discontinue use if frequent headaches or palpitations occur.
Orthostatic hypotension	May occur most commonly in patients with preexisting hypertension; when tranylcypromine is combined with phenothiazine derivatives or other compounds known to cause hypotension, the possibility of additive hypotensive effects should be considered
Elective surgery requiring general anesthesia	Discontinue use at least 7 days before surgery
Unwarranted uses	Severe endogenous depression and depressive reactions in which ECT or other antidepressant therapy may be the treatment of choice
Suicidal patients	Use only under strict medical supervision, preferably when patient is hospitalized

[1]Probably effective

Table continued on following page

PARNATE continued

WARNINGS/PRECAUTIONS continued

Patient instructions	Caution patients to avoid certain foods and proprietary cold, hay fever, or weight-reducing preparations (see CONTRAINDICATIONS), to reduce intake of alcohol and caffeine, and to report occurrence of headache or unusual symptoms
Influence on convulsive threshold	Has proved variable in animals; use with caution in epileptic patients
Hypoglycemia	May occur in diabetic patients receiving insulin or oral hypoglycemics
Anginal pain	May be suppressed, resulting in the masking of myocardial ischemia
Renal impairment	Use with caution and monitor for signs of excessive drug accumulation (see OVERDOSAGE)
Hyperthyroid patients	May show increased sensitivity to pressor amines; use with caution
Concomitant use of disulfiram	Use with caution
Excessive stimulation	May occur, including increased anxiety, agitation, and manic symptoms; reduce dosage or administer a phenothiazine sedative

ADVERSE REACTIONS

Central nervous system	Overstimulation, anxiety, agitation, mania, restlessness, insomnia, weakness, drowsiness, dizziness, headache (without hypertension), tinnitus, muscle spasm, tremor, paresthesia (causal relationship not established for last three)
Gastrointestinal	Dry mouth, nausea, diarrhea, abdominal pain, constipation, anorexia
Cardiovascular	Tachycardia, edema, palpitation, hypotension, hypertensive crisis
Ophthalmic	Blurred vision
Dermatological	Rash (rare)
Hepatic	Hepatitis (rare)
Genitourinary	Impotence, urinary retention (rare)
Other	Chills (causal relationship not established)

OVERDOSAGE

Signs and symptoms	See WARNINGS/PRECAUTIONS and ADVERSE REACTIONS. Insomnia, restlessness, and anxiety, progressing to agitation, mental confusion, and incoherence; or hypotension, dizziness, weakness, and drowsiness progressing to extreme dizziness or shock; or hypertension with severe headache, in rare cases accompanied by twitching or myoclonic fibrillation of skeletal muscles with hyperpyrexia progressing to generalized rigidity and coma.
Treatment	Empty stomach by gastric lavage. Employ general supportive measures. For hyperpyrexia, provide external cooling. Administer barbiturates with caution to control myoclonic reactions. For hypertensive crisis, administer phentolamine, 5 mg IV (slowly). *Do not use parenteral reserpine.* For hypotension, use standard measures for managing circulatory shock. If pressor agents are used, regulate rate of infusion carefully. Continue to observe patient closely for 1 wk.

DRUG INTERACTIONS

Alcohol, anesthetics, general narcotics (especially meperidine), other CNS depressants	Severe hypertension and hyperpyrexia; or severe hypotension
Anticonvulsants	Change in pattern of epileptiform seizures
Tricyclic antidepressants, MAO inhibitors	Hyperpyretic crises, severe convulsions, death
Antihistamines, antimuscarinics, antiparkinsonism agents	⇧ Antimuscarinic effects
Antihypertensives, especially thiazide diuretics	Severe hypotension
Caffeine	Cardiac arrhythmias, hypotension
Dopamine, guanethidine, levodopa, methyldopa, reserpine	Severe hypertension and hyperpyrexia, leading to crisis
Insulin, oral hypoglycemics	Hypoglycemia

Table continued on following page

PARNATE continued

DRUG INTERACTIONS continued

Indirect-acting sympathomimetics (amphetamines, ephedrine, methylphenidate, phenylpropanolamine, pseudoephedrine, tyramine, metaraminol, phenylephrine)	Severe hypertension and hyperpyrexia, leading to crisis
Direct-acting amines (epinephrine, isoproterenol, norepinephrine)	Hypertension, headache
Tyramine-containing foods and beverages	Hypertensive crisis

ALTERED LABORATORY VALUES

Blood/serum values	⇩ Glucose
Urinary values	⇩ 5-HIAA ⇩ VMA

Use in children

General guidelines not established

Use in pregnancy or nursing mothers

Safe use not established

SINEQUAN (Doxepin hydrochloride) Pfizer

Caps: 10, 25, 50, 75, 100, 150 mg **Conc:** 10 mg/ml

INDICATIONS	ORAL DOSAGE
Depression and/or anxiety in psychoneurotic patients; **depression and/or anxiety** associated with **alcoholism; depression and/or anxiety** associated with **organic disease; psychotic depressive disorders** associated with **anxiety,** including involutional depression and manic-depressive disorders	**Adult:** 75 mg/day in a single daily bedtime dose or div to start, followed by appropriate decreases or increases in dosage until optimal response is achieved; usual maintenance dosage: 75–150 mg/day. Oral concentrate should be diluted, just prior to administration, with 120 ml of water, milk, or fruit juice.

ADMINISTRATION/DOSAGE ADJUSTMENTS

Severely ill patients	May require up to 300 mg/day; increase dosage gradually
Mild symptoms	May be controlled with a dosage of 25–50 mg/day
Initial therapy	Do not use the 150-mg capsule strength
Once-daily dosage	Adjust dosage carefully in the elderly and in patients with intercurrent illness or in those taking other medications, especially other anticholinergic agents; once-daily dosage should not exceed 150 mg/day

CONTRAINDICATIONS

Hypersensitivity to doxepin or other dibenzoxepines ●	Glaucoma ●	Urinary retention ●

WARNINGS/PRECAUTIONS

Concomitant MAO inhibitor therapy	Wait at least 14 days after discontinuing MAO inhibitors before initiating therapy; start with low doses and increase dosage gradually with caution
Drowsiness	Performance of potentially hazardous activities may be impaired; caution patients accordingly and about potentiating effect on alcohol
Psychotic symptoms	May increase; manic-depressive patients may shift to manic phase; reduce dosage of doxepin or add an antipsychotic agent
Potentially suicidal patients	Should not have access to large quantities of doxepin; prescribe smallest amount feasible

ADVERSE REACTIONS[1]

Cardiovascular	Hypotension, tachycardia
Central nervous system and neuromuscular	Drowsiness, confusion, disorientation, hallucinations, numbness, paresthesias, ataxia, seizures, extrapyramidal symptoms, tinnitus, dizziness, weakness, fatigue, headache
Autonomic nervous system	Dry mouth, blurred vision, constipation, urinary retention
Hematological	Bone-marrow depression, including agranulocytosis, leukopenia, eosinophilia, purpura, and thrombocytopenia
Gastrointestinal	Nausea, vomiting, indigestion, anorexia, stomatitis, peculiar taste, diarrhea, jaundice
Endocrinological	Testicular swelling and gynecomastia (in males), breast enlargement and galactorrhea (in females), increased or decreased libido
Allergic	Skin rash, edema, photosensitization, pruritus
Other	Weight gain, diaphoresis, alopecia, chills, flushing

[1]Included are some tricyclic antidepressant adverse reactions not reported with this drug, but which must be considered before and during therapy

Table continued on following page

SINEQUAN continued

OVERDOSAGE

Signs and symptoms	Drowsiness, stupor, blurred vision, dry mouth, respiratory depression, hypotension, coma, tachycardia and other arrhythmias, hypothermia, hyperthermia, urinary retention, paralytic ileus, convulsions, hypertension, mydriasis, hyperactive reflexes
Treatment	Institute standard supportive measures. If patient is conscious, empty stomach by gastric lavage with saline, followed by activated charcoal. Obtain ECG and begin close monitoring of cardiac function if abnormalities appear. Maintain an open airway and adequate fluid intake; assist ventilation, if necessary. Regulate body temperature. Treat arrhythmias with an appropriate antiarrhythmic agent. Control convulsions with standard anticonvulsant therapy; however, barbiturates potentiate respiratory depression. Dialysis is of no value because of high tissue and protein binding.

DRUG INTERACTIONS

Alcohol, sedative-hypnotics, and other CNS depressants	⇧ CNS depression
Anticonvulsants	⇧ CNS depression
MAO inhibitors	Hyperpyrexia, excitability, severe convulsions, coma, death
Anticholinergic agents	Acute glaucoma, urinary retention, paralytic ileus
Ethchlorvynol	⇧ CNS depression
Guanethidine	⇩ Antihypertensive effect (at dosages above 150 mg/day)
Sympathomimetic agents	Severe hypertension, hyperpyrexia

ALTERED LABORATORY VALUES

Blood/serum	⇧ or ⇩ Glucose

No clinically significant alterations in urinary values occur at therapeutic dosages

Use in children	**Use in pregnancy or nursing mothers**
Not recommended for use in children under 12 yr of age	Safe use not established

Note: Doxepin hydrochloride also marketed as **ADAPIN** (Pennwalt)

SURMONTIL (Trimipramine maleate) Ives

Caps: 25, 50 mg

INDICATIONS	ORAL DOSAGE
Depression, especially endogenous depression	**Adult:** 75 mg/day div to start, followed by gradual increases in dosage up to 200 mg/day, if needed; usual maintenance dosage: 50–150 mg/day in a single daily dose at bedtime

ADMINISTRATION/DOSAGE ADJUSTMENTS	
Adolescent and elderly patients	Reduce initial dosage to 50 mg/day, followed by gradual increases in dosage up to 100 mg/day, depending on patient response and tolerance
Hospitalized patients	Give 100 mg/day div to start, followed in a few days by gradual increases in dosage up to 200 mg/day; if improvement does not occur in 2–3 wk, increase dosage to 250–300 mg/day. If dosage exceeds 2.5 mg/kg/day, monitor ECG when initiating therapy and at appropriate intervals during dosage stabilization phase.

CONTRAINDICATIONS	
Hypersensitivity	To trimipramine or other dibenzazepines
Concomitant MAO inhibitor therapy	Wait at least 14 days after discontinuing MAO inhibitors before initiating trimipramine therapy; start with low doses and increase dosage gradually with caution
Myocardial infarction	During acute recovery

WARNINGS/PRECAUTIONS	
Atropine-like action	Use with caution in patients with increased intraocular pressure, a history of urinary retention, or a history of narrow-angle glaucoma
Mental and/or physical impairment	Performance of potentially hazardous activities may be impaired; caution patients accordingly and about potentiating effect on alcohol
Cardiovascular disease	Use with extreme caution; conduction defects, arrhythmias, myocardial infarction, stroke, and tachycardia may occur
Cardiovascular toxicity	May be precipitated in patients with hyperthyroidism or those on thyroid medication; use with caution
Lowered seizure threshold	Use with caution in patients with a history of seizure disorder
Fever and sore throat developing during therapy	Discontinue therapy if leukocyte count and differential show evidence of pathologic neutrophil depression
Psychotic symptoms	May increase in schizophrenic patients; reduce dosage of trimipramine or add an antipsychotic agent
Manic or hypomanic episodes	May occur; if necessary, discontinue use of drug until episode is relieved and then reinstitute at a lower dosage
Potentially suicidal patients	Should not have access to large quantities of trimipramine; prescribe smallest amount feasible
Abrupt discontinuation of therapy	May produce nausea, headache, and malaise after prolonged administration; symptoms are not indicative of addiction
Elective surgery	If possible, discontinue medication several days prior to surgery
Electroconvulsive therapy (ECT)	Hazard may be increased; use ECT only when essential
Special-risk patients	Use with caution in patients with hepatic impairment and in those taking atropine or other anticholinergic agents, sympathomimetics, local decongestants, epinephrine-containing local anesthetics, clonidine, or guanethidine

ADVERSE REACTIONS[1]	
Cardiovascular	Hypotension, hypertension, tachycardia, palpitations, myocardial infarction, arrhythmias, heart block, stroke

[1]Included are some tricyclic antidepressant adverse reactions not reported with this drug, but which must be considered before and during therapy

Table continued on following page

ADVERSE REACTIONS continued

Central nervous system and neuromuscular	Confusion, hallucinations, disorientation, delusions, anxiety, restlessness, agitation, insomnia, nightmares, hypomania, exacerbated psychosis, numbness, tingling, paresthesias of the extremities, incoordination, ataxia, tremors, peripheral neuropathy, extrapyramidal symptoms, seizures, altered EEG patterns, tinnitus, drowsiness, dizziness, weakness, fatigue, headache
Autonomic nervous system	Dry mouth (rarely associated with sublingual adenitis), blurred vision, disturbance of accommodation, mydriasis, constipation, paralytic ileus, urinary retention, delayed micturition, dilatation of urinary tract
Hematological	Bone-marrow depression, including agranulocytosis, eosinophilia, purpura, and thrombocytopenia
Gastrointestinal	Nausea, vomiting, anorexia, epigastric distress, diarrhea, peculiar taste, stomatitis, abdominal cramps, black tongue, jaundice, altered liver function, parotid swelling
Endocrinological	Gynecomastia (in males), breast enlargement and galactorrhea (in females); increased or decreased libido; impotence; testicular swelling
Allergic	Skin rash, petechiae, urticaria, itching, photosensitization, edema of face and tongue
Other	Weight gain or loss, diaphoresis, flushing, urinary frequency, alopecia

OVERDOSAGE

Signs and symptoms	Drowsiness, stupor, coma, ataxia, restlessness, agitation, hyperactive reflexes, muscle rigidity, athetoid and choreiform movements, convulsions, tachycardia and other arrhythmias, ECG evidence of impaired conduction, congestive heart failure, respiratory depression, cyanosis, hypotention, vomiting, hyperpyrexia, mydriasis, diaphoresis, shock
Treatment	Admit patient to hospital. If patient is alert, empty stomach by induction of emesis, followed by gastric lavage. (In the obtunded patient, secure airway with a cuffed endotracheal tube before beginning lavage; do not induce emesis.) Administration of activated charcoal may be helpful. Obtain ECG and begin continuous monitoring of cardiac function for a minimum of 72 h if abnormalities appear. Maintain an open airway and adequate fluid intake. Regulate body temperature with ice packs and cooling sponge baths, if necessary. For cardiac arrhythmias and circulatory shock, institute standard supportive measures. If cardiac failure occurs, rapid digitalization may be necessary; use with extreme care. Minimize external stimulation to reduce convulsive tendency. If anticonvulsants are needed, use diazepam, short-acting barbiturates, paraldehyde, or methocarbamol. Dialysis, exchange transfusions, and forced diuresis are generally ineffective.

DRUG INTERACTIONS

Alcohol, sedative-hypnotics, and other CNS depressants	⇧ CNS depression
MAO inhibitors	Hyperpyrexia, excitability, severe convulsions, coma, death
Anticholinergic agents	Acute glaucoma, urinary retention, paralytic ileus
Guanethidine, clonidine	⇩ Antihypertensive effect
Sympathomimetic agents	Severe hypertension, hyperpyrexia
Thyroid preparations	⇧ Antidepressant effect and possible risk of arrhythmias

ALTERED LABORATORY VALUES

Blood/serum values	⇧ or ⇩ Glucose

No clinically significant alterations in urinary values occur at therapeutic dosages

Use in children

Not recommended for use in children

Use in pregnancy or nursing mothers

Safe use not established; general guidelines not established for use in nursing mothers.

TOFRANIL (Imipramine hydrochloride) Geigy

Tabs: 10, 25, 50 mg **Amps:** 25 mg/2 ml

INDICATIONS	ORAL DOSAGE	PARENTERAL DOSAGE
Depression, especially endogenous depression	**Adult:** 75 mg/day to start; followed by up to 200 mg/day, if needed; usual maintenance dosage: 50–150 mg/day	**Adult:** up to 100 mg/day IM div to start; switch to oral form as soon as possible
Childhood enuresis (adjunctive therapy)	**Child (>6 yr):** 25 mg/day 1 h before bedtime to start; increase dosage to 50 mg/day in children under 12 or up to 75 mg/day in children over 12 if no satisfactory response is attained after 1 wk; do not exceed 2.5 mg/kg/day	

ADMINISTRATION/DOSAGE ADJUSTMENTS

Hospitalized patients	Administer 100 mg/day orally or up to 100 mg/day IM div to start, followed by gradual increases up to 200 mg/day, as required; if no response is achieved after 2 wk, increase dosage to 250–300 mg/day. Switch to oral form as soon as possible.
Adolescent and elderly patients	Administer 30–40 mg/day to start; no more than 100 mg/day is generally necessary for maintenance

CONTRAINDICATIONS

Hypersensitivity	To imipramine or other dibenzazepines
Concomitant MAO inhibitor therapy	Wait at least 14 days after discontinuing MAO inhibitors before initiating imipramine therapy; start with low doses and increase dosage gradually with caution
Myocardial infarction	During acute recovery phase

WARNINGS/PRECAUTIONS

Atropine-like action	Use with extreme caution in patients with a history of urinary retention, narrow-angle glaucoma, or increased intraocular pressure
Cardiovascular disease	Use with extreme caution; conduction defects, congestive heart failure, arrhythmias, tachycardia, myocardial infarction, and stroke may occur, especially in the elderly and in patients with a history of cardiac disease
Mental and/or physical impairment	Performance of potentially hazardous activities may be impaired; caution patients accordingly and about potentiating effect on alcohol
Psychotic symptoms	May increase in schizophrenic patients; manic-depressive patients may shift to manic phase. Reduce dosage of imipramine or add a tranquilizing agent, or phenothiazine, as indicated.
Potentially suicidal patients	Should not have access to large quantities of imipramine; prescribe smallest amount feasible
Abrupt discontinuation of therapy	May produce nausea, headache, and malaise after prolonged administration; symptoms are not indicative of addiction
Elective surgery	If possible, discontinue medication several days prior to surgery
Electroconvulsive therapy (ECT)	Hazard may be increased; use ECT only when essential
Special-risk patients	Use with caution in patients with renal or hepatic impairment, hyperthyroidism, or a history of seizures and in those taking thyroid medication, anticholinergic agents, decongestants, guanethidine, clonidine, methylphenidate, or sympathomimetics (see DRUG INTERACTIONS)
Fever and sore throat developing during therapy	Discontinue therapy if leukocyte count and differential show evidence of pathologic neutrophil depression
Tartrazine sensitivity	Presence of FD&C Yellow No. 5 (tartrazine) in all tablets may cause allergic-type reactions, including bronchial asthma, in susceptible individuals

ADVERSE REACTIONS[1]

Cardiovascular	Orthostatic hypotension, hypertension, tachycardia, palpitations, myocardial infarction, arrhythmias, heart block, ECG changes, congestive heart failure, stroke
Central nervous system and neuromuscular	Confusion, disorientation, delusions, agitation, hallucinations, anxiety, restlessness, insomnia, nightmares, numbness, tingling and paresthesias of the extremities, peripheral neuropathy, incoordination, ataxia, tremors, seizures, alteration in EEG patterns, extrapyramidal symptoms, tinnitus, drowsiness, dizziness, weakness, fatigue, headache, hypomania, exacerbated psychosis
Autonomic nervous system	Dry mouth, sublingual adenitis (rare), blurred vision, disturbance of accommodation, constipation, paralytic ileus, urinary retention, dilatation of urinary tract, mydriasis, delayed micturition

[1]Included are some tricyclic antidepressant adverse reactions not reported with this drug, but which must be considered before and during therapy

Table continued on following page

ADVERSE REACTIONS continued

Hematological	Bone-marrow depression (including agranulocytosis), eosinophilia, purpura, thrombocytopenia
Gastrointestinal	Nausea, epigastric distress, vomiting, anorexia, stomatitis, peculiar taste, diarrhea, parotid swelling, black tongue, altered liver function, jaundice, abdominal cramps
Endocrinological	Testicular swelling and gynecomastia (in males), breast enlargement and galactorrhea (in females), increased or decreased libido, impotence
Allergic	Skin rash, petechiae, urticaria, photosensitization, edema, itching, drug fever, cross-sensitivity with desipramine
Other	Weight gain or loss, diaphoresis, urinary frequency, alopecia, flushing, proneness to falling

OVERDOSAGE

Signs and symptoms	Drowsiness, tachycardia and other arrhythmias, ECG evidence of impaired conduction, congestive heart failure, mydriasis, convulsions, severe hypotension, stupor, coma, agitation, hyperactive reflexes, muscle rigidity, vomiting, hyperpyrexia, ataxia, restlessness, athetoid and choreiform movements, respiratory depression, cyanosis, shock, diaphoresis (see also ADVERSE REACTIONS)
Treatment	Admit patient to hospital. If patient is alert, empty stomach by inducing emesis, followed by gastric lavage and activated charcoal. (In the obtunded patient, secure airway with a cuffed endotracheal tube before beginning lavage; do not induce emesis.) Continue lavage for 24 h or longer. Obtain ECG and begin close monitoring of cardiac function for at least 72 h if abnormalities appear. Maintain an open airway and adequate fluid intake. Regulate body temperature with ice packs and cooling sponge baths, if necessary. For circulatory shock, institute standard supportive measures. If cardiac failure occurs, rapid digitalization may be necessary; use with extreme care. Minimize external stimulation to reduce convulsive tendency. To control convulsions, use diazepam, paraldehyde, or methocarbamol; *do not use barbiturates.* Dialysis, exchange transfusions, and forced diuresis are generally ineffective because of low plasma drug concentrations and because of extensive tissue distribution of drug.

DRUG INTERACTIONS

Alcohol, sedative-hypnotics, and other CNS depressants	⇧ CNS depression
MAO inhibitors	Hyperpyrexia, excitability, severe convulsions, coma, death
Anticholinergic agents	Acute glaucoma, urinary retention, paralytic ileus
Epinephrine	⇧ Pressor response, arrhythmias
Ethchlorvynol	Transient delirium
Clonidine, guanethidine	⇩ Antihypertensive effect
Methylphenidate	⇧ Imipramine side effects
Sympathomimetic agents	Severe hypertension, hyperpyrexia
Thyroid preparations	⇧ Antidepressant effect and possible risk or arrhythmias

ALTERED LABORATORY VALUES

Blood/serum values	⇧ or ⇩ Glucose

No clinically significant alterations in urinary values occur at therapeutic dosages

Use in children

See INDICATIONS; not recommended for use in children under 6 yr of age. Rule out genitourinary disease before instituting therapy for enuresis. Safety of long-term chronic use has not been established.

Use in pregnancy or nursing mothers

Safe use not established

TOFRANIL-PM (Imipramine pamoate) Geigy

Caps: 75, 100, 125, 150 mg

INDICATIONS	ORAL DOSAGE
Depression, especially endogenous depression	**Adult:** 75 mg/day at bedtime to start, followed by up to 200 mg/day, if needed; usual maintenance dosage: 75–150 mg/day; some patients may require divided doses

ADMINISTRATION/DOSAGE ADJUSTMENTS	
Hospitalized patients	Administer 100–150 mg/day to start, followed by gradual increases up to 200 mg/day, as required; if no response is achieved after 2 wk, increase dosage to 250–300 mg/day
Adolescent and elderly patients	Use only after total daily dosage of imipramine pamoate is established at 75 mg or higher. It is generally unnecessary to exceed 100 mg/day for maintenance.

CONTRAINDICATIONS	
Hypersensitivity	To imipramine or other dibenzazepines
Concomitant MAO inhibitor therapy	Wait at least 14 days after discontinuing MAO inhibitors before initiating imipramine therapy; start with low doses and increase dosage gradually with caution
Myocardial infarction	During acute recovery phase

WARNINGS/PRECAUTIONS	
Atropine-like action	Use with extreme caution in patients with a history of urinary retention, narrow-angle glaucoma, or increased intraocular pressure
Cardiovascular disease	Use with extreme caution; conduction defects, congestive heart failure, arrhythmias, tachycardia, myocardial infarction, and stroke may occur, especially in the elderly and in patients with a history of cardiac disease
Mental and/or physical impairment	Performance of potentially hazardous activities may be impaired; caution patients accordingly and about potentiating effect on alcohol
Psychotic symptoms	May increase in schizophrenic patients; manic-depressive patients may shift to manic phase. Reduce dosage of imipramine or add a tranquilizing agent or phenothiazine, as indicated.
Potentially suicidal patients	Should not have access to large quantities of imipramine; prescribe smallest amount feasible
Abrupt discontinuation of therapy	May produce nausea, headache, and malaise after prolonged administration; symptoms are not indicative of addiction
Elective surgery	Discontinue medication several days prior to surgery, if possible
Electroconvulsive therapy (ECT)	May increase hazard; use ECT only when necessary
Special-risk patients	Use with caution in patients with renal or hepatic impairment, hyperthyroidism, or a history of seizures and in those taking thyroid medication, anticholinergic agents, decongestants, guanethidine, clonidine, methylphenidate, or sympathomimetics (see DRUG INTERACTIONS)
Fever and sore throat developing during therapy	Discontinue therapy if leukocyte count and differential show evidence of pathologic neutrophil depression
Tartrazine sensitivity	Presence of FD&C Yellow No. 5 (tartrazine) in 100- and 125-mg capsules may cause allergic-type reactions, including bronchial asthma, in susceptible individuals

ADVERSE REACTIONS[1]	
Cardiovascular	Orthostatic hypotension, hypertension, tachycardia, palpitations, myocardial infarction, arrhythmias, heart block, ECG changes, congestive heart failure, stroke
Central nervous system, neuromuscular	Confusion, disorientation, delusions, agitation, hallucinations, anxiety, restlessness, insomnia, nightmares, numbness, tingling and paresthesias of the extremities; peripheral neuropathy, incoordination, ataxia, tremors, seizures, alteration in EEG patterns, extrapyramidal symptoms, tinnitus, dizziness, weakness, fatigue, headache, hypomania, exacerbated psychosis

[1]Included are some tricyclic antidepressant adverse reactions not reported with this drug, but which must be considered before and during therapy

Table continued on following page

ADVERSE REACTIONS[1] continued

Autonomic nervous system	Dry mouth, sublingual adenitis (rare), blurred vision, disturbance of accommodation, constipation, paralytic ileus, urinary retention, dilatation of urinary tract, mydriasis, delayed micturition
Hematological	Bone-marrow depression (including agranulocytosis), eosinophilia, purpura, thrombocytopenia
Gastrointestinal	Nausea, epigastric distress, vomiting, anorexia, stomatitis, peculiar taste, diarrhea, parotid swelling, black tongue, altered liver function, jaundice, abdominal cramps
Endocrinological	Testicular swelling and gynecomastia (in males), breast enlargement and galactorrhea (in females), increased or decreased libido, impotence
Allergic	Skin rash, petechiae, photosensitization, edema, itching, drug fever, cross-sensitivity with desipramine
Other	Weight gain or loss, diaphoresis, urinary frequency, alopecia, flushing, proneness to falling

OVERDOSAGE

Signs and symptoms	Drowsiness, tachycardia and other arrhythmias, ECG evidence of impaired conduction, congestive heart failure, mydriasis, convulsions, severe hypotension, stupor, coma, agitation, hyperactive reflexes, muscle rigidity, vomiting, hyperpyrexia, ataxia, restlessness, athetoid and choreiform movements, respiratory depression, cyanosis, shock, diaphoresis (see also ADVERSE REACTIONS)
Treatment	Admit patient to hospital. If patient is alert, empty stomach by inducing emesis, followed by gastric lavage and activated charcoal. (In the obtunded patient, secure airway with a cuffed endotracheal tube before beginning lavage; do not induce emesis.) Continue lavage for 24 h or longer. Obtain ECG and begin close monitoring of cardiac function for at least 72 h if abnormalities appear. Maintain an open airway and adequate fluid intake. Regulate body temperature with ice packs and cooling sponge baths, if necessary. For circulatory shock, institute standard supportive measures. If cardiac failure occurs, rapid digitalization may be necessary; use with extreme care. Minimize external stimulation to reduce convulsive tendency. To control convulsions, use diazepam, paraldehyde, or methocarbamol; *do not use barbiturates.* Dialysis, exchange transfusions, and forced diuresis are generally ineffective because of low plasma drug concentrations and because of extensive tissue distribution of drug.

DRUG INTERACTIONS

Alcohol, sedative-hypnotics, and other CNS depressants	⇧ CNS depression
MAO inhibitors	Hyperpyrexia, excitability, severe convulsions, coma, death
Anticholinergic agents	Acute glaucoma, urinary retention, paralytic ileus
Epinephrine	⇧ Pressor response, arrhythmias
Ethchlorvynol	Transient delirium
Clonidine, guanethidine	⇩ Antihypertensive effect
Methylphenidate	⇧ Imipramine side effects
Sympathomimetic agents	Severe hypertension, hyperpyrexia
Thyroid preparations	⇧ Antidepressant effect and possible risk of arrhythmias

ALTERED LABORATORY VALUES

Blood/serum values	⇧ or ⇩ Glucose

No clinically significant alterations in urinary values occur at therapeutic dosages

Use in children	**Use in pregnancy or nursing mothers**
Not recommended for use in children	Safe use not established

TRIAVIL (Perphenazine and amitriptyline hydrochloride) **Merck Sharp & Dohme**

Tabs: 2 mg perphenazine and 25 mg amitriptyline hydrochloride (Triavil 2-25); 4 mg perphenazine and 25 mg amitriptyline hydrochloride (Triavil 4-25); 4 mg perphenazine and 50 mg amitriptyline hydrochloride (Triavil 4-50); 2 mg perphenazine and 10 mg amitriptyline hydrochloride (Triavil 2-10); 4 mg perphenazine and 10 mg amitriptyline hydrochloride (Triavil 4-10)

INDICATIONS	ORAL DOSAGE
Moderate to severe anxiety and/or agitation and depression or depressed mood; anxiety and depression associated with **chronic physical disease,** where depression and anxiety cannot be clearly differentiated **Depressive symptoms in schizophrenic patients, agitation, anxiety, insomnia, psychomotor retardation, functional somatic complaints, tiredness, loss of interest, anorexia**	**Adult:** 1 Triavil 2-25 or 4-25 tab tid or qid or 1 Triavil 4-50 tab bid to start, followed by decreases in dosage to the smallest amount necessary for symptom relief; usual maintenance dosage: 1 Triavil 2-25 or 4-25 tab bid to qid or 1 Triavil 4-50 tab bid. Total daily dose should not exceed 4 Triavil 4-50 tabs or 8 tabs of other dosage strengths.

ADMINISTRATION/DOSAGE ADJUSTMENTS

Schizophrenic patients	Give 2 Triavil 4-25 tabs tid or, if necessary, qid
Adolescents, elderly patients, and patients with predominant anxiety	Give 1 Triavil 4-10 tab tid or qid; adjust dosage as necessary to achieve desired response

CONTRAINDICATIONS

Bone-marrow depression	
Hypersensitivity	To phenothiazines or amitriptyline
CNS depression	Caused by barbiturates, alcohol, narcotics, analgesics, or antihistamines
Concomitant MAO inhibitor therapy	Wait at least 14 days after discontinuing MAO inhibitors before initiating therapy; start with low doses and increase dosage gradually with caution
Myocardial infarction	During acute recovery phase

WARNINGS/PRECAUTIONS

Atropine-like action	Use with caution in patients with a history of urinary retention, narrow-angle glaucoma, or increased intraocular pressure; even average doses may precipitate an attack in patients with narrow-angle glaucoma
Cardiovascular disease	May worsen; use with caution and keep patient under close supervision. Tricyclic antidepressants, especially in high doses, may produce arrhythmias, sinus tachycardia, and prolongation of conduction time; myocardial infarction and stroke have followed use of these agents.
Mental and/or physical impairment	Performance of potentially hazardous activities may be impaired; caution patients accordingly and about potentiating effect on alcohol
Psychotic symptoms	Paranoia may worsen, and manic-depressive patients may shift to manic phase; perphenazine component minimizes the occurrence of these effects
Potentially suicidal patients	Should not have access to large quantities of this drug; prescribe smallest amount feasible
Abrupt discontinuation of therapy	May produce nausea, headache, and malaise after prolonged administration; symptoms are not indicative of addiction
Elective surgery	If possible, discontinue medication several days prior to surgery
Electroconvulsive therapy (ECT)	Hazard may be increased; use ECT only when essential
Antiemetic effect	May mask signs of toxicity due to overdosage of other drugs or render more difficult the diagnosis of such disorders as brain tumors or intestinal obstruction
Unexplained fever	May suggest intolerance to perphenazine component; discontinue use if a significant rise occurs
Special-risk patients	Use with caution in patients with hepatic impairment, convulsive disorders, hyperthyroidism, or a history of adverse reaction to phenothiazines or amitriptyline; patients exposed to heat or phosphorus insecticides; and those taking thyroid medication, anticholinergic agents, or sympathomimetics (see DRUG INTERACTIONS)

ADVERSE REACTIONS[1]

Cardiovascular	Hypotension, hypertension, tachycardia, palpitations, myocardial infarction, arrhythmias, heart block, stroke, ECG abnormalities

[1]Included are some phenothiazine and tricyclic antidepressant adverse reactions not reported with this drug, but which must be considered before and during therapy

Table continued on following page

TRIAVIL continued

ADVERSE REACTIONS[1] continued

Central nervous system and neuromuscular	Confusion, disturbed concentration, disorientation, delusions, hallucinations, excitement, anxiety, restlessness, insomnia, nightmares, numbness, tingling, paresthesias of the extremities, peripheral neuropathy, incoordination, ataxia, tremors, seizures, alteration in EEG patterns, extrapyramidal reactions, tinnitus, inappropriate antidiuretic hormone (ADH) secretion syndrome, dizziness, weakness, fatigue, headache, tardive dyskinesia, reactivated psychotic symptoms, drowsiness, photophobia, catatonia, lassitude, grand mal seizures
Autonomic nervous system	Dry mouth, blurred vision, disturbance of accommodation, constipation, paralytic ileus, urinary retention, dilatation of urinary tract, salivation, nasal congestion, altered pulse rate
Hematological	Bone-marrow depression, including agranulocytosis, leukopenia, eosinophilia, purpura, thrombocytopenia, pancytopenia
Gastrointestinal	Nausea, epigastric distress, vomiting, anorexia, stomatitis, peculiar taste, diarrhea, parotid swelling, black tongue, hepatitis (including altered liver function and, rarely, jaundice), polyphagia, obstipation
Endocrinological	Testicular swelling and gynecomastia (in males), breast enlargement and galactorrhea (in females), increased or decreased libido, menstrual irregularities, failure of ejaculation, hyperglycemia, lactation
Allergic	Skin rash, urticaria, photosensitization, edema of face, tongue, and larynx, pruritus, eczema, erythema, exfoliative dermatitis, asthma, anaphylactoid reactions, angioneurotic edema, cerebral edema leading to circulatory collapse and death (rare), hyperpigmentation
Other	Weight gain or loss, diaphoresis, urinary frequency or retention, mydriasis, alopecia, biliary stasis, pigmentary retinopathy, pigmentation of cornea and lens

OVERDOSAGE

Signs and symptoms	Drowsiness, hypothermia, tachycardia and other arrhythmias, ECG evidence of impaired conduction, congestive heart failure, mydriasis, convulsions, severe hypotension, stupor, coma, agitation, hyperactive reflexes, muscle rigidity, vomiting, hyperpyrexia (see also ADVERSE REACTIONS)
Treatment	Admit patient to hospital. Empty stomach by inducing emesis, followed by gastric lavage and activated charcoal (20–30 g q4–6h during initial 24–48 h). Obtain ECG and begin close monitoring of cardiac function if abnormalities appear. Maintain an open airway and adequate fluid intake. Regulate body temperature. For cardiac arrhythmias, circulatory shock, and metabolic acidosis, institute standard supportive measures. Treat cardiac arrhythmias with neostigmine, pyridostigmine, or propranolol. If cardiac failure occurs, consider digitalization. (Cardiac function should be closely monitored for at least 5 days under these circumstances.) To control convulsions, use diazepam, paraldehyde, or an inhalation anesthetic; *do not use barbiturates.* Combat hypotension with levarterenol. not epinephrine. Administer benztropine mesylate or diphenhydramine for acute parkinsonian symptoms. Dialysis is of no value because of low plasma drug concentrations and because of extensive tissue distribution of drug. Continue treatment for at least 48 h in patients who do not respond earlier.

DRUG INTERACTIONS

Alcohol, sedative-hypnotics, and other CNS depressants	⇧ CNS depression
MAO inhibitors	Hyperpyrexia, excitability, severe convulsions, coma, death
Anticholinergic agents	Acute glaucoma, urinary retention, paralytic ileus
Epinephrine	⇧ Severe hypotension
Ethchlorvynol	Transient delirium
Guanethidine	⇩ Antihypertensive effect
Sympathomimetic agents	Severe hypertension, hyperpyrexia
Thyroid preparations	⇧ Antidepressant effect and possible risk of arrhythmias
Anticonvulsants	⇩ Convulsion threshold ⇧ CNS depression

ALTERED LABORATORY VALUES

Blood/serum values	⇧ or ⇩ Glucose

No clinically significant alterations in urinary values occur at therapeutic dosages

Use in children

Not recommended for use in children

Use in pregnancy or nursing mothers

Safe use not established

COMPAZINE (Prochlorperazine) Smith Kline & French

Tabs: 5, 10, 25 mg **Caps (sust rel):** 10, 15, 30, 75 mg **Amps:** 5 mg/ml (2 ml) **Vial:** 5 mg/ml (10 ml) **Syringe:** 5 mg/ml (2 ml)
Supp: 2½, 5, 25 mg **Syrup:** 5 mg/5 ml **Conc:** 10 mg/ml

INDICATIONS	ORAL DOSAGE	PARENTERAL DOSAGE
Severe nausea and vomiting, excessive anxiety in adults	**Adult:** 5–10 mg tid or qid; sust rel caps: 15 mg on arising or 10 mg q12h **Child (20–29 lb):** 2.5 mg qd or bid, or up to 7.5 mg/day **Child (30–39 lb):** 2.5 mg bid or tid, or up to 10 mg/day **Child (40–85 lb):** 2.5 mg tid or 5 mg bid, or up to 15 mg/day	**Adult:** 5–10 mg IM to start, repeated q3–4h, as needed, up to 40 mg/day **Child:** 0.06 mg/lb IM
Severe nausea and vomiting associated with anesthesia and surgery	—	**Adult:** 5–10 mg IM 1–2 h before induction of anesthesia (repeat once in 30 min, if needed), as well as during or after surgery, if needed (may be repeated once); 5–10 mg IV 15–30 min before anesthesia, as well as during or after surgery, if needed (may be repeated once); or 20 mg/liter of isotonic solution added to IV infusion 15–30 min before anesthesia
Relatively mild psychiatric conditions	**Adult:** 5–10 mg tid or qid	—
Moderate to severe psychiatric conditions, in hospitalized or supervised patients	**Adult:** 10 mg tid or qid; increase dosage in small increments every 2–3 days until symptoms are controlled or side effects become disturbing; some patients respond to 50–75 mg/day	—
Severe psychiatric conditions	**Adult:** 100–150 mg/day	**Adult:** 10–20 mg IM to start, repeated q2–4h (or in resistant cases every hour), as needed; prolonged therapy: 10–20 mg IM q4–6h
Pediatric psychiatric conditions	**Child (2–12 yr):** 2.5 mg bid or tid, up to 10 mg on 1st day, followed by increases in dosage up to 20 mg/day (2–5 yr) or 25 mg/day (6–12 yr), as needed	**Child (<12 yr):** 0.06 mg/lb IM

ADMINISTRATION/DOSAGE ADJUSTMENTS

Parenteral administration	Inject deeply into upper outer quadrant of buttock; total dosage should not exceed 40 mg/day; SC administration inadvisable because of local irritation
Rectal dosage	For severe nausea and vomiting in adults, give 25 mg bid; rectal dosages in children are the same as oral dosages
Debilitated or emaciated patients	Increase dosage gradually

CONTRAINDICATIONS

Coma •	Drug-induced CNS depression •	Bone-marrow depression •

WARNINGS/PRECAUTIONS

Drug-induced extrapyramidal symptoms	May mask signs of undiagnosed primary disease with CNS manifestations, such as Reye's syndrome or other encephalopathy
Mental impairment, reflex-slowing	Performance of potentially hazardous activities may be impaired, especially during first few days of therapy; caution patients accordingly
Disease, drug toxicity	Antiemetic effect may mask signs of overdosage or disease conditions, such as intestinal obstruction, brain tumor, or Reye's syndrome
Long-term therapy	Re-evaluate periodically to determine need and assess dosage
Phenothiazine hypersensitivity	Use with extreme caution in patients who have experienced blood dyscrasias, jaundice, or other hypersensitivity reactions to other phenothiazines

Table continued on following page

COMPAZINE continued

WARNINGS/PRECAUTIONS continued	
Elderly patients	May be more susceptible to hypotension and neuromuscular reactions; observe closely and use low dosages; if required, increase dosage gradually
Extrapyramidal tract symptoms	May occur; see ADVERSE REACTIONS. Depending on severity, dosage should be reduced or discontinued. Mild cases may be treated by administration of a barbiturate. Antiparkinsonism agents, except levodopa, will rapidly reverse symptoms in more severe cases.
ADVERSE REACTIONS[1]	
Neuromuscular	Neck-muscle spasm, torticollis, extensor rigidity of back muscles, opisthotonos, carpopedal spasm, trismus, swallowing difficulty, oculogyric crisis, tongue protrusion, hyperreflexia, dystonia, akathisia, dyskinesia, pseudo-parkinsonism, tardive dyskinesia
Central nervous system	Drowsiness, dizziness, agitation, jitteriness, insomnia, convulsions, altered cerebrospinal-fluid proteins, cerebral edema, headache, reactivated psychotic processes, catatonia
Gastrointestinal	Dry mouth, constipation, nausea, obstipation, adynamic ileus
Cardiovascular	ECG changes, hypotension, cardiac arrest, peripheral edema
Hepatic	Cholestatic jaundice, biliary stasis
Genitourinary	Urinary hesitancy and retention, inhibited ejaculation
Ophthalmic	Blurred vision, pigmentary retinopathy, lenticular and corneal deposits
Hematological	Leukopenia, pancytopenia, thrombocytopenic purpura, agranulocytosis, eosinophilia
Endocrinological	Amenorrhea, lactation suppression, galactorrhea, gynecomastia, menstrual irregularities
Dermatological	Skin reactions, contact dermatitis, photosensitivity, itching, erythema, urticaria, eczema, exfoliative dermatitis, skin pigmentation, epithelial keratopathy
Allergic	Asthma, laryngeal edema, angioneurotic edema, anaphylactoid reactions
Other	Hyperpyrexia, nasal congestion, lupus erythematosus-like syndrome
OVERDOSAGE	
Signs and symptoms	Extrapyramidal effects (see ADVERSE REACTIONS), CNS depression, deep sleep, coma, agitation, restlessness, convulsions, fever, hypotension, dry mouth, ileus
Treatment	Empty stomach by gastric lavage, repeated several times. *Do not induce emesis.* For respiratory depression, administer oxygen and, if needed, perform a tracheostomy, and assist ventilation. For extrapyramidal reactions, keep patient under observation and maintain open airway. Treat extrapyramidal symptoms with antiparkinsonism drugs (except levodopa), barbiturates, or diphenhydramine. For hypotension, employ standard measures. If a vasoconstrictor is indicated, use levarterenol or phenylephrine; other pressor agents may lower blood pressure further. Use saline cathartics to hasten evacuation of pellets that have not already released medication. Continue supportive therapy as long as overdosage symptoms remain.
DRUG INTERACTIONS	
Alcohol, tranquilizers, sedative-hypnotics, and other CNS depressants	⇧ CNS depression
Epinephrine	Severe hypotension

[1]Including reactions related to both phenothiazines in general and prochlorperazine

Table continued on following page

ALTERED LABORATORY VALUES

No clinically significant alterations in blood/serum or urinary values occur at therapeutic dosages

Use in children	Use in pregnancy or nursing mothers
See INDICATIONS; generally contraindicated in children under 2 yr of age. Children with acute illnesses (eg, chickenpox, CNS infection, measles, gastroenteritis) or dehydration are more susceptible to neuromuscular reactions, particularly dystonias, than adults. Use drug only under close supervision. Contraindicated for use in pediatric surgery. Avoid use in children and adolescents with signs and symptoms suggesting Reye's syndrome. The concentrate is not intended for use in children.	Safe use not established during pregnancy; general guidelines not established for use in nursing mothers

HALDOL (Haloperidol) **McNeil Laboratories**

Tabs: 0.5, 1, 2, 5, 10 mg **Conc:** 2 mg/ml **Amps:** 5 mg/ml (1 ml) **Vials:** 5 mg/ml (10 ml)

INDICATIONS	ORAL DOSAGE	PARENTERAL DOSAGE
Manifestations of **pyschotic disorders** Tics and vocal utterances of **Gilles de la Tourette's syndrome** in children and adults **Severe behavioral problems**, marked by combative, explosive behavior, in children Short-term treatment of hyperactive children with **excessive motor activity accompanied by conduct disorders**	**Adult:** 0.5–2.0 mg bid or tid; for severe symptoms, 3.0–5.0 mg bid or tid or more, if needed, to achieve prompt control; for maintenance therapy, reduce dosage to lowest effective level	**Adult:** for prompt control of moderate to severe symptoms, 2–5 mg IM q1–8h, as needed; switch to oral form as soon as possible

ADMINISTRATION/DOSAGE ADJUSTMENTS

Elderly or debilitated patients	Limit initial dosage to 0.5–2.0 mg bid or tid; titrate dosage gradually, as needed, for optimal response
Chronic or resistant patients	Administer 3.0–5.0 mg bid or tid; for severely resistant cases, increase dosage gradually up to a maximum of 100 mg/day
Initial dosage	Should be based on patient's age, severity of illness, previous response to other neuroleptic drugs, and any concomitant medication or disease
Prolonged high-dose therapy	The safety of prolonged use of haloperidol in dosages above 100 mg/day has not been established

CONTRAINDICATIONS

Severe toxic CNS depression or comatose states ●	Parkinson's disease ●	Hypersensitivity to haloperidol ●

WARNINGS/PRECAUTIONS

Concomitant lithium therapy	May result in an encephalopathic syndrome (causal relationship not established) characterized by weakness, lethargy, fever, tremulousness and confusion, extrapyramidal symptons, leukocytosis, elevated serum enzymes, BUN, and FBS, followed by irreversible brain damage. Monitor patients closely for early evidence of neurological toxicity and discontinue medication if such signs appear.
Bronchopneumonia	May occur; monitor patients, especially the elderly, and initiate remedial therapy promptly if signs of dehydration, hemoconcentration, or reduced pulmonary ventilation appear
Mental impairment, reflex-slowing	Performance of potentially hazardous activities may be impaired; caution patients accordingly, as well as about the additive CNS depressive and hypotensive effects of alcohol
Transient hypotension or angina pectoris	May occur or be precipitated; use with caution in patients with severe cardiovascular disorders
Convulsion threshold	May be reduced in patients receiving anticonvulsant medication; use haloperidol with caution and maintain adequate concomitant anticonvulsant therapy
Extrapyramidal symptoms	May occur with simultaneous discontinuation of concomitant antiparkinson and haloperidol therapy; discontinue antiparkinson therapy only after haloperidol is completely discontinued
Rapid mood swing to depression	May occur with haloperidol therapy of mania in cyclic disorders
Severe neurotoxicity	Rigidity and the inability to walk or talk may develop in patients with thyrotoxicosis
Abrupt discontinuation of therapy	May produce transient dyskinesia; withdraw medication gradually
Special-risk patients	Use with caution in patients with known allergies or a history of allergic reactions to drugs
Tartrazine sensitivity	Presence of FD&C Yellow No. 5 (tartrazine) in 1-, 5-, and 10-mg tablets may cause allergic-type reactions, including bronchial asthma, in susceptible individuals

ADVERSE REACTIONS

Central nervous system	Extrapyramidal reactions, including pseudoparkinsonism, motor restlessness, dystonia, akathisia, hyperreflexia, opisthotonos, and oculogyric crisis; transient dyskinesia, persistent tardive dyskinesia, insomnia, restlessness, anxiety, euphoria, agitation, drowsiness, depression, lethargy, headache, confusion, vertigo, grand mal seizures, and exacerbation of psychotic symptoms, including hallucinations

Table continued on following page

HALDOL continued

ADVERSE REACTIONS continued

Cardiovascular	Tachycardia, hypotension
Hematological	Leukopenia, leukocytosis, minimal decrease in red-blood-cell counts, anemia, lymphomonocytosis, agranulocytosis (rare)
Dermatological	Maculopapular and acneform skin reactions, photosensitivity, alopecia
Endocrinological	Lactation, breast engorgement, mastalgia, menstrual irregularities, gynecomastia, impotence, increased libido, hyperglycemia, hypoglycemia
Gastrointestinal	Anorexia, constipation, diarrhea, hypersalivation, dyspepsia, nausea, vomiting
Autonomic nervous system	Dry mouth, blurred vision, urinary retention, diaphoresis
Hepatic	Impaired function, jaundice
Respiratory	Laryngospasm, bronchospasm, increased depth of respiration

OVERDOSAGE

Signs and symptoms	Severe extrapyramidal reactions (muscular weakness or rigidity and tremor), hypotension, sedation, coma, respiratory depression (see ADVERSE REACTIONS)
Treatment	Empty stomach by emesis or gastric lavage, followed by activated charcoal. Institute supportive measures, as required. Establish patent airway by an oropharyngeal airway or endotracheal tube or, in prolonged cases of coma, by tracheostomy. For respiratory depression, employ artificial respiration and a mechanical respirator. Combat hypotension and circulatory collapse with IV fluids, plasma, or concentrated albumin and vasopressor agents, such as norepinephrine. *Do not use epinephrine.* For severe extrapyramidal symptoms, administer antiparkinson medication.

DRUG INTERACTIONS

Alcohol	Severe hypotension ⇧ Alcohol intoxication
CNS depressants	⇧ CNS depression
Anticonvulsants	⇩ Convulsion threshold
Epinephrine	Severe hypotension
Antihypertensives	Excessive hypotension
Antimuscarinics	⇧ Intraocular pressure ⇩ Effect of haloperidol in schizophrenic patients
Amphetamines	⇩ Amphetamine effect
Lithium	Possible neurological toxicity and irreversible brain damage

ALTERED LABORATORY VALUES

No clinically significant alterations in blood/serum or urinary values occur at therapeutic dosages

Use in children

General guidelines not established for oral dosage; parenteral form is not recommended for use in children[1]

Use in pregnancy or nursing mothers

Safe use has not been established during pregnancy; animal studies show an increased incidence of resorption, reduced fertility, delayed delivery, and pup mortality in rodents; cleft palate in mice; but no teratogenicity in rats, rabbits, or dogs. There are two reports of neonatal limb malformations following maternal use of haloperidol along with other drugs with suspected teratogenic potential. Patient should stop nursing if drug is prescribed.

[1]There is little evidence that behavioral improvement is further enhanced by dosages beyond 6 mg/day

LOXITANE (Loxapine succinate) **Lederle**

Caps: 5, 10, 25, 50 mg

LOXITANE C (Loxapine hydrochloride) **Lederle**

Conc: 25 mg/ml

LOXITANE IM (Loxapine hydrochloride) **Lederle**

Amps: 50 mg/ml (1 ml) **Vials:** 50 mg/ml (10 ml)

INDICATIONS	ORAL DOSAGE	PARENTERAL DOSAGE
Manifestations of **schizophrenia**	**Adult:** 10 mg bid to start, followed by a rapid increase in dosage over 7-10 days, up to 250 mg/day, until symptoms are controlled; usual maintenance dosage: 60-100 mg/day div; for severe symptoms, up to 50 mg/day to start. Mix concentrate with orange or grapefruit juice just before administration.	**Adult:** 12.5-50 mg IM (*not IV*) q4-6h or longer, adjusted according to patient response (many patients respond satisfactorily to bid dosing); replace with oral medication once acute symptoms are controlled and patient is able to take medication orally, usually within 5 days

CONTRAINDICATIONS

Hypersensitivity to loxapine	Drug-induced CNS depression	Comatose states

WARNINGS/PRECAUTIONS

Mental impairment, reflex-slowing	Performance of potentially hazardous activities may be impaired; caution patients accordingly, as well as about the additive effects of alcohol and other CNS depressants
Seizures	May occur in epileptic patients despite anticonvulsant therapy; use with caution in patients with a history of convulsive disorders
Antiemetic effect	May mask signs and symptoms of overdosage of other drugs and such conditions as intestinal obstruction and brain tumor
Transient hypotension and increased pulse rate	May occur; use with caution in patients with cardiovascular disease
Ocular changes	Have occurred during prolonged therapy with other antipsychotics; monitor patients for pigmentary retinopathy and lenticular pigmentation
Extrapyramidal symptoms	May be slightly more common with parenteral use than with oral administration due to higher plasma drug levels following IM injection
Special-risk patients	Use with caution in patients with glaucoma or tendency toward urinary retention, particularly with concomitant anticholinergic antiparkinson agents

ADVERSE REACTIONS

Central nervous system	Drowsiness; sedation; dizziness; faintness; staggering gait; muscle twitching; weakness; **extrapyramidal reactions, including pseudoparkinsonism, akathisia, and dystonia; persistent tardive dyskinesia**; headache; paresthesias; **hyperpyrexia**; light-headedness
Cardiovascular	Tachycardia, hypotension, hypertension, syncope, ECG changes
Dermatological	Dermatitis, edema, pruritus, seborrhea, photosensitivity, phototoxicity, skin rashes
Autonomic nervous system	Dry mouth, nasal congestion, constipation, blurred vision
Other	Nausea, vomiting, weight loss or gain, dyspnea, ptosis, flushed facies, polydipsia

OVERDOSAGE

Signs and symptoms	Varies from mild CNS and cardiovascular depression to profound hypotension, respiratory depression, and unconsciousness; extrapyramidal symptoms and/or convulsions may also occur
Treatment	Empty stomach by gastric lavage. Maintain patent airway. *Do not induce emesis.* Treat severe extrapyramidal symptoms with antiparkinson drugs or diphenhydramine, and initiate standard anticonvulsant therapy, if indicated. Avoid use of convulsion-inducing stimulants (eg, picrotoxin or pentylenetetrazol). Employ standard measures for circulatory shock. Restrict use of vasoconstrictors to levarterenol and phenylephrine; *do not use epinephrine.* Extended dialysis is likely to be beneficial. Additional supportive measures include oxygen and IV fluids.

DRUG INTERACTIONS

Epinephrine	Severe hypotension
Alcohol, anesthetics, barbiturates, narcotics, and other CNS depressants	⇧ CNS depression

Table continued on following page

LOXITANE continued

ALTERED LABORATORY VALUES

No clinically significant alterations in blood/serum or urinary values occur at therapeutic dosages

Use in children

Not recommended for use in children under 16 yr of age

Use in pregnancy or nursing mothers

Safe use has not been established during pregnancy. Animal studies have shown no embryotoxicity or teratogenic effects in rats, rabbits, or dogs. Renal papillary abnormalities have been observed in offspring of rats treated from midpregnancy on with doses that approximate the usual human dose. General guidelines not established for use in nursing mothers.

MELLARIL (Thioridazine hydrochloride) Sandoz

Tabs: 10, 15, 25, 50, 100, 150, 200 mg **Conc:** 30 mg/ml, 100 mg/ml

MELLARIL-S (Thioridazine) Sandoz

Susp: 25, 100 mg/5 ml

INDICATIONS	ORAL DOSAGE
Manifestations of **psychotic disorders**	**Adult:** 50–100 mg tid to start, followed by a gradual increase up to 800 mg/day for control, then 200–800 mg/day in 2–4 divided doses
Short-term treatment of **moderate to marked depression accompanied by anxiety** in adult patients **Agitation, anxiety, depressed mood, tension, sleep disturbances, fears, and other symptoms** in geriatric patients	**Adult:** 10 mg bid to qid for mild cases, or up to 50 mg tid or qid for more severe cases; usual starting dosage: 25 mg tid
Severe behavioral problems, marked by combativeness and/or explosive hyperexcitable behavior, in children Short-term treatment of hyperactive children with **excessive motor activity accompanied by conduct disorders**	**Child (2–12 yr):** 10 mg bid or tid to start; for severe symptoms, 25 mg bid or tid to start, followed by larger doses until optimum response is obtained or maximum dosage (3 mg/kg/day) is reached

CONTRAINDICATIONS

Extreme hypotensive or hypertensive heart disease ●	Severe CNS depression ●	Comatose states ●

WARNINGS/PRECAUTIONS

Hypersensitivity to phenothiazines	Use with caution in patients with past history of blood dyscrasias or jaundice or similar reactions to phenothiazines
Pigmentary retinopathy	May occur with larger than recommended doses; symptoms include diminished visual acuity, brownish coloring of vision, impaired night vision, and pigment deposits
Leukopenia and/or agranulocytosis	May occur infrequently
Convulsive seizures	May occur; patients taking anticonvulsant medication should continue their regimens
Orthostatic hypotension	Occurs more often in female patients
High-dose therapy	Daily dosages of 300 mg or more should be reserved for severe neuropsychiatric conditions
Mental impairment, reflex-slowing	Performance of potentially hazardous activities may be impaired; caution patients accordingly
Elderly patients	May have less tolerance for phenothiazines and may be more likely to develop agranulocytosis and leukopenia than younger patients

ADVERSE REACTIONS[1]

Central nervous system	Drowsiness, pseudoparkinsonism, extrapyramidal symptoms, nocturnal confusion, hyperactivity, lethargy, psychotic reactions, restlessness, headache
Autonomic nervous system	Dry mouth, blurred vision, constipation, nausea, vomiting, diarrhea, nasal stuffiness, pallor
Endocrinological	Galactorrhea, breast engorgement, amenorrhea, inhibition of ejaculation, peripheral edema
Dermatological	Dermatitis, urticarial skin eruptions, photosensitivity
Cardiovascular	ECG changes: Q-T prolongation, lowering and inversion of the T-wave, bifid T- or U-wave
Other	Parotid swelling

[1]Various other side effects common to phenothiazines in general may occur but have not been specifically reported with thioridazine

Table continued on following page

OVERDOSAGE

Signs and symptoms	See ADVERSE REACTIONS
Treatment	Discontinue medication; treat symptomatically and institute supportive measures, as required. Restrict use of vasoconstrictors to levarterenol and phenylephrine; *do not use epinephrine.*

DRUG INTERACTIONS

Alcohol, anesthetics, barbiturates, narcotics, and other CNS depressants	⇧ CNS depression
Anticonvulsants	⇩ Convulsion threshold
Epinephrine	Severe hypotension
Guanethidine	⇩ Antihypertensive effect
Antimuscarinics	⇧ Atropine-like effect ⇩ Thioridazine plasma level
Amphetamines	⇩ Amphetamine effect
Antacids containing aluminum and/or magnesium ions	⇩ Absorption of thioridazine
MAO inhibitors, tricyclic antidepressants	⇧ Sedation and antimuscarinic effects

ALTERED LABORATORY VALUES

Urinary values	False-positive or false-negative pregnancy tests ⇧ Bilirubin (false elevation)

No clinically significant alterations in blood/serum values occur at therapeutic dosages

Use in children

See INDICATIONS; not recommended for children under 2 yr of age

Use in pregnancy or nursing mothers

Safe use not established during pregnancy; general guidelines not established for use in nursing mothers

NAVANE (Thiothixene) **Roerig**

Caps: 1, 2, 5, 10, 20 mg

NAVANE (Thiothixene hydrochloride) **Roerig**

Conc: 5 mg/ml **Vials:** 2 mg/ml (2 ml), 5 mg/ml (2 ml)

INDICATIONS	ORAL DOSAGE	PARENTERAL DOSAGE
Manifestations of **psychotic disorders**	**Adult:** 2 mg tid to start, followed by up to 15 mg/day, if needed; for severe symptoms, 5 mg bid to start, followed by up to 60 mg/day; optimal maintenance dosage: 20–30 mg/day	**Adult:** for acute symptoms, 4 mg IM bid to qid, followed by up to 30 mg/day; usual maintenance dosage: 16–20 mg/day; switch to oral medication as soon as possible

ADMINISTRATION/DOSAGE ADJUSTMENTS

Maximum dosage — Carefully titrated dosages exceeding 60 mg/day may result in additional clinical improvement in schizophrenic patients

Parenteral administration — Inject deeply into relatively large muscle; preferred sites include the upper outer quadrant of the buttock and the mid-lateral thigh; do not inject into the lower and middle thirds of upper arm. Aspirate syringe before administration to avoid inadvertent injection into a blood vessel.

CONTRAINDICATIONS

Hypersensitivity to thiothixene ●	Blood dyscrasias ●	Comatose states ●
CNS depression ●	Circulatory collapse ●	

WARNINGS/PRECAUTIONS

Mental impairment, reflex-slowing — Performance of potentially hazardous activities may be impaired; caution patients accordingly, as well as about the possible additive effects of alcohol and other CNS depressants

Antiemetic action — May mask signs and symptoms of overdosage of other drugs or such conditions as intestinal obstruction and brain tumor

Special-risk patients — Use with caution in patients with cardiovascular disease or glaucoma (with IM use), in those receiving atropine or similar drugs and CNS depressants other than anticonvulsants, and in those exposed to extreme heat

Convulsions — May occur; use with extreme caution in patients with a history of convulsive disorders or those in a state of alcohol withdrawal; do not reduce dosage of concomitant anticonvulsant therapy

Ocular changes — May occur; monitor patients for pigmentary retinopathy and lenticular pigmentation

Photosensitivity — May occur; advise patients to avoid undue exposure to sunlight

Radial nerve injury — May result from IM injection into deltoid muscle; use the deltoid region with extreme caution and only if it is well developed (see ADMINISTRATION/DOSAGE ADJUSTMENTS)

Blood dyscrasias — Agranulocytosis, pancytopenia, and thrombocytopenic purpura have occurred with related drugs

Hepatic damage — Jaundice and biliary stasis have occurred with related drugs

Sudden death — Has occasionally occurred with phenothiazine therapy and, in some instances, was attributable to cardiac arrest or asphyxia due to failure of cough reflex

Table continued on following page

ADVERSE REACTIONS[1]

Central nervous system	Drowsiness, sedation, restlessness, agitation, insomnia, seizures, paradoxical exacerbation of psychotic symptoms, cerebral edema, CSF abnormalities; extrapyramidal symptoms, including pseudoparkinsonism, akathisia, and dystonia, persistent tardive dyskinesia, weakness, fatigue
Cardiovascular	Tachycardia, hypotension, lightheadedness, syncope, nonspecific ECG changes
Hematological	Leukopenia, leukocytosis
Allergic	Rash, pruritus, urticaria, photosensitivity, anaphylaxis (rare)
Endocrinological	Lactation, breast enlargement, amenorrhea
Autonomic nervous system	Dry mouth, blurred vision, nasal congestion, constipation, diaphoresis, increased salivation, impotence
Other	Hyperpyrexia, anorexia, nausea, vomiting, diarrhea, increased appetite and weight gain, polydipsia, peripheral edema

OVERDOSAGE

Signs and symptoms	Muscular twitching, drowsiness, dizziness, CNS depression, rigidity, weakness, torticollis, tremor, salivation, dysphagia, hypotension, disturbance of gait, coma
Treatment	Empty stomach by gastric lavage. Maintain patent airway. Treat extrapyramidal symptoms with antiparkinson drugs. Avoid use of convulsion-inducing stimulants (eg, picrotoxin or pentylenetetrazol). Employ standard measures for circulatory shock, including the use of IV fluids. Restrict use of vasoconstrictors to levarterenol and phenylephrine; *do not use epinephrine.* Peritoneal dialysis or hemodialysis is not helpful.

DRUG INTERACTIONS

Alcohol, anesthetics, barbiturates, narcotics, and other CNS depressants	⇧ CNS depression
Anticonvulsants	⇩ Convulsion threshold
Epinephrine	Severe hypotension
Guanethidine	⇩ Antihypertensive effect
Antimuscarinics	⇧ Atropine-like effect ⇩ Thiothixene plasma level
Amphetamines	⇩ Amphetamine effect
Antacids containing aluminum or magnesium ions	⇩ Absorption of thiothixene
MAO inhibitors, tricyclic antidepressants	⇧ Sedation and antimuscarinic effects

ALTERED LABORATORY VALUES

Blood/serum values	⇧ Alkaline phosphatase ⇧ SGOT ⇧ SGPT ⇩ Uric acid

No clinically significant alterations in urinary values occur at therapeutic dosages

Use in children

Safety and efficacy in children have not been established; not recommended for children under 12 yr of age

Use in pregnancy or nursing mothers

Safe use has not been established during pregnancy. Animal reproductive studies have not demonstrated teratogenicity, but some decrease in conception rate and litter size and an increase in resorption rate were observed in rats and rabbits. Hyperreflexia has occurred in infants of mothers receiving structurally related drugs. General guidelines not established for use in nursing mothers.

[1]Various other side effects common to phenothiazines in general may occur but have not been specifically reported with thiothixine, which is structurally related to these compounds

PROLIXIN (Fluphenazine hydrochloride) Squibb

Tabs: 1, 2.5, 5, 10 mg **Elixir:** 2.5 mg/5 ml[1] **Vial:** 2.5 mg/ml (10 ml)

INDICATIONS	ORAL DOSAGE	PARENTERAL DOSAGE
Manifestations of **psychotic disorders**	**Adult:** 2.5–10.0 mg/day div q6–8h to start, followed by up to 20 mg/day, if needed; reduce dosage gradually to 1.0–5.0 mg/day for maintenance	**Adult:** 1.25 mg IM to start, followed by 2.5–10.0 mg/day div q6–8h; switch to oral therapy for maintenance

PROLIXIN DECANOATE (Fluphenazine decanoate) Squibb

Vial: 25 mg/ml (5 ml) **Syringe:** 25 mg/ml (1 ml) **Cartridge-needle unit:** 25 mg/ml (1 ml)

INDICATIONS	PARENTERAL DOSAGE
Manifestations of **schizophrenia**	**Adult:** 12.5–25 mg SC or IM to start; adjust dosage and dosing interval in accordance with patient response; usual maintenance dosing interval: 4–6 wk

PROLIXIN ENANTHATE (Fluphenazine enanthate) Squibb

Vial: 25 mg/ml (5 ml) **Syringe:** 25 mg/ml (1 ml)

INDICATIONS	PARENTERAL DOSAGE
Manifestations of **psychotic disorders**	**Adult:** 25 mg SC or IM every 2 wk to start; adjust dosage and dosing interval in accordance with patient response; usual maintenance regimen: 12.5–100 mg every 1–3 wk

ADMINISTRATION/DOSAGE ADJUSTMENTS

Elderly patients	Administer 1.0–2.5 mg/day orally to start; adjust dosage according to patient response
Severe agitation	Initiate therapy with a rapid-acting phenothiazine. When acute symptoms subside, 25 mg of fluphenazine decanoate or enanthate may be administered; adjust subsequent dosage, as required.
Poor-risk patients	Dosage of fluphenazine decanoate or enanthate should not exceed 100 mg; if doses greater than 50 mg are needed, increase dosage cautiously in 12.5-mg increments
Parenteral administration	For SC or IM administration of fluphenazine decanoate or enanthate, use a dry syringe and needle of at least 21 gauge

CONTRAINDICATIONS

Subcortical brain damage ●	Severe CNS depression ●	Hypersensitivity to fluphenazine or phenothiazine derivatives ●
High-dose hypnotic therapy ●	Blood dyscrasias ●	
Comatose states ●	Hepatic disease ●	

WARNINGS/PRECAUTIONS

Initial therapy in patients with no history of taking phenothiazines	Begin with the shorter-acting form before administering the decanoate or enanthate to determine patient reponse and to establish appropriate dosage; switch from short-acting to long-acting forms of fluphenazine with caution, as dosage comparability is unknown
Mental impairment, reflex-slowing	Performance of potentially hazardous activities may be impaired; caution patients accordingly, as well as about the additive effects of alcohol
Cross-sensitivity	Use with caution in patients with a history of phenothiazine-related cholestatic jaundice, dermatoses, or other allergic reactions
Surgical patients	Monitor psychotic patients on high-dose phenothiazine therapy closely for hypotensive phenomena; administer reduced amounts of anesthetics or CNS depressants
Special-risk patients	Use with caution in patients with mitral insufficiency, other cardiovascular disease, pheochromocytoma, or a history of convulsive disorder, in those taking atropine, and in those exposed to extreme heat or phosphorus insecticides
Prolonged therapy	May cause liver damage, pigmentary retinopathy, lenticular and corneal deposits, and irreversible dyskinesia; monitor patients carefully
Abrupt discontinuation of therapy	May cause gastritis, nausea, vomiting, and dizziness; administer antiparkinson agents for several weeks after fluphenazine is discontinued to reduce withdrawal symptoms
Renal and hepatic function	Should be evaluated periodically; discontinue medication if BUN becomes abnormal
Silent pneumonia	May develop
Mammary neoplasms	Have been reported in rodents following chronic administration of antipsychotics that increase prolactin secretion; clinical significance is, at present, unknown

[1]Contains 14% alcohol

Table continued on following page

PROLIXIN continued

WARNINGS/PRECAUTIONS continued

Blood dyscrasias	Leukopenia, agranulocytosis, thrombocytopenic or nonthrombocytopenic purpura, eosinophilia, and pancytopenia have occurred with phenothiazine therapy; discontinue medication if soreness of the mouth, gums, or throat occurs, or if symptoms of upper respiratory infection and confirmatory leukocyte counts indicate bone-marrow depression
Tartrazine sensitivity	Presence of FD&C Yellow No. 5 (tartrazine) in 2.5-, 5-, and 10-mg tablets may cause allergic-type reactions, including bronchial asthma, in susceptible individuals

ADVERSE REACTIONS[2]

Central nervous system	Extrapyramidal symptoms, including pseudoparkinsonism, dystonia, dyskinesia, akathisia, oculogyric crises, opisthotonos, and hyperreflexia; persistent tardive dyskinesia; drowsiness; lethargy; catatonic-like states; restlessness; excitement; bizarre dreams; reactivation of psychotic processes
Cardiovascular	Hypertension, hypotension (rare), fluctuations in blood pressure, tachycardia
Autonomic nervous system	Nausea, loss of appetite, salivation, polyuria, perspiration, dry mouth, headache, constipation, blurred vision, glaucoma, bladder paralysis, fecal impaction, paralytic ileus, nasal congestion
Metabolic and endocrinological	Weight change, peripheral edema, abnormal lactation, gynecomastia, menstrual irregularities, false pregnancy tests, impotence, increased libido (in women)
Allergic	Itching, erythema, urticaria, seborrhea, photosensitivity, eczema, exfoliative dermatitis, anaphylactoid reactions
Hematological	Leukopenia, agranulocytosis, thrombocytopenic or nonthrombocytopenic purpura, eosinophilia, pancytopenia
Other	Cholestatic jaundice, flare-ups of psychotic behavior, sudden death

OVERDOSAGE

Signs and symptoms	See ADVERSE REACTIONS
Treatment	Discontinue medication; treat symptomatically and institute supportive measures, as required. Combat hypotension with levarterenol. *Do not use epinephrine.*

DRUG INTERACTIONS

Alcohol, anesthetics, barbiturates, narcotics, and other CNS depressants	⇧ CNS depression
Anticonvulsants	⇩ Convulsion threshold
Epinephrine	Severe hypotension
Guanethidine	⇩ Antihypertensive effect
Antimuscarinics	⇧ Atropine-like effect
Amphetamines	⇩ Amphetamine effect
Antacids containing aluminum and/or magnesium ions	⇩ Absorption of fluphenazine
Levodopa	⇩ Antiparkinsonian effect
MAO inhibitors, tricyclic antidepressants	⇧ Sedation and antimuscarinic effects

ALTERED LABORATORY VALUES

Urinary values	False-positive or false-negative pregnancy tests ⇧ Bilirubin (false elevation)

No clinically significant alterations in blood/serum values occur at therapeutic dosages

Use in children

Safety and efficacy of fluphenazine hydrochloride have not been established; fluphenazine decanoate and fluphenazine enanthate are not recommended for use in children under 12 yr of age

Use in pregnancy or nursing mothers

Safe use not established during pregnancy; general guidelines not established for use in nursing mothers

[2]Other reactions common to phenothiazines in general may occur but have not been specifically reported with fluphenazine

SERENTIL (Mesoridazine besylate) Boehringer Ingelheim

Tabs: 10, 25, 50, 100 mg **Conc:** 25 mg/ml **Amps:** 25 mg/ml (1 ml)

INDICATIONS	ORAL DOSAGE	PARENTERAL DOSAGE
Schizophrenia	**Adult:** 50 mg tid to start, followed by 100–400 mg/day	**Adult:** 25 mg IM to start; repeat dose in 30–60 min, if needed; usual maintenance dosage: 25–200 mg/day
Behavioral problems in mental deficiency and chronic brain syndrome	**Adult:** 25 mg tid to start, followed by 75–300 mg/day	**Adult:** same as above
Alcoholism	**Adult:** 25 mg bid to start, followed by 50–200 mg/day	**Adult:** same as above
Psychoneurotic manifestations	**Adult:** 10 mg tid to start, followed by 30–150 mg/day	**Adult:** same as above

ADMINISTRATION/DOSAGE ADJUSTMENTS

Maintenance regimen	When maximum effect is achieved, reduce dosage to lowest effective level for maintenance
Dilution of concentrate	May be done with distilled water, acidified tap water, orange juice, or grape juice; dilute just before administration

CONTRAINDICATIONS

Hypersensitivity to mesoridazine ●	Severe CNS depression ●	Comatose states ●

WARNINGS/PRECAUTIONS

Mental impairment, reflex-slowing	Performance of potentially hazardous activities may be impaired; caution patients accordingly, as well as about the additive effects of alcohol
Ocular changes	Have occurred with other drugs of this class
Leukopenia and/or agranulocytosis	May occur with mesoridazine therapy
Convulsive seizures	May occur; patients receiving anticonvulsant medication should be maintained on that regimen
Persistent tardive dyskinesia	May occur with prolonged mesoridazine use, especially in elderly patients on high-dose therapy; discontinue medication if symptoms appear
Hypotension	May occur following parenteral administration; reserve for bedridden or acute ambulatory patients. Keep patient recumbent for at least ½ h after injection.
Special-risk patients	Use with caution in patients exposed to organophosphorus insecticides or atropine, or related drugs
Tartrazine sensitivity	Presence of FD&C Yellow No. 5 (tartrazine) in tablets may cause allergic-type reactions, including bronchial asthma, in susceptible individuals

ADVERSE REACTIONS[1]

Central nervous system	Drowsiness, dizziness, Parkinson's syndrome, weakness, tremor, restlessness, ataxia, dystonia, faintness, rigidity, slurring, akathisia, opisthotonos
Cardiovascular	Hypotension, tachycardia
Gastrointestinal	Nausea, vomiting
Dermatological	Itching, rash, hypertrophic papillae of tongue, angioneurotic edema
Genitourinary	Inhibited ejaculation, impotence, enuresis, incontinence
Autonomic nervous system	Dry mouth, nasal congestion, photophobia, blurred vision, constipation

OVERDOSAGE

Signs and symptoms	See ADVERSE REACTIONS
Treatment	Discontinue medication, treat symptomatically, and institute supportive measures, as required

[1]Other side effects common to phenothiazines in general should be considered, but have not been specifically reported with mesoridazine

Table continued on following page

SERENTIL continued

DRUG INTERACTIONS

Alcohol, anesthetics, barbiturates, narcotics, and other CNS depressants	⇧ CNS depression
Anticonvulsants	⇩ Convulsion threshold
Epinephrine	Severe hypotension
Guanethidine	⇩ Antihypertensive effect
Antimuscarinics	⇧ Atropine-like effect ⇩ Mesoridazine plasma level
Amphetamines	⇩ Amphetamine effect
Antacids containing aluminum or magnesium ions	⇩ Absorption of mesoridazine
MAO inhibitors, tricyclic antidepressants	⇧ Sedation and antimuscarinic effects

ALTERED LABORATORY VALUES

Urinary values	False-positive or false-negative pregnancy tests ⇧ Bilirubin (false elevation)

No clinically significant alterations in blood/serum values occur at therapeutic dosages

Use in children

Safe use not established; not recommended for use in children under 12 yr of age

Use in pregnancy or nursing mothers

Safe use not established during pregnancy; general guidelines not established for use in nursing mothers

STELAZINE (Trifluoperazine hydrochloride) Smith Kline & French

Tabs: 1, 2, 5, 10 mg **Conc:** 10 mg/ml **Vial:** 2 mg/ml (10 ml)

INDICATIONS	ORAL DOSAGE	PARENTERAL DOSAGE
Manifestations of **psychotic disorders** **Excessive anxiety, tension, and agitation** associated with neurotic or somatic conditions[1]	**Adult:** 1–2 mg bid, up to 4 mg/day if needed; for hospitalized patients, 2–5 mg bid, or up to 40 mg/day if needed; usual maintenance dosage: 15–20 mg/day in the latter **Child (6–12 yr):** for hospitalized patients, 1 mg qd or bid to start, followed by up to 15 mg/day, if needed	**Adult:** 1–2 mg IM (deeply) q4–6h, as needed, up to 10 mg/24 h **Child (6–12 yr):** 1 mg IM (deeply) qd or bid

ADMINISTRATION/DOSAGE ADJUSTMENTS

Elderly, debilitated, or emaciated patients	Initiate therapy in lower dosage range and increase dosage more gradually than in younger adults; monitor patients carefully for hypotension and neuromuscular reactions
Oral concentrate	Should be added to 60 ml or more of diluent just before administration; suggested diluents include juice, milk, simple syrup, orange syrup, carbonated beverages, coffee, tea, water, or semi-solid foods

CONTRAINDICATIONS

Severe CNS depression ●	Bone-marrow depression ●	Liver damage ●
Comatose states ●	Blood dyscrasias ●	

WARNINGS/PRECAUTIONS

Hypersensitivity to phenothiazines	Use with extreme caution in patients with a history of phenothiazine-induced jaundice or blood dyscrasias
Mental impairment, reflex-slowing	Performance of potentially hazardous activities may be impaired; caution patients accordingly
Blood dyscrasias	Agranulocytosis, thrombocytopenia, pancytopenia, or anemia may occur; monitor patients carefully
Hepatic impairment	Cholestatic jaundice or liver damage may occur; monitor patients carefully
Anginal pain	Discontinue medication if anginal pain worsens
Hypotension	May occur; avoid high-dose parenteral administration in patients with impaired cardiovascular systems
Retinopathy	May occur; discontinue medication if ophthalmoscopic examination or visual-field studies reveal retinal changes
Prolonged high-dose therapy	May result in cumulative effects with sudden onset of severe CNS or vasomotor symptoms; evaluate patients periodically and adjust maintenance dosage or discontinue medication accordingly
Antiemetic effect	May mask signs and symptoms of overdosage of other drugs or such conditions as intestinal obstruction or brain tumor
Abrupt discontinuation	May cause temporary nausea, vomiting, dizziness, and tremulousness in patients on prolonged therapy
Special-risk patients	Use with caution in patients taking atropine and in those exposed to heat or organophosphorus insecticides
Sudden death	Has occasionally occurred with phenothiazine therapy and, in some instances, was attributable to asphyxia due to failure of cough reflex

ADVERSE REACTIONS

Cardiovascular	Hypotension (sometimes fatal), cardiac arrest, ECG changes
Hematological	Pancytopenia, thrombocytopenic purpura, leukopenia, agranulocytosis, eosinophilia

[1]Possibly effective

Table continued on following page

ADVERSE REACTIONS continued

Central nervous system	Drowsiness; dizziness; insomnia; fatigue; muscular weakness; motor restlessness; dystonia; pseudoparkinsonism; persistent tardive dyskinesia; extrapyramidal symptoms, including opisthotonos, oculogyric crisis, hyperreflexia, akathisia, dyskinesia, and parkinsonism; grand mal seizures; altered CSF proteins; cerebral edema; reactivation of psychotic symptoms; catatonic-like states
Autonomic nervous system	Dry mouth, anorexia, blurred vision, nasal congestion, headaches, nausea, constipation, obstipation, adynamic ileus, inhibited ejaculation
Hepatic	Jaundice, biliary stasis
Endocrinological	Lactation, galactorrhea, gynecomastia, menstrual irregularities
Dermatological	Photosensitivity, itching, erythema, urticaria, eczema, exfoliative dermatitis, skin pigmentation, epithelial keratopathy
Allergic	Asthma, laryngeal edema, angioneurotic edema, anaphylactoid reactions
Ophthalmic	Pigmentary retinopathy, lenticular and corneal deposits
Other	Peripheral edema, hyperpyrexia, systemic lupus erythematosus-like syndrome

OVERDOSAGE

Signs and symptoms	CNS depression, somnolence, coma, hypotension, extrapyramidal symptoms, agitation, restlessness, convulsions, fever, dry mouth, ileus,
Treatment	Empty stomach by gastric lavage. Maintain patent airway. *Do not induce emesis.* Treat extrapyramidal symptoms with antiparkinson drugs, barbiturates, or diphenhydramine. Avoid use of convulsion-Inducing stimulants (eg, picrotoxin or pentylenetetrazol). Employ standard measures for circulatory shock. Restrict use of vasoconstrictors to levarterenol and phenylephrine; *do not use epinephrine.* Dialysis is not helpful.

DRUG INTERACTIONS

Alcohol, anesthetics, barbiturates, narcotics, and other CNS depressants	⇧ CNS depression
Anticonvulsants	⇩ Convulsion threshold
Epinephrine	Severe hypotension
Guanethidine	⇩ Antihypertensive effect
Antimuscarinics	⇧ Atropine-like effect ⇩ Trifluoperazine plasma level
Amphetamines	⇩ Amphetamine effect
Antacids containing aluminum or magnesium ions	⇩ Absorption of trifluoperazine
MAO inhibitors, tricyclic antidepressants	⇧ Sedation and antimuscarinic effects

ALTERED LABORATORY VALUES

Urinary values	False-positive or false-negative pregnancy tests ⇧ Bilirubin (false elevation)

No clinically significant alterations in blood/serum values occur at therapeutic dosages

Use in children

See INDICATIONS.

Use in pregnancy or nursing mothers

Safe use not established during pregnancy; general guidelines not established for use in nursing mothers

THORAZINE (Chlorpromazine hydrochloride) Smith Kline & French

Tabs: 10, 25, 50, 100, 200 mg **Caps (sust rel):** 30, 75, 150, 200, 300 mg **Syrup:** 10 mg/5 ml **Supp:** 25, 100 mg
Conc: 30, 100 mg/ml **Amps:** 25 mg/ml (1,2 ml) **Vial:** 25 mg/ml (10 ml)

INDICATIONS	ORAL DOSAGE	PARENTERAL DOSAGE
Manifestations of psychotic disorders **Severe combative behavior, explosive hyperexcitability, and persistent hyperactivity in mentally retarded patients** **Moderate to severe agitation, hyperactivity, or aggressiveness in disturbed children**[1] **Excessive anxiety, tension, and agitation in adults**[2]	**Adult:** 10 mg tid or qid, or 25 mg bid or tid; for severe cases, 25 mg tid for 1-2 days, then increase dosage semi-weekly by 20-50 mg/day until symptoms subside, continue optimum dosage for 2 wk, and then reduce to maintenance level; maintenance dose range: 200-800 mg/day **Child:** 0.25 mg/lb q4-6h, as needed	**Adult:** For prompt control of severe symptoms, 25 mg IM; repeat 1 h later, if needed, followed by 25-50 mg orally tid **Child:** 0.25 mg/lb IM q6-8h, as needed
Acutely agitated, manic, or disturbed hospitalized patients	**Adult:** 25 mg tid; increase dosage gradually until effective dose is reached; usual maintenance dosage: 400 mg/day **Child:** start with low doses, then increase dosage gradually; for severe behavior disorders or psychoses, 50-100 mg/day in young children and 200 mg/day or more in older children may be necessary[3]	**Adult:** 25 mg IM, followed in 1 h by 25-50 mg IM, if needed; for exceptionally severe symptoms, increase doses gradually over several days up to 400 mg q4-6h; follow with oral regimen **Child:** same as oral, up to 40 mg/day IM (for children ≤5 yr or ≤50 lb) or 75 mg/day IM (for children 5-12 yr or 50-100 lb), except in unmanageable cases
Preoperative restlessness and apprehension	**Adult:** 25-50 mg 2-3 h before surgery **Child:** 0.25 mg/lb 2-3 h before surgery	**Adult:** 12.5-25 mg IM 1-2 h before surgery **Child:** 0.25 mg/lb IM 1-2 h before surgery
Postoperative medication	**Adult:** 10-25 mg q4-6h, as needed **Child:** 0.25 mg/lb q4-6h, as needed	**Adult:** 12.5-25 mg IM; repeat in 1 h, if needed and if no hypotension occurs **Child:** 0.25 mg/lb IM; repeat in 1 h, if needed and if no hypotension occurs
Nausea and vomiting	**Adult:** 10-25 mg q4-6h, as needed; increase dosage, if necessary **Child:** 0.25 mg/lb q4-6h	**Adult:** 25 mg IM to start; if no hypotension occurs, 25-50 mg q3-4h, as needed, until vomiting ceases; follow with oral regimen **Child (< 5 yr or 50 lb):** 0.25 mg/lb IM q6-8h, up to 40 mg/day, if needed **Child (5-12 yr or 50-100 lb):** 0.25 mg/lb IM q6-8h, up to 75 mg/day, if needed
Nausea and vomiting during surgery	—	**Adult:** 12.5 mg IM; repeat in ½ h, if needed and if no hypotension occurs; alternative regimen: 2 mg/fractional IV injection every 2 min, up to 25 mg; dilute to 1 mg/ml for IV administration **Child:** 0.125 mg/lb IM; repeat in ½ h if needed and if no hypotension occurs; alternative regimen: 1 mg/fractional IV injection every 2 min, up to 0.125 mg/lb; dilute to 1 mg/ml for IV administration
Intractable hiccoughs	**Adult:** 25-50 mg tid or qid; if symptoms persist for 2-3 days, switch to IM use	**Adult:** 25-50 mg IM, followed by 25-50 mg by slow IV infusion, if necessary, with patient flat in bed
Acute intermittent porphyria	**Adult:** 25-50 mg tid or qid	**Adult:** 25 mg IM tid or qid until patient can take oral therapy

[1]Probably effective
[2]Possibly effective
[3]There is little evidence that dosages greater than 500 mg/day further enhance behavioral improvement in severely disturbed mentally retarded patients

Table continued on following page

THORAZINE continued

INDICATIONS continued	ORAL DOSAGE	PARENTERAL DOSAGE
Tetanus (adjunctive therapy)	—	**Adult:** 25–50 mg IM tid or qid; alternative regimen: 25–50 mg IV (1 mg/min); dilute to at least 1 mg/ml for IV administration **Child:** 0.25 mg/lb IM or IV (2 mg/min) q6–8h, up to 40 mg/day (for children ≤50 lb) or 75 mg/day (for children 50–100 lb), except in severe cases; dilute to at least 1 mg/ml for IV administration
Mild alcohol withdrawal symptoms[4]	**Adult:** 50 mg to start, followed by 25–50 mg tid; alternative regimens: 10 mg tid or qid or 25 mg bid or tid	**Adult:** 25–50 mg IM (repeat, if needed), followed by 25–50 mg orally tid
Cancer and severe pain[5]	**Adult:** 10 mg tid or qid or 25 mg bid or tid	**Adult:** 25 mg IM bid or tid

ADMINISTRATION/DOSAGE ADJUSTMENTS

Psychiatric regimens	Increase dosage gradually until symptoms are controlled; maximum improvement may take weeks or even months. Continue optimum dosage for 2 wk, then gradually reduce to lowest effective level for maintenance.
Rectal use	For manifestations of psychiatric disorders in children, give 0.5 mg/lb q6–8h, as needed (if child is 20–30 lb, give ½ 25-mg supp q6–8h). For nausea and vomiting, give ½-1 100-mg supp to adult patients, or 0.5 mg/lb to children, q6–8h, as needed if child is 20–30 lb, give ½ 25-mg supp q6–8h.
Long-term therapy (>6 mo)	Temporarily discontinue therapy once or twice a year to assess effect on behavioral problems and to determine whether maintenance dosage should be lowered or therapy stopped
Elderly, malnourished, or debilitated patients	Reduce dosage to minimize hypotension and neuromuscular reactions, as well as anticholinergic and sedative effects[6]
Concomitant use of narcotics and sedatives	Reduce narcotic and sedative dosage by 50–75% normally, such CNS depressants should be discontinued before starting chlorpromazine therapy
Stuporous alcoholics	Should sleep off alcohol effects before therapy is initiated

CONTRAINDICATIONS

Comatose states ●	Bone-marrow depression ●	Hypersensitivity to phenothiazines ●
Presence of large amounts of CNS depressants ●		

WARNINGS/PRECAUTIONS

Extrapyramidal symptoms	May mask CNS symptoms of undiagnosed primary diseases; do not use chlorpromazine in children and adolescents with suspected Reye's syndrome or other encephalopathy
Mental impairment, reflex-slowing	Performance of potentially hazardous activities may be impaired; caution patients accordingly, as well as about the additive effects of alcohol
Special-risk patients	Use with caution in patients with cardiovascular disease, liver disease, hepatic encephalopathy due to cirrhosis, and chronic respiratory disorders (severe asthma, emphysema, and acute respiratory infections, especially in children), and in those exposed to extreme heat or organophosphorus insecticides, or in those receiving atropine or related drugs
Prolonged high-dose therapy	May lead to excessive drug accumulation (see OVERDOSAGE); monitor patients periodically
Hypotension	May result from parenteral administration; keep patient in reclining position for at least ½ h after injection
Antiemetic effect	May mask signs and symptoms of overdosage of other drugs or such conditions as intestinal obstruction, brain tumor, or Reye's syndrome

[4]Probably effective
[5]Possibly effective
[6]Shader RI: *Manual of Psychiatric Therapeutics*. Boston, Little Brown and Co, 1975

Table continued on following page

THORAZINE continued

WARNINGS/PRECAUTIONS continued

Abrupt discontinuation of therapy	May cause withdrawal symptoms, including gastritis, nausea, vomiting, dizziness, and tremulousness; reduce dosage gradually or administer concomitant antiparkinsonism agents for several weeks
Aspiration of vomitus	May result from suppression of cough reflex
Learning performance	May be impaired by high doses and/or prolonged therapy
Mentally retarded patients	May not report or effectively communicate adverse reactions; such patients may require special monitoring
Fever with grippe-like symptoms	May occur; discontinue therapy if serum bilirubin level is increased or bile is present in urine
Extrahepatic obstruction	May be mimicked in liver-function studies by drug-induced jaundice; withhold exploratory laparotomy until diagnosis is confirmed
Agranulocytosis	May occur; watch for sudden sore throat or other signs of infection and discontinue therapy if WBC count and differential indicate bone-marrow depression. Observe patient carefully between 4th and 10th wk of therapy, when most cases have occurred.

ADVERSE REACTIONS

Central nervous system	Drowsiness, dizziness, faintness, extrapyramidal reactions, hyperreflexia, tardive dyskinesia, psychotic symptoms, catatonic states, cerebral edema, grand mal or petit mal seizures, cerebrospinal-fluid abnormalities
Hematological	Agranulocytosis, eosinophilia, leukopenia, hemolytic anemia, thrombocytopenic purpura, pancytopenia
Cardiovascular	Postural hypotension, tachycardia, shock-like syndromes, ECG changes, cardiac arrest (causal relationship not established)
Hypersensitivity	Jaundice, urticaria, photosensitivity, exfoliative dermatitis, contact dermatitis
Dermatological	Skin pigmentation, lupus erythematosus
Endocrinological	Lactation and breast engorgement (in females), false-positive pregnancy tests, amenorrhea, gynecomastia, hyperglycemia, hypoglycemia, glycosuria
Ophthalmic	Particulate deposits in lens and cornea, lens opacities, epithelial keratopathy, pigmentary retinopathy
Autonomic nervous system	Dry mouth, nasal congestion, constipation, adynamic ileus, urinary retention, miosis, mydriasis
Other	Mild fever, hyperpyrexia, increased appetite and weight gain, peripheral edema, lupus erythematosus-like syndrome, failure of cough reflex

OVERDOSAGE

Signs and symptoms	CNS depression, somnolence, coma, hypotension, extrapyramidal symptoms, agitation, restlessness, convulsions, fever, dry mouth, ileus, ECG changes, cardiac arrhythmias
Treatment	Empty stomach by gastric lavage. Maintain patent airway. *Do not induce emesis.* Treat extrapyramidal symptoms with antiparkinsonism drugs, barbiturates, or diphenhydramine. Avoid use of convulsion-inducing stimulants (eg, picrotoxin or pentylenetetrazol). Employ standard measures for circulatory shock. Restrict use of vasoconstrictors to levarterenol and phenylephrine. Dialysis is not helpful. Use saline cathartics to hasten the evacuation of sustained-release pellets.

DRUG INTERACTIONS

Alcohol, anesthetics, barbiturates, narcotics, and other CNS depressants	⇧ CNS depression
Anticonvulsants	⇩ Convulsion threshold
Epinephrine	Severe hypotension
Guanethidine	⇩ Antihypertensive effect

Table continued on following page

THORAZINE continued

DRUG INTERACTIONS continued

Antimuscarinics	⇧ Atropine-like effect ⇩ Chlorpromazine plasma level
Amphetamines	⇩ Amphetamine effects
Antacids containing aluminum or magnesium ions	⇩ Absorption of chlorpromazine
MAO inhibitors, tricyclic antidepressants	⇧ Sedation and antimuscarinic effects

ALTERED LABORATORY VALUES

Urinary values	False-positive or false-negative pregnancy tests ⇧ Bilirubin (false elevation)

No clinically significant alterations in blood/serum values occur at therapeutic dosages

Use in children

See INDICATIONS; not recommended for use in children under 6 mo of age or for conditions in which children's dosages have not been established. After IM administration, the duration of activity may last up to 12 h.

Use in pregnancy or nursing mothers

Safe use not established during pregnancy; jaundice or prolonged extrapyramidal signs have occurred in newborn infants of mothers receiving chlorpromazine. Animal reproductive studies suggest a potential for embryotoxicity and increased neonatal mortality. Chlorpromazine is excreted in breast milk of nursing mothers.

TRILAFON (Perphenazine) Schering

Tabs: 2, 4, 8, 16 mg **Tabs (sust rel):** 8 mg **Conc:** 16 mg/5 ml **Amps:** 5 mg/ml (1 ml)

INDICATIONS	ORAL DOSAGE	PARENTERAL DOSAGE
Manifestations of **psychotic disorders**	**Adult:** 4–8 mg tid to start, followed by minimum effective dosage; sust-rel tabs: 1–2 tabs bid to start, followed by minimum effective dosage	**Adult:** 5–10 mg IM (deeply), repeated as necessary; switch to higher-dosage oral therapy and reduce dosage gradually
Severe nausea and vomiting	**Adult:** 8–16 mg/day div; sust-rel tabs: 1–2 tabs bid; for severe symptoms, up to 24 mg/day may be given	**Adult:** 5–10 mg IM

ADMINISTRATION/DOSAGE ADJUSTMENTS

Intravenous administration	For adult patients, give up to 5 mg by fractional injection or slow drip; when administered in divided doses, dilute to 0.5 mg/ml and give not more than 1 mg/injection at intervals of not less than 1–2 min
Hospitalized psychotic patients	For adult patients, give 8–16 mg of the tablets or concentrate bid to qid (or 1–4 sust-rel tabs bid); dilute each 5 ml (1 tsp) of the concentrate with 2 oz fruit juice, milk, coffee, carbonated beverage, or other suitable liquid; do not use tea as a diluent. Do not exceed 64 mg/day.

CONTRAINDICATIONS

Drug-induced CNS depression ●	Bone-marrow depression ●	Hypersensitivity to perphenazine ●
Blood dyscrasias ●	Liver damage ●	Coma or severed depression (with IM use) ●

WARNINGS/PRECAUTIONS

Intramuscular administration	The injection should be given with the patient seated or recumbent; observe the patient for a brief period after administration
Intravenous administration	Use with extreme caution and only in recumbent, hospitalized patients when it is essential to control severe vomiting, intractable hiccoughs, or acute conditions, such as retching during surgery (see ADMINISTRATION/DOSAGE ADJUSTMENTS)
Mental impairment, reflex-slowing	Performance of potentially hazardous activities may be impaired; caution patients accordingly
Convulsive threshold	May be lowered in susceptible individuals; use with caution in patients with convulsive disorders and increase dosage, if necessary,of concomitant anticonvulsant therapy
Severe, acute hypotension	May occur; monitor patients closely, especially those with mitral insufficiency or pheochromocytoma, and during IV administration
Potentially suicidal patients	Should not have access to large quantities of perphenazine; prescribe the smallest amount feasible
Prior hypersensitivity to phenothiazines or imipramine	Use with caution; monitor patient closely
Antiemetic effect	May mask signs and symptoms of overdosage of other drugs, or such conditions as intestinal obstruction and brain tumor
Contact dermatitis	May occur with perphenazine solution; contact with hands or clothing by those handling the solution should be avoided
Hyperthermia	May indicate an idiosyncratic reaction; discontinue medication if a significant rise in body temperature occurs
Potentiated CNS depression	Reduce dosage of narcotics, analgesics, antihistamines, and barbiturates when used concomitantly; caution patients about the additive effects of alcohol
Special-risk patients	Use with caution in patients with psychic depression and in those taking atropine or who may be exposed to heat or phosphorus insecticides

ADVERSE REACTIONS[1]

Central nervous system	Extrapyramidal reactions, including opisthotonos, trismus, torticollis, retrocollis, aching and numbness of limbs, motor restlessness, oculogyric crisis, hyperreflexia, dystonia, tonic spasm of masticatory muscles, tight feeling in throat, slurred speech, dysphagia, akathisia, dyskinesia, parkinsonism, ataxia, persistent tardive dyskinesia, altered CSF proteins, paradoxical excitement, headache, reactivated psychotic symptoms, paranoid-like reactions, catatonic-like states, grand mal seizures, lassitude, muscle weakness, mild insomnia, dizziness (with IM use)
Cardiovascular	Hypotension, hypertension, tachycardia, change in pulse rate, ECG abnormalities
Hypersensitivity	Photosensitivity, pruritus, erythema, urticaria, eczema, exfoliative dermatitis, asthma, anaphylactoid reactions, local and generalized edema, cerebral edema (extremely rare), circulatory collapse (extremely rare), death (extremely rare)

[1]Various other side effects common to phenothiazines in general may occur, but have not been specifically reported with perphenazine

Table continued on following page

TRILAFON continued

ADVERSE REACTIONS continued

Autonomic nervous system	Dry mouth, salivation, nausea, vomiting, anorexia, constipation, obstipation, blurred vision, nasal congestion
Endocrinological and genitourinary	Lactation, galactorrhea, gynecomastia, menstrual irregularities, failure of ejaculation, urinary frequency or incontinence
Hematological	Agranulocytosis
Other	Hyperglycemia, systemic lupus erythematosus-like syndrome, jaundice, hyperpigmentation of the skin

OVERDOSAGE

Signs and symptoms	Extrapyramidal symptoms, stupor, coma, convulsive seizures in children (see also ADVERSE REACTIONS)
Treatment	Empty stomach by induction of emesis with syrup of ipecac, followed by gastric lavage. Administer 20–30 g activated charcoal q4–6h for 24–48 h. Maintain patent airway. Employ standard measures (oxygen, IV fluids, corticosteroids) for circulatory shock or metabolic acidosis. Treat hypotension with levarterenol; *do not use epinephrine.* Control convulsions with an inhalation anesthetic, diazepam, or paraldehyde. Monitor cardic function closely; treat cardiac arrhythmias with neostigmine, pyridostigmine, or propranolol. Consider digitalis if cardiac failure occurs.

DRUG INTERACTIONS

Alcohol, anesthetics, barbiturates, narcotics, and other CNS depressants	⇧ CNS depression
Anticonvulsants	⇩ Convulsion threshold
Epinephrine	Severe hypotension
Guanethidine	⇩ Antihypertensive effect
Antimuscarinics	⇧ Atropine-like effect ⇩ Perphenazine plasma level
Amphetamines	⇩ Amphetamine effect
Antacids containing aluminum and/or magnesium ions	⇩ Absorption of perphenazine
MAO inhibitors, tricyclic antidepressants	⇧ Sedation and antimuscarinic effects

ALTERED LABORATORY VALUES

Blood/serum values	⇧ PBI ⇧ Glucose
Urinary values	False-positive or false-negative pregnancy tests ⇧ Bilirubin (false elevation)

Use in children

Not recommended for children under 12 yr of age

Use in pregnancy or nursing mothers

Safe use not established

Sleep Disorders

Sleep is generally regarded as a period of restorative repose and inaction that enables one to "recharge" for another day. How a person sleeps has a profound effect on happiness, mental and physical functioning, and general health and well-being. Although sleep is a vital function and something everyone needs in varying amounts, nearly half of all Americans complain of some sort of sleep disorder. Life problems of all kinds can haunt one at night, robbing the individual of peaceful sleep. Conversely, some problems may be rooted in the nature of sleep itself. Insomnia—the inability to fall or stay asleep—is the most common sleep complaint. Other sleep problems include frequent nighttime wakening, nightmares, sleep apnea (periods when a person stops breathing), and narcolepsy (an irresistible tendency to fall asleep, commonly referred to as "sleeping sickness"). These and various other sleep disorders, as well as the nature and function of sleep itself, will be reviewed in this section.

STAGES OF SLEEP

Sleep is divided into rapid eye movement (REM) periods and non-REM (NREM) periods. During the REM periods, in which the eyes move about beneath closed lids, the person dreams. These dreams can be recalled if the person awakens at this time, but tend to be forgotten otherwise. REM periods constitute about one fourth of total sleep; they last for about twenty minutes, and tend to recur approximately every ninety minutes. There are generally four or five such periods during a night's sleep.

Signs of sexual arousal are evident during almost all REM periods. Men have erections at this time and preliminary studies suggest that women also experience clitoral erections, pelvic engorgement, and vaginal lubrication. However, the accompanying dreams often are not of a sexual nature. Other physiological changes are increased during this period and include irregular respiration and pulse rates and loss of muscle tone.

NREM sleep is divided into four stages. Stages 3 and 4 represent the deepest states of sleep, in which people are most oblivious to their surroundings and least able to be aroused. Stage 4 tends to occur more regularly in children, and to be absent in the elderly, who may wake up often in the night and whose sleep may consist of a series of naps. Stage 4 sleep is associated with a number of sleep disorders.

INSOMNIA

Insomnia—the inability to sleep or to sleep to one's satisfaction—is the most common sleep disorder, with a multiplicity of causes. It is a completely subjective complaint since many people who need only a small amount of sleep may feel more energetic and rested than others who have slept longer, but fitfully. Also, sleep needs vary among people, with some persons requiring eight or more hours to feel rested, while others may need only four or six hours to achieve the same results.

Insomnia may take various forms: difficulty falling asleep; difficulty staying asleep; and waking up too early and being unable to return to sleep. Persons with painful medical conditions such as arthritis may be kept awake by discomfort; others with serious ailments such as asthma or heart disease may be unable to sleep for fear death will overcome them. For others, the cause of insomnia is to be found in their living habits. Older people, for example, often have particular trouble sleeping through the night because they have napped during the day and simply are not tired. Others become excited watching TV thrillers at bedtime or arguing with their spouses, and then naturally have trouble falling asleep. Caffeine in coffee or cola drinks before bedtime may interfere with sleep, as may a variety of medications.

For most, however, the core problem is one of agitation and psychologic conflict. Problems unresolved during the day preoccupy the individual at night. Those who internalize anger rather than express it are especially prone to sleeplessness. Insomnia is also a symptom of depression. As noted earlier, insomnia is a very subjective condition; many persons complain of sleep difficulties but when they are studied in a sleep laboratory, physicians find their sleep patterns are normal, or not as disturbed as perceived by the patient.

Treatment of Insomnia

At one time or another, virtually everyone experiences periods of sleeplessness or insomnia, and almost everyone has a number of remedies or routines to facilitate falling asleep. Counting sheep, reading a dull book, drinking warm milk, soaking in a hot tub, engaging in a tiring physical exercise, or listening to soothing music are common examples. If the problem is chronic, sleep medications (sedatives or hypnotics) may be tried. Insomniacs who suffer from depression may be helped by tricyclic antidepressant medications, such as doxepin (Sinequan, page 775), at bedtime. A number of nonprescription sleep medications are available, many of which contain antihistamines. While these may promote drowsiness in some persons, chronic insomnia may require stronger, prescription medication, preferably on a short-term basis.

The sleep-inducing drugs are classified as barbiturates and nonbarbiturates. The barbiturates have generally lost favor because they are addictive and can be used to commit suicide. Furthermore, they (and most other sleep medications) are effective only for limited periods, perhaps only two weeks, after which another solution must be sought for an ongoing sleep problem. Nonetheless, recent studies indicate that about 17 percent of prescriptions for insomnia are for the barbiturates, which include phenobarbital (Eskabarb, Luminal, and other brands), amobarbital (Amytal), pentobarbital (Nembutal), and secobarbital (Seconal).

More than half of the prescriptions for sleep-inducing drugs are now for flurazepam (Dalmane), It is less addictive than barbiturates and is effective for longer than two weeks. Other benzodiazepine drugs also may be prescribed for short-term treatment of insomnia, but only Ativan is specifically indicated for this purpose. Like the barbiturates, these drugs should not be combined with alcohol, nor should the user drive or operate machinery when on these medications.

The barbiturates suppress REM sleep as well as deep sleep (stages 3 and 4); suppression of REM dream sleep, if prolonged, may have a damaging effect on mental well-being, and the quality of sleep without stages 3 and 4 is poorer. When barbiturates, flurazepam, or the other sleep medications are withdrawn, there is sometimes a rebound effect that causes increased insomnia; withdrawal from barbiturates may also cause nightmares. Therefore, they should be withdrawn gradually, with tapering dosages.

Sleep-inducing medications should be considered a temporary measure, most suitable for short-lived conflicts in a person's life that will pass or for painful conditions such as a broken bone that also will heal with time. For chronic insomnia, treatment of the abiding problem is called for, or alteration of living habits to create patterns conducive to good sleep.

Some basic rules for insomniacs include no daytime naps, no late sleeping, no sleep-disturbing behavior near bedtime (e.g., bill paying, watching lively TV shows, or arguing), and no caffeinated beverages. Many physicians advise not going to bed until sleepy, no activity in the bedroom other than sleep or sex, and waking up at a fixed time in order to create a regular cycle. Other attempts at a long-lasting solution to insomnia have included a variety of relaxation techniques, such as biofeedback, meditation, and self-hypnosis.

MISCELLANEOUS SLEEP DISORDERS

Bedwetting

Nocturnal enuresis, commonly referred to as "bedwetting," is seen primarily in children, and tends to occur in the deepest stages of sleep when the child is least able to be aware of the sensations emanating from a distended bladder. Often the child will continue to sleep and only become aware of the wetness during an REM stage; then the wetness may be incorporated into a dream, with the child waking up thinking urination has just occurred. Among youngsters who have never achieved reliable bladder control, there tends to be a maturational lag, so that the nervous system has not yet reached the point of sophistication necessary to execute the various functions of perceiving a full bladder and responding appropriately to it despite sleep. This lag tends to run in families. The problem is not caused by psychological difficulties, although these can develop as a result of shame and ridicule. On the other hand, bedwetting that occurs after control had been established does tend to be associated with emotional conflicts.

In many instances, withholding water and other drinks in the evening and reminding the child to go to the bathroom before going to bed are sufficient to solve the problem. In other cases, treatments ranging from exercises in holding back a full bladder while awake to using bed pads that signal an alarm upon the first drops of urine, may help. In refractory cases, imipramine hydrochloride (Tofranil), an antidepressant drug sometimes used to treat urinary incontinence, may be prescribed. Although this drug reduces the frequency of bedwetting, some children relapse when the drug is stopped. A minority of cases are associated with urinary infections and other genitourinary conditions—a possibility that should be investigated and treated.

Sleepwalking and Night Terrors

Sleepwalking and night terrors, like enuresis, occur during stage 4 sleep. In fact, enuresis is not uncommon among sleepwalkers. People usually do not recall having sleepwalked, and are confused if awakened. Sleepwalking also may be a result of a maturational lag, since children tend to outgrow it; adults who sleepwalk usually have psychological disturbances. When the problem arises in the elderly, the possibility of nervous system disease should be investigated.

Drugs that suppress stages 3 and 4 of sleep have been tried in an effort to curb sleepwalking, but with poor results. Efforts should be made to create a safe environment, such as having the sleepwalker's bedroom on the first floor with no dangerous objects within reach.

Night terrors often occur only fifteen to thirty minutes after going to sleep—frequently to the same people who sleepwalk, and at the same time. During an episode of night terrors, there is accelerated heartbeat and breathing, accompanied by moans, gasps, or screams. The person has a sensation of doom, but it is not accompanied by a story line as in a nightmare. If anything is recalled, it is a single terrifying image. Night terrors are commonly outgrown and, in children, are not associated with psychological problems. Adult sufferers commonly exhibit anxiety and other psychological difficulties.

It is suspected that impaired deep sleep may cause confusion and subsequent terror. Treatment has been attempted with diazepam (Valium), presumably to suppress stage 4 sleep, although its general use—to calm anxiety—may be a factor. Such treatment seems to decrease the frequency of attacks.

Nightmares

Nightmares are frightening dreams, distinguished from night terrors in that they occur during REM sleep, later in the night, and involve less moving about and fewer utterances. They very often are associated with life conflicts and psychological disturbance, and tend to persist for many years.

Narcolepsy

Colloquially called "sleeping sickness," narcolepsy consists of "sleep attacks" in which the person falls asleep without the normal prelude of tiredness that enables most people to decide whether to resist or yield to the urge to sleep. These attacks often occur after meals, when the person is bored, and as the day progresses. Such episodes usually begin any time from just before adolescence until the mid-twenties and can create grave problems at school or work, since the young person may be suspected of goofing off or being drunk or on drugs.

Physicians often must distinguish narcolepsy from other conditions resembling sleep attacks, such as epilepsy or hypoglycemia. It must also be differentiated from hypersomnia—another sleep disorder involving excessive sleep. Narcolepsy is almost always associated with one or all of the following: *cataplexy,* a complete loss of muscle tone, frequently after laughing, which causes the person to go limp and fall; *sleep paralysis,* an inability to control one's movements (speak, move hands, or open eyes) during the twilight stage between wakefulness and sleep—usually when falling asleep, but also upon awakening; *hypnagogic hallucinations,* vivid and frightening hallucinations that are seen or heard, often during the sleep paralysis. Since the person is prone to fall asleep without warning, he should avoid driving cars or operating dangerous machinery.

Narcolepsy has been treated with a number of stimulant drugs; these include dextroamphetamine sulfate (Dexedrine), a stimulant used in the treatment of obesity, and methylphenidate hydrochloride (Ritalin), a stimulant that is often prescribed for hyperactivity in children.

Hypersomnia

Hypersomnia is an excessive need for sleep that is not marked by the irresistible attacks of narcolepsy. The sleep periods last much longer than in narcolepsy—from many hours to even days. It does not have the associated symptoms of cataplexy, sleep paralysis, or hypnagogic hallucinations; it can occur at any age, and is marked by confusion and inability to awaken completely ("sleep drunkenness") upon arising. Hypersomnia may be associated with extreme overeating (the Kleine-Levin syndrome) or with obesity and respiratory difficulty (Pickwickian syndrome). Occasionally it is associated with depression, the excessive sleeping representing the person's attempt to withdraw from life. Hypersomnia is treated with the same stimulant medications as narcolepsy.

Sleep Apnea

Some people experience a cessation of breathing during sleep, with the breathless episodes generally interspersed with bouts of difficult breathing. This condition, called apnea, is normal in newborn infants (one to three months of age), but requires careful attention if the interruptions of breathing are frequent and prolonged, since apnea is a suspected cause of "crib death" (sudden infant death syndrome).

Adults with sleep apnea may choke or gasp for breath during the night. The spouse can be helpful by reporting the intervals between breaths and the types of behavior that precede the breathing difficulty. Patients who snore may have silent periods punctuated by snorting sounds. A tape recording of the snorting may provide a doctor with clues as to the cause (e.g., obstructive malformation of the nose or throat). Apnea sufferers often awaken with headaches, a condition that is frequently associated with hypersomnia. Treatment often involves making an opening in the trachea (windpipe) to allow the patient to continue breathing even when an upper airway obstruction occurs.

IN CONCLUSION

Sleep problems, particularly insomnia, are among the most common health complaints voiced by Americans. In many instances, the problem is magnified by daytime problems; in others, the sleeplessness is not as marked in reality as it is in the mind of the insomniac. A number of sedative medications are available that can help ease the problem, but they generally should be used on a short-term or occasional basis. Other sleep problems, such as narcolepsy and sleep apnea, require careful medical evaluation and may be treated by drugs or other modalities.

The following charts cover the major presciption and nonprescription sleep or hypnotic medications. The complete charts for drugs prescribed for the treatment of narcolepsy, such as Dexedrine, are included in the sections on *Weight Control* (pages 620–640) and under Ritalin (page 829) in the section on *Childhood Emotional and Behavior Problems,* while medication prescribed for bedwetting (Tofranil) is included in the section on *Anxiety, Depression, and Psychotic Disorders* (pages 736–807).

BUTISOL SODIUM (Sodium butabarbital) **McNeil Pharmaceutical**

Tabs: 15, 30, 50, 100 mg **Elixir:** 30 mg/5 ml[1] *C-III*

BUTICAPS (Sodium butabarbital) **McNeil Pharmaceutical**

Caps: 15, 30 mg *C-III*

INDICATIONS	ORAL DOSAGE
Daytime sedation	**Adult:** 15–30 mg tid or qid **Child:** 7.5–30 mg, depending on age, weight, and degree of sedation desired
Preoperative sedation, insomnia	**Adult:** 50–100 mg before surgery or at bedtime **Child:** based on age and weight of patient

ADMINISTRATION/DOSAGE ADJUSTMENTS

Hypnotic use — Prolonged administration (more than 14 days) is not recommended; if insomnia persists, wait one or more weeks before re-treating

Discontinuation of therapy — Reduce dosage gradually after long use of high doses to avoid withdrawal symptoms

CONTRAINDICATIONS

Sensitivity or idiosyncratic reaction to barbiturates ●

Latent or active porphyria ●

Marked hepatic impairment ●

Respiratory disease with dyspnea or obstruction ●

Prior addiction to sedative-hypnotics ●

Acute or chronic pain ●

WARNINGS/PRECAUTIONS

Habit-forming — Psychic and/or physical dependence and tolerance may develop, especially in addiction-prone individuals

Mental impairment, reflex-slowing — Performance of potentially hazardous activities may be impaired; caution patients accordingly and about possible additive effect of alcohol and other CNS depressants

Withdrawal symptoms — May occur after chronic use of large doses, resulting in delirium, convulsions, or death

Edlerly or debilitated patients — May react with marked excitement or depression; use with caution

Borderline hypoadrenal function — Effects of cortisol may be diminished; use with caution

Hypersensitivity reactions — May occur, especially in patients with asthma, urticaria or angioneurotic edema,

ADVERSE REACTIONS

Central nervous system — Residual sedation (hangover), drowsiness, lethargy, headache

Respiratory — Depression, apnea

Cardiovascular — Circulatory collapse

Gastrointestinal — Nausea, vomiting

Hypersensitivity — Allergic reactions, skin eruptions

OVERDOSAGE

Signs and symptoms — Coma, early hypothermia, later fever, sluggish or absent reflexes, respiratory depression, circulatory collapse, pulmonary edema

Treatment — Maintain adequate airway, assist ventilation, and administer oxygen, as needed. Empty stomach by gastric lavage, taking care to avoid pulmonary aspiration. Monitor vital signs and fluid balance. Treat shock with fluids and other standard measures. If renal function is normal, force diuresis to help eliminate drug. Dialysis may be helpful.

DRUG INTERACTIONS

Alcohol, tranquilizers, and other CNS depressants — ⇧ CNS depression

Coumarin anticoagulants — ⇩ Prothrombin time

Hydrocortisone — ⇩ Systemic corticosteroid activity

ALTERED LABORATORY VALUES

No clinically significant alterations in blood/serum or urinary values occur at therapeutic dosages

Use in children	Use in pregnancy or nursing mothers
See INDICATIONS	Not recommended for use during pregnancy; general guidelines not established for use in nursing mothers

[1]Contains 7% alcohol

DALMANE (Flurazepam hydrochloride) Roche

Caps: 15, 30 mg *C-IV*

INDICATIONS	ORAL DOSAGE
Insomnia and in medical situations requiring restful sleep	**Adult:** 15–30 mg at bedtime

ADMINISTRATION/DOSAGE ADJUSTMENTS

Elderly and/or debilitated patients	Initiate therapy with 15 mg flurazepam until individual response is determined
Duration of therapy	Prolonged use is usually not indicated and should only be undertaken concomitantly with appropriate evaluation; effectiveness lasts for at least 28 consecutive nights of drug administration
Repeated use	Perform periodic blood counts and liver and kidney function tests if drug is used repeatedly

CONTRAINDICATIONS

Hypersensitivity to flurazepam

WARNINGS/PRECAUTIONS

Habit-forming	Psychic and/or physical dependence may develop, especially in addiction-prone individuals
Mental impairment, reflex-slowing	Performance of potentially hazardous activities may be impaired; caution patients accordingly and about possible additive effect of alcohol and other CNS depressants
Special-risk patients	Use with caution in elderly and/or depressed patients and in those with hepatic or renal functional impairment

ADVERSE REACTIONS

Central nervous system and neuromuscular	Dizziness, drowsiness, lightheadedness, staggering, ataxia, falling, headache, nervousness, talkativeness, apprehension, irritability, weakness, faintness, euphoria, depression, slurred speech, confusion, restlessness, hallucinations, excitement, stimulation, hyperactivity, body and joint pains
Ophthalmic	Difficulty focusing, blurred vision, burning eyes
Gastrointestinal	Heartburn, upset, nausea, vomiting, diarrhea, constipation, pain, excessive salivation, anorexia, dry mouth, bitter taste
Cardiovascular	Palpitations, chest pain, hypotension, shortness of breath
Hematological	Leukopenia, granulocytopenia
Dermatological	Pruritus, rash
Other	Genitourinary complaints, sweating, flushes

OVERDOSAGE

Signs and symptoms	Somnolence, sedation, lethargy, ataxia, disorientation, confusion, coma, hypotension, excitation
Treatment	Empty stomach immediately by gastric lavage. Maintain adequate airway, and administer IV fluids. Monitor respiration, pulse, and blood pressure. Treat hypotension with levarterenol or metaraminol. If excitation occurs, do *not* use barbiturates.

DRUG INTERACTIONS

Alcohol, tranquilizers, and other CNS depressants	⇧ CNS depression

ALTERED LABORATORY VALUES

Blood/serum values	⇧ SGOT ⇧ SGPT ⇧ Bilirubin (total and direct) ⇧ Alkaline phosphatase

No clinically significant alterations in urinary values occur at therapeutic dosages

Use in children

Not recommended for use in children under 15 yr of age

Use in pregnancy or nursing mothers

Use during pregnancy should almost always be avoided. Although flurazepam has not been studied adequately to determine whether it may be associated with fetal abnormalities, an increased risk of congenital malformations during the 1st trimester of pregnancy has been associated with the use of minor tranquilizers.
General guidelines not established for use in nursing mothers.

DORIDEN (Glutethimide) USV

Tabs: 0.25, 0.5 g **Caps:** 0.5 g *C-III*

INDICATIONS	ORAL DOSAGE
Temporary insomnia	**Adult:** 0.25–0.5 g at bedtime; some patients may require more or less

ADMINISTRATION/DOSAGE ADJUSTMENTS

Elderly or debilitated patients	To avoid oversedation, limit initial dosage to 0.5 g at bedtime
Persistent insomnia	Allow a drug-free interval of 1 wk or more to elapse before considering retreatment
Drug withdrawal	Withdrawal symptoms may be avoided by reducing glutethimide dosage gradually

CONTRAINDICATIONS

Hypersensitivity to glutethimide ●	Porphyria ●

WARNINGS/PRECAUTIONS

Habit-forming	Psychic and/or physical dependence may develop, especially in the addiction-prone
Mental impairment, reflex-slowing	Performance of potentially hazardous activities may be impaired; caution patients accordingly and about possible additive effect of alcohol and other CNS depressants
Abrupt discontinuation of therapy	May produce withdrawal symptoms, including nausea, abdominal discomfort, tremors, convulsions, and delirium in glutethimide-dependent individuals and newborn infants of dependent mothers

ADVERSE REACTIONS

Dermatological	Generalized rash, purpura, urticaria, exfoliative dermatitis (rare), porphyria (rare)
Gastrointestinal	Nausea
Central nervous system	Paradoxical excitation
Ophthalmic	Blurred vision
Hematological (rare)	Thrombocytopenic purpura, aplastic anemia, leukopenia
Other	Hangover, acute hypersensitivity (rare), osteomalacia (with prolonged use)

OVERDOSAGE

Signs and symptoms	CNS depression, coma, hypothermia, fever, depressed or lost deep-tendon reflexes, depressed or lost corneal and pupillary reflexes, mydriasis, depressed or absent pain response, inadequate ventilation, cyanosis, sudden apnea (especially with gastric lavage or endotracheal intubation), diminished or absent peristalsis, severe hypotension, tonic muscular spasms, twitching, convulsions
Treatment	Empty stomach immediately by gastric lavage with a 1:1 mixture of castor oil and water, leaving 50 ml of castor oil in stomach as a cathartic; employ precautionary measures to prevent aspiration of gastric contents or respiratory arrest. To remove unabsorbed drug from the intestine, perform intestinal lavage with 100–250 ml of 20–40% sorbitol or mannitol. Treat mild intoxication symptomatically. For moderate intoxication involving hypotension and deeper coma, maintain adequate respiratory exchange; monitor vital signs, level of consciousness, and ECG (for arrhythmias); and maintain blood pressure with plasma volume expanders and, if absolutely essential, vasopressor drugs. For prolonged coma, monitor and maintain urine output; overhydration must be avoided. For severe intoxication, employ more intensive supportive measures and consider hemodialysis or hemoperfusion. Combat supervening pulmonary or other infection with appropriate antibiotics.

DRUG INTERACTIONS

Alcohol, tranquilizers, and other CNS depressants	⇧ CNS depression
Coumarin anticoagulants	⇩ Prothrombin time

ALTERED LABORATORY VALUES

No clinically significant alterations in blood/serum or urinary values occur at therapeutic dosages

Use in children

Not recommended for use in children

Use in pregnancy or nursing mothers

Safe use not established; withdrawal symptoms may be exhibited by infants born to mothers dependent on glutethimide. General guidelines not established for use in nursing mothers.

MEQUIN (Methaqualone) Lemmon

Tabs: 300 mg *C-II*

INDICATIONS	ORAL DOSAGE
Insomnia and in medical situations requiring restful sleep	**Adult:** 150–300 mg at bedtime

ADMINISTRATION/DOSAGE ADJUSTMENTS

Elderly, debilitated, or highly agitated patients	Administer small doses to start; observe response and adjust dosage accordingly
Duration of therapy	Prolonged use is usually not indicated

CONTRAINDICATIONS

Hypersensitivity to methaqualone

WARNINGS/PRECAUTIONS

Habit-forming	Psychic and/or physical dependence and tolerance may develop, especially in addiction-prone individuals; if dependence develops, reduce dosage gradually
Mental impairment, reflex-slowing	Performance of potentially hazardous activities may be impaired; caution patients accordingly and about possible additive effect of alcohol and other CNS depressants
Hepatic impairment	Use with great caution and at reduced dosage

ADVERSE REACTIONS

Central nervous system	Headache, residual sedation ("hangover"), fatigue, dizziness, torpor, transient paresthesias in extremities, restlessness, anxiety
Hematological	Aplastic anemia
Gastrointestinal	Dry mouth, anorexia, nausea, vomiting, epigastric discomfort, diarrhea
Dermatological	Diaphoresis, bromhidrosis, exanthema, urticaria

OVERDOSAGE

Signs and symptoms	Delirium, coma, restlessness, and hypertonia, progressing to convulsions; vomiting and increased secretions leading to aspiration pneumonitis or respiratory obstruction; in cases of large acute ingestions: cutaneous and pulmonary edema, hepatic damage, renal insufficiency, mydriasis, tachycardia, hyperreflexia, bleeding, shock, respiratory arrest, coma (following acute ingestions of 2–4 g), and death
Treatment	Perform gastric lavage to empty stomach immediately. Maintain adequate ventilation and control blood pressure. Institute general supportive measures if patient is unconscious. Dialysis may be helpful. *Do not use analeptics.* Prolonged convulsions may require use of a muscle relaxant such as succinylcholine or tubocurarine, accompanied by assisted ventilation.

DRUG INTERACTIONS

Alcohol, tranquilizers, and other CNS depressants	⇧ CNS depression

ALTERED LABORATORY VALUES

No clinically significant alterations in blood/serum or urinary values occur at therapeutic dosages

Use in children

Not recommended; safety and effectiveness in pediatric age group have not been established

Use in pregnancy or nursing mothers

Contraindicated for women who are or who may become pregnant; minor, but clearcut, abnormalities have appeared in offspring of rats given methaqualone during gestation. General guidelines not established for use in nursing mothers.

NEMBUTAL (Pentobarbital) **Abbott**

Elixir: 18.2 mg (equivalent to 20 mg pentobarbital sodium) per 5 ml[1] *C-II*

NEMBUTAL SODIUM (Pentobarbital sodium) **Abbott**

Caps: 30, 50, 100 mg *C-II* **Amps:** 50 mg/ml (2 ml) *C-II* **Vials:** 50 mg/ml (20, 50 ml) *C-II* **Supp:** 30, 60, 120, 200 mg *C-III*

INDICATIONS	ORAL DOSAGE	PARENTERAL DOSAGE
Sedation	**Adult:** 5 ml (1 tsp) or 30 mg tid or qid **Child:** 8–30 mg, depending on age, weight, and desired degree of sedation	**Adult:** 150–200 mg IM (deeply) or 100 mg/70 kg IV (slowly) followed by small increments in dosage, as needed, up to a total of 200–500 mg IV **Child:** 25–80 mg IM (deeply) or proportional reduction in adult IV dosage
Hypnosis (preanesthetic medication)	**Adult:** 25 ml (5 tsp) or 100 mg **Child:** based on age and weight	**Adult:** same as adult's dosage above **Child:** same as child's dosage above
Acute convulsive conditions, including tetanus, status epilepticus, and toxic reactions to strychnine and local anesthetics	—	**Adult:** use minimum IV dose, allowing time for drug to penetrate blood/brain barrier **Child:** same as adult

ADMINISTRATION/DOSAGE ADJUSTMENTS

Intramuscular administration	Inject deeply into a large muscle mass (preferably the upper outer quadrant of the gluteus maximus); to preclude irritation, give no more than 5 ml at any one site. Exact dosage is determined by patient's age, weight, and condition.
Intravenous administration	Inject slowly in fractional doses, waiting at least 1 min between doses to determine full effect of dose; dosage is determined by clinical response and may be affected by patient's weight, age, state of health, and temperature
Elderly and/or debilitated patients	Reduce adult IV dosage proportionally
Rectal use	May be convenient for nauseated patients or small children or during preoperative fasting. For hypnosis in adults of average or above average weight, give one 120-mg or one 200-mg suppository. For hypnosis in infants 2 mo to 1 yr of age (10–20 lb), give one 30-mg suppository; for children 1–4 yr of age (20–40 lb), one 30-mg or one 60-mg suppository; for children 5–12 yr of age (40–80 lb), one 60-mg suppository; and for children 12–14 yr of age (80–110 lb), one 60-mg or one 120-mg suppository. For sedation in children 5–14 yr old or for adults, reduce hypnotic dose appropriately. Suppositories should not be divided.

CONTRAINDICATIONS

Porphyria ●	Sensitivity to barbiturates ●	Prior addiction to sedative/hypnotics ●

WARNINGS/PRECAUTIONS

Habit-forming	Psychic and/or physical dependence and tolerance may develop, especially in addiction-prone individuals
Mental impairment, reflex-slowing	Performance of potentially hazardous activities may be impaired; caution patients accordingly and about possible additive effect of alcohol and other CNS depressants
Abrupt discontinuation of therapy	May produce withdrawal symptoms after chronic use, resulting in delirium, convulsions, or death
Special-risk patients	Use with caution in patients with severe hepatic impairment or respiratory difficulty (particularly status asthmaticus), in the presence of shock or uremia, or soon after administration of other respiratory depressants
Hypotension	May result from too rapid IV administration, particularly in patients with hypertension; administer slowly and with caution
Perivascular extravasation	May cause local tissue damage with subsequent necrosis
Intra-arterial injection	May cause transient pain, delayed hypnosis, pallor and cyanosis of the extremity, and patchy discoloration of the skin; stop injection immediately if patient complains of pain in the limb
Tartrazine sensitivity	Presence of FD&C Yellow No. 5 (tartrazine) in 30- and 100-mg capsules may cause allergic-type reactions, including bronchial asthma, in susceptible individuals

[1]Contains 18% alcohol

Table continued on following page

NEMBUTAL/NEMBUTAL SODIUM continued

ADVERSE REACTIONS

Central nervous system	Severe depression, drowsiness, lethargy, residual sedation ("hangover"), paradoxical excitement
Respiratory	Depression, apnea; coughing, hiccoughing, laryngospasm, and bronchospasm (with IV use)
Cardiovascular	Circulatory collapse
Dermatological	Rash
Neuromuscular	Chest-wall spasm (with IV use)
Other	Allergic reactions, pain at injection site, injury to nerves adjacent to injection site, thrombophlebitis (with IV use)

OVERDOSAGE

Signs and symptoms	Coma, early hypothermia, fever, sluggish or absent reflexes, respiratory depression, circulatory collapse, pulmonary edema
Treatment	Following acute ingestion, empty stomach immediately by gastric lavage, taking care to avoid pulmonary aspiration. Maintain and assist respiration, as indicated. Support circulation with vasopressors and IV fluids. Administer an osmotic diuretic and measure fluid intake and output. Employ dialysis, if indicated. Control pulmonary complications with antibiotics.

DRUG INTERACTIONS

Alcohol, tranquilizers, and other CNS depressants	⇧ CNS depression
Coumarin anticoagulants	⇩ Prothrombin time

ALTERED LABORATORY VALUES

No clinically significant alterations in blood/serum or urinary values occur at therapeutic dosages

Use in children

See INDICATIONS and ADMINISTRATION/DOSAGE ADJUSTMENTS for rectal use

Use in pregnancy or nursing mothers

Safe use not established during fetal development; doses exceeding 200 mg given during labor may result in neonatal depression; premature infants are particularly susceptible, and hence, caution should be taken when delivery of a premature infant is anticipated. Reduce dosage if a narcotic analgesic is given concomitantly. General guidelines not established for use in nursing mothers.

NOCTEC (Chloral hydrate) Squibb

Caps: 250, 500 mg **Syrup:** 500 mg/5 ml *C-IV*

INDICATIONS	ORAL DOSAGE
Nocturnal sedation **Preoperative sedation** **Postoperative medication** as an adjunct to opiates and analgesics **First stage of labor** when combined with a barbiturate	**Adult:** for sedation, 250 mg tid after meals; for hypnosis, 500 mg to 1 g 15-30 min before bedtime or 30 min before surgery, up to 2 g/day in a single dose or div **Child:** for sedation, 25 mg/kg/day, up to 500 mg/day, in a single dose or div; for hypnosis, 50 mg/kg/day, up to 1 g/day in a single dose or div

ADMINISTRATION/DOSAGE ADJUSTMENTS

Administration with fluids	Caps should be taken with a full glass (8 oz) of liquid; syrup may be administered in half a glass of water, fruit juice, or ginger ale

CONTRAINDICATIONS

Marked hepatic or renal impairment	Idiosyncratic reaction or hypersensitivity to chloral hydrate

WARNINGS/PRECAUTIONS

Habit-forming	Psychic and/or physical dependence and tolerance may develop, especially in addiction-prone individuals
Concomitant use of alcohol	Caution patient about additive CNS depressant effect of alcohol
Severe cardiac disease	Large doses should be avoided

ADVERSE REACTIONS

Gastrointestinal	Gastric irritation
Central nervous system	Excitement (rare), delirium (rare)

OVERDOSAGE

Signs and symptoms	Somnolence, deep sedation, stupor
Treatment	Empty stomach by gastric lavage. Employ supportive measures, as indicated.

DRUG INTERACTIONS

Alcohol, tranquilizers, and other CNS depressants	⇧ CNS depression
Coumarin anticoagulants	⇧ Prothrombin time (transient)

ALTERED LABORATORY VALUES

Urinary values	⇧ Glucose (with Benedict's solution) ⇧ Catecholamines (with fluorometric tests) ⇧ 17-Hydroxycorticosteroids (with Reddy, Jenkins, and Thorn procedure)

No clinically significant alterations in blood/serum values occur at therapeutic dosages

Use in children	Use in pregnancy or nursing mothers
See INDICATIONS	General guidelines not established for use in pregnant women (except during labor; see INDICATIONS) or in nursing mothers

NOLUDAR (Methyprylon) **Roche**

Tabs: 50, 200 mg *C-III*

NOLUDAR 300 (Methyprylon) **Roche**

Caps: 300 mg *C-III*

INDICATIONS	ORAL DOSAGE
Insomnia	**Adult:** 200–400 mg at bedtime **Child(>12 yr):** 50 mg at bedtime, or up to 200 mg, if required

ADMINISTRATION/DOSAGE ADJUSTMENTS

Duration of therapy	Prolonged use is usually not indicated and should only be undertaken concomitantly with appropriate evaluation; effectiveness lasts for at least 7 consecutive nights of drug administration

CONTRAINDICATIONS

Hypersensitivity to methyprylon

WARNINGS/PRECAUTIONS

Habit-forming	Psychic and/or physical dependence and tolerance may develop, especially in addiction-prone individuals
Mental impairment, reflex-slowing	Performance of potentially hazardous activities may be impaired; caution patients accordingly and about possible additive effect of alcohol and other CNS depressants
Withdrawal symptoms	May occur, resembling those associated with barbiturate withdrawal; treat similarly
Special-risk patients	Use with caution in patients with hepatic or renal disorders
Repeated or prolonged use	Perform blood counts periodically (see ADVERSE REACTIONS)

ADVERSE REACTIONS

Central nervous system	Morning drowsiness, dizziness, headache, paradoxical excitation
Gastrointestinal	Diarrhea, esophagitis, nausea, vomiting
Dermatological	Rash
Hematological	Neutropenia, thrombocytopenia (causal relationship not established)

OVERDOSAGE

Signs and symptoms	Somnolence, confusion, coma, miosis, respiratory depression, hypotension, excitation, convulsions
Treatment	Empty stomach immediately by gastric lavage, taking steps to prevent pulmonary aspiration. Maintain adequate airway, and administer appropriate IV fluids. Combat hypotension with levarterenol or metaraminol. Analeptic agents can be hazardous and are of little or no value in treating respiratory depression. Hemodialysis may be useful. For excitation and convulsions, use barbiturates with great caution.

DRUG INTERACTIONS

Alcohol, tranquilizers, and other CNS depressants	⇧ CNS depression

ALTERED LABORATORY VALUES

No clinically significant alterations in blood/serum or urinary values occur at therapeutic dosages

Use in children	Use in pregnancy or nursing mothers
Not recommended for children under 12 yr of age	Safe use not established; general guidelines not established for use in nursing mothers

PHENOBARBITAL various manufacturers

Tabs: 8, 15, 16, 30, 32, 60, 65, 100 mg **Caps:** 16 mg **Drops:** 16 mg/ml **Elixir:** 20 mg/5 ml *C-IV*

PHENOBARBITAL SODIUM various manufacturers

Amps: 65 mg/ml (2 ml), 130 mg/ml (1 ml), 163 mg/ml (2 ml) **Vials:** 65, 120, 130, 325 mg **Syringes:** 65 mg/ml (1 ml), 130 mg/ml (1 ml)
Cartridge-needle units: 30 mg/ml (1 ml) *C-IV*

INDICATIONS	ORAL DOSAGE	PARENTERAL DOSAGE
Daytime and postoperative sedation	**Adult:** 30–120 mg/day in 2–3 divided doses **Child:** 6 mg/kg/day in 3 divided doses	**Adult:** 32–100 mg IM **Child:** 8–30 mg IM
Preoperative sedation	—	**Adult:** 100–200 mg IM 60–90 min before surgery **Child:** 16–100 mg IM 60–90 min before surgery
Hypnosis	**Adult:** 100–320 mg at bedtime **Child:** adjust according to age and weight	**Adult:** 100–320 mg IM or IV (slowly) **Child:** 3–6 mg/kg IM or IV (slowly)

Note: Full chart appears on page 580

PLACIDYL (Ethchlorvynol) Abbott

Caps: 100, 200, 500, 750 mg *C-IV*

INDICATIONS	ORAL DOSAGE
Insomnia	**Adult:** 500–750 mg at bedtime for not more than 1 wk

ADMINISTRATION/DOSAGE ADJUSTMENTS

Severe insomnia	Up to 1,000 mg may be given as a single bedtime dose
Persistent insomnia	Allow a drug-free interval of 1 wk or more to elapse and further evaluate patient before prescribing a second course
Untimely awakening	A single supplemental dose of 100–200 mg may be given to reinstitute sleep
Elderly and/or debilitated individuals	The lowest effective dose should be given

CONTRAINDICATIONS

Hypersensitivity to ethchlorvynol ●

Porphyria ●

WARNINGS/PRECAUTIONS

Habit-forming	Psychic and/or physical dependence and tolerance may develop, especially in addiction-prone individuals
Prolonged use	May lead to chronic intoxication (see OVERDOSAGE)
Mental impairment, reflex-slowing	Performance of potentially hazardous activities may be impaired; caution patients accordingly and about possible additive effect of alcohol and other CNS depressants
Pain	Administer ethchlorvynol only if insomnia persists after pain is controlled with analgesics
Special-risk patients	Use with caution in the elderly and/or debilitated and in those with hepatic or renal functional impairment
Abrupt discontinuation	May produce severe withdrawal symptoms, including convulsions, delirium, schizoid reactions, perceptual distortions, memory loss, ataxia, insomnia, slurred speech, anxiety, irritability, agitation, tremors, anorexia, nausea, vomiting, weakness, dizziness, diaphoresis, muscle twitching, and weight loss. These symptoms may appear as late as 9 days after sudden withdrawal (see OVERDOSAGE).
Idiosyncratic behavior	Patients who behave unpredictably in response to alcohol or barbiturates or who exhibit paradoxical restlessness or excitement may react similarly to ethchlorvynol
Transient giddiness and ataxia	May result from especially rapid absorption; may be controlled in some cases by taking drug with food
Tartrazine sensitivity	Presence of FD&C Yellow No. 5 (tartrazine) in 750-mg capsules may cause allergic-type reactions, including bronchial asthma, in susceptible individuals

ADVERSE REACTIONS

Gastrointestinal	Nausea, vomiting, upset, aftertaste
Hepatic	Cholestatic jaundice
Central nervous system and neuromuscular	Dizziness, facial numbness, giddiness, ataxia, residual sedation ("hangover")
Ophthalmic	Blurred vision
Cardiovascular	Hypotension
Dermatological	Rash, urticaria
Hematological	Thrombocytopenia
Idiosyncratic	Mild stimulation, marked excitement, hysteria, prolonged hypnosis, profound muscle weakness, syncope without hypotension

Table continued on following page

PLACIDYL continued

OVERDOSAGE

Signs and symptoms	*Acute toxicity:* prolonged deep coma, severe respiratory depression, hypothermia, hypotension, bradycardia, nystagmus, pancytopenia, death; *Chronic toxicity:* incoordination, tremors, ataxia, confusion, slurred speech, hyperreflexia, diplopia, muscle weakness, amblyopia, scotoma, nystagmus, peripheral neuropathy
Treatment	*Acute toxicity:* Empty stomach immediately by gastric lavage. (In the unconscious patient, precede lavage by tracheal intubation with a cuffed tube.) Assist ventilation, monitor vital signs, and control blood pressure. Hemodialysis or peritoneal dialysis may be of value. Forced diuresis may also be useful. *Chronic toxicity:* Reduce dosage gradually over a period of days or weeks. For psychotic symptoms, add a phenothiazine compound to the regimen. Provide supportive care as indicated. *Withdrawal symptoms:* Readminister ethchlorvynol to level of chronic toxicity that existed before abrupt discontinuation. Treat chronic toxicity as stated above.

DRUG INTERACTIONS

Alcohol, tranquilizers, and other CNS depressants	⇧ CNS depression
MAO inhibitors	⇧ CNS depression
Coumarin anticoagulants	⇩ Prothrombin time
Tricyclic antidepressants	Transient delirium

ALTERED LABORATORY VALUES

No clinically significant alterations in blood/serum or urinary values occur at therapeutic dosages

Use in children

Not recommended; safety and effectiveness in pediatric age group have not been established

Use in pregnancy or nursing mothers

Not recommended for use during the 1st and 2nd trimesters of pregnancy; when taken during the 3rd trimester of pregnancy, may produce CNS depression and transient withdrawal symptoms in newborns. Safe use during lactation has not been established.

SECONAL (Secobarbital) **Lilly**

Elixir: 22 mg/5 ml[1] *C-II*

SECONAL SODIUM (Secobarbital sodium) **Lilly**

Caps: 50, 100 mg *C-II* **Vial:** 50 mg/ml (20 ml) *C-II* **Supp:** 30, 60, 120, 200 mg *C-III*

INDICATIONS	ORAL DOSAGE	PARENTERAL DOSAGE
Sedation	**Adult:** 20–40 mg of the elixir bid or tid **Child:** 7.5–30 mg, depending on age, weight, and degree of sedation desired	—
Preoperative sedation	**Adult:** 200–300 mg (caps) 1–2 h before surgery **Child:** 50–100 mg (caps) 1–2 h before surgery	See ADMINISTRATION/DOSAGE ADJUSTMENTS
Insomnia	**Adult:** 100 mg (caps) at bedtime for not more than 14 days	—
Hypnosis (adjunctive therapy)	—	See ADMINISTRATION/DOSAGE ADJUSTMENTS
Acute convulsive conditions associated with tetanus, status epilepticus, and strychnine or local anesthetic poisoning	—	**Adult:** 5.5 mg/kg IM or IV, repeated q3–4h, as needed **Child:** 3–5 mg/kg IM or IV, repeated q3–4h, as needed[2]

ADMINISTRATION/DOSAGE ADJUSTMENTS

Persistent insomnia	Allow a drug-free interval of 1 wk or more to elapse before considering retreatment; alternative, nonpharmacologic therapy should be sought for chronic cases
Parenteral administration	May be used as supplied or diluted with Sterile Water for Injection, 0.9% Sodium Chloride Injection, or Ringer's Injection. If IM route is used, inject deeply into a large muscle mass and do not give more than 5 ml (regardless of dilution) at any one site.
Basal hypnosis for anesthesia or intubation procedures	Administer up to 250 mg IV at a rate not exceeding 50 mg/15 s. If hypnosis is inadequate with a total dose of 250 mg, a small quantity of meperidine may be added. As an adjunct to spinal or regional anesthesia, only 50–100 mg of secobarbital sodium is usually required.
Dental procedures	For sedation of apprehensive patients, both child and adult, administer 1 mg/lb IM 10–15 min before start of procedure. For light sedation, 0.5–0.75 mg/lb will suffice. For patients receiving nerve blocks, 100–150 mg IV may be given. If nitrous oxide is used, administer injection as suggested for anesthetic procedures.
Rectal use	For hypnosis in children prior to ear, nose, and throat procedures, the 5% solution should be diluted with lukewarm water to a concentration of 1–1.5%. Following a cleansing enema, a child weighing <40 kg may receive 5 mg/kg, along with atropine. Rectal suppositories may be employed for insomnia, preoperative sedation, or sedation in obstetrics. Suggested dosages are: infants (<6 mo), 15–60 mg; child (6 mo to 3 yr), 60 mg; older children, 60–120 mg; adults, 120–200 mg. These dosages should be adjusted according to the patient's general condition, degree of sedation or hypnosis desired, and clinical response.
Elderly or debilitated patients	Reduce dosage significantly

CONTRAINDICATIONS

Sensitivity to barbiturates	Prior addiction to sedative/hypnotics	Respiratory or cardiac disease (if more than minimal)
History of porphyria	Acute or chronic pain	

WARNINGS/PRECAUTIONS

Habit-forming	Psychic and/or physical dependence and tolerance may develop, especially in addiction-prone individuals
Mental impairment, reflex-slowing	Performance of potentially hazardous activities may be impaired; caution patients accordingly and about possible additive effect of alcohol and other CNS depressants
Hepatic or renal impairment	Use with extreme caution and observe for signs of excessive drug accumulation (see OVERDOSAGE)

[1]Contains 44 mg/ml methenamine, glycerin, and 12% alcohol
[2]*United States Pharmacopeia Dispensing Information 1980.* Rockville, Md, The United States Pharmacopeial Convention, Inc, 1980, p 456

Table continued on following page

WARNINGS/PRECAUTIONS continued

Excessive narcosis	May follow IM injection of large hypnotic doses; observe patients for 20–30 min after administration
Overly rapid IV administration	May cause respiratory depression or apnea, laryngospasm, or vasodilation with hypotension (see ADMINISTRATION/DOSAGE ADJUSTMENTS)
Withdrawal symptoms	May occur after chronic use of large doses, resulting in delirium, convulsions, or death
Hypersensitivity reactions	May occur, especially in patients with asthma, urticaria, or angioneurotic edema

ADVERSE REACTIONS

Central nervous system	Residual sedation ("hangover"), drowsiness, lethargy (with oral use)
Gastrointestinal	Nausea (with IV use), vomiting (with IV use)
Cardiorespiratory	Respiratory depression; apnea; laryngospasm (with IV use); rarely, postoperative atelectasis and circulatory disturbances (with IV use); vasodilation and hypotension following rapid IV administration
Allergic	Hypersensitivity reactions, skin eruptions (with oral use)
Idiosyncratic	Excitement, "hangover," and pain (with IV use)

OVERDOSAGE

Signs and symptoms	*Oral overdose:* hypothermia, followed by fever, sluggish or absent reflexes, respiratory depression, circulatory collapse, pulmonary edema, and coma; *parenteral overdose:* respiratory depression, depressed superficial and deep reflexes, miosis or (in severe cases) mydriasis, decreased urine formation, hypothermia, and coma
Treatment	Maintain patent airway, assist ventilation, and administer oxygen, as needed. Empty stomach by gastric lavage. Administer IV fluids, as needed. Control blood pressure and body temperature. Dialysis may be helpful. Antibiotics may be needed to control pulmonary complications.

DRUG INTERACTIONS

Alcohol, tranquilizers, and other CNS depressants	⇧ CNS depression
Coumarin anticoagulants	⇩ Prothrombin time

ALTERED LABORATORY VALUES

No clinically significant alterations in blood/serum or urinary values occur at therapeutic dosages

Use in children

See INDICATIONS and ADMINISTRATION/DOSAGE ADJUSTMENTS for dosage recommendations; safety and effectiveness of oral dosage forms in children have not been established

Use in pregnancy or nursing mothers

Safe use has not been established during pregnancy. If drug is administered, fetal heart should be monitored carefully and oxygen given to the mother if slowing or irregularities develop. The parenteral form is contraindicated in obstetric deliveries. Use with caution in nursing mothers.

Product (Manufacturer)	Ingredients	Actions
Compoz (Jeffrey Martin) Tablets **Dosage** 2 tabs at bedtime, or as directed by physician	15 mg Methapyrilene hydrochloride	Antihistamine
	10 mg Pyrilamine maleate	Antihistamine
Nervine (Miles) Tablets **Dosage** 2 tabs at bedtime, or as directed by physician	25 mg Methapyrilene hydrochloride	Antihistamine
Nytol (Block) Tablets **Dosage** 2 tabs or 1 cap 20 minutes before bedtime	Methapyrilene hydrochloride (tabs: 25 mg; caps: 50 mg)	Antihistamine
Sleep-Eze (Whitehall) Tablets **Dosage** 1-2 tabs with water at bedtime	25 mg Pyrilamine maleate	Antihistamine
Sominex (J.B. Williams) Tablets **Dosage** 2 tabs with water at bedtime	0.25 Aminoxide hydrobromide	Agent that blocks the parasympathetic nerves
	25 mg Methapyrilene hydrochloride	Antihistamine
	200 mg Salicylamide	Analgesic
Twilight (Pfeiffer) Tablets **Dosage** 2 caps at bedtime, or as directed by physician	25 mg Methapyrilene hydrochloride	Antihistamine
	300 mg Salicylamide	Analgesic

Childhood Emotional and Behavior Problems

In recent years, it has become increasingly evident that children, even very young ones, are as vulnerable to psychological problems like anxiety and depression as adolescents and adults. In addition, children are susceptible to other poorly understood disorders, such as hyperactivity, that may have an organic origin but may lead to psychological and behavioral problems. Two of the more common childhood emotional and behavioral disorders—depression and hyperactivity—are reviewed in this section.

CHILDHOOD DEPRESSION

Diagnosis

How can parents determine whether a child is suffering from depression or just having a "moody" spell that is simply a normal part of growing up? Dr. Aaron Beck, a psychiatrist at the University of Pennsylvania who has studied depression in children and adults for more than twenty years, concludes that children are clinically depressed if they are obviously sad over a period of weeks and this overriding sadness is accompanied by a sense of worthlessness and a feeling that no one cares whether they live or die. These feelings are usually combined with behavioral and other symptoms of depression: eating problems, fatigue, insomnia (or excessive sleeping), failure to develop or achieve at previous levels, periods of seemingly unprovoked agitation, and a withdrawal from friends and playmates. Family efforts to improve the situation often prove unsuccessful, and in many instances, the youngster may speak about or attempt suicide. In fact, suicide has become one of the leading causes of death among children ten years old and above.

Opinions differ about the cause or causes of childhood depression. Depression, as stressed in the earlier section on *Anxiety, Depression, and Psychotic Disorders*, is an organic illness that may be triggered by any of a number of life situations.

In classic cases of childhood depression, the youngster has been subject to a stressful situation such as the loss of a parent through death or divorce, a continuous feeling of inadequacy because of unachievable expectations, or a combination of factors, organic and circumstantial, that cause the child to see nothing ahead but defeat and failure.

Treatment of Childhood Depression

The most effective therapy seems to consist of the administration of antidepressant medication, closely monitored and adjusted to the child's physical and psychological responses, combined with some form of psychotherapy for the child and the family. Whatever underlying factors are brought to light by psychotherapy, the current prevailing opinion is that when depression is identified in children, the careful administration of antidepressant drugs makes a qualitative difference in their recovery.

HYPERACTIVITY

One of the most common childhood behavioral problems is a complex, little-understood disorder known as hyperactivity or hyperkinesis. (Hyperactivity until recently also was referred to as minimal brain dysfunction, but the currently preferred term is attention deficit disorder.) In many instances, what passes for hyperactivity is really depression—the agitated behavior is the child's way of masking the feelings of sadness or worthlessness. However, it is generally agreed that hyperactivity or hyperkinesis is an organic illness affecting an estimated two and a half million youngsters. Dr. Ronald Lipman of the National Institute of Mental Health has estimated that 1 to 5 percent of all American children suffer from the disorder. The symptoms of hyperactivity include a constant state of physical and emotional agitation, unusual impulsiveness, excitability, and above all, an inability to sit still and concentrate. In other words, these children cannot ignore distractions or focus on a particular circumstance or problem. These children have a profoundly disruptive effect in the classroom and at home, and they pose a challenge to medical and behavioral specialists. Parents often find it beneficial to exchange information and experiences with others with similar problems. To facilitate this, parents can contact The Association for Children with Learning Disabilities, 4156 Library Road, Pittsburgh, Pa. 15234.

In a significant number of cases, the disorder manifests itself in infancy with a pattern of restlessness and fretfulness so demanding that parents seek medical help. At any rate, it is almost always identified during the early school years. While no specific cause has yet been isolated and no single cure or treatment is effective in all cases, it is believed that early identification and a combination of therapies can keep the child functioning well enough to prevent the development of the low self-esteem that both results from and perpetuates the disorder.

Diagnosis

In attempting to make a correct diagnosis, it is extremely important that other physical or emotional causes of abnormal behavior be investigated and eliminated. Manifest brain damage, depression, specific learning disabilities, or a hearing loss can sometimes produce the erratic behavior that results from frustration rather than from true hyperkinesis.

Treatment

Once a diagnosis of hyperactivity has been established, treatment should begin without further delay. In many instances, a stimulant drug such as methylphenidate (Ritalin) will be prescribed. It is not fully understood why, in these circumstances, a stimulant should have a calming effect, but it does. The drugs do not cure the hyperactivity, but they modify behavior to the point where other functions improve. Since side effects of these drugs include possible interference with sleep and growth, constant supervision of dosage is critical.

If the full benefits of medication are to be realized, close attention should also be given to supportive therapies, such as a remedial learning program to help the child stay as close as possible to his or her classmates. Parents may also benefit from instruction in the techniques of behavior modification—a system of rewards and punishments to help the child understand why some types of behavior are not desirable.

Alternative Therapies

A number of alternative approaches to treating hyperactivity have been tried, often with mixed or controversial results. One that is a continuing source of controversy involves administering a diet free of all food additives, such as dyes and certain other substances. This approach, the Feingold diet, named for the physician who developed it, has never been proven effective by scientific studies, but there are numerous anecdotal accounts of improvement (as well as failure) attributed to its use. Various behavior modification techniques also have been attempted, with some individual successes, but again, none of these have been proved effective in large numbers of children.

IN CONCLUSION

Many children are susceptible to depression and other psychological disorders generally thought of as adult diseases. Parents and physicians should be particularly alert to the possibility of childhood depression—a disorder that appears to be increasingly common, as witnessed by the rising incidence of suicide among even young children. In most instances, carefully monitored doses of the antidepressant drugs used to treat adults produce cures. (See the section on *Anxiety, Depression, and Psychotic Disorders*, pages 736-807, for a listing of these agents.) The following drug charts cover the major agents prescribed to treat hyperactivity.

CYLERT (Pemoline) Abbott

Tabs: 18.75, 37.5, 75 mg **Tabs (chewable):** 37.5 mg *C-IV*

INDICATIONS

Attention deficit disorder (hyperkinetic syndrome, minimal brain dysfunction, hyperkinetic reaction of childhood, hyperactive child syndrome, minimal brain damage, minimal cerebral dysfunction, minor cerebral dysfunction)

ORAL DOSAGE

Child (>6 yr): 37.5 mg/day qd in AM to start, followed by weekly increments of 18.7 mg/day up to a total of 112.5 mg/day or until desired clinical response is achieved; usual maintenance dosage: 56.25–75 mg/day

ADMINISTRATION/DOSAGE ADJUSTMENTS

Onset of improvement	Significant benefit may not be evident until 3rd or 4th week of therapy
Duration of therapy	Interrupt therapy occasionally to determine whether symptoms recur, warranting continued therapy

CONTRAINDICATIONS

Hypersensitivity or idiosyncrasy to pemoline

WARNINGS/PRECAUTIONS

Psychotic children	Symptoms of behavior disturbance and thought disorder may be exacerbated
Growth inhibition	May occur during prolonged therapy, although present data are inadequate; monitor growth rate during treatment
Drug dependence	Psychic and/or physical dependence may occur; use with caution in emotionally unstable patients
Renal or hepatic impairment	Use with caution in patients with significant dysfunction
Hepatic abnormalities developing during therapy	Perform liver-function tests before and during therapy; if abnormalities are revealed and confirmed by follow-up tests, discontinue therapy

ADVERSE REACTIONS

Central nervous system	Insomnia; increased irritability; mild depression; dizziness; headache; drowsiness; hallucinations; dyskinetic movements of the tongue, lips, face, and extremities; nystagmus; nystagmoid eye movements; convulsive seizures (causal relationship of last four reactions not established)
Gastrointestinal	**Anorexia, weight loss, stomach ache, nausea, jaundice (causal relationship not established)**
Dermatological	Skin rash

OVERDOSAGE

Signs and symptoms	Agitation, restlessness, hallucinations, dyskinetic movements, tachycardia
Treatment	Induce emesis or perform gastric lavage to empty stomach, and institute appropriate supportive measures. Animal studies indicate that hemodialysis may be useful; forced diuresis and peritoneal dialysis are of little value.

DRUG INTERACTIONS

No clinically significant drug interactions have been observed

ALTERED LABORATORY VALUES

Blood/serum values	⇧ SGOT ⇧ SGPT ⇧ Lactate dehydrogenase

No clinically significant alterations in urinary values occur at therapeutic dosages

Use in children

See INDICATIONS; prescription of this drug should take into account the chronicity and severity of the child's symptoms and their appropriateness for his or her age. Pemoline should not be used in children under 6 yr of age or, in most cases, for symptoms associated with acute stress reactions. Long-term effects in children are unknown.

Use in pregnancy or nursing mothers

Safe use not established during pregnancy. Studies in rats have shown an increased incidence of stillbirths and cannibalization and reduced postnatal survival of offspring. General guidelines not established for use in nursing mothers.

DEXEDRINE (Dextroamphetamine sulfate) Smith Kline & French

Tabs: 5 mg **Caps (sust rel):** 5, 10, 15 mg **Elixir:** 5 mg/5 ml *C-II*

INDICATIONS	ORAL DOSAGE
Behavioral syndrome in children	**Child (3-5 yr):** 2.5 mg/day to start, followed by weekly increments of 2.5 mg/day until optimal response is obtained **Child (6-12 yr):** 5 mg qd or bid to start, followed by weekly increments of 5 mg/day until optimal response is obtained; sust-rel caps: 5 mg qd to start, followed by weekly increments of 5 mg/day, where appropriate

ADMINISTRATION/DOSAGE ADJUSTMENTS

Insomnia or anorexia	Dosage should be reduced if bothersome adverse reactions appear; late-evening doses tend to cause insomnia, particularly with sust-rel caps, and should be avoided
Child dosage intervals	With tablets or elixir, give 1st dose on awakening and 1-2 additional doses at intervals of 4-6 h
Duration of therapy for behavioral syndrome in children	Interrupt therapy occasionally to determine whether symptoms recur, warranting continued administration

Use in children

See INDICATIONS; prescription of this drug for behavioral syndrome in children should take into account the chronicity and severity of the child's symptoms and their appropriateness for his or her age. Dextroamphetamine should not be used in children under 3 yr of age or, in most cases, for symptoms associated with acute stress reactions. The drug is also not recommended for use as an anorectic in children under 12 yr of age. In psychotic children, use of amphetamines may exacerbate behavior disturbances and thought disorder. Growth should be monitored during treatment. Long-term effects in children are unknown.

Use in pregnancy or nursing mothers

Safe use has not been established. Animal reproductive studies have suggested embryotoxicity and teratogenicity. Drug should not be used by women who are or may become pregnant, especially during 1st trimester, unless potential benefit clearly outweighs possible risk to fetus. General guidelines not established for use in nursing mothers.

Note: Full chart appears on page 626.

RITALIN (Methylphenidate hydrochloride) **Ciba**

Tabs: 5, 10, 20 mg *C-II*

INDICATIONS	ORAL DOSAGE
Attention deficit disorder (minimal brain dysfunction, hyperkinetic child syndrome, minimal brain damage, minimal cerebral dysfunction, minor cerebral dysfunction) **Narcolepsy** **Mild depression**[1] **Apathetic or withdrawn senile behavior**[1]	**Adult:** 20–30 mg/day in 2–3 divided doses, preferably 30–45 min before meals; some patients may need only 10–15 mg/day, while others may require 40–60 mg/day **Child (>6 yr):** 5 mg before breakfast and lunch to start, followed by gradual increases of 5–10 mg/wk up to 60 mg/day; if no improvement after 1 mo, discontinue therapy

ADMINISTRATION/DOSAGE ADJUSTMENTS

Insomnia	Instruct patient to take last dose before 6 PM
Paradoxical aggravation of symptoms	Reduce dosage or, if necessary, discontinue drug
Duration of therapy	Interrupt therapy occasionally to determine whether symptoms recur, warranting continued therapy. Therapy should not be indefinite and may usually be discontinued in children after puberty.

CONTRAINDICATIONS

Severe exogenous or endogenous depression ●

Marked anxiety, tension, and agitation ●

Hypersensitivity to methylphenidate ●

Glaucoma ●

WARNINGS/PRECAUTIONS

Growth suppression	May occur with long-term therapy; weight gain and growth rate in children should be carefully monitored
Agitated patients	May react adversely; discontinue therapy if necessary
Psychotic children	Symptoms of behavior disturbance and thought disorder may be exacerbated
Seizures	May occur in patients with a history of seizures or EEG abnormalitites or, rarely, with neither; discontinue therapy
Blood pressure	Should be monitored, especially in hypertensive patients; use with caution in the presence of hypertension
Drug dependence	Marked tolerance and psychic dependence may develop with chronic abuse; use with caution in emotionally unstable individuals or where there is a history of drug dependence or alcoholism. Drug withdrawal may precipitate severe depression or unmask the effects of chronic overactivity; provide close supervision.
Prolonged therapy	Perform CBC, differential, and platelet count periodically
Tartrazine sensitivity	Presence of FD&C Yellow No. 5 (tartrazine) in 5- and 20-mg tablets may cause allergic-type reactions, including bronchial asthma, in susceptible individuals
Inappropriate indications	Methylphenidate should not be used to prevent or treat normal fatigue

ADVERSE REACTIONS

Central nervous system	Nervousness, insomnia,[2] dizziness, headache, dyskinesia, drowsiness, toxic psychosis
Ophthalmic	Accommodation difficulties and blurred vision (rare)
Gastrointestinal	Anorexia,[2] nausea, abdominal pain,[2] weight loss during prolonged therapy[2]
Cardiovascular	Palpitations, blood pressure and pulse changes, tachycardia,[2] angina, arrhythmias
Hematological	Leukopenia and/or anemia (causal relationship not established)
Hypersensitivity	Skin rash, urticaria, fever, arthralgia, exfoliative dermatitis, erythema multiforme with histopathologic findings of necrotizing vasculitis, thrombocytopenic purpura
Other	Scalp hair loss (causal relationship not established)

DRUG INTERACTIONS

Guanethidine	⇩ Antihypertensive effect
Vasopressors	⇧ Pressor effect
MAO inhibitors	⇧ Risk of hypertensive crisis
Oral anticoagulants	⇧ Prothrombin time
Phenobarbital, phenytoin, primidone	⇧ Anticonvulsant blood levels
Imipramine, desipramine	⇧ Antidepressant blood levels

[1]Possibly effective
[2]Occurs more frequently in children

Table continued on following page

RITALIN continued

ALTERED LABORATORY VALUES

No clinically significant alterations in blood/serum or urinary values occur at therapeutic dosages

OVERDOSAGE

Signs and symptoms	Vomiting, agitation, tremors, hyperreflexia, muscle twitching, convulsions (may be followed by coma), euphoria, confusion, hallucinations, delirium, sweating, flushing, headache, hyperpyrexia, tachycardia, palpitations, cardiac arrhythmias, hypertension, mydriasis, dryness of mucous membranes
Treatment	Institute appropriate supportive measures. Protect patient against self-injury and against external stimuli that would aggravate overstimulation. If signs and symptoms are not too severe and patient is conscious, induce emesis or perform gastric lavage to empty stomach. If severe, administer a carefully titrated dose of a *short-acting* barbiturate before performing gastric lavage. Maintain adequate circulation and respiratory exchange. External cooling procedures may be required for hyperpyrexia. Efficacy of hemodialysis or peritoneal dialysis has not been established.

Use in children

See INDICATIONS; prescription of this drug should take into account the chronicity and severity of the child's symptoms and their appropriateness for his or her age. Methylphenidate should not be used in children under 6 yr of age or, in most cases, for symptoms associated with acute stress reactions. Long-term effects in children are unknown.

Use in pregnancy or nursing mothers

Safe use not established during pregnancy; general guidelines not established for use in nursing mothers

Contraception

No single method of birth control is ideal for everyone—the best choice of a contraceptive depends on many factors, including age, frequency of sexual activity, number of sexual partners, general health, and desire for future parenthood.

In prescribing a contraceptive, physicians also consider the effectiveness, safety, and convenience of the method in addition to the patient's motivation, medical needs, personal habits, and life-style. The best choice is a contraceptive that is as effective and safe as possible, yet one that the person will use consistently and comfortably.

Although research efforts are aimed at developing new methods of birth control—including such things as a safe "morning-after pill," antipregnancy vaccines, and a pill for males—these are not on the immediate horizon. Presently available contraceptives fall into the following categories: (1) oral contraceptives or "the pill"; (2) intrauterine devices (IUD); (3) barrier methods, which include diaphragms and condoms; (4) chemical methods, which include jellies, creams, foams, and suppositories; (5) natural methods, such as rhythm and withdrawal; and (6) operative procedures, i.e., sterilization via tubal ligation or vasectomy. This discussion will focus on the various medical means of contraception, rather than the natural and operative procedures.

SAFETY, EFFECTIVENESS, AND CONVENIENCE

The major considerations in selecting a method of birth control are safety, effectiveness, and convenience. Effectiveness of a method depends highly upon the way in which it is used. A method may have a high degree of "theoretical" or potential effectiveness, yet may frequently fail, often because it is inconvenient. This is particularly true with the barrier methods, which may have a theoretical effectiveness of close to 99 percent, yet a failure rate in actual use of 30 percent or more. This disparity is explained primarily by inconsistent or improper use of the method.

When it comes to safety, the barrier contraceptives carry the least, if any, risk of medical complications of all contraceptive methods, while IUDs and oral contraceptives carry the greatest risk. Tables 1 and 2 summarize the comparative effectiveness and safety of the various methods of contraception.

ORAL CONTRACEPTIVES

Since the introduction of oral contraceptives more than twenty years ago, "the pill" has become the most widely used method of birth control among young American women. It is the most effective reversible contraceptive, with a generally reported annual failure rate of only one or two pregnancies per 100 users. Many of these pregnancies can be traced to skipped pills or a dosage that is too low.

Two types of oral contraceptives are now used: the combination pill, which contains both a synthetic estrogen (i.e., mestranol or ethinyl estradiol) and a progestogen (e.g., norethindrone), and the progestogen-only pill (the so-called minipill), which contains only progestogen, a synthetic progestational agent such as norethindrone or norgestrel. The combination pill is the more widely used oral contraceptive, as well as the more effective of the two types of pills.

Mechanisms of Action

The synthetic estrogen and progestogen in the combination oral contraceptives work primarily by inhibiting ovulation — the maturation and release of the egg from the ovary. The systemic effects of these pills simulate pregnancy; therefore, the pill may produce nausea, bloating, and some of the other side effects of early pregnancy. These effects usually diminish with continued use of the combination pill. An additional contraceptive effect results from an alteration in the mucous secretions, which creates a "hostile" environment for sperm.

The progestogen-only pills work primarily by altering mucous secretions from the cervix to form a physical barrier to sperm penetration and, by al-

Table 1: Comparative Rates of Effectiveness

Method	Number of Pregnancies per 100 Women During the First Year of Use
Oral Contraceptives	Less than 1 to 3
IUD	2 to 3
Condom	3 to 36
Diaphragm (with spermicidal cream or jelly)	2 to 20
Spermicidal foam	2 to 29
Spermicidal jelly or cream	4 to 36

Taken from Population Reports, Series B, No. 2; Series H, Nos. 2–4; and Series I, No. 1. *Population Information Program*, George Washington University Medical Center, Washington, D.C.

Table 2: Relative Risk of Death (per 100,000 Nonsterile Women per Year)

	Death Due to				
Age	**Pregnancy**	**Pill (Non-Smokers)**	**Pill (Smokers)**	**IUD**	**Barriers**
15–19	5.6	1.3	1.5	0.9	0
20–29	13.5	2.8	3.2	2.2	0
30–34	13.9	2.2	10.8	1.4	0
35–44	43.4	11.6	72.3	3.9	0

Taken from Tietze, C. *Family Planning Perspective* 9:74–76, 1977.

tering the lining of the uterus, to prevent implantation if fertilization does occur.

Dosages

The amounts of synthetic estrogen and progestogen vary among the different combination products. Since there have been reports of an increased risk of complications, such as blood clotting (thromboembolic) disorders, including stroke and heart attacks, with the higher estrogen dosage, those pills containing low amounts of estrogen are usually preferred as the initial choices of pills. Physicians usually recommend a combination pill containing 50 micrograms (μg), or less, of estrogen.

The major disadvantage to the low-estrogen combination pills is breakthrough bleeding (bleeding between periods), which is more frequent with the lower dosage of estrogen, but which usually lessens or ceases with continued use. Breakthrough bleeding, however, can lead some women to discontinue use or switch to a product containing more estrogen.

Combination pills are given for three weeks (twenty or twenty-one days). Menstrual-like bleeding usually occurs during the one week when the patient is off the pill. For convenience, some manufacturers also make a twenty-eight-day packet of pills, which contains twenty-one active pills and seven pills that contain iron or no active medication.

The progestogen-only pills are most frequently prescribed for women who, for medical reasons, avoid the combination pills. They are taken every day, without any period of cessation such as with combination pills. There is a higher incidence of irregular bleeding with these pills, and a pregnancy rate of about 2 to 8 percent a year.

Missed Pills

The risk of pregnancy increases with each pill missed. If one pill is missed, the user is usually advised to take that pill as soon as she remembers, in addition to her regular pill at the regular time for that day. A woman who misses two pills in a row is usually advised to take one extra pill per day until she "catches up," as well as to use an additional method of contraception for the remainder of the cycle.

Who Should Use Oral Contraceptives

Combination oral contraceptives are recommended primarily for young, healthy, sexually active women. They should not be used by women with a history of clotting disorder (thromboembolism) or coronary artery or cerebrovascular disease. They are also contraindicated for use by women with breast cancer, liver disorders, or any unexplained vaginal bleeding which might indicate the presence of a disease. Women who have diabetes, elevated cholesterol or other blood lipids, or who smoke, particularly those over the age of thirty-five, are usually advised not to use combination oral contraceptives. (More detailed information on hormone content and contraindications is provided in the individual drug charts.)

The potential side effects a woman may experience from oral contraceptives are related directly to her reaction to the progestogen and estrogen in the particular product. The synthetic progestogens may produce so-called androgenic (masculine) effects, such as acne, muscle cramps, weight gain, hairiness (hirsutism), and scanty periods. Norethindrone, the progestogen used in Ortho-Novum 135, Norlestrin, and Norinyl, tends to produce greater androgenic effects than norethynodrel or ethynodiol diacetate, the progestogens found in Enovid, Demulen, or Ovulen. Pills in which estrogenic (feminine) effects are dominant may produce heavier periods, nausea, and fluid retention, which may lead to swollen, tender breasts.

To some extent, side effects depend upon the woman's innate (endogenous) levels of estrogen and progesterone. If a woman normally has scanty periods and profuse hair, for example, it may be assumed that progesterone is dominant over estrogen. For such a woman, some physicians favor the estrogen-dominant pills to balance her natural excess of progesterone. (See Table 3.) Serious adverse reactions such as severe pain and swelling of the legs, severe headache, or blurred vision, should be reported to a physician immediately, as they may be signs of incipient thromboembolism. Minor side effects lasting more than two or three cycles should also be reported to the physician.

Reversibility

After discontinuing the pill, it may take several

Table 3: Oral Contraceptive Side Effects Caused by Hormonal Imbalances

Estrogen Excess	Estrogen Deficiency	Progesterone Excess	Progesterone Deficiency
Nausea	Breakthrough bleeding (days 1–14 of cycle)	Tiredness	Weight loss
Vomiting		Fatigue	Decreased breast size
Irritability		Depression	
Headache		Acne	Breakthrough bleeding (days 15–21 of cycle)
Edema		Lowered libido	
Leg cramps		Hairiness	
Bloating		Muscle cramps	
Clear vaginal discharge		Weight gain	
Hypertension			

Adapted from Dickey, R.P. *"The Pill—Physiology, Pharmacology and Clinical Use."* Chicago: Seminar in Family Planning, 1971, pp. 18-40.

months for a woman's reproductive cycle to return to its usual state. If menstruation does not resume within three months after cessation of pill use, the advice of a physician should be sought. In some cases, treatment may be required to induce ovulation, assuming that pregnancy is desired at that time.

Other Considerations

In recent years, there have been reports linking oral contraceptives to an increased risk of various types of cancer. This remains an area of considerable controversy and debate, with no conclusive answers. There are certain types of cancer that are triggered or stimulated by estrogen, and in these instances, oral contraceptives obviously should not be used. This is why they are contraindicated in women with a history of breast cancer. But there is no firm data indicating that oral contraceptives cause or increase the risk of cancer among women in general.

THE INTRAUTERINE DEVICE

IUDs are plastic devices of various shapes and sizes, designed to be inserted into the uterus by a physician to prevent conception. The IUDs appear to work by a variety of mechanisms to prevent a fertilized egg from becoming implanted in the uterus.

Types of IUDs

There are three types of IUDs in common use in the United States: (1) the inert IUDs (Saf-T-Coil and Lippes Loop), (2) the copper-bearing IUDs (Cu-7 and Tatum-T), and (3) the progestogen-releasing IUD (Progestasert). The copper-bearing IUDs have a copper wire wrapped around the plastic of their vertical limbs, which is believed to enhance the contraceptive effect. The progesterone-releasing IUD is a "T"-shaped plastic device, which releases small amounts of the hormone for up to about one year, altering the mucous secretions. Replacement after one year is usually recommended.

Special Considerations

Spontaneous expulsion is a potential drawback of the IUD, since the user may be unaware that the IUD is no longer in place. The IUD user should be taught, therefore, to check regularly—particularly after each menstural period—for the thread that is attached to the end of the IUD, to be certain that it is still in place.

Contraindications

The IUD is not recommended for women with endometriosis, venereal disease, a history of pelvic inflammatory disease, or for women with excessively heavy menstrual flow or cramping. The copper-bearing IUDs should not be used by women with a known allergy to copper, or those with a rare disorder known as Wilson's disease.

Possible Adverse Reactions

Major medical complications of the IUD include infection and, more rarely, perforation. There is an increased risk of both ectopic pregnancies and pelvic inflammatory diseases in women using IUDs. Perforations of the uterine and abdominal cavity have occurred either at the time of insertion or spontaneously at a later time.

Some women also experience considerable bleeding, cramping, and/or backache following insertion. There may be heavier and more irregular periods and/or more intense and prolonged cramps for the first three to six months, with bleeding possibly occurring between periods.

Should the IUD fail to provide contraceptive protection and the user become pregnant, the device should be removed as soon as possible to reduce the risk of sepsis (widespread infection) and spontaneous abortion (miscarriage). If the woman wishes to terminate the pregnancy, she should undergo induced abortion, with the removal of the IUD as soon as possible.

BARRIER METHODS

The barrier methods include the diaphragm (which should always be used with spermicidal cream or jelly) and the condom. These methods are among the safest means of birth control, and, if used properly and consistently, are highly effective.

The Condom

The condom (male sheath or "rubber") was first mass-produced as a contraceptive in about 1860, making it one of the early important methods of birth control. Condoms are usually made of a strong latex rubber, or, less commonly, of animal membranes, and are available with or without lubrication. They are designed to cover the erect penis, sometimes with a small outpouching at the closed end to collect the ejaculate and help keep the condom from bursting. Most are intended for one-time use, although high-quality products may be used several times, if they are well cared for.

Condoms have the distinct advantage of protecting against the spread of venereal disease, and it is for this reason that they are sometimes referred to as "prophylactics." Among the reputed disadvantages of condoms is that they reduce sensation and spontaneity of lovemaking. Condoms can be purchased in pharmacies and various nonprescription outlets, usually in packages of three or twelve, and they have a shelf life of two years. Condoms should never be used with any petroleum jelly products (e.g., Vaseline) since these will disintegrate rubber. Lubricated condoms, or surgical lubricating jellies (e.g., K-Y jelly), may be used.

The Diaphragm

The diaphragm is a shallow rubber cup with a flexible rim, designed to fit snugly in the vagina so as to cover the cervix (opening to the uterus). Diaphragms come in several sizes and require fitting by a physician or other family planning clinician.

There are several types of diaphragms with different degrees of rim flexibility. The clinician can usually judge which type of diaphragm is best for an individual woman, although some will have the patient try several and judge for herself which one is most comfortable and easiest to insert.

To be effective, the diaphragm must always be used with a spermicidal jelly or cream, which is spread around the dome and the rim. When in place, the diaphragm acts as a barrier keeping sperm from entering the cervical canal. The spermicidal jelly or cream acts as additional protection, killing any sperm that might get past the rim of the diaphragm. The diaphragm should remain in place at least six to eight hours following the last act of intercourse, since sperm can survive this long in the vagina.

When properly fitted, cared for, and used as directed, the diaphragm is highly effective. Failure may be the result of improper fit, faulty insertion, inadequate washing, ineffective cream or jelly, removal too soon after intercourse, or nonuse. The diaphragm user should be re-examined yearly, and she should be refitted after a pregnancy or after a gain or loss of ten or more pounds.

Disadvantages of the diaphragm are that the insertion, for some couples, interrupts the spontaneity of the sex act and the requirement that cream or jelly be added for each act of intercourse is felt by some women to be "messy."

CHEMICAL METHODS

Foams, Creams, Jellies, and Suppositories

There are many nonprescription products that, when inserted into the vagina, kill sperm on contact. The use of spermicide alone is not as effective in preventing pregnancy as when they are used with the diaphragm or condom. (Two methods are always more effective than one.) Foam may be slightly more effective than jelly or cream because it spreads more readily throughout the vagina.

Nonfoaming spermicides such as melting suppositories should be inserted at least fifteen minutes before intercourse so that the agent will disperse throughout the vagina. The application should be repeated with each act of intercourse. In addition, a woman should not douche for at least six hours to allow enough time for total immobilization of all sperm still in the vagina. Since each spermicide differs somewhat, the user should read the individual instructions carefully before using. On occasion, individuals misapply a method, such as inserting a vaginal suppository into the urethra.

A major advantage of spermicides is that they are readily available without a prescription or medical examination. They may also provide some degree of protection against contracting venereal disease.

IN CONCLUSION

Selection of a birth-control method depends upon a number of individual considerations. The following drug charts give detailed information on oral contraceptives, which are available only by prescription. The nonprescription contraceptives—condoms and chemical spermicides to be used alone or with a diaphragm—are summarized in the charts on Nonprescription Contraceptives. These latter charts give information on usage and list the major ingredients and their actions for each product. The IUDs and diaphragms, which are available only from a physician or family planning specialist, are not covered in these drug charts.

BREVICON 21-DAY (21-day regimen) **Syntex**
BREVICON 28-DAY (28-day regimen) **Syntex**

Tabs: 0.5 mg norethindrone and 35 μg ethinyl estradiol

INDICATIONS	ORAL DOSAGE
Contraception	**Adult:** 1 tab/day for 21 or 28 consecutive days of the menstrual cycle

ADMINISTRATION/DOSAGE ADJUSTMENTS

Initiating therapy	First tablet should be taken on the 5th day after the onset of menses
Subsequent cycles (21-day regimen)	First tablet is taken 8 days after last tablet was taken in preceding cycle
Subsequent cycles (28-day regimen)	First tablet is taken 1 day after last (placebo) tablet was taken in preceding cycle
Missed tablets	If one tablet is missed, it should be taken as soon as it is remembered, with the next tablet taken at the usual time. If two tablets are missed, one of them should be taken as soon as remembered and the other discarded. The remaining tablets should be taken as usual, but an additional form of contraception should be used for the remainder of the cycle. If three or more tablets in a row are missed, the tablet cycle should be discontinued and another form of contraception used until menses has appeared or pregnancy has been excluded.

CONTRAINDICATIONS

Past or present thrombophlebitis or thromboembolic disorders ●	Known or suspected breast cancer ●	Known or suspected pregnancy ●
Past or present coronary artery disease ●	Known or suspected estrogen-dependent neoplasia ●	Markedly impaired liver function ●
Past or present cerebrovascular disease ●	Undiagnosed abnormal vaginal bleeding ●	

WARNINGS/PRECAUTIONS

Cigarette smoking	Increases the risk of serious cardiovascular side effects, especially in women over 35 yr of age who smoke 15 or more cigarettes daily; patients who use oral contraceptives should be strongly urged not to smoke
Thromboembolic disease, thrombotic disorders, and other vascular problems	Risk is increased, becoming greater with age and the amount of estrogen present in the formulation. Discontinue oral contraception immediately if early signs of thromboembolic disease or thrombotic disorders (eg, thrombophlebitis, pulmonary embolism, cerebrovascular insufficiency, coronary occlusion, or retinal or mesenteric thrombosis) develop or are suspected.
Postsurgical thromboembolic complications	Risk is increased 4-6 times; if feasible, discontinue oral contraception at least 4 wk before elective surgery associated with an increased risk of thromboembolism or prolonged immobilization
Ocular lesions, including optic neuritis and retinal thrombosis	May occur; discontinue oral contraception in the presence of unexplained gradual or sudden, partial or complete loss of vision; proptosis or diplopia; papilledema; or retinal vascular lesions
Carcinoma	Closely monitor patients with a strong family history of breast cancer or with breast nodules, fibrocystic disease, or abnormal mammograms; investigate all cases of undiagnosed persistent or recurrent abnormal vaginal bleeding for malignancy (see CONTRAINDICATIONS)
Hepatic tumors	May occur and possibly rupture, resulting in intra-abdominal hemorrhage and death; investigate all cases of abdominal pain and tenderness, right upper quadrant mass, or shock for liver tumors
Gallbladder disease	Risk increases with duration of oral contraception
Hepatic impairment	Use with caution due to poor steroid hormone metabolism (see CONTRAINDICATIONS)
Jaundice	May recur in patients with a history of jaundice; discontinue oral contraception while cause is investigated
Glucose tolerance	May become impaired; closely monitor patients with latent or active diabetes
Hypertension	May be precipitated or may worsen with oral contraception, particularly with prolonged use and in older patients. Closely monitor patients with a history of hypertension, toxemia, or hypertension during pregnancy; excessive weight gain or fluid retention during the menstrual cycle; pre-existing renal disease; or a family history of hypertension or hypertensive complications.
Migraine headache	May develop or worsen; discontinue oral contraception and investigate cause of recurrent, persistent, or severe headaches
Bleeding irregularities, including breakthrough bleeding, spotting, and amenorrhea	May occur, necessitating either a change to a formulation with a higher estrogen content or discontinuation of therapy; higher amounts of estrogen, while potentially useful for minimizing menstrual irregularities, may increase the risk of thromboembolic disease

Table continued on following page

BREVICON continued

WARNINGS/PRECAUTIONS continued	
Mental depression	Risk is increased; discontinue oral contraception if serious depression develops or recurs in patients with a history of depression
Fluid retention	May occur; use with caution in patients with convulsive disorders, migraine, asthma, or cardiac, hepatic, or renal dysfunction
Vitamin deficiencies	May occur, particularly of pyridoxine and folic acid
Failure of withdrawal bleeding	If patient has not adhered to prescribed regimen, pregnancy should be considered after the first missed period and oral contraception withheld until pregnancy has been excluded; if patient has adhered to regimen and misses two consecutive periods, pregnancy should be ruled out before contraceptive regimen is continued
Postpill amenorrhea and anovulation	May occur, particularly in patients with a history of oligomenorrhea or secondary amenorrhea or in young women who have not established regular menstrual cycles; such patients should be encouraged to use alternative methods of contraception
Infertility	May occur following discontinuation of oral contraception, independent of its duration; diminishes with time but may still be apparent up to 30 mo in parous women and up to 42 mo in nulliparous women
ADVERSE REACTIONS	Frequent reactions are italicized
Genitourinary	*Breakthrough bleeding, spotting, menstrual irregularities, vaginal candidiasis,* postpill amenorrhea and infertility, dysmenorrhea, altered cervical erosion and secretion, enlargement of uterine leiomyomata, premenstrual-like syndrome, altered libido, cystitis-like syndrome, vaginitis
Cardiovascular	Thrombophlebitis, thrombosis, pulmonary embolism, coronary thrombosis, cerebral thrombosis, cerebral hemorrhage, hypertension, mesenteric thrombosis, edema
Gastrointestinal	*Nausea, vomiting,* gallbladder disease, abdominal cramps, bloating, change in appetite
Hepatic	Liver tumors, cholestatic jaundice
Metabolic and endocrinological	*Breast enlargement, tenderness, and/or secretion;* carbohydrate intolerance; increase or decrease in weight; hyperlipidemia
Central nervous system and neuromuscular	Migraine, depression, headache, nervousness, dizziness, chorea
Ophthalmic	Optic neuritis, retinal thrombosis, intolerance to contact lenses, altered corneal curvature, cataracts
Allergic and dermatological	Rash, melasma or chloasma, erythema multiforme, erythema nodosum, hirsutism, hair loss, hemorrhagic eruption, porphyria
Other	Congenital abnormalities, prolactin-secreting pituitary tumors, impaired renal function
OVERDOSAGE	
Signs and symptoms	Nausea, withdrawal bleeding
Treatment	Treat symptomatically
DRUG INTERACTIONS	
Ampicillin, penicillin V, neomycin, chloramphenicol, sulfonamides, nitrofurantoin, rifampin, isoniazid	⇩ Contraceptive effect ⇧ Breakthrough bleeding
Analgesics, phenylbutazone, antimigraine preparations	⇩ Contraceptive effect ⇧ Breakthrough bleeding
Phenytoin, primidone	⇩ Contraceptive effect ⇧ Breakthrough bleeding
Barbiturates, tranquilizers	⇩ Contraceptive effect ⇧ Breakthrough bleeding
Antihypertensive agents (eg, guanethidine)	⇩ Antihypertensive effect
Oral anticoagulants	⇩ Anticoagulant effect
Anticonvulsants	⇧ Seizure activity
Hypoglycemic agents	⇩ Glucose tolerance
Corticosteroids	⇧ Corticosteroid effects
Tricyclic antidepressants	⇧ Antidepressant side effects

Table continued on following page

BREVICON continued

ALTERED LABORATORY VALUES

Blood/serum values	⇧ Alkaline phosphatase ⇧ Bilirubin ⇧ Sulfobromophthalein retention ⇧ Prothrombin ⇧ Clotting factors VII, VIII, IX, and X ⇩ Antithrombin III ⇧ PBI ⇧ Thyroxine (T_4) ⇩ Triiodothyronine (T_3) uptake ⇧ Glucose ⇧ Cortisol ⇧ Transcortin ⇧ Ceruloplasmin ⇧ Triglycerides ⇧ Phospholipids ⇩ Folic acid ⇩ Pyridoxine
Urinary values	⇩ Pregnanediol

Use in children

No appropriate indications exist. Acute ingestion by young children has not been associated with serious ill effects.

Use in pregnancy or nursing mothers

Contraindicated if pregnancy is known or suspected, as serious fetal damage may occur during early pregnancy. Patient should discontinue oral contraception 3 mo before attempting to conceive. Postpartum use may interfere with lactation, causing a decrease in the quantity and quality of breast milk. Patient should use alternative form of contraception until infant is weaned.

DEMULEN (21-day regimen) **Searle**
DEMULEN-28 (28-day regimen) **Searle**
Tabs: 1 mg ethynodiol diacetate and 50 μg ethinyl estradiol

INDICATIONS	ORAL DOSAGE
Contraception	**Adult:** 1 tab/day for 21 or 28 consecutive days of the menstrual cycle

ADMINISTRATION/DOSAGE ADJUSTMENTS

Initiating therapy	First tablet should be taken on the 5th day (Demulen) or 1st Sunday (Demulen, Demulen-28) after the onset of menses; if menses begins on a Sunday, regimen is started the very same day
Subsequent cycles (21-day regimen)	First tablet is taken 8 days after last tablet was taken in preceding cycle
Subsequent cycles (28-day regimen)	First tablet is taken 1 day after last (placebo) tablet was taken in preceding cycle
Missed tablets	If one tablet is missed, it should be taken as soon as it is remembered, with the next tablet taken at the usual time. If two tablets are missed, the dosage should be doubled for the next 2 days. The remaining tablets should be taken as usual, but an additional form of contraception should be used for the remainder of the cycle.

CONTRAINDICATIONS

Past or present thrombophlebitis or thromboembolic disorders ●
Past or present myocardial infarction ●
Past or present coronary artery disease ●
Past or present cerebrovascular disease ●
Past or present benign or malignant liver tumors ●
Known or suspected breast cancer ●
Known or suspected estrogen-dependent neoplasia ●
Undiagnosed abnormal vaginal bleeding ●
Known or suspected pregnancy ●
Markedly impaired liver function ●

WARNINGS/PRECAUTIONS

Cigarette smoking	Increases the risk of serious cardiovascular side effects, especially in women over 35 yr of age who smoke 15 or more cigarettes daily; patients who use oral contraceptives should be strongly urged not to smoke
Thromboembolic disease, thrombotic disorders, and other vascular problems	Risk is increased, becoming greater with age and the amount of estrogen present in the formulation. Discontinue oral contraception immediately if early signs of thromboembolic disease or thrombotic disorders (eg, thrombophlebitis, pulmonary embolism, cerebrovascular insufficiency, coronary artery disease, myocardial infarction, or retinal or mesenteric thrombosis) develop or are suspected.
Postsurgical thromboembolic complications	Risk is increased 4–6 times; if feasible, discontinue oral contraception at least 4 wk before and for at least 4 wk after elective surgery or during periods of anticipated prolonged immobilization
Ocular lesions, including optic neuritis and retinal thrombosis	May occur; discontinue oral contraception in the presence of unexplained gradual or sudden, partial or complete loss of vision; proptosis or diplopia; papilledema; or retinal vascular lesions
Carcinoma	Closely monitor patients with a strong family history of breast cancer or with breast nodules, fibrocystic disease, recurrent cystic mastitis, abnormal mammograms, or cervical dysplasia; investigate all cases of undiagnosed persistent or recurrent abnormal vaginal bleeding for malignacy (see CONTRAINDICATIONS)
Hepatic lesions, including benign adenomas	May occur and possibly rupture, resulting in intra-abdominal hemorrhage and death; investigate all cases of abdominal pain and tenderness, abdominal mass, or shock for hepatic lesions
Gallbladder disease	Risk increases with duration of oral contraception
Hepatic impairment	Use with caution due to poor steroid hormone metabolism (see CONTRAINDICATIONS)
Jaundice	May recur in patients with a history of jaundice; discontinue oral contraception while cause is investigated
Glucose tolerance	May become impaired; closely monitor patients with latent or active diabetes
Hypertension	May be precipitated or may worsen with oral contraception, particularly with prolonged use and in older patients. Closely monitor patients with a history of hypertension, toxemia, hypertension during pregnacy, or excessive weight gain or fluid retention during the menstrual cycle; pre-existing renal disese; or a family history of hypertension or hypertensive complications.
Migraine headache	May develop or worsen; discontinue oral contraception and investigate cause of recurrent, persistent, or severe headaches
Bleeding irregularities, including breakthrough bleeding, spotting, and amenorrhea	May occur, necessitating either a change to a formulation with a higher estrogen content or discontinuation of therapy; higher amounts of estrogen, while potentially useful for minimizing menstrual irregularities, may increase the risk of thromboembolic disease

Table continued on following page

DEMULEN continued

WARNINGS/PRECAUTIONS continued	
Mental depression	Risk is increased; discontinue oral contraception if serious depression develops or recurs in patients with a history of depression.
Fluid retention	May occur; use with caution in patients with convulsive disorders, migrine, asthma, or cardiac, hepatic, or renal dysfunction
Vitamin deficiencies	May occur, particularly of pyridoxine and folic acid
Failure of withdrawal bleeding	If patient has not adhered to prescribed regimen, pregnancy should be considered after the first missed period and oral contraception withheld until pregnancy has been excluded; if patient has adhered to regimen and misses two consecutive periods, pregnancy should be ruled out before contraceptive regimen is continued
Postpill amenorrhea and anovulation	May occur, particularly in patients with a history of oligomenorrhea or secondary amenorrhea or in young women who have not established regular menstrual cycles; such patients should be encouraged to use alternative methods of contraception
Ectopic pregnancy	Risk may be increased after oral contraception is discontinued
Infertility	May occur following discontinuation of oral contraception, independent of its duration; diminishes with time but may still be apparent up to 30 mo in parous women and up to 42 mo in nulliparous women
Endocrine and liver-function studies	May be affected (see ALTERED LABORATORY VALUES); repeat any abnormal tests 2 mo after oral contraception is discontinued
ADVERSE REACTIONS	Frequent reactions are italicized
Genitourinary	*Breakthrough bleeding, spotting, menstrual irregularities, vaginal candidiasis,* postpill amenorrhea and infertility, dysmenorrhea, altered cervical erosion and secretion, endocervical hyperplasia, enlargement of uterine leiomyomata, premenstrual-like syndrome, altered libido, cystitis-like syndrome, vaginitis
Cardiovascular	Thrombophlebitis, thrombosis, pulmonary embolism, myocardial infarction, coronary thrombosis, cerebral thrombosis, cerebral hemorrhage, hypertension, mesenteric thrombosis, edema
Gastrointestinal	*Nausea, vomiting,* gallbladder disease, abdominal cramps, bloating, change in appetite, pancreatitis, colitis
Hepatic	Benign adenomas and other hepatic lesions, Budd-Chiari syndrome, cholestatic jaundice, hepatitis
Metabolic and endocrinological	*Breast enlargement, tenderness, and/or secretion;* carbohydrate intolerance; increase or decrease in weight; hyperlipidemia
Central nervous system and neuromuscular	Migraine, depression, headache, nervousness, dizziness, chorea, paresthesia, auditory disturbances, fatigue
Ophthalmic	Optic neuritis, retinal thrombosis, intolerance to contact lenses, altered corneal curvature, cataracts
Allergic and dermatological	Melasma or chloasma, rash, itching, rhinitis, erythema multiforme, erythema nodosum, hirsutism, hair loss, hemorrhagic eruption, porphyria
Other	Congenital anomalies, prolactin-secreting pituitary tumors, impaired renal function, backache, anemia, lupus erythematosus, rheumatoid arthritis
OVERDOSAGE	
Signs and symptoms	Nausea, withdrawal bleeding
Treatment	Treat symptomatically
DRUG INTERACTIONS	
Ampicillin, penicillin V, neomycin, chloramphenicol, sulfonamides, nitrofurantoin, rifampin, isoniazid	⇩ Contraceptive effect ⇧ Breakthrough bleeding
Analgesics, phenylbutazone, antimigraine preparations	⇩ Contraceptive effect ⇧ Breakthrough bleeding
Phenytoin, primidone	⇩ Contraceptive effect ⇧ Breakthrough bleeding
Barbiturates, tranquilizers	⇩ Contraceptive effect ⇧ Breakthrough bleeding
Antihypertensive agents (eg, guanethidine)	⇩ Antihypertensive effect
Oral anticoagulants	⇩ Anticoagulant effect
Anticonvulsants	⇧ Seizure activity
Hypoglycemic agents	⇩ Glucose tolerance
Corticosteroids	⇧ Corticosteroid effects
Tricyclic antidepressants	⇧ Antidepressant side effects

Table continued on following page

DEMULEN continued

ALTERED LABORATORY VALUES

Blood/serum values	⇧ Alkaline phosphatase ⇧ Bilirubin ⇧ Sulfobromophthalein retention ⇧ Prothrombin ⇧ Clotting factors VII, VIII, IX, and X ⇩ Antithrombin III ⇧ PBI ⇧ Thyroxine (T_4) ⇩ Triiodothyronine (T_3) uptake ⇧ Glucose ⇧ Cortisol ⇧ Transcortin ⇧ Ceruloplasmin ⇧ Triglycerides ⇧ Phospholipids ⇩ Folic acid ⇩ Pyridoxine
Urinary values	⇩ Pregnanediol

Use in children

No appropriate indications exist. Acute ingestion by young children has not been associated with serious ill effects.

Use in pregnancy or nursing mothers

Contraindicated if pregnancy is known or suspected, as serious fetal damage may occur during early pregnancy. Patient should discontinue oral contraception 3 mo before attempting to conceive. Postpartum use may interfere with lactation, causing a decrease in the quantity and quality of breast milk. Patient should use alternative form of contraception until infant is weaned.

LOESTRIN 21 1/20 (21-day regimen) **Parke-Davis**

Tabs: 1 mg norethindrone acetate and 20 μg ethinyl estradiol

LOESTRIN Fe 1/20 (28-day regimen) **Parke-Davis**

Tabs: 1 mg norethindrone acetate and 20 μg ethinyl estradiol (white); 75 mg ferrous fumarate (brown)

LOESTRIN 21 1.5/30 (21-day regimen) **Parke-Davis**

Tabs: 1.5 mg norethindrone acetate and 30 μg ethinyl estradiol

LOESTRIN Fe 1.5/30 (28-day regimen) **Parke-Davis**

Tabs: 1.5 mg norethindrone acetate and 30 μg ethinyl estradiol (green); 75 mg ferrous fumarate (brown)

INDICATIONS	**ORAL DOSAGE**
Contraception	**Adult:** 1 tab/day for 21 or 28 consecutive days of the menstrual cycle

ADMINISTRATION/DOSAGE ADJUSTMENTS

Initiating therapy	First tablet should be taken on the 5th day after the onset of menses
Subsequent cycles (21-day regimen)	First tablet is taken 8 days after last tablet was taken in preceding cycle
Subsequent cycles (28-day regimen)	First tablet is taken 1 day after last (placebo) tablet was taken in preceding cycle
Missed tablets	If one tablet is missed, it should be taken as soon as it is remembered or together with the next tablet on the following day. If two tablets are missed, the dosage should be doubled for the next 2 days but an additional form of contraception should be used for 7 consecutive days. If three tablets are missed, the tablet cycle should be discontinued and another form of contraception used until the start of the next menstrual period. Instruct the patient to start the next course of tablets 7 days after the last tablet was taken, even if she is still menstruating.

CONTRAINDICATIONS

Past or present thrombophlebitis or thromboembolic disorders ●	Known or suspected breast cancer ●	Known or suspected pregnancy ●
Coronary artery disease ●	Known or suspected estrogen-dependent neoplasia ●	
Cerebrovascular disease ●	Undiagnosed abnormal vaginal bleeding ●	

WARNINGS/PRECAUTIONS

Cigarette smoking	Increases the risk of serious cardiovascular side effects, especially in women over 35 yr of age who smoke 15 or more cigarettes daily; patients who use oral contraceptives should be strongly urged not to smoke
Thromboembolic disease, thrombotic disorders, and other vascular problems	Risk is increased, becoming greater with age and the amount of estrogen present in the formulation. Discontinue oral contraception immediately if early signs of thromboembolic disease or thrombotic disorders (eg, thrombophlebitis, pulmonary embolism, cerebrovascular insufficiency, coronary occlusion, or retinal or mesenteric thrombosis) develop or are suspected.
Postsurgical thromboembolic complications	Risk is increased 4-6 times; if feasible, discontinue oral contraception at least 4 wk before elective surgery associated with an increased risk of thromboembolism or prolonged immobilization
Ocular lesions, including optic neuritis and retinal thrombosis	May occur; discontinue oral contraception in the presence of unexplained gradual or sudden partial or complete loss of vision; proptosis or diplopia; papilledema; or retinal vascular lesions
Carcinoma	Closely monitor patients with a strong family history of breast cancer or with breast nodules, fibrocystic disease, or abnormal mammograms; investigate all cases of undiagnosed persistent or recurrent abnormal vaginal bleeding for malignancy (see CONTRAINDICATIONS)
Hepatic tumors, including benign adenomas	May occur and possibly rupture, resulting in intra-abdominal hemorrhage and death; investigate all cases of abdominal pain and tenderness, abdominal mass, or shock for hepatic adenoma
Gallbladder disease	Risk increases with duration of oral contraception
Hepatic impairment	Use with caution due to poor steroid hormone metabolism
Jaundice	May recur in patients with a history of jaundice; discontinue oral contraception while cause is investigated
Glucose tolerance	May become impaired; closely monitor patients with latent or active diabetes
Hypertension	May be precipitated or may worsen with oral contraception, particularly with prolonged use, in older patients, and in patients with a history of hypertension during pregnancy
Migraine headache	May develop or worsen; discontinue oral contraception and investigate cause of recurrent, persistent, or severe headaches

Table continued on following page

WARNINGS/PRECAUTIONS continued

Bleeding irregularities, including breakthrough bleeding, spotting, and amenorrhea	May occur, necessitating either a change to a formulation with a higher estrogen content or discontinuation of therapy; higher amounts of estrogen, while potentially useful for minimizing menstrual irregularities, may increase the risk of thromboembolic disease
Mental depression	Risk is increased; discontinue oral contraception if serious depression develops or recurs in patients with a history of depression
Fluid retention	May occur; use with caution in patients with convulsive disorders, migraine, asthma, or cardiac, hepatic, or renal dysfunction
Vitamin deficiencies	May occur, particularly of pyridoxine and folic acid
Failure of withdrawal bleeding	If patient has missed two consecutive periods, pregnancy should be ruled out before contraceptive regimen is continued; if patient has not adhered to prescribed regimen, pregnancy should be considered after the first missed period and oral contraception withheld until pregnancy has been excluded
Postpill amenorrhea and anovulation	May occur, particularly in patients with a history of oligomenorrhea or secondary amenorrhea or in young women who have not established regular menstrual cycles; such patients should be encouraged to use alternative methods of contraception

ADVERSE REACTIONS Frequent reactions are italicized

Genitourinary	*Breakthrough bleeding, spotting, menstrual irregularities, vaginal candidiasis,* postpill amenorrhea and infertility, dysmenorrhea, altered cervical erosion and secretion, enlargement of uterine leiomyomata, premenstrual-like syndrome, altered libido, cystitis-like syndrome, vaginitis
Cardiovascular	Thrombophlebitis, thrombosis, pulmonary embolism, coronary thrombosis, cerebral thrombosis, cerebral hemorrhage, hypertension, mesenteric thrombosis, edema
Gastrointestinal	*Nausea, vomiting,* gallbladder disease, abdominal cramps, bloating, change in appetite
Hepatic	Benign hepatomas, cholestatic jaundice
Metabolic and endocrinological	*Breast enlargement, tenderness, and/or secretion;* carbohydrate intolerance; increase or decrease in weight; hyperlipidemia
Central nervous system and neuromuscular	Migraine, depression, headache, nervousness, dizziness, chorea
Ophthalmic	Optic neuritis, retinal thrombosis, intolerance to contact lenses, altered corneal curvature, cataracts
Allergic and dermatological	Rash, melasma or chloasma, erythema multiforme, erythema nodosum, hirsutism, hair loss, hemorrhagic eruption, porphyria
Other	Congenital anomalies

OVERDOSAGE

Signs and symptoms	Nausea, withdrawal bleeding
Treatment	Treat symptomatically

DRUG INTERACTIONS

Ampicillin, penicillin V, heomycin, chloramphenicol, sulfonamides, nitrofurantoin, rifampin, isoniazid	⇩ Contraceptive effect ⇧ Breakthrough bleeding
Analgesics, phenylbutazone, antimigraine preparations	⇩ Contraceptive effect ⇧ Breakthrough bleeding
Phenytoin, primidone	⇩ Contraceptive effect ⇧ Breakthrough bleeding
Barbiturates, tranquilizers	⇩ Contraceptive effect ⇧ Breakthrough bleeding
Antihypertensive agents (eg, guanethidine)	⇩ Antihypertensive effect
Oral anticoagulants	⇩ Anticoagulant effect
Anticonvulsants	⇧ Seizure activity
Hypoglycemic agents	⇩ Glucose tolerance
Corticosteroids	⇧ Corticosteroid effects
Tricyclic antidepressants	⇧ Antidepressant side effects

Table continued on following page

ALTERED LABORATORY VALUES

Blood/serum values	⇧ Alkaline phosphatase ⇧ Bilirubin ⇧ Sulfobromophthalein retention ⇧ Prothrombin ⇧ Clotting factors VII, VIII, IX, and X ⇩ Antithrombin III ⇧ PBI ⇧ Thyroxine (T_4) ⇩ Triiodothyronine (T_3) uptake ⇧ Glucose ⇧ Cortisol ⇧ Transcortin ⇧ Ceruloplasmin ⇧ Triglycerides ⇧ Phospholipids ⇩ Folic acid ⇩ Pyridoxine
Urinary values	⇩ Pregnanediol

Use in children

No appropriate indications exist. Acute ingestion by young children has not been associated with serious ill effects.

Use in pregnancy or nursing mothers

Contraindicated if pregnancy is known or suspected, as serious fetal damage may occur during early pregnancy. Patient should discontinue oral contraception 3 mo before attempting to conceive. Postpartum use may interfere with lactation, causing a decrease in the quantity and quality of breast milk. Patient should use alternative form of contraception until infant is weaned.

LO-OVRAL (21-day regimen) **Wyeth**
LO-OVRAL-28 (28-day regimen) **Wyeth**
Tabs: 0.3 mg norgestrel and 30 μg ethinyl estradiol

INDICATIONS	ORAL DOSAGE
Contraception	**Adult:** 1 tab/day for 21 or 28 consecutive days of the menstrual cycle

ADMINISTRATION/DOSAGE ADJUSTMENTS

Initiating therapy	First tablet should be taken on the 5th day after the onset of menses
Subsequent cycles (21-day regimen)	First tablet is taken 8 days after last tablet was taken in preceding cycle
Subsequent cycles (28-day regimen)	First tablet is taken 1 day after last (placebo) tablet was taken in preceding cycle
Missed tablets	If one or two tablets are missed, they should be taken as soon as they are remembered, and an additional form of contraception should be used for 1 wk. If three tablets are missed, the tablet cycle should be discontinued; start the next tablet cycle 8 days after the last tablet was taken and instruct patient to use another form of contraception for the 7 days without tablets and until seven tablets are taken
Postpartum administration	For nonnursing mothers, may be started either immediately or after first postpartum examination, regardless of whether spontaneous menstruation has occurred

CONTRAINDICATIONS

Past or present thrombophlebitis or thromboembolic disorders ●	Known or suspected breast cancer ●	Known or suspected pregnancy ●
Coronary artery disease ●	Known or suspected estrogen-dependent neoplasia ●	
Cerebrovascular disease ●	Undiagnosed abnormal vaginal bleeding ●	

WARNINGS/PRECAUTIONS

Cigarette smoking	Increases the risk of serious cardiovascular side effects, especially in women over 35 yr of age who smoke 15 or more cigarettes daily; patients who use oral contraceptives should be strongly urged not to smoke
Thromboembolic disease, thrombotic disorders, and other vascular problems	Risk is increased, becoming greater with age and the amount of estrogen present in the formulation. Discontinue oral contraception immediately if early signs of thromboembolic disease or thrombotic disorders (eg, thrombophlebitis, pulmonary embolism, cerebrovascular insufficiency, coronary occlusion, or retinal or mesenteric thrombosis) develop or are suspected.
Postsurgical thromboembolic complications	Risk is increased 4–6 times; if feasible, discontinue oral contraception at least 4 wk before elective surgery associated with an increased risk of thromboembolism or prolonged immobilization
Ocular lesions, including optic neuritis and retinal thrombosis	May occur; discontinue oral contraception in the presence of unexplained gradual or sudden, partial or complete loss of vision; proptosis or diplopia; papilledema; or retinal vascular lesions
Carcinoma	Closely monitor patients with a strong family history of breast cancer or with breast nodules, fibrocystic disease, or abnormal mammograms; investigate all cases of undiagnosed persistent or recurrent abnormal vaginal bleeding for malignancy (see CONTRAINDICATIONS)
Hepatic tumors, including benign adenomas	May occur and possibly rupture, resulting in intra-abdominal hemorrhage and death; investigate all cases of abdominal pain and tenderness, abdominal mass, or shock for hepatic adenoma
Gallbladder disease	Risk increases with duration of oral contraception
Hepatic impairment	Use with caution due to poor steroid hormone metabolism
Jaundice	May recur in patients with a history of jaundice; discontinue oral contraception while cause is investigated
Glucose tolerance	May become impaired; closely monitor patients with latent or active diabetes
Hypertension	May be precipitated or may worsen with oral contraception, particularly with prolonged use in older patients, and in patients with a history of hypertension during pregnancy
Migraine headache	May develop or worsen; discontinue oral contraception and investigate cause of recurrent, persistent, or severe headaches
Bleeding irregularities, including breakthrough bleeding, spotting, and amenorrhea	May occur, necessitating either a change to a formulation with a higher estrogen content or discontinuation of therapy; higher amounts of estrogen, while potentially useful for minimizing menstrual irregularities, may increase the risk of thromboembolic disease
Mental depression	Risk is increased; discontinue oral contraception if serious depression develops or recurs in patients with a history of depression
Fluid retention	May occur; use with caution in patients with convulsive disorders, migraine, asthma, or cardiac, hepatic, or renal dysfunction

Table continued on following page

LO-OVRAL continued

WARNINGS/PRECAUTIONS continued

Vitamin deficiencies	May occur, particularly of pyridoxine and folic acid
Failure of withdrawal bleeding	If patient has missed two consecutive periods, pregnancy should be ruled out before contraceptive regimen is continued; if patient has not adhered to prescribed regimen, pregnancy should be considered after the first missed period and oral contraception withheld until pregnancy has been excluded
Postpill amenorrhea and anovulation	May occur, particularly in patients with a history of oligomenorrhea or secondary amenorrhea or in young women who have not established regular menstrual cycles; such patients should be encouraged to use alternative methods of contraception

ADVERSE REACTIONS	**Frequent reactions are italicized**
Genitourinary	*Breakthrough bleeding, spotting, menstrual irregularities, vaginal candidiasis,* postpill amenorrhea and infertility, dysmenorrhea, altered cervical erosion and secretion, enlargement of uterine leiomyomata, premenstrual-like syndrome, altered libido, cystitis-like syndrome, vaginitis
Cardiovascular	Thrombophlebitis, pulmonary embolism, coronary thrombosis, cerebral thrombosis, cerebral hemorrhage, hypertension, mesenteric thrombosis, edema
Gastrointestinal	*Nausea, vomiting,* gallbladder disease, abdominal cramps, bloating, change in appetite
Hepatic	Benign hepatomas, cholestatic jaundice
Metabolic and endocrinological	*Breast enlargement, tenderness, and/or secretion;* carbohydrate intolerance; increase or decrease in weight; hyperlipidemia
Central nervous system and neuromuscular	Migraine, depression, headache, nervousness, dizziness, chorea
Ophthalmic	Optic neuritis, retinal thrombosis, intolerance to contact lenses, altered corneal curvature, cataracts
Allergic and dermatological	Rash, melasma or chloasma, erythema multiforme, erythema nodosum, hirsutism, hair loss, hemorrhagic eruption, porphyria
Other	Congenital anomalies

OVERDOSAGE

Signs and symptoms	Nausea, withdrawal bleeding
Treatment	Treat symptomatically

DRUG INTERACTIONS

Ampicillin, penicillin V, neomycin, chloramphenicol, sulfonamides, nitrofurantoin, rifampin, isoniazid	⇩ Contraceptive effect ⇧ Breakthrough bleeding
Analgesics, phenylbutazone, antimigraine preparations	⇩ Contraceptive effect ⇧ Breakthrough bleeding
Phenytoin, primidone	⇩ Contraceptive effect ⇧ Breakthrough bleeding
Barbiturates, tranquilizers	⇩ Contraceptive effect ⇧ Breakthrough bleeding
Antihypertensive agents (eg, guanethidine)	⇩ Antihypertensive effect
Oral anticoagulants	⇩ Anticoagulant effect
Anticonvulsants	⇧ Seizure activity
Hypoglycemic agents	⇩ Glucose tolerance
Corticosteroids	⇧ Corticosteroid effects
Tricyclic antidepressants	⇧ Antidepressant side effects

ALTERED LABORATORY VALUES

Blood/serum values	⇧ Alkaline phosphatase ⇧ Bilirubin ⇧ Sulfobromophthalein retention ⇧ Prothrombin ⇧ Clotting factors VII, VIII, IX, and X ⇩ Antithrombin III ⇧ PBI ⇧ Thyroxine (T_4) ⇩ Triiodothyronine (T_3) uptake ⇧ Glucose ⇧ Cortisol ⇧ Transcortin ⇧ Ceruloplasmin ⇧ Triglycerides ⇧ Phospholipids ⇩ Folic acid ⇩ Pyridoxine
Urinary values	⇩ Pregnanediol

Use in children

No appropriate indications exist. Acute ingestion by young children has not been associated with serious ill effects.

Use in pregnancy or nursing mothers

Contraindicated if pregnancy is known or suspected, as serious fetal damage may occur during early pregnancy. Patient should discontinue oral contraception 3 mo before attempting to conceive. Postpartum use may interfere with lactation, causing a decrease in the quantity and quality of breast milk. Patient should use alternative form of contraception until infant is weaned.

MODICON (21-day regimen) **Ortho**
MODICON 28 (28-day regimen) **Ortho**

Tabs: 0.5 mg norethindrone and 35 μg ethinyl estradiol

INDICATIONS	**ORAL DOSAGE**
Contraception	**Adult:** 1 tab/day for 21 or 28 consecutive days of the menstrual cycle

ADMINISTRATION/DOSAGE ADJUSTMENTS

Initiating therapy	First tablet should be taken on the 5th day (Modicon) or 1st Sunday (Modicon 28) after the onset of menses; if menses begins on a Sunday, regimen is started the very same day
Subsequent cycles (21-day regimen)	First tablet is taken 8 days after last tablet was taken in preceding cycle
Subsequent cycles (28-day regimen)	First tablet is taken 1 day after last (placebo) tablet was taken in preceding cycle
Missed tablets	If more than one tablet is missed, instruct patient to resume taking tablets as soon as remembered, but to use an additional form of contraception for the remainder of the cycle

CONTRAINDICATIONS

Past or present thrombophlebitis or thromboembolic disorders ●	Known or suspected breast cancer ●	Known or suspected pregnancy ●
Coronary artery disease ●	Known or suspected estrogen-dependent neoplasia ●	
Cerebrovascular disease ●	Undiagnosed abnormal vaginal bleeding ●	

WARNINGS/PRECAUTIONS

Cigarette smoking	Increases the risk of serious cardiovascular side effects, especially in women over 35 yr of age who smoke 15 or more cigarettes daily; patients who use oral contraceptives should be strongly urged not to smoke
Thromboembolic disease, thrombotic disorders, and other vascular problems	Risk is increased, becoming greater with age and the amount of estrogen present in the formulation. Discontinue oral contraception immediately if early signs of thromboembolic disease or thrombotic disorders (eg, thrombophlebitis, pulmonary embolism, cerebrovascular insufficiency, coronary occlusion, or retinal or mesenteric thrombosis) develop or are suspected.
Postsurgical thromboembolic complications	Risk is increased 4–6 times; if feasible, discontinue oral contraception at least 4 wk before elective surgery associated with an increased risk of thromboembolism or prolonged immobilization
Ocular lesions, including optic neuritis and retinal thrombosis	May occur; discontinue oral contraception in the presence of unexplained gradual or sudden, partial or complete loss of vision; proptosis or diplopia; papilledema; or retinal vascular lesions
Carcinoma	Closely monitor patients with a strong family history of breast cancer or with breast nodules, fibrocystic disease, or abnormal mammograms; investigate all cases of undiagnosed persistent or recurrent abnormal vaginal bleeding for malignancy (see CONTRAINDICATIONS)
Hepatic tumors, including benign adenomas	May occur and possibly rupture, resulting in intra-abdominal hemorrhage and death; investigate all cases of abdominal pain and tenderness, abdominal mass, or shock for hepatic adenoma
Gallbladder disease	Risk increases with duration of oral contraception
Hepatic impairment	Use with caution due to poor steroid hormone metabolism
Jaundice	May recur in patients with a history of jaundice; discontinue oral contraception while cause is investigated
Glucose tolerance	May become impaired; closely monitor patients with latent or active diabetes
Hypertension	May be precipitated or may worsen with oral contraception, particularly with prolonged use, in older patients, and in patients with a history of hypertension during pregnancy
Migraine headache	May develop or worsen; discontinue oral contraception and investigate cause of recurrent, persistent, or severe headaches
Bleeding irregularities, including breakthrough bleeding, spotting, and amenorrhea	May occur, necessitating either a change to a formulation with a higher estrogen content or discontinuation of therapy; higher amounts of estrogen, while potentially useful for minimizing menstrual irregularities, may increase the risk of thromboembolic disease
Mental depression	Risk is increased; discontinue oral contraception if serious depression develops or recurs in patients with a history of depression
Fluid retention	May occur; use with caution in patients with convulsive disorders, migraine, asthma, or cardiac, hepatic, or renal dysfunction
Vitamin deficiencies	May occur, particularly of pyridoxine and folic acid

Table continued on following page

MODICON continued

WARNINGS/PRECAUTIONS continued

Failure of withdrawal bleeding	If patient has not adhered to prescribed regimen, pregnancy should be considered after the first missed period and oral contraception withheld until pregnancy has been excluded; if patient has adhered to regimen and misses two consecutive periods, pregnancy should be ruled out before contraceptive regimen is continued
Postpill amenorrhea and anovulation	May occur, particularly in patients with a history of oligomenorrhea or secondary amenorrhea or in young women who have not established regular menstrual cycles; such patients should be encouraged to use alternative methods of contraception

ADVERSE REACTIONS	Frequent reactions are italicized
Genitourinary	*Breakthrough bleeding, spotting, menstrual irregularities, vaginal candidiasis,* postpill amenorrhea and infertility, dysmenorrhea, altered cervical erosion and secretion, enlargement of uterine leiomyomata, premenstrual-like syndrome, altered libido, cystitis-like syndrome, vaginitis
Cardiovascular	Thrombophlebitis, pulmonary embolism, coronary thrombosis, cerebral thrombosis, cerebral hemorrhage, hypertension, mesenteric thrombosis, edema
Gastrointestinal	*Nausea, vomiting,* gallbladder disease, abdominal cramps, bloating, change in appetite
Hepatic	Hepatic tumors, cholestatic jaundice
Metabolic and endocrinological	*Breast enlargement, tenderness, and/or secretion;* carbohydrate intolerance; increase or decrease in weight; hyperlipidemia
Central nervous system and neuromuscular	Migraine, depression, headache, nervousness, dizziness, chorea
Ophthalmic	Optic neuritis, retinal thrombosis, intolerance to contact lenses, altered corneal curvature, cataracts
Allergic and dermatological	Rash, melasma or chloasma, erythema multiforme, erythema nodosum, hirsutism, hair loss, hemorrhagic eruption, porphyria
Other	Congenital anomalies; impaired renal function

OVERDOSAGE

Signs and symptoms	Nausea, withdrawal bleeding
Treatment	Treat symptomatically

DRUG INTERACTIONS

Ampicillin, penicillin V, neomycin, chloramphenicol, sulfonamides, nitrofurantoin, rifampin, isoniazid	⇩ Contraceptive effect ⇧ Breakthrough bleeding
Analgesics, phenylbutazone, antimigraine preparations	⇩ Contraceptive effect ⇧ Breakthrough bleeding
Phenytoin, primidone	⇩ Contraceptive effect ⇧ Breakthrough bleeding
Barbiturates, tranquilizers	⇩ Contraceptive effect ⇧ Breakthrough bleeding
Antihypertensive agents (eg, guanethidine)	⇩ Antihypertensive effect
Oral anticoagulants	⇩ Anticoagulant effect
Anticonvulsants	⇧ Seizure activity
Hypoglycemic agents	⇩ Glucose tolerance
Corticosteroids	⇧ Corticosteroid effects
Tricyclic antidepressants	⇧ Antidepressant side effects

ALTERED LABORATORY VALUES

Blood/serum values	⇧ Alkaline phosphatase ⇧ Bilirubin ⇧ Sulfobromophthalein retention ⇧ Prothrombin ⇧ Clotting factors VII, VIII, IX, and X ⇩ Antithrombin III ⇧ PBI ⇧ Thyroxine (T_4) ⇩ Triiodothyronine (T_3) uptake ⇧ Glucose ⇧ Cortisol ⇧ Transcortin ⇧ Ceruloplasmin ⇧ Triglycerides ⇧ Phospholipids ⇩ Folic acid ⇩ Pyridoxine
Urinary values	⇩ Pregnanediol

Use in children

No appropriate indications exist. Acute ingestion by young children has not been associated with serious ill effects.

Use in pregnancy or nursing mothers

Contraindicated if pregnancy is known or suspected, as serious fetal damage may occur during early pregnancy. Patient should discontinue oral contraception 3 mo before attempting to conceive. Postpartum use may interfere with lactation, causing a decrease in the quantity and quality of breast milk. Patient should use alternative form of contraception until infant is weaned.

NORINYL 1 + 35 21-DAY (21-day regimen) **Syntex**
NORINYL 1 + 35 28-DAY (28-day regimen) **Syntex**

Tabs: 1 mg norethindrone and 35 μg ethinyl estradiol

INDICATIONS	ORAL DOSAGE
Contraception	**Adult:** 1 tab/day for 21 or 28 consecutive days of the menstrual cycle

ADMINISTRATION/DOSAGE ADJUSTMENTS

Initiating therapy	First tablet should be taken on the 5th day after the onset of menses
Subsequent cycles (21-day regimen)	First tablet is taken 8 days after last tablet was taken in preceding cycle
Subsequent cycles (28-day regimen)	First tablet is taken 1 day after last (placebo) tablet was taken in preceding cycle
Missed tablets	If one tablet is missed, it should be taken as soon as it is remembered, with the next tablet taken at the usual time. If two tablets are missed, one of them should be taken as soon as remembered and the other discarded. The remaining tablets should be taken as usual, but an additional form of contraception should be used for the remainder of the cycle. If three or more tablets in a row are missed, the tablet cycle should be discontinued immediately and another form of contraception used until menses has appeared or pregnancy has been excluded.

CONTRAINDICATIONS

Past or present thrombophlebitis or thromboembolic disorders ●	Known or suspected breast cancer ●	Known or suspected pregnancy ●
Past or present coronary artery disease ●	Known or suspected estrogen-dependent neoplasia ●	Development of benign or malignant liver tumor during prior use of oral contraceptives or other estrogen-containing products ●
Past or present cerebrovascular disease ●	Undiagnosed abnormal vaginal bleeding ●	

WARNINGS/PRECAUTIONS

Cigarette smoking	Increases the risk of serious cardiovascular side effects, especially in women over 35 yr of age who smoke 15 or more cigarettes daily; patients who use oral contraceptives should be strongly urged not to smoke
Thromboembolic disease, thrombotic disorders, and other vascular problems	Risk is increased, becoming greater with age and the amount of estrogen present in the formulation. Discontinue oral contraception immediately if early signs of thromboembolic disease or thrombotic disorders (eg, thrombophlebitis, pulmonary embolism, cerebrovascular insufficiency, coronary occlusion, or retinal or mesenteric thrombosis) develop or are suspected.
Postsurgical thromboembolic complications	Risk is increased 4–6 times; if feasible, discontinue oral contraception at least 4 wk before elective surgery associated with an increased risk of thromboembolism or prolonged immobilization
Ocular lesions, including optic neuritis and retinal thrombosis	May occur; discontinue oral contraception in the presence of unexplained gradual or sudden, partial or complete loss of vision; proptosis or diplopia; papilledema; or retinal vascular lesions
Carcinoma	Closely monitor patients with a strong family history of breast cancer or with breast nodules, fibrocystic disease, or abnormal mammograms; investigate all cases of undiagnosed persistent or recurrent abnormal vaginal bleeding for malignancy (see CONTRAINDICATIONS)
Hepatic tumors	May occur and possibly rupture, resulting in intra-abdominal hemorrhage and death; investigate all cases of abdominal pain and tenderness, right upper quadrant mass, or shock for liver tumors
Gallbladder disease	Risk increases with duration of oral contraception
Hepatic impairment	Use with caution due to poor steroid hormone metabolism (see CONTRAINDICATIONS)
Jaundice	May recur in patients with a history of jaundice; discontinue oral contraception while cause is investigated
Glucose tolerance	May become impaired; closely monitor patients with latent or active diabetes
Hypertension	May be precipitated or may worsen with oral contraception, particularly with prolonged use and in older patients. Closely monitor patients with a history of hypertension, toxemia, hypertension during pregnancy, or excessive weight gain or fluid retention during the menstrual cycle; pre-existing renal disease; or a family history of hypertension or hypertensive complications.

Table continued on following page

NORINYL continued

WARNINGS/PRECAUTIONS continued	
Migraine headache	May develop or worsen; discontinue oral contraception and investigate cause of recurrent, persistent, or severe headaches
Bleeding irregularities, including breakthrough bleeding, spotting, and amenorrhea	May occur, necessitating either a change to a formulation with a higher estrogen content or discontinuation of therapy; higher amounts of estrogen, while potentially useful for minimizing menstrual irregularities, may increase the risk of thromboembolic disease
Mental depression	Risk is increased; discontinue oral contraception if serious depression develops or recurs in patients with a history of depression
Fluid retention	May occur; use with caution in patients with convulsive disorders, migraine, asthma, or cardiac, hepatic, or renal dysfunction
Vitamin deficiencies	May occur, particularly of pyridoxine and folic acid
Failure of withdrawal bleeding	If patient has not adhered to prescribed regimen, pregnancy should be considered after the first missed period and oral contraception withheld until pregnancy has been excluded; if patient has adhered to regimen and misses two consecutive periods, pregnancy should be ruled out before contraceptive regimen is continued
Postpill amenorrhea and anovulation	May occur, particularly in patients with a history of oligomenorrhea or secondary amenorrhea or in young women who have not established regular menstrual cycles; such patients should be encouraged to use alternative methods of contraception
Interfility	May occur following discontinuation of oral contraception, independent of its duration; diminishes with time but may still be apparent up to 30 mo in parous women and up to 42 mo in nulliparous women
ADVERSE REACTIONS	Frequent reactions are italicized
Genitourinary	*Breakthrough bleeding, spotting, menstrual irregularities, vaginal candidiasis,* postpill amenorrhea and infertility, dysmenorrhea, altered cervical erosion and secretion, enlargement of uterine leiomyomata, premenstrual-like syndrome, altered libido, cystitis-like syndrome, vaginitis
Cardiovascular	Thrombophlebitis, thrombosis, pulmonary embolism, coronary thrombosis, cerebral thrombosis, cerebral hemorrhage, hypertension, mesenteric thrombosis, edema
Gastrointestinal	*Nausea, vomiting,* gallbladder disease, abdominal cramps, bloating, change in appetite
Hepatic	Liver tumors, cholestatic jaundice
Metabolic and endocrinological	*Breast enlargement, tenderness, and/or secretion;* carbohydrate intolerance; increase or decrease in weight; hyperlipidemia
Central nervous system and neuromuscular	Migraine, depression, headache, nervousness, dizziness, chorea
Ophthalmic	Optic neuritis, retinal thrombosis, intolerance to contact lenses, altered corneal curvature, cataracts
Allergic and dermatological	Rash, melasma or chloasma, erythema multiforme, erythema nodosum, hirsutism, hair loss, hemorrhagic eruption, porphyria
Other	Congenital anomalies, prolactin-secreting pituitary tumors, impaired renal function
OVERDOSAGE	
Signs and symptoms	Nausea, withdrawal bleeding
Treatment	Treat symptomatically
DRUG INTERACTIONS	
Ampicillin, penicillin V, neomycin, chloramphenicol, sulfonamides, nitrofurantoin, rifampin, isoniazid	⇩ Contraceptive effect ⇧ Breakthrough bleeding
Analgesics, phenylbutazone, antimigraine preparations	⇩ Contraceptive effect ⇧ Breakthrough bleeding
Phenytoin, primidone	⇩ Contraceptive effect ⇧ Breakthrough bleeding
Barbiturates, tranquilizers	⇩ Contraceptive effect ⇧ Breakthrough bleeding
Antihypertensive agents (eg, guanethidine)	⇩ Antihypertensive effect
Oral anticoagulants	⇩ Anticoagulant effect
Anticonvulsants	⇧ Seizure activity
Hypoglycemic agents	⇩ Glucose tolerance
Corticosteroids	⇧ Corticosteroid effects
Tricyclic antidepressants	⇧ Antidepressant side effects

Table continued on following page

ALTERED LABORATORY VALUES

Blood/serum values	⇧ Alkaline phosphatase ⇧ Bilirubin ⇧ Sulfobromophthalein retention ⇧ Prothrombin ⇧ Clotting factors VII, VIII, IX, and X ⇩ Antithrombin III ⇧ PBI ⇧ Thyroxine (T_4) ⇩ Triiodothyronine (T_3) uptake ⇧ Glucose ⇧ Cortisol ⇧ Transcortin ⇧ Ceruloplasmin ⇧ Triglycerides ⇧ Phospholipids ⇩ Folic acid ⇩ Pyridoxine
Urinary values	⇩ Pregnanediol

Use in children

No appropriate indications exist. Acute ingestion by young children has not been associated with serious ill effects.

Use in pregnancy or nursing mothers

Contraindicated if pregnancy is known or suspected, as serious fetal damage may occur during early pregnancy. Patient should discontinue oral contraception 3 mo before attempting to conceive. Postpartum use may interfere with lactation, causing a decrease in the quantity and quality of breast milk. Patient should use alternative form of contraception until infant is weaned.

NORINYL 1+50 21-DAY (21-day regimen) **Syntex**
NORINYL 1+50 28-DAY (28-day regimen) **Syntex**

Tabs: 1 mg norethindrone and 50 μg mestranol

NORINYL 1+80 21-DAY (21-day regimen) **Syntex**
NORINYL 1+80 28-DAY (28-day regimen) **Syntex**

Tabs: 1 mg norethindrone and 80 μg mestranol

INDICATIONS	ORAL DOSAGE
Contraception	**Adult:** 1 tab/day for 21 or 28 consecutive days of the menstrual cycle

ADMINISTRATION/DOSAGE ADJUSTMENTS

Initiating therapy	First tablet should be taken on the 5th day after the onset of menses
Subsequent cycles (21-day regimen)	First tablet is taken 8 days after last tablet was taken in preceding cycle
Subsequent cycles (28-day regimen)	First tablet is taken 1 day after last (placebo) tablet was taken in preceding cycle
Missed tablets	If one tablet is missed, it should be taken as soon as it is remembered, with the next tablet taken at the usual time. If two tablets are missed, one of them should be taken as soon as remembered and the other discarded. The remaining tablets should be taken as usual, but an additional form of contraception should be used for the remainder of the cycle. If three or more tablets in a row are missed, the tablet cycle should be discontinued immediately and another form of contraception used until menses has appeared or pregnancy has been excluded.

CONTRAINDICATIONS

Past or present thrombophlebitis or thromboembolic disorders ●

Past or present coronary artery disease ●

Past or present cerebrovascular disease ●

Known or suspected breast cancer ●

Known or suspected estrogen-dependent neoplasia ●

Undiagnosed abnormal vaginal bleeding ●

Known or suspected pregnancy ●

Markedly impaired liver function ●

WARNINGS/PRECAUTIONS

Cigarette smoking	Increases the risk of serious cardiovascular side effects, especially in women over 35 yr of age who smoke 15 or more cigarettes daily; patients who use oral contraceptives should be strongly urged not to smoke
Thromboembolic disease, thrombotic disorders, and other vascular problems	Risk is increased, becoming greater with age and the amount of estrogen present in the formulation. Discontinue oral contraception immediately if early signs of thromboembolic disease or thrombotic disorders (eg, thrombophlebitis, pulmonary embolism, cerebrovascular insufficiency, coronary occlusion, or retinal or mesenteric thrombosis) develop or are suspected.
Postsurgical thromboembolic complications	Risk is increased 4-6 times; if feasible, discontinue oral contraception at least 4 wk before elective surgery associated with an increased risk of thromboembolism or prolonged immobilization
Ocular lesions, including optic neuritis and retinal thrombosis	May occur; discontinue oral contraception in the presence of unexplained gradual or sudden, partial or complete loss of vision; proptosis or diplopia; papilledema; or retinal vascular lesions
Carcinoma	Closely monitor patients with a strong family history of breast cancer or with breast nodules, fibrocystic disease, or abnormal mammograms; investigate all cases of undiagnosed persistent or recurrent abnormal vaginal bleeding for malignancy (see CONTRAINDICATIONS)
Hepatic tumors	May occur and possibly rupture, resulting in intra-abdominal hemorrhage and death; investigate all cases of abdominal pain and tenderness, right upper quadrant mass, or shock for liver tumors
Gallbladder disease	Risk increases with duration of oral contraception
Hepatic impairment	Use with caution due to poor steroid hormone metabolism (see CONTRAINDICATIONS)
Jaundice	May recur in patients with a history of jaundice; discontinue oral contraception while cause is investigated
Glucose tolerance	May become impaired; closely monitor patients with latent or active diabetes
Hypertension	May be precipitated or may worsen with oral contraception, particularly with prolonged use and in older patients. Closely monitor patients with a history of hypertension, toxemia, hypertension during pregnancy, or excessive weight gain or fluid retention during the menstrual cycle; pre-existing renal disease; or a family history of hypertension or hypertensive complications.

Table continued on following page

NORINYL continued

WARNINGS/PRECAUTIONS continued	
Migraine headache	May develop or worsen; discontinue oral contraception and investigate cause of recurrent, persistent, or severe headaches
Bleeding irregularities, including breakthrough bleeding, spotting, and amenorrhea	May occur, necessitating either a change to a formulation with a higher estrogen content or discontinuation of therapy; higher amounts of estrogen, while potentially useful for minimizing menstrual irregularities, may increase the risk of thromboembolic disease
Mental depression	Risk is increased; discontinue oral contraception if serious depression develops or recurs in patients with a history of depression
Fluid retention	May occur; use with caution in patients with convulsive disorders, migraine, asthma, or cardiac, hepatic, or renal dysfunction
Vitamin deficiencies	May occur, particularly of pyridoxine and folic acid
Failure of withdrawal bleeding	If patient has not adhered to prescribed regimen, pregnancy should be considered after the first missed period and oral contraception withheld until pregnancy has been excluded; if patient has adhered to regimen and misses two consecutive periods, pregnancy should be ruled out before contraceptive regimen is continued
Postpill amenorrhea and anovulation	May occur, particularly in patients with a history of oligomenorrhea or secondary amenorrhea or in young women who have not established regular menstrual cycles; such patients should be encouraged to use alternative methods of contraception
Interfility	May occur following discontinuation of oral contraception, independent of its duration; diminishes with time but may still be apparent up to 30 mo in parous women and up to 42 mo in nulliparous women

ADVERSE REACTIONS	Frequent reactions are italicized
Genitourinary	*Breakthrough bleeding, spotting, menstrual irregularities, vaginal candidiasis,* postpill amenorrhea and infertility, dysmenorrhea, altered cervical erosion and secretion, enlargement of uterine leiomyomata, premenstrual-like syndrome, altered libido, cystitis-like syndrome, vaginitis
Cardiovascular	Thrombophlebitis, thrombosis, pulmonary embolism, coronary thrombosis, cerebral thrombosis, cerebral hemorrhage, hypertension, mesenteric thrombosis, edema
Gastrointestinal	*Nausea, vomiting,* gallbladder disease, abdominal cramps, bloating, change in appetite
Hepatic	Liver tumors, cholestatic jaundice
Metabolic and endocrinological	*Breast enlargement, tenderness, and/or secretion;* carbohydrate intolerance; increase or decrease in weight; hyperlipidemia
Central nervous system and neuromuscular	Migraine, depression, headache, nervousness, dizziness, chorea
Ophthalmic	Optic neuritis, retinal thrombosis, intolerance to contact lenses, altered corneal curvature, cataracts
Allergic and dermatological	Rash, melasma or chloasma, erythema multiforme, erythema nodosum, hirsutism, hair loss, hemorrhagic eruption, porphyria
Other	Congenital anomalies, prolactin-secreting pituitary tumors, impaired renal function

OVERDOSAGE	
Signs and symptoms	Nausea, withdrawal bleeding
Treatment	Treat symptomatically

DRUG INTERACTIONS	
Ampicillin, penicillin V, neomycin, chloramphenicol, sulfonamides, nitrofurantoin, rifampin, isoniazid	⇩ Contraceptive effect ⇧ Breakthrough bleeding
Analgesics, phenylbutazone, antimigraine preparations	⇩ Contraceptive effect ⇧ Breakthrough bleeding
Phenytoin, primidone	⇩ Contraceptive effect ⇧ Breakthrough bleeding
Barbiturates, tranquilizers	⇩ Contraceptive effect ⇧ Breakthrough bleeding
Antihypertensive agents (eg, guanethidine)	⇩ Antihypertensive effect
Oral anticoagulants	⇩ Anticoagulant effect
Anticonvulsants	⇧ Seizure activity
Hypoglycemic agents	⇩ Glucose tolerance
Corticosteroids	⇧ Corticosteroid effects
Tricyclic antidepressants	⇧ Antidepressant side effects

Table continued on following page

NORINYL continued

ALTERED LABORATORY VALUES

Blood/serum values — ⇧ Alkaline phosphatase ⇧ Bilirubin ⇧ Sulfobromophthalein retention ⇧ Prothrombin ⇧ Clotting factors VII, VIII, IX, and X ⇩ Antithrombin III ⇧ PBI ⇧ Thyroxine (T_4) ⇩ Triiodothyronine (T_3) uptake ⇧ Glucose ⇧ Cortisol ⇧ Transcortin ⇧ Ceruloplasmin ⇧ Triglycerides ⇧ Phospholipids ⇩ Folic acid ⇩ Pyridoxine

Urinary values — ⇩ Pregnanediol

Use in children

No appropriate indications exist. Acute ingestion by young children has not been associated with serious ill effects.

Use in pregnancy or nursing mothers

Contraindicated if pregnancy is known or suspected, as serious fetal damage may occur during early pregnancy. Patient should discontinue oral contraception 3 mo before attempting to conceive. Postpartum use may interfere with lactation, causing a decrease in the quantity and quality of breast milk. Patient should use alternative form of contraception until infant is weaned.

NORLESTRIN 21 1/50 (21-day regimen) **Parke-Davis**
NORLESTRIN 28 1/50 (28-day regimen) **Parke-Davis**

Tabs: 1 mg norethindrone acetate and 50 μg ethinyl estradiol

NORLESTRIN Fe 1/50 (28-day regimen) **Parke-Davis**

Tabs: 1 mg norethindrone acetate and 50 μg ethinyl estradiol (yellow); 75 mg ferrous fumarate (brown)

NORLESTRIN 21 2.5/50 (21-day regimen) **Parke-Davis**

Tabs: 2.5 mg norethindrone acetate and 50 μg ethinyl estradiol

NORLESTRIN Fe 2.5/50 (28-day regimen) **Parke-Davis**

Tabs: 2.5 mg norethindrone acetate and 50 μg ethinyl estradiol (pink); 75 mg ferrous fumarate (brown)

INDICATIONS	ORAL DOSAGE
Contraception	**Adult:** 1 tab/day for 21 or 28 consecutive days of the menstrual cycle

ADMINISTRATION/DOSAGE ADJUSTMENTS

Initiating therapy	First tablet should be taken on the 5th day after the onset of menses
Subsequent cycles (21-day regimen)	First tablet is taken 8 days after last tablet was taken in preceding cycle
Subsequent cycles (28-day regimen)	First tablet is taken 1 day after last (placebo) tablet was taken in preceding cycle
Missed tablets	If one tablet is missed, it should be taken as soon as it is remembered or together with the next tablet on the following day. If two tablets are missed, the dosage should be doubled for the next 2 days. If three tablets are missed, the tablet cycle should be discontinued and another form of contraception used until the start of the next menstrual period. Instruct the patient to start the next course of tablets 7 days after the last tablet was taken, even if she is still menstruating.

CONTRAINDICATIONS

Past or present thrombophlebitis or thromboembolic disorders ●

Coronary artery disease ●

Cerebrovascular disease ●

Known or suspected breast cancer ●

Known or suspected estrogen-dependent neoplasia ●

Undiagnosed abnormal vaginal bleeding ●

Known or suspected pregnancy ●

WARNINGS/PRECAUTIONS

Cigarette smoking	Increases the risk of serious cardiovascular side effects, especially in women over 35 yr of age who smoke 15 or more cigarettes daily; patients who use oral contraceptives should be strongly urged not to smoke
Thromboembolic disease, thrombotic disorders, and other vascular problems	Risk is increased, becoming greater with age and the amount of estrogen present in the formulation. Discontinue oral contraception immediately if early signs of thromboembolic disease or thrombotic disorders (eg, thrombophlebitis, pulmonary embolism, cerebrovascular insufficiency, coronary occlusion, or retinal or mesenteric thrombosis) develop or are suspected.
Postsurgical thromboembolic complications	Risk is increased 4–6 times; if feasible, discontinue oral contraception at least 4 wk before elective surgery associated with an increased risk of thromboembolism or prolonged immobilization
Ocular lesions, including optic neuritis and retinal thrombosis	May occur; discontinue oral contraception in the presence of unexplained gradual or sudden, partial or complete loss of vision; proptosis or diplopia; papilledema; or retinal vascular lesions
Carcinoma	Closely monitor patients with a strong family history of breast cancer or with breast nodules, fibrocystic disease, or abnormal mammograms; investigate all cases of undiagnosed persistent or recurrent abnormal vaginal bleeding for malignancy (see CONTRAINDICATIONS)
Hepatic tumors, including benign adenomas	May occur and possibly rupture, resulting in intra-abdominal hemorrhage and death; investigate all cases of abdominal pain and tenderness, abdominal mass, or shock for hepatic adenoma
Gallbladder disease	Risk increases with duration of oral contraception
Hepatic impairment	Use with caution due to poor steroid hormone metabolism
Jaundice	May recur in patients with a history of jaundice; discontinue oral contraception while cause is investigated
Glucose tolerance	May become impaired; closely monitor patients with latent or active diabetes
Hypertension	May be precipitated or may worsen with oral contraception, particularly with prolonged use, in older patients, and in patients with a history of hypertension during pregnancy
Migraine headache	May develop or worsen; discontinue oral contraception and investigate cause of recurrent, persistent, or severe headaches

Table continued on following page

WARNINGS/PRECAUTIONS continued

Bleeding irregularities, including breakthrough bleeding, spotting, and amenorrhea	May occur, necessitating either a change to a formulation with a higher estrogen content or discontinuation of therapy; higher amounts of estrogen, while potentially useful for minimizing menstrual irregularities, may increase the risk of thromboembolic disease
Mental depression	Risk is increased; discontinue oral contraception if serious depression develops or recurs in patients with a history of depression
Fluid retention	May occur; use with caution in patients with convulsive disorders, migraine, asthma, or cardiac, hepatic, or renal dysfunction
Vitamin deficiencies	May occur, particularly of pyridoxine and folic acid
Failure of withdrawal bleeding	If patient has missed two consecutive periods, pregnancy should be ruled out before contraceptive regimen is continued; if patient has not adhered to prescribed regimen, pregnancy should be considered after the first missed period and oral contraception withheld until pregnancy has been excluded
Postpill amenorrhea and anovulation	May occur, particularly in patients with a history of oligomenorrhea or secondary amenorrhea or in young women who have not established regular menstrual cycles; such patients should be encouraged to use alternative methods of contraception

ADVERSE REACTIONS	Frequent reactions are italicized
Genitourinary	*Breakthrough bleeding, spotting, menstrual irregularities, vaginal candidiasis,* postpill amenorrhea and infertility, dysmenorrhea, altered cervical erosion and secretion, enlargement of uterine leiomyomata, premenstrual-like syndrome, altered libido, cystitis-like syndrome, vaginitis
Cardiovascular	Thrombophlebitis, pulmonary embolism, coronary thrombosis, cerebral thrombosis, cerebral hemorrhage, hypertension, mesenteric thrombosis, edema
Gastrointestinal	*Nausea, vomiting,* gallbladder disease, abdominal cramps, bloating, change in appetite
Hepatic	Benign hepatomas, cholestatic jaundice
Metabolic and endocrinological	*Breast enlargement, tenderness, and/or secretion;* carbohydrate intolerance; increase or decrease in weight; hyperlipidemia
Central nervous system and neuromuscular	Migraine, depression, headache, nervousness, dizziness, chorea
Ophthalmic	Optic neuritis, retinal thrombosis, intolerance to contact lenses, altered corneal curvature, cataracts
Allergic and dermatological	Rash, melasma or chloasma, erythema multiforme, erythema nodosum, hirsutism, hair loss, hemorrhagic eruption, porphyria
Other	Congenital anomalies

OVERDOSAGE

Signs and symptoms	Nausea, withdrawal bleeding
Treatment	Treat symptomatically

DRUG INTERACTIONS

Ampicillin, penicillin V, neomycin, chloramphenicol, sulfonamides, nitrofurantoin, rifampin, isoniazid	⇩ Contraceptive effect ⇧ Breakthrough bleeding
Analgesics, phenylbutazone, antimigraine preparations	⇩ Contraceptive effect ⇧ Breakthrough bleeding
Phenytoin, primidone	⇩ Contraceptive effect ⇧ Breakthrough bleeding
Barbiturates, tranquilizers	⇩ Contraceptive effect ⇧ Breakthrough bleeding
Antihypertensive agents (eg, guanethidine)	⇩ Antihypertensive effect
Oral anticoagulants	⇩ Anticoagulant effect
Anticonvulsants	⇧ Seizure activity
Hypoglycemic agents	⇩ Glucose tolerance
Corticosteroids	⇧ Corticosteroid effects
Tricyclic antidepressants	⇧ Antidepressant side effects

Table continued on following page

NORLESTRIN continued

ALTERED LABORATORY VALUES

Blood/serum values	⇧ Alkaline phosphatase ⇧ Bilirubin ⇧ Sulfobromophthalein retention ⇧ Prothrombin ⇧ Clotting factors VII, VIII, IX, and X ⇩ Antithrombin III ⇧ PBI ⇧ Thyroxine (T_4) ⇩ Triiodothyronine (T_3) uptake ⇧ Glucose ⇧ Cortisol ⇧ Transcortin ⇧ Ceruloplasmin ⇧ Triglycerides ⇧ Phospholipids ⇩ Folic acid ⇩ Pyridoxine
Urinary values	⇩ Pregnanediol

Use in children

No appropriate indications exist. Acute ingestion by young children has not been associated with serious ill effects.

Use in pregnancy or nursing mothers

Contraindicated if pregnancy is known or suspected, as serious fetal damage may occur during early pregnancy. Patient should discontinue oral contraception 3 mo before attempting to conceive. Postpartum use may interfere with lactation, causing a decrease in the quantity and quality of breast milk. Patient should use alternative form of contraception until infant is weaned.

ORTHO-NOVUM 1/35 ☐ 21 (21-day regimen) **Ortho**
ORTHO-NOVUM 1/35 ☐ 28 (28-day regimen) **Ortho**

Tabs: 1 mg norethindrone and 50 μg ethinyl estradiol

INDICATIONS	ORAL DOSAGE
Contraception	**Adult:** 1 tab/day for 21 or 28 consecutive days of the menstrual cycle

ADMINISTRATION/DOSAGE ADJUSTMENTS

Initiating therapy	First tablet should be taken on the 5th day (21-day regimen) or 1st Sunday (28-day regimen) after the onset of menses; if menses begins on a Sunday, regimen is started the very same day
Subsequent cycles (21-day regimen)	First tablet is taken 8 days after last tablet was taken in preceding cycle
Subsequent cycles (28-day regimen)	First tablet is taken 1 day after last (placebo) tablet was taken in preceding cycle
Missed tablets	If more than one tablet is missed, instruct patient to resume taking tablets as soon as remembered, but to use an additional form of contraception for the remainder of the cycle

CONTRAINDICATIONS

Past or present thrombophlebitis or thromboembolic disorders ●

Coronary artery disease ●

Cerebrovascular disease ●

Known or suspected breast cancer ●

Known or suspected estrogen-dependent neoplasia ●

Undiagnosed abnormal vaginal bleeding ●

Known or suspected pregnancy ●

WARNINGS/PRECAUTIONS

Cigarette smoking	Increases the risk of serious cardiovascular side effects, especially in women over 35 yr of age who smoke 15 or more cigarettes daily; patients who use oral contraceptives should be strongly urged not to smoke
Thromboembolic disease, thrombotic disorders, and other vascular problems	Risk is increased, becoming greater with age and the amount of estrogen present in the formulation. Discontinue oral contraception immediately if early signs of thromboembolic disease or thrombotic disorders (eg, thrombophlebitis, pulmonary embolism, cerebrovascular insufficiency, coronary occlusion, or retinal or mesenteric thrombosis) develop or are suspected.
Postsurgical thromboembolic complications	Risk is increased 4–6 times; if feasible, discontinue oral contraception at least 4 wk before elective surgery associated with an increased risk of thromboembolism or prolonged immobilization
Ocular lesions, including optic neuritis and retinal thrombosis	May occur; discontinue oral contraception in the presence of unexplained gradual or sudden, partial or complete loss of vision; proptosis or diplopia; papilledema; or retinal vascular lesions
Carcinoma	Closely monitor patients with a strong family history of breast cancer or with breast nodules, fibrocystic disease, or abnormal mammograms; investigate all cases of undiagnosed persistent or recurrent abnormal vaginal bleeding for malignancy (see CONTRAINDICATIONS)
Hepatic tumors, including benign adenomas	May occur and possibly rupture, resulting in intra-abdominal hemorrhage and death; investigate all cases of abdominal pain and tenderness, abdominal mass, or shock for hepatic adenoma
Gallbladder disease	Risk increases with duration of oral contraception
Hepatic impairment	Use with caution due to poor steroid hormone metabolism
Jaundice	May recur in patients with a history of jaundice; discontinue oral contraception while cause is investigated
Glucose tolerance	May become impaired; closely monitor patients with latent or active diabetes
Hypertension	May be precipitated or may worsen with oral contraception, particularly with prolonged use, in older patients and in patients with a history of hypertension during pregnancy
Migraine headache	May develop or worsen; discontinue oral contraception and investigate cause of recurrent, persistent, or severe headaches
Bleeding irregularities, including breakthrough bleeding, spotting, and amenorrhea	May occur, necessitating either a change to a formulation with a higher estrogen content or discontinuation of therapy; higher amounts of estrogen, while potentially useful for minimizing menstrual irregularities, may increase the risk of thromboembolic disease
Mental depression	Risk is increased; discontinue oral contraception if serious depression develops or recurs in patients with a history of depression
Fluid retention	May occur; use with caution in patients with convulsive disorders, migraine, asthma, or cardiac, hepatic, or renal dysfunction

Table continued on following page

WARNINGS/PRECAUTIONS continued	
Vitamin deficiencies	May occur, particularly of pyridoxine and folic acid
Failure of withdrawal bleeding	If patient has not adhered to prescribed regimen, pregnancy should be considered after the first missed period and oral contraception withheld until pregnancy has been excluded; if patient has adhered to regimen and misses two consecutive periods, pregnancy should be ruled out before regimen is continued
Postpill amenorrhea and anovulation	May occur, particularly in patients with a history of oligomenorrhea or secondary amenorrhea or in young women who have not established regular menstrual cycles; such patients should be encouraged to use alternative methods of contraception

ADVERSE REACTIONS	Frequent reactions are italicized
Genitourinary	*Breakthrough bleeding, spotting, menstrual irregularities, vaginal candidiasis,* postpill amenorrhea and infertility, dysmenorrhea, altered cervical erosion and secretion, enlargement of uterine leiomyomata, premenstrual-like syndrome, altered libido, cystitis-like syndrome, vaginitis
Cardiovascular	Thrombophlebitis, pulmonary embolism, coronary thrombosis, cerebral thrombosis, cerebral hemorrhage, hypertension, mesenteric thrombosis, edema
Gastrointestinal	*Nausea, vomiting,* gallbladder disease, abdominal cramps, bloating, change in appetite
Hepatic	Hepatic tumors, cholestatic jaundice
Metabolic and endocrinological	*Breast enlargement, tenderness, and/or secretion;* carbohydrate intolerance; increase or decrease in weight; hyperlipidemia
Central nervous system and neuromuscular	Migraine, depression, headache, nervousness, dizziness, chorea
Ophthalmic	Optic neuritis, retinal thrombosis, intolerance to contact lenses, altered corneal curvature, cataracts
Allergic and dermatological	Rash, melasma or chloasma, erythema multiforme, erythema nodosum, hirsutism, hair loss, hemorrhagic eruption, porphyria
Other	Congenital anomalies, impaired renal function

OVERDOSAGE	
Signs and symptoms	Nausea, withdrawal bleeding
Treatment	Treat symptomatically

DRUG INTERACTIONS	
Ampicillin, penicillin V, neomycin, chloramphenicol, sulfonamides, nitrofurantoin, rifampin, isoniazid	⇩ Contraceptive effect ⇧ Breakthrough bleeding
Analgesics, phenylbutazone, antimigraine preparations	⇩ Contraceptive effect ⇧ Breakthrough bleeding
Phenytoin, primidone	⇩ Contraceptive effect ⇧ Breakthrough bleeding
Barbiturates, tranquilizers	⇩ Contraceptive effect ⇧ Breakthrough bleeding
Antihypertensive agents	⇩ Antihypertensive effect
Oral anticoagulants	⇩ Anticoagulant effect
Anticonvulsants	⇧ Seizure activity
Hypoglycemic agents	⇩ Glucose tolerance
Corticosteroids	⇧ Corticosteroid effects
Tricyclic antidepressants	⇧ Antidepressant side effects

ALTERED LABORATORY VALUES	
Blood/serum values	⇧ Alkaline phosphatase ⇧ Bilirubin ⇧ Sulfobromophthalein retention ⇧ Prothrombin ⇧ Clotting factors VII, VIII, IX, and X ⇩ Antithrombin III ⇧ PBI ⇧ Thyroxine (T_4) ⇩ Triiodothyronine (T_3) uptake ⇧ Glucose ⇧ Cortisol ⇧ Transcortin ⇧ Ceruloplasmin ⇧ Triglycerides ⇧ Phospholipids ⇩ Folic acid ⇩ Pyridoxine
Urinary values	⇩ Pregnanediol

Use in children

No appropriate indications exist. Acute ingestion by young children has not been associated with serious ill effects.

Use in pregnancy or nursing mothers

Contraindicated if pregnancy is known or suspected, as serious fetal damage may occur during early pregnancy. Patient should discontinue oral contraception 3 mo before attempting to conceive. Postpartum use may interfere with lactation, causing a decrease in the quantity and quality of breast milk. Patient should use alternative form of contraception until infant is weaned.

ORTHO-NOVUM 1/50 □ 21 (21-day regimen) **Ortho**
ORTHO-NOVUM 1/50 □ 28 (28-day regimen) **Ortho**

Tabs: 1 mg norethindrone and 50 μg mestranol

ORTHO-NOVUM 1/80 □ 21 (21-day regimen) **Ortho**
ORTHO-NOVUM 1/80 □ 28 (21-day regimen) **Ortho**

Tabs: 1 mg norethindrone and 80 μg mestranol

INDICATIONS	ORAL DOSAGE
Contraception	**Adult:** 1 tab/day for 21 or 28 consecutive days of the menstrual cycle

ADMINISTRATION/DOSAGE ADJUSTMENTS

Initiating therapy	First tablet should be taken on the 5th day (21-day regimen) or 1st Sunday (28-day regimen) after the onset of menses; if menses begins on a Sunday, regimen is started the very same day
Subsequent cycles (21-day regimen)	First tablet is taken 8 days after last tablet was taken in preceding cycle
Subsequent cycles (28-day regimen)	First tablet is taken 1 day after last (placebo) tablet was taken in preceding cycle
Missed tablets	If more than one tablet is missed, instruct patient to resume taking tablets as soon as remembered, but to use an additional form of contraception for the remainder of the cycle

CONTRAINDICATIONS

Past or present thrombophlebitis or thromboembolic disorders ●	Known or suspected breast cancer ●	Known or suspected pregnancy ●
Coronary artery disease ●	Known or suspected estrogen-dependent neoplasia ●	
Cerebrovascular disease ●	Undiagnosed abnormal vaginal bleeding ●	

WARNINGS/PRECAUTIONS

Cigarette smoking	Increases the risk of serious cardiovascular side effects, especially in women over 35 yr of age who smoke 15 or more cigarettes daily; patients who use oral contraceptives should be strongly urged not to smoke
Thromboembolic disease, thrombotic disorders, and other vascular problems	Risk is increased, becoming greater with age and the amount of estrogen present in the formulation. Discontinue oral contraception immediately if early signs of thromboembolic disease or thrombotic disorders (eg, thrombophlebitis, pulmonary embolism, cerebrovascular insufficiency, coronary occlusion, or retinal or mesenteric thrombosis) develop or are suspected.
Postsurgical thromboembolic complications	Risk is increased 4–6 times; if feasible, discontinue oral contraception at least 4 wk before elective surgery associated with an increased risk of thromboembolism or prolonged immobilization
Ocular lesions, including optic neuritis and retinal thrombosis	May occur; discontinue oral contraception in the presence of unexplained gradual or sudden, partial or complete loss of vision; proptosis or diplopia; papilledema; or retinal vascular lesions
Carcinoma	Closely monitor patients with a strong family history of breast cancer or with breast nodules, fibrocystic disease, or abnormal mammograms; investigate all cases of undiagnosed persistent or recurrent abnormal vaginal bleeding for malignancy (see CONTRAINDICATIONS)
Hepatic tumors, including benign adenomas	May occur and possibly rupture, resulting in intra-abdominal hemorrhage and death; investigate all cases of abdominal pain and tenderness, abdominal mass, or shock for hepatic adenoma
Gallbladder disease	Risk increases with duration of oral contraception
Hepatic impairment	Use with caution due to poor steroid hormone metabolism
Jaundice	May recur in patients with a history of jaundice; discontinue oral contraception while cause is investigated
Glucose tolerance	May become impaired; closely monitor patients with latent or active diabetes
Hypertension	May be precipitated or may worsen with oral contraception, particularly with prolonged use, in older patients, and in patients with a history of hypertension during pregnancy
Migraine headache	May develop or worsen; discontinue oral contraception and investigate cause of recurrent, persistent, or severe headaches
Bleeding irregularities, including breakthrough bleeding, spotting, and amenorrhea	May occur, necessitating either a change to a formulation with a higher estrogen content or discontinuation of therapy; higher amounts of estrogen, while potentially useful for minimizing menstrual irregularities, may increase the risk of thromboembolic disease
Mental depression	Risk is increased; discontinue oral contraception if serious depression develops or recurs in patients with a history of depression

Table continued on following page

WARNINGS/PRECAUTIONS continued

Fluid retention	May occur; use with caution in patients with convulsive disorders, migraine, asthma, or cardiac, hepatic, or renal dysfunction
Vitamin deficiencies	May occur, particularly of pyridoxine and folic acid
Failure of withdrawal bleeding	If patient has not adhered to prescribed regimen, pregnancy should be considered after the first missed period and oral contraception withheld until pregnancy has been excluded; if patient has adhered to regimen and misses two consecutive periods, pregnancy should be ruled out before contraceptive regimen is continued
Postpill amenorrhea and anovulation	May occur, particularly in patients with a history of oligomenorrhea or secondary amenorrhea or in young women who have not established regular menstrual cycles; such patients should be encouraged to use alternative methods of contraception
Tartrazine sensitivity	Presence of FD&C Yellow No. 5 (tartrazine) in Ortho-Novum 1/50□21 and 1/50□28 tablets may cause allergic-type reactions, including bronchial asthma, in susceptible individuals

ADVERSE REACTIONS	Frequent reactions are italicized
Genitourinary	*Breakthrough bleeding, spotting, menstrual irregularities, vaginal candidiasis,* postpill amenorrhea and infertility, dysmenorrhea, altered cervical erosion and secretion, enlargement of uterine leiomyomata, premenstrual-like syndrome, altered libido, cystitis-like syndrome, vaginitis
Cardiovascular	Thrombophlebitis, pulmonary embolism, coronary thrombosis, cerebral thrombosis, cerebral hemorrhage, hypertension, mesenteric thrombosis, edema
Gastrointestinal	*Nausea, vomiting,* gallbladder disease, abdominal cramps, bloating, change in appetite
Hepatic	Hepatic tumors, cholestatic jaundice
Metabolic and endocrinological	*Breast enlargement, tenderness, and/or secretion;* carbohydrate intolerance; increase or decrease in weight; hyperlipidemia
Central nervous system and neuromuscular	Migraine, depression, headache, nervousness, dizziness, chorea
Ophthalmic	Optic neuritis, retinal thrombosis, intolerance to contact lenses, altered corneal curvature, cataracts
Allergic and dermatological	Rash, melasma or chloasma, erythema multiforme, erythema nodosum, hirsutism, hair loss, hemorrhagic eruption, porphyria
Other	Congenital anomalies, impaired renal function

OVERDOSAGE

Signs and symptoms	Nausea, withdrawal bleeding
Treatment	Treat symptomatically

DRUG INTERACTIONS

Ampicillin, penicillin V, neomycin, chloramphenicol, sulfonamides, nitrofurantoin, rifampin, isoniazid	⇩ Contraceptive effect ⇧ Breakthrough bleeding
Analgesics, phenylbutazone, antimigraine preparations	⇩ Contraceptive effect ⇧ Breakthrough bleeding
Phenytoin, primidone	⇩ Contraceptive effect ⇧ Breakthrough bleeding
Barbiturates, tranquilizers	⇩ Contraceptive effect ⇧ Breakthrough bleeding
Antihypertensive agents (eg, guanethidine)	⇩ Antihypertensive effect
Oral anticoagulants	⇩ Anticoagulant effect
Anticonvulsants	⇧ Seizure activity
Hypoglycemic agents	⇩ Glucose tolerance
Corticosteroids	⇧ Corticosteroid effects
Tricyclic antidepressants	⇧ Antidepressant side effects

Table continued on following page

ALTERED LABORATORY VALUES

Blood/serum values	⇧ Alkaline phosphatase ⇧ Bilirubin ⇧ Sulfobromophthalein retention ⇧ Prothrombin ⇧ Clotting factors VII, VIII, IX, and X ⇩ Antithrombin III ⇧ PBI ⇧ Thyroxine (T_4) ⇩ Triiodothyronine (T_3) uptake ⇧ Glucose ⇧ Cortisol ⇧ Transcortin ⇧ Ceruloplasmin ⇧ Triglycerides ⇧ Phospholipids ⇩ Folic acid ⇩ Pyridoxine
Urinary values	⇩ Pregnanediol

Use in children

No appropriate indications exist. Acute ingestion by young children has not been associated with serious ill effects.

Use in pregnancy or nursing mothers

Contraindicated if pregnancy is known or suspected, as serious fetal damage may occur during early pregnancy. Patient should discontinue oral contraception 3 mo before attempting to conceive. Postpartum use may interfere with lactation, causing a decrease in the quantity and quality of breast milk. Patient should use alternative form of contraception until infant is weaned.

OVCON-35 (21-day regimen) **Mead Johnson**
OVCON-35 (28-day regimen) **Mead Johnson**
Tabs: 0.4 mg norethindrone and 35 μg ethinyl estradiol

OVCON-50 (21-day regimen) **Mead Johnson**
OVCON-50 (28-day regimen) **Mead Johnson**
Tabs: 1 mg norethindrone and 50 μg ethinyl estradiol

INDICATIONS	ORAL DOSAGE
Contraception	**Adult:** 1 tab/day for 21 or 28 consecutive days of the menstrual cycle

ADMINISTRATION/DOSAGE ADJUSTMENTS

Initiating therapy	First tablet should be taken on the 5th day after the onset of menses
Subsequent cycles (21-day regimen)	First tablet is taken 8 days after last tablet was taken in preceding cycle
Subsequent cycles (28-day regimen)	First tablet is taken 1 day after last (placebo) tablet was taken in preceding cycle
Missed tablets	If the regimen is interrupted, an additional form of contraception should be used for the remainder of the cycle

CONTRAINDICATIONS

Past or present thrombophlebitis or thromboembolic disorders ●	Known or suspected breast cancer ●	Known or suspected pregnancy ●
Coronary artery disease ●	Known or suspected estrogen-dependent neoplasia ●	
Cerebrovascular disease ●	Undiagnosed abnormal vaginal bleeding ●	

WARNINGS/PRECAUTIONS

Cigarette smoking	Increases the risk of serious cardiovascular side effects, especially in women over 35 yr of age who smoke 15 or more cigarettes daily; patients who use oral contraceptives should be strongly urged not to smoke
Thromboembolic disease, thrombotic disorders, and other vascular problems	Risk is increased, becoming greater with age and the amount of estrogen present in the formulation. Discontinue oral contraception immediately if early signs of thromboembolic disease or thrombotic disorders (eg, thrombophlebitis, pulmonary embolism, cerebrovascular insufficiency, coronary occlusion, or retinal or mesenteric thrombosis) develop or are suspected.
Postsurgical thromboembolic complications	Risk is increased 4–6 times; if feasible, discontinue oral contraception at least 4 wk before elective surgery associated with an increased risk of thromboembolism or prolonged immobilization
Ocular lesions, including optic neuritis and retinal thrombosis	May occur; discontinue oral contraception in the presence of unexplained gradual or sudden, partial or complete loss of vision; proptosis or diplopia; papilledema; or retinal vascular lesions
Carcinoma	Closely monitor patients with a strong family history of breast cancer or with breast nodules, fibrocystic disease, or abnormal mammograms; investigate all cases of undiagnosed persistent or recurrent abnormal vaginal bleeding for malignancy (see CONTRAINDICATIONS)
Hepatic lesions, including benign adenomas	May occur and possibly rupture, resulting in intra-abdominal hemorrhage and death; investigate all cases of abdominal pain and tenderness, abdominal mass, or shock for hepatic adenoma
Gallbladder disease	Risk increases with duration of oral contraception
Hepatic impairment	Use with caution due to poor steroid hormone metabolism
Jaundice	May recur in patients with a history of jaundice; discontinue oral contraception while cause is investigated
Glucose tolerance	May become impaired; closely monitor patients with latent or active diabetes
Hypertension	May be precipitated or may worsen with oral contraception, particularly with prolonged use, in older patients, and in patients with a history of hypertension during pregnancy
Migraine headache	May develop or worsen; discontinue oral contraception and investigate cause of recurrent, persistent, or severe headaches
Bleeding irregularities, including breakthrough bleeding, spotting, and amenorrhea	May occur, necessitating either a change to a formulation with a higher estrogen content or discontinuation of therapy; higher amounts of estrogen, while potentially useful for minimizing menstrual irregularities, may increase the risk of thromboembolic disease
Mental depression	Risk is increased; discontinue oral contraception if serious depression develops or recurs in patients with a history of depression
Fluid retention	May occur; use with caution in patients with convulsive disorders, migraine, asthma, or cardiac, hepatic, or renal dysfunction

Table continued on following page

OVCON continued

WARNINGS/PRECAUTIONS continued

Vitamin deficiencies	May occur, particularly of pyridoxine and folic acid
Failure of withdrawal bleeding	If patient has not adhered to prescribed regimen, pregnancy should be considered after the first missed period and oral contraception withheld until pregnancy has been excluded; if patient has adhered to regimen and misses two consecutive periods, pregnancy should be ruled out before contraceptive regimen is reinstituted
Postpill amenorrhea and anovulation	May occur, particularly in patients with a history of oligomenorrhea or secondary amenorrhea or in young women who have not established regular menstrual cycles; such patients should be encouraged to use alternative methods of contraception
Tartrazine sensitivity	Presence of FD&C Yellow No. 5 (tartrazine) in 21-day Ovcon-35 tablets and 21- and 28-day Ovcon-50 tablets may cause allergic-type reactions, including bronchial asthma, in susceptible individuals

ADVERSE REACTIONS	Frequent reactions are italicized
Genitourinary	*Breakthrough bleeding, spotting, menstrual irregularities, vaginal candidiasis,* postpill amenorrhea and infertility, dysmenorrhea, altered cervical erosion and secretion, enlargement of uterine leiomyomata, premenstrual-like syndrome, altered libido, cystitis-like syndrome, vaginitis
Cardiovascular	Thrombophlebitis, pulmonary embolism, coronary thrombosis, cerebral thrombosis, cerebral hemorrhage, hypertension, mesenteric thrombosis, edema
Gastrointestinal	*Nausea, vomiting,* gallbladder disease, abdominal cramps, bloating, change in appetite
Hepatic	Benign hepatomas, cholestatic jaundice
Metabolic and endocrinological	*Breast enlargement, tenderness, and/or secretion;* carbohydrate intolerance; increase or decrease in weight; hyperlipidemia
Central nervous system and neuromuscular	Migraine, depression, headache, nervousness, dizziness, chorea
Ophthalmic	Optic neuritis, retinal thrombosis, intolerance to contact lenses, altered corneal curvature, cataracts
Allergic and dermatological	Rash, melasma or chloasma, erythema multiforme, erythema nodosum, hirsutism, hair loss, hemorrhagic eruption, porphyria
Other	Congenital anomalies

OVERDOSAGE

Signs and symptoms	Nausea, withdrawal bleeding
Treatment	Treat symptomatically

DRUG INTERACTIONS

Ampicillin, penicillin V, neomycin, chloramphenicol, sulfonamides, nitrofurantoin, rifampin, isoniazid	⇩ Contraceptive effect ⇧ Breakthrough bleeding
Analgesics, phenylbutazone, antimigraine preparations	⇩ Contraceptive effect ⇧ Breakthrough bleeding
Phenytoin, primidone	⇩ Contraceptive effect ⇧ Breakthrough bleeding
Barbiturates, tranquilizers	⇩ Contraceptive effect ⇧ Breakthrough bleeding
Antihypertensive agents (eg, guanethidine)	⇩ Antihypertensive effect
Oral anticoagulants	⇩ Anticoagulant effect
Anticonvulsants	⇧ Seizure activity
Hypoglycemic agents	⇩ Glucose tolerance
Corticosteroids	⇧ Corticosteroid effects
Tricyclic antidepressants	⇧ Antidepressant side effects

Table continued on following page

OVCON continued

ALTERED LABORATORY VALUES

Blood/serum values — ⇧ Alkaline phosphatase ⇧ Bilirubin ⇧ Sulfobromophthalein retention ⇧ Prothrombin ⇧ Clotting factors VII, VIII, IX, and X ⇩ Antithrombin III ⇧ PBI ⇧ Thyroxine (T_4) ⇩ Triiodothyronine (T_3) uptake ⇧ Glucose ⇧ Cortisol ⇧ Transcortin ⇧ Ceruloplasmin ⇧ Triglycerides ⇧ Phospholipids ⇩ Folic acid ⇩ Pyridoxine

Urinary values — ⇩ Pregnanediol

Use in children

No appropriate indications exist. Acute ingestion by young children has not been associated with serious ill effects.

Use in pregnancy or nursing mothers

Contraindicated if pregnancy is known or suspected, as serious fetal damage may occur during early pregnancy. Patient should discontinue oral contraception 3 mo before attempting to conceive. Postpartum use may interfere with lactation, causing a decrease in the quantity and quality of breast milk. Patient should use alternative form of contraception until infant is weaned.

OVRAL (21-day regimen) **Wyeth**
OVRAL-28 (28-day regimen) **Wyeth**

Tabs: 0.5 mg norgestrel and 50 μg ethinyl estradiol

INDICATIONS	ORAL DOSAGE
Contraception	**Adult:** 1 tab/day for 21 or 28 consecutive days of the menstrual cycle

ADMINISTRATION/DOSAGE ADJUSTMENTS

Initiating therapy	First tablet should be taken on the 5th day after the onset of menses
Subsequent cycles (21-day regimen)	First tablet is taken 8 days after last tablet was taken in preceding cycle
Subsequent cycles (28-day regimen)	First tablet is taken 1 day after last (placebo) tablet was taken in preceding cycle
Missed tablets	If one or two tablets are missed, they should be taken as soon as they are remembered, and an additional form of contraception should be used for 1 wk. If three tablets are missed, the tablet cycle should be discontinued; start the next tablet cycle 8 days after the last tablet was taken and instruct patient to use another form of contraception for the 7 days without tablets and until seven tablets have been taken.
Postpartum administration	For nonnursing mothers, may be started either immediately or after first postpartum examination, regardless of whether spontaneous menstruation has occurred

CONTRAINDICATIONS

Past or present thrombophlebitis or thromboembolic disorders ●	Known or suspected breast cancer ●	Known or suspected pregnancy ●
Coronary artery disease ●	Known or suspected estrogen-dependent neoplasia ●	
Cerebrovascular disease ●	Undiagnosed abnormal vaginal bleeding ●	

WARNINGS/PRECAUTIONS

Cigarette smoking	Increases the risk of serious cardiovascular side effects, especially in women over 35 yr of age who smoke 15 or more cigarettes daily; patients who use oral contraceptives should be strongly urged not to smoke
Thromboembolic disease, thrombotic disorders, and other vascular problems	Risk is increased, becoming greater with age and the amount of estrogen present in the formulation. Discontinue oral contraception immediately if early signs of thromboembolic disease or thrombotic disorders (eg, thrombophlebitis, pulmonary embolism, cerebrovascular insufficiency, coronary occlusion, or retinal or mesenteric thrombosis) develop or are suspected.
Postsurgical thromboembolic complications	Risk is increased 4–6 times; if feasible, discontinue oral contraception at least 4 wk before elective surgery associated with an increased risk of thromboembolism or prolonged immobilization
Ocular lesions, including optic neuritis and retinal thrombosis	May occur; discontinue oral contraception in the presence of unexplained gradual or sudden, partial or complete loss of vision; proptosis or diplopia; papilledema; or retinal vascular lesions
Carcinoma	Closely monitor patients with a strong family history of breast cancer or with breast nodules, fibrocystic disease, or abnormal mammograms; investigate all cases of undiagnosed persistent or recurrent abnormal vaginal bleeding for malignancy (see CONTRAINDICATIONS)
Hepatic tumors, including benign adenomas	May occur and possibly rupture, resulting in intra-abdominal hemorrhage and death; investigate all cases of abdominal pain and tenderness, abdominal mass, or shock for hepatic adenoma
Gallbladder disease	Risk increases with duration of oral contraception
Hepatic impairment	Use with caution due to poor steroid hormone metabolism
Jaundice	May recur in patients with a history of jaundice; discontinue oral contraception while cause is investigated
Glucose tolerance	May become impaired; closely monitor patients with latent or active diabetes
Hypertension	May be precipitated or may worsen with oral contraception, particularly with prolonged use, in older patients, and in patients with a history of hypertension during pregnancy
Migraine headache	May develop or worsen; discontinue oral contraception and investigate cause of recurrent, persistent, or severe headaches
Bleeding irregularities, including breakthrough bleeding, spotting, and amenorrhea	May occur, necessitating either a change to a formulation with a higher estrogen content or discontinuation of therapy; higher amounts of estrogen, while potentially useful for minimizing menstrual irregularities, may increase the risk of thromboembolic disease
Mental depression	Risk is increased; discontinue oral contraception if serious depression develops or recurs in patients with a history of depression
Fluid retention	May occur; use with caution in patients with convulsive disorders, migraine, asthma, or cardiac, hepatic, or renal dysfunction

Table continued on following page

OVRAL continued

WARNINGS/PRECAUTIONS continued

Vitamin deficiencies	May occur, particularly of pyridoxine and folic acid
Failure of withdrawal bleeding	If patient has missed two consecutive periods, pregnancy should be ruled out before contraceptive regimen is continued; if patient has not adhered to prescribed regimen, pregnancy should be considered after the first missed period and oral contraception withheld until pregnancy has been excluded
Postpill amenorrhea and anovulation	May occur, particularly in patients with a history of oligomenorrhea or secondary amenorrhea or in young women who have not established regular menstrual cycles; such patients should be encouraged to use alternative methods of contraception

ADVERSE REACTIONS Frequent reactions are italicized

Genitourinary	*Breakthrough bleeding, spotting, menstrual irregularities, vaginal candidiasis,* postpill amenorrhea and infertility, dysmenorhea, altered cervical erosion and secretion, enlargement of uterine leiomyomata, premenstrual-like syndrome, altered libido, cystitis-like syndrome, vaginitis
Cardiovascular	Thrombophlebitis, pulmonary embolism, coronary thrombosis, cerebral thrombosis, cerebral hemorrhage, hypertension, mesenteric thrombosis, edema
Gastrointestinal	*Nausea, vomiting,* gallbladder disease, abdominal cramps, bloating, change in appetite
Hepatic	Benign hepatomas, cholestatic jaundice
Metabolic and endocrinological	*Breast enlargement, tenderness, and/or secretion;* carbohydrate intolerance; increase or decrease in weight; hyperlipidemia
Central nervous system and neuromuscular	Migraine, depression, anxiety, headache, nervousness, dizziness, chorea
Ophthalmic	Optic neuritis, retinal thrombosis, intolerance to contact lenses, altered corneal curvature, cataracts
Allergic and dermatological	Rash, melasma or chloasma, erythema multiforme, erythema nodosum, hirsutism, hair loss, hemorrhagic eruption, porphyria
Other	Congenital anomalies,

OVERDOSAGE

Signs and symptoms	Nausea, withdrawal bleeding
Treatment	Treat symptomatically

DRUG INTERACTIONS

Ampicillin, penicillin V, neomycin, chloramphenicol, sulfonamides, nitrofurantoin, rifampin, isoniazid	⇩ Contraceptive effect ⇧ Breakthrough bleeding
Analgesics, phenylbutazone, antimigraine preparations	⇩ Contraceptive effect ⇧ Breakthrough bleeding
Phenytoin, primidone	⇩ Contraceptive effect ⇧ Breakthrough bleeding
Barbiturates, tranquilizers	⇩ Contraceptive effect ⇧ Breakthrough bleeding
Antihypertensive agents (eg, guanethidine)	⇩ Antihypertensive effect
Oral anticoagulants	⇩ Anticoagulant effect
Anticonvulsants	⇧ Seizure activity
Hypoglycemic agents	⇩ Glucose tolerance
Corticosteroids	⇧ Corticosteroid effects
Tricyclic antidepressants	⇧ Antidepressant side effects

ALTERED LABORATORY VALUES

Blood/serum values	⇧ Alkaline phosphatase ⇧ Bilirubin ⇧ Sulfobromophthalein retention ⇧ Prothrombin ⇧ Clotting factors VII, VIII, IX, and X ⇩ Antithrombin III ⇧ PBI ⇧ Thyroxine (T_4) ⇩ Triiodothyronine (T_3) uptake ⇧ Glucose ⇧ Cortisol ⇧ Transcortin ⇧ Ceruloplasmin ⇧ Triglycerides ⇧ Phospholipids ⇩ Folic acid ⇩ Pyridoxine
Urinary values	⇩ Pregnanediol

Use in children

No appropriate indications exist. Acute ingestion by young children has not been associated with serious ill effects.

Use in pregnancy or nursing mothers

Contraindicated if pregnancy is known or suspected, as serious fetal damage may occur during early pregnancy. Patient should discontinue oral contraception 3 mo before attempting to conceive. Postpartum use may interfere with lactation, causing a decrease in the quantity and quality of breast milk. Patient should use alternative form of contraception until infant is weaned.

OVULEN (20-day regimen) **Searle**
OVULEN-21 (21-day regimen) **Searle**
OVULEN-28 (28-day regimen) **Searle**

Tabs: 1 mg ethynodiol diacetate and 100 μg mestranol

INDICATIONS	**ORAL DOSAGE**
Contraception	**Adult:** 1 tab/day for 20, 21, or 28 consecutive days of the menstrual cycle

ADMINISTRATION/DOSAGE ADJUSTMENTS

Initiating therapy	First tablet should be taken on the 5th day (Ovulen, Ovulen-21) or 1st Sunday (Ovulen-28) after the onset of menses; if menses begins on a Sunday, regimen is started the very same day
Subsequent cycles (20- or 21-day regimen)	First tablet is taken 8 days after last tablet was taken in preceding cycle
Subsequent cycles (28-day regimen)	First tablet is taken 1 day after last (placebo) tablet was taken in preceding cycle
Missed tablets	If one tablet is missed, it should be taken as soon as it is remembered, with the next tablet taken at the usual time. If two tablets are missed, the dosage should be doubled for the next 2 days. The remaining tablets should be taken as usual, but an additional form of contraception should be used for the remainder of the cycle.
Postpartum administration	For nonnursing mothers, may be started (1) immediately after delivery, (2) on first Sunday after delivery, (3) when patient leaves hospital, or (4) after first postpartum examination, regardless of whether spontaneous menstruation has occurred

CONTRAINDICATIONS

Past or present thrombophlebitis or thromboembolic disorders ●
Past or present myocardial infarction ●
Past or present coronary artery disease ●
Past or present cerebrovascular disease ●
Past or present benign or malignant liver tumors ●
Known or suspected breast cancer ●
Known or suspected estrogen-dependent neoplasia ●
Undiagnosed abnormal vaginal bleeding ●
Known or suspected pregnancy ●
Markedly impaired liver function ●

WARNINGS/PRECAUTIONS

Cigarette smoking	Increases the risk of serious cardiovascular side effects, especially in women over 35 yr of age who smoke 15 or more cigarettes daily; patients who use oral contraceptives should be strongly urged not to smoke
Thromboembolic disease, thrombotic disorders, and other vascular problems	Risk is increased, becoming greater with age and the amount of estrogen present in the formulation. Discontinue oral contraception immediately if early signs of thromboembolic disease or thrombotic disorders (eg, thrombophlebitis, pulmonary embolism, cerebrovascular insufficiency, coronary artery disease, myocardial infarction, or retinal or mesenteric thrombosis) develop or are suspected.
Postsurgical thromboembolic complications	Risk is increased 4-6 times; if feasible, discontinue oral contraception at least 4 wk before and for at least 4 wk after elective surgery or during periods of anticipated prolonged immobilization
Ocular lesions, including optic neuritis and retinal thrombosis	May occur; discontinue oral contraception in the presence of unexplained gradual or sudden, partial or complete loss of vision; proptosis or diplopia; papilledema; or retinal vascular lesions
Carcinoma	Closely monitor patients with a strong family history of breast cancer or with breast nodules, fibrocystic disease, recurrent cystic mastitis, abnormal mammograms, or cervical dysplasia; investigate all cases of undiagnosed persistent or recurrent abnormal vaginal bleeding for malignancy (see CONTRAINDICATIONS)
Hepatic lesions, including benign adenomas	May occur and possibly rupture, resulting in intra-abdominal hemorrhage and death; investigate all cases of abdominal pain and tenderness, abdominal mass, or shock for hepatic lesions
Gallbladder disease	Risk increases with duration of oral contraception
Hepatic impairment	Use with caution due to poor steroid hormone metabolism (see CONTRAINDICATIONS)
Jaundice	May recur in patients with a history of jaundice; discontinue oral contraception while cause is investigated
Glucose tolerance	May become impaired; closely monitor patients with latent or active diabetes
Hypertension	May be precipitated or may worsen with oral contraception, particularly with prolonged use, and in older patients. Closely monitor patients with a history of hypertension, toxemia, hypertension during pregnancy, or excessive weight gain or fluid retention during the menstrual cycle; pre-existing renal disease; or a family history of hypertension or hypertensive complications.

Table continued on following page

WARNINGS/PRECAUTIONS continued	
Migraine headache	May develop or worsen; discontinue oral contraception and investigate cause of recurrent, persistent, or severe headaches
Bleeding irregularities, including breakthrough bleeding, spotting, and amenorrhea	May occur, necessitating either a change to a formulation with a higher estrogen content or discontinuation of therapy; higher amounts of estrogen, while potentially useful for minimizing menstrual irregularities, may increase the risk of thromboembolic disease
Mental depression	Risk is increased; discontinue oral contraception if serious depression develops or recurs in patients with a history of depression
Fluid retention	May occur; use with caution in patients with convulsive disorders, migraine, asthma, or cardiac, hepatic, or renal dysfunction
Vitamin deficiencies	May occur, particularly of pyridoxine and folic acid
Failure of withdrawal bleeding	If patient has not adhered to prescribed regimen, pregnancy should be considered after the first missed period and oral contraception withheld until pregnancy has been excluded; if patient has adhered to regimen and misses two consecutive periods, pregnancy should be ruled out before contraceptive regimen is reinstituted
Postpill amenorrhea and anovulation	May occur, particularly in patients with a history of oligomenorrhea or secondary amenorrhea or in young women who have not established regular menstrual cycles; such patients should be encouraged to use alternative methods of contraception
Ectopic pregnancy	Risk may be increased after oral contraception is discontinued
Infertility	May occur following discontinuation of oral contraception, independent of its duration; diminishes with time but may still be apparent up to 30 mo in parous women and up to 42 mo in nulliparous women
Endocrine and liver-function tests	May be affected (see ALTERED LABORATORY VALUES); repeat any abnormal tests 2 mo after oral contraception is discontinued
ADVERSE REACTIONS	Frequent reactions are italicized
Genitourinary	*Breakthrough bleeding, spotting, menstrual irregularities, vaginal candidiasis,* postpill amenorrhea and infertility, dysmenorrhea, altered cervical erosion and secretion, endocervical hyperplasia, enlargement of uterine leiomyomata, premenstrual-like syndrome, altered libido, cystitis-like syndrome, vaginitis
Cardiovascular	Thrombophlebitis, thrombosis, pulmonary embolism, myocardial infarction, coronary thrombosis, cerebral thrombosis, cerebral hemorrhage, hypertension, mesenteric thrombosis, edema
Gastrointestinal	*Nausea, vomiting,* gallbladder disease, abdominal cramps, bloating, change in appetite, pancreatitis, colitis
Hepatic	Benign adenomas and other hepatic lesions, Budd-Chiari syndrome, cholestatic jaundice, hepatitis
Metabolic and endocrinological	*Breast enlargement, tenderness, and/or secretion;* carbohydrate intolerance; increase or decrease in weight; hyperlipidemia
Central nervous system and neuromuscular	Migraine, depression, headache, nervousness, dizziness, chorea, paresthesia, auditory disturbances, fatigue
Ophthalmic	Optic neuritis, retinal thrombosis, intolerance to contact lenses, altered corneal curvature, cataracts
Allergic and dermatological	Melasma or chloasma, rash, itching, rhinitis, erythema multiforme, erythema nodosum, hirsutism, hair loss, hemorrhagic eruption, porphyria
Other	Congenital anomalies, prolactin-secreting pituitary tumors, impaired renal function, backache, anemia, lupus erythematosus, rheumatoid arthritis
OVERDOSAGE	
Signs and symptoms	Nausea, withdrawal bleeding
Treatment	Treat symptomatically
DRUG INTERACTIONS	
Ampicillin, penicillin V, neomycin, chloramphenicol, sulfonamides, nitrofurantoin, rifampin, isoniazid	⇩ Contraceptive effect ⇧ Breakthrough bleeding
Analgesics, phenylbutazone, antimigraine preparations	⇩ Contraceptive effect ⇧ Breakthrough bleeding

Table continued on following page

DRUG INTERACTION continued

Phenytoin, primidone	⇩ Contraceptive effect ⇧ Breakthrough bleeding
Barbiturates, tranquilizers	⇩ Contraceptive effect ⇧ Breakthrough bleeding
Antihypertensive agents (eg, guanethidine)	⇩ Antihypertensive effect
Oral anticoagulants	⇩ Anticoagulant effect
Anticonvulsants	⇧ Seizure activity
Hypoglycemic agents	⇩ Glucose tolerance
Corticosteroids	⇧ Corticosteroid effects
Tricyclic antidepressants	⇧ Antidepressant side effects

ALTERED LABORATORY VALUES

Blood/serum values	⇧ Alkaline phosphatase ⇧ Bilirubin ⇧ Sulfobromophthalein retention ⇧ Prothrombin ⇧ Clotting factors VII, VIII, IX, and X ⇩ Antithrombin III ⇧ PBI ⇧ Thyroxine (T_4) ⇩ Triiodothyronine (T_3) uptake ⇧ Glucose ⇧ Cortisol ⇧ Transcortin ⇧ Ceruloplasmin ⇧ Triglycerides ⇧ Phospholipids ⇩ Folic acid ⇩ Pyridoxine
Urinary values	⇩ Pregnanediol

Use in children

No appropriate indications exist. Acute ingestion by young children has not been associated with serious ill effects.

Use in pregnancy or nursing mothers

Contraindicated if pregnancy is known or suspected, as serious fetal damage may occur during early pregnancy. Patient should discontinue oral contraception 3 mo before attempting to conceive. Postpartum use may interfere with lactation, causing a decrease in the quantity and quality of breast milk. Patient should use alternative form of contraception until infant is weaned.

VAGINAL SPERMICIDES USED WITHOUT DIAPHRAGM

Product (Manufacturer)	Ingredients	Actions
Because (Emko) Foam **Dosage** Insert 1 applicatorful into vagina no more than 1 h prior to intercourse; repeat prior to each act of intercourse. Do not douche for at least 6 h.	8% Nonoxynol 9	Immobilizes sperm, thereby preventing conception
	0.2% Benzethonium chloride	Preservative
Conceptrol (Ortho) Cream **Dosage** Insert 1 applicatorful into vagina no more than 1 h prior to intercourse; repeat prior to each act of intercourse. Do not douche for at least 6 h.	5% Nonoxynol 9	Immobilizes sperm, thereby preventing conception
Delfen (Ortho) Foam **Dosage** Insert 1 applicatorful into vagina no more than 1 h prior to intercourse; repeat prior to each act of intercourse. Do not douche for at least 6 h.	12.5% Nonoxynol 9	Immobilizes sperm, thereby preventing conception
Emko (Shering) Foam **Dosage** Insert 1 applicatorful into vagina no more than 1 h prior to intercourse; repeat prior to each act of intercourse. Do not douche for at least 6 h.	8% Nonoxynol 9	Immobilizes sperm, thereby preventing conception
	0.2% Benzethonium chloride	Preservative
	Stearic acid	Foam base
	Triethanolamine	Buffer
	Glyceryl monostearate	Foam base
	Poloxamer 188	Surfactant
	Polyethylene glycol 600	Foam base
	Substituted adamantane	Preservative
	Dichlorodifluoromethane	Aerosol propellant
	Dichlorotetrafluoroethane	Aerosol propellant
Encare Oval (Norwich-Eaton) Suppository **Dosage** Insert 1 suppository into vagina no more than 1 h prior to intercourse; repeat prior to each act of intercourse. Do not douche for at least 6 h.	2.27% Nonoxynol 9	Immobilizes sperm, thereby preventing conception
	Water-soluble base	

VAGINAL SPERMICIDES USED WITHOUT DIAPHRAGM (continued)

Product (Manufacturer)	Ingredients	Actions
Koromex (Holland-Rantos) Foam **Dosage** Insert 1 applicatorful into vagina no more than 1 h prior to intercourse; repeat prior to each act of intercourse. Do not douche for at least 6 h.	12.5% Nonoxynol 9	Immobilizes sperm, thereby preventing conception
	Propylene glycol	Solvent
	Isopropyl alcohol	Solvent
	Laureth 4	Surfactant and emulsifier
	Cetyl alcohol	Emulsifier
	Polyethylene glycol stearate	Foam base
	Fragrance	Aesthetic
	Dichlorodifluoromethane	Aerosol propellant
	Dichlorotetrafluoroethane	Aerosol propellant
	Water-soluble base	
Koromex[11]-A (Holland-Rantos) Jelly **Dosage** Insert 1 applicatorful into vagina no more than 1 h prior to intercourse; repeat prior to each act of intercourse. Do not douche for at least 6 h.	2% Nonoxynol 9	Immobilizes sperm, thereby preventing conception
	Propylene glycol	Solvent
	Cellulose gum	Maintains moisture
	Boric acid	Astringent and antiseptic
	Sorbitol	Maintains moisture
	Starch	Thickening agent
	Simethicone	Gel base
	Fragrance	Aesthetic
	Water-soluble base	
Ramses "10-Hour" (Schmid) Jelly **Dosage** Insert 1 applicatorful into vagina no more than 1 h prior to intercourse; repeat prior to each act of intercourse. Do not douche for at least 6 h.	5% Dodecaethylene glycol monolaurate	Immobilizes sperm, thereby preventing conception
	5% Ethyl alcohol	Solvent
	1% Boric acid	Astringent and antiseptic

VAGINAL SPERMICIDES USED WITH DIAPHRAGM

Product (Manufacturer)	Ingredients	Actions
Koromex[11] (Holland-Rantos) Jelly **Dosage** Spread approx. ½ tsp jelly over dome surface of diaphragm coming in direct contact with cervix and spread small amount around rim of diaphragm no more than 6 h prior to intercourse; insert 1 applicatorful prior to each subsequent act of intercourse. Leave diaphragm in place at least 8 h after last act of intercourse. Do not douche for at least 6 h.	1% Octoxynol	Immobilizes sperm, thereby preventing conception
	Water-soluble base	

VAGINAL SPERMICIDES USED WITH DIAPHRAGM (continued)

Product (Manufacturer)	Ingredients	Actions
Koromex[11] (Holland-Rantos) Cream **Dosage** Spread approx. ½ tsp cream over dome surface of diaphragm coming in direct contact with cervix and spread small amount around rim of diaphragm no more than 6 h prior to intercourse; insert 1 applicatorful prior to each subsequent act of intercourse. Leave diaphragm in place at least 8 h after last act of intercourse. Do not douche for at least 6 h.	3% Octoxynol	Immobilizes sperm, thereby preventing conception
	Water-soluble base	
Koromex[11]-A (Holland-Rantos) Jelly **Dosage** Spread approx. ½ tsp jelly over dome surface of diaphragm coming in direct contact with cervix and spread small amount around rim of diaphragm no more than 6 h prior to intercourse; insert 1 applicatorful prior to each subsequent act of intercourse. Leave diaphragm in place at least 8 h after last act of intercourse. Do not douche for at least 6 h.	2% Nonoxynol 9	Immobilizes sperm, thereby preventing conception
	Cellulose gum	Builds viscosity
	Boric acid	Astringent and antiseptive
	Sorbitol	Maintains moisture
	Starch	Thickening agent
	Simethicone	Gel base
	Fragrance	Aesthetic
	Water-soluble base	
Ortho-Creme (Ortho) Cream **Dosage** Spread approx. 1 tsp cream over dome surface of diaphragm coming in direct contact with cervix and spread small amount around rim of diaphragm no more than 6 h prior to intercourse; insert 1 applicatorful prior to each subsequent act of intercourse. Leave diaphragm in place at least 8 h after last act of intercourse. Do not douche for at least 6 h.	2% Nonoxynol 9	Immobilizes sperm, thereby preventing conception
Ortho-Gynol (Ortho) Jelly **Dosage** Spread approx. 1 tsp jelly over dome surface of diaphragm coming in direct contact with cervix and spread small amount around rim of diaphragm no more than 6 h prior to intercourse; insert 1 applicatorful prior to each subsequent act of intercourse. Leave diaphragm in place at least 8 h after last act of intercourse. Do not douche for at least 6 h.	p-Diisobutylphenoxy-polyethoxy-ethanol	Immobilizes sperm, thereby preventing conception
	Water-soluble base	

VAGINAL SPERMICIDES USED WITH DIAPHRAGM (continued)

Product (Manufacturer)	Ingredients	Actions
Ramses "10-Hour" (Schmid) Jelly **Dosage** Spread approx. 1 tsp jelly over dome surface of diaphragm coming in direct contact with cervix and spread small amount around rim of diaphragm no more than 6 h prior to intercourse; insert 1 applicatorful prior to each subsequent act of intercourse. Leave diaphragm in place at least 8 h after last act of intercourse. Do not douche for at least 6 h.	5% Dodecaethylene glycol monolaurate	Immobilizes sperm, thereby preventing conception
	5% Ethyl alcohol	Solvent
	1% Boric acid	Astringent and antiseptic

CONDOMS

Product (Manufacturer)	Ingredients
Conceptrol Shields (Lubricated or Nonlubricated) (Ortho) Shaped and/or ribbed, reservoir tip	Rubber, packaged dry or with lubricant
Conture (Akwell) Shaped and/or ribbed	Rubber, packaged with lubricant
Excita Sensitor (Schmid) Shaped and/or ribbed, regular tip	Rubber, packaged with lubricant
Featherlite (Schmid) Shaped and/or ribbed	Rubber, packaged dry or with lubricant
Fiesta Sensi-Color (Schmid) Shaped, regular tip	Rubber, packaged with lubricant
Fourex (Schmid) Shaped, regular tip	Lamb cecum, packaged with lubricant
Guardian (Youngs) Shaped, reservoir tip	Rubber, packaged with lubricant
Naturalamb (Youngs) Shaped, regular tip	Lamb cecum, packaged with lubricant
Nuda (Akwell) Shaped, reservoir tip	Rubber, packaged with lubricant
Nuform Sensi-Shaped, Lubricated or Nonlubricated (Schmid) Shaped, and/or ribbed	Rubber, packaged dry or with lubricant
Prime; Prime Nonlubricated Shaped, reservoir tip	Rubber, packaged dry or with lubricant
Ramses (Schmid) Shaped, plain tip	Rubber, packaged dry
Sheik (Plain End; Reservoir End, Lubricated; or Reservoir, Nonlubricated) (Schmid) Shaped, regular tip	Rubber, packaged dry or with lubricant

CONDOMS (continued)

Product (Manufacturer)	Ingredients
Stimula (Akwell) Shaped, and/or ribbed	Rubber, packaged with lubricant
Tahiti (Akwell) Shaped, reservoir	Rubber, packaged with lubricant
Trojan-Enz (Lubricated or Nonlubricated) (Youngs) Shaped, reservoir tip	Rubber, packaged dry or with lubricant
Trojans (Youngs) Shaped, plain end	Rubber, packaged dry or with lubricant
Trojans Plus (Youngs) Shaped, and/or ribbed	Rubber, packaged with lubricant
Trojans Ribbed (Youngs) Shaped, and/or ribbed	Rubber, packaged with lubricant

Infertility

Although most people regard contraception as the major concern in fertility control, for one out of every eight American couples, the problem is quite the opposite—infertility. Infertility is defined as failure to conceive after at least one year of repeated attempts to achieve pregnancy.

CAUSES OF INFERTILITY

In about 30 to 40 percent of all cases, infertility can be traced to the male partner; the remainder are attributed to the female. There are numerous causes of infertility for both sexes. In women, the most common causes are a number of specific hormonal defects, failure to ovulate (produce eggs), scarring or other defects of the fallopian tubes, pelvic inflammatory disease or other infections, endometriosis (a disorder characterized by the abnormal growth of endometrial cells both inside and outside the uterus), and a cervical environment that is "hostile" to sperm. In men, the cause often involves impaired production or transport of sperm, hormonal disorders affecting sperm production, genital disease or injury, or developmental abnormalities. Venereal disease, marital and psychological problems, nutritional deficiencies, sexual ignorance or dysfunction, and the use of certain drugs are among the many factors influencing fertility in both sexes.

Diagnosing Infertility

Because diagnosing infertility is often costly, time-consuming, and complex, it is wise to start by consulting a physician who is knowledgeable in this area. Many obstetrician-gynecologists specialize in the treatment of infertility or can refer a couple to an appropriate physician. The American Fertility Society (1608 Thirteenth Avenue South, Suite 101, Birmingham, Alabama, Tel: 205-934-7222) maintains a roster of physicians who treat infertility throughout the United States.

INFERTILITY IN MEN

Unless the cause is readily apparent, an investigation of infertility usually begins with a study of the male's gonadal function, a simpler process than the studies often required to diagnose female infertility. The physician begins with a physical examination and then an analysis of the semen for shape, quantity, and motility of sperm. This is particularly important, since infertility may be the result of an abnormally large number of deformed or defective sperm, or a low count of viable sperm.

Male infertility may also be caused by a number of diseases or anatomical or metabolic disorders that disrupt the development or transport of sperm. For example, elevated testicular temperatures interfere with the production of sperm—a process that requires the temperature within the scrotum to be

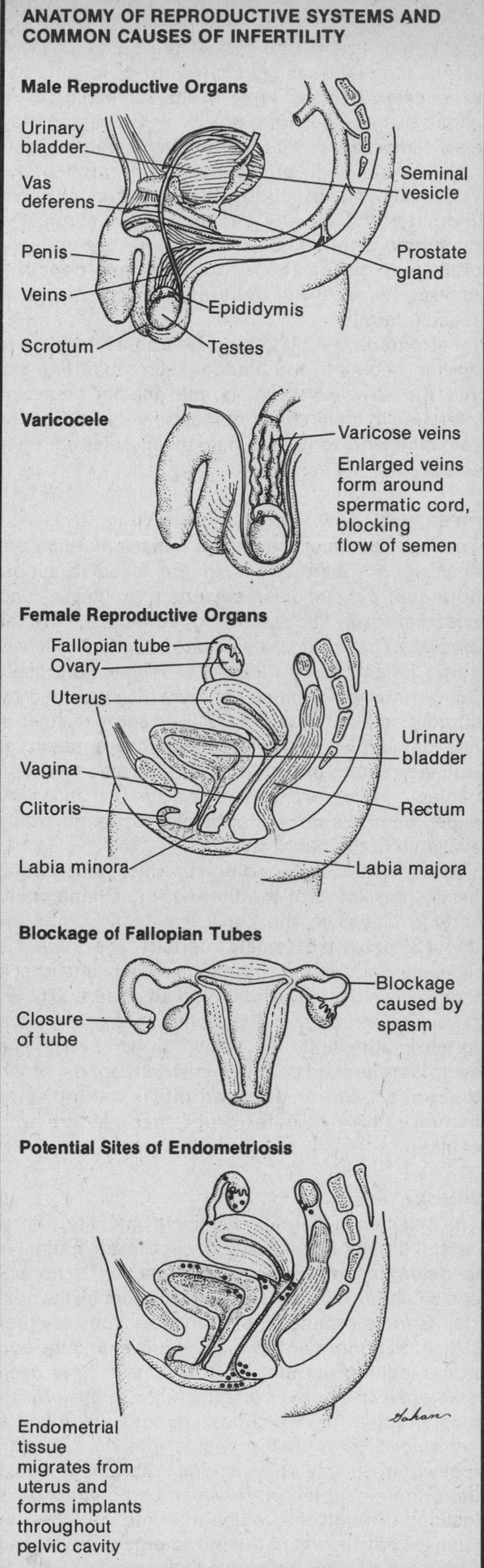

lower than that of the rest of the body. Elevated scrotal temperatures are usually due to infection or varicocele (varicose veins of the spermatic cord), although frequent hot baths or tight clothing may also temporarily raise scrotal temperatures and have a transient effect on sperm production. Varicocele causes about 30 percent of all male infertility, and usually can be treated surgically. Endocrine disorders, such as underactive pituitary or thyroid glands (hypopituitarism and hypothyroidism, respectively) or adrenal tumors, may also cause infertility.

Retrograde ejaculation, in which the ejaculate is pushed back into the bladder rather than forward into the female vagina, is still another cause of infertility. In these cases, epinephrine-like drugs are sometimes prescribed to help the muscles contract and project the semen.

INFERTILITY IN WOMEN

The most common causes of female infertility are scarring or obstructions in the fallopian tubes, hormone deficiencies, ovulation problems, and endometriosis. Tubal scarring, adhesions, or other blockages can often be traced to infections, such as pelvic inflammatory disease or venereal diseases. Some tubal deformities can now be corrected by surgery. Implantation of a fertilized egg in the uterus has gained widespread publicity as a result of isolated reports of success (the so-called test-tube babies). However, this technique is still very experimental and is not likely to be generally available in the near future.

Endometriosis, a condition in which endometrial tissue (the lining of the uterus) forms implants in various places in the pelvic cavity, accounts for about 30 percent of female infertility. The process is not fully understood, but as these implants attach themselves to the ovaries, fallopian tubes, and other organs or structures, they continue to grow, often forming adhesions or large, brown cysts. The symptoms include painful menstrual periods, which disappear when the patient is taking oral contraceptives or other drugs that interfere with ovulation.

Infertility Tests

The first step in diagnosing female infertility, after a careful patient history and physical examination, is to determine whether ovarian function is normal and ovulation occurs. If ovulation is normal, the next step is to determine whether obstructions or other structural abnormalities may be preventing the egg from reaching the uterus. Several tests have been developed to discover this, including a hysterosalpingography, in which an opaque solution is introduced through the vagina into the fallopian tubes to make any obstructions visible on an x-ray; uterotubal insufflation, in which carbon dioxide is instilled through the vagina and into the tubes; or laparoscopy, in which the pelvic organs are viewed through a flexible tube called a laparoscope that is inserted via a small abdominal incision. A number of other examinations and tests are available; the decision of which tests to perform depends upon individual patient considerations and the availability of testing facilities.

In a significant number of cases, no reason for the apparent infertility can be found. In some instances, both partners may have normal fertility, but for poorly understood reasons, may be unable to conceive with each other. In some, the cervical secretions may prove "hostile" to the sperm. In other couples, there may be an immunological incompatibility, in which antibodies to the sperm are produced in the female partner. Anxiety, stress, and other psychological factors also may make conception difficult or impossible.

DRUGS TO INDUCE FERTILITY

The treatment of infertility is a growing field with many promising experimental approaches under investigation. Improved surgical techniques, for instance, are succeeding in restoring fertility to many women with scarred or blocked fallopian tubes, ovarian cysts, or endometriosis. This discussion, however, will focus primarily on the drugs used to treat infertility.

Fertility drugs, which are used most often to treat female infertility but in some cases also are given to men, act by stimulating the gonads (the sex organs, specifically ovaries and testes). All of these drugs should be administered only under very close supervision of a physician experienced in the treatment of infertility.

Endometriosis

When endometriosis is not treated surgically, danazol (Danocrine), an androgen derivative, may be administered. This drug inhibits the production of ovarian hormones, inducing a temporary or pseudomenopause. Without ovarian hormones, the endometrial tissue stops growing and the endometriosis regresses. Once the drug is stopped and ovarian function resumes, fertility is restored in about 50 to 70 percent of women with endometriosis.

Ovulation Failure

Three drugs are used to achieve ovulation in women whose infertility is traced to ovulatory failure: clomiphene citrate (Clomid), menotropins (Pergonal), and human chorionic gonadotropin (HCG, which is marketed as Antuitrin-S, A.P.L., Pregnyl, and Follutein). Sex hormones, such as estrogen and progesterone, may also be indicated, particularly in cases of hostile cervical mucus, which is treated with estrogen, or luteal phase (the portion of the menstrual cycle following ovulation) dysfunction, which is treated with progesterone.

Clomid, the most frequently used fertility-inducing drug, may also be given in conjunction with other fertility-inducing agents, particularly the gonadotropins (drugs that stimulate gonadal function). It is believed to work by stimulating the hypothalamus and pituitary glands, which in turn stimulate the release of follicle-stimulating hormone and luteinizing hormone, which are necessary for ovulation and sperm production.

After therapy with Clomid, ovulation occurs in about 70 percent of properly selected patients, and 40 percent of these women achieve pregnancy. About 3 to 8 percent of these women will have multiple births, usually twins. Although instances of larger multiple births have gained considerable publicity, they are rare. The incidence of multiple births also is lower with Clomid than with other fertility-inducing drugs.

The major gonadotropins are human menopausal gonadotropin, which is extracted and purified from the urine of postmenopausal women, and human chorionic gonadotropin, which is extracted and purified from the urine of pregnant women. The two substances are usually administered together.

Approximately 90 percent of properly selected patients appear to ovulate with the use of these two gonadotropins, and about two thirds of these achieve pregnancy. About 20 percent of the pregnancies result in multiple births, with twins accounting for three fourths of this number. This rate of multiple births is much higher for the gonadotropins than for Clomid.

The spontaneous abortion (miscarriage) rate for all the fertility-inducing drugs is about 20 percent—a figure comparable to that of the general population. There is no increase in the incidence of congenital abnormalities, and there appear to be few significant side effects associated with these drugs. Of the adverse effects, overstimulation of the ovaries is the most serious, but it occurs in only about 1 percent of the women who use these drugs, and usually subsides when the drugs are stopped.

IN CONCLUSION

Infertility is a complex problem both to diagnose and to treat. The use of fertility-inducing drugs and other recent advances in surgical correction of certain malformations and conditions leading to infertility, such as endometriosis, makes conception possible for increasing numbers of previously infertile couples.

The following charts give specific prescribing information for the major drugs used to treat infertility. Information on estrogen and progesterone, as well as the androgens used to treat some types of male infertility, is in the section on *Sex Hormones* (pages 296–323). All of these agents should be used under close medical supervision, and the regimens must be determined individually for each patient.

CLOMID (Clomiphene citrate) **Merrell-National**

Tabs: 50 mg

INDICATIONS	ORAL DOSAGE
Induction of ovulation in patients with secondary anovulatory infertility	**Adult:** 50 mg/day for 5 days, beginning on or about the 5th day of the menstrual cycle if spontaneous uterine bleeding occurs, or at any time if there has been no recent history of bleeding; repeat course up to two more times if ovulation but not conception occurs during first cycle

ADMINISTRATION/DOSAGE ADJUSTMENTS

Pretreatment evaluation	Perform a complete pelvic examination prior to treatment and before each subsequent course; in addition, obtain an endometrial biopsy and evaluate liver function before initiating therapy. If abnormal vaginal bleeding is present, full diagnostic measures are mandatory; do not overlook neoplastic lesions (see CONTRAINDICATIONS).
Lack of response to initial course of therapy	If ovulation does not occur, increase dosage during next course to 100 mg/day for 5 days, beginning as early as 30 days after previous course; if ovulation but not conception occurs at this dosage, course may be repeated once
Patients with unusual sensitivity to pituitary gonadotropins	Reduce dosage or duration of treatment course (see WARNINGS/PRECAUTIONS)

CONTRAINDICATIONS

Hepatic disease or history of hepatic dysfunction●	Abnormal bleeding of unknown origin●	Thyroid or adrenal dysfunction●
Primary ovarian failure●	Ovarian cysts●	
Primary pituitary failure●	Infertility not caused by anovulation●	

WARNINGS/PRECAUTIONS

Visual symptoms	Blurring and other visual disturbances (see ADVERSE REACTIONS) may occur, depending on dose; discontinue use and perform a complete ophthalmological evaluation. Caution patients that performance of potentially hazardous activities may be impaired if vision is affected, particularly under variable lighting.
Ovarian overstimulation	Abnormal ovarian enlargement and cyst formation, possibly accompanied by pain, may occur, especially in patients with polycystic ovary syndrome; to reduce the hazard, the lowest dose consistent with expectation of good results should be used. Maximal enlargement of the ovary, whether physiological or abnormal, does not occur until 7 days after discontinuation of therapy; patients who complain of pelvic pain after clomiphene treatment should be carefully examined. If ovarian enlargement does occur, stop treatment until the ovaries have returned to pretreatment size, and reduce the dosage or duration of the next course; manage cystic enlargement conservatively, unless surgical indication for laparotomy exists.
Inadvertent use during early pregnancy	May be avoided by recording the basal body temperature throughout all treatment cycles and by observing patient carefully to determine whether ovulation has occurred; if basal body temperature following clomiphene treatment is biphasic and followed by menses, examine patient for an ovarian cyst and perform a pregnancy test. Delay the next course of therapy until it is determined that the patient is not pregnant.
Multiple pregnancy	The prospective parents should be advised of the frequency and potential hazards of multiple pregnancy before starting treatment; 7.9% of the pregnancies following the use of clomiphene in clinical trials were multiple pregnancies

ADVERSE REACTIONS[1]	Frequent reactions are italicized
Vasomotor	*Flushes (10%)*
Gastrointestinal	*Abdominal or pelvic discomfort (including distention, bloating, pain, or soreness) (5.5%), nausea and vomiting (2.2%),* increased appetite, acute abdomen, constipation, diarrhea
Endocrinological	*Ovarian enlargement (14%), breast discomfort (2.1%),* menorrhagia, intermenstrual spotting, dry vaginal mucosa
Ophthalmic	Phosphenes, blurred vision, diplopia, scotomata, afterimages, photophobia, lights, floaters, waves, other visual complaints; posterior capsular cataract, detachment of posterior vitreous, spasm of retinal arteriole, and thrombosis of temporal arteries of retina (causal relationship not established)
Central nervous system	*Headache (1.3%),* dizziness, lightheadedness, vertigo, nervous tension, insomnia, fatigue, depression
Genitourinary	Increased urinary frequency and/or volume

[1]Adverse effects appear to be dose-dependent

Table continued on following page

CLOMID continued

ADVERSE REACTIONS continued

Dermatological	Dermatitis, rash, hair loss, dry hair
Birth defects	Congenital heart lesions, Down's syndrome, clubfoot, congenital gut lesions, hypospadias, microcephaly, harelip, cleft palate, congential hip, hemangioma, undescended testes, polydactyly, conjoined twins with teratomatous malformation, patent ductus arteriosus, amaurosis, arteriovenous fistula, inguinal hernia, umbilical hernia, syndactyly, pectus excavatum, myopathy, dermoid cyst of scalp, omphalocele, spina bifida occulta, icthyosis, persistent lingual frenulum, multiple somatic defects
Other	Weight gain or loss, cholestatic jaundice (1 case), ascites (2 cases); hydatiform mole (causal relationship not established)

OVERDOSAGE

Signs and symptoms	See WARNINGS/PRECAUTIONS and ADVERSE REACTIONS
Treatment	Discontinue use; treat symptomatically and institute supportive measures, as required

DRUG INTERACTIONS

No clinically significant drug interactions have been reported

ALTERED LABORATORY VALUES

Blood/serum values	⇧ Sulfobromophthalein (BSP) retention ⇧ FSH ⇧ LH ⇧ Desmosterol ⇧ Transcortin ⇧ Thyroxine ⇧ Sex hormone-binding globulin ⇧ Thyroxine-binding globulin
Urinary values	⇧ FSH ⇧ LH ⇧ Estrogen

Use in children

No indication exists for use in children

Use in pregnancy or nursing mothers

Do not administer during pregnancy (see WARNINGS/PRECAUTIONS); general guidelines not established for use in nursing mothers

DANOCRINE (Danazol) Winthrop

Caps: 200 mg

INDICATIONS	ORAL DOSAGE
Endometriosis in patients who cannot tolerate or fail to respond to adequate doses of other effective medications or in whom other effective drugs are contraindicated	**Adult:** 400 mg bid for 3–6 mo, or up to 9 mo, if necessary; may be reinstituted if symptoms recur after therapy is terminated

ADMINISTRATION/DOSAGE ADJUSTMENTS

Initiating therapy	Begin therapy during menstruation, unless appropriate tests have been performed to rule out pregnancy

CONTRAINDICATIONS

Undiagnosed abnormal genital bleeding	Markedly impaired hepatic, renal, or cardiac function

WARNINGS/PRECAUTIONS

Virilization	Monitor patient closely for signs of virilization (see ADVERSE REACTIONS); some androgenic effects may not be reversible even when therapy is stopped
Fluid retention	May occur; patients with epilepsy, migraine, or cardiac or renal dysfunction should be closely observed

ADVERSE REACTIONS

Dermatological	Acne, mild hirsutism, and oily skin or hair; loss of hair (causal relationship not established)
Endocrinological and metabolic	Decrease in breast size, deepening of the voice, edema, and weight gain; changes in libido (causal relationship not established)
Genitourinary	Vaginitis, including itching, dryness, burning, and vaginal bleeding; clitoral hypertrophy (rare); hematuria (rare; causal relationship not established)
Central nervous system	Nervousness and emotional lability; dizziness, headache, sleep disorders, fatigue, tremor, and, rarely, paresthesia in extremities, visual disturbances, changes in appetite, and chills (causal relationship not established)
Musculoskeletal	Muscle cramps or spasms and pain in back, neck, or legs (causal relationship not established)
Gastrointestinal	Gastroenteritis and, rarely, nausea, vomiting, and constipation (causal relationship not established)
Allergic	Skin rash and, rarely, nasal congestion (causal relationship not established)
Other	Flushing; sweating; elevation in blood pressure and, rarely, pelvic pain (causal relationship not established)

OVERDOSAGE

Signs and symptoms	See ADVERSE REACTIONS
Treatment	Discontinue medication; treat symptomatically

DRUG INTERACTIONS

No clinically significant drug interactions have been observed

ALTERED LABORATORY VALUES

No clinically significant alterations in blood/serum or urinary values occur at therapeutic dosages

Use in children

General guidelines not established

Use in pregnancy or nursing mothers

Contraindicated during pregnancy and for use in nursing mothers; if patient becomes pregnant during treatment, medication should be discontinued

PERGONAL (Menotropins) Serono

Amps: 75 IU follicle-stimulating hormone (FSH), 75 IU luteinizing hormone (LH), and 10 mg lactose

INDICATIONS	PARENTERAL DOSAGE
Induction of ovulation and pregnancy in patients with secondary anovulatory infertility	**Adult:** 1 ampule/day IM for 9–12 days followed by 10,000 IU HCG 1 day after last dose; if there is evidence of ovulation but pregnancy does not ensue, repeat same course twice before increasing dose to 2 ampules

ADMINISTRATION/DOSAGE ADJUSTMENTS

Use of urinary estrogen determinations — If total estrogen excretion $<100\ \mu g/24$ h or estriol excretion $<50\ \mu g/24$ h prior to HCG administration, hyperstimulation syndrome is less likely to occur. If estrogen or estriol values are higher than these values, or if ovarian enlargement is present, do not administer HCG.

CONTRAINDICATIONS

Primary ovarian failure●

Thyroid and adrenal dysfunction●

Organic intracranial lesion (eg, pituitary tumor)●

Infertility not caused by anovulation●

Abnormal bleeding of unknown origin●

Ovarian cysts or enlargement not due to polycystic ovary syndrome●

WARNINGS/PRECAUTIONS

Ovarian overstimulation — Mild to moderate uncomplicated ovarian enlargement, possibly accompanied by abdominal distention and/or pain, occurs in ~20% of patients; to reduce the hazard, the lowest dose consistent with expectation of good results should be used. If hyperstimulation occurs (see ADVERSE REACTIONS), stop treatment, hospitalize patient, and determine if hemoconcentration associated with abdominal fluid loss exists. Treat symptomatically; *do not remove ascitic fluid.*

Hemoperitoneum — May occur from ruptured ovarian cysts, usually as a result of pelvic examination; to lessen the danger of hemoperitoneum in patients with significant ovarian enlargement occurring after ovulation, prohibit intercourse

Multiple births — The prospective parents should be advised of the frequency and potential hazards of multiple births before the patient begins therapy; 20% of the pregnancies following treatment with menotropins and HCG have resulted in multiple births

ADVERSE REACTIONS

Frequent reactions are italicized

Genitourinary — *Ovarian enlargement (20%), hyperstimulation syndrome characterized by sudden ovarian enlargement accompanied by ascites with or without pain and/or pleural effusion (1.3%)*

Congenital anomalies[1] — Imperforated anus, sigmoid colon aplasia, third-degree hypospadias, cecovesicle fistula, bifid scrotum, meningocele, bilateral internal tibial torsion, right metatarsus adductus, heart lesion, supernumerary digit, bladder exstrophy, Down's syndrome

Hypersensitivity — Febrile reactions

Other — Hemoperitoneum, arterial thromboembolism (two cases)

OVERDOSAGE

Sigs and symptoms — Hyperstimulation syndrome characterized by sudden ovarian enlargement accompanied by ascites, with or without pain and/or pleural effusion

Treatment — Treat symptomatically with bed rest, fluid and electrolyte replacement, and analgesics, as needed. Do not remove ascitic fluid.

DRUG INTERACTIONS

No clinically significant drug interactions have been observed

ALTERED LABORATORY VALUES

Urinary values — ⇧ Estrogen ⇧ Estriol ⇧ Pregnanediol

No clinically significant alterations in blood/serum values occur at therapeutic dosages

Use in children

No appropriate indication exists in children

Use in pregnancy or nursing mothers

Contraindicated during pregnancy; general guidelines not established for use in nursing mothers

[1]Causal relationship not established; probably not drug-related

Respiratory and Allergic Disorders

Asthma

More than 600,000 Americans suffer from asthma, a chronic condition marked by episodes of wheezing (dyspnea). The disease often begins in childhood, but in many other persons, it starts in adulthood. In some cases, no apparent reason can be found for the periodic attacks, while in many others, various identifiable stimuli appear to trigger an episode of asthma. Between acute episodes, most asthma sufferers have no symptoms, although shortness of breath upon mild exertion is sometimes noted.

In many cases, there appears to be an inherited tendency to develop the disease, with affected families tending to have a high incidence of allergic disorders, including asthma. The stresses or stimuli that are known to precipitate asthmatic attacks include allergenic factors, such as pollens, dusts, and animal dander, and nonallergenic irritants and situations, including exposure to dry, cold air, tobacco smoke, noxious fumes, exercise, viral respiratory infection, and emotional upset. Some patients have extrinsic, or allergic, asthma, in which attacks are brought about by exposure to various allergens. Avoidance of these stimuli can minimize the severity of the disease. Other asthmatics, however, are thought to have intrinsic (nonallergic) asthma, marked by attacks due to many types of nonallergenic stimuli. Most patients exhibit a mixed type of asthma, with both allergenic and nonallergenic stimuli causing attacks.

GENERAL CONSIDERATIONS

Three events occur during asthma attacks, each contributing to the characteristic dyspnea and wheezing, and each the "target" of anti-asthma medication. The process is initiated with bronchospasm, or constriction of the smooth muscle that lines the progressively narrowed airway—starting with the trachea and terminating in the thousands of tiny bronchioles that make up the lungs. This makes inhalation and exhalation difficult, producing the panicked feeling of suffocation that occurs during attacks. The airways are further narrowed by swelling and inflammation of the bronchial mucosal walls and increased production of viscid mucus in these passages. In its severest, most intractable form, status asthmaticus, an attack can last for days or even weeks, and is often complicated by pulmonary failure. Emergency medical treatment is always necessary on such occasions. Most asthma attacks, however, are readily controlled with proper medication that relaxes bronchiolar smooth muscle, reduces swelling of inflamed mucous tissue, and then loosens viscid mucus plugs.

The onset of an acute attack may be very rapid, with paroxysms of coughing and wheezing. More often, however, the attack begins insidiously, with increasing difficulty in breathing and feelings of tightness or pressure in the chest. As the attack progresses, signs of cyanosis (oxygen deprivation), manifested by a bluish coloration of the lips and hands, may appear. In prolonged or severe attacks, the patient may become very fatigued, confused, or lethargic. An attack may end within minutes; others may persist for hours or longer. In any case, pulmonary function tests may not return to normal for weeks after an episode. The cough during an attack is usually dry and hacking; following an attack, however, large amounts of mucus may be coughed up.

Anyone who suspects he or she has asthma should consult a physician rather than resort to self-medication with nonprescription medications, even though many of these are effective in controlling an occasional mild episode of asthma. These medications may, however, contain drug combinations or dosages that are inappropriate for many individuals. Moreover, the physician may be able to identify allergenic and nonallergenic stimuli that the patient should avoid as well as assess pulmonary function, evaluate the severity of the disease, and rule out other conditions that can mimic asthma, including bronchitis, emphysema, cancer, and some forms of pneumonia and heart disease. Awareness of these factors, along with knowledge of the patient's total health profile, can help the physician design an individual treatment regimen that is both effective and safe.

TREATMENT OF ASTHMA

Asthma is complicated by many factors, including psychological or emotional stresses and a variety of allergens. In some instances, the disease can be controlled by identifying and eliminating as many of the precipitating factors as possible, but in most cases, asthma is a chronic, lifelong disease with unpredictable flare-ups.

Asthma can be a particularly trying disease to children. They often are prevented from joining many childhood activities because of their illness, and thus are singled out as being "different." In addition, school absenteeism runs high in many of these children, causing them to fall behind their peers or develop learning and related emotional problems. In addition, many myths about asthma still prevail (e.g., "It's all in the mind" or "Asthma is not really serious"), making life for the asthmatic even more difficult. Very often, the entire family is affected and in need of counseling or other forms of help. For information and listings of local resources, persons with asthma or their families can contact the Asthma and Allergy Foundation, 19 West 44th Street, New York, N.Y. 10036 (212/921-9100).

Drugs to Treat Asthma

Drugs used in the treatment of asthma fall into four therapeutic classes, each with a specific function or mode of action.

Adrenergic bronchodilators (or sympathomimetic agents) These agents reverse bronchospasm by relaxing bronchiolar smooth muscle. Many drugs in this category contain ephedrine, a common ingredient in nonprescription asthma medications, and epinephrine, which is available in both injectable and inhalant forms for use during asthmatic episodes. Other drugs in this class include isoproterenol (Isuprel, Medihaler-Iso, and other brands), metaproterenol (Alupen and Metaprel), terbutaline (Brethine and Bricanyl), and isoetharine (Bronkometer, Bronkosol, and other brands). When taken in tablet, capsule, or liquid form, adrenergic agents can reduce the frequency and intensity of asthmatic attacks. Quicker-acting aerosols containing these agents are used to stop an attack, or at least limit its severity. Intravenous epinephrine may be administered in emergency rooms to reverse the severe distress of status asthmaticus.

Most adrenergic agents stimulate the central nervous and cardiovascular systems, causing excitability, nervousness, tremors, palpitations, and loss of appetite. These symptoms are dose-related and may appear in mild form when these agents are taken within prescribed doses. In cases of overdose, beta-adrenergic agents can be fatal, producing convulsions and cardiac arrest. Due to the stimulatory effects of beta-adrenergic agents on the cardiovascular and central nervous systems, patients with heart disease, hypertension, diabetes,

12

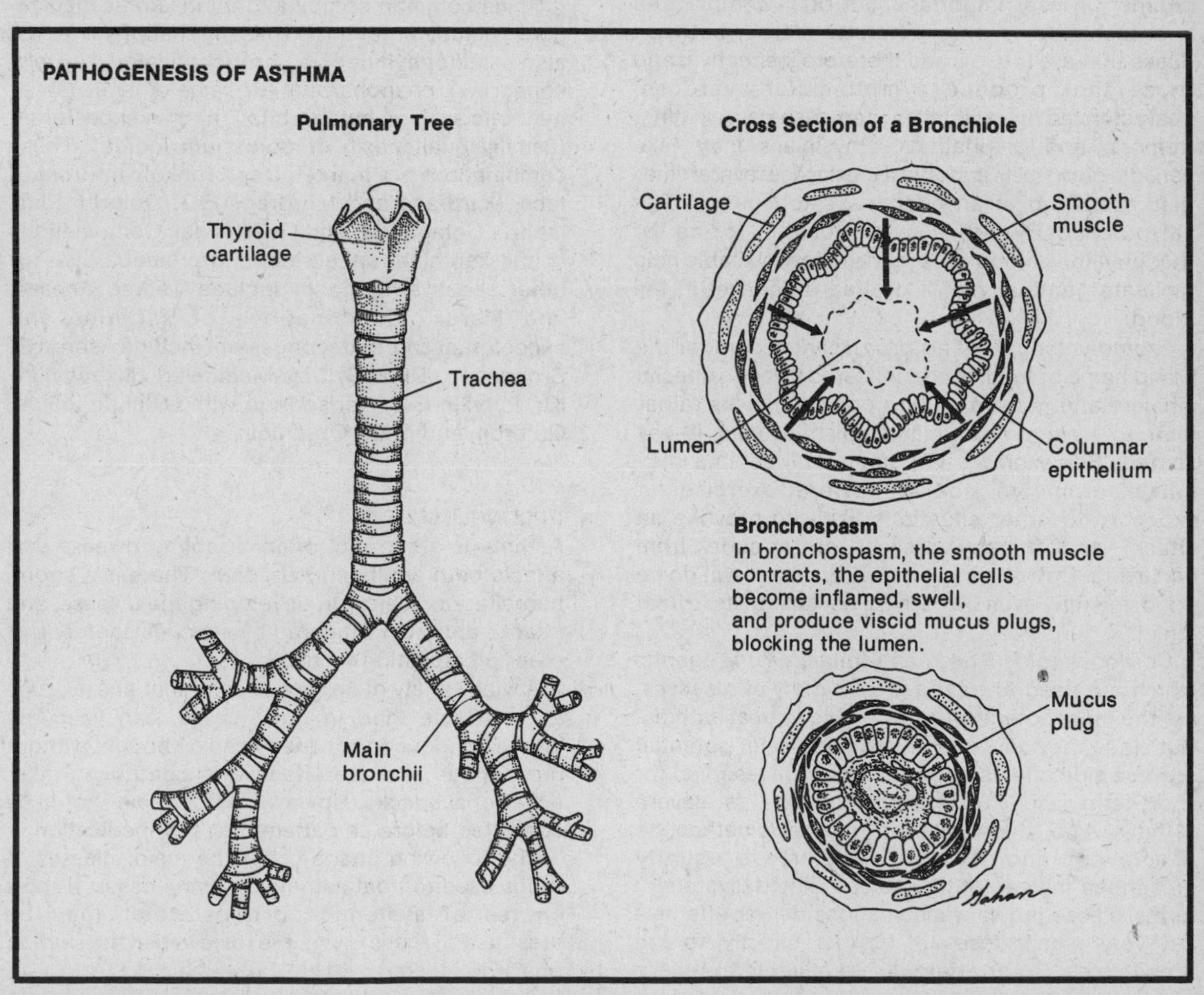

Bronchospasm
In bronchospasm, the smooth muscle contracts, the epithelial cells become inflamed, swell, and produce viscid mucus plugs, blocking the lumen.

and thyroid disease should consult a physician before taking any product containing a beta-adrenergic agent.

Xanthine compounds The xanthines are substances such as theophylline or aminophpylline that occur naturally in coffee, colas, and teas. This group of agents, best represented by theophylline (Bronkodyl, Slo-Phyllin, Elixophyllin, and other brands), relaxes bronchiolar smooth muscle and, as with beta-adrenergic agents, also stimulates the cardiovascular and central nervous systems. Most xanthines are mild diuretics, increasing urine output by the kidney. Theophylline and other xanthines, such as aminophylline (sold under the same brand name), are available in injectable forms for use during an asthmatic attack and in capsule, tablet (both regular and sustained-release), and liquid forms for daily use to prevent attacks. The drug is also available as suppositories, but absorption of this form is often erratic.

The modes and speed with which the body absorbs, uses, and excretes theophylline compounds vary from person to person, and dosages must be carefully tailored to the individual patient. Drug levels in the blood are affected by the patient's metabolism, dosage route and form, frequency of administration, and concomitant food intake and cigarette smoking. Establishing a proper dosage regimen is very important, but often complicated because there is a very narrow margin between doses that are too low and therefore ineffective, and those that produce symptoms of overdose, characterized by excitability, nervousness, sweating, tremors, and palpitations. Physicians may take periodic blood tests and adjust the dosage several times before arriving at an effective, safe regimen. The various sustained-release dosage forms of theophylline compounds that are now available help facilitate continuity of a desired drug level in the blood.

Cromolyn sodium This drug, marketed under the brand name of Intal, is administered through special inhalers and is used only to prevent attacks rather than to treat an asthmatic episode once it has started. For example, a person with asthma may inhale cromolyn sodium before exercise or exposure to other situations likely to provoke an attack, and thereby prevent an episode from occurring. But inhaling it during an attack will do no good and may even be harmful because of its irritant effect.

Corticosteroids These anti-inflammatory agents, which are used to treat a great variety of diseases, are the most potent drugs available to treat asthma. But since they also carry a high degree of potential adverse side effects, they generally are reserved for short-term use in treating moderate to severe asthma. Also, the inhalant form—beclomethasone (Beclovent and Vanceril Inhaler)—is usually prescribed instead of the tablet or liquid (systemic) forms. These inhalant medications deliver effective but very small doses of steroid directly to the bronchioles. Corticosteroids are believed to relieve asthma by reducing the inflammatory process in asthma, which causes swelling and irritation of mucous tissue in the airways. When judiciously administered, aerosolized microdoses of corticosteroids can reduce both the number and severity of asthma attacks without producing significant side effects. These drugs require a prescription and should only be taken upon a physician's specific recommendation.

Combination of Drugs

Many of the medications used to treat asthma are combinations of agents, usually a combination of bronchodilators with an expectorant and/or decongestant. Other combinations add an antianxiety agent or a barbiturate to the bronchodilators. The use of various combinations is controversial, with some authorities contending that there is no evidence that expectorants or antianxiety agents are useful in treating asthma, and indeed, may have an adverse effect in some patients. Combinations of adrenergic and theophylline agents, however, may be more effective than either ingredient taken alone.

Many of the combination drugs are nonprescription; therefore, close attention should be paid to the listing of ingredients and a physician should be consulted before they are used.

Some common combination antiasthma medications include a xanthine (usually theophylline, but also aminophylline), a bronchodilator (usually ephedrine), phenobarbital (or some other sedative-hypnotic such as butabarbital), and an expectorant (usually guaifenesin or potassium iodide). These combinations are marketed as Bronkolixir, Bronkotabs, Murdrane and Murdrane GG, Quibron Plus, Isuprel Compound, and Quandrinal. Combinations of the xanthine, ephedrine, and phenobarbital (or other sedative-hypnotic) include Tedral, Anesec, and Marax. Combinations of xanthine and expectorant and/or decongestant include Asbron G, Brondecon, Dilor-G, Duo-Medihaler, Elixophyllin-KL, Lufyllin-GG, Norisodrine with Calcium Iodide, Quibron, and Theo-Organidin.

IN CONCLUSION

Asthma is a chronic, often disabling disease that affects both adults and children. There is a strong hereditary tendency in developing the disease, and attacks are often triggered by specifiic allergens or other precipitating factors.

A wide variety of drugs and combinations of drugs are available that, in most cases, can keep the disease under control. Many can be bought without prescription and are effective in controlling mild, occasional attacks. However, a physician should be consulted before any attempt at self-medication.

The following charts cover the major classes of drugs used to treat asthma. In some cases, a short course of systemic corticosteroids may be prescribed. These drugs are reviewed in the section on *Corticosteroids* (pages 1038-66).

ALUPENT (Metaproterenol sulfate) Boehringer Ingelheim

Tabs: 10, 20 mg **Syrup:** 10 mg/5 ml

INDICATIONS	ORAL DOSAGE
Bronchial asthma **Reversible bronchospasm** associated with bronchitis and emphysema	**Adult:** 20 mg or 10 ml (2 tsp) tid or qid **Child (6–9 yr or <60 lb):** 10 mg or 5 ml (1 tsp) tid or qid **Child (9–12 yr or >60 lb):** 20 mg or 10 ml (2 tsp) tid or qid

ALUPENT Metered Dose Inhaler (Metaproterenol sulfate) Boehringer Ingelheim

Metered-dose inhaler: 0.65 mg/inhalation

INDICATIONS	ORAL DOSAGE
Bronchial asthma **Reversible bronchospasm** associated with bronchitis and emphysema	**Adult:** 2–3 inhalations q3–4h, up to 12 inhalations/day if needed

CONTRAINDICATIONS

Cardiac arrhythmias associated with tachycardia

WARNINGS/PRECAUTIONS

Excessive aerosol use	May be dangerous; cardiac arrest and fatalities have occurred. Repeated excessive administration may lead to paradoxical bronchoconstriction.
Additional sympathomimetic agents	Use with extreme caution; allow sufficient time before administering another sympathomimetic agent
Paradoxical bronchoconstriction	Has occurred with excessive use of other sympathomimetic agents; advise patient to report any failure to respond to usual doses
Special-risk patients	Use with great caution in patients with hypertension, coronary artery disease, congestive heart failure, hyperthyroidism, diabetes, or hypersensitivity to sympathomimetic amines

ADVERSE REACTIONS

Cardiovascular	Tachycardia, hypertension, palpitations
Central nervous system	Nervousness, tremor
Gastrointestinal	Nausea, vomiting, bad taste

OVERDOSAGE

Signs and symptoms	Excessive beta-adrenergic stimulation (see ADVERSE REACTIONS)
Treatment	Discontinue medication; treat symptomatically

DRUG INTERACTIONS

Sympathomimetic bronchodilators	⇧ Adrenergic effects
Nonselective beta blockers	⇩ Bronchodilation

ALTERED LABORATORY VALUES

No clinically significant alterations in blood/serum or urinary values occur at therapeutic dosages

Use in children

See INDICATIONS; tablets are not recommended for use in children under 6 yr of age

Use in pregnancy or nursing mothers

Safe use not established during pregnancy; general guidelines not established for use in nursing mothers

AMINOPHYLLIN (Aminophylline) Searle

Tabs: 100, 200 mg **Amps:** 500 mg/2 ml (for IM use); 250 mg/10 ml, 500 mg/20 ml (for IV use)

INDICATIONS	ORAL DOSAGE	PARENTERAL DOSAGE
Acute bronchial asthma **Reversible bronchospasm** associated with chronic bronchitis and emphysema	**Adult:** 600–1,600 mg in 3–4 divided doses **Child:** 12 mg/kg/24 h in 4 divided doses	——
Bronchial asthma; status asthmaticus; congestive heart failure; Cheyne-Stokes respiration; reduction of exertional dyspnea in emphysema; cardiac paroxysmal dyspnea; diuresis	——	**Adult:** 5–6 mg/kg IM q6–8h, as needed, or 250–500 mg (5–6 mg/kg) IV, injected slowly over a period of 20 min, to start, followed (if desired) by ~0.9 mg/kg/h by continuous IV infusion; adjust subsequent dosage according to clinical response **Child:** may require somewhat higher IM doses, on a mg/kg basis, than adults; for IV use, give ~6 mg/kg, injected slowly over a period of 20 min, to start; base subsequent dosage on clinical response and serum theophylline level, if available; usual maintenance dosage: 3.5–4.0 mg/kg IV q6–8h

ADMINISTRATION/DOSAGE ADJUSTMENTS

Use of serum theophylline levels	Adjust dosage to maintain serum theophylline level between 10 and 20 μg/ml; levels >20 μg/ml may produce toxicity. Ingestion of coffee, tea, cola beverages, chocolate, and acetaminophen may result in falsely high serum values when spectrophotometric methods are used to measure theophylline blood levels.
Patients with congestive heart failure or hepatic impairment	Serum theophylline level may persist longer than expected. Reduce initial and subsequent dosage by 20–25% if congestive heart failure is present; patients with impaired hepatic function may also require lower than usual doses.
Parenteral administration	Undiluted solution can either be injected very slowly by syringe or, more conveniently, infused IV in a small quantity (usually 100–200 ml) of 5% dextrose-in-water or saline or delivered in "piggyback" fashion through an existing IV system. Aminophylline should not be mixed with other drugs in a syringe or added to IV solutions of alkali-labile drugs, including isoproterenol, epinephrine, levarterenol, and penicillin G potassium. IM administration is painful. The dosages suggested above apply to patients with normal cardiac and hepatic function who have not been treated with aminophylline or theophylline for at least 24 h.

CONTRAINDICATIONS

Active peptic ulcer disease[1]	Hypersensitivity to aminophylline or theophylline

WARNINGS/PRECAUTIONS

Special-risk patients	Use with caution in patients with severe cardiac or hepatic disease, hypertension, hyperthyroidism, or acute myocardial injury
Peptic ulcer	May be exacerbated in patients with a history of peptic ulcer; use with caution. Chronic oral administration of high doses may result in GI irritation.

ADVERSE REACTIONS

Gastrointestinal	Nausea, vomiting, anorexia, GI distress; bitter aftertaste, dyspepsia, and heavy feeling in the stomach (with oral use)
Central nervous system	Dizziness, vertigo, light-headedness, headache, nervousness, agitation; insomnia (with oral use)
Cardiovascular	Palpitations, tachycardia, flushing; extrasystoles (with oral use); other arrhythmias and hypotension (with parenteral use)
Respiratory	Increase in respiration rate
Dermatological	Urticaria; rash (with parenteral use)

[1]If need is urgent, parenteral aminophylline may be given with appropriate concomitant therapy for peptic ulcer disease

Table continued on following page

AMINOPHYLLIN continued

OVERDOSAGE

Signs and symptoms	Nausea, vomiting, epigastric pain, hematemesis, diarrhea, hyperreflexia, fasciculations, clonic and tonic convulsions (especially in infants and small children), marked hypotension, circulatory failure, tachypnea, respiratory arrest, albuminuria, microhematuria, increased excretion of renal tubular cells, syncope, collapse, fever and dehydration, hyperthermia (see also ADVERSE REACTIONS)
Treatment	Discontinue drug immediately; use gastric lavage and emetic medication following acute oral overdosage. Avoid use of sympathomimetic drugs. Administer fluids, oxygen, and other supportive measures to prevent hypotension, overcome dehydration, and correct acid/base imbalance. Control seizures with short-acting barbiturates, diazepam, or phenytoin. For hyperthermia, use a cooling blanket or give sponge baths, as needed. If respiratory depression occurs, maintain patent airway and institute artificial respiration. Monitor theophylline serum levels until they fall below 20 μg/ml.

DRUG INTERACTIONS

Epinephrine and other sympathomimetic agents	⇧ Risk of toxicity
Other xanthine derivatives	⇧ Risk of toxicity; do not administer concurrently
Erythromycin, clindamycin, lincomycin, troleandomycin	⇧ Theophylline serum levels and/or toxicity
Lithium	⇧ Lithium excretion
Propranolol	Antagonism of propranolol effect ⇩ Bronchodilation

ALTERED LABORATORY VALUES

Blood/serum values	⇧ Glucose ⇧ Uric acid (with Bittner and colorimetric methods) ⇧ Bilirubin (with diazo tablet method)
Urinary values	⇧ Albumin ⇧ Catecholamines

Use in children

Use with caution; some children may be unusually sensitive to aminophylline

Use in pregnancy or nursing mothers

Safe use not established during pregnancy; general guidelines not established for use in nursing mothers

BRETHINE (Terbutaline sulfate) Geigy

Tabs: 2.5, 5 mg **Amps:** 1 mg/ml (2 ml)

INDICATIONS	ORAL DOSAGE	PARENTERAL DOSAGE
Bronchial asthma **Reversible bronchospasm** associated wth bronchitis and emphysema	**Adult:** 5 mg tid, during waking hours, up to 15 mg/24 h **Child (12-15 yr):** 2.5 mg tid, during waking hours, up to 7.5 mg/24 h	**Adult:** 0.25 mg SC, repeated after 15-30 min, if needed, up to 0.5 mg/4 h

ADMINISTRATION/DOSAGE ADJUSTMENTS

Presence of disturbing side effects — Reduce oral dosage in adults to 2.5 mg tid

CONTRAINDICATIONS

Hypersensitivity to sympathomimetic amines

WARNINGS/PRECAUTIONS

Special-risk patients — Use with caution in patients with diabetes, hypertension, hyperthyroidism, or a history of seizures and in cardiac patients, especially when arrhythmias are present

Concomitant use with other sympathomimetics — Not recommended except to relieve acute bronchospasm in patients on chronic oral terbutaline therapy

ADVERSE REACTIONS Frequent reactions are italicized

With oral use

Cardiovascular — Increase in heart rate, palpitations

Central nervous system — *Nervousness, tremor,* headache, drowsiness

Gastrointestinal — Nausea, vomiting

Other — Sweating, muscle cramps

With SC use

Cardiovascular — *Increase in heart rate, palpitations*

Central nervous system — *Nervousness, tremor, dizziness,* headache, anxiety

Gastrointestinal — Nausea, vomiting

Other — Muscle cramps

OVERDOSAGE

Signs and symptoms — Excessive beta-adrenergic stimulation (see ADVERSE REACTIONS)

Treatment — If patient is alert, induce emesis, followed by gastric lavage. If patient is unconscious, use a cuffed endotracheal tube to secure airway before starting gastric lavage; *do not induce emesis.* Instill a slurry of activated charcoal; provide cardiac and respiratory support, and maintain respiratory exchange. Monitor patient until asymptomatic.

DRUG INTERACTIONS

Other sympathomimetic agents — ⇧ Sympathomimetic effect

ALTERED LABORATORY VALUES

No clinically significant alterations in blood/serum or urinary values occur at therapeutic dosages

Use in children

Not recommended for use in children under 12 yr of age

Use in pregnancy or nursing mothers

Safe use not established, although no adverse effects on fetal development have been observed in animal studies

BRICANYL (Terbutaline sulfate) Astra

Tabs: 2.5, 5 mg **Amps:** 1 mg/ml (2 ml)

INDICATIONS	ORAL DOSAGE	PARENTERAL DOSAGE
Bronchial asthma **Reversible bronchospasm** associated with bronchitis and emphysema	**Adult:** 5 mg q6h during waking hours, up to 15 mg/24 h **Child (12–15 yr):** 2.5 mg tid, up to 7.5 mg/24 h	**Adult:** 0.25 mg SC, repeated after 15–30 min, if needed, up to 0.5 mg/4h

ADMINISTRATION/DOSAGE ADJUSTMENTS

Presence of disturbing side effects — Reduce oral dosage in adults to 2.5 mg tid

CONTRAINDICATIONS

Hypersensitivity to sympathomimetic amines

WARNINGS/PRECAUTIONS

Special-risk patients — Use with caution in patients with diabetes, hypertension, hyperthyroidism, or (if given SC) a history of seizures, and in cardiac patients, especially those with arrhythmias

Concomitant use with other sympathomimetics — Not recommended except to relieve acute bronchospasm in patients on chronic oral terbutaline therapy

ADVERSE REACTIONS

Frequent reactions are italicized

With oral use

Cardiovascular — Increase in heart rate, palpitations

Central nervous system — *Nervousness, tremor*, headache, drowsiness

Gastrointestinal — Nausea, vomiting

Other — Sweating

With SC use

Cardiovascular — *Increase in heart rate, palpitations*

Central nervous system — *Nervousness, tremor, dizziness*, headache, anxiety

Gastrointestinal — Nausea, vomiting

Other — Muscle cramps

OVERDOSAGE

Signs and symptoms — Symptoms of excessive beta-adrenergic stimulation (see ADVERSE REACTIONS)

Treatment — If patient is alert, induce emesis, followed by gastric lavage. If patient is unconscious, use a cuffed endotracheal tube to secure airway before starting gastric lavage; *do not induce emesis.* Instill a slurry of activated charcoal; provide cardiac and respiratory support, and maintain respiratory exchange. Monitor patient until asymptomatic.

DRUG INTERACTIONS

Other sympathomimetic agents — ⇧ Sympathomimetic effect

ALTERED LABORATORY VALUES

No clinically significant alterations in blood/serum or urinary values occur at therapeutic dosages

Use in children

Not recommended for use in children under 12 yr of age

Use in pregnancy or nursing mothers

Safe use not established, although no adverse effects on fetal development have been observed in animal studies

BRONDECON (Oxtriphylline and guaifenesin) Parke-Davis

Tabs: 200 mg oxtriphylline and 100 mg guaifenesin **Elixir:** 100 mg oxtriphylline and 50 mg guaifenesin per 5 ml[1]

INDICATIONS	ORAL DOSAGE
Bronchitis, bronchial asthma, asthmatic bronchitis, pulmonary emphysema, other chronic obstructive pulmonary diseases (adjunctive therapy)	**Adult:** 1 tab or 10 ml (2 tsp) qid; some patients may require higher or lower doses **Child (2–12 yr):** 5 ml (1 tsp)/60 lb qid; some patients may require higher or lower doses

CONTRAINDICATIONS

None

WARNINGS/PRECAUTIONS

Concurrent use of other xanthine-containing preparations	May lead to adverse reactions, particularly CNS stimulation in children

ADVERSE REACTIONS

Gastrointestinal	Gastric distress
Cardiovascular	Palpitations (occasional)
Central nervous system	CNS stimulation (occasional)

OVERDOSAGE

Signs and symptoms	See ADVERSE REACTIONS
Treatment	Discontinue medication; treat symptomatically

DRUG INTERACTIONS

Other xanthine derivatives	⇧ Risk of toxicity
Erythromycin, clindamycin, lincomycin, troleandomycin	⇧ Serum theophylline level and/or toxicity
Nonselective beta blockers	Antagonism of propranolol effect ⇩ Bronchodilation
Lithium	⇧ Lithium excretion

ALTERED LABORATORY VALUES

Blood/serum values	⇧ Glucose ⇧ Uric acid (with Bittner and colorimetric methods) ⇧ Bilirubin (with diazo tablet method)
Urinary values	⇧ Albumin ⇧ Catecholamines ⇧ 5-HIAA (with nitrosonaphthol reagent method) ⇧ VMA (with colorimetric methods)

Use in children	Use in pregnancy or nursing mothers
See INDICATIONS; general guidelines not established for use in children under 2 yr of age	General guidelines not established

[1]Contains 20% alcohol

BRONKOMETER (Isoetharine mesylate) Breon

Metered-dose inhaler: 340 μg/inhalation

INDICATIONS	ORAL DOSAGE
Bronchial asthma **Reversible bronchospasm** associated with bronchitis and emphysema	**Adult:** 1-2 inhalations q4h; some patients may require more inhalations (wait 1 full min after initial dose before readministering) or, in severe cases, more frequent administration may be needed

CONTRAINDICATIONS

Hypersensitivity to isoetharine mesylate or other components

WARNINGS/PRECAUTIONS

Excessive aerosol use	May lead to loss of effectiveness; discontinue medication immediately if severe paradoxical airway resistance develops and institute alternative therapy; cardiac arrest has also occurred
Concomitant sympathomimetic therapy	May cause excessive tachycardia; however, isoetharine may be alternated with epinephrine or other sympathomimetic amines, if desired
Special-risk patients	Adjust dosage carefully in patients with hyperthyroidism, hypertension, acute coronary artery disease, cardiac asthma, limited cardiac reserve, or sensitivity to sympathomimetic amines

ADVERSE REACTIONS

Essentially none at therapeutic dosages

OVERDOSAGE

Signs and symptoms	Tachycardia, palpitations, nausea, headache, changes in blood pressure, anxiety, tension, restlessness, insomnia, tremor, weakness, dizziness, excitement
Treatment	Discontinue medication; treat symptomatically and institute supportive measures, as required

DRUG INTERACTIONS

Epinephrine and other sympathomimetic agents	⇧ Sympathomimetic effect
Nonselective beta blockers	⇩ Bronchodilation

ALTERED LABORATORY VALUES

No clinically significant alterations in blood/serum or urinary values occur at therapeutic dosages

Use in children

General guidelines not established

Use in pregnancy or nursing mothers

Safe use not established, although there has been no evidence of teratogenicity

BRONKOSOL (Isoetharine hydrochloride) Breon

Sol: 1% (10, 30 ml)

INDICATIONS	ORAL DOSAGE
Bronchial asthma **Reversible bronchospasm** associated with bronchitis and emphysema	**Adult:** 3–7 inhalations of undiluted solution q4h via hand nebulizer

ADMINISTRATION/DOSAGE ADJUSTMENTS

Oxygen aerosolization	Administer 0.25–0.5 ml, diluted 1:3 with saline or other diluent, over a period of 15–20 min q4h, with oxygen flow adjusted to deliver 4–6 liters/min
IPPB	Administer 0.25–1.0 ml, diluted 1:3 with saline or other diluent, q4h at a usual inspiratory flow rate of 15 liters/min with a cycling pressure of 15 cm H_2O; depending on the type of apparatus used, some patients may require an inspiratory flow rate of 6–30 liters/min, a cycling pressure of 10–15 cm H_2O, or further dilution of the solution

CONTRAINDICATIONS

Hypersensitivity to isoetharine hydrochloride or other components

WARNINGS/PRECAUTIONS

Excessive aerosol use	May lead to loss of effectiveness; discontinue medication immediately if severe paradoxical airway resistance develops and institute alternative therapy; cardiac arrest has also occurred
Concomitant sympathomimetic therapy	May cause excessive tachycardia; however, isoetharine may be alternated with epinephrine or other sympathomimetic amines, if desired
Special-risk patients	Adjust dosage carefully in patients with hyperthyroidism, hypertension, acute coronary artery disease, cardiac asthma, limited cardiac reserve, or sensitivity to sympathomimetic amines

ADVERSE REACTIONS

Essentially none at therapeutic dosages

OVERDOSAGE

Signs and symptoms	Tachycardia, palpitations, nausea, headache, changes in blood pressure, anxiety, tension, restlessness, insomnia, tremor, weakness, dizziness, excitement
Treatment	Discontinue medication; treat symptomatically and institute supportive measures, as required

DRUG INTERACTIONS

Epinephrine, other sympathomimetic agents	⇧ Sympathomimetic effect
Nonselective beta blockers	⇩ Bronchodilation

ALTERED LABORATORY VALUES

No clinically significant alterations in blood/serum or urinary values occur at therapeutic dosages

Use in children	Use in pregnancy or nursing mothers
General guidelines not established	Safe use not established, although there has been no evidence of teratogenicity

CHOLEDYL (Oxtriphylline) Parke-Davis

Tabs: 100, 200 mg **Elixir:** 100 mg oxtriphylline/5 ml[1]

INDICATIONS	ORAL DOSAGE
Acute bronchial asthma **Reversible bronchospasm** associated with chronic bronchitis and emphysema	**Adult:** 200 mg or 10 ml (2 tsp) qid **Child (2–12 yr):** 5 ml (1 tsp)/60 lb qid

CONTRAINDICATIONS

None

WARNINGS/PRECAUTIONS

Concurrent use of other xanthine-containing preparations	May lead to adverse reactions, particularly CNS stimulation in children

ADVERSE REACTIONS

Gastrointestinal	Gastric distress
Cardiovascular	Palpitations (occasional)
Central nervous system	Stimulation (occasional)

OVERDOSAGE

Signs and symptoms	*Cardiovascular:* precordial pain, tachycardia, ventricular and other arrhythmias, hypotension, and, in extreme cases, severe shock, cardiovascular collapse, and death. *Gastrointestinal:* abdominal pain, nausea, persistent vomiting, and hematemesis. *Central nervous system:* headache, dizziness, restlessness, irritability, tremors, hyperactivity, and agitation, followed, in severe cases, by convulsions, drowsiness, coma, and death.
Treatment	If patient is conscious and seizure has not occurred, induce emesis and administer a cathartic and activated charcoal. If patient is convulsing, establish an airway and administer oxygen and IV diazepam (0.1–0.3 mg/kg, up to 10 mg). If patient is comatose following the occurrence of seizures, intubate immediately, using an endotracheal tube with an inflated cuff, and perform gastric lavage; introduce the cathartic and activated charcoal through a large-bore gastric-lavage tube. Monitor vital signs, maintain blood pressure, and provide adequate hydration. Treat hypotension and shock by appropriate fluid replacement, avoiding the use of vasopressors, if possible. In general, the drug is metabolized sufficiently rapidly to preclude any additional benefit from dialysis; however, dialysis may be useful in the presence of congestive heart failure or hepatic dysfunction. Serial monitoring of the serum theophylline level is helpful in following the patient's course and in guiding further management.

DRUG INTERACTIONS

Other xanthine derivatives	⇧ Risk of toxicity; do not administer concurrently
Lithium	⇧ Lithium excretion
Propranolol	Antagonism of propranolol effect ⇩ Bronchodilation
Erythromycin, clindamycin, lincomycin, troleandomycin	⇧ Theophylline serum level

ALTERED LABORATORY VALUES

Blood/serum values	⇧ Glucose ⇧ Uric acid (with Bittner and colorimetric methods) ⇧ Bilirubin (with diazo tablet method)
Urinary values	⇧ Albumin ⇧ Catecholamines

Use in children

See INDICATIONS

Use in pregnancy or nursing mothers

Safe use not established, although there has been no evidence of teratogenicity in animal studies

[1]Contains 20% alcohol

CHOLEDYL Pediatric Syrup (Oxtriphylline) Parke-Davis

Pediatric syrup: 50 mg/5 ml (equivalent to 32 mg anhydrous theophylline)

INDICATIONS	ORAL DOSAGE
Acute bronchial asthma **Reversible bronchospasm** associated with chronic bronchitis and emphysema	**Adult, nonsmoker:** 9.4 mg/kg to start, followed by 4.7 mg/kg q6h for the next 12 h; thereafter, 4.7 mg/kg q8h for maintenance **Infant and child (6 mo to 9 yr):** 9.4 mg/kg to start, followed by 6.2 mg/kg q4h for the next 12 h; thereafter, 6.2 mg/kg q6h for maintenance **Child (9–16 yr) and young adult smoker:** 9.4 mg/kg to start, followed by 4.7 mg/kg q4h for the next 12 h; thereafter, 4.7 mg/kg q6h for maintenance
Chronic asthma	**Adult:** 6.2 mg/kg q6h or 625 mg/day, whichever is less, to start, followed, if tolerated, by an approximately 25% increase in dosage every 2–3 days, up to 5 mg/kg q6h or 1,400 mg/day, whichever is less **Infant and child (<9 yr):** 6.2 mg/kg q6h or 625 mg/day, whichever is less, to start, followed, if tolerated, by an approximately 25% increase in dosage every 2–3 days, up to 9.4 mg/kg q6h or 1,400 mg/day, whichever is less **Child (9–12 yr):** 6.2 mg/kg q6h or 625 mg/day, whichever is less, to start, followed, if tolerated, by an approximately 25% increase in dosage every 2–3 days, up to 7.8 mg/kg q6h or 1,400 mg/day, whichever is less **Child (12–16 yr):** 6.2 mg/kg q6h or 625 mg/day, whichever is less, to start, followed, if tolerated, by an approximately 25% increase in dosage every 2–3 days, up to 7 mg/kg q6h or 1,400 mg/day, whichever is less

ADMINISTRATION/DOSAGE ADJUSTMENTS

Use of serum theophylline levels	Adjust dosage to maintain serum theophylline level between 10 and 20 µg/ml; levels >20 µg/ml may produce toxicity. Check serum level 1–1½ h after last dose; medication must have been taken at typical intervals, with no missed or added doses, for a period of 48 h prior to measurement.
Older patients and patients with cor pulmonale	For acute asthmatic symptoms requiring rapid theophyllinization, give 9.4 mg/kg to start, followed by 3.1 mg/kg q6h for the next 12 h and q8h thereafter for maintenance
Patients with congestive heart failure or hepatic failure	For acute asthmatic symptoms requiring rapid theophyllinization, give 9.4 mg/kg to start, followed by 3.1 mg/kg q8h for the next 12 h and 1.6–3.1 mg/kg q12h thereafter for maintenance
Patients currently receiving theophylline products	Loading dose is based on the principle that 0.8 mg/kg of oxtriphylline will increase the serum theophylline concentration by 1 µg/ml. A loading dose should be deferred if therapeutic serum levels are rapidly obtained. When respiratory distress is sufficient to warrant a small risk, a 4 mg/kg loading dose (which will raise the serum theophylline level by 5 µg/ml) may be safely used, unless the patient is experiencing theophylline toxicity.
Gastric irritation	May be prevented by giving medication with food; although absorption may be delayed, it is still complete
Concomitant bronchodilator therapy	Reduce dosage of oxtriphylline when administered concomitantly with other bronchodilating agents, such as beta-adrenergic receptor agonists

CONTRAINDICATIONS

Hypersensitivity to theophylline or oxtriphylline

WARNINGS/PRECAUTIONS

Status asthmaticus	If patient does not rapidly respond to bronchodilating agents, additional medication, including corticosteroids, may be required
Cigarette smoking	Decreases serum half-life of theophylline; heavy smokers (1–2 packs/day) may require larger doses
Gastric irritation	Use with caution in patients with a history of peptic ulcer (see ADMINISTRATION/DOSAGE ADJUSTMENTS)
Cardiac disease	Careful reduction of dosage and monitoring of serum levels are particularly important in the presence of cardiac decompensation, owing to a reduction in theophylline clearance rate; use with caution in patients with severe cardiac disease, acute myocardial injury, or cor pulmonale and with great caution in patients with congestive heart failure, since theophylline blood-level curves may be markedly prolonged, with theophylline persisting in the serum long after the drug is discontinued
Hepatic or renal impairment	Use with caution and at reduced dosage in patients with liver disease or renal failure, owing to increase in serum half-life of theophylline; monitoring of serum theophylline levels is advisable

Table continued on following page

WARNINGS/PRECAUTIONS continued

Other special-risk patients	Theophylline clearance rate is decreased in neonates, patients over 55 yr of age (especially males), debilitated or alcoholic patients, and patients with severe or acute hypoxia or chronic obstructive pulmonary disease; use with caution at reduced dosage, if necessary, and monitor serum theophylline levels, if feasible. Oxtriphylline should also be used with caution in patients with hypertension, hyperthyroidism, or pre-existing arrhythmias.

ADVERSE REACTIONS

Gastrointestinal	Nausea, vomiting, epigastric pain, hematemesis, diarrhea
Central nervous system and neuromuscular	Headache, irritability, restlessness, insomnia, reflex hyperexcitability, muscle twitching, clonic and tonic generalized convulsions
Cardiovascular	Palpitations, tachycardia, extrasystoles, flushing, hypotension, circulatory failure, life-threatening ventricular arrhythmias
Respiratory	Tachypnea
Renal	Albuminuria, increased excretion of renal tubule cells and red blood cells, potentiation of diuresis
Metabolic and endocrinological	Hyperglycemia, inappropriate antidiuretic hormone secretion syndrome

OVERDOSAGE

Signs and symptoms[1]	*Cardiovascular:* precordial pain, tachycardia, ventricular and other arrhythmias, hypotension, and, in extreme cases, severe shock, cardiovascular collapse, and death. *Gastrointestinal:* abdominal pain, nausea, persistent vomiting, and hematemesis. *Central nervous system:* headache, dizziness, restlessness, irritability, tremors, hyperactivity, and agitation, followed, in severe cases, by convulsions, drowsiness, coma, and death.
Treatment	If patient is conscious and seizure has not occurred, induce emesis and administer a cathartic and activated charcoal. If patient is convulsing, establish an airway and administer oxygen and IV diazepam (0.1–0.3 mg/kg, up to 10 mg). If patient is comatose following the occurrence of seizures, intubate immediately, using an endotracheal tube with an inflated cuff, and perform gastric lavage; introduce the cathartic and activated charcoal through a large-bore gastric-lavage tube. Monitor vital signs, maintain blood pressure, and provide adequate hydration. Treat hypotension and shock by appropriate fluid replacement, avoiding the use of vasopressors, if possible. In general, the drug is metabolized sufficiently rapidly to preclude any additional benefit from dialysis; however, dialysis may be useful in the presence of congestive heart failure or hepatic dysfunction. Serial monitoring of the serum theophylline level is helpful in following the patient's course and in guiding further management.

DRUG INTERACTIONS

Other xanthine derivatives	⇧ Risk of toxicity; do not administer concurrently
Lithium	⇧ Lithium excretion
Propranolol	Antagonism of propranolol effect ⇩ Bronchodilation
Erythromycin, clindamycin, lincomycin, troleandomycin	⇧ Theophylline serum level

ALTERED LABORATORY VALUES

Blood/serum values	⇧ Glucose ⇧ Uric acid (with Bittner and colorimetric methods) ⇧ Bilirubin (with diazo tablet method)
Urinary values	⇧ Albumin ⇧ Catecholamines

Use in children

See INDICATIONS. Children may exhibit marked sensitivity to CNS stimulation. Use with caution in neonates, owing to reduced theophylline clearance rate.

Use in pregnancy or nursing mothers

Safe use not established during pregnancy or in nursing mothers

[1]Serious toxicity may occur suddenly and may or may not be preceded by minor adverse effects such as nausea, vomiting, or restlessness; convulsions, tachycardia, or ventricular arrhythmias may be the first signs of toxicity

DUO-MEDIHALER (Isoproterenol hydrochloride and phenylephrine bitartrate) **Riker**

Metered-dose inhaler: 0.16 mg isoproterenol hydrochloride and 0.24 mg phenylephrine bitartrate per dose

INDICATIONS	ORAL DOSAGE
Bronchospasm associated with acute and chronic bronchial asthma, pulmonary emphysema, bronchitis, and bronchiectasis	**Adult:** for acute episodes, 1 inhalation to start, repeated after 2–5 min, if necessary, not to exceed 2 inhalations at any one time or 6 inhalations/h during any 24-h period; for maintenance, 1–2 inhalations 4–6 times/day

CONTRAINDICATIONS

Hypersensitivity to either component ● Pre-existing cardiac arrhythmias associated with tachycardia ●

WARNINGS/PRECAUTIONS

Excessive use	May lead to loss of effectiveness; discontinue medication immediately if severe paradoxical airway resistance develops and institute alternative therapy; cardiac arrest and death have also occurred
Special-risk patients	Use with caution in patients with cardiovascular disorders (including coronary insufficiency), diabetes, or hyperthyroidism and in patients sensitive to sympathomimetic amines
Concurrent use of epinephrine	May result in serious arrhythmias; however, if desired, both drugs may be alternated, provided that at least 4 h have elapsed between doses

ADVERSE REACTIONS

Essentially none at therapeutic dosages

OVERDOSAGE

Signs and symptoms	*Isoproterenol-related effects:* palpitations, tachycardia, tremulousness, flushing, anginal-type pain, nausea, dizziness, weakness, sweating; *phenylephrine-related effects:* cardiac irregularities, CNS disturbances, reflex bradycardia
Treatment	Discontinue medication; treat symptomatically and institute supportive measures, as required

DRUG INTERACTIONS

Epinephrine	⇧ Cardiac stimulation and risk of arrhythmias

ALTERED LABORATORY VALUES

No clinically significant alterations in blood/serum or urinary values occur at therapeutic dosages

Use in children

General guidelines not established

Use in pregnancy or nursing mothers

Safe use not established, although there has been no evidence of teratogenicity

ELIXOPHYLLIN (Theophylline) Berlex

Caps: 100, 200 mg **Caps (sust rel):** 125, 250 mg (Elixophyllin SR) **Elixir:** 80 mg/15 ml[1]

INDICATIONS	ORAL DOSAGE
Acute bronchial asthma **Reversible bronchospasm** associated with chronic bronchitis and emphysema	**Adult, nonsmoker:** 6 mg/kg to start, followed by 3 mg/kg q6h for the next 12 h; thereafter, 3 mg/kg q8h for maintenance **Infant and child (6 mo to 9 yr):** 6 mg/kg to start, followed by 4 mg/kg q4h for the next 12 h; thereafter, 4 mg/kg q6h for maintenance **Child (9–16 yr) and young adult smoker:** 6 mg/kg to start, followed by 3 mg/kg q4h for the next 12 h; thereafter, 3 mg/kg q6h for maintenance
Chronic asthma	**Adult:** 16 mg/kg/day or 400 mg/day, whichever is less, in 3–4 divided doses q6–8h to start, followed, if tolerated, by an approximately 25% increase in dosage every 2–3 days, up to 13 mg/kg/day or 900 mg/day, whichever is less **Infant and child (<9 yr):** 16 mg/kg/day or 400 mg/day, whichever is less, in 3–4 divided doses q6–8h to start, followed, if tolerated, by an approximately 25% increase in dosage every 2–3 days, up to 24 mg/kg/day or 900 mg/day, whichever is less **Child (9–12 yr):** 16 mg/kg/day or 400 mg/day, whichever is less, in 3–4 divided doses q6–8h to start, followed, if tolerated, by an approximately 25% increase in dosage every 2–3 days, up to 20 mg/kg/day or 900 mg/day, whichever is less **Child (12–16 yr):** 16 mg/kg/day or 400 mg/day, whichever is less, in 3–4 divided doses q6–8h to start, followed, if tolerated, by an approximately 25% increase in dosage every 2–3 days, up to 18 mg/kg/day or 900 mg/day, whichever is less

ADMINISTRATION/DOSAGE ADJUSTMENTS

Use of serum theophylline levels	Adjust dosage to maintain serum theophylline level between 10 and 20 µg/ml; levels > 20 µg/ml may produce toxicity. Check serum level 1–2 h after last dose if elixir or capsules that undergo rapid dissolution are used and 3–5 h after last dose if sustained-release capsules are used. Medication must have been taken at typical intervals, with no missed or added doses, for a period of 48 h prior to measurement. If peak serum level is less than 5 µg/ml, increase the total daily dose by 100% and recheck blood level; if between 5 and 7.5 µg/ml, increase dose by 50% and recheck blood level; if between 8 and 10 µg/ml, increase dose by 20% even if patient is asymptomatic; if between 11 and 13 µg/ml and patient is asymptomatic, no adjustment is needed; if between 11 and 13 µg/ml and symptoms are present during upper respiratory infection or exercise, cautiously increase dose by 10%; if between 14 and 20 µg/ml and asthmatic symptoms break through at end of dosing interval, switch to sustained-release capsules and recheck blood level; if between 14 and 20 µg/ml and side effects are present, decrease dose by 10%; if between 21 and 25 µg/ml, decrease dose by 10% even if side effects are absent; if between 26 and 34 µg/ml, omit the next dose even if side effects are absent, decrease the total daily dose by 25–33%, and recheck blood level; if equal to or greater than 35 µg/ml, omit the next two doses, decrease the total daily dose by 50%, and recheck blood level.
Use of sustained-release capsules	During chronic therapy may allow longer dosing intervals and/or less fluctuation in serum levels between doses. For adults and children over 12 yr of age, give 250 mg q12h or, in severe cases, q8h; for children 6–12 yr old, give 125 mg q12h or, in severe cases, q8h.
Older patients and patients with cor pulmonale	For acute asthmatic symptoms requiring rapid theophyllinization, give 6 mg/kg to start, followed by 2 mg/kg q6h for the next 12 h and q8h thereafter for maintenance
Patients with congestive heart failure or hepatic failure	For acute asthmatic symptoms requiring rapid theophyllinization, give 6 mg/kg to start, followed by 2 mg/kg q8h for the next 12 h and 1–2 mg/kg q12h thereafter for maintenance
Patients currently receiving theophylline products	Loading dose is based on the principle that 0.5 mg/kg of theophylline will increase the serum theophylline concentration by 1 µg/ml. A loading dose should be deferred if therapeutic serum levels are rapidly obtained. When respiratory distress is sufficient to warrant a small risk, a 2.5 mg/kg loading dose (which will raise the serum theophylline level by 5 µg/ml) may be safely used, unless the patient is experiencing theophylline toxicity.
Gastric irritation	May be prevented by giving medication with food; although absorption may be delayed, it is still complete

CONTRAINDICATIONS

Hypersensitivity to theophylline

WARNINGS/PRECAUTIONS

Status asthmaticus	If patient does not rapidly respond to bronchodilating agents, additional medication, including corticosteroids, may be required

Table continued on following page

ELIXOPHYLLIN continued

WARNINGS/PRECAUTIONS continued	
Cardiac disease	Use with caution in patients with severe cardiac disease, acute myocardial injury, or cor pulmonale and with great caution in patients with congestive heart failure, since theophylline blood-level curves may be markedly prolonged, with theophylline persisting in the serum long after the drug is discontinued
Hepatic or renal impairment	Use with caution and at reduced dosage in patients with liver disease or renal failure, owing to increase in serum half-life of theophylline; monitoring of serum theophylline levels is advisable
Other special-risk patients	Theophylline clearance rate is decreased in neonates, patients over 55 yr of age (especially males), and patients with severe hypoxia or chronic obstructive pulmonary disease; use with caution at reduced dosage, if necessary, and monitor serum theophylline levels, if feasible. Theophylline should also be used with caution in patients with hypertension, hyperthyroidism, or pre-existing arrhythmias.

ADVERSE REACTIONS	
Gastrointestinal	Nausea, vomiting, epigastric pain, hematemesis, diarrhea
Central nervous system and neuromuscular	Headache, irritability, restlessness, insomnia, reflex hyperexcitability, muscle twitching, clonic and tonic generalized convulsions
Cardiovascular	Palpitations, tachycardia, extrasystoles, flushing, hypotension, circulatory failure, life-threatening ventricular arrhythmias
Respiratory	Tachypnea
Renal	Albuminuria, increased excretion of renal tubule cells and red blood cells, potentiation of diuresis
Metabolic and endocrinological	Hyperglycemia, inappropriate antidiuretic hormone secretion syndrome

OVERDOSAGE	
Signs and symptoms[2]	*Cardiovascular:* precordial pain, tachycardia, ventricular and other arrhythmias, hypotension, and, in extreme cases, severe shock, cardiovascular collapse, and death. *Gastrointestinal:* abdominal pain, nausea, persistent vomiting, and hematemesis. *Central nervous system:* headache, dizziness, restlessness, irritability, tremors, hyperactivity, and agitation, followed, in severe cases, by convulsions, drowsiness, coma, and death.
Treatment	If patient is conscious and seizure has not occurred, induce emesis and administer a cathartic and activated charcoal. If patient is convulsing, establish an airway and administer oxygen and IV diazepam (0.1–0.3 mg/kg, up to 10 mg). If patient is comatose following the occurrence of seizures, intubate immediately, using an endotracheal tube with an inflated cuff, and perform gastric lavage; introduce the cathartic and activated charcoal through a large-bore gastric-lavage tube. Monitor vital signs, maintain blood pressure, and provide adequate hydration. Treat hypotension and shock by appropriate fluid replacement, avoiding the use of vasopressors, if possible. In general, the drug is metabolized sufficiently rapidly to preclude any additional benefit from dialysis; however, dialysis may be useful in the presence of congestive heart failure or hepatic dysfunction.

DRUG INTERACTIONS	
Other xanthine derivatives	⇧ Risk of toxicity; do not administer concurrently
Lithium	⇧ Lithium excretion
Propranolol	Antagonism of propranolol effect ⇩ Bronchodilation
Erythromycin, clindamycin, lincomycin, troleandomycin	⇧ Theophylline serum level

ALTERED LABORATORY VALUES	
Blood/serum values	⇧ Glucose ⇧ Uric acid ⇧ Bilirubin
Urinary values	⇧ Albumin ⇧ Catecholamines

Use in children

See INDICATIONS; use with caution in neonates, owing to reduced theophylline clearance rate. A nonalcoholic suspension is available for use in children under 6 yr of age.

Use in pregnancy or nursing mothers

Safe use not established during pregnancy; general guidelines not established for use in nursing mothers

NOTE: Theophylline also marketed as **BRONKODYL** (Breon); **SLO-PHYLLIN** (Dooner); **THEO-DUR** (Key); **THEOLAIR** (R. Ker); and **THEOPHYL** (Knoll).

INTAL (Cromolyn sodium) Fisons

Caps (for inhalation): 20 mg

INDICATIONS	ORAL DOSAGE
Severe bronchial asthma (adjunctive therapy)	**Adult:** 20 mg inhaled qid at regular intervals **Child (>5 yr):** same as adult

ADMINISTRATION/DOSAGE ADJUSTMENTS

Introduction into regimen	May be undertaken after acute episode is controlled and patient can inhale adequately
Downward dosage titration	May be undertaken gradually when patient is stabilized on cromolyn and if steroids are not needed; usual decrease: from 4 caps to 3 caps/day. If clinical condition worsens, increase dosage gradually.
Concomitant use of corticosteroids, bronchodilators	Should be continued; if patient improves, gradual tapering of steroid therapy or institution of an alternate-day regimen should be attempted. However, if patient undergoes significant stress during treatment (eg, a severe asthma attack, surgery, trauma, or severe illness) or within 1 (or sometimes 2) yr of terminating steroid treatment, corticosteroid therapy may need to be resumed. Also, if cromolyn inhalation is impaired (eg, as in a severe exacerbation of asthma), the dosage of steroids and/or other agents may need to be temporarily increased.
Withdrawal of cromolyn when steroid dosage has been reduced	Requires continued close monitoring of patient; sudden reappearance of severe asthma may necessitate immediate treatment and possible reintroduction of steroids

CONTRAINDICATIONS

Hypersensitivity to cromolyn sodium ●	During an acute asthmatic attack, especially status asthmaticus ●

WARNINGS/PRECAUTIONS

Special-risk patients	Use with caution when considering long-term therapy, especially in patients with impaired renal or hepatic function
Eosinophilic pneumonia	May occur; discontinue therapy
Cough, bronchospasm	May occur in some patients following inhalation of drug; if not reversed by prior bronchodilator administration, discontinue therapy
Asthmatic symptoms	May recur if dosage is reduced below recommended levels or drug is discontinued

ADVERSE REACTIONS

Respiratory	Bronchospasm, cough, laryngeal edema (rare), nasal congestion, pharyngeal irritation, wheezing (rare and possibly not drug-related: hoarseness, hemoptysis, pulmonary infiltrates with eosinophilia)
Cardiovascular	Angioedema, periarteritic vasculitis (rare), pericarditis (rare)
Central nervous system	Dizziness, headache, peripheral neuritis (rare), vertigo (rare)
Gastrointestinal	Nausea
Dermatological and hypersensitivity	Rash, urticaria, anaphylaxis (rare), exfoliative dermatitis (rare), photodermatitis (rare)
Other	Dysuria and urinary frequency, joint swelling and pain, lacrimation, swollen parotid glands, anemia (rare), myalgia (rare), nephrosis (rare), polymyositis (rare), inhalation of gelatin particles, mouthpiece, or propeller

OVERDOSAGE

Signs and symptoms	See ADVERSE REACTIONS
Treatment	Discontinue medication; treat symptomatically and institute supportive measures, as required

DRUG INTERACTIONS

No clinically significant drug interactions have been observed

ALTERED LABORATORY VALUES

No clinically significant alterations in blood/serum or urinary values occur at therapeutic dosages

Use in children	Use in pregnancy or nursing mothers
Not recommended for children under 5 yr of age; use with caution in older children (possible adverse effects may not be manifested for many years)	Not recommended during pregnancy; general guidelines not established for use in nursing mothers

ISUPREL (Isoproterenol hydrochloride) Breon

Metered-dose inhaler: 0.125 mg/inhalation

INDICATIONS	ORAL DOSAGE
Bronchospasm associated with acute and chronic bronchial asthma, pulmonary emphysema, bronchitis, and bronchiectasis	**Adult:** for acute episodes, 1 inhalation to start, repeated after 1 min, if necessary, not to exceed 5 doses/day; for chronic conditions, 1-2 inhalations not less than 3-4 h apart **Child:** same as adult

CONTRAINDICATIONS

Pre-existing cardiac arrhythmias associated with tachycardia

WARNINGS/PRECAUTIONS

Excessive use	May lead to loss of effectiveness; discontinue medication immediately if severe paradoxical airway resistance develops and institute alternative therapy; cardiac arrest and death have also occurred
Special-risk patients	Use with caution in patients with cardiovascular disorders (including coronary insufficiency), diabetes, hyperthyroidism, or sensitivity to sympathomimetic agents
Status asthmaticus, abnormal blood-gas tensions	Relief of bronchospasm may not be accompanied by improved vital capacity and blood-gas tensions; oxygen-mixture administration and ventilatory assistance are necessary
Concurrent use of epinephrine	May result in serious arrhythmias; however, if desired, both drugs may be alternated, provided that at least 4 h have elapsed between doses

ADVERSE REACTIONS

Respiratory	Throat irritation

OVERDOSAGE

Signs and symptoms	Tachycardia, palpitations, nervousness, nausea, vomiting; rarely: headache, flushing of skin, tremor, dizziness, weakness, sweating, precordial distress, anginal-type pain
Treatment	Discontinue medication; treat symptomatically and institute supportive measures, as required

DRUG INTERACTIONS

Epinephrine	⇧ Cardiac activity and risk of arrhythmias
Nonselective beta blockers	⇩ Bronchodilation

ALTERED LABORATORY VALUES

No clinically significant alterations in blood/serum or urinary values occur at therapeutic dosages

Use in children	Use in pregnancy or nursing mothers
See INDICATIONS	Safe use not established, although there has been no evidence of teratogenicity

LUFYLLIN (Dyphylline) Wallace

Tabs: 200 mg (Lufyllin), 400 mg (Lufyllin-400) **Elixir:** 100 mg/15 ml (1 tbsp) **Amps:** 250 mg/ml

INDICATIONS	ORAL DOSAGE	PARENTERAL DOSAGE
Acute bronchial asthma **Reversible bronchospasm** associated with chronic bronchitis and emphysema	**Adult:** 15 mg/kg q6h on an empty stomach, up to 4 doses/day	**Adult:** 250–500 mg IM (very slowly) q6h, as needed

ADMINISTRATION/DOSAGE ADJUSTMENTS

Prolonged or repeated therapy	Monitor theophylline blood levels: therapeutic range, 10–20 μg/ml

CONTRAINDICATIONS

Hypersensitivity to dyphylline ●	Concurrent use with other xanthines ●

WARNINGS/PRECAUTIONS

Status asthmaticus	Inappropriate indication; toxicity may occur with excessive doses
Special-risk patients	Use with caution in patients with severe cardiac disease, hypertension, hyperthyroidism, or acute myocardial injury; use with great caution in patients with congestive heart failure, since dyphylline blood-level curves may be markedly prolonged, with dyphylline persisting in the serum long after the drug is discontinued
Peptic ulcer	May be exacerbated; use with particular caution; gastrointestinal irritation may occur at chronic oral dosage levels of 500–1,000 mg/day
Toxicity	May occur with theophylline blood levels >20 μg/ml

ADVERSE REACTIONS

Gastrointestinal	Irritation, nausea, vomiting, and epigastric pain, generally preceded by headache, hematemesis, and diarrhea
Central nervous system and neuromuscular	Stimulation, irritability, restlessness, insomnia, reflex hyperexcitability, muscle twitching, clonic and tonic generalized convulsions, agitation
Cardiovascular	Palpitations, tachycardia, extrasystoles, flushing, marked hypotension, and circulatory failure
Respiratory	Tachypnea, respiratory arrest
Genitourinary	Albuminuria, increased excretion of renal tubule cells and red blood cells
Other	Fever, dehydration

OVERDOSAGE

Signs and symptoms	*In infants and small children:* agitation, headache, hyperreflexia, fasciculations, clonic and tonic convulsions; *in adults:* nervousness, insomnia, nausea, vomiting, tachycardia, extrasystoles
Treatment	Discontinue drug immediately. No specific treatment is available. Avoid sympathomimetics. Institute supportive treatment for hypotension, seizures, arrhythmias, and dehydration. Use of sedatives such as short-acting barbiturates will help control CNS stimulation. Restore the acid-base balance with lactate or bicarbonate. Administer oxygen and antibiotics to provide supportive treatment, as indicated.

DRUG INTERACTIONS

Ephedrine and other sympathomimetic agents	⇧ Risk of toxicity
Other xanthine derivatives	⇧ Risk of toxicity; do not administer concurrently
Propranolol	Antagonism of propranolol effect ⇩ Bronchodilation
Lithium	⇧ Lithium excretion

ALTERED LABORATORY VALUES

No clinically significant alterations in blood/serum or urinary values have been reported at therapeutic dosages

Use in children	Use in pregnancy or nursing mothers
General guidelines not established	Safe use not established during pregnancy; general guidelines not established for use in nursing mothers

MARAX (Ephedrine sulfate, theophylline, and hydroxyzine hydrochloride) Roerig

Tabs: 25 mg ephedrine sulfate, 130 mg theophylline, and 10 mg hydroxyzine hydrochloride **Syrup:** 6.25 mg ephedrine sulfate, 32.5 mg theophylline, and 2.5 mg hydroxyzine hydrochloride per 5 ml

INDICATIONS	ORAL DOSAGE
Bronchospastic disorders[1]	**Adult:** 1 tab bid to qid, allowing at least 4 h between doses **Child (2-5 yr):** 2.5-5 ml (½ to 1 tsp) tid or qid **Child (>5 yr):** ½ tab bid to qid, allowing at least 4 h between doses, or 5 ml (1 tsp) tid or qid

ADMINISTRATION/DOSAGE ADJUSTMENTS

Adults sensitive to ephedrine	Give ½ the usual adult dose
Bedtime dosage	Some patients may be adequately controlled with ½-1 tab at bedtime
Gastric irritation	Upper abdominal discomfort, nausea, and vomiting often occur when theophylline is taken on an empty stomach; advise patient to take medication after meals to minimize irritation

CONTRAINDICATIONS

Cardiovascular disease ● Hypersensitivity ● Hyperthyroidism ● Hypertension ●

WARNINGS/PRECAUTIONS

Special-risk patients	Use with caution in elderly men or in those with prostatic hypertrophy
Drowsiness	Performance of potentially hazardous activities may be impaired; caution patients
Tolerance	May occur when ephedrine is given 3 or more times daily for several weeks

ADVERSE REACTIONS

Central nervous system and neuromuscular	Excitation, tremulousness, insomnia, nervousness, vertigo, headache, drowsiness; with extremely high doses: involuntary motor activity, unsteady gait, weakness
Cardiovascular	Palpitations, tachycardia, precordial pain, arrhythmias, cardiac stimulation
Gastrointestinal	Gastric irritation, upper abdominal discomfort, nausea, vomiting
Genitourinary	Vesical sphincter spasm and resultant urinary hesitation, acute urinary retention (occasional), diuresis
Other	Sweating, warmth, dry mouth and throat

OVERDOSAGE

Signs and symptoms	See ADVERSE REACTIONS
Treatment	Discontinue medication or reduce dosage of drug; treat symptomatically

DRUG INTERACTIONS

Other xanthine derivatives	⇧ CNS stimulation and toxicity
Erythromycin, clindamycin, lincomycin, troleandomycin	⇧ Theophylline serum level and/or toxicity
Propranolol	Antagonism of propranolol effect ⇩ Bronchodilation
Lithium	⇧ Lithium excretion
Sympathomimetic agents	⇧ Sympathomimetic effects
Alcohol, tranquilizers, sedative-hypnotics, and other CNS depressants	⇧ CNS depression
MAO inhibitors	Hypertensive crisis
General anesthetics, digitalis	Cardiac arrhythmias

ALTERED LABORATORY VALUES

Blood/serum values	⇧ Glucose ⇧ Uric acid (with Bittner and colorimetric methods) ⇧ Bilirubin (with diazo tablet method)
Urinary values	⇧ Albumin ⇧ Catecholamines ⇧ 17-Hydroxycorticosteroids

Use in children	Use in pregnancy or nursing mothers
Not recommended for use in children under 2 yr of age	Contraindicated in early pregnancy; general guidelines not established for use during later pregnancy and lactation

[1]Possibly effective

MEDIHALER-ISO (Isoproterenol sulfate) Riker

Metered-dose inhaler: 0.075 mg/inhalation

INDICATIONS	ORAL DOSAGE
Bronchospasm associated with acute and chronic bronchial asthma, pulmonary emphysema, bronchitis, and bronchiectasis	**Adult:** for acute episodes, 1 inhalation to start, repeated after 2–5 min, if necessary, not to exceed 2 inhalations at any one time or 6 inhalations/h during any 24-h period; for maintenance, 1–2 inhalations 4–6 times/day

CONTRAINDICATIONS

Pre-existing cardiac arrhythmias associated with tachycardia

WARNINGS/PRECAUTIONS

Excessive use	May lead to loss of effectiveness; discontinue medication immediately if severe paradoxical airway resistance develops and institute alternative therapy; cardiac arrest and death have also occurred
Special-risk patients	Use with great caution in patients with cardiovascular disorders (including coronary insufficiency and hypertension), hyperthyroidism, diabetes, or sensitivity to sympathomimetic amines
Concurrent use of epinephrine	May result in serious arrhythmias; however, if desired, both drugs may be alternated, provided that at least 4 h have elapsed between doses

ADVERSE REACTIONS

Essentially none at therapeutic dosages

OVERDOSAGE

Signs and symptoms	Tachycardia with resultant coronary insufficiency, palpitations, vertigo, nausea, tremors, headache, insomnia, central excitation, blood-pressure changes
Treatment	Discontinue medication; treat symptomatically and institute supportive measures, as required

DRUG INTERACTIONS

Epinephrine	⇧ Cardiac activity and risk of arrhythmias
Nonselective beta blockers	⇩ Bronchodilation

ALTERED LABORATORY VALUES

No clinically significant alterations in blood/serum or urinary values occur at therapeutic dosages

Use in children	Use in pregnancy or nursing mothers
General guidelines not established	Safe use not established, although there has been no evidence of teratogenicity

MUCOMYST (Acetylcysteine) Mead Johnson

Vials: 10%, 20% (4, 10, 30 ml)

INDICATIONS

Adjuvant therapy for patients with **abnormal, viscid, or inspissated mucous secretions** in such conditions as chronic and acute bronchopulmonary disease; pulmonary complications of cystic fibrosis; tracheostomy care; pulmonary complications with surgery; use during anesthesia, posttraumatic chest conditions; atelectasis due to mucous obstruction; diagnostic bronchial studies (bronchograms, bronchospirometry, bronchial wedge catheterization)

ORAL DOSAGE

Adult: when nebulized into a face mask, mouthpiece, or tracheostomy, administer 1–10 ml of 20% solution or 2–20 ml of 10% solution q2–6h (usual dose: 3–5 ml of 20% solution or 6–10 ml of 10% solution tid or qid); when nebulized into a tent or Croupette, give enough solution to maintain a very heavy mist for the desired period (up to 300 ml/treatment period); for direct instillation, 1–2 ml of 10% or 20% solution may be given as often as every hour, if needed

ADMINISTRATION/DOSAGE ADJUSTMENTS

Direct instillation — Usual dosage for patients with a tracheostomy: 1–2 ml of 10% or 20% solution q1–4h; via intratracheal catheterization: 2–5 ml of 20% solution; via percutaneous intratracheal catheterization: 1–2 ml of 20% solution or 2–4 ml of 10% solution q1–4h

Diagnostic bronchograms — Administer 1–2 ml of 20% solution or 2–4 ml of 10% solution 2–3 times by nebulization or intratracheal instillation prior to procedure

CONTRAINDICATIONS

Hypersensitivity to acetylcysteine

WARNINGS/PRECAUTIONS

Increased liquified bronchial secretions — May appear after administration; maintain open airway, by mechanical suction if necessary, if cough is inadequate

Mechanical block from foreign body or local accumulation — Clear airway by endotracheal aspiration, with or without bronchoscopy

Asthmatic patients — Monitor carefully; if bronchospasm progresses, discontinue acetylcysteine therapy immediately

Slight odor — May be observed initially, but soon becomes unnoticeable

Stickiness — May develop on the patient's face with use of a face mask; remove with water

Purple discoloration of solution — Does not significantly affect safety or mucolytic effectiveness

Drug concentration after prolonged nebulization — May be prevented by dilution with an equal volume of Sterile Water for Injection USP when ¾ of the initial volume has been nebulized

Hand bulbs — Deliver particles that are larger than optimum for inhalation therapy and at too small an output; not recommended for routine nebulization

ADVERSE REACTIONS

Gastrointestinal — Stomatitis, nausea

Bronchopulmonary — Rhinorrhea, reversible bronchospasm

OVERDOSAGE

Signs and symptoms — See ADVERSE REACTIONS

Treatment — Discontinue medication; treat symptomatically

DRUG INTERACTIONS

No clinically significant drug interactions have been observed

ALTERED LABORATORY VALUES

No clinically significant alterations in blood/serum or urinary values occur at therapeutic dosages

Use in children

General guidelines not established

Use in pregnancy or nursing mothers

General guidelines not established

QUADRINAL (Ephedrine hydrochloride, phenobarbital, theophylline calcium salicylate, and potassium iodide) Knoll

Tabs: 24 mg ephedrine hydrochloride, 24 mg phenobarbital, 130 mg theophylline calcium salicylate, and 320 mg potassium iodide
Susp: 12 mg ephedrine hydrochloride, 12 mg phenobarbital, 65 mg theophylline calcium salicylate, and 160 mg potassium iodide per 5 ml

INDICATIONS

Chronic respiratory diseases, such as bronchial asthma, chronic bronchitis, and pulmonary emphysema, in which tenacious mucus and bronchospasm are dominant symptoms

ORAL DOSAGE

Adult: 1 tab or 10 ml (2 tsp) tid or qid
Child (<6 yr): proportionately smaller dose than for older children
Child (6–12 yr): ½ tab or 5 ml (1 tsp) tid

ADMINISTRATION/DOSAGE ADJUSTMENTS

Nighttime relief	Give patients over 12 yr of age an additional 1 tab or 10 ml (2 tsp) at bedtime, if needed
Gastric irritation	May be minimized by taking medication with or after meals

CONTRAINDICATIONS

Concomitant use of other theophylline preparations

WARNINGS/PRECAUTIONS

Habit-forming	Psychic and/or physical dependence and tolerance may develop,
Hypothyroidism	May occur in some patients after prolonged use due to iodide component
Special-risk patients	Use with caution in patients sensitive to iodides, in patients receiving potassium-sparing diuretics or potassium supplements, and in patients with cardiovascular disease, hyperthyroidism, or diabetes
Gouty patients	Uricosuric action of antigout agents may be blocked; use with caution
Peptic ulcer	May be exacerbated; use with caution

ADVERSE REACTIONS

Gastrointestinal	Irritation (rare)

OVERDOSAGE

Signs and symptoms	Palpitations, tachycardia, tremulousness, flushing, anginal-type pain, nausea, dizziness, weakness, sweating, cardiac irregularities, CNS disturbances, reflex bradycardia, respiratory depression, ataxia, miosis, decreased urine formation, hypothermia, shock
Treatment	Empty stomach by gastric lavage, followed by activated charcoal. Maintain patent airway and provide assisted ventilation, as needed. Maintain body temperature.

DRUG INTERACTIONS

Other xanthine derivatives	⇧ Risk of toxicity
Lithium	⇧ Lithium excretion
Erythromycin, clindamycin, lincomycin, troleandomycin	⇧ Serum theophylline level and/or clearance
Propranolol	Antagonism of propranolol effect ⇩ Bronchodilation
Sympathomimetic agents	⇧ Sympathomimetic effect
Alcohol, tranquilizers, sedative-hypnotics, and other CNS depressants	⇧ CNS depression
MAO inhibitors	Hypertensive crisis
Probenecid, sulfinpyrazone	⇩ Uricosuric effect

ALTERED LABORATORY VALUES

Blood/serum values	⇧ Glucose ⇧ Uric acid ⇧ Bilirubin
Urinary values	⇧ Albumin ⇧ Catecholamines

Use in children

See INDICATIONS

Use in pregnancy or nursing mothers

Use with caution during pregnancy; although extremely rare, iodide-induced goiter and hypothyroidism has been reported. General guidelines not established for use in nursing mothers.

QUIBRON (Theophylline and guaifenesin) Mead Johnson

Caps: 150 mg theophylline and 90 mg guaifenesin (Quibron); 300 mg theophylline and 180 mg guaifenesin (Quibron-300)
Liq: 150 mg theophylline and 90 mg guaifenesin per 15 ml

INDICATIONS	ORAL DOSAGE
Bronchospasm associated, eg, with bronchial asthma, chronic bronchitis, and pulmonary emphysema	**Adult:** 150 mg q6h to start, followed, if tolerated, by an increase in dosage of not more than 25% every 2–3 days, up to 13 mg/kg/day or 900 mg/day, whichever is less, until desired clinical response is achieved **Child (<9 yr):** 4 mg/kg q6h to start, followed, if tolerated, by an increase in dosage of not more than 25% every 2–3 days, up to 24 mg/kg/day or 900 mg/day, whichever is less, until desired clinical reponse is achieved **Child (9–12 yr):** 4 mg/kg q6h to start, followed, if tolerated, by an increase in dosage of not more than 25% every 2–3 days, up to 20 mg/kg/day or 900 mg/day, whichever is less, until desired clinical response is achieved **Child (12–16 yr):** 150 mg q6h to start, followed, if tolerated, by an increase in dosage of not more than 25% every 2–3 days, up to 18 mg/kg/day or 900 mg/day, whichever is less, until desired clinical response is achieved

ADMINISTRATION/DOSAGE ADJUSTMENTS

Use of serum theophylline levels	Adjust dosage to maintain serum theophylline level between 10 and 20 μg/ml; levels >20 μg/ml may produce toxicity. Check serum level ~2 h after last dose; medication must have been taken at typical intervals, with no missed or added doses, for a period of 72 h prior to measurement.
Use of Quibron-300 capsules	When higher theophylline dosages are required in adults, give 1 cap q6–8h after dosage has been adjusted upward to achieve therapeutic serum levels
Gastric irritation	May be prevented by giving medication with food; although absorption may be delayed, it is still complete

CONTRAINDICATIONS

Hypersensitivity to guaifenesin, theophylline, or other xanthine derivatives

WARNINGS/PRECAUTIONS

Hepatic or renal impairment	Use with caution and at reduced dosage in patients with liver disease or renal failure, owing to increase in serum half-life of theophylline; monitoring of serum theophylline levels is advisable
Special-risk patients	Use with caution in patients with severe cardiac disease, hypertension, acute myocardial injury, congestive heart failure, cor pulmonale, severe hypoxemia, hyperthyroidism, preexisting arrhythmias, or a history of peptic ulcer, and in elderly patients (especially males) and alcoholics

ADVERSE REACTIONS

Gastrointestinal	Nausea, vomiting, epigastric pain, hematemesis, diarrhea
Central nervous system and neuromuscular	Headache, irritability, restlessness, insomnia, reflex hyperexcitability, muscle twitching, clonic and tonic generalized convulsions
Cardiovascular	Palpitations, tachycardia, extrasystoles, flushing, hypotension, circulatory failure, ventricular arrhythmias
Respiratory	Tachypnea
Genitourinary	Albuminuria, increased excretion of renal tubule cells and red blood cells, diuresis
Other	Hyperglycemia, inappropriate antidiuretic hormone secretion syndrome

OVERDOSAGE

Signs and symptoms[1]	*Cardiovascular:* precordial pain, tachycardia, ventricular and other arrhythmias, hypotension, and, in extreme cases, severe shock, cardiovascular collapse, and death. *Gastrointestinal:* abdominal pain, nausea, persistent vomiting, and hematemesis. *Central nervous system:* headache, dizziness, restlessness, irritability, tremors, hyperactivity, and agitation, followed, in severe cases, by convulsions, drowsiness, coma, and death.

[1]Serious taxicity may or may not be preceded by less-serious side effects, such as nausea, irritability, or restlessness

Table continued on following page

QUIBRON continued

OVERDOSAGE continued

Treatment	If patient is conscious and seizure has not occurred, induce emesis and administer a cathartic and activated charcoal. If patient is convulsing, establish an airway and administer oxygen and IV diazepam (0.1–0.3 mg/kg, up to 10 mg). If patient is comatose following the occurrence of seizures, intubate immediately, using an endotracheal tube with an inflated cuff, and perform gastric lavage; introduce the cathartic and activated charcoal through a large-bore gastric-lavage tube. Monitor vital signs, maintain blood pressure, and provide adequate hydration. Treat hypotension and shock by appropriate fluid relacement, avoiding the use of vasopressors, if possible. In general, the drug is metabolized sufficiently rapidly to preclude any additional benefit from dialysis; however, dialysis may be useful in the presence of congestive heart failure or hepatic dysfunction. Serial monitoring of the serum theophylline level is helpful in following the patient's course and in guiding further management.

DRUG INTERACTIONS

Other xanthine derivatives	⇧ Risk of toxicity; do not administer concurrently
Propranolol	Antagonism of propranolol effect ⇩ Bronchodilation
Lithium	⇧ Lithium excretion
Erythromycin, clindamycin, lincomycin, troleandomycin	⇧ Serum theophylline level and/or toxicity

ALTERED LABORATORY VALUES

Blood/serum values	⇧ Prothrombin activity ⇧ Coagulation factor V ⇧ Glucose ⇧ Uric acid (with Bittner and colorimetric methods) ⇧ Bilirubin (with diazo tablet method)
Urinary values	⇧ Albumin ⇧ Catecholamines ⇧ 5-HIAA (with nitrosonaphthol reagent method) ⇧ VMA (with colorimetric methods)

Use in children

See INDICATIONS

Use in pregnancy or nursing mothers

Safe use not established. Use with caution in nursing mothers.

RESPIHALER DECADRON PHOSPHATE (Dexamethasone sodium phosphate) Merck Sharp & Dohme

Metered-dose inhaler: 0.1 mg/inhalation

INDICATIONS	ORAL DOSAGE
Bronchial asthma and related corticosteroid-responsive bronchospastic states intractable to an adequate trial of conventional therapy	**Adult:** 3 inhalations tid or qid, not to exceed 3 inhalations/dose or 12 inhalations/day **Child:** 2 inhalations tid or qid, not to exceed 2 inhalations/dose or 8 inhalations/day

ADMINISTRATION/DOSAGE ADJUSTMENTS

Selection of patients	Consider use only for (1) patients not on corticosteroid therapy who have not responded adequately to other treatment and (2) patients on systemic steroid therapy in an attempt to reduce or eliminate systemic administration
Concomitant use of systemic corticosteroids	Reduce or eliminate systemic corticosteroids before reducing Respihaler dosage; to avoid withdrawal symptoms, reduce systemic steroid therapy gradually

CONTRAINDICATIONS

Persistently positive *Candida albicans* sputum cultures ●	Systemic fungal infections ●	Hypersensitivity to any component ●

WARNINGS/PRECAUTIONS

Unwarranted uses	Not recommended for the treatment of occasional, mild, isolated asthmatic attacks responsive to epinephrine, isoproterenol, aminophylline, or other drugs, or for severe status asthmaticus requiring intensive measures
Laryngeal and pharyngeal fungal infections	May occur on rare occasions; discontinue medication and institute antifungal therapy
Systemic absorption	Although low, may lead to adrenal suppression or other systemic effects
Patients subjected to unusual stress	Require increased dosage of rapidly acting corticosteroids before, during, and after emotionally or physically stressful situations
Infection	Clinical signs may be masked, new infections may appear, resistance may be decreased, and infections may be difficult to localize; false-negative results may be obtained with nitroblue-tetrazolium test for bacterial infection
Latent amebiasis	May be activated; before instituting therapy, rule out latent or active amebiasis in any patient with unexplained diarrhea or who has spent time in the tropics
Ocular damage	Prolonged use may produce posterior subcapsular cataracts and glaucoma, with possible damage to optic nerves, and may enhance development of secondary fungal or viral ocular infections
Dietary salt restriction and potassium supplementation	May be necessary to combat blood-pressure elevation, salt and water retention, and increased potassium excretion with average- and high-dose therapy
Immunization procedures	Especially against smallpox, should not be undertaken because of possible neurological complications and lack of antibody response
Latent tuberculosis or tuberculin reactivity	Observe patient closely, since reactivation of the disease may occur during prolonged therapy; employ antituberculous chemoprophylactic measures
Secondary adrenocortical insufficiency	May be minimized by gradual dosage reduction; since insufficiency may persist for months, reinstitute corticosteroid therapy in any stressful situation during this period, and administer salt and/or a mineralocorticoid concurrently to correct impaired mineralocorticoid secretion
Withdrawal symptoms	Including fever, myalgia, arthralgia, and malaise, may occur when drug is withdrawn following prolonged therapy, even in the absence of adrenal insufficiency
Hypothyroidism, hepatic cirrhosis	May enhance effects of dexamethasone
Corneal perforation	May occur in patients with ocular herpes simplex; use with caution
Special-risk patients	Use with caution in patients with nonspecific ulcerative colitis if impending perforation, abscess, or other pyogenic infection is likely, as well as in patients with diverticulitis, fresh intestinal anastomoses, active or latent peptic ulcer, renal insufficiency, hypertension, osteoporosis, or myasthenia gravis
Psychic derangements	May appear, ranging from euphoria, insomnia, mood swings, personality changes, and severe depression to frank psychotic manifestations; existing emotional instability or psychotic tendencies may be aggravated

Table continued on following page

RESPIHALER DECADRON PHOSPHATE continued

WARNINGS/PRECAUTIONS continued

Concomitant use with aspirin	Use with caution in patients with hypoprothrombinemia during therapy
Concomitant use with oral anticoagulants	Check prothrombin time frequently; anticoagulant effect may be increased or decreased
Concomitant use with potassium-depleting diuretics	Monitor serum potassium level periodically; risk of hypokalemia is increased
Fertility	Motility and number of spermatozoa may be increased or decreased

ADVERSE REACTIONS

Respiratory	Throat irritation, hoarseness, cough, laryngeal and pharyngeal fungal infections
Fluid and electrolyte disturbances	Sodium retention, fluid retention, congestive heart failure in susceptible patients, loss of potassium, hypokalemic alkalosis, hypertension
Musculoskeletal	Muscle weakness, steroid myopathy, loss of muscle mass, osteoporosis, vertebral compression fractures, aseptic necrosis of femoral and humeral heads, pathological fracture of long bones, tendon rupture
Gastrointestinal	Peptic ulcer with possible perforation and hemorrhage, pancreatitis, abdominal distention, ulcerative esophagitis, increased appetite, nausea
Dermatological	Impaired wound healing, thin fragile skin, petechiae and ecchymoses, erythema, increased sweating, suppressed reaction to skin tests, allergic dermatitis, urticaria, angioneurotic edema
Neurological	Convulsions, increased intracranial pressure with papilledema (pseudotumor cerebri), vertigo, headache
Endocrinological	Menstrual irregularities, Cushingoid state, growth suppression in children, secondary adrenocortical and pituitary unresponsiveness, decreased carbohydrate tolerance, latent diabetes mellitus, increased insulin or oral hypoglycemic requirements
Ophthalmic	Posterior subcapsular cataracts, increased intraocular pressure, glaucoma, exophthalmos
Metabolic	Negative nitrogen balance, weight gain
Other	Hypersensitivity reactions, thromboembolism, malaise

OVERDOSAGE

Signs and symptoms	See ADVERSE REACTIONS
Treatment	Discontinue medication; treat symptomatically and institute supportive measures, as required

DRUG INTERACTIONS

Insulin, oral hypoglycemics	⇩ Hypoglycemic effect
Phenytoin, phenobarbital, ephedrine, rifampin	⇧ Metabolic clearance of dexamethasone ⇩ Steroid blood level and physiological activity
Oral anticoagulants	⇧ or ⇩ Prothrombin time
Potassium-depleting diuretics	⇧ Risk of hypokalemia
Cardiac glycosides	⇧ Risk of arrhythmias or digitalis toxicity secondary to hypokalemia
Skin-test antigens	⇩ Reactivity
Immunizations	⇩ Antibody response

ALTERED LABORATORY VALUES

Blood/serum values	⇧ Glucose ⇧ Cholesterol ⇧ Sodium ⇩ Potassium ⇩ Calcium ⇩ PBI ⇩ Thyroxine (T_4) ⇩ ^{131}I thyroid uptake ⇩ Uric acid
Urinary values	⇧ Glucose ⇧ Potassium ⇧ Calcium ⇧ Uric acid ⇩ 17-Hydroxycorticosteroids (17-OHCS) ⇩ 17-Ketosteroids

Use in children

Growth and development should be carefully observed in infants and children on prolonged therapy

Use in pregnancy or nursing mothers

Safe use has not been established during pregnancy. Infants born of mothers who have received substantial doses of corticosteroids during pregnancy should be carefully observed for signs of hypoadrenalism. Corticosteroids appear in breast milk and may suppress growth, interfere with endogenous corticosteroid production, or cause other untoward effects. Patient should stop nursing if drug is prescribed.

TEDRAL-25 (Theophylline, ephedrine hydrochloride, and butabarbital) **Parke-Davis**

Tabs: 130 mg theophylline, 24 mg ephedrine hydrochloride, and 25 mg butabarbital

TEDRAL EXPECTORANT (Theophylline, ephedrine hydrochloride, phenobarbital, and guaifenesin) **Parke-Davis**

Tabs: 130 mg theophylline, 24 mg ephedrine hydrochloride, 8 mg phenobarbital, and 100 mg guaifenesin

INDICATIONS	ORAL DOSAGE
Bronchial asthma; asthmatic bronchitis and other bronchospastic disorders; occasional, seasonal, or perennial **asthma** (adjunctive therapy)	**Adult:** 1–2 Tedral tabs,10–20 ml (2–4 tsp) of the suspension, or 15–30 ml (1–2 tbsp) of the elixir q4h, or 1 Tedral SA (sustained action) tab upon arising and a 2nd tab 12 h later **Child:** 5 ml (1 tsp) of the suspension or 10 ml (2 tsp) of the elixir per 60 lb q4–6h; alternatively, children weighing >60 lb may be given ½–1 Tedral tab q4h

ADMINISTRATION/DOSAGE ADJUSTMENTS	
Excessive nervousness or apprehension, sensitivity to ephedrine	Administer 1 Tedral-25 tab q4h; child (6–12 yr): ½ tab q4h
Expectorant formulation	When both bronchodilation and expectoration are required, adults and patients over 12 yr of age may be given 1–2 tabs qid

CONTRAINDICATIONS	
Hypersensitivity to any component	Porphyria

WARNINGS/PRECAUTIONS	
Habit-forming	Psychic and/or physical dependence and tolerance may develop, especially in addiction-prone individuals
Drowsiness	Performance of potentially hazardous activities may be impaired; caution patients accordingly
Special-risk patients	Use with caution in patients with cardiovascular disease, severe hypertension, hyperthyroidism, prostatic hypertrophy, or glaucoma

ADVERSE REACTIONS	
Gastrointestinal	Mild epigastric distress
Cardiovascular	Palpitations
Central nervous system	Tremulousness, insomnia, stimulation
Genitourinary	Difficult micturition

OVERDOSAGE	
Signs and symptoms	Palpitations, tachycardia, tremulousness, flushing, anginal-type pain, nausea, dizziness, weakness, sweating, cardiac irregularities, CNS disturbances, reflex bradycardia, respiratory depression, ataxia, miosis, decreased urine formation, hypothermia, shock
Treatment	Empty stomach by gastric lavage, followed by activated charcoal. Maintain patent airway and provide assisted ventilation, as needed. Maintain body temperature. Institute supportive measures, as required.

DRUG INTERACTIONS	
Other xanthine derivatives	⇧ Risk of toxicity
Lithium	⇧ Lithium excretion
Erythromycin, clindamycin, lincomycin, troleandomycin	⇧ Serum theophylline level and/or clearance
Propranolol	⇩ Bronchodilation
Sympathomimetic agents	⇧ Sympathomimetic effect
Alcohol, tranquilizers, sedative-hypnotics, and other CNS depressants	⇧ CNS depression
MAO inhibitors	Hypertensive crisis

Table continued on following page

TEDRAL/TEDRAL-25/TEDRAL EXPECTORANT continued

ALTERED LABORATORY VALUES

Blood/serum values	⇧ Glucose ⇧ Uric acid (with Bittner and colorimetric methods) ⇧ Bilirubin (with diazo tablet method)
Urinary values	⇧ Albumin ⇧ Catecholamines

Use in children

See INDICATIONS; suspension and elixir formulations should be used with extreme caution in children under 2 yr of age. Dosage of sustained-release and expectorant formulations has not been established for children under 12 yr of age.

Use in pregnancy or nursing mothers

General guidelines not established

VANCERIL (Beclomethasone dipropionate) Schering

Metered-dose inhaler: 42 μg/inhalation

INDICATIONS	ORAL DOSAGE
Bronchial asthma requiring chronic corticosteroid therapy	**Adult:** 2 inhalations tid or qid, or up to 20 inhalations/24 h, if needed **Child (6–12 yr):** 1–2 inhalations tid or qid, or up to 10 inhalations/24 h, if needed

ADMINISTRATION/DOSAGE ADJUSTMENTS

Patients with severe asthma (adults)	Initiate therapy with 12–16 inhalations/day and adjust dosage downward according to response
Concomitant use of inhalant bronchodilators	Use of bronchodilator before inhaler administration of beclomethasone enhances penetration of beclomethasone into bronchial tree. Allow several minutes to elapse before using beclomethasone inhaler to avoid toxicity from fluorocarbon propellants in both drugs.
Patients receiving systemic corticosteroids	Initially, use inhaler concurrently with usual dosage of systemic steroid. After 1 wk, *gradually* withdraw systemic steroid by reducing daily or alternate-day dose. Depending on response, continue gradually to withdraw systemic steroid by reducing dosage every 1–2 wk. Decrements generally should not exceed 2.5 mg of prednisone or its equivalent.
Patients experiencing steroid withdrawal symptoms (eg, joint or muscle pain, lassitude, depression)	Continue use of inhaler and observe patient closely for objective signs of adrenal insufficiency (eg, hypotension, weight loss); if signs appear, increase dose of systemic steroid temporarily and taper dosage more gradually
Exacerbation of asthma	Give short course of systemic steroid therapy; taper dosage gradually as symptoms subside

CONTRAINDICATIONS

Primary treatment of status asthmaticus or other acute asthmatic episodes requiring intensive measures ●	Hypersensitivity to beclomethasone or other components ●

WARNINGS/PRECAUTIONS

Deaths due to adrenal insufficiency	Have occurred in asthmatic patients during and after transfer from systemic corticosteroids to beclomethasone inhaler therapy
Recovery of hypothalamic-pituitary-adrenal (HPA) function	Requires many months after withdrawal from systemic corticosteroids; during this HPA-suppressed period, signs and symptoms of adrenal insufficiency may appear in the presence of trauma, surgery, or infection, especially gastroenteritis
During stress or severe asthma attack	Patients withdrawn from systemic steroids should immediately resume large doses of corticosteroids; these patients should carry a warning card indicating their need of supplementary systemic steroid therapy in case of stress or severe asthma attack
Assessing risk of adrenal insufficiency	Tests of adrenocortical function should be performed periodically, including measurement of early-morning resting cortisol levels
Fungal infections *(Candida albicans, Aspergillus niger)*	Frequently occur in mouth and pharynx and occasionally in larynx; up to 75% of patients may have positive oral *Candida* cultures. Antifungal treatment and discontinuation of inhaler therapy may be necessary.
Episodes of asthma unresponsive to treatment	Patients should report immediately any such episode during treatment; systemic corticosteroid therapy may be needed
Transfer of patients from systemic corticosteroids	May unmask previously suppressed allergic conditions (eg, rhinitis, conjunctivitis, eczema)
Systemic steroid withdrawal symptoms	May occur during withdrawal from oral corticosteroid therapy (see ADMINISTRATION/DOSAGE ADJUSTMENTS)

ADVERSE REACTIONS[1]

Respiratory	Pulmonary infiltrates with eosinophilia (causal relationship not established); bronchospasm (rare)
Endocrinological	Suppression of hypothalamic-pituitary-adrenal function
Other	Hoarseness, dry mouth; rash (rare)

[1]Long-term effects in humans are unknown

Table continued on following page

VANCERIL continued

OVERDOSAGE

Signs and symptoms ——— See WARNINGS/PRECAUTIONS

Treatment ——— Discontinue medication; reinstitute systemic steroid therapy, if needed

DRUG INTERACTIONS

No clinically significant drug interactions have been observed

ALTERED LABORATORY VALUES

No clinically significant alterations in blood/serum or urinary values occur at therapeutic dosages

Use in children

See INDICATIONS; not recommended for use in children under 6 yr of age

Use in pregnancy or nursing mothers

Safe use has not been established. Glucocorticoids, including beclomethasone, are known teratogens in rodent species. Infants born to mothers who received substantial corticosteroid dosages during pregnancy should be carefully observed for hypoadrenalism. Glucocorticoids are excreted in human milk.

NOTE: Belclomethasone dipropionate also marketed as **BECLOVANT** (Glaxo).

NONPRESCRIPTION ASTHMA MEDICATIONS

Product (Manufacturer)	Ingredients	Actions
AsthmaHaler (Norcliff Thayer) Inhaler **Dosage** 1 inhalation to start, repeated after 1 min, if needed	7 mg/ml Epinephrine bitartrate	Bronchodilator
AsthmaNefrin (Norcliff Thayer) Inhaler **Dosage** 2-3 inhalations to start, repeated after 5 min, if needed. Procedure may be repeated up to a maximum of 4–6 times/day.	2.25% Racemic epinephrine hydrochloride	Bronchodilator
	0.5% Chlorobutanol	Antibacterial (preservative)
Bronkaid Mist (Winthrop) Inhaler **Dosage** 1 inhalation to start, repeated after ≥1 min, if needed. Do not repeat for at least 4 h.	0.5% Epinephrine	Bronchodilator
	0.07% Ascorbic acid	Preservative
	34% Alcohol	Vehicle
Bronkotabs (Breon) Tablets **Dosage** **Adult:** 1 tab q3–4h, 4–5 times/day **Child (under 6 yr):** as directed by physican **Child (over 6 yr):** ½ tab q3–4h, 4–5 times/day	24 mg Ephedrine sulfate	Bronchodilator and decongestant
	100 mg Theophylline	Bronchodilator
	100 mg Guaifenesin	Expectorant
	8 mg Phenobarbital	Sedative
Primatene M (Whitehall) Tablets **Dosage** **Adult:** 1–2 tabs to start, followed by 1 tab q4h, as needed, up to 6 tabs/day **Child (under 6 yr):** consult physican **Child (over 6 yr):** ½–1 tab to start, followed by ½ tab q4h, as needed up to 3 tabs/day	24 mg Ephedrine hydrochloride	Bronchodilator and decongestant
	130 mg Theophylline	Bronchodilator
	16 mg Pyrilamine maleate	Antihistamine
Primatene Mist (Whitehall) Inhaler **Dosage** 1 inhalation to start, repeated after ≥1 min, if needed. Do not repeat for at least 4 h.	0.5% Epinephrine	Bronchodilator
	Ascorbic acid	Preservative
	34% Alcohol	Vehicle
Primatene P (Whitehall) Tablets **Dosage** **Adult:** 1–2 tabs to start, and then 1 q4h, as needed, up to 6 tabs/day **Child (under 6 yr):** consult physician **Child (over 6 yr):** ½ the adult dose.	24 mg Ephedrine hydrochloride	Bronchodilator and decongestant
	130 mg Theophylline	Bronchodilator
	8 mg Phenobarbital	Sedative
Vaponefrin Solution (Fisons) Inhaler **Dosage** 2-3 inhalations to start, repeated after 5 min, if needed. Use of nebulizer 4–6 times/day is usually sufficient.	2.25% Racemic epinephrine hydrochloride	Bronchodilator
	0.5% Chlorobutanol	Antibacterial (preservative)

Table continued on following page

Product (Manufacturer)	Ingredients	Actions
Verequad Suspension (Knoll) Liquid **Dosage** **Adult:** 10 ml (2 tsp) 3–4 times/day; give additional 2 tsp at bedtime, if needed **Child (6–12 yr):** 5 ml (1 tsp) 3 times/day	12 mg Ephedrine hydrochloride per 5 ml (1 tsp)	Bronchodilator and decongestant
	65 mg Theophylline calcium salicylate per 5 ml (1 tsp)	Bronchodilator
	50 mg Guaifenesin per 5 ml (1 tsp)	Expectorant
	4 mg Phenobarbital per 5 ml (1 tsp)	Sedative
Verequad Tablets (Knoll) Tablets **Dosage** **Adult:** 1 tab 3–4 times/day; give additional tab at bedtime, if needed **Child (6–12 yr):** ½ tab 3 times/day	24 mg Ephedrine hydrochloride	Bronchodilator and decongestant
	130 mg Theophylline calcium salicylate	Bronchodilator
	100 mg Guaifenesin	Expectorant
	8 mg Phenobarbital	Sedative

Allergic Disorders

Hay fever and other allergies affecting the upper respiratory tract are by far the most common type of allergic disease. (Dermatological allergies are discussed in the section on *Dermatitis and Psoriasis,* page 1079.) Allergic rhinitis or pollinosis caused by pollens of grasses, trees, flowers, ragweed, and other plants affects some sufferers during specific seasons. For example, those afflicted during the spring are usually allergic to the tree pollens and flowers and are said to have rose fever, while hay fever sufferers are allergic to the grass and weed pollens prevalent in late summer and throughout the fall. Other people suffer from respiratory allergies throughout the year (perennial or chronic allergic rhinitis), mainly due to various inhalants, such as house dust, molds, or animal dander.

DIAGNOSIS

Most people with respiratory allergies develop them in childhood, the severity diminishing with age, although many individuals remain allergic throughout life. Allergies tend to run in families—the offspring of two allergic parents have an 80 percent chance of having allergies themselves—but most allergies are not, strictly speaking, inherited. Rather, the tendency to allergic response is genetically transmitted, and may be variably expressed in the child, depending on a host of environmental and other factors.

As allergy sufferers know, sneezing, nasal congestion, watery, itchy eyes, and dry cough follow within minutes (sometimes seconds) of exposure to the offending allergen. Discomfort can be considerable, with paroxysms—veritable volleys—of sneezing heralding the onslaught of a severe allergic attack. Almost one-third of patients with allergic rhinitis have extrinsic asthma as well, brought on by exposure to the same allergens. (See the section on *Asthma,* page 882.)

In many instances, the specific allergen or allergens can be identified simply by noting what appears to trigger an attack of sneezing and other symptoms. In other instances, however, the causes may not be readily apparent, and specific tests may be needed to confirm sensitivity to particular substances. These tests usually involve exposing (challenging) a person to specific allergens, and then noting whether they provoke a reaction. One of the most common tests is the direct skin test, in which extracts of allergens are prepared and introduced just under the skin in shallow scratches, pricks, or injections. The development of a wheal-

ANATOMY OF AN ALLERGIC REACTION

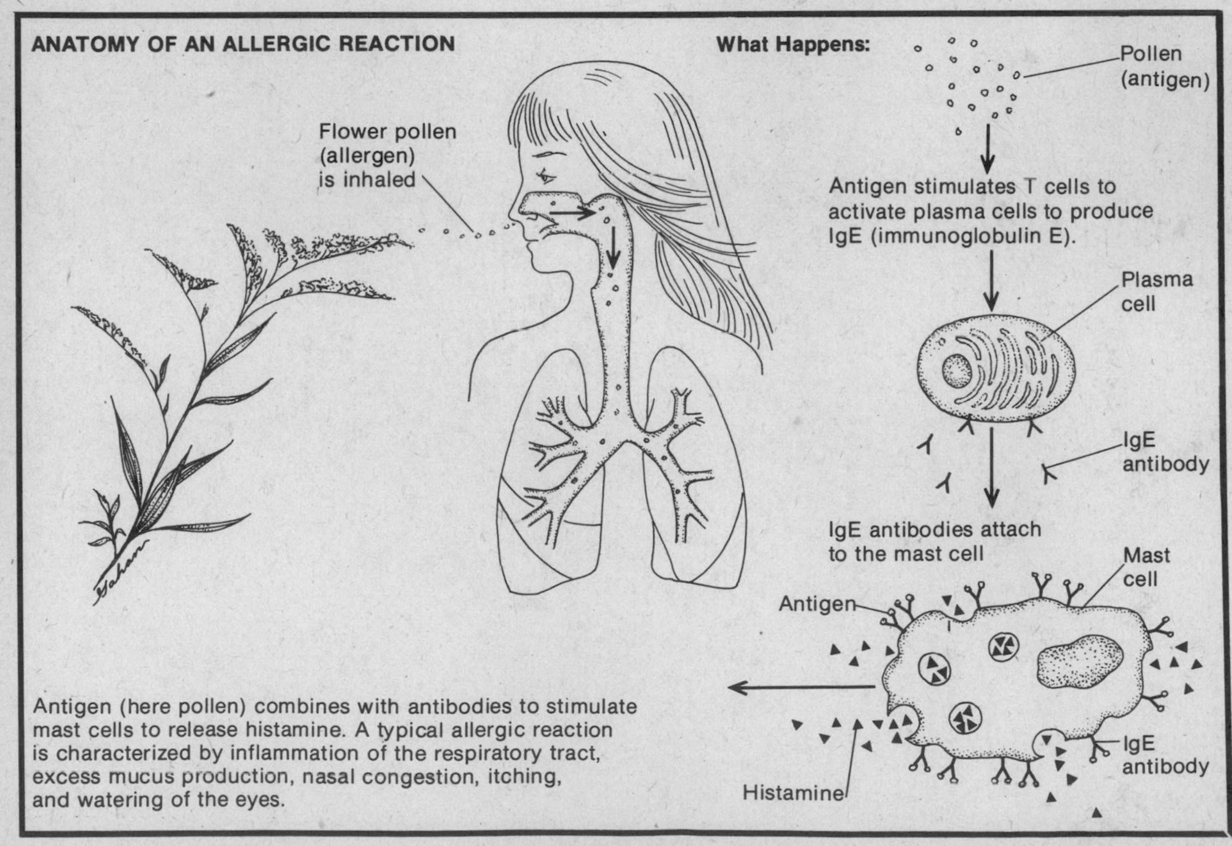

Antigen (here pollen) combines with antibodies to stimulate mast cells to release histamine. A typical allergic reaction is characterized by inflammation of the respiratory tract, excess mucus production, nasal congestion, itching, and watering of the eyes.

and-flare reaction (a reddish, burning, or itching welt) usually confirms sensitivity to the specific allergen. Blood tests may also be used to identify allergens. When food allergies are suspected, an elimination diet may be recommended in which the suspected foods are eliminated from the diet for a specific period, and then reintroduced one at a time every three to seven days to see which ones provoke an allergic reaction.

PREVENTION AND TREATMENT

Treatment

Aside from avoidance of known allergens, which is usually difficult, if not impossible, two modes of treatment are available to the allergic patient. One is immunotherapy, which involves repeated injection of known allergens to increase the patient's tolerance to these substances. This approach produces gradual relief from allergy attacks in 70 to 80 percent of patients. The second approach is to prescribe symptomatic treatment aimed at suppressing the allergic response.

The primary ingredient in almost all allergy medications is some type of antihistamine. In an allergic individual, exposure to an allergen causes histamine to be released by specialized cells in the respiratory tract (mast cells). It is the histamine release, rather than the allergen per se, that produces the swelling of mucous tissue and watery discharge typical of respiratory allergy. Antihistamine compounds block the effects of histamines in the body.

Common antihistamines found in both nonprescription and prescription products include diphenhydramine, methapyrilene, brompheniramine, tripelennamine, and chlorpheniramine. Most products (either in tablet or liquid form) are taken every four to six hours as needed, although some sustained-release preparations may be taken only once or twice daily. Many nonprescription allergy products also contain a decongestant, which helps to shrink mucous tissue and reduce discharge.

The major drawbacks to antihistamines are twofold: All agents tend to produce some degree of drowsiness, and most become less effective when taken over long periods of time. Most people also experience anticholinergic effects, such as dry mouth. Some drugs (e.g., chlorpheniramine) are reported to produce less drowsiness than others, although individual response should govern the choice of antihistamine.

In children, it should be noted, antihistamines can produce a stimulating rather than sedating effect. Children with convulsive disorders should be given antihistamines only after consultation with a physician.

Tolerance to a particular antihistamine—producing less effect at the same dosage over time—may be minimized by switching preparations periodically. Patients should *never* exceed the maximum dosages listed on the package directions.

ALLERGIC REACTIONS TO INSECT STINGS

A small minority of the general population (about 1 percent) is hypersensitive to the stings of bees, hornets, wasps, and yellow jackets (hymenopteran insects). Whereas, in most people, a sting by a hymenopteran insect produces pain, localized redness, swelling, and itching, which subside in a few hours, the same occurrence in an allergic individual may be a life-threatening medical emergency. In such a case, a single sting may cause an anaphylactic reaction, producing serious generalized effects, including rash, asthma, shortness of breath, swelling of the face and throat, abdominal pain, and, if untreated, shock and death.

Prevention and Treatment

Unfortunately, a hypersensitivity reaction may occur in a person with *no* history of excessive reaction to hymenopteran venom. Once an allergic episode has occurred, there are two measures—aside from avoidance of insects—for protection against similar future events.

Immunotherapy As with other forms of allergy (asthma, hay fever), severe allergic response to insect venom *may* be lessened by a course of antigen injections.

Bee sting kits Whenever there is a tangible risk of bee sting (e.g., when attending an outdoor picnic during summer), hypersensitive individuals should bring with them a sting kit, with instructions for use by the prescribing physician, that contains a premeasured syringe of epinephrine solution. Subcutaneous injection of this substance *immediately after* the sting can help stem the allergic response, giving the patient time to seek professional aid. In many patients, repeated epinephrine injections at 30-minute intervals are necessary.

Other measures include evaluation of the affected extremity and application of ice packs to reduce pain and swelling. In addition to epinephrine, the physician may administer corticosteroids.

IN CONCLUSION

Hay fever and other respiratory allergies afflict millions of Americans, but in most instances, control can be achieved through judicious use of antihistamines. In severe cases, desensitization treatments may be recommended. The following charts give information on the major prescription antihistamines, as well as prescription bee and insect sting medications. Numerous nonprescription products are also available to treat the rhinitis, congestion, and other cold-like symptoms of respiratory allergies. Representative products are included in the chart on Nonprescription Cold, Cough, and Respiratory Allergy Medications, page 992. For information on skin allergies, including nonprescription medications for bee and other insect stings, see the section on *Dermatitis and Psoriasis* (page 1079). Allergic asthma and its treatment are covered in the section on *Asthma* (page 882-915).

ANA-KIT (Epinephrine hydrochloride; chlorpheniramine maleate) **Hollister-Stier**

Kit: syringe, 1 mg/ml epinephrine hydrochloride (1 ml)[1]; tabs (chewable), 2 mg chlorpheniramine maleate; impregnated pads, 70% isopropyl alcohol; and tourniquet

INDICATIONS	ORAL DOSAGE	PARENTERAL DOSAGE
Emergency treatment of **severe systemic allergic reaction caused by the sting of bees, wasps, hornets, yellow jackets, or bumble bees** when medical attention or hospital care is not immediately available	**Adult:** 8 mg chlorpheniramine **Child (<6 yr):** 2 mg chlorpheniramine **Child (6–12 yr):** 4 mg chlorpheniramine	**Adult:** 0.3 ml epinephrine 1:1000 SC or IM, repeated in 10 min, if necessary **Child (infant to 2 yr):** 0.05–0.10 ml epinephrine 1:1000 SC or IM, repeated in 10 min, if necessary **Child (2–6 yr):** 0.15 ml epinephrine 1:1000 SC or IM, repeated in 10 min, if necessary **Child (6–12 yr):** 0.2 ml epinephrine 1:1000 SC or IM, repeated in 10 min, if necessary

ADMINISTRATION/DOSAGE ADJUSTMENTS

Instructions for use	Instruct the patient in the use of the syringe and explain use of the drugs and other components of the kit: (1) remove stinger; (2) apply tourniquet if sting is on arm or leg and tighten; (3) swab 4-inch area on upper arm or thigh with alcohol-impregnated swab; (4) remove rubber needle protector and expel air and excess epinephrine from syringe; (5) inject epinephrine (see PARENTERAL DOSAGE); (6) chew and swallow chlorpheniramine tablets (see ORAL DOSAGE); (7) apply ice packs, if available, to stung area; (8) keep warm and still; (9) prepare syringe for possible second injection (see PARENTERAL DOSAGE). Consult manufacturer's literature for further details, particularly in regard to use of specially constructed syringe.

CONTRAINDICATIONS[2]

Hypertension ●	Diabetes ●	Hyperthyroidism ●
Coronary artery disease ●		

WARNINGS/PRECAUTIONS

Intra-arterial injection of epinephrine	Is contraindicated, as marked vasoconstriction may result in gangrene
Improper storage or handling	May reduce the efficacy of this preparation or result in an ill effect following its use; caution patient to store the syringe in the box provided in a dark, cool place and not to force air out of the syringe until ready to use the epinephrine. Instruct patient also to check periodically contents of syringe; if discolored or a precipitate is present, the syringe should be discarded. Removal of the rubber protector over the needle may cause contamination of the needle and contents of the syringe.
Expiration date on syringe	Should be checked periodically; if expiration date is near, reorder new syringe and discard outdated syringe after new syringe has been received
Drowsiness	Performance of potentially hazardous activities may be impaired by chlorpheniramine; caution patients accordingly
Individuals highly sensitive to insect stings	Should keep kit readily available at all times
External cardiac massage or mouth-to-mouth breathing	Is required if breathing and/or pulse ceases

ADVERSE REACTIONS

Central nervous system	Excessive sympathetic stimulation, anxiety, tremor, headache, depression, convulsions, drowsiness, dizziness, blurred vision
Cardiovascular	Palpitation, acute hypertension, cardiac arrhythmias
Gastrointestinal	Upset, dry mouth
Other	Hematological disorders (rare)

OVERDOSAGE

Signs and symptoms	*Epinephrine-related effects:* cerebrovascular hemorrage due to sharp rise in blood pressure; pulmonary edema resulting from peripheral constriction and cardiac stimulation; *chlorpheniramine-related effects:* CNS depression, tremors, convulsions
Treatment	Counteract excessive pressor effects with rapidly acting vasodilators, such as nitrites, or alpha-adrenergic blocking agents. For acute toxic manifestations of chlorpheniramine overdosage, treat symptomatically and institute supportive measures, as required.

[1]Also contains 5 mg chlorobutanol, 8.5 mg sodium chloride, and not more than 1.5 mg sodium bisulfate per ml

[2]Relative contraindications ("probably contraindicated")

Table continued on following page

ANA-KIT continued

DRUG INTERACTIONS

With epinephrine

Sympathomimetics	⇧ Pressor effects
Beta-adrenergic blocking agents	Antagonism of cardiac and bronchodilating effects of epinephrine
Alpha-adrenergic blocking agents	Antagonism of epinephrine-induced vasoconstriction and hypertension
Ergot alkaloids	⇩ Pressor response
Cyclopropane and halogenated hydrocarbon anesthetics, digitalis glycosides, mercurial diuretics	Risk of cardiac arrhythmias
Tricyclic antidepressants, antihistamines, thyroid hormones	⇧ Heart rhythm and rate
Phenothiazines	⇧ Hypotension

With chlorpheniramine

Alcohol, tranquilizers, or other CNS depressants	⇧ CNS depression
Tricyclic antidepressants	⇧ CNS depression ⇧ Antidepressant effect
MAO inhibitors	⇧ Antimuscarinic effects

ALTERED LABORATORY VALUES

Blood serum values	⇧ Glucose (with epinephrine)

No clinically significant alterations in urinary values occur at therapeutic dosages

Use in children

See INDICATIONS

Use in pregnancy or nursing mothers

General guidelines not established

BENADRYL (Diphenhydramine hydrochloride) Parke-Davis

Caps: 25, 50 mg **Elixir:** 12.5 mg/5 ml[1] **Vials:** 10 mg/ml (10, 30 ml) **Amps:** 50 mg/ml (1 ml) **Syringe:** 50 mg/ml (1 ml)

INDICATIONS	ORAL DOSAGE	PARENTERAL DOSAGE
Seasonal and perennial **allergic rhinitis; vasomotor rhinitis; allergic conjunctivitis** due to inhalant allergens and foods; mild, uncomplicated **urticaria** and **angioedema;** and **dermatographism**	**Adult:** 50 mg or 20 ml (4 tsp) tid or qid **Child:** 5 mg/kg/day or 150 mg/m²/day, up to 300 mg/day **Child (>20 lb):** 12.5–25 mg tid or qid	—
Allergic reactions to blood or plasma and in **anaphylactic reactions,** as an adjunct to epinephrine and other standard measures after acute symptoms have been controlled	**Adult:** same as above **Child:** same as above	**Adult:** 10–50 mg IM (deeply) or IV (100 mg, if needed), up to 400 mg/day **Child:** 5 mg/kg/day or 150 mg/m²/day, up to 300 mg/day, IM (deeply) or IV, divided into 4 doses
Uncomplicated, **immediate-type allergic reactions,** when oral therapy is impossible or contraindicated	—	**Adult:** same as above **Child:** same as above
Motion sickness	**Adult:** same as above, 30 min before anticipated travel, before meals, and before bedtime **Child:** same as above, 30 min before exposure to motion, before meals, and before bedtime	**Adult:** same as above, 30 min before exposure to motion, before meals, and before bedtime **Child:** same as above, 30 min before exposure to motion, before meals, and before bedtime
Parkinsonism (including drug-induced extrapyramidal symptoms) in elderly patients unable to tolerate more potent agents, and in other age groups for mild symptoms or in combination with centrally acting anticholinergic agents	**Adult:** same as above **Child:** same as above	—
Parkinsonism (as above), when oral therapy is impossible or contra-indicated	—	**Adult:** same as above **Child:** same as above

CONTRAINDICATIONS

Hypersensitivity	To diphenhydramine and structurally related compounds
Lower-respiratory-tract symptoms	Including asthma
Concomitant MAO-inhibitor therapy	Anticholinergic (drying) effect of diphenhydramine is intensified and prolonged

WARNINGS/PRECAUTIONS

Drowsiness, disturbed coordination	Performance of potentially hazardous activities may be impaired; caution patients accordingly
Elderly patients	Dizziness, sedation, and hypotension occur more frequently in patients over 60 yr of age
Atropine-like, anticholinergic activity	Use with caution in patients with a history of bronchial asthma, increased intraocular pressure, hyperthyroidism, cardiovascular disease, or hypertension
Special-risk patients	Use with caution in patients with narrow-angle glaucoma, stenosing peptic ulcer, pyloroduodenal obstruction, symptomatic prostatic hypertrophy, or bladder-neck obstruction

ADVERSE REACTIONS

Frequent reactions are italicized

Cardiovascular	Hypotension, headache, palpitations, tachycardia, extrasystoles
Hematological	Hemolytic anemia, thrombocytopenia, agranulocytosis

[1]Contains 14% alcohol

Table continued on following page

ADVERSE REACTIONS continued

Central nervous system	*Sedation, sleepiness, dizziness, disturbed coordination,* fatigue, confusion, restlessness, excitation, nervousness, tremor, irritability, insomnia, euphoria, paresthesias, vertigo, tinnitus, acute labyrinthitis, hysteria, neuritis, convulsions
Ophthalmic	Blurred vision, diplopia
Gastrointestinal	*Epigastric distress,* anorexia, nausea, vomiting, diarrhea, constipation
Genitourinary	Urinary frequency, difficult urination, urinary retention, early menses
Respiratory	*Thickening of bronchial secretions,* tightness in the chest and wheezing, nasal stuffiness
Dermatological	Urticaria, drug rash, photosensitivity
Hypersensitivity	Anaphylactic shock
Other	Dry mouth, nose, and throat, chills, excessive perspiration

OVERDOSAGE

Signs and symptoms	Varies from CNS depression (drowsiness, sedation, diminished mental alertness, apnea, cardiovascular collapse) to CNS stimulation (insomnia, excitement, hallucinations, ataxia, incoordination, athetosis, tremors, convulsions) and may include dizziness, tinnitus, blurred vision, and hypotension; CNS stimulation, followed by postictal depression, and atropine-like symptoms (dry mouth; fixed, dilated pupils; fever; flushing; GI disturbances) are particularly likely in children
Treatment	If patient is conscious, induce emesis with syrup of ipecac, even though vomiting may have occurred spontaneously. If vomiting is unsuccessful or contraindicated, perform gastric lavage with isotonic or ½ isotonic saline solution. Remove any remaining drug in the stomach by instillation of activated charcoal. Administer a saline cathartic to rapidly dilute bowel content. Treatment is symptomatic and supportive. If breathing is significantly impaired, maintain an adequate airway and provide mechanically assisted ventilation; *do not use analeptics.* Vasopressors (eg, levarterenol) may be used for significant hypotension. Treat hyperpyrexia by sponging with tepid water or use of ice packs or a hypothermal blanket. For seizures, administer a short-acting barbiturate, diazepam, or paraldehyde.

DRUG INTERACTIONS

Alcohol, tranquilizers, sedative-hypnotics, and other CNS depressants	⇧ CNS depression
MAO inhibitors	⇧ Anticholinergic effects

ALTERED LABORATORY VALUES

No clinically significant alterations in blood/serum or urinary values occur at therapeutic dosages

Use in children

See INDICATIONS; contraindicated for use in newborn or premature infants. May produce excitation in young children. Overdosage may cause hallucinations, convulsions, or death.

Use in pregnancy or nursing mothers

Safe use has not been established during pregnancy. Contraindicated in nursing mothers due to increased risk of antihistamine side effects in newborns and infants; patient should stop nursing if drug is essential.

CHLOR-TRIMETON (Chlorpheniramine maleate) Schering

Tabs: 4 mg *OTC* **Tabs (sust rel):** 8 mg *OTC*, 12 mg **Syrup:** 2 mg/5 ml[1] *OTC* **Amps:** 10 mg/ml (1 ml)
Vial: 100 mg/ml (2 ml) for SC or IM use only

INDICATIONS	ORAL DOSAGE	PARENTERAL DOSAGE
Seasonal and perennial **allergic rhinitis; vasomotor rhinitis; allergic conjunctivitis** due to inhalant allergens and foods; mild, uncomplicated **urticaria** and **angioedema;** and **dermatographism**	**Adult:** 4 mg or 10 ml (2 tsp) q4-6h, up to 24 mg or 60 ml (12 tsp)/24 h; sust-rel tabs: 8 mg q8-12h, up to 24 mg/24 h, or 12 mg q8-10h or at bedtime **Child (2-5 yr):** 1 mg or 2.5 ml (½ tsp) q4-6h, up to 6 mg or 15 ml (3 tsp)/24 h **Child (6-11 yr):** 2 mg or 5 ml (1 tsp) q4-6h, up to 12 mg or 30 ml (6 tsp)/24 h; sust-rel tabs (6-12 yr): 8 mg at bedtime, or as needed	—
Allergic reactions to blood or plasma	**Adult:** same as above **Child (>2 yr):** same as above	**Adult:** 10-20 mg SC, IM, or IV, or up to 40 mg/24 h, if needed
In **anaphylactic reactions** as an adjunct to epinephrine and other standard measures after acute symptoms have been controlled	**Adult:** same as above **Child (>2 yr):** same as above	**Adult:** 10-20 mg IV
Uncomplicated, **immediate-type allergic reactions,** when oral therapy is impossible or contraindicated	—	**Adult:** 5-20 mg SC, IM, or IV

CONTRAINDICATIONS

Hypersensitivity	To chlorpheniramine and structurally related compounds
Lower-respiratory-tract symptoms	Including asthma
Concomitant MAO-inhibitor therapy	Anticholinergic (drying) effect of chlorpheniramine is intensified and prolonged

WARNINGS/PRECAUTIONS

Drowsiness, disturbed coordination	Performance of potentially hazardous activities may be impaired; caution patients accordingly
Elderly patients	Dizziness, sedation, and hypotension occur more frequently in patients over 60 yr of age
Atropine-like, anticholinergic activity	Use with caution in patients with history of bronchial asthma, increased intraocular pressure, hyperthyroidism, cardiovascular disease, or hypertension
Special-risk patients	Use with caution in patients with narrow-angle glaucoma, stenosing peptic ulcer, pyloroduodenal obstruction, symptomatic prostatic hypertrophy, or bladder-neck obstruction

ADVERSE REACTIONS[2]

Cardiovascular	Hypotension, headache, palpitations, tachycardia, extrasystoles
Hematological	Hemolytic anemia, thrombocytopenia, agranulocytosis
Central nervous system	Drowsiness, sedation, dizziness, disturbed coordination, fatigue, confusion, restlessness, excitation, nervousness, tremor, irritability, insomnia, euphoria, paresthesias, vertigo, tinnitus, acute labyrinthitis, hysteria, neuritis, convulsions
Ophthalmic	Blurred vision, diplopia
Gastrointestinal	Epigastric distress, anorexia, nausea, vomiting, diarrhea, constipation
Genitourinary	Urinary frequency, difficult urination, urinary retention, early menses
Respiratory	Thickened bronchial secretions, tightness in the chest and wheezing, nasal stuffiness

[1]Contains 7% alcohol
[2]Including reactions common to antihistamines in general

Table continued on following page

CHLOR-TRIMETON continued

ADVERSE REACTIONS continued

Dermatological	Urticaria, rash, photosensitivity
Hypersensitivity	Anaphylactic shock
Other	Excessive perspiration, chills, dry mouth, nose, and throat

OVERDOSAGE

Signs and symptoms	Varies from CNS depression (drowsiness, sedation, diminished mental alertness, apnea, cardiovascular collapse) to CNS stimulation (insomnia, excitement, hallucinations, ataxia, incoordination, athetosis, tremors, convulsions) and may include dizziness, tinnitus, blurred vision, and hypotension; CNS stimulation, followed by postictal depression, and atropine-like symptoms (dry mouth; fixed, dilated pupils; fever; flushing; GI disturbances) are particularly likely in children
Treatment	If patient is conscious, induce emesis with syrup of ipecac, even though vomiting may have occurred spontaneously. If vomiting is unsuccessful or contraindicated, perform gastric lavage with isotonic or ½ isotonic saline solution. Remove any remaining drug in the stomach by instillation of activated charcoal. Administer a saline cathartic to rapidly dilute bowel content. Treatment is symptomatic and supportive. If breathing is significantly impaired, maintain an adequate airway and provide mechanically assisted ventilation; *do not use analeptics.* Vasopressors (eg, levarterenol) may be used for significant hypotension. Treat hyperpyrexia by sponging with tepid water or use of ice packs or a hypothermal blanket. For seizures, administer a short-acting barbiturate, diazepam, or paraldehyde.

DRUG INTERACTIONS

Alcohol, tranquilizers, sedative-hypnotics, and other CNS depressants	⇧ CNS depression
MAO inhibitors	⇧ Anticholinergic effects

ALTERED LABORATORY VALUES

No clinically significant alterations in blood/serum or urinary values occur at therapeutic dosages

Use in children

See INDICATIONS; contraindicated for use in newborn and premature infants. May produce excitation in young children. Overdosage may cause hallucinations, convulsions, or death.

Use in pregnancy or nursing mothers

Safe use during pregnancy has not been established. Contraindicated for use in nursing mothers due to increased risk of antihistamine side effects in newborns and infants; patient should stop nursing if drug is essential.

DIMETANE (Brompheniramine maleate) **Robins**

Tabs: 4 mg *OTC* **Tabs (sust rel):** 8, 12 mg **Elixir:** 2 mg/5 ml[1] *OTC*

DIMETANE-TEN (Brompheniramine maleate) **Robins**

Amps: 10 mg/ml (1 ml)

INDICATIONS	ORAL DOSAGE	PARENTERAL DOSAGE
Seasonal and perennial **allergic rhinitis; vasomotor rhinitis; allergic conjunctivitis** due to inhalant allergens and foods; mild, uncomplicated **urticaria** and **angioedema;** and **dermatographism**	**Adult:** 4 mg or 10 ml (2 tsp) q4-6h, up to 24 mg or 60 ml (12 tsp)/24 h; sust-rel tabs: 8-12 mg q8-12h or bid **Child (2-6 yr):** 2.5 ml (½ tsp) q4-6h, up to 15 ml (3 tsp)/24 h **Child (6-12 yr):** 2 mg or 5 ml (1 tsp) q4-6h, up to 12 mg or 30 ml (6 tsp)/24 h; sust-rel tabs: 8-12 mg q12h	—
Allergic reactions to blood or plasma and in **anaphylactic reactions,** as an adjunct to epinephrine and other standard measures after acute symptoms have been controlled	**Adult:** same as above **Child (<12 yr):** same as above	**Adult:** 5-20 mg SC, IM, or IV (slowly) bid, up to 40 mg/24 h **Child (<12 yr):** 0.5 mg/kg/24 h or 15 mg/m^2/24 h SC, IM, or IV (slowly), divided into 3-4 doses
Uncomplicated, **immediate-type allergic reactions,** when oral therapy is impossible or contraindicated	—	**Adult:** same as above **Child: (<12 yr):** same as above

CONTRAINDICATIONS

Hypersensitivity	To brompheniramine and structurally related compounds
Lower-respiratory-tract symptoms	Including asthma
Concomitant MAO-inhibitor therapy	Anticholinergic (drying) effect of brompheniramine is intensified and prolonged

WARNINGS/PRECAUTIONS

Drowsiness, disturbed coordination	Performance of potentially hazardous activities may be impaired; caution patients accordingly
Elderly patients	Dizziness, sedation, and hypotension occur more frequently in patients over 60 yr of age
Atropine-like, anticholinergic activity	Use with caution in patients with a history of bronchial asthma, increased intraocular pressure, hyperthyroidism, cardiovascular disease, or hypertension
Special-risk patients	Use with caution in patients with narrow-angle glaucoma, stenosing peptic ulcer, pyloroduodenal obstruction, symptomatic prostatic hypertrophy, or bladder-neck obstruction

ADVERSE REACTIONS
Frequent reactions are italicized

Cardiovascular	Hypotension, headache, palpitations, tachycardia, extrasystoles
Hematological	Hemolytic anemia, thrombocytopenia, agranulocytosis
Central nervous system	*Sedation, sleepiness, dizziness, disturbed coordination,* fatigue, confusion, restlessness, excitation, nervousness, tremor, irritability, insomnia, euphoria, paresthesias, vertigo, tinnitus, acute labyrinthitis, hysteria, neuritis, convulsions
Ophthalmic	Blurred vision, diplopia
Gastrointestinal	*Epigastric distress,* anorexia, nausea, vomiting, diarrhea, constipation
Genitourinary	Urinary frequency, difficult urination, urinary retention, early menses
Respiratory	*Thickening of bronchial secretions,* tightness in the chest and wheezing, nasal stuffiness

[1]Contains 3% alcohol

Table continued on following page

ADVERSE REACTIONS continued

Dermatological	Urticaria, drug rash, photosensitivity
Hypersensitivity	Anaphylactic shock
Other	Dry mouth, nose, and throat, chills, excessive perspiration

OVERDOSAGE

Signs and symptoms	Varies from CNS depression (drowsiness, sedation, diminished mental alertness, apnea, cardiovascular collapse) to CNS stimulation (insomnia, excitement, hallucinations, ataxia, incoordination, athetosis, tremors, convulsions) and may include dizziness, tinnitus, blurred vision, and hypotension; CNS stimulation, followed by postictal depression, and atropine-like symptoms (dry mouth; fixed, dilated pupils; fever; flushing; GI disturbances) are particularly likely in children
Treatment	If patient is conscious, induce emesis with syrup of ipecac, even though vomiting may have occurred spontaneously. If vomiting is unsuccessful or contraindicated, perform gastric lavage with isotonic or ½ isotonic saline solution. Remove any remaining drug in the stomach by instillation of activated charcoal. Administer a saline cathartic to rapidly dilute bowel content. Treatment is symptomatic and supportive. If breathing is significantly impaired, maintain an adequate airway and provide mechanically assisted ventilation; *do not use analeptics.* Vasopressors (eg, levarterenol) may be used for significant hypotension. Treat hyperpyrexia by sponging with tepid water or use of ice packs or a hypothermal blanket. For seizures, administer a short-acting barbiturate, diazepam, or paraldehyde.

DRUG INTERACTIONS

Alcohol, tranquilizers, sedative-hypnotics, and other CNS depressants	⇧ CNS depression
MAO inhibitors	⇧ Anticholinergic effects

ALTERED LABORATORY VALUES

No clinically significant alterations in blood/serum or urinary values occur at therapeutic dosages

Use in children

See INDICATIONS. Contraindicated in newborn or premature infants; sust-rel tabs specifically are contraindicated in children under 6 yr of age. May produce excitation in young children. Overdosage may cause hallucinations, convulsions, or death.

Use in pregnancy or nursing mothers

Safe use has not been established during pregnancy. Contraindicated in nursing mothers due to increased risk of antihistamine side effects in newborns and infants; patient should stop nursing if drug is essential.

OPTIMINE (Azatadine maleate) Schering

Tabs: 1 mg

INDICATIONS	ORAL DOSAGE
Seasonal and perennial **allergic rhinitis;** chronic **urticaria**	**Adult:** 1-2 mg bid

CONTRAINDICATIONS	
Hypersensitivity	To azatadine and structurally related compounds
Lower-respiratory-tract symptoms	Including asthma
Concomitant MAO-inhibitor therapy	Anticholinergic effect of azatadine is intensified and prolonged

WARNINGS/PRECAUTIONS	
Drowsiness, disturbed coordination	Performance of potentially hazardous activities may be impaired; caution patients accordingly
Elderly patients	Dizziness, sedation, and hypotension occur more frequently in patients over 60 yr of age
Atropine-like, anticholinergic activity	Use with caution in patients with a history of bronchial asthma, increased intraocular pressure, hyperthyroidism, cardiovascular disease, or hypertension
Special-risk patients	Use with caution in patients with narrow-angle glaucoma, stenosing peptic ulcer, pyloroduodenal obstruction, symptomatic prostatic hypertrophy, or bladder-neck obstruction

ADVERSE REACTIONS	Frequent reactions are italicized
Cardiovascular	Hypotension, headache, palpitations, tachycardia, extrasystoles
Hematological	Hemolytic anemia, thrombocytopenia, agranulocytosis
Central nervous system	*Sedation, sleepiness, dizziness, disturbed coordination,* fatigue, confusion, restlessness, excitation, nervousness, tremor, irritability, insomnia, euphoria, paresthesias, vertigo, tinnitus, acute labyrinthitis, hysteria, neuritis, convulsions
Ophthalmic	Blurred vision, diplopia
Gastrointestinal	*Epigastric distress,* anorexia, nausea, vomiting, diarrhea, constipation
Genitourinary	Urinary frequency, difficult urination, urinary retention, early menses
Respiratory	*Thickening of bronchial secretions*, tightness in the chest and wheezing, nasal stuffiness
Dermatological	Urticaria, drug rash, photosensitivity
Hypersensitivity	Anaphylactic shock
Other	Dry mouth, nose, and throat, chills, excessive perspiration

OVERDOSAGE	
Signs and symptoms	Varies from CNS depression (drowsiness, sedation, diminished mental alertness, apnea, cardiovascular collapse) to CNS stimulation (insomnia, excitement, hallucinations, ataxia, incoordination, athetosis, tremors, convulsions) and may include dizziness, tinnitus, blurred vision, and hypotension; CNS stimulation, followed by postictal depression, and atropine-like symptoms (dry mouth; fixed, dilated pupils; fever; flushing; GI disturbances) are particularly likely in children
Treatment	If patient is conscious, induce emesis with syrup of ipecac, even though vomiting may have occurred spontaneously. If vomiting is unsuccessful or contraindicated, perform gastric lavage with isotonic or ½ isotonic saline solution. Remove any remaining drug in the stomach by instillation of activated charcoal. Administer a saline cathartic to rapidly dilute bowel content. Treatment is symptomatic and supportive. If breathing is significantly impaired, maintain an adequate airway and provide mechanically assisted ventilation; *do not use analeptics.* Vasopressors (eg, levarterenol) may be used for significant hypotension. Treat hyperpyrexia by sponging with tepid water or use of ice packs or a hypothermal blanket. For seizures, administer a short-acting barbiturate, diazepam, or paraldehyde.

Table continued on following page

OPTIMINE continued

DRUG INTERACTIONS

Alcohol, tranquilizers, sedative-hypnotics, and other CNS depressants	⇧ CNS depression
MAO inhibitors	⇧ Anticholinergic effects

ALTERED LABORATORY VALUES

No clinically significant alterations in blood/serum or urinary values occur at therapeutic dosages

Use in children

Contraindicated for use in children under 12 yr of age

Use in pregnancy or nursing mothers

Safe use has not been established during pregnancy. Contraindicated for use in nursing mothers due to increased risk of antihistamine side effects in newborns and infants; patient should stop nursing if drug is essential.

PBZ (Tripelennamine) **Geigy**

Tabs: 25, 50 mg tripelennamine hydrochloride **Tabs (sust rel):** 50 mg tripelennamine hydrochloride
Elixir: 37.5 mg tripelennamine citrate (equivalent to 25 mg tripelennamine hydrochloride)/5 ml

PBZ-SR (Tripelennamine hydrochloride) **Geigy**

Tabs (sust rel): 100 mg

INDICATIONS	ORAL DOSAGE
Seasonal and perennial **allergic rhinitis; vasomotor rhinitis, allergic conjunctivitis** due to inhalant allergens and foods; mild, uncomplicated **urticaria** and **angioedema; allergic reactions to blood or plasma; dermatographism;** in **anaphylactic reactions,** as an adjunct to epinephrine and other standard measures after acute symptoms have been controlled[1]	**Adult:** 25–50 mg q4–6h, up to 600 mg/day; sust-rel tabs: 100 mg bid or q8h, if needed **Infant:** 5 mg/kg/24 h or 150 mg/m²/24 h, up to 300 mg/24 h, in 4–6 divided doses **Child:** same as infant; sust-rel tabs: 50 mg bid or q8h, if needed

CONTRAINDICATIONS

Hypersensitivity	To tripelennamine and structurally related compounds
Lower-respiratory-tract symptoms	Including asthma
Concomitant MAO-inhibitor therapy	Anticholinergic effect of tripelennamine is intensified and prolonged
Conditions aggravated by anticholinergic action of drug	Narrow-angle glaucoma, stenosing peptic ulcer, pyloroduodenal obstruction, symptomatic prostatic hypertrophy, or bladder-neck obstruction

WARNINGS/PRECAUTIONS

Drowsiness, disturbed coordination	Performance of potentially hazardous activities may be impaired; caution patients accordingly
Elderly patients	Dizziness, sedation, and hypotension occur more frequently in patients over 60 yr of age
Atropine-like, anticholinergic activity	Use with caution in patients with a history of bronchial asthma, increased intraocular pressure, hyperthyroidism, cardiovascular disease, or hypertension
Tartrazine sensitivity	Presence of FD&C Yellow No. 5 (tartrazine) in 25-mg tablets and 50-mg sustained release tablets may cause allergic-type reactions, including bronchial asthma, in susceptible individuals

ADVERSE REACTIONS[2]
Frequent reactions are italicized

Cardiovascular	Hypotension, palpitations, tachycardia, extrasystoles
Hematological	Leukopenia, hemolytic anemia, thrombocytopenia, agranulocytosis, aplastic anemia
Central nervous system	*Sedation, sleepiness, dizziness, disturbed coordination,* fatigue, confusion, restlessness, excitation, hysteria, nervousness, irritability, insomnia, euphoria, vertigo, tinnitus, convulsions, headache, tremor, paresthesias, acute labyrinthitis, neuritis
Ophthalmic	Blurred vision, diplopia
Gastrointestinal	*Epigastric distress,* anorexia, nausea, vomiting, diarrhea, constipation
Genitourinary	Urinary frequency, difficult urination, urinary retention, early menses
Respiratory	*Thickened bronchial secretions,* tightness in the chest and wheezing, nasal stuffiness
Dermatological	Urticaria, rash, photosensitivity
Hypersensitivity	Anaphylactic shock
Other	*Dry mouth, nose, and throat,* chills, excessive perspiration

[1]Probably effective (50-mg sust rel tabs only)
[2]Including reactions common to antihistamines in general

Table continued on following page

PBZ/PBZ-SR continued

OVERDOSAGE

Signs and symptoms	Varies from CNS depression (drowsiness, sedation, diminished mental alertness, apnea, cardiovascular collapse) to CNS stimulation (insomnia, excitement, hallucinations, ataxia, incoordination, athetosis, tremors, convulsions) and may include dizziness, tinnitus, blurred vision, and hypotension; CNS stimulation, followed by postictal depression, and atropine-like symptoms (dry mouth; fixed, dilated pupils; fever; flushing; GI disturbances) are particularly likely in children
Treatment	If patient is conscious, induce emesis with syrup of ipecac, even though vomiting may have occurred spontaneously. If vomiting is unsuccessful or contraindicated, perform gastric lavage with isotonic or ½ isotonic saline solution. Remove any remaining drug in the stomach by instillation of activated charcoal. Administer a saline cathartic to rapidly dilute bowel content. Treatment is symptomatic and supportive. If breathing is significantly impaired, maintain an adequate airway and provide mechanically assisted ventilation; *do not use analeptics.* Vasopressors (eg, levarterenol) may be used for significant hypotension. Treat hyperpyrexia by sponging with tepid water or use of ice packs or a hypothermal blanket. For seizures, administer a short-acting barbiturate, diazepam, or paraldehyde.

DRUG INTERACTIONS

Alcohol, tranquilizers, sedative-hypnotics, and other CNS depressants	⇧ CNS depression
MAO inhibitors	⇧ Anticholinergic effects

ALTERED LABORATORY VALUES

No clinically significant alterations in blood/serum or urinary values occur at therapeutic dosages

Use in children

See INDICATIONS; contraindicated for use in newborn and premature infants. May produce excitation in children. Overdosage in infants and children may cause hallucinations, convulsions, or death.

Use in pregnancy or nursing mothers

Safe use has not been established during pregnancy. Contraindicated for use in nursing mothers; increased risk of antihistamine side effects in newborns and infants; patient should stop nursing if drug is essential.

PERIACTIN (Cyproheptadine hydrochloride) **Merck Sharp & Dohme**

Tabs: 4 mg **Syrup:** 2 mg/5 ml[1]

INDICATIONS	ORAL DOSAGE
Perennial and seasonal **allergic rhinitis; vasomotor rhinitis; allergic conjunctivitis** due to inhalant allergens and foods; mild, uncomplicated **urticaria** and **angioedema; cold urticaria; dematographism; allergic reactions to blood or plasma;** and in **anaphylactic reactions,** as an adjunct to epinephrine and other standard measures after acute symptoms have been controlled	**Adult:** 4 mg or 10 ml (2 tsp) tid to start; adjust dosage according to response up to 0.5 mg/kg/day; usual dosage range: 4–20 mg/day **Child (2–6 yr):** 2 mg or 5 ml (1 tsp) bid or tid, or up to 12 mg/day, if needed **Child (7–14 yr):** 4 mg or 10 ml (2 tsp) bid or tid, or up to 16 mg/day, if needed

CONTRAINDICATIONS

Hypersensitivity	To cyproheptadine and structurally related compounds
Lower-respiratory-tract symptoms	Including asthma
Concomitant MAO-inhibitor therapy	Anticholinergic effects are prolonged and intensified
Conditions aggravated by anticholinergic action of drug	Narrow-angle glaucoma, stenosing peptic ulcer, symptomatic prostatic hypertrophy, bladder neck obstruction, or pyloroduodenal obstruction
Elderly, debilitated patients	Dizziness, sedation, and hypotension occur more frequently

WARNINGS/PRECAUTIONS

Drowsiness, disturbed coordination	Performance of potentially hazardous activities may be impaired; caution patients accordingly
Atropine-like effect, anticholinergic activity	Use with caution in patients with a history of bronchial asthma, increased intraocular pressure, hyperthyroidism, cardiovascular disease, or hypertension

ADVERSE REACTIONS[2]
Frequent reactions are italicized

Cardiovascular	Faintness, hypotension, headache, palpitations, tachycardia, extrasystoles
Hematological	Hemolytic anemia, leukopenia, thrombocytopenia, agranulocytosis
Central nervous svstem	*Sedation, sleepiness, dizziness, disturbed coordination,* fatigue, confusion restlessness, excitation, nervousness, tremor, irritability, insomnia, euphoria, paresthesias, vertigo, tinnitus, acute labyrinthitis, hysteria, neuritis, convulsions, hallucinations
Ophthalmic	Blurred vision, diplopia
Gastrointestinal	*Epigastric distress,* anorexia, nausea, vomiting, diarrhea, constipation
Genitourinary	Urinary frequency, difficult urination, urinary retention, early menses
Respiratory	*Thickened bronchial secretions,* tightness in the chest and wheezing, nasal stuffiness
Dermatological	Urticaria, rash, photosensitivity
Hypersensitivity	Anaphylactic shock
Other	*Dry mouth, nose, and throat,* chills, excessive perspiration, edema

OVERDOSAGE

Signs and symptoms	Varies from CNS depression (drowsiness, sedation, diminished mental alertness, apnea, cardiovascular collapse) to CNS stimulation (insomnia, excitement, hallucinations, ataxia, incoordination, athetosis, tremors, convulsions) and may include dizziness, tinnitus, blurred vision, and hypotension; CNS stimulation, followed by postictal depression, and atropine-like symptoms (dry mouth; fixed, dilated pupils; fever; flushing; GI disturbances) are particularly likely in children

[1]Contains 5% alcohol
[2]Including reactions common to antihistamines in general

Table continued on following page

OVERDOSAGE continued

Treatment	If patient is conscious, induce emesis with syrup of ipecac, even though vomiting may have occurred spontaneously. If vomiting is unsuccessful or contraindicated, perform gastric lavage with isotonic or ½ isotonic saline solution. Remove any remaining drug in the stomach by instillation of activated charcoal. Administer a saline cathartic to rapidly dilute bowel content. Treatment is symptomatic and supportive. If breathing is significantly impaired, maintain an adequate airway and provide mechanically assisted ventilation; *do not use analeptics.* Vasopressors (eg, levarterenol) may be used for significant hypotension. Treat hyperpyrexia by sponging with tepid water or use of ice packs or a hypothermal blanket. For seizures, administer a short-acting barbiturate, diazepam, or paraldehyde.

DRUG INTERACTIONS

Alcohol, tranquilizers, sedative-hypnotics, and other CNS depressants	⇧ CNS depression
MAO inhibitors	⇧ Anticholinergic effects

ALTERED LABORATORY VALUES

No clinically significant alterations in blood/serum or urinary values occur at therapeutic dosages

Use in children

See INDICATIONS; contraindicated for use in newborn and premature infants. May produce excitation in young children. Overdosage may cause hallucinations, CNS depression, convulsions, or death.

Use in pregnancy or nursing mothers

Safe use during pregnancy has not been established. Contraindicated for use in nursing mothers due to increased risk of antihistamine side effects in newborns and infants; patient should stop nursing if drug is essential.

PHENERGAN (Promethazine hydrochloride) Wyeth

Tabs: 12.5, 25, 50 mg **Syrup:** 6.25 mg/5 ml,[1] 25 mg/5 ml[1] **Supp:** 12.5, 25, 50 mg

INDICATIONS	ORAL DOSAGE	RECTAL DOSAGE
Seasonal and perennial **allergic rhinitis; vasomotor rhinitis; allergic conjunctivitis** due to inhalant allergens and foods; mild, uncomplicated **urticaria** and **angioedema; dermatographism;** and in **anaphylactic reactions,** as an adjunct to epinephrine and other standard measures after acute symptoms have been controlled	**Adult:** 25 mg at bedtime or 12.5 mg before meals and at bedime, if necessary **Child:** 25 mg before bedtime or 6.25–12.5 mg tid	**Adult:** 25 mg, repeated 2 h later if necessary **Child:** same as adult
Allergic reactions to blood or plasma	**Adult:** 25 mg, as needed **Child:** 25 mg, as needed	—
Nausea and vomiting associated with anesthesia and surgery	**Adult:** for treatment, 25 mg to start, followed by 12.5–25 mg q4–6h, as needed; for prophylaxis, 25 mg q4–6h **Child:** adjust dosage based on child's weight and age and on the severity of the condition	**Adult:** for treatment, 12.5–25 mg q4–6h, as needed; for prophylaxis, 25 mg q4–6h **Child:** adjust dosage based on child's weight and age and on the severity of the condition
Sedation	**Adult:** 25–50 mg at bedtime **Child:** 12.5–25 mg at bedtime	**Adult:** 25–50 mg at bedtime **Child:** 12.5–25 mg at bedtime
Preoperative medication	**Adult:** 50 mg with an equal amount of meperidine and the required amount of belladonna alkaloids **Child:** 0.5 mg/lb with an equal dose of meperidine and the appropriate dose of an atropine-like drug	**Child (<3 yr):** 25 mg **Child (3–12 yr):** 50 mg
Postoperative pain, as an adjunct to analgesia, and for **postoperative sedation**	**Adult:** 25–50 mg, as needed **Child:** 12.5–25 mg, as needed	—
Motion sickness	**Adult:** 25 mg ½–1 h before anticipated travel, repeated 8–12 h later, if necessary; then 25 mg on arising in AM and again before evening meal **Child:** 12.5–25 mg bid	**Child:** 12.5–25 mg bid

ADMINISTRATION/DOSAGE ADJUSTMENTS

Concomitant therapy — Reduce usual dose of barbiturates by at least ½ and that of narcotic analgesics, such as morphine or meperidine, by ¼ to ½ when given concomitantly with promethazine

CONTRAINDICATIONS

Hypersensitivity to hydroxyzine

WARNINGS/PRECAUTIONS

Drowsiness, dizziness — Performance of potentially hazardous activities may be impaired; caution patients accordingly

Diagnostic interference — Antiemetic effects may mask signs and symptoms of unrecognized disease

[1]Contains 1.5% alcohol

Table continued on following page

PHENERGAN continued

ADVERSE REACTIONS

Central nervous system	Paradoxical hyperexcitability and nightmares (in children receiving single doses of 75–125 mg), dizziness (rare)
Ophthalmic	Blurred vision
Hematological	Leukopenia (rare), agranulocytosis (one case)
Cardiovascular	Mild hypotension or hypertension
Hypersensitivity	Photosensitivity (extremely rare)
Other	Dry mouth, local discomfort (with rectal suppositories in the presence of abraded or denuded rectal lesions)

OVERDOSAGE

Signs and symptoms	Varies from CNS depression (drowsiness, sedation, diminished mental alertness, apnea, cardiovascular collapse) to CNS stimulation (insomnia, excitement, hallucinations, ataxia, incoordination, athetosis, tremors, convulsions) and may include dizziness, tinnitus, blurred vision, and hypotension; CNS stimulation, followed by postictal depression, and atropine-like symptoms (dry mouth; fixed, dilated pupils; fever; flushing; GI disturbances) are particularly likely in children
Treatment	If patient is conscious, induce emesis with syrup of ipecac, even though vomiting may have occurred spontaneously. If vomiting is unsuccessful or contraindicated, perform gastric lavage with isotonic or ½ isotonic saline solution. Remove any remaining drug in the stomach by instillation of activated charcoal. Administer a saline cathartic to rapidly dilute bowel content. Treatment is symptomatic and supportive. If breathing is significantly impaired, maintain an adequate airway and provide mechanically assisted ventilation; *do not use analeptics.* Vasopressors (eg, levarterenol) may be used for significant hypotension. Treat hyperpyrexia by sponging with tepid water or use of ice packs or a hypothermal blanket. For seizures, administer a short-acting barbiturate, diazepam, or paraldehyde.

DRUG INTERACTIONS

Narcotic analgesics, barbiturates, and alcohol	⇧ CNS depression

ALTERED LABORATORY VALUES

Blood/serum values	⇧ Glucose tolerance
Urinary values	False-negative and false-positive pregnancy tests

Use in children

See INDICATIONS

Use in pregnancy or nursing mothers

General guidelines not established

POLARAMINE (Dexchlorpheniramine maleate) Schering

Tabs: 2 mg **Tabs (sust rel):** 4, 6 mg **Syrup:** 2 mg/5 ml[1]

INDICATIONS	ORAL DOSAGE
Allergic conditions, including hay fever, urticaria, angioedema, vasomotor rhinitis, allergic eczema, atopic dermatitis, contact dermatitis (eg, reactions to poison ivy and poison oak), drug and serum reactions (eg, injections of allergic substances), insect bites, pruritus ani and vulvae, and nonspecific pruritus; **allergic migraine and asthma** (sometimes beneficial)	**Adult:** 1–2 mg or 5 ml (1 tsp) tid or qid; sust-rel tabs: 4–6 mg bid (in AM and at bedtime) or, if needed, 8 mg bid or 6 mg q8h **Infant:** 0.5 mg or 1.25 ml (¼ tsp) tid or qid **Child (<12 yr):** 1 mg or 2.5 ml (½ tsp) tid or qid
Prophylaxis and treatment of **allergic reactions to injected substances;** some cases of **asthma, spasmodic bronchial cough, and migraine**	**Adult:** 1–2 mg or 5 ml (1 tsp) tid or qid **Infant:** same as infant dosage above **Child (<12 yr):** same as child dosage above

CONTRAINDICATIONS

None

WARNINGS/PRECAUTIONS

Drowsiness	Performance of potentially hazardous activities may be impaired; caution patients accordingly

ADVERSE REACTIONS

Central nervous system	Drowsiness, dizziness, restlessness, weakness, headache, nervousness
Gastrointestinal	Nausea, dry mouth, anorexia, heartburn
Genitourinary	Polyuria, dysuria
Dermatological	Dermatitis (rare)
Other	Diaphoresis, diplopia

OVERDOSAGE

Signs and symptoms	Varies from CNS depression (drowsiness, sedation, diminished mental alertness, apnea, cardiovascular collapse) to CNS stimulation (insomnia, excitement, hallucinations, ataxia, incoordination, athetosis, tremors, convulsions) and may include dizziness, tinnitus, blurred vision, and hypotension; CNS stimulation, followed by postictal depression, and atropine-like symptoms (dry mouth; fixed, dilated pupils; fever; flushing; GI disturbances) are particularly likely in children
Treatment	If patient is conscious, induce emesis with syrup of ipecac, even though vomiting may have occurred spontaneously. If vomiting is unsuccessful or contraindicated, perform gastric lavage with isotonic or ½ isotonic saline solution. Remove any remaining drug in the stomach by instillation of activated charcoal. Administer a saline cathartic to rapidly dilute bowel content. Treatment is symptomatic and supportive. If breathing is significantly impaired, maintain an adequate airway and provide mechanically assisted ventilation; *do not use analeptics.* Vasopressors (eg, levarterenol) may be used for significant hypotension. Treat hyperpyrexia by sponging with tepid water or use of ice packs or a hypothermal blanket. For seizures, administer a short-acting barbiturate, diazepam, or paraldehyde.

DRUG INTERACTIONS

Alcohol, tranquilizers, sedative-hypnotics, and other CNS depressants	⇧ CNS depression
MAO inhibitors	⇧ Anticholinergic effects

ALTERED LABORATORY VALUES

No clinically significant alterations in blood/serum or urinary values occur at therapeutic dosages

Use in children	Use in pregnancy or nursing mothers
See INDICATIONS	General guidelines not established

[1]Contains 6% alcohol

TAVIST (Clemastine fumarate) Dorsey

Tabs: 2.68 mg

INDICATIONS	ORAL DOSAGE
Allergic rhinitis; mild, uncomplicated **urticaria** and **angioedema**	**Adult:** 2.68 mg qd, bid, or tid, as needed

TAVIST-1 (Clemastine fumarate) Dorsey

Tabs: 1.34 mg

INDICATIONS	ORAL DOSAGE
Allergic rhinitis	**Adult:** 1.34 mg bid to start, followed by up to 8 mg (6 tabs)/day, if needed

CONTRAINDICATIONS

Hypersensitivity	To clemastine and structurally related compounds
Lower-respiratory-tract symptoms	Including asthma
Concomitant MAO-inhibitor therapy	Anticholinergic (drying) effect of clemastine is intensified and prolonged

WARNINGS/PRECAUTIONS

Drowsiness, disturbed coordination	Performance of potentially hazardous activities may be impaired; caution patients accordingly
Elderly patients	Dizziness, sedation, and hypotension occur more frequently in patients over 60 yr of age
Atropine-like, anticholinergic activity	Use with caution in patients with a history of bronchial asthma, increased intraocular pressure, hyperthyroidism, cardiovascular disease, or hypertension
Special-risk patients	Use with caution in patients with narrow-angle glaucoma, stenosing peptic ulcer, pyloroduodenal obstruction, symptomatic prostatic hypertrophy, or bladder-neck obstruction

ADVERSE REACTIONS[1]
Frequent reactions are italicized

Cardiovascular	Hypotension, headache, palpitations, tachycardia, extrasystoles
Hematological	Hemolytic anemia, thrombocytopenia, agranulocytosis
Central nervous system	*Sedation, sleepiness, dizziness, disturbed coordination,* fatigue, confusion, restlessness, excitation, nervousness, tremor, irritability, insomnia, euphoria, paresthesias, vertigo, tinnitus, acute labyrinthitis, hysteria, neuritis, convulsions
Ophthalmic	Blurred vision, diplopia
Gastrointestinal	*Epigastric distress,* anorexia, nausea, vomiting, diarrhea, constipation
Genitourinary	Urinary frequency, difficult urination, urinary retention, early menses
Respiratory	Thickened bronchial secretions, tightness in the chest and wheezing, nasal stuffiness
Dermatological	Urticaria, rash, photosensitivity
Hypersensitivity	Anaphylactic shock
Other	Dry mouth, nose, and throat, chills, excessive perspiration

OVERDOSAGE

Signs and symptoms	Varies from CNS depression (drowsiness, sedation, diminished mental alertness, apnea, cardiovascular collapse) to CNS stimulation (insomnia, excitement, hallucinations, ataxia, incoordination, athetosis, tremors, convulsions) and may include dizziness, tinnitus, blurred vision, and hypotension; CNS stimulation, followed by postictal depression, and atropine-like symptoms (dry mouth; fixed, dilated pupils; fever; flushing; GI disturbances) are particularly likely in children

[1]Including reactions common to antihistamines in general

Table continued on following page

TAVIST/TAVIST-1 continued

OVERDOSAGE continued

Treatment	If patient is conscious, induce emesis with syrup of ipecac, even though vomiting may have occurred spontaneously. If vomiting is unsuccessful or contraindicated, perform gastric lavage with isotonic or ½ isotonic saline solution. Remove any remaining drug in the stomach by instillation of activated charcoal. Administer a saline cathartic to rapidly dilute bowel content. Treatment is symptomatic and supportive. If breathing is significantly impaired, maintain an adequate airway and provide mechanically assisted ventilation; *do not use analeptics*. Vasopressors (eg, levarterenol) may be used for significant hypotension. Treat hyperpyrexia by sponging with tepid water or use of ice packs or a hypothermal blanket. For seizures, administer a short-acting barbiturate, diazepam, or paraldehyde.

DRUG INTERACTIONS

Alcohol, tranquilizers, sedative-hypnotics, and other CNS depressants	⇧ CNS depression
MAO inhibitors	⇧ Anticholinergic effects

ALTERED LABORATORY VALUES

No clinically significant alterations in blood/serum or urinary values occur at therapeutic dosages

Use in children

Safe use not established in children under 12 yr of age

Use in pregnancy or nursing mothers

Safe use during pregnancy has not been established. Contraindicated for use in nursing mothers due to increased risk of antihistamine side effects in newborns and infants; patient should stop nursing if drug is essential.

TEMARIL (Trimeprazine tartrate) **Smith Kline & French**

Tabs: 2.5 mg **Caps (sust rel):** 5 mg **Syrup:** 2.5 mg/5 ml[1]

INDICATIONS	ORAL DOSAGE
Pruritus associated with urticaria, neurodermatitis,[2] allergic dermatitis,[2] contact dermatitis,[2] atopic dermatitis,[2] varicella,[2] and pruritus ani and vulvae[2]	**Adult:** 2.5 mg or 5 ml (1 tsp) qid; sust-rel caps: 5 mg q12h **Child (6 mo to 3 yr):** 2.5 ml (½ tsp) at bedtime or tid, if needed **Child (3-6 yr):** 2.5 mg or 5 ml (1 tsp) at bedtime or tid, if needed **Child (>6 yr):** 2.5 mg or 5 ml (1 tsp) at bedtime or tid, if needed; sust-rel caps: 5 mg qd

ADMINISTRATION/DOSAGE ADJUSTMENTS

Concomitant therapy	Reduce dose of concomitantly administered narcotics or barbiturates to ¼ or ½ the usual amount; use with extreme caution in patients receiving MAO inhibitor therapy

CONTRAINDICATIONS

Drug-induced CNS depression ●

Hypersensitivity or idiosyncracy to phenothiazines ●

Bone-marrow depression ●

Comatose states ●

WARNINGS/PRECAUTIONS

Mental impairment, reflex-slowing	Performance of potentially hazardous tasks may be impaired; caution patient accordingly and about additive effect of alcohol and other CNS depressants
Antiemetic action	May mask signs and symptoms of overdosage of other drugs or such conditions as intestinal obstruction or brain tumor
Suppression of cough reflex	May occur; use with caution in patients with acute or chronic respiratory impairment, especially children
Special-risk patients	Use with caution in patients with cardiovascular disease, hepatic impairment, or a history of ulcer disease, and with extreme caution in patients with asthmatic attacks, narrow-angle glaucoma, prostatic hypertrophy, stenosing peptic ulcer, pyloroduodenal obstruction, or bladder-neck obstruction

ADVERSE REACTIONS[3]	Frequent reactions are italicized
Central nervous system	*Drowsiness,* extrapyramidal reactions (including opisthotonos, dystonia, akathisia, dyskinesia, and parkinsonism), dizziness, headache, lassitude, tinnitus, incoordination, fatigue, euphoria, nervousness, insomnia, tremors, grand mal seizures, excitation, catatonic-like states, neuritis, hysteria, disturbing dreams/nightmares, pseudoschizophrenia
Cardiovascular	*Postural hypotension,* reflex tachycardia, bradycardia, syncope, cardiac arrest, ECG changes (including blunting of T waves and prolongation of Q-T interval)
Gastrointestinal	Anorexia, nausea, vomiting, epigastric distress, diarrhea, constipation, dry mouth
Endocrinological	Early menses, induced lactation, gynecomastia, decreased libido
Genitourinary	Urinary frequency, urinary retention, dysuria, inhibition of ejaculation
Respiratory	Thickening of bronchial secretions, tightness in the chest, wheezing, nasal stuffiness
Allergic	Urticaria, dermatitis, asthma, laryngeal edema, angioneurotic edema, photosensitivity, lupus erythematosus-like syndrome, anaphylactoid reactions
Hematological	Leukopenia, agranulocytosis, pancytopenia, hemolytic anemia, thrombocytopenic purpura
Dermatological	Erythema; pigmentation of skin, especially exposed skin (with prolonged high-dose therapy)
Ophthalmic	Diplopia; blurred vision; oculogyric crises; lenticular and corneal opacities, epithelial keratopathies, pigmentary retinopathy, and impaired vision (with prolonged high-dose therapy)
Other	Obstructive jaundice, increased appetite, weight gain, peripheral edema, stomatitis, high or prolonged glucose tolerance curves, elevated spinal-fluid proteins

OVERDOSAGE

Signs and symptoms	CNS depression, cardiovascular depression, severe hypotension, respiratory depression, unconsciousness, stimulation (especially in children and the elderly), dry mouth, fixed dilated pupils, flushing, GI disturbances
Treatment	Early gastric lavage may be useful; *do not induce emesis.* Treat extrapyramidal symptoms with antiparkinsonism drugs, barbiturates, or diphenhydramine. Avoid analeptics. Severe hypotension may be treated with levarterenol or phenylephrine; do not administer epinephrine. Institute additional symptomatic and supportive measures, including the use of oxygen and IV fluids, as indicated. Saline cathartics are useful for hastening evacuation of sustained-release pellets.

[1]Contains 5.7% alcohol
[2]Possibly effective
[3]Includes reactions common to phenothiazines in general

Table continued on following page

TEMARIL continued

DRUG INTERACTIONS

Narcotics	⇧ CNS depression and analgesia Restlessness and motor hyperactivity with excessive amounts of trimeprazine
Barbiturates, anesthetics, alcohol, and other CNS depressants	⇧ CNS depression
Epinephrine	Hypotension
Atropine	⇧ Anticholinergic effects
MAO inhibitors	⇧ Anticholinergic effects, hypertension, extrapyramidal reactions
Thiazide diuretics	⇧ Anticholinergic effects
Oral contraceptives, progesterone, reserpine, nylidrin hydrochloride	⇧ Phenothiazine activity

ALTERED LABORATORY VALUES

Blood/serum values	⇧ Cholesterol
Urinary values	⇧ Glucose False-positive tests for bilirubin and pregnancy

Use in children

See INDICATIONS; contraindicated for use in newborn or premature infants, as well as acutely ill or dehydrated children due to increased susceptibility to dystonias. May produce paradoxical excitation in children. Overdosage may cause hallucinations, convulsions, and sudden death.

Use in pregnancy or nursing mothers

Safe use not established during pregnancy. Jaundice, hyperreflexia, and prolonged extrapyramidal symptoms have occurred in infants born to mothers who received phenothiazines during pregnancy. Contraindicated for use in nursing mothers.

Common Cold and Influenza

Virtually everyone suffers an occasional cold or, less frequently, a bout of influenza. Both are viral infections of the upper airway, which includes the nose, sinuses, throat, and larynx. More than a hundred different rhinoviruses are responsible for the common cold, whose medical name is coryza or acute rhinitis. In many instances, the infection begins in or spreads to the lower airway—the trachea (windpipe) and bronchi—causing the mucus-producing cough and congestion typical of a chest cold. These viruses spread from person to person and are almost always present in the environment, but the factors that predispose an individual to contract a cold infection are not clearly understood. In contrast, influenza is caused by three major forms of myxoviruses—types A, B, and C—and the infection is spread from person to person.

THE COMMON COLD

For the vast majority of the 100 million Americans who suffer at least one cold annually, the common cold is rarely more than a nuisance. Colds may be serious, however, in children under five years old, the very old, and in patients with asthma, chronic bronchitis, or emphysema. In these individuals, the primary viral infection can give way to a secondary bacterial invasion, leading to a more serious illness requiring treatment by a physician.

A cold is easy to diagnose. After an incubation period of one to three days, a vague malaise and scratchy throat are followed by sneezing, a runny nose, feverishness, and nasal and sinus congestion. Mucous debris that accumulate in the trachea and bronchi usually produce the cough that marks the beginning of the cold's resolution. Most uncomplicated colds last a week to ten days. Although feverishness may accompany the infection, true fever (greater than 99° F when measured orally) is rare. Fever is an indication for bed rest, and, if it persists for more than a day, a physician should be consulted because it may signal the presence of a more serious infection.

Because of the anatomy of the ears and throat of children under age five, secondary bacterial infection is common. Similarly, chest congestion in patients with chronic pulmonary diseases can significantly impair breathing; cold sufferers in this group should consult a physician, especially before beginning self-medication.

Prevention and Treatment

There is no cure for the common cold, although preventive measures of varying merit abound. Adequate protection against cold, damp weather may have some usefulness. However, chilling does not bring on a cold, as is popularly assumed. Susceptibility may be enhanced by fatigue or close contact with an infected person. However, it is difficult to avoid exposure since most cold viruses are spread readily before symptoms develop. The notion that megadoses of vitamin C taken during the "cold seasons" (spring, fall, and winter) can prevent colds has not been borne out by controlled scientific studies, although there is some evidence that large doses of vitamin C taken when symptoms appear may reduce the severity and duration of the cold. Since over 100 viruses have been implicated in the disease, comprehensive vaccination or inoculation seems impossible at this time.

Most cold sufferers treat the symptoms of infection to lessen discomfort. However, aside from bed rest, mild analgesics and antipyretics (e.g., aspirin or acetaminophen) to reduce discomfort and lower fever, and increased fluid intake for patients with chest congestion, there is little to be gained by self-medication.

Cold Preparations

According to recent reports, cold sufferers spend over $700 million annually on the dozens of cough/cold preparations available in drugstores and supermarkets. These products exist in myriad dosage forms and drug combinations, and the consumer may wish to seek a pharmacist's assistance in choosing an appropriate product. For otherwise healthy individuals, cold preparations are safe *when taken according to package directions.* Warnings regarding maximum dosage and use in children, pregnant women, and patients with certain chronic diseases should always be heeded. Patients with glaucoma, hypertension, diabetes, and heart disease should always consult their physician or pharmacist before taking *any* nonprescription drug product. Caution also should be exercised by persons who are on other medications, since some of the ingredients in cold products, such as alcohol in many cough preparations and antihistamines in cold pills, may interact with other drugs. Also, antihistamines should not be mixed with alcoholic beverages, since this can result in dangerous depression of the central nervous system.

Dosage Forms and Ingredient Combinations

Depending on their purpose, cold preparations come in a variety of dosage forms, including sustained-release capsules, pills, syrups, lozenges, nasal sprays, and inhalants. Some preparations treat only one symptom, while the vast majority contain drugs with multiple effects. Since it is always unwise to take unnecessary medication, patients should choose a product judiciously, so that they treat only the symptoms they are experiencing.

Every cough/cold preparation has at least one of the following six classes of agents:

Antihistamines Commonly found in allergy medications, antihistamines help to reduce mucus production and consequent sneezing and runny nose. Antihistamines are of limited value in colds, however. They produce drowsiness in adults, making driving or operating heavy machinery dangerous. Alcohol should not be taken while using antihistamines. In children, antihistamines can produce insomnia, nervousness, and excitability, making home care even more difficult. Patients with chronic pulmonary disease should consult a physician before taking antihistamines, since these drugs may be present in medicines already being taken. In some asthma patients, antihistamines may worsen breathing ability.

Antitussives Antitussives reduce cough while sometimes producing considerable drowsiness. Both narcotic (e.g., codeine) and nonnarcotic (e.g., dextromethorpan) antitussives are available.

Decongestants The primary ingredient in nasal sprays (topical decongestants), alpha-adrenergic agonists, shrink swollen and inflamed mucous tissues that line the nose, sinuses, and throat. Excessive use of nasal sprays (for more than two or three days) can lead to "rebound" congestion, making nasal stuffiness much worse in the long run. Patients with heart disease, hypertension, or glaucoma should consult a physician before using a decongestant.

Expectorants Expectorants (e.g., guaifenesin) help to saturate and thus loosen mucus plugs in bronchi and bronchioles, facilitating a productive cough that can clear chest congestion.

Analgesics/Antipyretics Aspirin and acetaminophen are common constituents of many cold preparations. They reduce fever and diminish malaise and muscle aches that accompany colds. Patients taking anticoagulants or those with bleeding disorders should not take aspirin without consulting a physician.

Anticholinergics Anticholinergic agents (e.g., atropine) help to dry up "boggy" nasal and sinus tissue by reducing mucus secretion. They may worsen breathing ability, however, in patients with significant chest congestion. Moreover, anticholinergic agents are often contraindicated in patients with glaucoma, hypertension, heart disease, asthma, and prostatic hypertrophy.

INFLUENZA

Like the common cold, influenza (also known as flu, grippe, or grip) strikes the upper respiratory tract, producing symptoms that mimic those of a cold. Illness caused by type A virus is the most common, with acute epidemics occurring about every three years. This type of influenza virus periodically changes—with new strains emerging and the older ones disappearing—which is why new epidemics appear every few years. In addition, a marked change in the type A virus occurs about every decade, producing major worldwide outbreaks or pandemics. Recent examples include the pandemics of so-called Asian and Hong Kong flus. To a lesser extent, the B viruses also undergo change, leading

Table 1: COMMON INGREDIENTS OF COLD/COUGH MEDICATIONS

Analgesics/Antipyretics
Acetaminophen
Aspirin
Phenacetin
Salicylamide
Sodium salicylate

Anesthetics
Benzocaine
Benzyl alcohol
Phenol
Sodium phenolate

Antibacterials
Calcium-iodine complex
Cetalkonium chloride
Cetylpyridinium chloride
Hexylresorcinol
Meralein sodium
Phenol
Sodium phenolate

Anticholinergics
Atropine sulfate
Belladonna alkaloids
Homatropine methylbromide

Antihistamines
Brompheniramine maleate
Chlorcyclizine hydrochloride
Chlorpheniramine maleate
Diphenhydramine hydrochloride
Doxylamine succinate
Methapyrilene fumarate
Methapyrilene hydrochloride
Phenindamine tartrate
Pheniramine maleate
Phenyltoloxamine citrate
Phenyltoloxamine dihydrogen citrate
Pyrilamine maleate
Thenyldiamine hydrochloride
Thonzylamine hydrochloride

Antitussives
Carbetapentane citrate
Codeine phosphate
Dextromethorphan hydrobromide
Noscapine
Potassium iodide
Sodium citrate
Terpin hydrate

Decongestants
Ephedrine (various salts)
Epinephrine hydrochloride
Etafedrine hydrochloride
Levodesoxyephedrine
Methoxyphenamine hydrochloride
Naphazoline hydrochloride
Oxymetazoline hydrochloride
Phenylephrine hydrochloride
Phenylpropanolamine bitartrate
Phenylpropanolamine hydrochloride
Propylhexedrine
Pseudoephedrine hydrochloride
Tuaminoheptane sulfate
Xylometazoline hydrochloride

Expectorants
Ammonium chloride
Cephaeline hydrochloride
Citric acid
Creosote
Guaifenesin
Hydrogen iodide
Ipecac syrup
Potassium citrate
Potassium guaiacolsulfonate

to acute epidemics about every five years. Type C is an endemic virus (native to particular locales) and causes only sporadic mild respiratory illness.

Prevention and Treatment

Influenza infection is spread from person to person by inhalation of aerosolized droplets from sneezes and coughs. Following exposure, the incubation period ranges from eighteen hours to three days. The onset of active disease is characterized by cough, malaise, and a feeling of chilliness. In many patients, respiratory symptoms are accompanied by headache and generalized muscle pain. Fever, sometimes reaching 103° F, is usually present and may persist for five to seven days. A painful, hacking cough develops in many patients, along with considerable sinus and chest congestion. Complete resolution of symptoms may take as long as ten days to two weeks.

Widespread outbreaks of influenza often occur during winter, and vaccines that provide immunity to the prevailing types of viruses are sometimes given to protect persons who are at high risk of developing complications to influenza infection. Since the viruses constantly change, revaccination is needed every year or two. The very young and very old, along with patients with chronic respiratory disease or certain autoimmune diseases, are prone to develop pneumonia—either from secondary bacterial invaders or the influenza virus itself—following a serious bout with the flu. Secondary bacterial infections are treated with antibiotics.

Fever lasting more than one day is an indication to seek a physician's care. Treatment usually includes bed rest, increased fluid intake, and aspirin or acetaminophen for fever and pain. Family members should avoid close contact with the infected person, although the virus can be spread by infected individuals before symptoms are apparent.

IN CONCLUSION

Colds and influenza are among our most common viral illnesses. Most persons recover without incident, but for the very young or old or persons with chronic lung disorders or other debilitating illness, a cold or bout of flu may be a serious, even life-threatening illness.

Although there is no specific cure other than time for either the common cold or influenza, there are hundreds of medications promoted to ease their symptoms. The following charts list the ingredients and actions of these substances for the most common cold and cough medications. Information on influenza vaccines is included in the section on *Childhood and Adult Immunization* (pages 490-494).

Since hundreds of these products are available, it is impossible to include them all. By using Table 1, which lists the ingredients used in the various nonprescription cold and cough medications and their functions, and then referring to the listings in the product label, one can identify the actions of products not included in the following charts.

ACTIFED (Triprolidine hydrochloride and pseudoephedrine hydrochloride) **Burroughs Wellcome**

Tabs: 2.5 mg triprolidine hydrochloride and 60 mg pseudoephedrine hydrochloride **Syrup:** 1.25 mg triprolidine hydrochloride and 30 mg pseudoephedrine hydrochloride per 5 ml

INDICATIONS	ORAL DOSAGE
Symptomatic relief of seasonal and perennial **allergic rhinitis and vasomotor rhinitis**[1]; **cold symptoms**[2]	**Adult:** 1 tab or 10 ml (2 tsp) tid or qid **Infant (4 mo to 2 yr):** 1.25 ml (¼ tsp) tid or qid **Child (2-4 yr):** 2.5 ml (½ tsp) tid or qid **Child (4-6 yr):** 3.75 ml (¾ tsp) tid or qid **Child (6-12 yr):** ½ tab or 5 ml (1 tsp) tid or qid

CONTRAINDICATIONS

Hypersensitivity to triprolidine, chemically related antihistamines, pseudoephedrine, or other sympathomimetic amines ●	Lower respiratory disease symptoms, including asthma ●	MAO-inhibitor therapy ●

WARNINGS/PRECAUTIONS

Drowsiness	Performance of potentially hazardous activities may be impaired; caution patients accordingly
Special-risk patients	Use with caution in patients with increased intraocular pressure (narrow-angle glaucoma), stenosing peptic ulcer, pyloroduodenal obstruction, symptomatic prostatic hypertrophy, bladder-neck obstruction, hypertension, diabetes mellitus, ischemic heart disease, hyperthyroidism, or in patients with a history of bronchial asthma, increased intraocular pressure, hyperthyroidism, cardiovascular disease, or hypertension
Elderly patients	Dizziness, sedation, and hypotension are more likely to occur in patients over 60 yr of age

ADVERSE REACTIONS

	Frequent reactions are italicized
Central nervous system	*Sedation, sleepiness, dizziness, disturbed coordination,* fatigue, confusion, headache, restlessness, excitation, nervousness, tremor, irritability, insomnia, euphoria, paresthesias, blurred vision, diplopia, vertigo, tinnitus, acute labyrinthitis, hysteria, neuritis, convulsions, CNS depression, hallucinations
Cardiovascular	Hypotension, palpitations, tachycardia, extrasystoles, circulatory collapse
Hematological	Hemolytic anemia, thrombocytopenia, agranulocytosis
Gastrointestinal	*Epigastric distress,* anorexia, nausea, vomiting, diarrhea, constipation, dry mouth
Genitourinary	Urinary frequency, difficult urination, urinary retention, early menses
Respiratory	*Thickened bronchial secretions,* tightness in the chest and wheezing, nasal stuffiness, dry nose and throat
Dermatological	Urticaria, drug rash, photosensitivity
Other	Anaphylactic shock, diaphoresis, chills

OVERDOSAGE

Signs and symptoms	CNS depression or stimulation (particularly in children), atropine-like effects (dry mouth; fixed, dilated pupils; flushing; GI symptoms); *in infants, children, and elderly patients:* hallucinations, convulsions, CNS depression, death
Treatment	Empty stomach by emesis, taking precautions against aspiration. If unsuccessful, use gastric lavage. Follow with a saline cathartic. Treat hypotension by elevating feet and administering fluids IV; if necessary, administer a vasopressor. Do not use stimulants.

DRUG INTERACTIONS

Alcohol, tranquilizers, sedative-hypnotics, and other CNS depressants	⇧ CNS depression
MAO inhibitors	⇧ Sympathomimetic and anticholinergic effects
Methylodopa, mecamylamine, reserpine, *Veratrum* alkaloids	⇩ Antihypertensive effect

[1]Probably effective
[2]Lacks substantial evidence of effectiveness as a fixed combination for this indication

Table continued on following page

ACTIFED continued

ALTERED LABORATORY VALUES

No clinically significant alterations in blood/serum or urinary values occur at therapeutic dosages

Use in children

See INDICATIONS; contraindicated in newborns and premature infants. Mild stimulation is seen more often than sedation in young children.

Use in pregnancy or nursing mothers

Safe use not established during pregnancy; contraindicated for use in nursing mothers due to higher risk of antihistaminic and sympathomimetic side effects for infants in general and for newborn and premature infants in particular

Note: Actifed with codeine phosphate and guaifenesin added is marketed as **ACTIFED-C** (Burroughs Wellcome)

AMBENYL EXPECTORANT (Codeine sulfate, bromodiphenhydramine hydrochloride, diphenhydramine hydrochloride, ammonium chloride, potassium guaiacolsulfonate, and menthol) **Marion**

Liq: 10 mg codeine sulfate, 3.75 mg bromodiphenhydramine hydrochloride, 8.75 mg diphenhydramine hydrochloride, 80 mg ammonium chloride, 80 mg potassium guaiacolsulfonate, 0.5 mg menthol, and 5% alcohol per 5 ml *C-V*

INDICATIONS	ORAL DOSAGE
Cough due to colds or allergy[1]	**Adult:** 5–10 ml (1–2 tsp) q4–6h, up to 60 ml (12 tsp)/24 h **Child (2–6 yr):** 1.25–2.5 ml (¼–½ tsp) q6h **Child (6–12 yr):** 2.5–5 ml (½–1 tsp) q6h, up to 1 mg codeine sulfate/kg/24 h

CONTRAINDICATIONS

Asthmatic attack ●	Stenosing peptic ulcer ●	MAO-inhibitor therapy ●
Narrow-angle glaucoma ●	Pyloroduodenal obstruction ●	Hypersensitivity to any of the components ●
Prostatic hypertrophy ●	Bladder-neck obstruction ●	

WARNINGS/PRECAUTIONS

Habit-forming	Psychic and/or physical dependence and tolerance may develop, especially in addiction-prone individuals
Drowsiness	Performance of potentially hazardous activities may be impaired; caution patients accordingly
Special-risk patients	Use with caution in patients with a history of asthma or in those who might otherwise be adversely affected by the atropine-like action of this drug

ADVERSE REACTIONS

Central nervous system and neuromuscular	Drowsiness, confusion, nervousness, restlessness, vertigo, headache, insomnia, tingling, heaviness and weakness in hands
Gastrointestinal	Nausea, vomiting, diarrhea, constipation, dry mouth, epigastric distress
Ophthalmic	Blurred vision, diplopia
Genitourinary	Difficult urination
Respiratory	Nasal stuffiness, tightness in the chest, wheezing, thickened bronchial secretions, dry nose and throat
Dermatological	Urticaria, rash, photosensitivity
Cardiovascular	Palpitations, hypotension
Hematological	Hemolytic anemia

OVERDOSAGE

Signs and symptoms	*Toxic effects primarily attributable to codeine:* respiratory depression, somnolence, stupor, coma, skeletal-muscle flaccidity, cold and clammy skin, bradycardia, hypotension, apnea, circulatory collapse, and cardiac arrest, leading to death
Treatment	Re-establish adequate airway and institute artificial respiration. For respiratory depression, administer a narcotic antagonist (eg, naloxone) along with attempts at resuscitation. Empty stomach by emesis or gastric lavage. Employ supportive measures, as indicated.

DRUG INTERACTIONS

Alcohol, tranquilizers, sedative-hypnotics, and other CNS depressants	⇧ CNS depression

ALTERED LABORATORY VALUES

No clinically significant alterations in blood/serum or urinary values occur at therapeutic dosages

Use in children

See INDICATIONS. Contraindicated for use in children under 2 yr of age. For older children, limit total intake of codeine sulfate to 1 mg/kg/day. Overdosage or accidental ingestion of large quantities of antihistamines may produce convulsions or death, especially in infants and children.

Use in pregnancy or nursing mothers

Safe use not established; may inhibit lactation

[1]Lacks substantial evidence of effectiveness as a fixed combination for indicated use

CALCIDRINE (Codeine and calcium iodide) Abbott

Syrup: 8.4 mg codeine, 152 mg calcium iodide, and 6% alcohol per 5 ml *C-V*

INDICATIONS	ORAL DOSAGE
Cough, mucus in respiratory tract	**Adult:** 5–10 ml (1–2 tsp) q4h **Child (2–6 yr):** 2.5 ml (½ tsp) q4h **Child (6–10 yr):** 2.5–5 ml (½–1 tsp) q4h **Child (>10 yr):** same as adult

CONTRAINDICATIONS

History of iodism ●	Hypersensitivity to iodides or codeine ●

WARNINGS/PRECAUTIONS

Habit-forming	Psychic and/or physical dependence and tolerance may develop, especially in addiction-prone individuals
Long-term therapy	Evaluate periodically for possible depression of thyroid function
Severe skin eruptions	May occur with prolonged iodide administration and may be fatal

ADVERSE REACTIONS[1]

Dermatological	Acneform skin lesions, ioderma
Gastrointestinal	Nausea, vomiting, constipation, metallic taste, gastric distress
Other	Mucous-membrane irritation, salivary gland swelling

OVERDOSAGE

Signs and symptoms	*Codeine-related effects:* respiratory and CNS depression, miosis, coma, fall in blood pressure, hypothermia; *iodide-related effects:* GI irritation, angioedema with laryngeal swelling, shock
Treatment	Establish patent airway and institute artificial respiration, if needed. Empty stomach by inducing emesis or gastric lavage, followed by activated charcoal. Treat for shock. Institute general supportive measures, including replacement of fluids and electrolytes, as indicated. For respiratory depression, administer naloxone (0.4 mg, preferably IV), along with attempts at resuscitation.

DRUG INTERACTIONS

Alcohol, tranquilizers, sedative-hypnotics, and other CNS depressants	⇧ CNS depression
Lithium	⇧ Hypothyroid and goitrogenic effects

ALTERED LABORATORY VALUES

Blood/serum values	⇧ PBI ⇩ ^{131}I thyroid uptake
Urinary values	+ Occult blood (with guaiac and benzidine test methods)

Use in children

See INDICATIONS

Use in pregnancy or nursing mothers

Contraindicated for long-term use during pregnancy; maternal ingestion of large amounts of iodides is associated with development of fetal goiter and resultant acute respiratory distress in neonates. Iodine is excreted in breast milk; use with caution in nursing mothers.

[1]For other possible side effects, see codeine

DILAUDID COUGH SYRUP (Hydromorphone hydrochloride and guaifenesin) Knoll

Syrup: 1 mg hydromorphone hydrochloride, 100 mg guaifenesin, and 5% alcohol per 5 ml *C-II*

INDICATIONS	ORAL DOSAGE
Cough (nonproductive)	**Adult:** 5 ml (1 tsp) q3–4h

CONTRAINDICATIONS

Intracranial lesion associated with increased intracranial pressure ●

Depressed ventilatory function ●

Hypersensitivity to either component ●

WARNINGS/PRECAUTIONS

Habit-forming	Psychic and/or physical dependence and tolerance may develop, especially in addiction-prone individuals
Drowsiness	Performance of potentially hazardous activities may be impaired; caution patients accordingly
Respiratory depression	May occur in susceptible individuals or when excessive doses are taken
Head injury, intracranial lesion	Narcotic-induced CSF elevation may be exaggerated or clinical course may be obscured
Acute abdominal conditions	Diagnosis or clinical course may be obscured
Special-risk patients	Use with caution in elderly or debilitated patients and in patients with impaired renal or hepatic function, hypothyroidism, Addison's disease, prostatic hypertrophy, or urethral stricture
Tartrazine sensitivity	Presence of FD&C Yellow No. 5 (tartrazine) may cause allergic-type reactions, including bronchial asthma, in susceptible individuals

ADVERSE REACTIONS

Central nervous system	Dizziness, somnolence, drowsiness, mood changes, mental clouding, respiratory depression, elevated CSF pressure, anxiety, fear, dysphoria
Gastrointestinal	Nausea, vomiting, constipation, increased biliary pressure
Genitourinary	Ureteral spasm, vesical sphincter spasm, urinary retention

OVERDOSAGE

Signs and symptoms	*Toxic effects primarily attributable to hydromorphone:* respiratory depression, somnolence, stupor, coma, skeletal-muscle flaccidity, cold and clammy skin, bradycardia, hypotension, apnea, circulatory collapse, and cardiac arrest, leading to death
Treatment	Re-establish adequate airway and institute artificial respiration. For clinically significant respiratory depression, administer a narcotic antagonist (eg, naloxone) along with attempts at resuscitation. Empty stomach by emesis or gastric lavage. Employ supportive measures, as indicated.

DRUG INTERACTIONS

Alcohol, tranquilizers, sedative-hypnotics, and other CNS depressants	⇧ CNS depression

ALTERED LABORATORY VALUES

Blood/serum values	⇧ Glucose
Urinary values	⇧ 5-HIAA (colorimetric interference) ⇧ VMA (colorimetric interference)

Use in children

Safety and efficacy in children not established

Use in pregnancy or nursing mothers

Safe use not established during pregnancy. Teratogenicity has been reported in hamsters at doses 600 times the human dose. Infants born to mothers taking opioids regularly prior to delivery will be physically dependent; those born to mothers taking opioids shortly before delivery may experience respiratory depression. Because of potential for serious adverse effects in nursing infants, patient should either discontinue breast-feeding or discontinue use of the drug.

DIMETANE EXPECTORANT (Brompheniramine maleate, guaifenesin, phenylephrine hydrochloride, and phenylpropanolamine hydrochloride) Robins

Liq: 2 mg brompheniramine maleate, 100 mg guaifenesin, 5 mg phenylephrine hydrochloride, 5 mg phenylpropanolamine hydrochloride, and 3.5% alcohol per 5 ml

INDICATIONS	ORAL DOSAGE
Cough and **allergic manifestations** for which an expectorant is desirable[1]	**Adult:** 5–10 ml (1–2 tsp) qid **Child:** 2.5–5 ml (½–1 tsp) tid or qid

CONTRAINDICATIONS

Hypersensitivity to any component or related compound ●	Lower respiratory disease, including asthma ●	MAO-inhibitor therapy ●

WARNINGS/PRECAUTIONS

Sedation, sleepiness, disturbed coordination	Performance of potentially hazardous activities may be impaired; caution patients accordingly
Atropine-like activity	Use with caution in patients with a history of bronchial asthma, increased intraocular pressure, hyperthyroidism, cardiovascular disease, or hypertension
Elderly patients	Dizziness, sedation, and hypotension are more likely to occur in patients over 60 yr of age
Special-risk patients	Administer with considerable caution to patients with narrow-angle glaucoma, stenosing peptic ulcer, symptomatic prostatic hypertrophy, bladder-neck obstruction, or pyloroduodenal obstruction

ADVERSE REACTIONS

Central nervous system and neuromuscular	Sedation, drowsiness, dizziness, disturbed coordination, fatigue, confusion, restlessness, excitation, nervousness, tremor, irritability, insomnia, euphoria, paresthesias, vertigo, tinnitus, acute labyrinthitis, hysteria, neuritis, convulsions, headache
Ophthalmic	Blurred vision, diplopia
Cardiovascular	Hypotension, hypertension, palpitations, tachycardia, extrasystoles
Hematological	Hemolytic anemia, thrombocytopenia, agranulocytosis
Dermatological	Urticaria, rash, photosensitivity, diaphoresis
Gastrointestinal	Epigastric distress, dry mouth, anorexia, nausea, vomiting, diarrhea, constipation
Genitourinary	Urinary frequency and retention, difficult urination, early menses
Respiratory	Thickened bronchial secretions, tightness in the chest, wheezing, nasal stuffiness, dry nose and throat
Other	Anaphylactic shock, chills

OVERDOSAGE

Signs and symptoms	Dry mouth, fixed, dilated pupils, flushing, GI symptoms, dizziness, somnolence, hallucinations, CNS depression, stimulation, and convulsions, leading to death
Treatment	Induce vomiting with water, milk, or syrup of ipecac, taking precautions against aspiration, especially in infants and children. If vomiting is unsuccessful, empty stomach contents by gastric lavage within 3 h after ingestion and later if large amounts of milk were given beforehand. Dilute bowel contents with a saline cathartic. **Do *not* administer stimulants. Treat hypotension with vasopressors.**

[1]Lacks substantial evidence of effectiveness as a fixed combination for indicated use

Table continued on following page

DIMETANE EXPECTORANT continued

DRUG INTERACTIONS

Alcohol, sedative-hypnotics, tranquilizers, and other CNS depressants	⇧ CNS depression
MAO inhibitors	⇧ Anticholinergic effect

ALTERED LABORATORY VALUES

Urinary values	⇧ 5-HIAA (with colorimetric methods) ⇧ VMA (with colorimetric methods)

No clinically significant alterations in blood/serum values occur at therapeutic dosages

Use in children

Contraindicated for use in newborn or premature infants. Overdosage may cause hallucinations, convulsions, or death. As in adults, mental alertness may be impaired. In young children particularly, excitation may be produced.

Use in pregnancy or nursing mothers

Contraindicated during pregnancy and in nursing mothers. A high risk of adverse effects from antihistamines exists for infants generally and newborn and premature infants in particular; patient should stop nursing if drug is prescribed.

DIMETANE EXPECTORANT-DC (Codeine phosphate, brompheniramine maleate, guaifenesin, phenylephrine hydrochloride, and phenylpropanolamine hydrochloride) **Robins**

Liq: 10 mg codeine phosphate, 2 mg brompheniramine maleate, 100 mg guaifenesin, 5 mg phenylephrine hydrochloride, 5 mg phenylpropanolamine hydrochloride, and 3.5% alcohol per 5 ml *C-V*

INDICATIONS	ORAL DOSAGE
Cough and **allergic states** for which an expectorant and antitussive are desired[1]	**Adult:** 5–10 ml (1–2 tsp) qid **Child:** 2.5–5 ml (½–1 tsp) tid or qid

CONTRAINDICATIONS

Hypersensitivity to any component or to related antihistamines ●	MAO-inhibitor therapy ●	Lower respiratory-tract symptoms, including asthma ●

WARNINGS/PRECAUTIONS

Habit-forming	Psychic and/or physical dependence and tolerance may develop, especially in addiction-prone individuals
Drowsiness	Performance of potentially hazardous activities may be impaired; caution patients accordingly
Elderly patients	Dizziness, sedation, and hypotension are more likely to occur in patients over 60 yr of age
Special-risk patients	Use with caution in patients with narrow-angle glaucoma, stenosing peptic ulcer, pyloroduodenal obstruction, prostatic hypertrophy, bladder-neck obstruction, bronchial asthma, increased intraocular pressure, hyperthyroidism, cardiovascular disease, peripheral vascular disease, or hypertension

ADVERSE REACTIONS

Central nervous system and neuromuscular	Headache, sedation, sleepiness, dizziness, disturbed coordination, fatigue, confusion, restlessness, excitation, nervousness, tremor, irritability, insomnia, euphoria, paresthesias, vertigo, tinnitus, acute labyrinthitis, hysteria, neuritis, convulsions
Gastrointestinal	Dry mouth, epigastric distress, anorexia, nausea, vomiting, diarrhea, constipation
Dermatological	Urticaria, rash, photosensitivity
Cardiovascular	Hypotension, hypertension, palpitations, tachycardia, extrasystoles
Hematological	Hemolytic anemia, thrombocytopenia, agranulocytosis
Ophthalmic	Blurred vision, diplopia
Genitourinary	Urinary frequency, difficult urination, urinary retention, early menses
Respiratory	Dry nose and throat, thickened bronchial secretions, tightness in the chest and wheezing, nasal stuffiness
Other	Diaphoresis, chills, anaphylactic shock

OVERDOSAGE

Signs and symptoms	Toxic effects primarily attributable to codeine: respiratory depression, somnolence, stupor, coma, skeletal-muscle flaccidity, cold and clammy skin, bradycardia, hypotension, apnea, circulatory collapse, and cardiac arrest, leading to death; *atropine-like effects:* dry mouth, mydriasis, flushing, epigastric distress, anorexia, nausea, vomiting, diarrhea, constipation
Treatment	Re-establish adequate airway and institute artificial respiration. For respiratory depression, administer a narcotic antagonist (eg, naloxone), along with attempts at resuscitation. Induce emesis if the patient has not vomited spontaneously, or use gastric lavage within 3 h of ingestion; in addition, administer a saline cathartic, such as milk of magnesia, to dilute bowel contents. Employ supportive measures, as indicated. Treat hypotension with a vasopressor. *Do not use stimulants.*

[1]Lacks substantial evidence of effectiveness as a fixed combination for indicated use

Table continued on following page

DIMETANE EXPECTORANT-DC continued

DRUG INTERACTIONS

Alcohol, tranquilizers, sedative-hypnotics, and other CNS depressants	⇧ CNS depression
MAO inhibitors	⇧ Sympathomimetic and anticholinergic effects

ALTERED LABORATORY VALUES

Urinary values	⇧ 5-HIAA (with colorimetric methods) ⇧ VMA (with colorimetric methods)

No clinically significant alterations in blood/serum values occur at therapeutic dosages

Use in children

See INDICATIONS; contraindicated in newborn or premature infants. Antihistamines may diminish mental alertness in children and, in young children particularly, produce excitation. Overdosage may cause hallucinations, convulsions, and death.

Use in pregnancy or nursing mothers

Contraindicated both during pregnancy and in nursing mothers

DIMETAPP (Brompheniramine maleate, phenylephrine hydrochloride, and phenylpropanolamine hydrochloride) Robins

Tabs (sust rel): 12 mg brompheniramine maleate, 15 mg phenylephrine hydrochloride, and 15 mg phenylpropanolamine hydrochloride **Elixir:** 4 mg brompheniramine maleate, 5 mg phenylephrine hydrochloride, 5 mg phenylpropanolamine hydrochloride, and 2.3% alcohol per 5 ml

INDICATIONS	ORAL DOSAGE
Seasonal and perennial **allergic rhinitis and vasomotor rhinitis**[1] **Allergic manifestations** of upper-respiratory illnesses, acute sinusitis, nasal congestion, and otitis[2]	**Adult:** 1 tab q8–12h or 5–10 ml (1–2 tsp) tid or qid **Infant (1–6 mo):** 1.25 ml (¼ tsp) tid or qid **Infant (7 mo to 2 yr):** 2.5 ml (½ tsp) tid or qid **Child (2–4 yr):** 3.75 ml (¾ tsp) tid or qid **Child (4–12 yr):** 5 ml (1 tsp) tid or qid

CONTRAINDICATIONS

Hypersensitivity to chemically related antihistamines ●

Bronchial asthma ●

MAO-inhibitor therapy ●

WARNINGS/PRECAUTIONS

Drowsiness	Performance of potentially hazardous activities may be impaired; caution patients accordingly
Special-risk patients	Use with caution in patients with cardiac or peripheral vascular disease or hypertension

ADVERSE REACTIONS

Hypersensitivity	Rash, urticaria, leukopenia, agranulocytosis, thrombocytopenia
Central nervous system	Drowsiness, lassitude, giddiness, headache, faintness, dizziness, tinnitus, incoordination, depression, stimulation, irritability, excitement
Ophthalmic	Visual disturbances, mydriasis
Gastrointestinal	Dry mouth, anorexia, nausea, vomiting, diarrhea, constipation, epigastric distress
Respiratory	Tightness in the chest, thickening of bronchial secretions, mucous-membrane dryness
Cardiovascular	Palpitations, hypotension, hypertension
Genitourinary	Urinary frequency, dysuria

OVERDOSAGE

Signs and symptoms	Convulsions and death, particularly in children
Treatment	Induce emesis or use gastric lavage to empty stomach. Activated charcoal may be helpful. Treat convulsions with IV diazepam.

DRUG INTERACTIONS

Alcohol, sedatives, and other CNS depressants	⇧ CNS depression
MAO inhibitors	⇧ Sympathomimetic and anticholinergic effects

ALTERED LABORATORY VALUES

No clinically significant alterations in blood/serum or urinary values occur at therapeutic dosages

Use in children

See INDICATIONS; sustained-release tablets are contraindicated for children under 12 yr of age

Use in pregnancy or nursing mothers

Contraindicated for use during pregnancy; general guidelines not established for use in nursing mothers

[1]Elixir is classified as probably effective and sustained-release tablets as lacking substantial evidence of effectiveness as a fixed combination for this indication
[2]Both elixir and sustained-release tablets are classified as lacking substantial evidence of effectiveness as a fixed combination for this indication

EMPRAZIL (Pseudoephedrine hydrochloride, aspirin, phenacetin, and caffeine) **Burroughs Wellcome**

Tabs: 20 mg pseudoephedrine hydrochloride, 150 mg phenacetin, 200 mg aspirin, and 30 mg caffeine

INDICATIONS	ORAL DOSAGE
Symptomatic relief of **upper-respiratory-tract infections** and prevention of **secondary otitis media** or **sinusitis**	**Adult:** 1-2 tabs tid **Child (6–12 yr):** 1 tab tid

CONTRAINDICATIONS

For possible contraindications, see aspirin

WARNINGS/PRECAUTIONS[1]

Pressor effect — Use with caution in patients with hypertension

ADVERSE REACTIONS[1]

Central nervous system — Mild stimulation

OVERDOSAGE

Signs and symptoms — Hypertension, hyperventilation, CNS depression

Treatment — Induce emesis or use gastric lavage to empty stomach. Activated charcoal may be helpful. Treat symptomatically.

DRUG INTERACTIONS

Oral anticoagulants — ⇧ Risk of bleeding

ALTERED LABORATORY VALUES

No clinically significant alterations in blood/serum or urinary values occur at therapeutic dosages

Use in children	**Use in pregnancy or nursing mothers**
See INDICATIONS	General guidelines not established

[1]For other possible WARNINGS/PRECAUTIONS and ADVERSE REACTIONS, see aspirin

HYCODAN (Hydrocodone bitartrate and homatropine methylbromide) Endo

Tabs, syrup (per 5 ml): 5 mg hydrocodone bitartrate and 1.5 mg homatropine methylbromide *C-III*

INDICATIONS	ORAL DOSAGE
Cough[1]	**Adult:** 1 tab or 5 ml (1 tsp) to start, then up to 3 tabs or 15 ml (1 tbsp) after meals and at bedtime (not less than 4 h apart) **Infant (<2 yr):** ¼ tab or 1.25 ml (¼ tsp) to start, then continue same dose after meals and at bedtime (not less than 4 h apart) **Child (2-12 yr):** ½ tab or 2.5 ml (½ tsp) to start, then up to 1 tab or 5 ml (1 tsp) after meals and at bedtime (not less than 4 h apart) **Child (>12 yr):** 1 tab or 5 ml (1 tsp) to start, then up to 2 tabs or 10 ml (2 tsp) after meals and at bedtime (not less than 4 h apart)

ADMINISTRATION/DOSAGE ADJUSTMENTS

Initiating therapy — Symptomatic treatment of cough should be initiated only when the underlying cause has been identified and appropriate therapy, when available, has been provided, and when the risk of complications resulting from cough suppression is not increased

CONTRAINDICATIONS

Hypersensitivity to hydrocodone or homatropine methylbromide ●

Glaucoma ●

WARNINGS/PRECAUTIONS

Habit-forming — Psychic and/or physical dependence and tolerance to hydrocodone may develop, especially in addiction-prone individuals

Drowsiness — Performance of hazardous activites may be impaired; caution patients accordingly

ADVERSE REACTIONS

Gastrointestinal — Nausea, vomiting, constipation

Central nervous system — Sedation

OVERDOSAGE

Signs and symptoms — Respiratory depression, extreme somnolence progressing to stupor or coma, skeletal-muscle flaccidity, cold and clammy skin, occasional bradycardia and hypotension; *severe toxicity:* apnea, circulatory collapse, cardiac arrest, death; ingestion of very large amounts may result in paralytic ileus, blurred vision, dry mouth, pupillary dilatation, urinary retention, and tachycardia

Treatment — Re-establish adequate respiratory exchange. Provide a patent airway and begin assisted or controlled ventilation, if indicated. For respiratory depression, administer naloxone or another narcotic antagonist IV. Employ oxygen, IV fluids, vasopressors, and other supportive measures, as indicated, including treatment for anticholinergic drug intoxication. Gastric emptying and activated charcoal may be useful.

DRUG INTERACTIONS

Alcohol, tranquilizers, sedative-hypnotics, and other CNS depressants — ⇧ CNS depression

ALTERED LABORATORY VALUES

No clinically significant alterations in blood/serum or urinary values occur at therapeutic dosages

Use in children

See INDICATIONS

Use in pregnancy or nursing mothers

General guidelines not established

[1]Probably effective

HYCOMINE (Hydrocodone bitartrate and phenylpropanolamine hydrochloride) Endo

Syrup: 5 mg hydrocodone bitartrate and 25 mg phenylpropanolamine hydrochloride per 5 ml *C-III*

INDICATIONS	ORAL DOSAGE
Cough and **congestion** due to colds, pharyngitis, tracheitis, or bronchitis	**Adult:** 5 ml (1 tsp) after meals and at bedtime, not more than q4h or up to 30 ml (6 tsp)/24 h

ADMINISTRATION/DOSAGE ADJUSTMENTS

Initiating therapy	Symptomatic treatment of cough should be initiated only when the underlying cause has been identified and appropriate therapy, when available, has been provided, and when the risk of complications resulting from cough suppression is not increased

CONTRAINDICATIONS

MAO-inhibitor therapy	Sympathomimetic component may increase blood pressure
Hypersensitivity	To hydrocodone or phenylpropanolamine

WARNINGS/PRECAUTIONS

Habit-forming	Psychic and/or physical dependence and tolerance may develop, especially in addiction-prone individuals
Drowsiness, dizziness	Performance of potentially hazardous activities may be impaired; caution patients accordingly
Special-risk patients	Use with caution in the elderly and in patients with diabetes mellitus, hyperthyroidism, hypertension, or cardiovascular disease

ADVERSE REACTIONS

Central nervous system	Drowsiness, dizziness, nervousness
Cardiovascular	Palpitations
Gastrointestinal	Upset

OVERDOSAGE

Signs and symptoms	Toxic effects primarily attributable to hydrocodone: respiratory depression, somnolence, stupor, coma, skeletal-muscle flaccidity, cold and clammy skin, bradycardia, hypotension, apnea, circulatory collapse, and cardiac arrest, leading to death
Treatment	Re-establish adequate airway and institute artificial respiration. For respiratory depression, administer a narcotic antagonist (eg, naloxone), along with attempts at resuscitation. Empty stomach by emesis or gastric lavage. Employ supportive measures, as indicated.

DRUG INTERACTIONS

Alcohol, tranquilizers, sedative-hypnotics, and other CNS depressants	⇧ CNS depression
MAO inhibitors	⇧ Sympathomimetic effect

ALTERED LABORATORY VALUES

No clinically significant alterations in blood/serum or urinary values occur at therapeutic dosages

Use in children	Use in pregnancy or nursing mothers
General guidelines not established	General guidelines not established

HYCOMINE PEDIATRIC (Hydrocodone bitartrate and phenylpropanolamine hydrochloride) Endo

Syrup: 2.5 mg hydrocodone bitartrate and 12.5 mg phenylpropanolamine hydrochloride per 5 ml *C-III*

INDICATIONS	ORAL DOSAGE
Cough and congestion due to colds, pharyngitis, tracheitis, or bronchitis	**Child (6–12 yr):** 5 ml (1 tsp) after meals and at bedtime, not more than q4h or up to 30 ml (6 tsp)/24 h

ADMINISTRATION/DOSAGE ADJUSTMENTS

Initiating therapy — Symptomatic treatment of cough should be initiated only when the underlying cause has been identified and appropriate therapy, when available, has been provided, and when the risk of complications resulting from cough suppression is not increased

CONTRAINDICATIONS

Hypersensitivity to hydrocodone or phenylpropanolamine

WARNINGS/PRECAUTIONS

Habit-forming — Psychic and/or physical dependence and tolerance may develop, especially in addiction-prone individuals

Special-risk patients — Use with caution in patients with diabetes, hyperthyroidism, hypertension, or cardiovascular disease

Drowsiness, dizziness — Performance of potentially hazardous activities may be impaired; caution patients accordingly

ADVERSE REACTIONS

Central nervous system — Drowsiness, dizziness, nervousness

Gastrointestinal — Upset

Cardiovascular — Palpitations

OVERDOSAGE

Signs and symptoms — Toxic effects primarily attributable to hydrocodone: respiratory depression, somnolence, stupor, coma, skeletal-muscle flaccidity, cold and clammy skin, bradycardia, hypotension, apnea, circulatory collapse, and cardiac arrest, leading to death

Treatment — Re-establish adequate airway and institute artificial respiration. For respiratory depression, administer a narcotic antagonist (eg, naloxone) along with attempts at resuscitation. Empty stomach by emesis or gastric lavage. Employ supportive measures, as indicated.

DRUG INTERACTIONS

Narcotic analgesics, general anesthetics, sedative-hypnotics, and other CNS depressants — ⇧ CNS depression

MAO inhibitors — ⇧ Sympathomimetic effect

ALTERED LABORATORY VALUES

No clinically significant alterations in blood/serum or urinary values occur at therapeutic dosages

Use in children

See INDICATIONS; general guidelines not established for use in children under 6 yr of age

Use in pregnancy or nursing mothers

General guidelines not established

NALDECON (Phenylpropanolamine hydrochloride, phenylephrine hydrochloride, phenyltoloxamine citrate, and chlorpheniramine maleate) Bristol

Tabs (sust rel): 40 mg phenylpropanolamine hydrochloride, 10 mg phenylephrine hydrochloride, 15 mg phenyltoloxamine citrate, and 5 mg chlorpheniramine maleate **Syrup:** 20 mg phenylpropanolamine hydrochloride, 5 mg phenylephrine hydrochloride, 7.5 mg phenyltoloxamine citrate, and 2.5 mg chlorpheniramine maleate per 5 ml **Pediatric syrup (per 5 ml), drops (per 1 ml):** 5 mg phenylpropanolamine hydrochloride, 1.25 mg phenylephrine hydrochloride, 2.0 mg phenyltoloxamine citrate, and 0.5 mg chlorpheniramine maleate

INDICATIONS	ORAL DOSAGE
Symptomatic relief of **colds** and other **upper-respiratory-tract infections, acute and chronic sinusitis, hay fever,** and other **pollen allergies**	**Adult:** 1 tab tid or 5 ml syrup (1 tsp) q3–4h, up to 4 doses/24 h **Infant (3–6 mo):** ¼ ml drops q3–4h, up to 4 doses/24 h **Infant (6–12 mo):** ½ ml drops or 2.5 ml ped syrup (½ tsp) q3–4h, up to 4 doses/24 h **Child (1–6 yr):** 1 ml drops or 5 ml ped syrup (1 tsp) q3–4h, up to 4 doses/24 h **Child (6–12 yr):** ½ tab tid or 10 ml (2 tsp) ped syrup or 2.5 ml (½ tsp) syrup q3–4h, up to 4 doses/24 h **Child (>12 yr):** same as adult

CONTRAINDICATIONS

Hypersensitivity to any component

WARNINGS/PRECAUTIONS

Drowsiness — Performance of potentially hazardous activities may be impaired; caution patients accordingly

Special-risk patients — Use with care in patients with hypertension, heart disease, diabetes mellitus, thyroid disease, glaucoma, peripheral vascular disease, or prostatic hypertrophy

ADVERSE REACTIONS

Central nervous system — Drowsiness, anxiety

Gastrointestinal — Mild upset

OVERDOSAGE

Signs and symptoms — Hypertension, hyperventilation, CNS depression

Treatment — Induce emesis or use gastric lavage to empty stomach. Activated charcoal may be helpful. Treat symptomatically.

DRUG INTERACTIONS

Alcohol, tranquilizers, sedative-hypnotics, and other CNS depressants — ⇧ CNS depression

MAO inhibitors — ⇧ Sympathomimetic and anticholinergic effects

ALTERED LABORATORY VALUES

No clinically significant alterations in blood/serum or urinary values occur at therapeutic dosages

Use in children

See INDICATIONS

Use in pregnancy or nursing mothers

General guidelines not established

NOVAFED A (Pseudoephedrine hydrochloride and chlorpheniramine maleate) Dow

Caps (sust rel): 120 mg pseudoephedrine hydrochloride and 8 mg chlorpheniramine maleate **Liq:** 30 mg pseudoephedrine hydrochloride, 2 mg chlorpheniramine maleate, and 5% alcohol per 5 ml

INDICATIONS	ORAL DOSAGE
Symptomatic relief of **nasal and eustachian-tube congestion** associated with common colds and other acute upper-respiratory infections, sinusitis, hay fever, and other upper-respiratory allergies, acute eustachian salpingitis, aerotitis media, acute otitis media, and serous otitis media	**Adult:** 1 cap q12h or 10 ml (2 tsp) q4h, up to 4 doses/24 h **Child (<6 yr):** 2.5 ml (½ tsp) q4h, up to 4 doses/24 h **Child (6–12 yr):** 5 ml (1 tsp) q4h, up to 4 doses/24 h **Child (>12 yr):** same as adult
Symptomatic relief of **seasonal and perennial allergic rhinitis; vasomotor rhinitis; allergic conjunctivitis** due to inhalant allergens and foods; and mild, uncomplicated **allergic skin manifestations of urticaria and angioedema**	**Adult:** 1 cap q12h

CONTRAINDICATIONS

Severe hypertension ●	Narrow-angle glaucoma ●	During an asthmatic attack ●
Severe coronary-artery disease ●	Urinary retention ●	Hypersensitivity or idiosyncratic reaction to any component ●
MAO-inhibitor therapy ●	Peptic ulcer ●	

WARNINGS/PRECAUTIONS

Drowsiness	Performance of potentially hazardous activities may be impaired; caution patients accordingly
Special-risk patients	Use sparingly and with caution in patients with hypertension, diabetes mellitus, ischemic heart disease, cardiovascular disease, increased intraocular pressure, prostatic hypertrophy, hyperthyroidism, a history of bronchial asthma, or hyperreactivity to ephedrine
Elderly patients	Sympathomimetic effects are more likely to occur in patients over 60 yr of age; demonstrate safe use of short-acting form before giving sustained-release capsules

ADVERSE REACTIONS

Central nervous system	Drowsiness, sedation, headache, dizziness, fear, anxiety, tension, restlessness, nervousness, tremor, weakness, insomnia, hallucinations, convulsions, CNS depression
Ophthalmic	Blurred vision
Cardiovascular	Tachycardia, palpitations, arrhythmias, collapse with hypotension
Gastrointestinal	Dry mouth, nausea, vomiting, anorexia, heartburn
Dermatological	Pallor, dermatitis (rare)
Respiratory	Difficult breathing
Genitourinary	Dysuria, polyuria

OVERDOSAGE

Signs and symptoms	Hypertension, stimulation, depression, convulsions; *in elderly patients:* hallucinations, convulsions, CNS depression, death
Treatment	Induce emesis or use gastric lavage to empty stomach. Activated charcoal may be helpful. Institute supportive measures, as indicated. Treat symptomatically.

DRUG INTERACTIONS

Alcohol, tranquilizers, sedative-hypnotics, and other CNS depressants	⇧ CNS depression
MAO inhibitors	⇧ Sympathomimetic and anticholinergic effects
Beta-adrenergic blockers	⇧ Sympathomimetic effect
Methyldopa	⇩ Antihypertensive effect
Mecamylamine	⇩ Antihypertensive effect
Reserpine	⇩ Antihypertensive effect
Veratrum alkaloids	⇩ Antihypertensive effect

Table continued on following page

NOVAFED A continued

ALTERED LABORATORY VALUES

No clinically significant alterations in blood/serum or urinary values occur at therapeutic dosages

Use in children

See INDICATIONS; sustained-release capsules contraindicated in children under 12 yr of age

Use in pregnancy or nursing mothers

Safe use not established during pregnancy. Contraindicated in nursing mothers; patient should stop nursing if drug is prescribed

NOVAHISTINE DH (Codeine phosphate, phenylpropanolamine hydrochloride, and chlorpheniramine maleate) Dow

Liq: 10 mg codeine phosphate, 18.75 mg phenylpropanolamine hydrochloride, 2 mg chlorpheniramine maleate, and 5% alcohol per 5 ml *C-V*

INDICATIONS	ORAL DOSAGE
Cough associated with minor throat and bronchial irritation **Nasal congestion** due to colds, sinusitis, and allergic rhinitis **Acute otitis media** (adjunctive therapy) **Mild otalgia** (adjunctive therapy)	**Adult:** 10 ml (2 tsp) q4h, up to 40 ml (8 tsp)/day **Infant (<2 yr):** 3 drops/kg q4h, up to 12 drops/kg/day **Child (25-50 lb):** 1.25–2.5 ml (¼–½ tsp) q4h, up to 5–10 ml (1–2 tsp)/day **Child (50-90 lb):** 2.5–5 ml (½–1 tsp) q4h, up to 10–20 ml (2–4 tsp)/day

CONTRAINDICATIONS

Severe hypertension ●	Urinary retention ●	MAO-inhibitor therapy ●
Severe coronary-artery disease ●	Peptic ulcer ●	Hypersensitivity or idiosyncratic reactions to any of the components ●
Narrow-angle glaucoma ●	During an asthmatic attack ●	

WARNINGS/PRECAUTIONS

Habit-forming	Psychic and/or physical dependence and tolerance may develop, especially in addiction-prone individuals
Unwarranted uses	Discontinue treatment if cough persists for more than 1 wk, tends to recur, or is accompanied by fever, rash, or headache
Elderly patients	Sympathomimetic side effects are more likely to occur in patients over 60 yr of age
Drowsiness	Performance of hazardous activities may be impaired; caution patients accordingly
Special-risk patients	Use with caution in patients with hypertension, diabetes mellitus, ischemic heart disease, thyroid disease (especially hyperthyroidism), increased intraocular pressure, prostatic hypertrophy, asthma, or emphysema
Excitability	May occur, especially in children

ADVERSE REACTIONS

Gastrointestinal	Nausea, vomiting, constipation, dry mouth, heartburn
Central nervous system	Dizziness, sedation, fear, anxiety, tension, restlessness, tremor, weakness, insomnia, hallucinations, convulsions, CNS depression, anorexia, headache, nervousness
Ophthalmic	Diplopia
Dermatological	Pruritus, dermatitis
Cardiovascular	Palpitations, arrhythmias, cardiovascular collapse, pallor, hypotension, hypertension
Respiratory	Depression, difficulty
Genitourinary	Dysuria, polyuria

OVERDOSAGE

Signs and symptoms	Respiratory depression (especially in patients with respiratory disease associated with CO_2 retention), nausea, vomiting, hallucinations, CNS depression, hypotension, cardiovascular collapse, convulsions
Treatment	Empty stomach by gastric lavage or emesis, followed by activated charcoal. For respiratory depression, administer a narcotic antagonist (eg, naloxone).

DRUG INTERACTIONS

Alcohol, tranquilizers, sedative-hypnotics, and other CNS depressants	⇧ CNS depression	
MAO inhibitors	⇧ Sympathomimetic effect	
Beta-adrenergic blockers	⇩ Antihypertensive effect	⇧ Sympathomimetic effect
Methyldopa	⇩ Antihypertensive effect	
Mecamylamine	⇩ Antihypertensive effect	
Reserpine	⇩ Antihypertensive effect	
Veratrum alkaloids	⇩ Antihypertensive effect	

Table continued on following page

NOVAHISTINE DH continued

ALTERED LABORATORY VALUES

Urinary values —— ⇧ 5-HIAA (with colorimetric methods) ⇧ VMA (with colorimetric methods)

No clinically significant alterations in blood/serum values occur at therapeutic dosages

Use in children

See INDICATIONS

Use in pregnancy or nursing mothers

Safe use has not been established during pregnancy. Codeine is excreted in breast milk; patient should stop nursing if drug is prescribed.

NOVAHISTINE EXPECTORANT (Codeine phosphate, phenylpropanolamine hydrochloride, and guaifenesin) Dow

Liq: 10 mg codeine phosphate, 18.75 mg phenylpropanolamine hydrochloride, 100 mg guaifenesin, and 7.5% alcohol per 5 ml *C-V*

INDICATIONS	ORAL DOSAGE
Tenacious pulmonary secretions associated with cough and respiratory congestion **Acute otitis media** and **mild otalgia** (adjunctive therapy)	**Adult:** 10 ml (2 tsp) q4h, up to 4 doses/24 h **Infant (<2 yr):** 3 drops/kg q4h, up to 4 doses/24 h **Child (25–50 lb):** 1.25–2.5 ml (¼–½ tsp) q4h, up to 4 doses/24 h **Child (50–90 lb):** 2.5–5 ml (½–1 tsp) q4h, up to 4 doses/24 h

CONTRAINDICATIONS	
Severe hypertension	
Severe coronary-artery disease	
MAO-inhibitor therapy	Concomitant therapy may enhance sympathomimetic effects
Hypersensitivity or idiosyncracy	To codeine, phenylpropanolamine, or guaifenesin

WARNINGS/PRECAUTIONS	
Habit-forming	Psychic and/or physical dependence and tolerance may develop, especially in addiction-prone individuals
Elderly patients	Adverse reactions to sympathomimetics are more likely to occur in patients over 60 yr of age
Special-risk patients	Use with caution in patients with hypertension, diabetes mellitus, ischemic heart disease, hyperthyroidism, increased intraocular pressure, prostatic hypertrophy, asthma, or emphysema
Unwarranted use	Discontinue treatment if cough persists for more than 1 wk, tends to recur, or is accompanied by fever, rash, or headache

ADVERSE REACTIONS[1]	
Central nervous system and neuromuscular	Dizziness, sedation, fear, anxiety, tension, restlessness, tremor, weakness, insomnia, hallucinations, convulsions, CNS depression
Gastrointestinal	Nausea, vomiting, constipation
Cardiovascular	Palpitations, pallor, arrhythmias, cardiovascular collapse with hypotension, hypertensive crises
Dermatological	Pruritus
Respiratory	Respiratory difficulty and depression (especially in patients with respiratory disease associated with CO_2 retention)
Genitourinary	Dysuria

OVERDOSAGE	
Signs and symptoms	See ADVERSE REACTIONS
Treatment	Induce emesis or use gastric lavage, followed by activated charcoal, to empty stomach. For respiratory depression, administer a narcotic antagonist (eg, naloxone). Administer oxygen and pressor agents, as needed.

DRUG INTERACTIONS	
MAO inhibitors	⇧ Sympathomimetic effect
Alcohol, tranquilizers, sedative-hypnotics, and other CNS depressants	⇧ CNS depression
Beta-adrenergic blockers	⇧ Sympathomimetic effect
Methyldopa	⇩ Antihypertensive effect
Mecamylamine	⇩ Antihypertensive effect
Reserpine	⇩ Antihypertensive effect
Veratrum alkaloids	⇩ Antihypertensive effect

[1] Including reactions common to sympathomimetic amines in general

Table continued on following page

ALTERED LABORATORY VALUES

No clinically significant alterations in blood/serum or urinary values occur at therapeutic dosages

Use in children

See INDICATIONS

Use in pregnancy or nursing mothers

Safe use has not been established during pregnancy. Contraindicated for use in nursing mothers; codeine is excreted in breast milk.

OMNI-TUSS SUSPENSION (Ephedrine, chlorpheniramine, phenyltoloxamine, codeine phosphate, guaiacol carbonate) Pennwalt

Liq: 25 mg ephedrine, 3 mg chlorpheniramine, 5 mg phenyltoloxamine, 10 mg codeine phosphate, and 20 mg guaiacol carbonate per 5 ml *C-V*

INDICATIONS	ORAL DOSAGE
Cough associated with upper respiratory infection, bronchitis, bronchiectasis, bronchial asthma, emphysema, sinusitis, rhinitis, hay fever, and other allergic conditions	**Adult:** 5 ml (1 tsp) q12h **Child (6–12 yr):** 2.5 ml (½ tsp) q12h

CONTRAINDICATIONS

Hypersensitivity to any of the components ●

Hypertension ●

Cardiovascular disease ●

Coronary-artery disease ●

Hyperthyroidism ●

Pyloroduodenal obstruction ●

Prostatic hypertrophy ●

Bladder-neck obstruction ●

WARNINGS/PRECAUTIONS

Habit-forming	Psychic and/or physical dependence and tolerance may develop, especially in addiction-prone individuals
Drowsiness	Performance of potentially hazardous activities may be impaired; caution patients accordingly

ADVERSE REACTIONS

Central nervous system	Jitteriness, insomnia
Gastrointestinal	Nausea, dry mouth, constipation

OVERDOSAGE

Signs and symptoms	Toxic effects primarily attributable to codeine: respiratory depression, somnolence, stupor, coma, skeletal-muscle flaccidity, cold and clammy skin, bradycardia, hypotension, apnea, circulatory collapse, and cardiac arrest, leading to death
Treatment	Re-establish adequate airway and institute artificial respiration. For respiratory depression, administer a narcotic antagonist (eg, naloxone), along with attempts at resuscitation. Empty stomach by emesis or gastric lavage. Employ supportive measures, as indicated.

DRUG INTERACTIONS

Alcohol, tranquilizers, sedative-hypnotics, and other CNS depressants	⇧ CNS depression
MAO inhibitors	⇧ Sympathomimetic and anticholinergic effects
Beta-adrenergic blockers	⇧ Sympathomimetic effect
Methyldopa	⇩ Antihypertensive effect
Mecamylamine	⇩ Antihypertensive effect
Reserpine	⇩ Antihypertensive effect
Veratrum alkaloids	⇩ Antihypertensive effect

ALTERED LABORATORY VALUES

No clinically significant alterations in blood/serum or urinary values occur at therapeutic dosages

Use in children

See INDICATIONS; general guidelines not established for use in children under 6 yr of age

Use in pregnancy or nursing mothers

Safe use not established

ORGANIDIN (Iodinated glycerol) Wallace

Tabs: 30 mg **Sol:** 50 mg/ml **Elixir:** 60 mg/5 ml

INDICATIONS	ORAL DOSAGE
Respiratory-tract conditions, including bronchitis, bronchial asthma, pulmonary emphysema, cystic fibrosis, and chronic sinusitis (adjunctive therapy) **Prevention of postoperative atelectasis**	**Adult:** 60 mg (2 tabs) with liquid, 5 ml (1 tsp) with liquid, or 20 drops (60 mg) qid **Child:** up to 30 mg (1 tab) with liquid, 2.5 ml (½ tsp) with liquid, or 10 drops (30 mg), based on child's weight, qid

CONTRAINDICATIONS

Hypersensitivity to iodinated glycerol or related compounds ●

History of marked sensitivity to inorganic iodides ●

WARNINGS/PRECAUTIONS

Iodism — Discontinue use if dermatitis or other manifestations of hypersensitivity develop

ADVERSE REACTIONS

Gastrointestinal — Irritation

Dermatological — Rash, other hypersensitivity manifestations

OVERDOSAGE

Signs and symptoms — See ADVERSE REACTIONS

Treatment — Empty stomach by inducing emesis; treat symptomatically

DRUG INTERACTIONS

No clinically significant drug interactions have been observed

ALTERED LABORATORY VALUES

Blood/serum values — ⇧ PBI ⇩ ^{131}I thyroid uptake

No clinically significant alterations in urinary values occur at therapeutic dosages

Use in children

See INDICATIONS

Use in pregnancy or nursing mothers

Iodides have been associated with abnormal thyroid function and/or goiter in newborns. General guidelines not established for use in nursing mothers

ORNADE (Chlorpheniramine maleate, phenylpropanolamine hydrochloride, and isopropamide iodide) **Smith Kline & French**

Caps (sust rel): 8 mg chlorpheniramine maleate, 50 mg phenylpropanolamine hydrochloride, and 2.5 mg isopropamide iodide

INDICATIONS	ORAL DOSAGE
Relief of **upper respiratory-tract congestion and hypersecretion** associated with vasomotor rhinitis and allergic rhinitis, and for prolonged relief[1] Relief of **nasal congestion and hypersecretion** associated with the common cold and sinusitis[2]	**Adult:** 1 cap q12h **Child (6–12 yr):** same as adult

CONTRAINDICATIONS

Hypersensitivity to any component ●	Coronary-artery disease ●	Bladder-neck obstruction ●
Severe hypertension ●	Stenosing peptic ulcer ●	MAO-inhibitor therapy ●
Bronchial asthma ●	Pyloroduodenal obstruction ●	

WARNINGS/PRECAUTIONS

Drowsiness	Performance of potentially hazardous activities may be impaired; caution patients accordingly
Concurrent therapy	Caution patients about the possible additive effects of alcohol and other CNS depressants
Special-risk patients	Use with caution in patients with cardiovascular disease, glaucoma, prostatic hypertrophy, or hyperthyroidism

ADVERSE REACTIONS

Central nervous system	Drowsiness, nervousness, insomnia, dizziness, weakness, irritability, headache, incoordination, tremor, convulsions
Ophthalmic	Visual disturbances
Gastrointestinal	Dry mouth, nausea, vomiting, epigastric pain, diarrhea, abdominal pain, anorexia, constipation, parotitis
Respiratory	Dry nose and throat, tightness in the chest
Cardiovascular	Anginal pain, palpitations, hypertension, hypotension
Genitourinary	Difficult urination, dysuria
Hematological	Thrombocytopenia, leukopenia
Dermatological	Rash, acne

OVERDOSAGE

Signs and symptoms	Dry mouth, dysphagia, thirst, blurred vision, dilated pupils, photophobia, fever, rapid pulse and respiration, disorientation, CNS depression or excitation
Treatment	Use gastric lavage to empty stomach, repeating several times. Administer saline cathartics to hasten evacuation of pellets. Treat respiratory depression with oxygen and stimulants. For marked excitement, use a short-acting barbiturate or chloral hydrate.

DRUG INTERACTIONS

Alcohol, tranquilizers, sedative-hypnotics, and other CNS depressants	⇧ CNS depression
MAO inhibitors	⇧ Sympathomimetic and anticholinergic effects

ALTERED LABORATORY VALUES

Blood/serum values	⇧ PBI ⇩ ^{131}I thyroid uptake

No clinically significant alterations in urinary values occur at therapeutic dosages

Use in children	Use in pregnancy or nursing mothers
See INDICATIONS; contraindicated for use in children under 6 yr of age	Safe use not established; lactation may be inhibited

[1]Possibly effective
[2]Lacks substantial evidence of effectiveness for this indication

PEDIACOF (Codeine phosphate, phenylephrine hydrochloride, chlorpheniramine maleate, and potassium iodide) Breon

Liq: 5 mg codeine phosphate, 2.5 mg phenylephrine hydrochloride, 0.75 mg chlorpheniramine maleate, 75 mg potassium iodide, and 5% alcohol per 5 ml *C-V*

INDICATIONS	ORAL DOSAGE
Cough and congestion due to colds and upper-respiratory-tract infections	**Infant (6 mo to 1 yr):** 1.25 ml (¼ tsp) q4–6h **Child (1–3 yr):** 2.5–5 ml (½–1 tsp) q4–6h **Child (3–6 yr):** 5–10 ml (1–2 tsp) q4–6h **Child (6–12 yr):** 10 ml (2 tsp) q4–6h

CONTRAINDICATIONS

Tuberculosis ●	Sensitivity to iodides ●

WARNINGS/PRECAUTIONS

Habit-forming	Psychic and/or physical dependence and tolerance may develop, especially in addiction-prone individuals
Special-risk patients	Use with caution in patients with cardiac disorders, hypertension, or hyperthyroidism

ADVERSE REACTIONS

Central nervous system	Drowsiness
Gastrointestinal	Anorexia, constipation

OVERDOSAGE

Signs and symptoms	Toxic effects primarily attributable to codeine: respiratory depression, somnolence, stupor, coma, skeletal-muscle flaccidity, cold and clammy skin, bradycardia, hypotension, apnea, circulatory collapse, and cardiac arrest, leading to death
Treatment	Re-establish adequate airway and institute artificial respiration. For respiratory depression, administer a narcotic antagonist (eg, naloxone) along with attempts at resuscitation. Empty stomach by emesis or gastric lavage. Employ supportive measures, as indicated.

DRUG INTERACTIONS

Narcotic analgesics, general anesthetics, sedative-hypnotics, and other CNS depressants	⇧ CNS depression

ALTERED LABORATORY VALUES

Blood/serum values	⇧ PBI ⇩ ^{131}I thyroid uptake

No clinically significant alterations in urinary values occur at therapeutic dosages

Use in children	Use in pregnancy or nursing mothers
See INDICATIONS; general guidelines not established for use in infants under 6 mo of age	General guidelines not established

PERCOGESIC with CODEINE (Codeine phosphate, acetaminophen, and phenyltoloxamine citrate) Endo

Tabs: 32.4 mg codeine phosphate, 325 mg acetaminophen, and 30 mg phenyltoloxamine citrate *C-III*

INDICATIONS	ORAL DOSAGE
Moderate acute pain **Temporary relief of cold symptoms, fever, and other discomforts** accompanying systemic viral infections	**Adult:** 1–2 tabs q4h, as needed **Child (5–12 yr):** ½–1 tab q4h, as needed

CONTRAINDICATIONS

Hypersensitivity to codeine, acetaminophen, or phenyltoloxamine

WARNINGS/PRECAUTIONS

Habit-forming	Psychic and/or physical dependence and tolerance may develop, especially in addiction-prone individuals
Drowsiness	Performance of potentially hazardous activities may be impaired; caution patients accordingly
Productive cough suppression	May occur, owing to codeine component; use with caution

ADVERSE REACTIONS

Gastrointestinal	Nausea, vomiting, constipation
Central nervous system	Drowsiness
Ophthalmic	Miosis

OVERDOSAGE

Signs and symptoms	Toxic effects primarily attributable to acetaminophen and codeine components: cyanosis, tachycardia, anemia, pancytopenia, neutropenia, jaundice, leukopenia, skin eruptions, chills, fever, vomiting, CNS stimulation, excitement, delirium, depression, coma, vascular collapse, convulsions, skeletal-muscle flaccidity, hypotension, bradycardia, apnea, circulatory collapse, and cardiac arrest; hepatotoxicity may occur, although laboratory and clinical evidence may be delayed. Serial hepatic enzyme determinations are recommended. Hepatic failure may be severe, leading to encephalopathy, coma, and death.
Treatment	Maintain patent airway and institute artificial respiration. Gastric lavage or emesis, followed by activated charcoal, may be indicated. For respiratory depression, administer a narcotic antagonist (eg, naloxone). An anticonvulsant may be necessary. Avoid analeptic drugs.

DRUG INTERACTIONS

Warfarin	⇧ Hypoprothrombinemia (slight)
Alcohol, tranquilizers, sedative-hypnotics, and other CNS depressants	⇧ CNS depression (reduce dosage when using more than one agent)

ALTERED LABORATORY VALUES

Blood/serum values	⇧ Prothrombin time ⇧ Uric acid (with phosphotungstate method)

No clinically significant alterations in urinary values occur at therapeutic dosages

Use in children	Use in pregnancy or nursing mothers
See INDICATIONS; general guidelines not established for use in children under 5 yr of age	General guidelines not established

PHENERGAN EXPECTORANT PLAIN (Promethazine hydrochloride, fluidextract ipecac, potassium guaiacolsulfonate, citric acid, and sodium citrate) **Wyeth**

Liq: 5 mg promethazine hydrochloride, 0.17 min fluidextract ipecac, 44 mg potassium guaiacolsulfonate, 60 mg citric acid, 197 mg sodium citrate, and 7% alcohol per 5 ml

INDICATIONS	ORAL DOSAGE
Cough due to colds and minor upper-respiratory-tract infections, as well as **allergic cough** associated with vasomotor rhinitis, pollen hay fever, and food or dust sensitivity	**Adult:** 5 ml (1 tsp) q4–6h

ADMINISTRATION/DOSAGE ADJUSTMENTS

Concomitant use of CNS depressants —— Administer CNS depressants in reduced dosages, with caution

CONTRAINDICATIONS

None

WARNINGS/PRECAUTIONS

Drowsiness, dizziness —— Performance of potentially hazardous activities may be impaired; caution patients accordingly. May be advisable to administer medication only at bedtime.

ADVERSE REACTIONS

Central nervous system —— Sedation, dizziness, paradoxical hyperexcitability and nightmares (in children receiving single doses of 75–125 mg)

Ophthalmic —— Blurred vision

Hematological —— Leukopenia (rare), agranulocytosis (one case)

Other —— Dry mouth

OVERDOSAGE

Signs and symptoms —— Range from mild CNS and cardiovascular depression to profound hypotension, respiratory depression, and unconsciousness. Stimulation may be present, especially in children and in geriatric patients. Atropine-like symptoms (eg, dry mouth; fixed, dilated pupils; flushing), and GI disturbances may occur.

Treatment —— Generally supportive and symptomatic. Early gastric lavage may be helpful. *Do not use stimulants.* Treat severe hypotension with levarterenol or phenylephrine; *do not use epinephrine or other pressor agents.* Treat extrapyramidal reactions with anticholinergic antiparkinsonism agents, diphenhydramine, or barbiturates. Additional measures include administration of oxygen and IV fluids. Dialysis does *not* seem to be beneficial.

DRUG INTERACTIONS

Alcohol, sedative-hypnotics, tranquilizers, and other CNS depressants —— ⇧ CNS depression

ALTERED LABORATORY VALUES

No clinically significant alterations in blood/serum or urinary values occur at therapeutic dosages

Use in children

General guidelines not established

Use in pregnancy or nursing mothers

General guidelines not established

PHENERGAN EXPECTORANT with CODEINE (Promethazine hydrochloride, codeine phosphate, fluidextract ipecac, potassium guaiacolsulfonate, sodium citrate, and citric acid) Wyeth

Syrup: 5 mg promethazine hydrochloride, 10 mg codeine phosphate, 0.17 min fluidextract ipecac, 44 mg potassium guaiacolsulfonate, 197 mg sodium citrate, 60 mg citric acid, and 7% alcohol per 5 ml *C-V*

INDICATIONS	ORAL DOSAGE
Cough due to cold, minor upper-respiratory-tract infections, or allergy	**Adult:** 5 ml (1 tsp) q4-6h

CONTRAINDICATIONS

None

WARNINGS/PRECAUTIONS

Habit-forming — Psychic and/or physical dependence and tolerance may develop, especially in addiction-prone individuals

Drowsiness — Performance of potentially hazardous activities may be impaired; caution patients accordingly

ADVERSE REACTIONS

Central nervous system — Sedation, dizziness

Gastrointestinal — Dry mouth

Ophthalmic — Blurred vision

Hematological — Leukopenia (rare), agranulocytosis (very rare)

OVERDOSAGE

Signs and symptoms — *Promethazine-related effects:* deep sedation, coma, convulsions, cardiorespiratory symptoms; *codeine-related effects:* respiratory depression, somnolence, stupor, coma, skeletal-muscle flaccidity, cold and clammy skin, bradycardia, hypotension, apnea, circulatory collapse, and cardiac arrest, leading to death

Treatment — Re-establish adequate airway and institute artificial respiration. For respiratory depression, administer a narcotic antagonist (eg, naloxone) along with attempts at resuscitation. Empty stomach by emesis or gastric lavage. To control convulsions, administer diazepam. Employ supportive measures as indicated. Hypotension may respond to position, fluids, and, in severe cases, vasopressor agents (eg, levarterenol or phenylephrine); do not use epinephrine.

DRUG INTERACTIONS

Alcohol, tranquilizers, sedative-hypnotics, and other CNS depressants — ⇧ CNS depression

MAO inhibitors — ⇧ Anticholinergic effect

ALTERED LABORATORY VALUES

No clinically significant alterations in blood/serum or urinary values occur at therapeutic dosages

Use in children	Use in pregnancy or nursing mothers
Doses of 75–125 mg of promethazine may cause a paradoxical reaction, characterized by hyperexcitability and nightmares. General guidelines not established for dosage recommendations.	General guidelines not established

PHENERGAN EXPECTORANT with DEXTROMETHORPHAN (Dextromethorphan hydrobromide, promethazine hydrochloride, fluidextract ipecac, potassium guaiacolsulfonate, citric acid, and sodium citrate) Wyeth

Syrup: 7.5 mg dextromethorphan hydrobromide, 5 mg promethazine hydrochloride, 0.17 min fluidextract ipecac, 44 mg potassium guaiacolsulfonate, 60 mg citric acid, 197 mg sodium citrate, and 7% alcohol per 5 ml

INDICATIONS	ORAL DOSAGE
Cough due to colds, minor upper-respiratory-tract infections, or allergy	**Child (3 mo to 4 yr):** 2.5 ml (½ tsp) in 1–4 daily doses, not less than 3 h apart **Child (>4 yr):** 5–10 ml (1–2 tsp) in 1–4 daily doses, not less than 3 h apart

CONTRAINDICATIONS

None

WARNINGS/PRECAUTIONS

Antiemetic effect	May mask toxicity of other drugs or obscure underlying disease, such as GI obstruction
Drowsiness	Performance of potentially hazardous activities may be impaired; caution patients accordingly
Dehydration, oliguria	May potentiate toxicity; reducc dosage if these conditions exist
Hyperexcitability, nightmares	May occur following a single dose of 75–125 mg; discontinue therapy

ADVERSE REACTIONS

Central nervous system	Drowsiness, dizziness
Gastrointestinal	Dry mouth
Ophthalmic	Blurred vision
Hematological	Leukopenia (rare), agranulocytosis (very rare)

OVERDOSAGE

Signs and symptoms	Deep sedation, coma, convulsions, cardiac and respiratory depression
Treatment	Treat symptomatically; employ general measures to support adequate ventilation, blood pressure, and urine output. Gastric lavage and/or activated charcoal may be useful. To control convulsions, administer diazepam. Hypotension may respond to position, IV fluids, and, in severe cases, vasopressor agents (eg, levarterenol or phenylephrine); *do not use epinephrine.*

DRUG INTERACTIONS

Anesthetics, narcotic analgesics, sedative-hypnotics, and other CNS depressants	⇧ CNS depression
Epinephrine	⇩ Pressor effect

ALTERED LABORATORY VALUES

No clinically significant alterations in blood/serum or urinary values occur at therapeutic dosages

Use in children

Not recommended for use in infants under 3 mo of age

Use in pregnancy or nursing mothers

General guidelines not established

PHENERGAN VC EXPECTORANT with CODEINE (Promethazine hydrochloride, phenylephrine hydrochloride, codeine phosphate, fluidextract ipecac, potassium guaiacolsulfonate, citric acid, and sodium citrate) **Wyeth**

Syrup: 5 mg promethazine hydrochloride, 5 mg phenylephrine hydrochloride, 10 mg codeine phosphate, 0.17 min fluidextract ipecac, 44 mg potassium guaiacolsulfonate, 60 mg citric acid, 197 mg sodium citrate, and 7% alcohol per 5 ml *C-V*

INDICATIONS	ORAL DOSAGE
Cough due to colds, minor upper-respiratory infections, or allergy	**Adult:** 5 ml (1 tsp) q4–6h

CONTRAINDICATIONS

None

WARNINGS/PRECAUTIONS

Habit-forming	Psychic and/or physical dependence and tolerance may develop, especially in addiction-prone individuals
Drowsiness	Performance of potentially hazardous activities may be impaired; caution patients accordingly. May be advisable to administer medication only at bedtime.
Special-risk patients	Administer with caution to patients with hypertension, cardiac or peripheral vascular disease, hyperthyroidism, or diabetes

ADVERSE REACTIONS

Central nervous system	Drowsiness, sedation, dizziness (rare)
Gastrointestinal	Dry mouth
Ophthalmic	Blurred vision
Hematological	Leukopenia (rare), agranulocytosis (very rare)

OVERDOSAGE

Signs and symptoms	*Promethazine-related effects:* deep sedation, coma, convulsions, cardiorespiratory symptoms; *codeine-related effects:* respiratory depression, somnolence, stupor, coma, skeletal-muscle flaccidity, cold and clammy skin, bradycardia, hypotension, apnea, circulatory collapse, and cardiac arrest, leading to death
Treatment	Re-establish adequate airway and institute artificial respiration. For respiratory depression, administer a narcotic antagonist (eg, naloxone), along with attempts at resuscitation. Empty stomach by emesis or gastric lavage. To control convulsions, administer diazepam. Employ supportive measures, as indicated. Hypotension may respond to position, IV fluids, and, in severe cases, vasopressor agents (eg, levarterenol or phenylephrine); do not use epinephrine.

DRUG INTERACTIONS

Alcohol, tranquilizers, sedative-hypnotics, and other CNS depressants	⇧ CNS depression
MAO inhibitors	⇧ Anticholinergic effect

ALTERED LABORATORY VALUES

No clinically significant alterations in blood/serum or urinary values occur at therapeutic dosages

Use in children

Doses of 75–125 mg may cause a paradoxical reaction, characterized by hyperexcitability and nightmares. General guidelines not established for dosage recommendations.

Use in pregnancy or nursing mothers

General guidelines not established

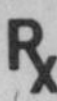

ROBITUSSIN A-C (Guaifenesin and codeine phosphate) Robins

Syrup: 100 mg guaifenesin, 10 mg codeine phosphate, and 3.5% alcohol per 5 ml *C-V*

INDICATIONS	ORAL DOSAGE
Cough due to colds, bronchitis, laryngitis, tracheitis, pharyngitis, pertussis, influenza, or measles	**Adult:** 10 ml (2 tsp) q4h, up to 60 ml (12 tsp)/24 h **Child (2–6 yr):** 2.5 ml (½ tsp) q4h, up to 15 ml (3 tsp)/24 h **Child (6–12 yr):** 5 ml (1 tsp) q4h, up to 30 ml (6 tsp)/24 h

CONTRAINDICATIONS

Hypersensitivity to guaifenesin or codeine

WARNINGS/PRECAUTIONS

Habit-forming — Psychic and/or physical dependence and tolerance may develop, especially in addiction-prone individuals

Drowsiness — Performance of potentially hazardous activities may be impaired; caution patients accordingly

ADVERSE REACTIONS

Central nervous system — Drowsiness

Gastrointestinal — Nausea, upset, constipation

OVERDOSAGE

Signs and symptoms — Toxic effects primarily attributable to codeine: respiratory depression, somnolence, stupor, coma, skeletal-muscle flaccidity, cold and clammy skin, bradycardia, hypotension, apnea, circulatory collapse, and cardiac arrest, leading to death

Treatment — Re-establish adequate airway and institute artificial respiration. For respiratory depression, administer a narcotic antagonist (eg, naloxone), along with attempts at resuscitation. Empty stomach by emesis or gastric lavage. Employ supportive measures, as indicated.

DRUG INTERACTIONS

Alcohol, tranquilizers, sedative-hypnotics, and other CNS depressants — ⇧ CNS depression

ALTERED LABORATORY VALUES

Urinary values — ⇧ 5-HIAA (colorimetric interference) ⇧ VMA (colorimetric interference)

No clinically significant alterations in blood/serum values occur at therapeutic dosages

Use in children

See INDICATIONS. For use in children under 2 yr of age, general guidelines not established.

Use in pregnancy or nursing mothers

General guidelines not established

ROBITUSSIN-DAC (Guaifenesin, pseudoephedrine hydrochloride, and codeine phosphate) Robins

Syrup: 100 mg guaifenesin, 30 mg pseudoephedrine hydrochloride, 10 mg codeine phosphate, and 1.4%, alcohol per 5 ml *C-V*

INDICATIONS	ORAL DOSAGE
Cough and **nasal congestion** associated with colds and inhaled irritants	**Adult:** 5–10 ml (1–2 tsp) q4h, up to 60 ml (12 tsp)/24 h **Child (2–6 yr):** 2.5 ml (½ tsp) q4h, up to 15 ml (3 tsp)/24h **Child (6–12 yr):** 5 ml (1 tsp) q4h, up to 30 ml (6 tsp)/24 h

CONTRAINDICATIONS

Marked hypertension ●	MAO-inhibitor therapy ●	Hypersensitivity to guaifenesin, pseudoephedrine, or codeine ●
Hyperthyroidism ●	Antihypertensive medication ●	

WARNINGS/PRECAUTIONS

Habit-forming	Psychic and/or physical dependence may occur, especially in addiction-prone individuals
Persistent or chronic cough, or cough accompanied by excessive secretions	Use with caution
Special-risk patients	Use with caution in patients with hypertension, heart disease, diabetes mellitus, chronic pulmonary disease, shortness of breath, prostatic hypertrophy, or glaucoma

ADVERSE REACTIONS

Central nervous system	Agitation, dizziness, insomnia
Gastrointestinal	Nausea, constipation
Cardiovascular	Palpitations

OVERDOSAGE

Signs and symptoms	Nervousness, dizziness, and sleeplessness, progressing to somnolence, respiratory depression, stupor, and coma
Treatment	Induce emesis or use gastric lavage, followed by activated charcoal, to empty stomach. Maintain patent airway and ventilatory exchange. For respiratory depression, administer a narcotic antagonist (eg, naloxone). Administer oxygen and pressor agents, as needed.

DRUG INTERACTIONS

Alcohol, tranquilizers, sedative-hypnotics, and other CNS depressants	⇧ CNS depression
MAO inhibitors	⇧ Sympathomimetic and anticholinergic effects
Methyldopa, mecamylamine, reserpine, *Veratrum* alkaloids	⇩ Antihypertensive effect

ALTERED LABORATORY VALUES

Urinary values	⇧ 5-HIAA (with colorimetric methods) ⇧ VMA (with colorimetric methods)

No clinically significant alterations in blood/serum values occur at therapeutic dosages

Use in children

Sèe INDICATIONS; use with caution in children < 2 yr of age or those taking another drug. General guidelines not established for dosage recommendations.

Use in pregnancy or nursing mothers

General guidelines not established

RONDEC-DM (Carbinoxamine maleate, pseudoephedrine hydrochloride, and dextromethorphan hydrobromide) Ross

Syrup: 4 mg carbinoxamine maleate, 60 mg pseudoephedrine hydrochloride, and 15 mg dextromethorphan hydrobromide per 5 ml **Drops:** 2 mg carbinoxamine maleate, 25 mg pseudoephedrine hydrochloride, and 4 mg dextromethorphan hydrobromide per 1 ml

INDICATIONS	ORAL DOSAGE
Nasopharyngitis with postnasal drip; **colds; bronchitis; bronchial cough; recurrent cough** due to recurrent respiratory infection	**Adult:** 5 ml (1 tsp) qid **Infant (1-3 mo):** 0.25 ml (¼ dropperful) qid **Infant (4-6 mo):** 0.5 ml (½ dropperful) qid **Infant (7-9 mo):** 0.75 ml (¾ dropperful) qid **Infant (10-18 mo):** 1 ml (1 dropperful) qid **Child (18 mo to 5 yr):** 2.5 ml (½ tsp) qid **Child (6-12 yr):** same as adult

ADMINISTRATION/DOSAGE ADJUSTMENTS

Mild cough — Less frequent doses may be adequate

CONTRAINDICATIONS

None

WARNINGS/PRECAUTIONS

Drowsiness — Performance of potentially hazardous activities may be impaired; caution patients accordingly

Special-risk patients — Use with caution in patients with hypertension and in those hypersensitive to any of the components

ADVERSE REACTIONS

Central nervous system — Stimulation, sedation, moderate to severe drowsiness

Gastrointestinal — Mild GI disturbances

OVERDOSAGE

Signs and symptoms — Stimulation, nervousness, drowsiness, sedation, or convulsions

Treatment — Induce emesis or use gastric lavage to empty stomach, followed by activated charcoal. Treat symptomatically.

DRUG INTERACTIONS

No clinically significant drug interactions have been observed

ALTERED LABORATORY VALUES

No clinically significant alterations in blood/serum or urinary values occur at therapeutic dosages

Use in children

See INDICATIONS

Use in pregnancy or nursing mothers

Safe use has not been established during pregnancy. General guidelines not established for use in nursing mothers.

RONDEC Tablets/RONDEC Syrup/RONDEC Drops (Carbinoxamine maleate and pseudoephedrine hydrochloride) Ross

Tabs, syrup (per 5 ml): 4 mg carbinoxamine maleate and 60 mg pseudoephedrine hydrochloride **Drops:** 2 mg carbinoxamine maleate and 25 mg pseudoephedrine hydrochloride per 1 ml (1 dropperful)

INDICATIONS	ORAL DOSAGE
Symptomatic relief of seasonal and perennial **allergic rhinitis** and **vasomotor rhinitis**	**Adult:** 1 tab or 5 ml (1 tsp) qid **Infant (1-3 mo):** ¼ dropperful qid **Infant (4-6 mo):** ½ dropperful qid **Infant (7-9 mo):** ¾ dropperful qid **Infant (10-17 mo):** 1 dropperful qid **Child (18 mo to 5 yr):** 2.5 ml (½ tsp) qid **Child (6-12 yr):** same as adult

CONTRAINDICATIONS

None

WARNINGS/PRECAUTIONS

Pressor effect	Use with caution in patients with hypertension
Drowsiness	Performance of potentially hazardous activities may be impaired; caution patients accordingly
Sensitivity or idiosyncratic reactions	Withdraw drug

ADVERSE REACTIONS

Central nervous system	Stimulation, sedation, drowsiness

OVERDOSAGE

Signs and symptoms	Hypertension, stimulation, CNS depression, convulsions
Treatment	Induce emesis or use gastric lavage to empty stomach. Activated charcoal may be helpful. Institute supportive measures, as indicated. Treat symptomatically.

DRUG INTERACTIONS

Alcohol, tranquilizers, sedative-hypnotics, and other CNS depressants	⇧ CNS depression
MAO inhibitors	⇧ Sympathomimetic and anticholinergic effects

ALTERED LABORATORY VALUES

No clinically significant alterations in blood/serum or urinary values occur at therapeutic dosages

Use in children

See INDICATIONS; general guidelines not established for use in neonates

Use in pregnancy or nursing mothers

Safe use not established; general guidelines not established for use in nursing mothers

RYNATUSS (Carbetapentane tannate, chlorpheniramine tannate, ephedrine tannate, and phenylephrine tannate) **Wallace**

Tabs: 60 mg carbetapentane tannate, 5 mg chlorpheniramine tannate, 10 mg ephedrine tannate, and 10 mg phenylephrine tannate **Susp (ped):** 30 mg carbetapentane tannate, 4 mg chlorpheniramine tannate, 5 mg ephedrine tannate, and 5 mg phenylephrine tannate per 5 ml

INDICATIONS	ORAL DOSAGE
Cough (nonproductive) due to colds, asthma, and acute and chronic bronchitis	**Adult:** 1–2 tabs q12h **Infant (<2 yr):** 1.7 ml (1/3 tsp) q12h **Child (2–6 yr):** 2.5–5 ml (½–1 tsp) q12h **Child (>6 yr):** 5–10 ml (1–2 tsp) q12h

CONTRAINDICATIONS

Hypersensitivity to sympathomimetic drugs

WARNINGS/PRECAUTIONS

Drowsiness — Performance of potentially hazardous activites may be impaired; caution patients accordingly

Special-risk patients — Use with caution in patients with hypertension, hyperthyroidism, diabetes, or coronary-artery disease

Tartrazine sensitivity — Presence of FD&C Yellow No. 5 (tartrazine) in suspension form may cause allergic-type reactions, including bronchial asthma, in susceptible individuals

ADVERSE REACTIONS

Gastrointestinal — Dry mouth

Central nervous system — Drowsiness

OVERDOSAGE

Signs and symptoms — Stimulation, somnolence, drowsiness, convulsions

Treatment — Induce emesis or use gastric lavage to empty stomach; treat symptomatically

DRUG INTERACTIONS

No clinically significant drug interactions have been observed

ALTERED LABORATORY VALUES

No clinically significant alterations in blood/serum or urinary values occur at therapeutic dosages

Use in children

See INDICATIONS

Use in pregnancy or nursing mothers

General guidelines not established

RYNATUSS Pediatric Suspension (Carbetapentane tannate, chlorpheniramine tannate, ephedrine tannate, and phenylephrine tannate) **Wallace**

Susp: 30 mg carbetapentane tannate, 4 mg chlorpheniramine tannate, 5 mg ephedrine tannate, and 5 mg phenylephrine tannate per 5 ml

INDICATIONS	ORAL DOSAGE
Cough due to colds, asthma, or bronchitis	**Infant (<2 yr):** 1.7 ml (1/3 tsp) q12h **Child (2-6 yr):** 2.5-5 ml (½-1 tsp) q12h **Child (>6 yr):** 5-10 ml (1-2 tsp) q12h

CONTRAINDICATIONS

Hypersensitivity to sympathomimetic agents

WARNINGS/PRECAUTIONS

Special-risk patients — Use with caution in patients with hypertension, hyperthyroidism, diabetes, or coronary artery disease

Drowsiness — Performance of potentially hazardous activities may be impaired; caution patients accordingly

Tartrazine sensitivity — Presence of FC&C Yellow No. 5 (tartrazine) may cause allergic-type reactions, including bronchial asthma, in susceptible individuals

ADVERSE REACTIONS

Central nervous system — Drowsiness

Gastrointestinal — Dry mouth

OVERDOSAGE

Signs and symptoms — Depression, excitation, hypertension, hypotension

Treatment — Induce emesis or use gastric lavage to empty stomach, followed by activated charcoal. Careful observation and symptomatic treatment are advised.

DRUG INTERACTIONS

Narcotic analgesics, general anesthetics, sedative-hypnotics, and other CNS depressants — ⇧ CNS depression

ALTERED LABORATORY VALUES

No clinically significant alterations in blood/serum or urinary values occur at therapeutic dosages

Use in children

See INDICATIONS

Use in pregnancy or nursing mothers

General guidelines not established

SINGLET (Phenylephrine hydrochloride, chlorpheniramine maleate, and acetaminophen) **Dow**

Tabs: 40 mg phenylephrine hydrochloride, 8 mg chlorpheniramine maleate, and 500 mg acetaminophen

INDICATIONS	ORAL DOSAGE
Nasal and eustachian-tube congestion, sneezing, runny nose, watery eyes, myalgia, headache, and fever associated with colds and other viral infections, sinusitis, influenza, and seasonal and perennial nasal allergies	**Adult:** 1 tab tid or qid, not less than 6 h apart

CONTRAINDICATIONS

Hypersensitivity to any component ●	Severe hypertension ●	Peptic ulcer ●
Narrow-angle glaucoma ●	Severe coronary-artery disease ●	During an asthmatic attack ●
Urinary retention ●	MAO-inhibitor therapy ●	Serious liver or kidney dysfunction ●

WARNINGS/PRECAUTIONS

Drowsiness	Performance of potentially hazardous activities may be impaired; caution patients accordingly
Special-risk patients	Administer with caution to patients with increased intraocular pressure (narrow-angle glaucoma), prostatic hypertrophy, bladder-neck obstruction, hypertension, diabetes mellitus, ischemic heart disease, hyperthyroidism, liver and kidney disease, anemia, history of bronchial asthma, or hyperreactivity to ephedrine
Elderly patients	Adverse reactions to sympathomimetics and antihistamines are more likely to occur in patients over 60 yr of age

ADVERSE REACTIONS

Central nervous system	Fear, anxiety, tension, restlessness, tremor, weakness, insomnia, hallucinations, convulsions, CNS depression, drowsiness, dizziness, headache, nervousness
Ophthalmic	Blurred vision
Gastrointestinal	Dry mouth, anorexia, nausea, heartburn
Dermatological	Dermatitis (rare)
Cardiovascular	Pallor, arrhythmias, cardiovascular collapse with hypotension
Respiratory	Difficult breathing
Genitourinary	Dysuria

OVERDOSAGE

Signs and symptoms	Somnolence, tremor, weakness, dyspnea, pallor, hallucinations, convulsions, CNS depression; acetaminophen overdosage may result in liver damage and fatal hepatic necrosis
Treatment	Induce emesis or use gastric lavage to empty stomach, followed by activated charcoal. Institute supportive measures, as needed. Treat symptomatically.

DRUG INTERACTIONS

Alcohol, tranquilizers, sedative-hypnotics, and other CNS depressants	⇧ CNS depression
MAO inhibitors	⇧ Sympathomimetic and anticholinergic effects
Beta-adrenergic blockers	⇧ Sympathomimetic and antichlolinergic effects
Methyldopa	⇩ Antihypertensive effect
Mecamylamine	⇩ Antihypertensive effect
Reserpine	⇩ Antihypertensive effect
Veratrum alkaloids	⇩ Antihypertensive effect

ALTERED LABORATORY VALUES

No clinically significant alterations in blood/serum or urinary values occur at therapeutic dosages

Use in children

Contraindicated in children under 12 yr of age

Use in pregnancy or nursing mothers

Safe use not established during pregnancy; contraindicated for use in nursing mothers

SINUBID (Acetaminophen, phenacetin, phenylpropanolamine hydrochloride, and phenyltoloxamine citrate) **Parke-Davis**

Tabs: 300 mg acetaminophen, 300 mg phenacetin, 100 mg phenylpropanolamine hydrochloride, and 66 mg phenyltoloxamine citrate

INDICATIONS	ORAL DOSAGE
Nasal congestion, sinusitis, allergic and vasomotor rhinitis, coryza, facial pain and "pressure" of sinusitis, fever	**Adult:** 1 tab q12h **Child (6-12 yr):** ½ tab q12h

CONTRAINDICATIONS

Hypersensitivity to sympathomimetic amines	Manifested by sleepiness, dizziness, lightheadedness, weakness, tremulousness, or cardiac arrhythmias
Hypersensitivity to any component	

WARNINGS/PRECAUTIONS

Drowsiness	Performance of potentially hazardous activities may be impaired; caution patients accordingly
Special-risk patients	Use with caution in patients with hypertension, heart disease, diabetes mellitus, chronic renal disease, or thyroid disease
Excessive or prolonged use	May result in cyanosis, methemoglobinemia, hemolytic anemia, dyspnea, headache, vascular collapse, and kidney damage, owing to phenacetin component
Concomitant medication	Avoid concurrent use of MAO inhibitors or barbiturates, or ingestion of alcoholic beverages

ADVERSE REACTIONS

Central nervous system	Dizziness, headache, anxiety, restlessness, tension, insomnia, tremor, weakness, nervousness, vertigo, drowsiness, disturbed coordination, poor concentration, convulsions
Gastrointestinal	Epigastric distress, nausea, vomiting, diarrhea, intestinal cramps, dry mouth
Ophthalmic	Blurred vision
Hematological	Cyanosis with methemoglobinemia, hemolytic anemia
Respiratory	Dyspnea, dry nose and throat
Cardiovascular	Palpitations, vascular collapse, arrhythmias, hypotension
Dermatological	Urticaria, diaphoresis
Genitourinary	Renal damage, urinary retention

OVERDOSAGE

Signs and symptoms	Somnolence, tremor, weakness, dyspnea, pallor, hallucinations, convulsions, CNS depression; acetaminophen overdosage may result in liver damage and fatal hepatic necrosis
Treatment	Induce emesis or use gastric lavage to empty stomach, followed by activated charcoal. Institute supportive measures, as needed. Treat symptomatically.

DRUG INTERACTIONS

Alcohol, tranquilizers, sedative-hypnotics, and other CNS depressants	⇧ CNS depression
MAO inhibitors	⇧ Sympathomimetic and anticholinergic effects

ALTERED LABORATORY VALUES

No clinically significant alterations in blood/serum or urinary values occur at therapeutic dosages

Use in children

See INDICATIONS; general guidelines not established for use in children under 6 yr of age

Use in pregnancy or nursing mothers

Safe use not established during pregnancy; contraindicated for use in nursing mothers

TERPIN HYDRATE with CODEINE ELIXIR (various manufacturers)

Elixir: 85 mg terpin hydrate and 10 mg codeine per 5 ml *C-V*

INDICATIONS	ORAL DOSAGE
Cough	**Adult:** 5 ml (1 tsp) tid or qid

CONTRAINDICATIONS

Hypersensitivity to terpin hydrate or codeine

WARNINGS/PRECAUTIONS

Habit-forming	Psychic and/or physical dependence and tolerance may develop, especially in addiction-prone individuals
Drowsiness	Performance of hazardous activities may be impaired; caution patients accordingly

ADVERSE REACTIONS

Gastrointestinal	Nausea, constipation, epigastric pain, vomiting
Central nervous system	Drowsiness, dizziness, sedation, respiratory depression
Ophthalmic	Miosis

OVERDOSAGE

Signs and symptoms	Toxic effects primarily attributable to codeine: respiratory depression, somnolence, stupor, coma, skeletal-muscle flaccidity, cold and clammy skin, bradycardia, hypotension, apnea, circulatory collapse, and cardiac arrest, leading to death
Treatment	Re-establish adequate airway and institute artificial respiration. For respiratory depression, administer a narcotic antagonist (eg, naloxone) along with attempts at resuscitation. Empty stomach by emesis or gastric lavage. Employ supportive measures, as indicated.

DRUG INTERACTIONS

Alcohol, tranquilizers, sedative-hypnotics, and other CNS depressants	⇧ CNS depression

ALTERED LABORATORY VALUES

No clinically significant alterations in blood/serum or urinary values occur at therapeutic dosages

Use in children

General guidelines not established

Use in pregnancy or nursing mothers

Safe use has not been established during pregnancy. Codeine is excreted in breast milk; patient should stop nursing if drug is prescribed.

TRIAMINIC (Phenylpropanolamine hydrochloride, pheniramine maleate, and pyrilamine maleate) Dorsey

Tabs (sust rel): 50 mg phenylpropanolamine hydrochloride, 25 mg pheniramine maleate, and 25 mg pyrilamine maleate
Ped tabs (sust rel): 25 mg phenylpropanolamine hydrochloride, 12.5 mg pheniramine maleate, and 12.5 mg pyrilamine maleate
Drops: 20 mg phenylpropanolamine hydrochloride, 10 mg pheniramine maleate, and 10 mg pyrilamine maleate per 1 ml

INDICATIONS

Symptomatic relief of **nasal congestion, profuse nasal discharge and post-nasal drip** associated with colds, nasal allergies, sinusitis, and rhinitis

ORAL DOSAGE

Adult: 1 tab or 2 ped tabs tid (in AM, in midafternoon, and at bedtime)
Infant (<1 yr): 1 drop/2 lb qid
Child (6–12 yr): 1 ped tab tid (in AM, in midafternoon, and at bedtime)

CONTRAINDICATIONS

None

WARNINGS/PRECAUTIONS

Drowsiness	Performance of potentially hazardous activities may be impaired; caution patients accordingly
Special-risk patients	Use with caution in patients with hypertension, cardiovascular disease, diabetes mellitus, and hyperthyroidism

ADVERSE REACTIONS

Central nervous system	Drowsiness, dizziness, nervousness
Ophthalmic	Blurred vision
Cardiovascular	Palpitations, flushing
Gastrointestinal	Upset

OVERDOSAGE

Signs and symptoms	Hypertension, stimulation, CNS depression, convulsions
Treatment	Induce emesis or use gastric lavage to empty stomach. Activated charcoal may be helpful. Institute supportive measures, as indicated. Treat symptomatically.

DRUG INTERACTIONS

Alcohol, tranquilizers, sedative-hypnotics, and other CNS depressants	⇧ CNS depression
MAO inhibitors	⇧ Sympathomimetic and anticholinergic effects

ALTERED LABORATORY VALUES

No clinically significant alterations in blood/serum or urinary values occur at therapeutic dosages

Use in children

See INDICATIONS; a nonprescription syrup form is available for use in children 1–6 yr of age, as well as for other pediatric patients and adults

Use in pregnancy or nursing mothers

General guidelines not established

TRIAMINIC EXPECTORANT DH (Hydrocodone bitartrate, phenylpropanolamine hydrochloride, pheniramine maleate, pyrilamine maleate, and guaifenesin) **Dorsey**

Liq: 1.67 mg hydrocodone bitartrate, 12.5 mg phenylpropanolamine hydrochloride, 6.25 mg pheniramine maleate, 6.25 mg pyrilamine maleate, 100 mg guaifenesin, and 5% alcohol per 5 ml *C-III*

INDICATIONS	ORAL DOSAGE
Cough, nasal congestion due to colds, nasal allergies, sinusitis, or postnasal drip **Severe, prolonged, refractory cough** associated with other respiratory infections	**Adult:** 10 ml (2 tsp) q4h **Child (1–6 yr):** 2.5 ml (½ tsp) q4h **Child (6–12 yr):** 5 ml (1 tsp) q4h

CONTRAINDICATIONS

None

WARNINGS/PRECAUTIONS

Habit-forming — Psychic and/or physical dependence and tolerance may develop, especially in addiction-prone individuals

Drowsiness — Performance of potentially hazardous activities may be impaired; caution patients accordingly

Special-risk patients — Use with caution in patients with hypertension, hyperthyroidism, cardiovascular disease, or diabetes

ADVERSE REACTIONS

Central nervous system — Drowsiness, dizziness, nervousness

Ophthalmic — Blurred vision

Cardiovascular — Palpitations

Gastrointestinal — Upset

Other — Flushing

OVERDOSAGE

Signs and symptoms — Toxic effects primarily attributable to hydrocodone: respiratory depression, somnolence, stupor, coma, skeletal-muscle flaccidity, cold and clammy skin, bradycardia, hypotension, apnea, circulatory collapse, and cardiac arrest, leading to death

Treatment — Re-establish adequate airway and institute artificial respiration. For respiratory depression, administer a narcotic antagonist (eg, naloxone), along with attempts at resuscitation. Empty stomach by emesis or gastric lavage. Employ supportive measures, as indicated.

DRUG INTERACTIONS

Alcohol, tranquilizers, sedative-hypnotics, and other CNS depressants — ⇧ CNS depression

ALTERED LABORATORY VALUES

Urinary values — ⇧ 5-HIAA (with colorimetric methods) ⇧ VMA (with colorimetric methods)

No clinically significant alterations in blood/serum values occur at therapeutic dosages

Use in children	**Use in pregnancy or nursing mothers**
See INDICATIONS; general guidelines not established for use in infants under 1 yr of age	General guidelines not established

TRIAMINIC EXPECTORANT with CODEINE (Codeine phosphate, phenylpropanolamine hydrochloride, and guaifenesin) Dorsey

Liq: 10 mg codeine phosphate, 12.5 mg phenylpropanolamine hydrochloride, 100 mg guaifenesin, and 5% alcohol per 5 ml *C-V*

INDICATIONS	ORAL DOSAGE
Cough and **nasal congestion** due to colds	**Adult:** 10 ml (2 tsp) q4h **Infant (3 mo to 2 yr):** 2 drops/kg q4h **Child (2–6 yr):** 2.5 ml (½ tsp) q4h **Child (6–12 yr):** 5 ml (1 tsp) q4h

CONTRAINDICATIONS

Hypersensitivity to any component ●	MAO-inhibitor therapy ●

WARNINGS/PRECAUTIONS

Habit-forming	Psychic and/or physical dependence and tolerance may develop, especially in addiction-prone individuals
Drowsiness	Performance of potentially hazardous activities may be impaired; caution patients accordingly
Special-risk patients	Use with caution in patients with persistent or chronic cough, hypertension, hyperthyroidism, cardiovascular disease, diabetes, chronic pulmonary disease, or shortness of breath

ADVERSE REACTIONS

Central nervous system	Drowsiness, dizziness, nervousness, insomnia
Ophthalmic	Blurred vision
Cardiovascular	Palpitations
Gastrointestinal	Upset, constipation
Other	Flushing

OVERDOSAGE

Signs and symptoms	Toxic effects primarily attributable to codeine: respiratory depression, somnolence, stupor, coma, skeletal-muscle flaccidity, cold and clammy skin, bradycardia, hypotension, apnea, circulatory collapse, and cardiac arrest, leading to death
Treatment	Re-establish adequate airway and institute artificial respiration. For respiratory depression, administer a narcotic antagonist (eg, naloxone), along with attempts at resuscitation. Empty stomach by emesis or gastric lavage. Employ supportive measures, as indicated.

DRUG INTERACTIONS

Alcohol, tranquilizers, sedative-hypnotics, and other CNS depressants	⇧ CNS depression

ALTERED LABORATORY VALUES

Urinary values	⇧ 5-HIAA (with colorimetric methods) ⇧ VMA (with colorimetric methods)

No clinically significant alterations in blood/serum values occur at therapeutic dosages

Use in children	**Use in pregnancy or nursing mothers**
See INDICATIONS; general guidelines not established for use in infants under 3 mo of age	General guidelines not established

TUSSEND (Hydrocodone bitartrate and pseudoephedrine hydrochloride) **Dow**

Tabs: 5 mg hydrocodone bitartrate and 60 mg pseudoephedrine hydrochloride **Liq:** 5 mg hydrocodone bitartrate, 60 mg pseudoephedrine hydrochloride, and 5% alcohol per 5 ml *C-III*

INDICATIONS	ORAL DOSAGE
Exhausting cough spasms accompanying **upper-respiratory-tract congestion** due to colds, influenza, bronchitis, or sinusitis	**Adult:** 1 tab or 5 ml (1 tsp) qid, as needed **Child (25–50 lb):** 1.25 ml (¼ tsp) qid, as needed **Child (50–90 lb):** 2.5 ml (½ tsp) qid, as needed **Child (>90 lb):** same as for adult

CONTRAINDICATIONS	
Severe hypertension	
Severe coronary-artery disease	
MAO-inhibitor therapy	Sympathomimetic effects of pseudoephedrine may be exacerbated
Idiosyncratic reaction to adrenergic agents	Manifested by insomnia, dizziness, weakness, tremor, or arrhythmias
Hypersensitivity	To sympathomimetic amines, phenanthrene derivatives, or any component

WARNINGS/PRECAUTIONS	
Habit-forming	Psychic and/or physical dependence and tolerance may develop, especially in addiction-prone individuals
Drowsiness	Performance of potentially hazardous activities may be impaired; caution patients accordingly
Elderly patients	Adverse reactions to sympathomimetics are more likely to occur in patients over 60 yr of age
Special-risk patients	Use with caution in patients with diabetes mellitus, hypertension, ischemic heart disease, hyperthyroidism, increased intraocular pressure, prostatic hypertrophy, or in those with a history of hyperreactivity to ephedrine (see CONTRAINDICATIONS)

ADVERSE REACTIONS[1]	
Gastrointestinal	Upset, nausea, constipation
Central nervous system and neuromuscular	Drowsiness, headache, dizziness, fear, anxiety, tension, restlessness, tremor, weakness, insomnia, hallucinations, convulsions, depression
Cardiovascular	Tachycardia, palpitations, pallor, arrhythmias, cardiovascular collapse with hypotension
Respiratory	Difficult breathing
Genitourinary	Dysuria

OVERDOSAGE	
Signs and symptoms	*Toxic effects primarily attributable to hydrocodone:* respiratory depression, somnolence, stupor, coma, skeletal-muscle flaccidity, cold and clammy skin, bradycardia, hypotension, apnea, circulatory collapse, and cardiac arrest, leading to death
Treatment	**Re-establish adequate airway and institute artificial respiration. For respiratory** depression, administer a narcotic antagonist (eg, naloxone) along with attempts at resuscitation. Empty stomach by emesis or gastric lavage. Employ supportive measures, as indicated.

DRUG INTERACTIONS	
Alcohol, tranquilizers, sedative-hypnotics, and other CNS depressants	⇧ CNS depression
MAO inhibitors	⇧ Sympathomimetic effect
Beta-adrenergic blockers	⇧ Sympathomimetic effect
Methylodopa, mecamylamine, reserpine, *Veratrum* alkaloids	⇩ Antihypertensive effect

[1]Including reactions common to sympathomimetic amines in general and to pseudoephedrine in particular

Table continued on following page

TUSSEND continued

ALTERED LABORATORY VALUES

Blood/serum values ——— ⇧ SGOT ⇧ SGPT

No clinically significant alterations in urinary values occur at therapeutic dosages

Use in children

See INDICATIONS. General guidelines not established for use in children under 25 lb.

Use in pregnancy or nursing mothers

Safe use in pregnancy not established. Contraindicated for use in nursing mothers, due to higher than usual risk for infants from sympathomimetic amines.

TUSSEND EXPECTORANT (Hydrocodone bitartrate, pseudoephedrine hydrochloride, and guaifenesin) Dow

Liq: 5 mg hydrocodone bitartrate, 60 mg pseudoephedrine hydrochloride, 200 mg guaifenesin, and 12.5% alcohol per 5 ml *C-III*

INDICATIONS	ORAL DOSAGE
Cough (nonproductive) accompanying respiratory tract congestion due to colds, influenza, sinusitis, and bronchitis	**Adult:** 5 ml (1 tsp) qid, as needed **Child (25–50 lb):** 1.25 ml (¼ tsp) qid, as needed **Child (50–90 lb):** 2.5 ml (½ tsp) qid, as needed

CONTRAINDICATIONS	
Severe hypertension	
Severe coronary-artery disease	
MAO-inhibitor therapy	
Idiosyncratic reactions to adrenergic agents	Manifested by insomnia, dizziness, weakness, tremors, or arrhythmias
Hypersensitivity	To sympathomimetic amines, phenanthrene derivatives, or any component

WARNINGS/PRECAUTIONS	
Habit-forming	Psychic and/or physical dependence and tolerance may develop, especially in addiction-prone individuals
Drowsiness	Performance of potentially hazardous activities may be impaired; caution patients accordingly
Elderly patients	Sympathomimetic side effects are more likely to occur in patients over 60 yr of age
Special-risk patients	Use with caution in patients with hypertension, diabetes mellitus, ischemic heart disease, hyperthyroidism, increased intraocular pressure, prostatic hypertrophy, or hypersensitivity to ephedrine (see CONTRAINDICATIONS)

ADVERSE REACTIONS[1]	
Gastrointestinal	Upset, nausea, constipation
Central nervous system and neuromuscular	Drowsiness, dizziness, headache, fear, anxiety, tension, restlessness, tremor, weakness, insomnia, hallucinations, convulsions, CNS depression
Cardiovascular	Tachycardia, palpitations, pallor, arrhythmias, cardiovascular collapse with hypotension
Respiratory	Difficult breathing
Genitourinary	Dysuria

OVERDOSAGE	
Signs and symptoms	*Toxic effects primarily attributable to hydrocodone:* respiratory depression, somnolence, stupor, coma, skeletal-muscle flaccidity, cold and clammy skin, bradycardia, hypotension, apnea, circulatory collapse, and cardiac arrest, leading to death
Treatment	**Re-establish adequate airway and institute artificial respiration.** For respiratory depression, administer a narcotic antagonist (eg, naloxone) along with attempts at resuscitation. Empty stomach by emesis or gastric lavage. Employ supportive measures, as indicated.

DRUG INTERACTIONS	
Alcohol, tranquilizers, sedative-hypnotics, and other CNS depressants	⇧ CNS depression
MAO inhibitors	⇧ Blood pressure
Beta-adrenergic blockers	⇧ Sympathomimetic effect
Methylodopa, mecamylamine, reserpine, *Veratrum* alkaloids	⇩ Antihypertensive effect

[1]Including reactions common to sympathomimetic amines in general and to pseudoephedrine in particular

ALTERED LABORATORY VALUES

Blood/serum values	⇧ SGOT ⇧ SGPT
Urinary values	⇧ 5-HIAA (colorimetric interference) ⇧ VMA (colorimetric interference)

Use in children

See INDICATIONS. General guidelines not established for use in children under 25 lb.

Use in pregnancy or nursing mothers

Safe use has not been established during pregnancy. Contraindicated for use in nursing mothers, due to higher than usual risk from sympathomimetic agents for infants; patient should stop breast feeding if drug is prescribed.

TUSSIONEX (Hydrocodone and phenyltoloxamine) Pennwalt

Tabs, caps, susp (per 5 ml): 5 mg hydrocodone and 10 mg phenyltoloxamine *C-III*

INDICATIONS	ORAL DOSAGE
Cough (nonproductive)	**Adult:** 1 tab or cap or 5 ml (1 tsp) q8–12h **Infant (<1 yr):** 1.25 ml (¼ tsp) q12h **Child (1–5 yr):** 2.5 ml (½ tsp) q12h **Child (6–12 yr):** 5 ml (1 tsp) q12h

CONTRAINDICATIONS

None

WARNINGS/PRECAUTIONS

Habit-forming — Psychic and/or physical dependence and tolerance may develop, especially in addiction-prone individuals

ADVERSE REACTIONS

Gastrointestinal — Mild constipation, nausea

Central nervous system — Drowsiness

Dermatological — Facial pruritus

OVERDOSAGE

Signs and symptoms — Respiratory depression, convulsions (sometimes seen in children), hypothermia

Treatment — Immediately empty the stomach. To counteract respiratory depression, use respiratory stimulants. Administer short-acting barbiturates to treat convulsions. Hypothermia can be controlled by usual supportive methods.

DRUG INTERACTIONS

Alcohol, tranquilizers, sedative-hypnotics, and other CNS depressants — ⇧ CNS depression

ALTERED LABORATORY VALUES

No clinically significant alterations in blood/serum or urinary values occur at therapeutic dosages

Use in children

See INDICATIONS. Respiratory depression may be precipitated in children with compromised respiration; young children are especially susceptible to the depressant action of narcotic cough suppressants.

Use in pregnancy or nursing mothers

General guidelines not established

TUSSI-ORGANIDIN DM (Iodinated glycerol, chlorpheniramine maleate, and dextromethorphan hydrobromide) Wallace

Liq: 30 mg iodinated glycerol, 2 mg chlorpheniramine maleate, 10 mg dextromethorphan hydrobromide, and 15% alcohol per 5 ml

INDICATIONS	ORAL DOSAGE
Cough (nonproductive) due to colds or allergic respiratory conditions or accompanying other respiratory-tract conditions (eg, laryngitis, pharyngitis, croup, pertussis, and emphysema)	**Adult:** 5–10 ml (1–2 tsp) q4h **Child:** 2.5–5 ml (½–1 tsp) q4h

CONTRAINDICATIONS

Hypersensitivity to components or related compounds ●	History of marked sensitivity to inorganic iodides ●

WARNINGS/PRECAUTIONS

Drowsiness	Performance of potentially hazardous activities may be impaired; caution patients accordingly
Rash	Discontinue use if evidence of hypersensitivity occurs
Iodism	Dermatitis and other reversible manifestations may occur

ADVERSE REACTIONS

Central nervous system	Drowsiness, sedation, restlessness, dizziness, headache, excitation (particularly in children)
Ophthalmic	Visual disturbances
Gastrointestinal	Dry mouth, nausea, heartburn, GI irritation
Genitourinary	Dysuria, polyuria
Hypersensitivity	Rash
Other	Drying of mucous membranes

OVERDOSAGE

Signs and symptoms	Somnolence, drowsiness, excitation, respiratory depression
Treatment	Induce emesis or use gastric lavage, followed by activated charcoal, to empty stomach. Monitor vital signs and provide supportive measures, as indicated.

DRUG INTERACTIONS

Alcohol, tranquilizers, sedative-hypnotics, and other CNS depressants	⇧ CNS depression

ALTERED LABORATORY VALUES

Blood/serum values	⇧ PBI

No clinically significant alterations in urinary values occur at therapeutic dosages

Use in children	Use in pregnancy or nursing mothers
See INDICATIONS. Antihistamines may produce excitation in children.	General guidelines not established

TUSS-ORNADE (Phenylpropanolamine hydrochloride, chlorpheniramine maleate, caramiphen edisylate, and isopropamide iodide) **Smith Kline & French**

Caps (sust rel): 50 mg phenylpropanolamine hydrochloride, 8 mg chlorpheniramine maleate, 20 mg caramiphen edisylate, and 2.5 mg isopropamide iodide **Liq:** 15 mg phenylpropanolamine hydrochloride, 2 mg chlorpheniramine maleate, 5 mg caramiphen edisylate, 0.75 mg isopropamide iodide, and 7.5% alcohol per 5 ml

INDICATIONS	ORAL DOSAGE
Cough; upper respiratory congestion and hypersecretion associated with colds; **sinusitis; vasomotor rhinitis;** and **allergic rhinitis**[1]	**Adult:** 1 cap q12h or 5–10 ml (1–2 tsp) tid or qid **Child (15–25 lb):** 2.5 ml (½ tsp) tid or qid **Child (>25 lb):** 5 ml (1 tsp) tid or qid

CONTRAINDICATIONS

Hypersensitivity to any of the components ●

Concurrent MAO-inhibitor therapy ●

Severe hypertension ●

Bronchial asthma ●

Coronary-artery disease ●

Stenosing peptic ulcer ●

Pyloroduodenal or bladder-neck obstruction ●

WARNINGS/PRECAUTIONS

Drowsiness	Performance of potentially hazardous activities may be impaired; caution patients accordingly
Special-risk patients	Use with caution in patients with cardiovascular disease, glaucoma, prostatic hypertrophy, or hyperthyroidism

ADVERSE REACTIONS

Central nervous system	Drowsiness, nervousness, insomnia, irritability, dizziness, weakness, headache, incoordination, tremor, convulsions, visual disturbances
Gastrointestinal	Nausea, vomiting, epigastric distress, diarrhea, abdominal pain, anorexia, constipation, parotitis
Dermatological	Rash, acne
Cardiovascular	Angina pain, palpitations, hypertension, hypotension
Respiratory	Excessive dryness of nose, throat, or mouth, tightness in the chest
Genitourinary	Difficulty in urination, dysuria
Hematological	Thrombocytopenia, leukopenia

OVERDOSAGE

Signs and symptoms	Dryness of mouth, dysphagia, thirst, blurred vision, dilated pupils, photophobia, fever, rapid pulse and respiration, disorientation, dizziness, nausea, fainting, tachycardia, CNS excitation or depression
Treatment	Empty stomach by gastric lavage, repeated several times. Administer saline cathartics to hasten evacuation of unused capsules. For respiratory depression, administer oxygen and stimulants. Use a short-acting barbiturate or chloral hydrate to treat marked excitement.

DRUG INTERACTIONS

Alcohol, tranquilizers, sedative-hypnotics, and other CNS depressants	⇧ CNS depression

ALTERED LABORATORY VALUES

Blood/serum values	⇧ PBI ⇩ ^{131}I thyroid uptake

No clinically significant alterations in urinary values occur at therapeutic dosages

Use in children

See INDICATIONS. Contraindicated for use in children less than 15 lb or in children less than 6 mo of age; sustained-release capsules are contraindicated in children under 12 yr of age

Use in pregnancy or nursing mothers

Safe use has not been established during pregnancy or in nursing mothers; lactation may be inhibited

[1] Lacks substantial evidence of effectiveness as a fixed combination for indicated uses

VOXIN-PG (Phenylpropanolamine hydrochloride and guaifenesin) Norwich-Eaton

Tabs: 75 mg phenylpropanolamine hydrochloride and 400 mg guaifenesin

INDICATIONS	ORAL DOSAGE
Respiratory conditions complicated by tenacious mucous plugs and congestion, including sinusitis, pharyngitis, bronchitis, and asthma **Serous otitis media** (adjunctive therapy **Prevention of secondary middle-ear complications of nasopharyngeal congestion accompanying coryza and rhinitis**[1]	**Adult:** 1 tab bid

ADMINISTRATION/DOSAGE ADJUSTMENTS

Oral administration	Tablets may be broken in half to ease administration

CONTRAINDICATIONS

Hypersensitivity to sympathomimetics ●	Severe hypertension ●	MAO-inhibitor therapy ●

WARNINGS/PRECAUTIONS

Special-risk patients	Use with caution in patients with hypertension, hyperthyroidism, diabetes, heart disease, or peripheral vascular disease
Urinary retention	May occur in patients with benign prostatic hypertrophy

ADVERSE REACTIONS

Central nervous system	Stimulation
Genitourinary	Urinary retention

OVERDOSAGE

Signs and symptoms	See ADVERSE REACTIONS
Treatment	Treat symptomatically and institute supportive measures, as required, for at least 12 h after ingestion. Administer a saline cathartic to hasten evacuation of unreleased medication.

DRUG INTERACTIONS

MAO inhibitors	⇧ Sympathomimetic effects

ALTERED LABORATORY VALUES

Urinary values	⇧ 5-HIAA (colorimetric interference)	⇧ VMA (colorimetric interference)

No clinically significant alterations in blood/serum values occur at therapeutic dosages

Use in children	Use in pregnancy or nursing mothers
Not recommended for use in children under 12 yr of age	General guidelines not established

[1]Possibly effective

Composition of Nonprescription Cold, Cough, and Respiratory Allergy Medications

	Antihistamine	Antitussive	Decongestant	Expectorant	Analgesic/Antipyretic	Antibacterial
Afrin Nasal Spray (Schering)			X			
Afrin Nose Drops (Schering)			X			
Afrin Pediatric Nose Drops (Schering)			X			
Alka-Seltzer Plus Tablets (Miles)	X		X		AS	
Allerest (Children's) Chewable Tablets (Pharmacraft)	X		X			
Allerest Nasal Spray (Pharmacraft)			X			
Allerest Tablets (Pharmacraft)	X		X			
Allerest Time Capsules (Pharmacraft)	X		X			
A.R.M. Tablets (Menley & James)	X		X			
Benylin DM Cough Syrup (Parke-Davis)		X				
Benzedrex Inhaler (Menley & James)			X			
Cepacol Lozenges (Merrell-National)[1]						X
Cepacol Troches (Merrell-National)[1]						X
Cheracol D Cough Syrup (Upjohn)		X		X		
Chexit Tablets (Dorsey)	X	X	X	X	AC	
Chloraseptic DM Cough Control Lozenges (Norwich-Eaton)		X				
Chlor-Trimeton Decongestant Tablets (Schering)	X		X			
Chlor-Trimeton Expectorant (Schering)	X		X	X		
Comtrex (Bristol-Myers)	X	X	X		AC	
Conar-A Tablets (Beecham)		X	X	X	AC	
Conar Expectorant (Beecham)		X	X	X		
Conar Suspension (Beecham)		X	X			
Congespirin Chewable Tablets (Bristol-Myers)			X		AS	
Consotuss Antitussive Syrup (Merrell-National)	X	X				
Contac Capsules (Menley & James)	X		X			
Contac Nasal Mist (Menley & James)			X			
Coricidin Cough Syrup (Schering)	X		X	X		
Coricidin Medilets (Schering)	X				AS	
Coricidin Tablets (Schering)	X				AS	
Coryban-D Capsules (Pfipharmecs)	X		X			
Coryban-D Cough Syrup (Pfipharmecs)		X	X	X	AC	
Coricidin D Decongestant Tablets (Schering)	X		X		AS	
CoTylenol Liquid (McNeil)	X	X	X		AC	

Key: X = present in preparation
AS = aspirin
AC = acetaminophen

[1]Also contains an anesthetic

Table continued on following page

Composition of Nonprescription Cold, Cough, and Respiratory Allergy Medications continued

	Antihistamine	Antitussive	Decongestant	Expectorant	Analgesic/Antipyretic	Antibacterial
CoTylenol Tablets (McNeil)	X		X		AC	
Demazin Repetabs (Schering)	X		X			
Demazin Syrup (Schering)	X		X			
Dimacol Capsules (Robins)		X	X	X		
Dimacol Liquid (Robins)		X	X	X		
Dimetane Decongestant Elixir (Robins)	X		X			
Dimetane Decongestant Tablets (Robins)	X		X			
Dorcol Pediatric Cough Syrup (Dorsey)		X	X	X		
Dristan Cough Formula Liquid (Whitehall)	X	X	X	X		
Dristan Nasal Mist (Whitehall)	X		X			
Dristan Tablets (Whitehall)	X		X		AS	
Dristan Time Capsules (Whitehall)	X		X			
Dristan Vapor Mist (Whitehall)	X		X			
Endotussin-NN Pediatric Syrup (Endo)		X		X		
Endotussin-NN Syrup (Endo)	X	X		X		
Ephedrine (various manufacturers)			X			
Fedrazil Tablets (Burroughs Wellcome)	X		X			
Flogesic Tablets (Sandoz)	X		X		AS	
Formula 44 Cough Control Discs (Vicks)		X				
2/G Syrup (Dow)				X		
Listerine Lozenges (Parke-Davis)						X
Naldetuss Syrup (Bristol)	X	X	X		AC	
Neo-Synephrine Compound Tablets (Winthrop)	X		X		AC	
Neo-Synephrine Drops (Winthrop)			X			
Neo-Synephrine Jelly (Winthrop)			X			
Neo-Synephrine Spray (Winthrop)			X			
Neo-Synephrine II Long-Acting Drops (Winthrop)			X			
Neo-Synephrine II Long-Acting Pediatric Drops (Winthrop)			X			
Neo-Syneprine II Long-Acting Spray (Winthrop)			X			
Novafed Liquid (Dow)			X			
Novafed A Liquid (Dow)	X		X			
Novahistine Elixir (Dow)	X		X			
Novahistine Melet Tablets (Dow)	X		X			

Key: X = present in preparation
AS = aspirin
AC = acetaminophen

Table continued on following page

Composition of Nonprescription Cold, Cough, and Respiratory Allergy Medications continued

	Antihistamine	Antitussive	Decongestant	Expectorant	Analgesic/Antipyretic	Antibacterial
Novahistine Sinus Tablets (Dow)	X		X		AC	
Novahistine Tablets (Dow)	X		X			
Novahistine DMX Liquid (Dow)		X	X	X		
Novahistine Fortis Capsules (Dow)	X		X			
Novahistine LP Tablets (Dow)	X		X			
NTZ Nasal Drops (Winthrop)	X		X			
NTZ Nasal Spray (Winthrop)	X		X			
NyQuil Liquid (Vicks)	X	X	X		AC	
Ornade 2 Liquid for Children (Smith Kline & French)	X		X			
Ornex Capsules (Menley & James)			X		AC	
Orthoxicol Cough Syrup (Upjohn)		X	X			
Otrivin (Geigy)			X			
Percogesic Tablets (Endo)	X				AC	
Pertussin Cough Syrup for Children (Chesebrough-Ponds)		X		X		
Pertussin 8 Hour Cough Formula (Chesebrough-Ponds)		X				
Privine Drops (Ciba)			X			
Privine Spray (Ciba)			X			
Quelidrine Syrup (Abbott)	X	X	X	X		
Robitussin Syrup (Robins)				X		
Robitussin-CF Liquid (Robins)		X	X	X		
Robitussin-DM Cough Calmers (Robins)		X		X		
Robitussin-DM Syrup (Robins)		X		X		
Robitussin-PE Syrup (Robins)			X	X		
Romilar CF 8 Hour Formula (Block)		X				
Romilar Children's Cough Syrup (Block)		X				
Romilar III Decongestant Cough Syrup (Block)		X	X			
Sine-off AF Extra Strength Tablets (Menley & James)	X		X			
Sinutab Extra Strength Capsules (Parke-Davis)	X		X		AC	
Sinutab Extra Strength Tablets (Parke-Davis)	X		X		AC	
Sinutab Tablets (Parke-Davis)	X		X		AC	
Sinutab II Tablets (Parke-Davis)			X		AC	
Spec-T Sore Throat/Decongestant Lozenges (Squibb)[1]			X			
Sucrets Lozenges (Beecham)						X

Key: X = present in preparation
AS = aspirin
AC = acetaminophen

[1]Also contains an anesthetic

Table continued on following page

Composition of Nonprescription Cold, Cough, and Respiratory Allergy Medications continued

	Antihistamine	Antitussive	Decongestant	Expectorant	Analgesic/Antipyretic	Antibacterial
Sudafed (Burroughs Wellcome)			X			
Sudafed Cough Syrup (Burroughs Wellcome)		X	X	X		
Sudafed Plus Syrup (Burroughs Wellcome)	X		X			
Sudafed Plus Tablets (Burroughs Wellcome)	X		X			
Symptom 1 Liquid (Parke-Davis)		X				
Triaminic Syrup (Dorsey)	X		X			
Triaminicin Allergy Tablets (Dorsey)	X		X			
Triaminicin Chewable Tablets (Dorsey)	X		X			
Triaminicin Nasal Spray (Dorsey)	X		X			
Triaminicol Cough Syrup (Dorsey)	X	X	X	X		
Trind Syrup (Mead Johnson)		X	X	X	AC	
Trind-DM Syrup (Mead Johnson)			X	X	AC	
Tuamine Sulfate (Lilly)			X			
Tussagesic Suspension (Dorsey)	X	X	X	X	AC	
Tussagesic Time Tablets (Dorsey)	X	X	X	X	AC	
Tussar DM Cough Syrup (Armour)	X	X	X			
Tusscapine Chewable Tablets (Fisons)		X				
Tusscapine Syrup (Fisons)		X				
Vicks Cough Silencer Tablets (Vicks)		X				
Vicks Cough Syrup (Vicks)		X		X		X
Vicks Inhaler (Vicks)			X			
4-Way Cold Tablets (Bristol-Myers)	X		X		AS	

Key: X = present in preparation
AS = aspirin
AC = acetaminophen

Rheumatic Diseases

Arthritis and Gout

Arthritis is an umbrella term used to categorize over 100 diverse diseases of the bones, joints, and muscles that are characterized by swollen, painful joints, stiffness, and—in the more severe forms—limitation of motion and deformity. Although arthritic diseases vary markedly in terms of incidence, cause (which is often unknown in arthritis), and symptoms, each disorder has a common underlying mechanism: inflammation of the affected structure or system. This inflammatory process produces the pain of arthritic disease and is responsible for the breakdown and destruction of tissues, which, if unchecked, can lead to disability.

Most of the drugs described in this chapter are designed to control inflammation, thereby reducing pain and preventing irreversible tissue damage. Indeed, the widespread use of effective and generally safe nonsteroidal anti-inflammatory drugs (of which the most well known is aspirin) has vastly improved the quality of life for people with arthritis. The chronic pain and disability of arthritis can usually be controlled or overcome with the judicious use of drugs, patient education, exercise and rehabilitation, and, in severe cases, with innovative surgical procedures such as prosthetic joint replacement. The following discussion will present a brief overview of the most common types of arthritis and the drugs used to treat them.

RHEUMATOID ARTHRITIS

Rheumatoid arthritis afflicts at least one million Americans and is considered one of the most painful and potentially limiting of the arthritic disorders. It may occur in people of any age or sex, although it is most frequently encountered in women over age forty. Although rheumatoid arthritis does result in disability in some persons, this aspect is often exaggerated; the disease is rarely severe enough to warrant the fear engendered among many newly diagnosed patients. Most cases of rheumatoid arthritis can be controlled with a therapeutic program that includes some type of anti-inflammatory drug. As in many chronic diseases, successful therapy depends upon active patient participation in a program of physical rehabilitation and adjustment of life-style and attitude.

Synovitis, in which the synovium (the tissue that lines the fluid-filled space found in many of the body's joints) is painfully inflamed, is the hallmark of rheumatoid arthritis. This inflammation of the synovial tissue produces the pain, stiffness, reddened overlying skin, and swelling that are typical of the disease. Before a definite diagnosis of rheumatoid arthritis can be established, a number of symptoms and signs (based on standards set by the American Rheumatism Association) must be present. These criteria form an accurate profile of the rheumatoid arthritis patient. They include:

- Unusual stiffness in the morning or after any long period of immobilization.
- Tender joints or painful joint motion.
- Swelling in symmetrical joints (e.g., both wrists, both knees, etc.).

These symptoms must be present for at least six weeks and should be confirmed by typical x-ray and blood tests. Other tests are often performed to rule out disorders that may mimic rheumatoid arthritis, such as gout.

The joints are not the only sites of inflammation in rheumatoid arthritis: Some patients, in addition to joint symptoms, develop small bumps (rheumatic nodules) in characteristic locations. Lymph glands may swell, and cysts that rupture behind the knee (popliteal cysts) are occasionally found. It is important to understand that rheumatoid arthritis is a systemic disease that may involve the heart, lungs, blood vessels, eyes, throat, and other organs.

Rheumatoid arthritis is usually a chronic disease and requires regular therapeutic measures. In many patients, alternating periods of active disease (during which symptoms flare up) and relatively quiescent periods are observed, whereas in a smaller fraction of patients an acute attack may be followed by complete remission.

Juvenile rheumatoid arthritis (Still's disease) presents a somewhat different clinical profile than does rheumatoid arthitis in adults. High fever and skin rash may accompany the synovitis. Eye inflammation, which is often difficult to detect because of the absence of symptoms, can also occur. Complete remission after adolescence is common, although some degree of deformity may persist throughout life.

ANKYLOSING SPONDYLITIS

As in rheumatoid arthritis, the basic disease mechanism in ankylosing spondylitis is chronic inflammation. Spondylitis is much less common than rheumatoid arthritis and is a hereditary ailment that usually afflicts men, generally in young adulthood. The inflammation and degenerative changes occur primarily in the spinal joints; in about 20 percent of patients, the disease affects some large joints (knees, hips, shoulders) as well. The eyes and heart may also be involved.

Spondylitis does not produce synovial inflammation; instead, the inflammatory process affects the connecting ligaments of the spinal vertebrae. If spondylitis goes untreated, these flexible tissues are eroded by the disease, eventually turning to bone (ossification) and fusing the spinal joints—producing a characteristic stiff back and deformity of posture. In severe cases, this loss of spinal flexibility restricts chest wall expansion and contributes to the development of restrictive lung disease due to incomplete exhalation.

Treatment involves a program of anti-inflammatory drugs, spinal exercise, and, if respiration is compromised, deep-breathing exercise.

REITER'S SYNDROME

An acute episode of asymmetrical joint synovitis (i.e., one knee, one ankle), along with inflammation of the eyes, skin, and urinary tract, are the main features of Reiter's syndrome. As in ankylosing spondylitis, the majority of sufferers are young men. Reiter's syndrome is relatively rare, and the exact cause of the disease is unclear, although it is commonly associated with a sexually transmitted infection (usually gonorrhea). Treatment is aimed at decreasing the synovitis and other inflammatory manifestations with anti-inflammatory drugs.

PSORIATIC ARTHRITIS

This form of arthritis is similar in some respects to rheumatoid arthritis, except that bouts of synovitis occur more often in finger joints in an asymmetrical pattern. It is accompanied by psoriasis, a skin disorder characterized by patches of small, reddened bumps (papules), shiny, flaking skin, and pitted nails.

Joint involvement in psoriatic arthritis tends to be less severe than that of rheumatoid arthritis. Both the psoriasis and synovitis are treated with appropriate drugs. One note of caution, however: Antimalarial drugs (second-line agents for arthritis, discussed later in this chapter), sometimes used to treat synovitis, are contraindicated in patients with psoriatic arthritis, since many of these agents can worsen the accompanying skin lesions.

OSTEOARTHRITIS

Osteoarthritis or degenerative joint disease—the most common form of arthritis—is usually not an inflammatory disease. This disorder usually afflicts older people, although it is sometimes seen in the middle-aged and, more rarely, in younger persons.

JOINT CHANGES CHARACTERISTIC OF ARTHRITIS

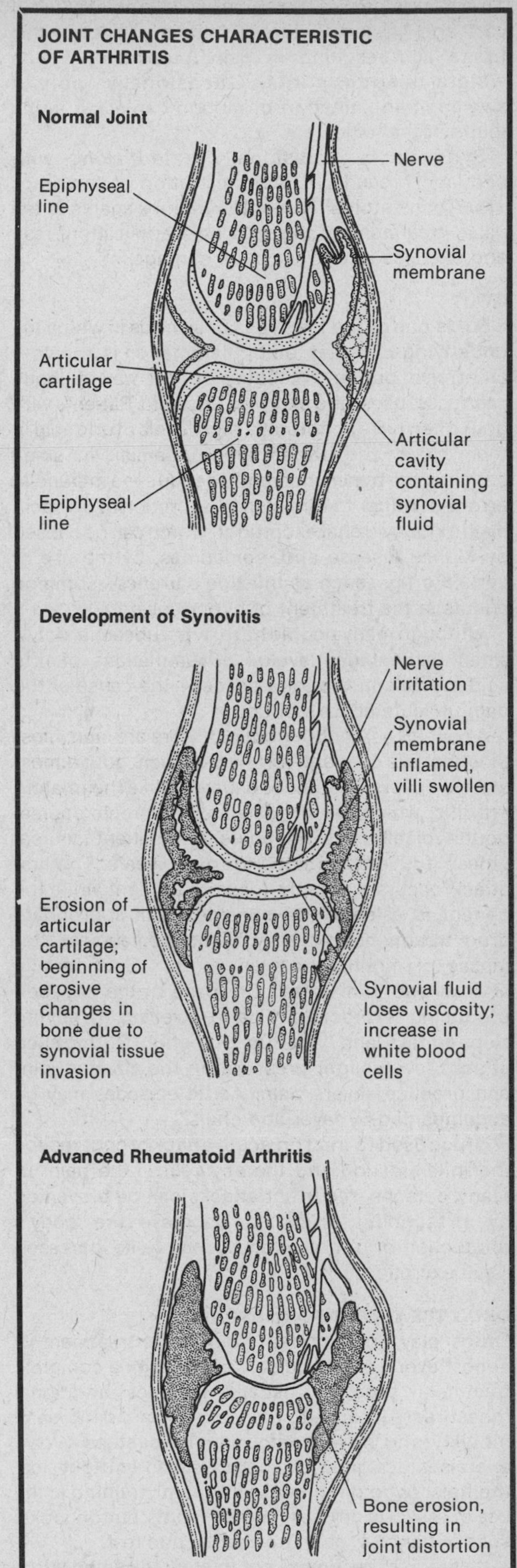

13

The disease causes degeneration and breakdown of cartilage, lessening the cushioning effect of this tissue and resulting in pain, particularly in the weight-bearing joints. Occasionally, painful swelling and limitation of motion can occur in the joints of the hands.

Synovitis is occasionally noted along with cartilage breakdown. Administration of aspirin or other nonsteroidal anti-inflammatory agents is the usual treatment, along with heat application, rest, and exercise to prevent bone damage.

GOUT

Gout is one of the few types of arthritis in which the underlying cause of joint inflammation is known—an error of purine metabolism, or the way the body produces, uses, and excretes uric acid. Patients with gout often have abnormally high levels of uric acid in their blood and urine (hyperuricemia). In some patients, the hyperuricemia is not due to a metabolic error but rather to diminished excretion of uric acid by the kidney (renal excretion), which can be caused by kidney disease and, sometimes, by the use of certain drugs, such as thiazide diuretics—common agents in the treatment of hypertension.

Although many people have hyperuricemia, only a small percentage develop accumulations of uric acid crystals in the joint spaces—the cause of the painful acute attacks of gout.

About 95 percent of gout sufferers are men, most of whom are over age forty. In women, gout almost always occurs after menopause. Unlike rheumatoid arthritis, which usually assumes a chronic course, gout typically has an acute intermittent course, unless it is left untreated for many years. The first attack occurs suddenly (usually at night while the patient is asleep) and subsides with appropriate drug treatment, but may recur, sometimes after lapses of months or even years. Gout usually attacks one joint (often the base of the big toe), producing excruciating pain, swelling, overlying skin redness, and limitation of motion. During such attacks, even slight pressure on the affected joint can produce severe pain. Acute episodes may be accompanied by fever and chills.

Drugs used to treat an acute attack of gout reduce the inflammation and thereby relieve the pain. In many persons, recurrent attacks can be prevented by prescribing drugs to decrease the body's production of uric acid and promote its increased renal excretion.

DRUG TREATMENT FOR ARTHRITIS

Drugs play an important role in the treatment of almost every arthritic disease, although a complete treatment program usually includes additional measures designed to lessen pain, increase mobility, and prevent deformity. These steps involve exercises designed by the physician and physical therapist (who often work as a team), training in the use of assistive devices (canes, splints, buttonhooks, special handles, etc.), hot baths, and rest.

If a joint becomes completely disabled from arthritis, surgical replacement with a prosthetic joint may be possible, particularly for the hip and, to a lesser extent, the knee and finger joints. Moreover, surgical fusion of an unstable joint can eliminate pain and inflammation, but at the expense of full joint motion.

Nonsteroidal Anti-Inflammatory Drugs

In all but the most severe or unusually refractory (unresponsive) cases, physicians rely on anti-inflammatory drugs for their arthritic patients. Sometimes referred to as "first-line" agents, the nonsteroidal anti-inflammatory drugs are used primarily because they are highly effective in many patients, with a relatively low risk of producing side effects. The physician must always balance the anticipated efficacy of the prescribed medication with the concomitant potential for unpleasant—and sometimes dangerous—side effects and toxic reactions. It should be remembered, however, that no drug, including aspirin—the leading antiarthritic medication—is entirely safe. Therefore, untoward effects should always be reported to the physician.

Aspirin (acetylsalicylic acid or ASA) not only reduces the pain and fever of arthritis, but also fights the inflammatory process typical of most arthritic conditions. To accomplish this effect, however, aspirin must be taken in doses considerably higher than those recommended for mild pain or fever. This may involve taking as many as sixteen to twenty tablets, or three to six grams a day.

Aspirin in such high doses can cause unpleasant and sometimes harmful side effects. These include tinnitus (ringing in the ears), heartburn, stomach pain, nausea, and vomiting. Occasionally, stomach bleeding and the development or worsening of gastric ulcer can occur—sometimes without warning symptoms. Other nonsteroidal anti-inflammatory drugs do not cause these problems and may be recommended instead of aspirin. These agents include sulindac (Clinoril), ibuprofen (Motrin), fenoprofen (Nalfon), naproxen (Naprosyn), tolmetin (Tolectin), indomethacin (Indocin), phenylbutazone (Azolid, Butazolidin), oxyphenbutazone (Oxalid, Tandearil), and nonacetylated salicylates. Potential side effects that may occur with this group of drugs include ear problems (salicylates), blood disorders (phenylbutazone and oxyphenbutazone), and fluid retention, which may be dangerous in patients with hypertension or heart disease.

The individual response to these drugs is variable. Therefore, a number of agents may be prescribed in succession before patient and physician agree on the best choice.

Second-Line Drugs

"Second-line" drugs are used when the nonsteroidal anti-inflammatory agents do not provide adequate relief or when their use is contraindicated. They include penicillamine (Cuprimine, Depen), gold salt injections (Myochrysine, Solganal), and antimalarial drugs, such as hydroxychloroquine (Plaquenil Sulfate).

Usually, these drugs are reserved for patients with severe disease; each agent is effective but can cause numerous side effects. Whenever a second-line agent is used, the course of therapy must be followed very closely to monitor adverse effects and adjust dosage accordingly.

Third-Line Drugs

"Third-line" drugs include the corticosteroids and certain suppressors of the immune system, including anticancer drugs. The corticosteroids, a group of chemicals that are naturally produced in very small quantities by the body (mostly in the adrenal glands) are excellent anti-inflammatory agents and highly effective in combating the arthritic disease process. However, their use is associated with a score or more of harmful adverse reactions ranging from edema to psychosis, and their administration, at least in oral form, has become limited to severely ill patients with refractory disease. When oral corticosteroids are given, the physician keeps the dose as low as possible to avoid harmful reactions.

Corticosteroids, such as methylprednisolone (Depo-Medrol) or triamcinolone diacetate (Aristocort), are sometimes injected into severely affected joints (intra-articular corticosteroids) to reduce pain and increase mobility. This allows the patient to perform exercises that both strengthen surrounding muscle and stop joint erosion, helping to prevent deformity. The danger of side effects is much reduced by this method, although joint infection is a risk.

Immunosuppressive agents are sometimes used for patients with severe, life-threatening arthritic disease, such as systemic lupus erythematosus. These agents are considered drugs of last resort for the severely ill patient.

Anti-Gout Drugs

The main goal of drug treatment for gout is the reduction of uric acid levels in the blood and urine, thereby preventing crystal accumulation in the joint space and the resultant synovitis.

Colchicine—a drug derived from a type of crocus plant—is taken during an acute attack to lessen the severity and duration of the episode. It is given in multiple daily doses with a lot of fluid (sometimes one pill each hour for a maximum of six hours) until the gout attack subsides or side effects appear. Unfortunately, relief of joint pain may be accompanied by equally unpleasant diarrhea and cramps. Even so, colchicine is extremely effective in shortening the length of the gout attack.

Probenecid (Benemid and other brand names), allopurinol (Zyloprim), and sulfinpyrazone (Anturane) are given prophylactically (that is, as a preventive measure, even when the patient is asymptomatic) to lessen the number and severity of acute attacks. Most often, these drugs must be taken every day to keep blood uric acid levels within the normal range. They are not recommended for immediate relief of acute attacks, nor are they routinely taken by patients with high uric acid levels who have *not* experienced a gouty episode. Colchicine also may be administered on a regular basis to prevent attacks of gout.

Some special precautions: Since aspirin blocks the effect of probenecid, these two drugs should not be taken together. Allopurinol causes skin rash and stomach upset in a small percentage of patients.

IN CONCLUSION

Most forms of arthritis can be controlled, but this often requires a multifaceted approach that includes drug therapy, rest, exercise, and life-style adjustments. The following drug charts cover the common prescription drugs used in the treatment of arthritis and gout. Aspirin, the most commonly used drug to treat rheumatoid arthritis, is included in the *Pain* section (page 641), as are other nonprescription analgestics used for arthritis pain. The section on *Corticosteroids* (page 1038) lists still other drugs that may be prescribed for refractory arthritis.

BUTAZOLIDIN (Phenylbutazone) Geigy

Tabs: 100 mg

BUTAZOLIDIN ALKA (Phenylbutazone with aluminum hydroxide and magnesium trisilicate) Geigy

Caps: 100 mg phenylbutazone, 100 mg dried aluminum hydroxide gel, and 150 mg magnesium trisilicate

INDICATIONS	ORAL DOSAGE
Rheumatoid arthritis, ankylosing spondylitis, acute attacks of **degenerative joint disease, painful shoulder**	**Adult:** 300–600 mg/day in 3–4 divided doses to start, followed, when improvement is noted, by a prompt reduction to minimum effective level for maintenance, as low as 100–200 mg/day or up to 400 mg/day, if needed
Acute gouty arthritis	**Adult:** 400 mg to start, followed by 100 mg q4h for not more than 1 wk

ADMINISTRATION/DOSAGE ADJUSTMENTS

Initiating therapy	Use only in patients unresponsive to other therapies. Begin therapy only after a careful, detailed history and a complete physical and laboratory examination (including a complete hemogram and urinalysis) have been made. Repeat examinations frequently. Warn patients not to exceed dosage and to immediately report fever, sore throat, skin rashes, dyspepsia, epigastric pain, unusual bleeding, unusual bruising, black or tarry stools, weight gain, or edema.
Duration of therapy	Trial period of 1 wk is adequate to determine therapeutic effect of drug; discontinue in absence of favorable response; aim for short-term use at lowest possible dose
Elderly patients	Not recommended for chronic therapy in patients over 60 yr of age; duration of therapy should not exceed 1 wk, if possible; discontinue if signs of fluid retention develop in patients at risk for cardiac decompensation
Gastric irritation	May be minimized by administering drug immediately before or after meals or with a full glass (8 oz) of milk

CONTRAINDICATIONS

Prior toxicity, sensitivity, or idiosyncratic reaction	To phenylbutazone or oxyphenbutazone
High-risk conditions	Senility, drug allergy, blood dyscrasias, severe renal, hepatic, or cardiac disease, parotitis, stomatitis, polymyalgia rheumatica, temporal arteritis, pancreatitis, incipient cardiac failure, symptoms of GI inflammation or active ulceration, or a history of peptic ulcer disease
Concomitant therapy	With other potent drugs (see DRUG INTERACTIONS)

WARNINGS/PRECAUTIONS

Drug toxicity	Severe or fatal reactions may occur, especially in patients over 40 yr of age; elderly are at greatest risk (see ADMINISTRATION/DOSAGE ADJUSTMENTS)
Upper GI tests	Should be performed in patients with persistent or severe dyspepsia; peptic ulcer (new or reactivated), bleeding, and perforation may occur
Blood dyscrasias	May occur suddenly and sometimes fatally. Perform frequent regular hematologic evaluations in patients receiving drug for >1 wk. Appearance may be delayed weeks after discontinuing therapy. Significant changes in total leukocyte count, relative decrease in granulocytes, appearance of immature cell forms, or fall in hematocrit requires cessation of therapy and full investigation.
Thyroid inhibition	Reduced iodine uptake may occur
Visual disturbances	May be a manifestation of phenylbutazone toxicity; discontinue treatment and perform a complete ophthalmologic workup
Systemic lupus erythematosus	Discontinue drug if symptoms are activated
Mental impairment, reflex-slowing	Performance of potentially hazardous activities may be impaired; caution patients accordingly and about additive effects of alcohol
Leukemia	Causal relationship has not been firmly established, but cases have been reported
Acute asthma attacks	May occur in asthmatic patients
Tartrazine sensitivity	Presence of FD&C Yellow No. 5 (tartrazine) may cause allergic-type reactions, including bronchial asthma, in susceptible individuals

Table continued on following page

ADVERSE REACTIONS	Frequent reactions are italicized
Gastrointestinal	*Distress (3-9%), nausea (1-2%), dyspepsia (1-2%), abdominal discomfort (1-2%),* vomiting, abdominal distention with flatulence, constipation, diarrhea, esophagitis, gastritis, salivary gland enlargement, stomatitis (sometimes with ulceration), ulceration and perforation of the intestinal tract (including acute and reactivated peptic ulcer with perforation, hemorrhage, and hematemesis), anemia from GI bleeding (may be occult), fatal and nonfatal hepatitis (sometimes with cholestasis)
Hematological	Anemia; leukopenia; thrombocytopenia with purpura, petechiae, and hemorrhage; pancytopenia; aplastic anemia; bone-marrow depression; agranulocytosis and agranulocytic anginal syndrome; hemolytic anemia; leukemia (causal relationship not established)
Hypersensitivity	Urticaria, anaphylactic shock, arthralgia, drug fever, hypersensitivity angiitis (polyarteritis) and vasculitis, Lyell's syndrome, serum sickness, Stevens-Johnson syndrome, activation of systemic lupus erythematosus, aggravation of temporal arteritis in patients with polymyalgia rheumatica
Dermatological	*Rash (1-2%),* pruritis, erythema nodosum, erythema multiforme, nonthrombocytopenic purpura
Cardiovascular, fluid and electrolyte	*Edema and water retention (3-9%),* sodium and chloride retention, fluid retention and plasma dilution, cardiac decompensation with edema and dyspnea, metabolic acidosis, respiratory alkalosis, hypertension, pericarditis, interstitial myocarditis with muscle necrosis and perivascular granulomata
Renal	Hematuria, proteinuria, ureteral obstruction with uric acid crystals, anuria, glomerulonephritis, acute tubular necrosis, cortical necrosis, lithiasis, nephrotic syndrome, impairment and failure with azotemia
Central nervous system	Headache, drowsiness, agitation, confusion, lethargy, tremors, numbness, weakness
Metabolic and endocrinological	Hyperglycemia; thyroid hyperplasia, goiter with hyper- and hypothyroidism, and pancreatitis (causal relationship not established)
Ophthalmic	Blurred vision, optic neuritis, toxic amblyopia, scotomata, retinal detachment, retinal hemorrhage, and oculomotor palsy (causal relationship not established)
Otic	Hearing loss, tinnitus

OVERDOSAGE	
Signs and symptoms	Nausea, vomiting, epigastric pain, excessive sweating, euphoria, psychosis, headache, giddiness, vertigo, hyperventilation, insomnia, tinnitus, hearing difficulties, edema, hypertension, cyanosis, respiratory depression, agitation, hallucinations, stupor, convulsions, coma, hematuria, oliguria, respiratory or metabolic acidosis, impaired hepatic or renal function, abnormalities of formed blood elements; *late manifestations of massive overdosage:* hepatomegaly, jaundice, ulceration of buccal or GI mucosa
Treatment	Induce emesis, followed by gastric lavage, to empty stomach. In obtunded patients, secure airway with cuffed endotracheal tube before starting lavage *(do not induce emesis).* Maintain adequate respiratory exchange; avoid respiratory stimulants. Treat shock with supportive measures. Control seizures with IV diazepam or short-acting barbiturates. Dialysis may be helpful if renal function is impaired.

DRUG INTERACTIONS	
Alcohol	⇧ Risk of ulcer
Other anti-inflammatory agents	⇧ Risk of ulcer
Digitoxin	⇩ Serum digitoxin levels
Heparin	⇧ Risk of hemorrhage
Amodiaquine, chloroquine, gold salts, hydroxychloroquine	⇧ Risk of skin toxicity
Insulin	⇧ Hypoglycemia
Sulfonylureas	⇧ Sulfonylurea effect
Sulfonamides	⇧ Sulfonamide effect
Phenytoin	⇧ Phenytoin serum level
Coumarin anticoagulants	⇧ Prothrombin time

[1]Discontinue therapy immediately and do not reinstitute

Table continued on following page

ALTERED LABORATORY VALUES

Blood/serum values	⇧ Sodium	⇩ Chloride	⇧ T_3 uptake	⇩ ^{131}I uptake	⇩ Uric acid
Urinary values	⇧ Protein	⇧ Uric acid			

Use in children

Contraindicated in children under 14 yr of age

Use in pregnancy or nursing mothers

Animal reproduction studies have provided inconclusive evidence of embryotoxicity; therefore, use with caution in pregnancy if drug is deemed essential. Drug may appear in cord blood and breast milk; use with caution in nursing mothers.

CLINORIL (Sulindac) Merck Sharp & Dohme

Tabs: 150, 200 mg

INDICATIONS	ORAL DOSAGE
Osteoarthritis, rheumatoid arthritis,[1] ankylosing spondylitis	**Adult:** 150 mg bid with food to start, followed by up to 400 mg/day, as needed
Acute painful shoulder, acute gouty arthritis	**Adult:** 200 mg bid with food to start, followed by lower doses, as needed

ADMINISTRATION/DOSAGE ADJUSTMENTS	
Duration of therapy in acute conditions	Generally 7–14 days for acute painful shoulder, 1 wk for acute gouty arthritis
Combination therapy	May allow reduction in dosage or elimination of corticosteroids

CONTRAINDICATIONS	
Hypersensitivity	To sulindac or to aspirin and other nonsteroidal, anti-inflammatory agents when manifested by asthma, rhinitis, or urticaria

WARNINGS/PRECAUTIONS	
Peptic ulceration, GI bleeding	May occur or be aggravated; use with extreme caution in patients with a history of upper-GI-tract disease or with active peptic ulcer
Prolonged bleeding time	May occur due to inhibition of platelet function; monitor patients, especially those with coagulation abnormalities
Hepatic impairment	Abnormalities in liver-function tests may occur; if significant, discontinue therapy
Renal damage	Mild renal toxicity (papillary edema, interstitial nephritis) has occurred in animal studies; dosage may need to be reduced to avoid excessive drug accumulation in patients with significant renal impairment
Visual impairment	May occur; perform ophthalmologic testing periodically
Peripheral edema	May occur; use with caution in patients with compromised cardiac function, hypertension, or other conditions predisposing to fluid retention
Corticosteroid therapy	If discontinued, taper dosage gradually over several months to avoid disease flare-up or signs and symptoms of adrenal insufficiency

ADVERSE REACTIONS Frequent reactions are italicized	
Gastrointestinal	*Pain (10%), dyspepsia (3–9%), nausea (3–9%), vomiting (1–3%), diarrhea (3–9%), constipation (3–9%), flatulence (1–3%), anorexia (1–3%), cramps (1–3%),* gastritis or gastroenteritis, peptic ulcer (0.4%), bleeding (0.2%), perforation (rare)
Dermatological	*Rash (3–9%), pruritus (1–3%),* stomatitis, sore or dry mucous membranes, toxic epidermal necrolysis, erythema multiforme, Stevens-Johnson syndrome (rare)
Central nervous system	*Dizziness (3–9%), headache (3–9%), nervousness (1–3%), tinnitus (1–3%),* vertigo, blurred vision, paresthesias, neuritis, transient visual disturbances, decreased hearing, depression psychosis (causal relationship of last six reactions not established)
Hepatic	Jaundice, cholestasis, hepatitis
Hematologic	Thrombocytopenia, leukopenia; bone marrow depression including aplastic anemia (causal relationship not established)
Hypersensitivity	Anaphylaxis, angioneurotic edema, fever, chills, rash, liver function changes, jaundice, leukopenia, eosinophilia
Genitourinary	Vaginal bleeding, hematuria, azotemia (causal relationship not established)
Cardiovascular	Hypertension (causal relationship not established), congestive heart failure, palpitation
Other	*Edema (1–3%),* epistaxis

[1]Safety and effectiveness have not been established for rheumatoid arthritis patients designated by the American Rheumatism Association as Functional Class IV (incapacitated, largely or wholly bedridden or confined to a wheelchair, little or no self-care)

Table continued on following page

OVERDOSAGE

Signs and symptoms	See ADVERSE REACTIONS
Treatment	Induce emesis or use gastric lavage to empty stomach. Observe patient, and give symptomatic and supportive treatment, as needed.

DRUG INTERACTIONS

Oral anticoagulants	Use with caution
Oral hypoglycemics	Use with caution
Aspirin	⇩ Plasma level of active sulfide metabolite of sulindac; do not use concomitantly
Probenecid	⇧ Plasma levels of sulindac and sulfone metabolite ⇩ Uricosuric effect
Alcohol	⇧ Risk of ulcer
Other anti-inflammatory agents	⇧ Risk of ulcer

ALTERED LABORATORY VALUES

Blood/serum values	⇧ Alkaline phosphatase (discontinue if persistent)

No clinically significant alterations in urinary values occur at therapeutic dosages

Use in children

General guidelines not established

Use in pregnancy or nursing mothers

Not recommended during pregnancy; patient should stop nursing if drug is prescribed

CUPRIMINE (Penicillamine) Merck Sharp & Dohme

Caps: 125, 250 mg

INDICATIONS	ORAL DOSAGE
Severe, active rheumatoid arthritis in patients refractory to conventional therapy	**Adult:** 125–250 mg/day, at least 1 h before eating or 1 h apart from other drugs, followed by increases of 125–250 mg/day every 1–3 mo until satisfactory remission occurs or patient has failed to respond to 1,000–1,500 mg/day for 3–4 mo; average maintenance dosage: 500–750 mg/day
Wilson's disease	**Adult:** 250 mg qid, ½–1 h before meals and at bedtime (at least 2 h after evening meal), increased if needed up to 2 g/day **Child:** same as adult
Cystinuria	**Adult:** 250 mg/day at bedtime to start, followed by gradual increases to 1–4 g/day in 4 divided doses; usual maintenance dosage: 2 g/day **Child:** 30 mg/kg/day in 4 divided doses

ADMINISTRATION/DOSAGE ADJUSTMENTS

Rheumatoid arthritis	Response may not be apparent for 2-3 mo after each dosage adjustment
Concomitant antiarthritic therapy	Do not use with gold, antimalarials, immunosuppressives, phenylbutazone, or oxyphenbutazone; salicylates, other nonsteroidal anti-inflammatory drugs, or steroids may be continued or withdrawn gradually; exacerbations may be managed with addition of nonsteroidal anti-inflammatory drugs
Wilson's disease	For patients unable to tolerate 1 g/day to start, therapy may be initiated with 250 mg/day and dosage gradually increased to recommended level. Dosage should be titrated according to urinary copper excretion and therapy monitored every 3 mo according to 24-h copper analysis.
Cystinuria	Individualize dosage to limit cystine excretion to 100–200 mg/day in patients with no history of stones and <100 mg/day in those with stones and/or pain; instruct patients to drink 1 pt of fluid at bedtime and during the night, since greater fluid intake will allow lower dosages

CONTRAINDICATIONS

History of penicillamine-related aplastic anemia or agranulocytosis •

History or evidence of renal insufficiency •

WARNINGS/PRECAUTIONS

Blood dyscrasias	May occur and can be fatal; monitor hemoglobin, WBC, differential count, and direct platelet count every 2 wk for first 6 mo of therapy and monthly thereafter, and instruct patients to report signs such as fever, sore throat, chills, bruising, or bleeding. If WBC falls below 3,500, discontinue therapy; if platelet count falls below 100,000, temporarily suspend therapy.
Renal impairment	May occur; perform routine urinalysis every two weeks for first 6 mo of therapy and monthly thereafter. Proteinuria and/or hematuria may indicate incipient membranous glomerulopathy; if proteinuria exceeds 1 g/24 h or increases progressively, reduce dosage or discontinue therapy; in rheumatoid arthritis patients, if gross hematuria develops or microscopic hematuria persists, discontinue therapy.
Intrahepatic cholestasis and toxic hepatitis	May occur rarely; perform liver-function tests every 6 mo during first 1½ yr of therapy
Goodpasture's syndrome	May occur rarely; if urinary findings are abnormal in conjunction with hemoptysis and pulmonary infiltrates on x-ray, discontinue therapy
Myasthenic syndrome	May occur; discontinue therapy
Pemphigoid-type reactions	May occur; discontinue therapy and treat with corticosteroids
Interruption of therapy in Wilson's disease or cystinuria	May be followed by sensitivity reactions after reinstitution of therapy
Positive ANA test	May occur and may foreshadow development of lupus erythematosus-like syndrome
Oral ulcerations	May occur; reduce dosage or discontinue therapy
Collagen changes	May occur, resulting in increased skin friability at sites subject to pressure or trauma, extravasation of blood, and development of papules at venipuncture and surgical sites; reduce dosage to 250 mg/day prior to surgery and until wound healing is complete
Drug fever	May occur, sometimes accompanied by macular cutaneous eruptions; in Wilson's disease and cystinuria, suspend therapy temporarily and reinstitute at lower dosage level when reaction has subsided; in rheumatoid arthritis, discontinue therapy

Table continued on following page

CUPRIMINE continued

WARNINGS/PRECAUTIONS continued

Dietary supplements	Pyridoxine 25 mg/day is necessary in patients with Wilson's disease or cystinuria and in rheumatoid arthritis patients with impaired nutrition; short courses of iron supplements may be necessary, especially in children and menstruating women
Unwarranted uses	Ankylosing spondylitis

ADVERSE REACTIONS — Frequent reactions are italicized

Allergic	*Early and late rashes (5%);* generalized pruritus; pemphigoid-type reactions; eruptions accompanied by fever, arthralgia, or lymphadenopathy; urticaria; exfoliative dermatitis; thyroiditis (rare); migratory polyarthralgia, often with objective synovitis
Gastrointestinal	*Anorexia (17%), epigastric pain (17%), nausea (17%), vomiting (17%), diarrhea (17%), decreased taste perception (12%),* reactivated peptic ulcer, hepatic dysfunction, cholestatic jaundice, pancreatitis, oral ulcerations, cheilosis, glossitis, gingivostomatitis
Hematological	*Leukopenia (2%), thrombocytopenia (4%),* agranulocytosis, aplastic anemia, thrombocytopenic purpura, hemolytic anemia, red cell aplasia, monocytosis, leukocytosis, eosinophilia, thrombocytosis
Renal	*Proteinuria (6%)* and/or hematuria progressing to nephrotic syndrome, Goodpasture's syndrome
Central nervous system	Tinnitus, optic neuritis (with administration of racemic form)
Dermatological	Elastosis perforans serpiginosa; toxic epidermal necrolysis, anetoderma, increased skin friability, excessive wrinkling, white papules at venipuncture sites
Other	Thrombophlebitis (rare), hyperpyrexia, hair loss, myasthenic syndrome, polymyositis, mammary hyperplasia, allergic alveolitis, obliterative bronchiolitis

OVERDOSAGE

Signs and symptoms	See ADVERSE REACTIONS
Treatment	Treat symptomatically and institute supportive measures, as needed. Reduce dosage or discontinue therapy (see WARNINGS/PRECAUTIONS).

DRUG INTERACTIONS

Gold salts	⇧ Risk of toxicity
Antimalarials	⇧ Risk of toxicity
Cytotoxic drugs	⇧ Risk of toxicity
Phenylbutazone, oxyphenbutazone	⇧ Risk of toxicity

ALTERED LABORATORY VALUES

Urinary values	⇩ Cystine ⇧ Copper ⇧ Zinc ⇧ Mercury ⇧ Lead

No clinically significant alterations in blood/serum values occur at therapeutic dosages

Use in children

See INDICATIONS; efficacy in juvenile rheumatoid arthritis not established

Use in pregnancy or nursing mothers

Contraindicated in pregnant women with rheumatoid arthritis. In pregnant women with Wilson's disease, limit dosage to 1 g/day; if cesarean section is planned, reduce dosage to 250 mg/day during last 6 wk of pregnancy and postoperatively until wound healing is completed. Not recommended for use in pregnant women with cystinuria. General guidelines not established for use in nursing mothers.

DEPEN (Penicillamine) Wallace

Tabs: 250 mg

INDICATIONS	ORAL DOSAGE
Severe, active rheumatoid arthritis in patients refractory to conventional therapy	**Adult:** 125–250 mg/day, at least 1 h before eating or 1 h apart from other drugs, followed by increases of 125–250 mg/day every 1–3 mo until satisfactory remission occurs or patient has failed to respond to 1,000–1,500 mg/day for 3–4 mo; average maintenance dosage: 500–750 mg/day
Wilson's disease	**Adult:** 250 mg qid, ½–1 h before meals and at bedtime (at least 2 h after evening meal); increase if needed up to 2 g/day **Child:** same as adult
Cystinuria	**Adult:** 250 mg/day at bedtime to start, followed by gradual increases to 1–4 g/day in 4 divided doses; usual maintenance dosage: 2 g/day **Child:** 30 mg/kg/day in 4 divided doses

ADMINISTRATION/DOSAGE ADJUSTMENTS

Rheumatoid arthritis	Response may not be apparent for 2–3 mo after each dosage adjustment
Wilson's disease	For patients unable to tolerate 1 g/day to start, therapy may be initiated with 250 mg/day and dosage gradually increased to recommended level. Dosage should be titrated according to urinary copper excretion and therapy monitored every 3 mo according to 24-h copper analysis.
Concomitant antiarthritic therapy	Do not use with gold, antimalarials, immunosuppressives, phenylbutazone, or oxyphenbutazone; salicylates, other nonsteroidal anti-inflammatory drugs, or steroids may be continued or withdrawn gradually; exacerbations may be managed with addition of nonsteroidal anti-inflammatory drugs
Cystinuria	Individualize dosage to limit cystine excretion to 100–200 mg/day in patients with no history of stones and <100 mg/day in those with stones and/or pain; instruct patients to drink 1 pt of fluid at bedtime and during the night, since greater fluid intake will allow lower dosages

CONTRAINDICATIONS

History of penicillamine-related aplastic anemia or agranulocytosis ●	History or evidence of renal insufficiency ●

WARNINGS/PRECAUTIONS

Blood dyscrasias	May occur and can be fatal; monitor hemoglobin, WBC, differential count, and direct platelet count every 2 wk for first 6 mo of therapy and monthly thereafter, and instruct patients to report signs such as fever, sore throat, chills, bruising, or bleeding. If WBC falls below 3,500, discontinue therapy; if platelet count falls below 100,000, temporarily suspend therapy.
Renal impairment	May occur; perform routine urinalysis every two weeks for first 6 mo of therapy and monthly thereafter. Proteinuria or hematuria may indicate incipient membranous glomerulopathy; if proteinuria exceeds 1 g/24 h or increases progressively, reduce dosage or discontinue therapy; in rheumatoid arthritis patients, if gross hematuria develops or microscopic hematuria persists, discontinue therapy.
Intrahepatic cholestasis and toxic hepatitis	May occur rarely; perform liver-function tests every 6 mo during first 1½ yr of therapy
Drug fever	May occur, sometimes accompanied by macular cutaneous eruptions; in Wilson's disease and cystinuria, suspend therapy temporarily and reinstitute at lower dosage level when reaction has subsided; in rheumatoid arthritis, discontinue therapy
Dietary supplements	Pyridoxine 25 mg/day is necessary in patients with Wilson's disease or cystinuria and in rheumatoid arthritis patients with impaired nutrition; short courses of iron supplements may be necessary, especially in children and menstruating women
Unwarranted uses	Ankylosing spondylitis
Goodpasture's syndrome	May occur rarely; if urinary findings are abnormal in conjunction with hemoptysis and pulmonary infiltrates on x-ray, discontinue therapy
Myasthenic syndrome	May occur; discontinue therapy
Pemphigoid-type reactions	May occur; discontinue therapy and treat with corticosteroids
Interruption of therapy in Wilson's disease or cystinuria	May be followed by sensitivity reactions after reinstitution of therapy
Positive ANA test	May occur and may foreshadow development of lupus erythematosus-like syndrome

Table continued on following page

DEPEN continued

WARNINGS/PRECAUTIONS continued

Oral ulcerations	May occur; reduce dosage or discontinue therapy
Collagen changes	May occur, resulting in increased skin friability at sites subject to pressure or trauma, extravasation of blood, and development of papules at venipuncture and surgical sites; reduce dosage to 250 mg/day prior to surgery and until wound healing is complete

ADVERSE REACTIONS — Frequent reactions are italicized

Allergic	*Early and late rashes (5%);* generalized pruritus; pemphigoid-type reactions; eruptions accompanied by fever, arthralgia, or lymphadenopathy; urticaria; exfoliative dermatitis; thyroiditis (rare); migratory polyarthralgia, often with objective synovitis
Gastrointestinal	*Anorexia (17%), epigastric pain (17%), nausea (17%), vomiting (17%), diarrhea (17%), decreased taste perception (12%),* reactivated peptic ulcer, hepatic dysfunction, cholestatic jaundice, pancreatitis, oral ulcerations, cheilosis, glossitis, gingivostomatitis
Hematological	*Leukopenia (2%), thrombocytopenia (4%),* agranulocytosis, aplastic anemia, thrombocytopenic purpura, hemolytic anemia, red cell aplasia, monocytosis, leukocytosis, eosinophilia, thrombocytosis
Renal	*Proteinuria (6%)* and/or hematuria progressing to nephrotic syndrome, Goodpasture's syndrome
Central nervous system	Tinnitus, optic neuritis (with administration of racemic form)
Dermatological	Elastosis perforans serpiginosa, toxic epidermal necrolysis, anetoderma, increased skin friability, excessive wrinkling, white papules at venipuncture sites
Other	Allergic alveolitis, obliterative bronchiolitis

OVERDOSAGE

Signs and symptoms	See ADVERSE REACTIONS
Treatment	Treat symptomatically and institute supportive measures, as needed. Reduce dosage or discontinue therapy (see WARNINGS/PRECAUTIONS).

DRUG INTERACTIONS

Gold salts	⇧ Risk of toxicity
Antimalarials	⇧ Risk of toxicity
Cytotoxic drugs	⇧ Risk of toxicity
Phenylbutazone, oxyphenbutazone	⇧ Risk of toxicity

ALTERED LABORATORY VALUES

Urinary values	⇩ Cystine ⇧ Copper ⇧ Zinc ⇧ Mercury ⇧ Lead

No clinically significant alterations in blood/serum values occur at therapeutic dosages

Use in children

See INDICATIONS; efficacy in juvenile rheumatoid arthritis not established

Use in pregnancy or nursing mothers

Contraindicated in pregnant women with rheumatoid arthritis. In pregnant women with Wilson's disease, limit dosage to 1 g/day; if cesarean section is planned, reduce dosage to 250 mg/day during last 6 wk of pregnancy and postoperatively until wound healing is completed. Not recommended for use in pregnant women with cystinuria. General guidelines not established for use in nursing mothers.

INDOCIN (Indomethacin) **Merck Sharp & Dohme**

Caps: 25, 50 mg

INDICATIONS	ORAL DOSAGE
Moderate to severe **rheumatoid arthritis,** including acute episodes; moderate to severe **ankylosing spondylitis;** moderate to severe **osteoarthritis**	**Adult:** 25 mg bid or tid to start, followed by increases of 25-50 mg/day at weekly intervals, as needed, up to 150-200 mg/day
Acute gouty arthritis	**Adult:** 50 mg tid, as needed

ADMINISTRATION/DOSAGE ADJUSTMENTS

Persistent night pain and/or morning stiffness	Up to 100 mg of the total daily dose may be given at bedtime
Acute flare-ups of chronic rheumatoid arthritis	Increase dosage temporarily by 25-50 mg/day until acute phase is under control. If minor adverse reactions occur, reduce dosage rapidly to a tolerable level. If severe adverse reactions occur, discontinue therapy.
Therapeutic response of acute gouty arthritis	Pain is generally relieved within 2-4 h, tenderness and heat usually subside in 24-36 h, and swelling gradually disappears in 3-5 days. Reduce dosage rapidly until drug is withdrawn completely.
Combination therapy	May allow reduction in dosage or elimination of corticosteroids
Gastric irritation	May be minimized by administering drug after meals, with food, or with antacids

CONTRAINDICATIONS

Nasal polyps associated with angioedema	
Hypersensitivity	To indomethacin or to aspirin and other nonsteroidal, anti-inflammatory agents when manifested by bronchospastic reactions

WARNINGS/PRECAUTIONS

Elderly patients	Are more likely to experience adverse reactions; use with caution
High doses(>150-200 mg/day)	Increase the risk of adverse effects without increasing clinical benefits and are not recommended
GI reactions	Can be severe and even fatal (see ADVERSE REACTIONS); use with extreme caution in patients with a history of recurrent GI lesions or with active GI-tract disease
Ocular-corneal deposits and reticular disturbances (including macular disorders)	May occur without warning after prolonged use; examine eyes periodically, especially if blurred vision occurs
Psychiatric disturbances, epilepsy, and parkinsonism	May be aggravated; if CNS reactions are severe, discontinue therapy
Drowsiness	Performance of potentially hazardous activities may be impaired; caution patients accordingly
Headache	Reduce dosage; if headache persists, discontinue therapy
Infection	Signs and symptoms may be masked
Prolonged bleeding time	May occur due to inhibition of platelet aggregation; use with caution in patients with coagulation defects or in those on anticoagulant therapy
Severe renal impairment	May worsen; use with caution
Acute renal failure	May occur in patients with sodium retention associated with hepatic disease or congestive heart failure

ADVERSE REACTIONS	Frequent reactions are italicized
Central nervous system and neuromuscular	*Headache (>10%), dizziness (3-9%),* vertigo, somnolence, depression and fatigue, anxiety, muscle weakness, involuntary muscle activity, insomnia, muzziness, psychic disturbances, mental confusion, drowsiness, lightheadedness, syncope, parasthesias, aggravation of epilepsy and parksinsonism, depersonalization, coma, peripheral neuropathy, convulsions

Table continued on following page

INDOCIN continued

ADVERSE REACTIONS continued

Otic	*Tinnitus (1-2%)*, hearing disturbances, deafness
Gastrointestinal	*Nausea (with or without vomiting) (3-9%), dyspepsia (indigestion, heartburn, epigastric pain) (3-9%)*, diarrhea, abdominal distress or pain, constipation, anorexia, bloating, flatulence, peptic ulcer, gastroenteritis, rectal bleeding, proctitis, perforation and hemorrhage of the esophagus, stomach, duodenum, or small intestine, intestinal ulceration associated with stenosis and obstruction, bleeding without obvious ulceration, perforation of pre-existing sigmoid lesions, ulcerative colitis, regional ileitis, ulcerative stomatitis
Cardiovascular	Hypertension, tachycardia, chest pain, arrhythmia, palpitations
Dermatological	Pruritus, rash, urticaria, petechiae or ecchymosis, exfoliative dermatitis, erythema nodosum, hair loss
Hepatic	Toxic hepatitis, jaundice
Ophthalmic	Ocular-corneal deposits, retinal disturbances (including macular disturbances), blurred vision
Hematological	Leukopenia, bone-marrow depression anemia secondary to GI bleeding, aplastic or hemolytic anemia, agranulocytosis, thrombocytopenic purpura; leukemia (causal relationship not established)
Metabolic and endocrinological	Edema, weight gain, flushing or sweating, hyperglycemia, glycosuria, hyperkalemia; breast tenderness and/or enlargement (causal relationship not established)
Genitourinary	Hematuria, vaginal bleeding, urinary frequency (causal relationship not established)
Hypersensitivity	Acute respiratory distress, shock-like hypotension, angioedema, dyspnea, asthma, purpura, angiitis
Other	Epistaxis

OVERDOSAGE

Signs and symptoms	See ADVERSE REACTIONS
Treatment	Immediately discontinue drug; treat symptomatically and institute supportive measures, as indicated

DRUG INTERACTIONS

Aspirin	⇩ Indomethacin plasma level ⇧ GI side effects
Probenecid	⇧ Indomethacin plasma level
Furosemide	⇩ Natriuretic effect ⇩ Antihypertensive effect
Lithium	⇧ Plasma lithium level

ALTERED LABORATORY VALUES

Blood/serum values	⇧ Glucose ⇧ BUN ⇧ Potassium
Urinary values	⇧ Glucose

Use in children

Not recommended for children under 14 yr of age unless lack of efficacy or toxicity of other drugs warrants the risk; such patients should be closely monitored

Use in pregnancy or nursing mothers

Not recommended; retarded fetal ossification has been noted in animal reproductive studies at a dosage of 4.0 mg/kg/day. Drug is excreted in human breast milk.

MECLOMEN (Meclofenamate sodium) Parke-Davis

Caps: equivalent to 50 or 100 mg meclofenamic acid

INDICATIONS	ORAL DOSAGE
Acute and chronic rheumatoid arthritis[1] and osteoarthritis	**Adult:** 200–400 mg/day in 3–4 equally divided doses; optimum therapeutic benefit may not be obtained for 2–3 wk

ADMINISTRATION/DOSAGE ADJUSTMENTS

Gastrointestinal complaints	Diarrhea. irritation. or abdominal pain may be minimized by administering meclofenamate with meals; concomitant use of an antacid (ie. aluminum or magnesium hydroxide) does not interfere with absorption of the drug
Initiating therapy of arthritis	Meclofenamate is not recommended as the initial drug for treatment because of gastrointestinal side effects (see ADVERSE REACTIONS)

CONTRAINDICATIONS

Hypersensitivity	To meclofenamate or to aspirin or other nonsteroidal and inflammatory drugs, when manifested by bronchospasm, allergic rhinitis, or urticaria

WARNINGS/PRECAUTIONS

Peptic ulceration, GI bleeding	May occur and can be severe or even fatal (one case); use with extreme caution in patients with a history of upper GI-tract disease
Diarrhea, GI irritation, abdominal pain	May occur; reduce dosage or temporarily discontinue use
Long-term therapy	Determine hemoglobin and hematocrit values if anemia is suspected
Opthalmic studies	Should be performed if visual symptoms develop; adverse eye findings have been reported in animal studies with other nonsteroidal anti-inflammatory drugs
Corticosteroid therapy	If discontinued, reduce dosage gradually to avoid possible complications
Persistent leukopenia	May occur (rarely) and warrants further clinical evaluation

ADVERSE REACTIONS

	Frequent reactions are italicized
Gastrointestinal	*Diarrhea (10–33%), nausea with or without vomiting (11%), other GI disorders (10%), abdominal pain (3–9%), pyrosis (3–9%), flatulence (3–9%), anorexia (1–3%), constipation (1–3%), stomatitis (1–3%), peptic ulcer (1–3%),* bleeding without ulcer
Cardiovascular	*Edema (1–3%),* palpitations (causal relationship not established)
Dermatological	*Rash (3–9%), urticaria (1–3%), pruritus (1–3%)*
Central nervous system	*Headache (3–9%), dizziness (3–9%), tinnitus (1–3%),* malaise, fatigue, paresthesia, insomnia, depression, blurred vision (causal relationship not established for last six)
Other	Nocturia, taste disturbances (causal relationship not established)

OVERDOSAGE

Signs and symptoms	See ADVERSE REACTIONS
Treatment	Empty stomach by emesis or gastric lavage, followed by activated charcoal. Institute supportive measures and careful monitoring. Hemodialysis and peritoneal dialysis are of little value.

DRUG INTERACTIONS

Warfarin	⇧ Anticoagulant effect
Aspirin	⇧ Fecal blood loss ⇩ Plasma meclofenamate level

ALTERED LABORATORY VALUES

Blood/serum values	⇧ Transaminase ⇧ Alkaline phosphatase ⇧ BUN ⇧ Creatinine

No clinically significant alterations in urinary values occur at therapeutic dosages

Use in children

Safety and efficacy not established in children under 14 yr of age

Use in pregnancy or nursing mothers

Not recommended for use during pregnancy, particularly the 1st and 3rd trimesters, because of potential risk to the fetus; not recommended for use in nursing mothers.

[1]Safety and efficacy not established in patients with rheumatoid arthritis who are designated by the American Rheumatism Association as Functional Class IV (incapacitated, largely or wholly bedridden or confined to a wheelchair, little or no self-care)

MOTRIN (Ibuprofen) **Upjohn**

Tabs: 300, 400, 600 mg

INDICATIONS	ORAL DOSAGE
Rheumatoid arthritis,[1] osteoarthritis	**Adult:** 300–600 mg tid or qid
Mild to moderate pain	**Adult:** 400 mg q4–6h, as needed, up to 2,400 mg/day

ADMINISTRATION/DOSAGE ADJUSTMENTS

Rheumatoid arthritis	Higher doses than for osteoarthritis may be required
Therapeutic response	May not be observed for up to 2 wk, after which optimal dosage should be determined
Gastric irritation	May be minimized by administering drug with meals or milk
Combination therapy	Additional symptomatic relief has been obtained in combination with gold salts. Neither benefits nor harmful interactions have been demonstrated with corticosteroids. Use with salicylates is not recommended.

CONTRAINDICATIONS

Hypersensitivity	To ibuprofen or to aspirin and other nonsteroidal, anti-inflammatory drugs when manifested by nasal polyps, angioedema, or bronchospasm

WARNINGS/PRECAUTIONS

Anaphylactoid reactions	May occur in patients hypersensitive to aspirin (see CONTRAINDICATIONS)
Peptic ulceration, perforation, GI bleeding	May occur and can be severe or even fatal; use with extreme caution in patients with a history of upper-GI-tract disease or with active peptic ulcer
Ophthalmic changes	May occur (see ADVERSE REACTIONS); discontinue drug and perform ophthalmologic testing, including examination of central fields
Fluid retention and edema	May occur; use with caution in patients with a history of cardiac decompensation
Prolonged bleeding time	May occur due to inhibition of platelet aggregation; use with caution in patients with coagulation defects or with those on anticoagulant therapy
Corticosteroid therapy	If discontinued, reduce dosage gradually to avoid complications of sudden steroid withdrawal

ADVERSE REACTIONS
Frequent reactions are italicized

Gastrointestinal	*Nausea (3–9%), epigastric pain (3–9%), heartburn (3–9%), diarrhea (1–2%), abdominal distress (1–2%), nausea and vomiting (1–2%), indigestion (1–2%), constipation (1–2%), abdominal cramps or pain (1–2%), bloating and flatulence (1–2%),* gastric or duodenal-ulcer bleeding and/or perforation, GI hemorrhage, melena
Hepatic	Hepatitis, jaundice, abnormal liver function (causal relationship of these reactions not established)
Central nervous system	*Dizziness (3–9%), headache (1–2%), nervousness (1–2%),* depression, insomnia, hallucinations, paresthesias, dream abnormalities (causal relationship of last three reactions not established)
Ophthalmic	Blurred and/or diminished vision, scotomata, changes in color vision, conjunctivitis, diplopia, optic neuritis (causal relationship of last three reactions not established)
Otic	*Tinnitus (1–2%)*
Dermatological	*Rash (including maculopapular rash) (3–9%), pruritus (1–2%),* vesiculobullous eruptions, urticaria, erythema multiforme, alopecia, Stevens-Johnson syndrome (causal relationship of last two reactions not established)

[1]Safety and effectiveness have not been established for rheumatoid arthritis patients designated by the American Rheumatism Association as Functional Class IV (incapacitated, largely or wholly bedridden or confined to a wheelchair; little or no self-care).

Table continued on following page

ADVERSE REACTIONS continued

Metabolic and endocrinological	*Decreased appetite (1-2%), edema (1-2%), fluid retention (1-2%)*, gynecomastia, hypoglycemia (causal relationship of last two reactions not established)
Cardiovascular	Congestive heart failure in patients with marginal cardiac function, elevated blood pressure, arrhythmias (causal relationship of last reaction not established)
Hematological	Leukopenia, decreased hemoglobin and hematocrit, hemolytic anemia, thrombocytopenia, granulocytopenia, bleeding episodes (causal relationship of last four reactions not established)
Renal	Decreased creatinine clearance, polyuria, azotemia (causal relationship of these reactions not established)
Allergic	Fever, serum sickness, lupus erythematosus syndrome (causal relationship of these reactions not established)

OVERDOSAGE

Signs and symptoms	Apnea, cyanosis, dizziness, nystagmus
Treatment	Following recent ingestion (<1 h), remove drug by induced emesis or gastric lavage. Activated charcoal may be helpful. If drug is already absorbed, it may be useful to induce diuresis and alkalinize the urine.

DRUG INTERACTIONS

Coumarin anticoagulants	⇧ Risk of bleeding; use with caution
Aspirin	⇩ Anti-inflammatory activity (potential)

ALTERED LABORATORY VALUES

No clinically significant alterations in blood/serum or urinary values occur at therapeutic dosages

Use in children	Use in pregnancy or nursing mothers
Safety and effectiveness have not been established	Not recommended

MYOCHRYSINE (Gold sodium thiomalate) Merck Sharp & Dohme

Amps: 10, 25, 50, 100 mg/ml (1 ml) **Vial:** 50 mg/ml (10 ml)

INDICATIONS	PARENTERAL DOSAGE
Active rheumatoid arthritis (adjunctive therapy)	**Adult:** 10 mg IM (preferably intragluteally), followed in 1 wk by 25 mg IM, and subsequently by 25–50 mg/wk IM until toxicity or major improvement occurs or total cumulative dose reaches 1 g; for maintenance: 25–50 mg IM every 2 wk for 2–20 wk, followed by 25–50 mg IM every 3–4 wk **Child:** 10 mg IM (preferably intragluteally), followed by 1 mg/kg/wk IM up to 50 mg/dose; other guidelines: same as for adult

ADMINISTRATION/DOSAGE ADJUSTMENTS

Position during injections	Patient should be lying down and should remain recumbent for 10 min after injection
Failure of initial therapy	Discontinue therapy, continue 25–50 mg/wk for 10 wk, or increase dose by 10 mg every 1–4 wk, up to 100 mg/dose
Exacerbations during maintenance therapy	Resume weekly injections until disease activity is suppressed

CONTRAINDICATIONS

Previous toxicity from gold or other heavy metals ●	Severe debilitation ●	Systemic lupus erythematosus ●
Sjögren's syndrome in rheumatoid arthritis ●		

WARNINGS/PRECAUTIONS

Hematological, renal, and dermatological toxicity	May occur; obtain baseline hemoglobin, erythrocyte, WBC, differential, and platelet counts and urinalysis; analyze urine for protein and sediment changes prior to each injection and repeat complete blood and platelet counts before every second injection, and whenever purpura or ecchymoses develop. If hemoglobin drops rapidly, WBC falls below 4,000, platelet count falls below 100,000, or albuminuria, hematuria, pruritus, skin eruption, or stomatitis develops, discontinue therapy until another cause of abnormality can be determined.
Special-risk patients	Use with caution in patients with history of drug-related blood dyscrasias, allergy, or hypersensitivity; skin rashes; previous kidney or liver disease; marked hypertension; or compromised cerebral or cardiovascular circulation
Diabetes mellitus, congestive heart failure	Must be under control before instituting gold therapy
Pruritus	May occur as a warning signal of impending dermatological reaction (see ADVERSE REACTIONS)
Metallic taste	May occur as warning signal of impending oral mucous membrane reactions (see ADVERSE REACTIONS)

ADVERSE REACTIONS

Dermatological	Dermatitis, pruritus, exfoliative dermatitis (aggravated by sunlight) leading to alopecia and nail shedding, actinic rash
Mucous membrane	Stomatitis, buccal ulceration, glossitis, gingivitis
Renal	Nephrotic syndrome, glomerulitis with hematuria
Hematological	Granulocytopenia, thrombocytopenia (with or without purpura), hypoplastic and aplastic anemia
Nitritoid and allergic	Flushing, fainting, dizziness, sweating, anaphylactic shock, syncope, bradycardia, swallowing difficulty and angioneurotic edema
Gastrointestinal	Nausea, vomiting, anorexia, abdominal cramps, diarrhea, ulcerative enterocolitis
Ophthalmological	Iritis, corneal ulcers, gold deposits in ocular tissues, conjunctivitis (rare)
Other	Hepatitis with jaundice, peripheral neuritis, gold bronchitis, interstitial pneumonitis and fibrosis, alopecia, fever, arthralgia

Table continued on following page

MYOCHRYSINE continued

OVERDOSAGE	
Signs and symptoms	See ADVERSE REACTIONS
Treatment	Discontinue treatment immediately. Severe dermatitis or stomatitis may benefit from prednisone 10-40 mg/day div. Less severe skin and mucous-membrane reactions often benefit from topical corticosteroids, oral antihistaminics, or anesthetic lotions. For serious renal, hematological, pulmonary, and enterocolitic complications, high doses of systemic corticosteroids (40-100 mg/day prednisone div) are recommended. The chelating agent dimercaprol may be given in addition to corticosteroids to enhance gold excretion in patients who do not improve on steroids alone, but careful monitoring is required.

DRUG INTERACTIONS	
Antimalarial agents	⇧ Risk of toxicity
Immunosuppressives	⇧ Risk of toxicity
Phenylbutazone, oxyphenbutazone	⇧ Risk of toxicity
Penicillamine	⇧ Risk of toxicity
Other dermatitis-causing drugs	⇧ Risk of skin reactions

ALTERED LABORATORY VALUES	
Blood/serum values	⇧ or ⇩ PBI

No clinically significant alterations in urinary values occur at therapeutic dosages

Use in children

See INDICATIONS

Use in pregnancy or nursing mothers

Contraindicated for pregnancy; general guidelines not established for use in nursing mothers

NALFON (Fenoprofen calcium) Dista

Caps: 300 mg **Tabs:** 600 mg

INDICATIONS	ORAL DOSAGE
Rheumatoid arthritis **Osteoarthritis**	**Adult:** 300–600 mg tid or qid, or up to 3,200 mg/day, if needed

ADMINISTRATION/DOSAGE ADJUSTMENTS	
Timing of administration	Since food decreases fenoprofen blood levels, administer 30 min before or 2 h after meals; if gastrointestinal complaints occur, administer with meals or milk
Combination therapy	Neither benefits nor harmful interactions have been demonstrated with gold salts or corticosteroids. Concomitant therapy with salicylates is not recommended; aspirin may increase excretion rate of fenoprofen, and no additional benefit is obtained beyond the effect of aspirin alone.

CONTRAINDICATIONS	
Hypersensitivity	To fenoprofen or to aspirin and other nonsteroidal, anti-inflammatory drugs when manifested by asthma, rhinitis, or urticaria
Significantly impaired renal function	Drug may accumulate, since it is eliminated primarily by the kidneys

WARNINGS/PRECAUTIONS	
Peptic ulcer, perforation, GI bleeding	May occur and can be severe; use with extreme caution in patients with a history of upper-GI-tract disease or with active peptic ulcer
Genitourinary tract problems	Have been reported (see ADVERSE REACTIONS); do not use in patients who have had such reactions with other nonsteroidal anti-inflammatory drugs. In patients with possibly compromised renal function, examine renal function periodically.
Liver function	Test periodically for alterations (see ALTERED LABORATORY VALUES); discontinue therapy if significant abnormalities appear
Corticosteroid therapy	If discontinued, reduce dosage gradually to avoid complications of sudden steroid withdrawal
Initial low hemoglobin values	Obtain periodic hemoglobin determinations during long-term therapy
Peripheral edema	May occur; use with caution in patients with compromised cardiac function or hypertension
Prolonged bleeding time	May occur due to inhibition of platelet aggregation
Impaired hearing	Monitor auditory function periodically
Mental impairment	Performance of potentially hazardous activities may be impaired; caution patients accordingly
Visual impairment	May occur with some nonsteroidal anti-inflammatory drugs; perform ophthalmologic studies periodically

ADVERSE REACTIONS	Frequent reactions are italicized
Gastrointestinal	*Dyspepsia (3-9%), constipation (3-9%), nausea (3-9%), vomiting (3-9%), abdominal pain (1-2%), anorexia (1-2%), occult blood loss (1-2%), diarrhea (1-2%), flatulence (1-2%), dry mouth (1-2%),* gastritis, peptic ulcer with or without perforation and/or GI hemorrhage; aphthous ulcerations or the buccal mucosa, metallic taste, and pancreatitis (causal relationship not established)
Hepatic	Jaundice, cholestatic hepatitis
Central nervous system	*Headache (15%), somnolence (15%), dizziness (3-9%), nervousness (3-9%), asthenia (3-9%), tremor (1-2%), confusion (1-2%), insomnia (1-2%), fatigue (1-2%), malaise (1-2%);* depression, disorientation, seizures, trigeminal neuralgia, and personality change (causal relationship not established)
Dermatological	*Pruritus (3-9%), rash (1-2%), increased sweating (1-2%), urticaria (1-2%);* Stevens-Johnson syndrome, angioneurotic edema, exfoliative dermatitis, and alopecia (causal relationship not established)
Cardiovascular	*Palpitations (3-9%), tachycardia (1-2%);* atrial fibrillation, pulmonary edema, ECG changes, and supraventricular tachycardia (causal relationship not established)
Ophthalmic	*Blurred vision (1-2%);* diplopia and optic neuritis (causal relationship not established)
Otic	*Tinnitus (1-2%), decreased hearing (1-2%)*
Genitourinary	Dysuria, cystitis, hematuria, oliguria, azotemia, anuria, allergic nephritis, nephrosis, papillary necrosis

Table continued on following page

NALFON continued

ADVERSE REACTIONS continued

Hematological	Purpura, bruising, hemorrhage, thrombocytopenia, hemolytic anemia, agranulocytosis, pancytopenia; aplastic anemia (causal relationship not established)
Other	*Dyspnea (1-2%)*, peripheral edema, anaphylaxis; lymphadenopathy, mastodynia, and fever (causal relationship not established)

OVERDOSAGE

Signs and symptoms	See ADVERSE REACTIONS
Treatment	Induce emesis or use gastric lavage to empty stomach, followed by activated charcoal. Employ supportive measures, as indicated. Urinary alkalinization and forced diuresis may be helpful. Furosemide does *not* lower blood levels of fenoprofen.

DRUG INTERACTIONS

Albumin-bound drugs	Displacement of either drug
Hydantoins	⇧ Hydantoin plasma level; observe for signs of toxicity
Sulfonamides	⇧ Sulfonamide plasma level; observe for signs of toxicity
Sulfonylureas	⇧ Sulfonylurea plasma level; observe for signs of toxicity
Coumarin anticoagulants	⇧ Prothrombin time; observe patient carefully
Aspirin	⇩ Plasma half-life of fenoprofen; do not use concomitantly
Phenobarbital	⇩ Plasma half-life of fenoprofen; if necessary, adjust fenoprofen dosage

ALTERED LABORATORY VALUES

Blood/serum values	⇧ Alkaline phosphatase ⇧ SGOT ⇧ Lactate dehydrogenase ⇧ BUN

No clinically significant alterations in urinary values occur at therapeutic dosages

Use in children

Safety and effectiveness have not been established

Use in pregnancy or nursing mothers

Not recommended due to lack of proof that use is safe in pregnant patients and nursing mothers

NAPROSYN (Naproxen) Syntex

Tabs: 250, 375 mg

INDICATIONS	ORAL DOSAGE
Rhematoid arthritis,[1] osteoarthritis	**Adult:** 250–375 mg bid (in AM and PM)
Mild to moderate pain, dysmenorrhea	**Adult:** 500 mg to start, followed by 250 mg q6–8h, as needed; maximum daily dose: 1250 mg

ADMINISTRATION/DOSAGE ADJUSTMENTS	
Therapeutic response	Should be observed within 2 wk ; in some patients, symptomatic improvement may not be seen for up to 4 wk
Combination therapy	Added benefits in arthritis have not been demonstrated with corticosteroids; however, use with gold salts has resulted in greater improvement. Use with salicylates is not recommended. Use with related drug naproxen sodium not recommended.
Adrenal function tests	Discontinue naproxen therapy 72 h prior to testing

CONTRAINDICATIONS	
Hypersensitivity	To naproxen or aspirin and other nonsteroidal, anti-inflammatory drugs when manifested by asthma, rhinitis, or urticaria

WARNINGS/PRECAUTIONS	
Peptic ulcer, perforation, GI bleeding	May occur and can be severe or even fatal; use with caution in patients with a history of upper-GI-tract disease or with active peptic ulcer
Renal damage	High doses have caused nephritis in animal studies; use with great caution in patients with significant renal functional impairment, and monitor serum creatinine and/or creatinine clearance periodically
Corticosteroid therapy	If discontinued, reduce dosage gradually to avoid complications of sudden steroid withdrawal
Impaired vision	May occur with some nonsteroidal antiinflammatory drugs; perform ophthalmologic studies periodically
Drowsiness, dizziness, vertigo, depression	Performance of potentially hazardous activities may be impaired; caution patients accordingly
Peripheral edema	May occur, especially in patients with questionable or compromised cardiac function
Prolonged bleeding time	May occur due to inhibition of platelet aggregation; use with caution in patients with coagulation defects or in those on anticoagulant therapy
Initial low hemoglobin values (≤10 g)	Obtain periodic hemoglobin determinations during long-term therapy

ADVERSE REACTIONS[2]	Frequent reactions are italicized
Gastrointestinal (14%)	*Heartburn, nausea, dyspepsia, abdominal pain, constipation, stomatitis, diarrhea, vomiting, melena, bleeding,* peptic ulceration; jaundice (rare)
Central nervous system (8.3%)	*Headache, drowsiness, dizziness, lightheadedness, vertigo, inability to concentrate, depression*
Dermatological (5%)	*Pruritus, skin eruptions, sweating, ecchymoses, rashes, urticaria, purpura*
Cardiovascular (2%)	*Edema, palpitations, dyspnea*
Other	*Tinnitus (5%), visual and hearing disturbances (5%), thirst (1%);* angioneurotic edema, thrombocytopenia, agranulocytosis (rare)

[1]Safety and effectiveness have not been established for rheumatoid arthritis patients designated by the American Rheumatism Association as Functional Class IV (incapacitated, largely or wholly bedridden or confined to a wheelchair, little or no self-care)

[2]Adverse reactions are 2–10 times more frequent in patients treated for arthritis than for pain or dysmenorrhea

Table continued on following page

NAPROSYN continued

OVERDOSAGE

Signs and symptoms	See ADVERSE REACTIONS
Treatment	Induce emesis or use gastric lavage to empty stomach, and institute supportive measures. Activated charcoal may be helpful

DRUG INTERACTIONS

Albumin-bound drugs	Displacement of either drug
Coumarin anticoagulants	⇧ Prothrombin time
Hydantoins	⇧ Hydantoin plasma level
Sulfonylureas	⇧ Sulfonylurea plasma level
Sulfonamides	⇧ Sulfonamide plasma level
Aspirin	⇧ Excretion of naproxen
Probenecid	⇧ Naproxen plasma half-life

ALTERED LABORATORY VALUES

Blood/serum values	⇧ BUN
Urinary values	⇧ 17-Ketogenic steroids Interference with 5-HIAA

Use in children

Safety and effectiveness have not been established

Use in pregnancy or nursing mothers

Not recommended; naproxen readily crosses the placental barrier and appears in breast milk at a concentration of 1% of that in the maternal plasma

TANDEARIL (Oxyphenbutazone) Geigy

Tabs: 100 mg

INDICATIONS	ORAL DOSAGE
Rheumatoid arthritis, ankylosing spondylitis, acute attacks of **degenerative joint disease, painful shoulder**	**Adult:** 300–600 mg/day in 3–4 divided doses to start, followed, when improvement is noted, by a prompt reduction to minimum effective level for maintenance, as low as 100–200 mg/day or up to 400 mg/day, if needed
Acute gouty arthritis	**Adult:** 400 mg to start, followed by 100 mg q4h for not more than 1 wk

ADMINISTRATION/DOSAGE ADJUSTMENTS	
Initiating therapy	Use only in patients unresponsive to other therapies. Begin therapy only after a careful, detailed history and a complete physical and laboratory examination (including a complete hemogram and urinalysis) have been made. Repeat examinations frequently. Warn patients not to exceed dosage and to immediately report fever, sore throat, skin rashes, dyspepsia, epigastric pain, unusual bleeding, unusual bruising, black or tarry stools, weight gain, or edema.
Duration of therapy	Trial period of 1 wk is adequate to determine therapeutic effect of drug; discontinue in absence of favorable response; aim for short-term use at lowest possible dose
Elderly patients	Not recommended for chronic therapy in patients over 60 yr of age; duration of therapy should not exceed 1 wk, if possible; discontinue if signs of fluid retention develop in patients at risk for cardiac decompensation
Gastric irritation	May be minimized by administering drug immediately before or after meals or with a full glass (8 oz) of milk

CONTRAINDICATIONS	
Prior toxicity, sensitivity, or idiosyncratic reaction	To phenylbutazone or oxyphenbutazone
High-risk conditions	Senility, drug allergy, blood dyscrasias, severe renal, hepatic, or cardiac disease, parotitis, stomatitis, polymyalgia rheumatica, temporal arteritis, pancreatitis, incipient cardiac failure, symptoms of GI inflammation or active ulceration, or a history of peptic ulcer disease
Concomitant therapy	With other potent drugs (see DRUG INTERACTIONS)

WARNINGS/PRECAUTIONS	
Drug toxicity	Severe or fatal reactions may occur, especially in patients over 40 yr of age; elderly are at greatest risk (see ADMINISTRATION/DOSAGE ADJUSTMENTS)
Upper GI tests	Should be performed in patients with persistent or severe dyspepsia; peptic ulcer (new or reactivated), bleeding, and perforation may occur
Blood dyscrasias	May occur suddenly and sometimes fatally. Perform frequent regular hematologic evaluations in patients receiving drug for >1 wk. Appearance may be delayed weeks after discontinuing therapy. Significant changes in total leukocyte count, relative decrease in granulocytes, appearance of immature cell forms, or fall in hematocrit requires cessation of therapy and full investigation.
Thyroid inhibition	Reduced iodine uptake may occur
Blurred vision	May be a manifestation of oxyphenbutazone toxicity; discontinue treatment and perform a complete ophthalmologic workup
Systemic lupus erythematosus	Discontinue drug if symptoms are activated
Mental impairment, reflex-slowing	Performance of potentially hazardous activities may be impaired; caution patients accordingly and about additive effects of alcohol
Leukemia	Causal relationship has not been firmly established, but cases have been reported
Acute asthma attacks	May occur in asthmatic patients

ADVERSE REACTIONS	Frequent reactions are italicized
Gastrointestinal	*GI upset, nausea, dyspepsia, abdominal and epigastric distress,* vomiting, abdominal distention with flatulence, constipation, diarrhea, esophagitis, gastritis, salivary-gland enlargement, stomatitis (sometimes with ulceration), ulceration and perforation of the intestinal tract (including acute and reactivated peptic ulcer with perforation, hemorrhage, and hematemesis), anemia from GI bleeding (may be occult), fatal and nonfatal hepatitis (sometimes with chloestasis)

Table continued on following page

ADVERSE REACTIONS continued

Hematological	Anemia; leukopenia; thrombocytopenia with purpura, petechiae, and hemorrhage; pancytopenia; aplastic anemia; bone-marrow depression; agranulocytosis and agranulocytic anginal syndrome; hemolytic anemia; leukemia (causal relationship not established)
Hypersensitivity	Urticaria, anaphylactic shock, arthralgia, drug fever, hypersensitivity angiitis (polyarteritis) and vasculitis, Lyell's syndrome, serum sickness, Stevens-Johnson syndrome, activation of systemic lupus erythematosus, aggravation of temporal arteritis in patients with polymyalgia rheumatica
Dermatological	Pruritus, rash, erythema nodosum, erythema multiforme, nonthrombocytopenic purpura
Cardiovascular, fluid and electrolyte	Sodium and chloride retention, fluid retention and plasma dilution, cardiac decompensation with edema and dyspnea, metabolic acidosis, respiratory alkalosis, hypertension, pericarditis, interstitial myocarditis with muscle necrosis, and perivascular granulomata
Renal	Hematuria, proteinuria, ureteral obstruction with uric acid crystals, anuria, glomerulonephritis, acute tubular necrosis, cortical necrosis, lithiasis, nephrotic syndrome, impairment and failure with azotemia
Central nervous system	Headache, drowsiness, agitation, confusion, lethargy, tremors, numbness, weakness
Metabolic and endocrinological	Thyroid hyperplasia, goiter with hyper- and hypothyroidism, pancreatitis, and hyperglycemia (causal relationship not established)
Ophthalmic	Blurred vision, optic neuritis, toxic amblyopia, scotomata, retinal detachment, retinal hemorrhage, and oculomotor palsy (causal relationship not established)
Otic	Hearing loss, tinnitus

OVERDOSAGE

Signs and symptoms	Nausea, vomiting, epigastric pain, excessive sweating, euphoria, psychosis, headache, giddiness, vertigo, hyperventilation, insomnia, tinnitus, hearing difficulties, edema, hypertension, cyanosis, respiratory depression, agitation, hallucinations, stupor, convulsions, coma, hematuria, oliguria, respiratory or metabolic acidosis, impaired hepatic or renal function, abnormalities of formed blood elements; *late manifestations of massive overdosage:* hepatomegaly, jaundice, ulceration of buccal or GI mucosa
Treatment	Induce emesis, followed by gastric lavage, to empty stomach. In obtunded patients, secure airway with cuffed endotracheal tube before starting lavage *(do not induce emesis).* Maintain adequate respiratory exchange; avoid respiratory stimulants. Treat shock with supportive measures. Control seizures with IV diazepam or short-acting barbiturates. Dialysis may be helpful if renal function is impaired.

DRUG INTERACTIONS

Alcohol	⇧ Risk of ulcer
Other anti-inflammatory agents	⇧ Risk of ulcer
Digitoxin	⇩ Serum digitoxin levels
Heparin	⇧ Risk of hemorrhage
Amodiaquine, chloroquine, gold salts, hydroxychloroquine	⇧ Risk of skin toxicity
Insulin	⇧ Hypoglycemia
Sulfonylureas	⇧ Sulfonylurea effect
Sulfonamides	⇧ Sulfonamide effect
Phenytoin	⇧ Phenytoin serum level
Coumarin anticoagulants	⇧ Prothrombin time

ALTERED LABORATORY VALUES

Blood/serum values	⇧ Sodium ⇩ Chloride ⇧ T_3 uptake ⇩ ^{131}I uptake ⇩ Uric acid
Urinary values	⇧ Protein ⇧ Uric acid

Use in children

Contraindicated in children under 14 yr of age

Use in pregnancy or nursing mothers

Animal reproduction studies have provided inconclusive evidence of embryotoxicity; therefore, use with caution in pregnancy if drug is deemed essential. Drug may appear in cord blood and breast milk; use with caution in nursing mothers.

TOLECTIN (Tolmetin sodium) McNeil Pharmaceutical

Tabs: 200 mg

TOLECTIN DS (Tolmetin sodium) McNeil Pharmaceutical

Caps: 400 mg

INDICATIONS	ORAL DOSAGE
Rheumatoid arthritis[1]	**Adult:** 400 mg tid to start, followed by 600–1,800 mg/day div, or up to 2,000 mg/day, if needed
Osteoarthritis	**Adult:** 400 mg tid to start, followed by 600–1,600 mg/day div
Juvenile rheumatoid arthritis[1]	**Child (≥2 yr):** 20 mg/kg/day div (tid or qid) to start, followed by 15–30 mg/kg/day div

ADMINISTRATION/DOSAGE ADJUSTMENTS

Combination therapy	Additional therapeutic benefits have been produced when added to a gold salt or corticosteroid regimen; use with salicylates is not recommended
Gastric irritation	May be avoided by giving drug with meals, milk, or antacids other than sodium bicarbonate
Therapeutic response	Should be observed within a few days to a week; progressive improvement can be expected during succeeding weeks

CONTRAINDICATIONS

Hypersensitivity	To tolmetin or to aspirin and other nonsteroidal, anti-inflammatory agents when manifested by asthma, rhinitis, or urticaria

WARNINGS/PRECAUTIONS

Peptic ulceration, GI bleeding	May occur and can be severe; use with extreme caution in patients with a history of upper-GI-tract disease or with active peptic ulcer
Renal impairment	Use with caution; monitor renal function closely and reduce dosage if necessary
Corticosteroid therapy	If discontinued, reduce dosage gradually to avoid complications of sudden steroid withdrawal
Peripheral edema	May occur; use with caution in patients with compromised cardiac function
Prolonged bleeding time	May occur due to inhibition of platelet aggregation; use with caution in patients with coagulation defects or in those on anticoagulant therapy
Impaired vision	May occur with some nonsteroidal anti-inflammatory drugs; perform ophthalmologic studies periodically

ADVERSE REACTIONS
Frequent reactions are italicized

Gastrointestinal	*Nausea (11%), dyspepsia (10%), abdominal pain (6.7%), gastrointestinal distress (6.7%), flatulence (4%), diarrhea (4%), vomiting (3.3%), constipation (2.5%), peptic ulcer (2%), gastritis (1.8%),* GI bleeding without peptic ulcer (0.4%)
Central nervous system	*Headache (10%), dizziness or lightheadedness (5%), tension or nervousness (2%), drowsiness (1.7%),* insomnia, depression
Cardiovascular	*Edema (6.7%),* hypertension
Dermatological	*Rash (2.5%), skin irritation (1.8%), pruritus (1.7%)*
Hematological	Small, transient decreases in hemoglobin and hematocrit, granulocytopenia
Other	*Tinnitus (1.5%),* asthenia, chest pain; anaphylactoid reactions (rare)

[1]Safety and effectiveness have not been established for rheumatoid arthritis patients designated by the American Rheumatism Association as Functional Class IV (incapacitated, largely or wholly bedridden or confined to a wheelchair, little or no self-care)

Table continued on following page

OVERDOSAGE

Signs and symptoms	See ADVERSE REACTIONS
Treatment	Induce vomiting or use gastric lavage, followed by activated charcoal. Alkalinization of urine with sodium bicarbonate may enhance excretion of drug.

DRUG INTERACTIONS

Anticoagulants	⇧ Bleeding time
Alcohol	⇧ Risk of ulcer
Other anti-inflammatory agents	⇧ Risk of ulcer
Sodium bicarbonate	⇧ Tolmetin excretion

ALTERED LABORATORY VALUES

Blood/serum values	⇧ Sodium
Urinary values	⇧ Protein (when assayed by acid precipitation tests)

Use in children

Safety and effectiveness have not been established in children under 2 yr of age

Use in pregnancy or nursing mothers

Not recommended

TRILISATE (Choline magnesium trisalicylate) Purdue Frederick

Tabs: 500 mg

INDICATIONS	ORAL DOSAGE
Rheumatoid arthritis,[1] osteoarthritis, and other severe arthritides	**Adult:** 1,000–1,500 mg q12h or 500–1,000 mg tid
Mild to moderate arthritis	**Adult:** 500–1,000 mg q12h or tid

ADMINISTRATION/DOSAGE ADJUSTMENTS

Onset of action	Some patients may require 2–3 wk of therapy for optimal effect
Combination therapy	May be used in combination with gold salts

CONTRAINDICATIONS

Hypersensitivity to salicylates

WARNINGS/PRECAUTIONS

Special-risk patients	Use with caution in patients with chronic renal insufficiency, active erosive gastritis, or peptic ulcer
Salicylism and/or salicylate intoxication	May occur if taken in large doses or for a prolonged period; reduce dosage if tinnitus develops (see ADVERSE REACTIONS and OVERDOSAGE)

ADVERSE REACTIONS

Central nervous system	Salicylism, including tinnitus, vertigo, headache, confusion, drowsiness (see WARNINGS/PRECAUTIONS)
Gastrointestinal	Salicylism, including vomiting, diarrhea (see WARNINGS/PRECAUTIONS)
Other	Salicylism, including diaphoresis, hyperventilation (see WARNINGS/PRECAUTIONS)

OVERDOSAGE

Signs and symptoms	*Early:* rapid and deep breathing, hyperventilation, nausea, vomiting, vertigo, tinnitus, flushing, sweating, thirst, headache, drowsiness, diarrhea, tachycardia; *late:* fever, hemorrhage, excitement, confusion, convulsions, vasomotor depression, coma, respiratory failure, and respiratory alkalosis followed by respiratory and metabolic acidosis (primarily in children)
Treatment	If less than 4 h have elapsed since ingestion, induce emesis or perform gastric lavage, followed by activated charcoal, to remove any remaining drug from the stomach. Initial therapy should be directed at reducing hyperthermia by external sponging with tepid water, correcting dehydration by appropriate IV fluid replacement, and maintaining adequate cardiorespiratory and renal function. In moderately severe cases of salicylate poisoning, cautiously administer sodium bicarbonate IV in sufficient quantity, if possible, to maintain an alkaline diuresis; intermittent peritoneal dialysis may also be helpful. In severe cases, hemodialysis should be seriously considered. Potassium should be added to the repair solution to compensate for potassium losses once urine formation is deemed adequate. Glucose may be provided to correct ketosis and hypoglycemia. Plasma transfusion may be beneficial if shock intervenes. Hemorrhagic phenomena may necessitate whole-blood transfusions and phytonadione (vitamin K). Do not administer barbiturates to treat excitement or convulsions.

DRUG INTERACTIONS

Corticosteroids	⇧ Risk of GI ulceration
Phenylbutazone, oxyphenbutazone	⇧ Risk of GI ulceration
Alcohol	⇧ Risk of GI ulceration
Anticoagulants	⇧ Anticoagulant effect
Antacids, urinary alkalizers	⇩ Plasma salicylate levels
Oral hypoglycemics	⇧ Hypoglycemic effect
Methotrexate	⇧ Plasma methotrexate plasma level and risk of toxicity
Probenecid, sulfinpyrazone	⇩ Uricosuric effect
Urinary acidifiers	⇧ Plasma salicylate levels

[1]Safety and effectiveness have not been established for rheumatoid arthritis patients designated by the American Rheumatism Association as Functional Class IV (incapacitated, largely or wholly bedridden or confined to a wheelchair, little or no self-care)

Table continued on following page

ALTERED LABORATORY VALUES

Blood/serum values	⇧ or ⇩ Uric acid
Urinary values	⇧ or ⇩ VMA

Use in children

Not recommended for use in children

Use in pregnancy or nursing mothers

Use with caution during pregnancy. Because of possible prostaglandin inhibition with high doses of salicylates, do not administer prior to parturition. General guidelines not established for use in nursing mothers.

ANTURANE (Sulfinpyrazone) Ciba

Tabs: 100 mg **Caps:** 200 mg

INDICATIONS	ORAL DOSAGE
Chronic or intermittent gouty arthritis	**Adult:** 200–400 mg/day in 2 divided doses, with milk or meals, followed by 400 mg/day in 2 divided doses

ADMINISTRATION/DOSAGE ADJUSTMENTS

Initiating therapy	Increase initial dosage gradually within 1 wk up to maintenance dosage; use full maintenance dosage when transferring patients previously controlled by other uricosuric agents
Maintenance	Dosage may be increased to 800 mg/day, if needed; after blood urate level has been controlled, dosages as low as 200 mg/day may be adequate
Gastric irritation	May be minimized by administering drug with food, milk, or antacids

CONTRAINDICATIONS

Active peptic ulcer ●

GI inflammation ●

GI ulceration ●

Hypersensitivity to phenylbutazone or other pyrazole compounds ●

Blood dyscrasias (past or present) ●

WARNINGS/PRECAUTIONS

Acute gouty attacks	May be precipitated in initial stages of therapy; treat with colchicine or phenylbutazone while therapy continues
Renal colic, urolithiasis	May result, especially in initial stages of therapy; maintain an adequate fluid intake and alkaline urine
Renal impairment	Requires periodic assessment; renal failure has been reported but causal relationship not established
Past peptic ulcer	May be reactivated; use with caution in patients with healed ulcers
Blood counts	Monitor perodically (see ADVERSE REACTIONS)
Tartrazine sensitivity	Presence of FD&C Yellow No. 5 (tartrazine) in capsules may cause allergic-type reactions, including bronchial asthma, in susceptible individuals

ADVERSE REACTIONS

Gastrointestinal	Various upper-GI-tract disturbances
Dermatological	Rash
Hematological	Anemia, leukopenia, agranulocytosis, thrombocytopenia, aplastic anemia, leukemia (two cases; causal relationship not established)

OVERDOSAGE

Signs and symptoms	Nausea, vomiting, diarrhea, epigastric pain, ataxia, labored respiration, convulsions, coma (also anemia, jaundice, ulceration[1])
Treatment	No specific antidote. Induce emesis or use gastric lavage to empty stomach. Treat symptomatically and institute supportive measures, as needed.

DRUG INTERACTIONS

Salicylates	⇩ Uricosuria
Sulfonamides	⇧ Sulfonamide effect
Oral sulfonylureas	⇧ Hypoglycemia
Insulin	⇧ Hypoglycemia
Coumarin anticoagulants	⇧ Prothrombin time

ALTERED LABORATORY VALUES

No clinically significant alterations in blood/serum or urinary values occur at therapeutic dosages

Use in children

General guidelines not established

Use in pregnancy or nursing mothers

Safe use not established; results from animal reproductive studies have been inconclusive. May be used with caution during pregnancy; General guidelines not established for use in nursing mothers.

[1]Possible symptoms, seen after overdosage with other pyrazolone derivatives

BENEMID (Probenecid) **Merck Sharp & Dohme**

Tabs: 0.5 g

INDICATIONS	ORAL DOSAGE
Gout and gouty arthritis	**Adult:** 0.25 g bid for 1 wk, followed by 0.5 g bid
Adjuvant to penicillin therapy	**Adult:** 2 g/day div **Child (2–14 yr):** 25 mg/kg to start, followed by 40 mg/kg/day in 4 divided doses **Child (>110 lb):** same as adult

ADMINISTRATION/DOSAGE ADJUSTMENTS

Initiating therapy	Wait until acute gouty attack subsides. Acute attacks arising during therapy may be controlled with colchicine while probenecid is continued.
Maintenance regimen	Maintain a liberal fluid intake and alkaline urine until serum urate levels are normal and tophaceous deposits disappear. Continue dosage for 6 mo after urate levels have normalized and acute attacks have subsided, then decrease daily dosage by 0.5 g every 6 mo, unless serum urate levels rise.
Renal impairment	Begin with 1 g/day and increase dosage by 0.5 g/day every 4 wk, as needed (especially if 24-h urate excretion < 700 mg) and tolerated, up to 2 g/day (increased dosage may not be effective if GFR ≤ 30 ml/min)
Uncomplicated gonorrhea	Administer 4.8 million units of aqueous procaine penicillin G in 2 IM doses at different sites with 1 g probenecid just prior to injection, or give 3.5 g ampicillin orally with 1 g probenecid simultaneously
Penicillin adjuvant	Reduce probenecid dosage in the elderly due to possible renal impairment. Do not use concomitantly in patients with known renal impairment. When probenecid dosage is adequate, renal clearance of PSP is reduced to ~1/5 normal rate.

CONTRAINDICATIONS

Uric-acid kidney stones •	During acute gouty attack •
Blood dyscrasias •	Hypersensitivity to probenecid •

WARNINGS/PRECAUTIONS

Exacerbation of gout	Add colchicine or other appropriate therapy
Hypersensitivity reactions	Necessitate discontinuation of drug
Hematuria, renal colic, costovertebral pain, uric-acid stone formation	May be prevented in gouty patients by alkalinization of urine and liberal fluid intake; monitor acid-base balance periodically
Special-risk patients	Use with caution in patients with a history of peptic ulcer or G6PD deficiency
Renal impairment	Do not use concomitantly with penicillin
Concomitant methotrexate therapy	Reduce dosage of methotrexate to avoid toxicity and monitor serum methotrexate level
Theophylline blood levels	May appear falsely elevated when determined by Schack and Waxler method

ADVERSE REACTIONS

Gastrointestinal	Anorexia, nausea, vomiting, hepatic necrosis (rare)
Central nervous system	Headache, dizziness
Hematological	Anemia, aplastic anemia (rare), hemolytic anemia
Genitourinary	Urinary frequency, hematuria, uric-acid stones, renal colic
Hypersensitivity	Anaphylaxis, dermatitis, pruritus, fever
Other	Sore gums, flushing, exacerbation of gout, nephrotic syndrome (rare), costovertebral pain

Table continued on following page

BENEMID continued

OVERDOSAGE

Signs and symptoms	See ADVERSE REACTIONS
Treatment	Decrease dosage or discontinue drug; treat symptomatically

DRUG INTERACTIONS

Penicillin	⇧ Penicillin plasma level
Salicylates	⇩ Uricosuria
Pyrazinamide	⇩ Uricosuria
Sulfonamides	⇧ Sulfonamide plasma level
Oral sulfonylureas	⇧ Hypoglycemia
Indomethacin	⇧ Indomethacin plasma level
Rifampin	⇧ Rifampin plasma level
Methotrexate	⇧ Methotrexate plasma level and risk of toxicity
Para-aminohippuric acid (PAH)	⇩ Excretion of PAH
Para-aminosalicylic acid (PAS)	⇩ Excretion of PAS
Sodium iodomethamate	⇩ Excretion of sodium iodomethamate
Pantothenic acid	⇩ Excretion of pantothenic acid
Phenolsulfonphthalein	⇩ Excretion of phenolsulfonphthalein

ALTERED LABORATORY VALUES

Blood/serum values	⇩ Uric acid
Urinary values	⇧ Uric acid ⇧ Glucose (with Clinitest tablets; transient) ⇩ 17-Ketosteroids

Use in children

Contraindicated in children under 2 yr of age. General guidelines not established for use in children with gouty arthritis.

Use in pregnancy or nursing mothers

Safe use not established; probenecid crosses the placental barrier and appears in cord blood. General guidelines not established for use in nursing mothers.

ColBENEMID (Probenecid and colchicine) Merck Sharp & Dohme

Tabs: 0.5 g probenecid and 0.5 mg colchicine

INDICATIONS	ORAL DOSAGE
Chronic gouty arthritis complicated by frequent, recurrent gouty attacks	**Adult:** 1 tab/day for 1 wk, followed by 1 tab bid

ADMINISTRATION/DOSAGE ADJUSTMENTS

Initiating therapy	Wait until acute attack subsides; acute attacks arising during therapy may be controlled with additional colchicine while drug is continued
Maintenance	Maintain a liberal fluid intake and alkaline urine until serum uric-acid levels are normal and tophaceous deposits disappear. Reduce daily dosage by 1 tab every 6 mo if attacks have subsided for at least 6 mo and serum uric-acid levels have normalized.
Renal impairment	Increase daily dosage by 1 tab every 4 wk, as needed (especially if 24-h urate excretion $<$ 700 mg) and tolerated, up to generally no more than 4 tabs/day (increased dosage may not be effective if GFR $\leq$ 30 ml/min)

CONTRAINDICATIONS

Blood dyscrasias ●	Hypersensitivity to probenecid or colchicine, alone or in combination ●
Uric-acid kidney stones ●	During acute gouty attack ●

WARNINGS/PRECAUTIONS

Exacerbation of gout	Add colchicine or other appropriate therapy
Hypersensitivity reactions	Necessitate discontinuation of drug
Impaired spermatogenesis	May result; reversible azoospermia has occurred in one patient
Hematuria, renal colic, costovertebral pain, uric-acid stone formation	May be prevented by alkalinization of urine and liberal fluid intake; monitor acid-base balance periodically
Concomitant methotrexate therapy	Reduce dosage of methotrexate to avoid toxicity and monitor serum methotrexate level
Special-risk patients	Use with caution in patients with a history of peptic ulcer or active peptic ulcer disease, spastic colon, hepatic dysfunction, or G6PD deficiency
Theophylline blood levels	May appear falsely elevated when determined by Schack and Waxler method

ADVERSE REACTIONS

Gastrointestinal	Anorexia, nausea, vomiting, abdominal pain, diarrhea, hepatic necrosis (rare)
Central nervous system and neuromuscular	Headache, dizziness, weakness, peripheral neuritis (with prolonged use)
Renal and genitourinary	Urinary frequency, hematuria, renal colic, nephrotic syndrome (rare), oliguria
Dermatological	Urticaria, dermatitis, purpura, hair loss
Hematological	Anemia, aplastic anemia, hemolytic anemia, agranulocytosis (with prolonged use)
Hypersensitivity	Anaphylaxis, dermatitis, pruritus, fever
Other	Sore gums, flushing, exacerbation of gout, costovertebral pain, generalized vascular damage

OVERDOSAGE

Signs and symptoms	See ADVERSE REACTIONS
Treatment	Decrease dosage or discontinue therapy

Table continued on following page

DRUG INTERACTIONS

Penicillin	⇧ Penicillin plasma level
Salicylates	⇩ Uricosuria
Pyrazinamide	⇩ Uricosuria
Sulfonamides	⇧ Sulfonamide plasma level
Oral sulfonylureas	⇧ Hypoglycemia
Indomethacin	⇧ Indomethacin plasma level
Rifampin	⇧ Rifampin plasma level
Methotrexate	⇧ Methotrexate plasma level and risk of toxicity
Para-aminohippuric acid (PAH)	⇩ Excretion of PAH
Para-aminosalicylic acid (PAS)	⇩ Excretion of PAS
Sodium iodomethamate	⇩ Excretion of sodium iodomethamate
Pantothenic acid	⇩ Excretion of pantothenic acid
Phenolsulfonphthalein	⇩ Excretion of phenolsulfonphthalein

ALTERED LABORATORY VALUES

Blood/serum values	⇩ Uric acid
Urinary values	⇧ Glucose (with Clinitest tablets; transient) ⇧ Uric acid ⇩ 17-Ketosteroids

Use in children

Contraindicated in children under 2 yr of age. General guidelines not established for dosage recommendations for older children.

Use in pregnancy or nursing mothers

Contraindicated during pregnancy. Probenecid crosses placental barrier and appears in cord blood. Colchicine can arrest cell division and has proved teratogenic in certain animals under certain conditions. General guidelines not established for use in nursing mothers.

COLCHICINE Lilly

Tabs: 0.6 mg **Amps:** 0.5 mg/ml (2 ml)

INDICATIONS	ORAL DOSAGE	PARENTERAL DOSAGE
Acute gouty arthritis	**Adult:** 0.6–1.2 mg to start, followed by 0.6 mg q1–2h until pain ceases or nausea, vomiting, or diarrhea starts; alternative regimen: 1.2 mg bid, as needed	**Adult:** 2 mg IV to start, followed by 0.5 mg IV q6h, as needed, up to 4 mg/24 h; alternative regimens: 3 mg IV in a single dose or 1 mg IV to start, followed by 0.5 mg IV qd or bid, as needed

ADMINISTRATION/DOSAGE ADJUSTMENTS

Initiating therapy — Begin treatment at first sign of attack; if second course is required, wait 3 days[1]

Parenteral indications — Use IV route for acute attacks only and replace with oral form when attack subsides. IV route may also be used when GI effects interfere with oral use, or when tablets are ineffective. IM or SC use causes severe local irritation.

Prophylaxis (interval therapy) — Oral route is preferred, in conjunction with a uricosuric agent. For mild to moderate cases, give 0.6 mg orally one to four times a week; for severe cases, give 0.6 mg qd or bid. If IV route is used, give 0.5–1 mg qd or bid.

CONTRAINDICATIONS

None

WARNINGS/PRECAUTIONS

Special-risk patients — Use with caution in elderly or debilitated patients, especially if renal, gastrointestinal, or heart disease is present; reduce dosage or discontinue drug if such symptoms as weakness, anorexia, nausea, vomiting, or diarrhea appear

Thrombophlebitis (rare) — May occur at injection site

Toxicity — As little as 8 mg may be fatal (see OVERDOSAGE)

Diarrhea — May be severe, even with IV route; administer paregoric

ADVERSE REACTIONS

Frequent reactions are italicized

Gastrointestinal — *Abdominal pain, nausea, vomiting, diarrhea*

Dermatological — Hair loss

Neuromuscular — Peripheral neuritis

Hematological — Bone-marrow depression with agranulocytosis, thrombocytopenia, aplastic anemia

OVERDOSAGE

Signs and symptoms — Onset is usually delayed, regardless of route. Symptoms include nausea, vomiting, abdominal pain, diarrhea (possibly severe and bloody), burning sensations in the throat, stomach, and skin, vascular damage (shock), oliguria, hematuria, marked muscular weakness, ascending paralysis, delirium, convulsions, and death due to respiratory depression.

Treatment — Remove drug by gastric lavage, combined with hemodialysis or peritoneal dialysis. Establish a patent airway and provide respiratory assistance, if needed. Observe for signs of shock and provide appropriate supportive measures. Atropine or morphine may relieve abdominal pain.

DRUG INTERACTIONS

No clinically significant drug interactions have been observed

ALTERED LABORATORY VALUES

No clinically significant alterations in blood/serum or urinary values occur at therapeutic dosages

Use in children

General guidelines not established

Use in pregnancy or nursing mothers

General guidelines not established; possibly teratogenic, although evidence is slight in humans[1]

[1]Nicholson HO: *J Obstet Gynaec Br Commonw* 75:307, 1968

[1]Goodman LS, Gilman A: *The Pharmacological Basis of Therapeutics,* 5th ed, New York, Macmillan, 1975, p 352

ZYLOPRIM (Allopurinol) Burroughs Wellcome

Tabs: 100, 300 mg

INDICATIONS	ORAL DOSAGE
Gout, either primary or secondary to hyperuricemia associated with blood dyscrasias or their treatment **Primary or secondary uric acid nephropathy,** with or without gouty symptoms **Recurrent uric acid stone formation**	**Adult:** 100 mg/day to start, preferably after meals, followed by weekly increases of 100 mg/day, as needed, until serum uric acid level falls to 6 mg/dl or less or until a maximum of 800 mg/day is reached (divide doses exceeding 300 mg/day); average dosage is 200–300 mg/day for mild gout and 400–600 mg/day for moderately severe tophaceous gout
Prevention of uric acid nephropathy during cancer chemotherapy	**Adult:** 600–800 mg/day div, preferably after meals, for 2–3 days, together with a high fluid intake
Hyperuricemia secondary to neoplastic disease in children	**Child (<6 yr):** 150 mg/day; after 48 h, adjust dosage as needed **Child (6–10 yr):** 300 mg/day; after 48 h, adjust dosage as needed

ADMINISTRATION/DOSAGE ADJUSTMENTS

Maintenance therapy	After serum uric acid level is controlled, it may be possible to lower dosage using serum uric acid level as a guide; minimum effective dosage is 100–200 mg/day
Renal impairment	If creatinine clearance is 10–20 ml/min, give 200 mg/day; if less than 10 ml/min, give 100 mg/day; and if less than 3 ml/min, lengthen dosage interval
Transferring from colchicine and/or anti-inflammatory agents	Continue these agents until freedom from gouty attacks and normal serum uric acid levels are maintained for several months
Transferring from uricosuric agents	Gradually reduce uricosuric dose over several weeks while increasing dose of allopurinol
Combination therapy	May be used with salicylates and uricosuric agents

CONTRAINDICATIONS

Immediate relatives of patients with idiopathic hemochromatosis ●	Hypersensitivity to allopurinol ●

WARNINGS/PRECAUTIONS

Acute gouty attacks	May increase in frequency during initial stages of therapy; start with low doses (see ORAL DOSAGE) and administer colchicine prophylactically (0.5 mg bid) for the first 3–6 mo. Therapeutic doses of cochicine or anti-inflammatory drugs may be required in some cases to suppress acute attacks; do *not* discontinue allopurinol or alter dosage.
Fluid intake	Advise patient to drink sufficient fluids (10–12 full glasses of water daily) to yield a daily urinary output of 2 liters or more and maintain a neutral or preferably slightly alkaline urine to avoid possible formation of xanthine calculi and to help prevent renal precipitation of urates in patients receiving concomitant uricosuric therapy
Rash, adverse reactions	May be followed by more severe hypersensitivity reactions (see ADVERSE REACTIONS), including generalized vasculitis, hepatotoxicity, or death; stop therapy immediately and do not reinstitute after reaction clears
Clinical hepatotoxicity	May occur; monitor liver function periodically, especially in patients with pre-existing liver disease
Drowsiness	Performance of potentially hazardous activities may be impaired; caution patients accordingly
Renal impairment or poor urate clearance	Reduce dosage (see ADMINISTRATION/DOSAGE ADJUSTMENTS); stop therapy if renal functional abnormalities increase
Mild reticulocytosis	May occur; causal relationship has not been established
Renal/hepatic function, complete blood counts	Monitor regularly, especially during first few months of therapy
Concomitant use of thiazide diuretics	May be associated with renal failure (rare); hypersensitivity may occur in patients with renal compromise receiving this combination; use with caution

Table continued on following page

ZYLOPRIM continued

ADVERSE REACTIONS	Frequent reactions are italicized
Dermatological	*Rash (usually maculopapular);* exfoliative, urticarial, and purpuric lesions; Stevens-Johnson syndrome; toxic epidermal necrolysis; alopecia, with or without dermatitis
Gastrointestinal	Nausea, vomiting, diarrhea, abdominal pain
Cardiovascular	Vasculitis, necrotizing angiitis
Hematological	Agranulocytosis, anemia, aplastic anemia, bone-marrow depression, leukopenia, pancytopenia, thrombocytopenia (causal relationship not established)
Central nervous system and neurological	Peripheral neuritis, drowsiness
Ophthalmic	Cataracts (causal relationship not established)
Hepatic	Granulomatous hepatitis, necrosis (both rare)
Renal	Failure (with concomitant thiazide use; rare)
Idiosyncratic	Fever, chills, leukopenia or leukocytosis, eosinophilia, arthralgias, skin rash, pruritus, nausea, vomiting

OVERDOSAGE	
Signs and symptoms	Skin rash or any sign of adverse reaction
Treatment	Immediately discontinue drug

DRUG INTERACTIONS	
Azathioprine, mercaptopurine	⇧ Azathioprine or mercaptopurine toxicity; if given concomitantly, reduce dosage of azothioprine or mercaptopurine to 1/3 to 1/4 of usual dose
Dicumarol	⇧ Half-life of dicumarol
Other oral anticoagulants	⇧ Risk of bleeding (possible)
Uricosurics	⇩ Urinary excretion of oxypurines
Iron salts	⇧ Hepatic iron concentration (possible); do not give concomitantly

ALTERED LABORATORY VALUES	
Blood/serum values	⇧ Alkaline phosphatase ⇧ SGOT ⇧ SGPT ⇧ or ⇩ BUN ⇩ Uric acid
Urinary values	⇩ Uric acid

Use in children

Indicated only for secondary hyperuricemia associated with malignancies

Use in pregnancy or nursing mothers

Safe use during pregnancy has not been established, although reproductive studies have shown no adverse effect on animal litters. Patient should stop nursing if drug is prescribed.

Product (Manufacturer)	Ingredients	Actions
Absorbine Arthritic (W.F. Young) Lotion **Dosage** Apply evenly over affected area. Repeat as often as every 2 h if needed.	Methyl salicylate	Counterirritant
	Menthol	Counterirritant and mild local anesthetic
	Methyl nicotinate	Counterirritant and local vasodilator
	Greaseless emulsion base	
Absorbine Jr. (W.F. Young) Lotion **Dosage** **For overexertion:** rub in freely and promptly. Repeat 3–4 times daily. **For strains and bruises:** apply generously over feet and ankles	Wormwood oil	Counterirritant
	Thymol	Counterirritant
	Menthol	Counterirritant and mild local anesthetic
	Chlorocylenol	Counterirritant
	Acetone	Solvent
Analgesic Balm (Lilly) Ointment **Dosage** Apply locally 2–3 times daily by massaging gently into affected area	15% Methyl salicylate	Counterirritant
	15% Menthol	Counterirritant and mild local anesthetic
	Hydrocarbon waxes	Hardening agents
	Lanolin	Ointment base
	Petrolatum	Ointment base
	Sorbitan sesquioleate	Stabilizer
	Water-soluble base	
Ben-Gay (Leeming) Lotion **Dosage** Rub generously into painful area, then massage gently until product disappears. Repeat as needed.	15% Methyl salicylate	Counterirritant
	7% Menthol	Counterirritant and mild local anesthetic
	Greaseless base	
Ben-Gay Extra Strength Balm (Leeming) Ointment **Dosage** Rub generously into painful area, then massage gently until product disappears. Repeat as needed.	30% Methyl salicylate	Counterirritant
	8% Menthol	Counterirritant and mild local anesthetic
	Greaseless base	
Ben-Gay Gel (Leeming) Gel **Dosage** Rub generously into painful area, then massage gently until product disappears. Repeat as needed.	15% Methyl salicylate	Counterirritant
	7% Menthol	Counterirritant and mild local anesthetic
	Hydroalcoholic gel base	
Ben-Gay Greaseless/Stainless (Leeming) Ointment **Dosage** Rub generously into painful area, then massage gently until product disappears. Repeat as needed.	15% Methyl salicylate	Counterirritant
	10% Menthol	Counterirritant and mild local anesthetic
	Greaseless base	

Table continued on following page

Product (Manufacturer)	Ingredients	Actions
Ben-Gay Original Ointment (Leeming) Ointment **Dosage** Rub generously into painful area, then massage gently until product disappears. Repeat as needed.	16.3% Methyl salicylate	Counterirritant
	16% Menthol	Counterirritant and mild local anesthetic
	Oleginous base	
Counterpain Rub (Squibb) Ointment **Dosage** Massage into affected area. Repeat 1–3 times daily as needed.	10.2% Methyl salicylate	Counterirritant
	5.4% Menthol	Counterirritant and mild local anesthetic
	1.4% Eugenol	Counterirritant
Dencorub (Roberts) Lotion **Dosage** Apply freely, then massage gently until product disappears. Repeat as needed.	Methyl salicylate	Counterirritant
	Menthol	Counterirritant and mild local anesthetic
	Camphor	Counterirritant and mild local anesthetic
	Eucalyptus oil	Counterirritant
Doan's Rub (Purex) Cream **Dosage** **For adults and children over 2 yr:** rub generously into painful area. Massage gently. Use up to 3–4 times daily.	25% Methyl salicylate	Counterirritant
	10% Menthol	Counterirritant and mild local anesthetic
Emul-O-Balm (Pennwalt) Lotion **Dosage** Rub into painful area. Repeat every 3–4 h if needed.	22.45 mg Methyl salicylate per ml	Counterirritant
	22.45 mg Menthol per ml	Counterirritant and mild local anesthetic
	11.22 mg Camphor per ml	Counterirritant and mild local anesthetic
	8.37 mg Ribbon gum tragacanth per ml	Suspending agent
	1.50 mg Methylparaben per ml	Antifungal agent (preservative)
	0.30 mg Propylparaben per ml	Antifungal agent (preservative)
Heat Liniment (Whitehall) Liniment **Dosage** Using applicator, brush freely over and around sore areas. Repeat 15 min later if needed. If pain persists, apply every 2 h.	15% Methyl salicylate	Counterirritant
	0.025% Capsicum	Counterirritant
	3.6% Camphor	Counterirritant and mild local anesthetic
	70% Alcohol	Vehicle
Heet Spray (Whitehall) Spray **Dosage** Spray affected area, let dry, then spray again. May be reapplied every 2–3 h.	25% Methyl salicylate	Counterirritant
	3% Menthol	Counterirritant and mild local anesthetic
	1.5% Camphor	Counterirritant and mild local anesthetic
	1% Methyl nicotinate	Counterirritant and local vasodilator
	29.5% Alcohol	Vehicle

Table continued on following page

Product (Manufacturer)	Ingredients	Actions
Icy Hot (Searle) Ointment **Dosage** Apply to painful area, then massage gently until product is completely absorbed. Repeat as needed.	29% Methyl salicylate	Counterirritant
	8% Menthol	Counterirritant and mild local anesthetic
Mentholatum (Mentholatum) Ointment **Dosage** Spread on affected areas. Cover areas with warm cloth. Repeat up to 3 times daily.	9% Camphor	Counterirritant and mild local anesthetic
	1.3% Menthol	Counterirritant and mild local anesthetic
	Aromatic oils	Fragrance
	Petrolatum	Ointment base
Mentholatum Deep Heating Lotion (Mentholatum) Lotion **Dosage** Apply to affected area. Massage gently until lotion is absorbed into the skin. Repeat as needed.	20% Methyl salicylate	Counterirritant
	6% Menthol	Counterirritant and mild local anesthetic
	Lanolin oil	Lotion base
	Greaseless base	
Mentholatum Deep Heating Rub (Mentholatum) Ointment **Dosage** Massage into affected area until product is absorbed into the skin. Repeat as needed.	12.7% Methyl salicylate	Counterirritant
	5.8% Menthol	Counterirritant and mild local anesthetic
	Eucalyptus oil	Fragrance
	Turpentine oil	Fragrance
	Anhydrous lanolin	Ointment base
	Greaseless base	
Minit-Rub (Bristol-Myers) Ointment **Dosage** Apply small amount to affected area. Massage lightly until ointment vanishes. Repeat as needed.	10% Methyl salicylate	Counterirritant
	3.54% Menthol	Counterirritant and mild local anesthetic
	4.44% Camphor	Counterirritant and mild local anesthetic
	1.77% Eucalyptus oil	Counterirritant
	4.44% Anhydrous lanolin	Ointment base
Musterole Deep Strength (Plough) Ointment **Dosage** Rub freely on affected areas until absorbed. Repeat as needed.	Methyl salicylate	Counterirritant
	Menthol	Counterirritant and mild local anesthetic
	Methyl nicotinate	Counterirritant and local vasodilator
Musterole Regular, Extra, and Children's Strength (Plough) Ointment **Dosage** Rub well on affected areas	Camphor	Counterirritant and mild local anesthetic
	Menthol	Counterirritant and mild local anesthetic
	Methyl salicylate	Counterirritant
	Mustard oil	Counterirritant
	Glycol monosalicylate	Analgesic and mild counterirritant

Table continued on following page

Product (Manufacturer)	Ingredients	Actions
Sloan's (Warner-Lambert) Liniment	4.76% Turpentine oil	Counterirritant
	6.74% Pine oil	Counterirritant
Dosage Apply freely 1 or more times daily. Do not rub after applying. For milder action, mix with equal parts of cooking or mineral oil before applying, and use once or twice daily.	3.35% Camphor oil	Counterirritant and mild local anesthetic
	2.66% Methyl salicylate	Counterirritant
	0.62% Capsicum oleoresin	Counterirritant
	39.88% Kerosene	Solvent

Corticosteroids

Corticosteroids are a group of substances made in the outer part (cortex) of the adrenal gland, a small organ that lies above the kidney. They belong to the larger family of steroid hormones, which includes the male sex hormone testosterone, made primarily in the testes, and the female sex hormones progesterone and estradiol, made primarily in the ovaries. The term corticosteroid also refers to chemically modified forms of the naturally occurring compounds.

There are two types of adrenal cortical steroid hormones, the mineralocorticoids and the glucocorticoids. The term mineralocorticoid refers to the fact that these substances regulate the concentration of sodium and potassium salts in the body. By increasing the amount of sodium in the body, mineralocorticoids increase both retention of water and, ultimately, blood pressure. The most important natural human mineralocorticoid is aldosterone.

The glucocorticoids, named for the fact that one of their chief effects is to alter glucose metabolism, have a much wider range of activities. They affect metabolism of sugars, fats, and proteins; alter secretion in the stomach; change the types of cells in the blood; and inhibit some aspects of immune and allergic responses. The chief natural human glucocorticoid is cortisol, or hydrocortisone.

It is their range of effects that makes the glucocorticoids important therapeutic agents. Paradoxically, this wide spectrum of activities is also their greatest drawback, since unwanted effects accompanying the desired therapeutic effect can harm the patient. For this reason, steroids are generally used only when other treatments have failed; they are considered first-line therapy only for diseases for which no other effective treatment is known. When employed, they must be used with the greatest caution and for the shortest time necessary to achieve therapeutic effects. When used for the proper indications and with due caution, glucocorticoids can bring about dramatic improvement in disabling diseases. In this section, some of the more important conditions for which corticosteroids are used will be reviewed, as well as the precautions that should be followed during steroid therapy.

HORMONE DEFICIENCY STATES

The most obvious and appropriate use of adrenal cortical steroid hormones is in replacement therapy when a person's own adrenal glands are not functioning correctly. Adrenal dysfunction can result from a number of causes, and although these conditions are not common, they are usually life-threatening.

Adrenal cortical insufficiency, commonly referred to as Addison's disease, after the British physician who first described it in 1855, is characterized by lowered blood pressure, low blood sugar, loss of appetite, vomiting and diarrhea, rapid weight loss, depression and irritability, vulnerability to infection, anemia, and intensification of pigmentation. Three types of adrenal cortical insufficiency may occur: primary, secondary, and congenital.

Primary adrenal insufficiency results from a loss of adrenal cortical tissue because of a tumor or other cause. Since both glucocorticoid and mineralocorticoid hormones are lost, the functions of both must be replaced. This is usually done with the natural steroid hormones cortisol or cortisone, since each possesses both activities. Therapy is accomplished with small doses of the hormone and is continued for life.

Secondary insufficiency results from disturbance of the pituitary gland. Adrenocorticotrophic hormone (ACTH or corticotropin), which is secreted by the pituitary, stimulates production of adrenal steroid hormones. If the pituitary gland produces too little ACTH, not enough corticosteroids will be made. Replacement therapy is usually the same as for primary adrenal insufficiency.

Congenital adrenal hyperplasia (CAH) is caused by an inherited defect in synthesis of corticosteroid hormones. Any of several steps in hormone biosynthesis can be affected. Hyperplasia of the adrenal results from the feedback loop between the pituitary and the adrenal. The pituitary senses when sufficient cortisol is present in the blood and shuts off production of ACTH. If production of cortisol is deficient as a result of an enzymatic block, secretion of ACTH will increase, thus greatly increasing activity in the adrenal cortex, a situation referred to as hyperplasia. The result will be greatly increased synthesis of steroid hormones that are normally secreted only in very small amounts by the adrenal gland. In the most common form of congenital hyperplasia, androgenic hormones increase to very high levels. Since this condition is present from birth, the outcome is excessive virilization in infant girls and precocious sexual development in infant boys. Replacement therapy with cortisol restores ACTH levels to normal and reverses adrenal hyperplasia and its effects.

NONENDOCRINE DISORDERS

The beneficial effects of corticosteroids in disorders not related to the adrenal gland itself are usually based on the ability of these compounds to inhibit certain aspects of inflammatory and immunological responses. Only the glucocorticoid activity is needed for these purposes; therefore, synthetic corticosteroids that have little effect on salt and water retention are preferred.

AUTOIMMUNE DISORDERS

Corticosteroids are used to treat several conditions thought to result from the body's mounting an immune reaction against its own tissues (autoimmune response). These include neuromuscular disorders such as myasthenia gravis and multiple sclerosis (see the section on *Movement Disorders*, page 531). Corticosteroids may be used to achieve a remission in myasthenia gravis after other therapeutic approaches fail. They also may be of temporary benefit in multiple sclerosis.

Severe allergic disorders such as bronchial asthma may be treated with corticosteroids if other medications are inadequate. Corticosteroids are also useful as an adjunct to epinephrine in the treatment of severe acute allergic reactions (anaphylaxis) to drugs such as penicillin and with theophylline for the life-threatening condition called status asthmaticus. (See the section on *Asthma*, page 882, for a more detailed discussion.)

Connective Tissue Diseases

Connective tissue diseases are poorly understood disorders that affect many parts of the body. In the most studied connective tissue disease—systemic lupus erythematosus—the skin, kidney, heart, brain, and other organs may be damaged. Antibodies against many components of normal tissue have been detected in the blood of lupus patients, but their relation to the disease is not yet clear. Polymyositis is characterized by inflammation and pain in muscles throughout the body. If the skin is also involved, it is called dermatomyositis. A similar but less severe disease in older persons is polymyalgia rheumatica. Large doses of corticosteroids can alleviate acute attacks of these conditions, and long-term maintenance is useful in some cases. For skin manifestations topical steroid preparations are helpful.

Autoimmune Blood Disorders

Autoimmune hemolytic anemia The condition known as autoimmune hemolytic anemia, in which the body makes an antibody to its own red blood cells, often responds to prednisone, one of the more commonly prescribed corticosteroids.

Idiopathic thrombocytopenic purpura Steroids are the first-line treatment for idiopathic thrombocytopenic purpura, which involves destruction of the platelets, the cells in the blood that mediate clotting. Steroids are beneficial, particularly in the early stages of disease, to reduce intracranial hemorrhage.

Inflammatory Bowel Disease

Inflammatory bowel disorders such as ulcerative colitis and Crohn's disease have both an autoimmune and an inflammatory component. Local application, either by enema or rectal drip of corticosteroids, is sometimes useful in both acute and long-term therapy of ulcerative colitis. Steroids are less helpful for Crohn's disease, with alteration of diet and activity being the preferred first step to disease control.

INFLAMMATORY CONDITIONS

Dermatologic Problems

Steroids are helpful in preventing the swelling and tissue damage associated with many diseases, especially dermatologic problems.

Dermatoses Many skin lesions are complicated by both allergic and inflammatory components. Topical steroid creams and ointments are helpful for these conditions, including those associated with fungal infections. Injection of steroids directly into the sores of psoriasis or keloids often brings relief. (See the section on *Dermatitis and Psoriasis*, page 1079.)

Pemphigus vulgaris Rare and potentially fatal, pemphigus vulgaris is a disease in which groups of vesicles repeatedly erupt within the skin and mucous membranes. Massive doses of steroids can bring about remission of acute attacks, and lower maintenance doses can prevent recurrences.

Arthritis and Rheumatic Disorders

Perhaps the most common disease treated with steroids is arthritis (see the section on *Arthritis and Gout*, page 996.) Corticosteroids are employed for rheumatic diseases only when reduced activity, physical therapy, and use of aspirin or other nonsteroidal anti-inflammatory agents bring no relief of pain and immobility. Even then, steroids are used only during the acute phase of the disease. Systemic therapy can sometimes be avoided by injecting the preparation directly into the affected joint (intra-articular injection). However, this route is not used when the arthritis is thought to be due to infection (septic arthritis), since steroids reduce resistance to infection.

Miscellaneous Inflammatory Diseases

Liver disorders Steroids are used chiefly in inflammatory conditions such as severe alcoholic hepatitis and as the initial therapy for chronic active hepatitis. They are not appropriate, however, for the acute phase of viral hepatitis.

Idiopathic nephrotic syndrome A form of kidney damage in which protein is lost in the urine and body tissues swell with water is known as idiopathic nephrotic syndrome. In some children with an early form of this disease, steroid treatment induces a remission that is frequently permanent.

Eye diseases Allergic responses frequently involve inflammation of the eyelid or the conjunctiva, the membrane lining the underside of the eyelid. The sclera, the outermost surface of the eyeball, may also become red and swollen. Topical and injectable steroids are used to reduce these inflammations, but only if they are not associated with infection.

MISCELLANEOUS CONDITIONS

Cancer

For some cancers of the blood and lymph cells, prednisone is among the combination of drugs used to induce remissions. Cancers treated in this manner include acute lymphocytic leukemia, chronic lymphocytic leukemia, multiple myeloma, and Hodgkin's lymphoma. Prednisone is also included in some of the important chemotherapy regimens for breast cancer. In rare instances, steroids are able to induce remission in aplastic anemia, a condition in which primitive blood cells proliferate at the expense of mature, functional blood cells.

Cerebral Edema

Swelling of the brain caused by brain tumors or abscesses often responds to large doses of the synthetic corticosteroid dexamethasone (Decadron). This treatment is less successful for edema after stroke.

Respiratory Distress Syndrome

In premature infants, pulmonary function is often impaired due to lack of a substance called surfactant that allows expansion and contraction of the lungs. This condition can be fatal, or at least require extended hospitalization and ventilatory support. If delivery appears imminent before the thirty-fourth week of pregnancy, the obstetrician may administer an agent that inhibits labor for twenty-four to forty-eight hours and inject betamethasone (Celestone) or dexamethasone (Decadron) into the mother's circulation. These drugs enter the fetal circulation and in many cases induce production of mature surfactant, thereby preventing respiratory distress syndrome.

ORGAN TRANSPLANTATION

Immunological rejection is one of the major obstacles to successful transplantation of kidneys and other organs. The body's natural immunological system can recognize and destroy alien tissue, a defense function that is vital in maintaining health. On the other hand, there are instances in which the immune system goes awry (autoimmune disease) or in which its actions must be moderated or suppressed for other purposes. Organ transplantation falls into the latter category. This is why steroids are administered to patients undergoing kidney and other transplants; otherwise, the immune system would destroy these organs in much the same manner that it destroys invading bacteria and other foreign organisms.

MECHANISMS OF ACTION

Most observed effects of steroids in the body are probably secondary to some basic effect on cellular metabolism. At present, this basic mechanism is thought to involve an interaction of the hormones with the DNA in the cell's nucleus, resulting in increased synthesis of many different enzymes by the cell.

Measurable results of administration of steroids include increased glucose released from the liver, increased glucose formation from amino acids, and decreased utilization of glucose by the tissues. This results in increased glucose levels in the blood and a greater demand for insulin. Corticosteroids also decrease the synthesis of protein from amino acids, so that muscle and collagen are depleted.

During steroid therapy, the number of red blood cells increases and the number of lymphocytes is reduced, perhaps by direct destruction of lymphocytes. The ability of white blood cells to migrate to areas of tissue damage is decreased and the permeability of blood vessels to these cells is also reduced.

Corticosteroids increase secretion of acid by the stomach and of enzymes by the stomach and pancreas. They also produce mood changes, probably through their metabolic effects on the central nervous system.

SPECIAL PRECAUTIONS

As a direct result of the actions described above, long-term administration of adrenal corticosteroids can produce many undesired physiological changes. The use of steroids leads to insulin resistance, and the resulting increased demand for insulin, for example, can deplete the pancreas and lead to a diabetic state, which will aggravate any preexisting diabetes.

Breakdown of protein may lead to muscle wasting and weakness. Loss of bone tissue (osteoporosis) can reduce resistance to fractures, especially in children with nephrotic syndrome and people with arthritis.

Destruction of lymphocytes and decreased migratory capacity of these cells mediate the anti-immune and anti-inflammatory effects of steroids. But they also lead to a generalized susceptibility to infection, especially from viruses and fungi. Steroids can also reactivate latent tuberculosis. Decreased resistance to infection is particularly pronounced in cancer patients, transplant recipients, and people using topical steroids for eye conditions. In addition, because inflammatory responses are suppressed, infections may go undetected.

Increase in gastric secretions sometimes results in ulcers. Again, because of the masking of pain and inflammation, the ulcers may go undetected.

Large doses of steroids for prolonged periods may cause mental symptoms, such as euphoria, irritability, or hyperkinesia (excessive movement or restlessness). Steroids are not recommended for persons with preexisting mental problems unless they are a result of systemic lupus erythematosus, which may improve with steroid therapy.

Dosage Adjustments

Total steroid dosage can be reduced by employing alternate-day therapy. This has been used in psoriasis, ulcerative colitis, the skin condition pemphigus, and myasthenia gravis, and is being tested for kidney transplantation.

Administration of high doses of steroids can greatly suppress ACTH production via the natural feedback mechanism. If the steroid is suddenly stopped, there will not be enough ACTH to stimulate the adrenal glands and the patient will go into functional adrenal insufficiency, which can be fatal.

Therefore, after achieving the remission of a disease, steroids should be gradually tapered. This caution should also be followed in transferring asthma patients from systemic corticosteroids to an inhalant such as beclomethasone (Beclovent or Vanceril inhalers).

Because of the decreased immunity that steroids produce, they should not be used in patients with infections unless absolutely necessary. In these cases, antibiotics should be given simultaneously. A tuberculin skin test should be administered before using systemic steroids to guard against possible reactivation of tuberculosis. Persons with a positive tuberculin test may be given prophylactic drug therapy during steroid administration.

In an attempt to prevent ulcers in patients on long-term, high-dose steroids, some physicians prescribe concomitant use of an antacid. Even so, stools should be periodically examined for occult (microscopic) blood to detect bleeding ulcers.

There are several important interactions between metabolism of steroids and of other drugs. The anticonvulsants phenytoin (Dilantin or Phenytoin Sodium) and phenobarbital and the antibiotic rifampin (Rifadin, Rifamate, and Rimactane) enhance excretion of steroids, sometimes necessitating increased doses of the hormones. Breakdown of the steroid dexamethasone (Decadron) is increased by ephedrine, a compound used in many asthma drugs. Because they increase blood glucose, steroids can increase the requirement for insulin in diabetics. Steroids also enhance clearance of salicylates, which is important since both drugs may be used to treat patients with arthritis.

IN CONCLUSION

Corticosteroids are potent drugs, producing dramatic improvement in a wide variety of diseases. By the same token, they also affect many organ systems and body functions; therefore, they are usually reserved for use after other approaches have failed. They should always be used under the close supervision of a physician, and patients on steroids should be aware of possible signs warning of serious side effects. The following charts cover the major systemic corticosteroids. Topical steroids are in the section on *Dermatitis and Psoriasis* (page 1079) and steroids in inhalant forms are included in the section on *Asthma* (page 882 .)

ARISTOCORT (Triamcinolone) Lederle

Tabs: 1, 2, 4, 8, 16 mg

ARISTOCORT (Triamcinolone diacetate) Lederle

Vials: 40 mg/ml (1, 5 ml) (Aristocort Forte); 25 mg/ml (5 ml) for intralesional use **Syrup:** 2 mg/5 ml

INDICATIONS	ORAL DOSAGE	PARENTERAL DOSAGE
Endocrine disorders, including congenital adrenal hyperplasia, nonsuppurative thyroiditis, and hypercalcemia associated with cancer	**Adult:** 4–48 mg/day to start, followed by gradual reductions in dosage to lowest level consistent with maintaining an adequate clinical response; dosage must be individualized on the basis of the specific disease being treated, its severity, and clinical response	**Adult:** 3–48 mg in a single weekly IM dose to start, followed by gradual dosage adjustments to the point where adequate, but not necessarily complete, relief of symptoms is obtained
Primary or secondary adrenocortical insufficiency	**Adult:** 4–12 mg/day in addition to mineralocorticoid therapy	**Adult:** same as above, as well as preoperatively and in the event of serious trauma or illness
Rheumatic disorders, including psoriatic arthritis, rheumatoid arthritis, juvenile rheumatoid arthritis, ankylosing spondylitis, acute and subacute bursitis, acute nonspecific tenosynovitis, acute gouty arthritis, post-traumatic osteoarthritis, synovitis of osteoarthritis, and epicondylitis (adjunctive, short-term therapy)	**Adult:** ordinarily, 8–16 mg/day, given in a single morning dose daily or every other day, to start, followed by maintenance doses adjusted to keep symptoms to a tolerable level; some patients may require higher doses or may obtain greater relief on divided doses (bid or qid)	**Adult:** see ADMINISTRATION/ DOSAGE ADJUSTMENTS
Collagen diseases, including systemic lupus erythematosus	**Adult:** 20–32 mg/day to start, followed by maintenance therapy as above; patients with severe symptoms may require 48 mg/day or more and higher daily maintenance doses for 3–4 consecutive days, followed by a rest period of several days; repeat regimen weekly	**Adult:** same as above
Acute rheumatic carditis	**Adult:** 20–60 mg/day to start, followed by maintenance therapy, as above, for at least 6–8 wk (but seldom beyond 3 mo)	—
Dermatological diseases, including pemphigus, bullous dermatitis herpetiformis, severe erythema multiforme (Stevens-Johnson syndrome), exfoliative dermatitis, mycosis fungoides, and severe seborrheic dermatitis	**Adult:** 8–16 mg/day to start, followed by maintenance therapy as above; in these conditions, as well as in certain allergic dermatoses, alternate-day administration is effective and less likely to produce adverse effects	**Adult:** same as above (see also ADMINISTRATION/DOSAGE ADJUSTMENTS)
Severe psoriasis	**Adult:** 8–16 mg/day to start, followed by maintenance therapy as above	**Adult:** same as above
Acute seasonal or perennial allergic rhinitis	**Adult:** 8–12 mg/day; intractable cases may require high initial and maintenance doses; maintenance therapy should be limited in duration	**Adult:** same as above
Bronchial asthma	**Adult:** 8–16 mg/day; maintenance therapy should be limited in duration	**Adult:** same as above
Contact dermatitis, atopic dermatitis	**Adult:** short courses of 8–16 mg/day (supplementing topical therapy)	**Adult:** same as above
Serum sickness (adjunctive therapy); **drug hypersensitivity reactions; urticarial transfusion reactions** (IM use only); **acute noninfectious laryngeal edema** (IM use only)	**Adult:** determine dosage by severity of the disorder, the speed with which the therapeutic response is desired, and the response of the patient to initial therapy	**Adult:** same as above
Ophthalmic diseases, including allergic conjunctivitis, keratitis, allergic corneal marginal ulcers, herpes zoster ophthalmicus, iritis and iridocyclitis, chorioretinitis, anterior segment inflammation, diffuse posterior uveitis and choroiditis, optic neuritis, and sympathetic ophthalmia	**Adult:** 12–40 mg/day to start (depending on the severity of the condition, the nature, and degree of involvement of ocular structure), followed by maintenance therapy as above	**Adult:** same as above

Table continued on following page

ARISTOCORT continued

INDICATIONS continued	ORAL DOSAGE	PARENTERAL DOSAGE
Respiratory diseases, including symptomatic sarcoidosis, Loeffler's syndrome not manageable by other means, berylliosis, fulminating or disseminated pulmonary tuberculosis (with appropriate antituberculous chemotherapy), or aspiration pneumonitis	**Adult:** 16–48 mg/day to start, followed by maintenance therapy as above	**Adult:** same as above
Hematological disorders, including idiopathic thrombocytopenic purpura in adults (oral use only), secondary thrombocytopenia in adults, acquired (autoimmune) hemolytic anemia, erythroblastopenia (RBC anemia), and congenital (erythroid) hypoplastic anemia	**Adult:** 16–60 mg/day, followed by lower doses after adequate clinical response is obtained	**Adult:** same as above
Palliative management of **neoplastic diseases,** including leukemias and lymphomas in adults	**Adult:** 16–40 mg/day, or up to 100 mg/day for leukemia, if needed	**Adult:** same as above
Acute **leukemia** of childhood	**Child:** 1–2 mg/kg/day	—
To induce a diuresis or remission of proteinuria in the **nephrotic syndrome,** without uremia, of the idiopathic type or that due to lupus erythematosus	**Adult:** 16–20 mg/day (or up to 48 mg/day, if needed) until diuresis occurs; then continued treatment until maximal or complete chemical and clinical remission occurs; reduce dosage gradually and then discontinue; in less severe cases, as little as 4 mg/day may be adequate for maintenance	**Adult:** same as above
Tuberculous meningitis with subarachnoid block or impending block (with appropriate antituberculous chemotherapy)	**Adult:** 32–48 mg/day as a single dose or div	**Adult:** same as above
Gastrointestinal diseases, including ulcerative colitis and regional enteritis **Trichinosis** associated with neurological or myocardial involvement Acute exacerbations of **multiple sclerosis**		

ADMINISTRATION/DOSAGE ADJUSTMENTS

Suppression of autogenous pituitary function	May be minimized by administering a single daily dose at or after 8:00 AM or by use of alternate-day or intermittent dosage regimens if long-term therapy or high doses are needed
Alternate-day regimen	Once minimum effective dose has been established, administer total 48-h dose at 8:00 AM every other day
Intermittent therapy	When long-term administration of medium or high doses is required, the usual daily maintenance dose may be given for 3–4 consecutive days, followed by a 3-day "rest period" during which no corticosteroid is given; continue giving the drug in this fashion as long as it is therapeutically indicated
Intra-articular or intrasynovial administration	The usual dose varies from 5 to 40 mg, depending on the size of the joint; duration of effect varies from 1 wk to 2 mo. Acutely inflamed joints may require more frequent injections.
Intralesional administration (eg, keloids, lichen planus lesions, psoriatic plaques, ganglia)	The total amount of drug, the concentration, and the number and pattern of injection sites utilized depend on the size of the lesion. No more than 12.5 mg should be injected per injection site or 25 mg per lesion. For many conditions 2–3 injections at intervals of 1–2 wk are sufficient. Injections may be repeated, as needed, but probably no more than 75 mg/wk should be given to any one patient.

CONTRAINDICATIONS

Sensitivity to triamcinolone (oral only) •	Injection into infected or unstable joints •	Systemic fungal infections •

Table continued on following page

ARISTOCORT continued

WARNINGS/PRECAUTIONS	
Patients subjected to unusual stress	Require increased dosage of rapidly acting corticosteroids before, during, and after emotionally or physically stressful situations
Infection	Clinical signs may be masked, new infections may appear, resistance may be decreased, and infections may be difficult to localize
Ocular damage	Prolonged use may produce posterior subcapsular cataracts and glaucoma, with possible damage to optic nerves, and may enhance development of secondary fungal or viral ocular infections
Dietary salt restriction and potassium supplementation	May be necessary to combat blood pressure elevation, salt and water retention, and increased potassium excretion with high-dose therapy
Immunization procedures	Especially against smallpox, should not be undertaken because of possible neurological complications and lack of antibody response
Active tuberculosis	Restrict use to fulminating or disseminated cases, as an adjunct to appropriate antituberculous therapy
Latent tuberculosis or tuberculin reactivity	Observe patient closely, since reactivation of the disease may occur; during prolonged therapy, employ antituberculous chemoprophylactic measures
Secondary adrenocortical insufficiency	May be minimized by gradual dosage reduction; since insufficiency may persist for months, reinstitute corticosteroid therapy in any stressful situation during this period, and administer salt and/or a mineralocorticoid concurrently to correct impaired mineralocorticoid secretion
Hypothyroidism, hepatic cirrhosis	May enhance effects of triamcinolone
Corneal perforation	May occur in patients with ocular herpes simplex; use with caution
Special-risk patients	Use with caution in patients with nonspecific ulcerative colitis if impending perforation, abscess, or other pyogenic infection is likely, as well as in patients with diverticulitis, fresh intestinal anastomoses, active or latent peptic ulcer, renal insufficiency, hypertension, osteoporosis, or myasthenia gravis
Psychic derangements	May appear, ranging from euphoria, insomnia, mood swings, personality changes, and severe depression to frank psychotic manifestations; existing emotional instability or psychotic tendencies may be aggravated
Concomitant use with aspirin	Use with caution in patients with hypoprothrombinemia during therapy
Septic arthritis	May occur with intra-articular injection and require appropriate antimicrobial therapy; observe patient for suggestive symptoms (eg, increased pain, local swelling, further restrictions of joint mobility, fever, malaise) and examine joint fluid microscopically
Anaphylactoid reactions	Have occurred following parenteral corticosteroid administration; take appropriate precautionary measures before injecting triamcinolone diacetate, especially in patients with a history of drug allergy
ADVERSE REACTIONS	
Fluid and electrolyte disturbances	Sodium retention, fluid retention, congestive heart failure in susceptible patients, loss of potassium, hypokalemic alkalosis, hypertension
Musculoskeletal	Muscle weakness, steroid myopathy, loss of muscle mass, osteoporosis, vertebral compression fractures, aseptic necrosis of femoral and humeral heads, pathological fracture of long bones
Gastrointestinal	Peptic ulcer with possible perforation and hemorrhage, pancreatitis, abdominal distention, ulcerative esophagitis
Dermatological	Impaired wound healing, thin fragile skin, petechiae and ecchymoses, facial erythema, increased sweating, suppressed reaction to skin tests
Neurological	Convulsions, increased intracranial pressure with papilledema (pseudotumor cerebri), vertigo, headache
Endocrinological	Menstrual irregularities, Cushingoid state, growth suppression in children, secondary adrenocortical and pituitary unresponsiveness, decreased carbohydrate tolerance, latent diabetes mellitus, increased insulin or oral hypoglycemic requirements
Ophthalmic	Posterior subcapsular cataracts, increased intraocular pressure, glaucoma, exophthalmos
Metabolic	Negative nitrogen balance
Additional reactions to parenteral therapy only	Hyperpigmentation and hypopigmentation, subcutaneous and cutaneous atrophy, sterile abscess, postinjection flare (following intra-articular use), Charcot-like arthropathy, and blindness (rare) associated with intralesional therapy around the face and head

Table continued on following page

ARISTOCORT continued

OVERDOSAGE

Signs and symptoms	CNS changes, GI bleeding, hyperglycemia, hypertension, edema
Treatment	Discontinue medication; institute supportive measures, as required

DRUG INTERACTIONS

Insulin, oral hypoglycemics	⇩ Hypoglycemic effect
Phenytoin, phenobarbital, ephedrine, rifampin	⇧ Metabolic clearance of triamcinolone ⇩ Steroid blood level and physiological activity
Oral anticoagulants	⇧ or ⇩ Prothrombin time
Potassium-depleting diuretics	⇧ Risk of hypokalemia
Cardiac glycosides	⇧ Risk of arrhythmias or digitalis toxicity secondary to hypokalemia
Skin-test antigens	⇩ Reactivity
Immunizations	⇩ Antibody response

ALTERED LABORATORY VALUES

Blood/serum values	⇧ Glucose ⇧ Cholesterol ⇧ Sodium ⇩ Potassium ⇩ Calcium ⇩ PBI ⇩ Thyroxine (T_4) ⇩ ^{131}I thyroid uptake ⇩ Uric acid
Urinary values	⇧ Glucose ⇧ Potassium ⇧ Calcium ⇧ Uric acid ⇩ 17-Hydroxycorticosteroids (17-OHCS) ⇩ 17-Ketosteroids

Use in children

Growth and development should be carefully observed in infants and children on prolonged therapy; general guidelines not established for dosage recommendations

Use in pregnancy or nursing mothers

Safe use has not been established during pregnancy or for nursing mothers. Infants born of mothers who have received substantial doses of corticosteroids during pregnancy should be carefully observed for signs of hypoadrenalism.

Note: Triamcinolone also marketed as **KENACORT** (Squibb); triamcinolone acetonide is marketed as **KENALOG** (Squibb).

CELESTONE (Betamethasone) Schering

Tabs: 0.6 mg **Syrup:** 0.6 mg/5 ml

CELESTONE PHOSPHATE (Betamethasone sodium phosphate suspension) Schering

Amps: 4 mg/ml (1 ml) **Vial:** 4 mg/ml (5 ml)

CELESTONE SOLUSPAN (Betamethasone sodium phosphate and betamethasone acetate) Schering

Vial: 3.0 mg betamethasone (as betamethasone sodium phosphate) and 3.0 mg betamethasone acetate (5 ml)

INDICATIONS

Endocrine disorders, including primary or secondary adrenocortical insufficiency, congenital adrenal hyperplasia, nonsuppurative thyroiditis, and hypercalcemia associated with cancer (oral only), acute adrenocortical insufficiency (IM, IV only), preoperatively and in the event of serious trauma or illness in patients with known adrenal insufficiency or when adrenocortical reserve is doubtful (IM, IV only), and shock unresponsive to conventional therapy in patients with known or suspected adrenocortical insufficiency (IM, IV only)
Rheumatic disorders, including psoriatic arthritis, rheumatoid arthritis, juvenile rheumatoid arthritis, ankylosing spondylitis, acute and subacute bursitis, acute nonspecific tenosynovitis, acute gouty arthritis, posttraumatic osteoarthritis, synovitis of osteoarthritis, and epicondylitis (adjunctive, short-term therapy)
Collagen diseases, including systemic lupus erythematosus and acute rheumatic carditis
Dermatological diseases, including pemphigus, bullous dermatitis herpetiformis, severe erythema multiforme (Stevens-Johnson syndrome), exfoliative dermatitis, mycosis fungoides (oral only), severe psoriasis, and severe seborrheic dermatitis
Severe or incapacitating **allergic conditions** intractable to adequate trials of conventional treatment, including seasonal or perennial allergic rhinitis, bronchial asthma, contact dermatitis, atopic dermatitis, serum sickness, drug hypersensitivity reactions, urticarial transfusion reactions (IM, IV only), and acute noninfectious laryngeal edema (IM, IV only)
Opthalmic diseases, including allergic conjunctivitis (oral only), keratitis (oral only), allergic corneal marginal ulcers (oral), herpes zoster opthalmicus, iritis and iridocyclitis, chorioretinitis, anterior segment inflammation, diffuse posterior uveitis and choroiditis, optic neuritis, and sympathetic ophthalmia
Respiratory diseases, including symptomatic sarcoidosis, Loeffler's syndrome not manageable by other means (oral only), berylliosis, fulminating or disseminated pulmonary tuberculosis (with appropriate antituberculous chemotherapy), and aspiration pneumonitis
Hematological disorders, including idiopathic thrombocytopenic purpura (oral, IV only) and secondary thrombocytopenia in adults, acquired (autoimmune) hemolytic anemia, erythroblastopenia (RBC anemia) (oral only), and congenital (erythroid) hypoplastic anemia (oral only)
Palliative management of **neoplastic diseases,** including leukemias and lymphomas in adults and acute leukemia of childhood
To induce a diuresis or remission of proteinuria in the **nephrotic syndrome,** without uremia, of the idiopathic type or that due to lupus erythematosus
Gastrointestinal diseases, including ulcerative colitis and regional enteritis
Tuberculous meningitis with subarachnoid block or impending block (with appropriate antituberculous chemotherapy)
Trichinosis associated with neurological or myocardial involvement

ORAL DOSAGE

Adult: 0.6–7.2 mg/day to start, followed by gradual reductions in dosage to lowest level possible consistent with maintaining an adequate clinical response; dosage must be individualized on the basis of the specific disease being treated, its severity, and clinical response

PARENTERAL DOSAGE

Adult: 0.5–9.0 mg/day IM (Celestone Phosphate, Celestone Soluspan) or IV (Celestone Phosphate only) to start, followed by gradual reductions in dosage to lowest level possible consistent with maintaining an adequate clinical response; dosage must be individualized on the basis of the specific disease being treated, its severity, and clinical response; larger than usual doses may be justified in certain overwhelming, acute, life-threatening situations

ADMINISTRATION/DOSAGE ADJUSTMENTS

Intra-articular administration in rheumatoid arthritis and osteoarthritis	Dose of suspension is dependent on joint size, as follows: very large (hip), 1.0–2.0 ml; large, (eg, knee, ankle, shoulder), 1.0 ml; medium (eg, elbow, wrist), 0.5–1.0 ml; small (eg, metacarpophalangeal, interphalangeal, sternoclavicular), 0.25–0.5 ml. Systemic absorption of suspension following intra-articular administration should be considered in determining dosage in patients receiving concomitant oral or parenteral corticosteroids, especially in high doses.
Bursitis	For acute subdeltoid, subacromial, olecranon, and prepatellar bursitis, administer a single 1-ml dose of the suspension directly into the bursa; several intrabursal injections are usually required for recurrent acute bursitis and acute exacerbations of chronic bursitis. Once acute condition is controlled, lower doses may be given intrabursally to treat chronic bursitis.
Tenosynovitis and tendinitis	Inject 1.0 ml of the suspension into affected tendon sheath three or four times at intervals of 1–2 wk
Ganglia of joint capsules and tendon sheaths	Inject 0.5 ml of the suspension directly into ganglion cysts
Intralesional treatment of dermatologic conditions	Inject 0.2 ml/cm² of the suspension intradermally (not subcutaneously); up to a total of 1.0 ml may be given at weekly intervals

Table continued on following page

CELESTONE continued

ADMINISTRATION/DOSAGE ADJUSTMENTS continued	
Injections into the foot	Dose of suspension is dependent on disorder and location, as follows: bursitis under heloma durum or heloma molle, 0.25–0.5 ml; bursitis under calcaneal spur or over hallux rigidus or digiti quinti varus, 0.5 ml; tenosynovitis or periostitis of cuboid, 0.5 ml; acute gouty arthritis, 0.5–1.0 ml; injection may be repeated at 3- to 7-day intervals
Concomitant use of local anesthetics	Suspension may be mixed in a syringe with 1 or 2% lidocaine hydrochloride or similar local anesthetic solutions without parabens (avoid diluents containing methylparaben, propylparaben, phenol, etc); do not inject local anesthetics into Celestone Soluspan vial

CONTRAINDICATIONS

Systemic fungal infections ●	Injection into unstable or previously infected joints ●

WARNINGS/PRECAUTIONS	
Patients subjected to unusual stress	Require increased dosage of rapidly acting corticosteroids before, during, and after emotionally or physically stressful situations
Infection	Clinical signs may be masked, new infections may appear, resistance may be decreased, and infections may be difficult to localize
Ocular damage	Prolonged use may produce posterior subcapsular cataracts and glaucoma with possible damage to optic nerves, and may enhance development of secondary fungal or viral ocular infections
Dietary salt restriction and potassium supplementation	May be necessary to combat blood pressure elevation, salt and water retention, and increased potassium excretion with average- and high-dose therapy
Immunization procedures	Especially against smallpox, should not be undertaken because of possible neurological complications and lack of antibody response
Active tuberculosis	Restrict use to fulminating or disseminated cases, as an adjunct to appropriate antituberculous therapy
Latent tuberculosis or tuberculin reactivity	Observe patient closely, since reactivation of the disease may occur; during prolonged therapy, employ antituberculous chemoprophylactic measures
Secondary adrenocortical insufficiency	May be minimized by gradual dosage reduction; since insufficiency may persist for months, reinstitute corticosteroid therapy in any stressful situation during this period, and administer salt and/or a mineralocorticoid concurrently to correct impaired mineralocorticoid secretion
Hypothyroidism, hepatic cirrhosis	May enhance effects of betamethasone
Corneal perforation	May occur in patients with ocular herpes simplex; use with caution
Special-risk patients	Use with caution in patients with nonspecific ulcerative colitis if impending perforation, abscess, or other pyogenic infection is likely, as well as in patients with diverticulitis, fresh intestinal anastomoses, active or latent peptic ulcer, renal insufficiency, hypertension, osteoporosis, or myasthenia gravis
Psychic derangements	May appear, ranging from euphoria, insomnia, mood swings, personality changes, and severe depression to frank psychotic manifestations; existing emotional instability or psychotic tendencies may be aggravated
Concomitant use with aspirin	Use with caution in patients with hypoprothrombinemia during therapy
Septic arthritis	May occur with intra-articular injection and require appropriate antimicrobial therapy; observe patient for suggestive symptoms (eg, increased pain, local swelling, further restrictions of joint mobility, fever, malaise) and examine joint fluid microscopically
Anaphylactoid reactions	Have occurred following parenteral corticosteroid administration; take appropriate precautionary measures before injecting betamethasone sodium phosphate, especially in patients with a history of drug allergy

ADVERSE REACTIONS	
Fluid and electrolyte disturbances	Sodium retention, fluid retention, congestive heart failure in susceptible patients, loss of potassium, hypokalemic alkalosis, hypertension
Musculoskeletal	Muscle weakness, steroid myopathy, loss of muscle mass, osteoporosis, vertebral compression fractures, aseptic necrosis of femoral and humeral heads, pathological fracture of long bones
Gastrointestinal	Peptic ulcer with possible perforation and hemorrhage, pancreatitis, abdominal distention, ulcerative esophagitis
Dermatological	Impaired wound healing, thin fragile skin, petechiae and ecchymoses, facial erythema, increased sweating, suppressed reaction to skin tests

Table continued on following page

ADVERSE REACTIONS continued

Neurological	Convulsions, increased intracranial pressure with papilledema (pseudotumor cerebri), vertigo, headache
Endocrinological	Menstrual irregularities, Cushingoid state, growth suppression in children, secondary adrenocortical and pituitary unresponsiveness, decreased carbohydrate tolerance, latent diabetes mellitus, increased insulin or oral hypoglycemic requirements
Ophthalmic	Posterior subcapsular cataracts, increased intraocular pressure, glaucoma, exophthalmos
Metabolic	Negative nitrogen balance
Additional reactions to parenteral therapy only	Hyperpigmentation and hypopigmentation, subcutaneous and cutaneous atrophy, sterile abscess, postinjection flare (following intra-articular use), Charcot-like arthropathy, and blindness (rare) associated with intralesional therapy around face and head

OVERDOSAGE

Signs and symptoms	CNS changes, GI bleeding, hyperglycemia, hypertension, edema
Treatment	Discontinue medication; institute supportive measures, as required

DRUG INTERACTIONS

Insulin, oral hypoglycemics	⇩ Hypoglycemic effects
Phenytoin, phenobarbital, ephedrine, rifampin	⇧ Metabolic clearance of betamethasone ⇩ Steroid blood level and physiological activity
Oral anticoagulants	⇧ or ⇩ Prothrombin time
Potassium-depleting diuretics	⇧ Risk of hypokalemia
Cardiac glycosides	⇧ Risk of arrhythmias or digitalis toxicity secondary to hypokalemia
Skin-test antigens	⇩ Reactivity
Immunizations	⇩ Antibody response

ALTERED LABORATORY VALUES

Blood/serum values	⇧ Glucose ⇧ Cholesterol ⇧ Sodium ⇩ Potassium ⇩ Calcium ⇩ PBI ⇩ Thyroxine (T_4) ⇩ ^{131}I thyroid uptake ⇩ Uric acid
Urinary values	⇧ Glucose ⇧ Potassium ⇧ Calcium ⇧ Uric acid ⇩ 17-Hydroxycorticosteroids (17-OHCS) ⇩ 17-Ketosteroids

Use in children

Growth and development should be carefully observed in infants and children on prolonged therapy; general guidelines not established for dosage recommendations

Use in pregnancy or nursing mothers

Safe use has not been established during pregnancy or for nursing mothers. Infants born of mothers who have received substantial doses of corticosteroids during pregnancy should be carefully observed for signs of hypoadrenalism.

CORTEF (Hydrocortisone) **Upjohn**

Tabs: 5, 10, 20 mg **Vial:** 50 mg/ml (5 ml) for IM use only

CORTEF ACETATE (Hydrocortisone acetate suspension) **Upjohn**

Vial: 50 mg/ml (5 ml) for local injection only

CORTEF Fluid (Hydrocortisone cypionate) **Upjohn**

Oral susp: 13.4 mg (equivalent to 10 mg hydrocortisone)/5 ml

SOLU-CORTEF (Hydrocortisone sodium succinate) **Upjohn**

Vials: 100 mg (2 ml), 250 mg (2 ml), 500 mg (4 ml), 1 g (8 ml)

INDICATIONS

Endocrine disorders, including primary or secondary adrenocortical insufficiency, congenital adrenal hyperplasia, nonsuppurative thyroiditis, hypercalcemia associated with cancer, acute adrenocortical insufficiency (IM, IV only), and preoperatively and in the event of serious trauma or illness in patients with known adrenal insufficiency or when adrenocortical reserve is doubtful (IM, IV only)
Rheumatic disorders, including psoriatic arthritis, rheumatoid arthritis, juvenile rheumatoid arthritis, ankylosing spondylitis, acute and subacute bursitis, acute nonspecific tenosynovitis, acute gouty arthritis, posttraumatic osteoarthritis, synovitis of osteoarthritis, and epicondylitis (adjunctive, short-term therapy)
Collagen diseases, including systemic lupus erythematosus, acute rheumatic carditis, and systemic dermatomyositis (polymyositis)
Dermatological diseases, including pemphigus, bullous dermatitis herpetiformis, severe erythema multiforme (Stevens-Johnson syndrome), exfoliative dermatitis, mycosis fungoides, severe psoriasis, and severe seborrheic dermatitis
Severe or incapacitating **allergic conditions** intractable to adequate trials of conventional treatment, including seasonal or perennial allergic rhinitis, bronchial asthma, contact dermatitis, atopic dermatitis, serum sickness, drug hypersensitivity reactions, urticarial transfusion reactions (IM, IV only), and acute noninfectious laryngeal edema (IM, IV only)
Ophthalmic diseases, including allergic conjunctivitis, keratitis, allergic corneal marginal ulcers, herpes zoster ophthalmicus, iritis and iridocyclitis, chorioretinitis, anterior segment inflammation, diffuse posterior uveitis and choroiditis, optic neuritis, and sympathetic ophthalmia
Respiratory diseases, including symptomatic sarcoidosis, Loeffler's syndrome not manageable by other means, berylliosis, fulminating or disseminated pulmonary tuberculosis (with appropriate antituberculous chemotherapy), and aspiration pneumonitis
Hematological disorders, including idiopathic thrombocytopenic purpura (oral, IV only) and secondary thrombocytopenia in adults, acquired (autoimmune) hemolytic anemia, erythroblastopenia (RBC anemia), and congenital (erythroid) hypoplastic anemia
Palliative management of **neoplastic diseases,** including leukemias and lymphomas in adults and acute leukemia of childhood
To induce diuresis or remission of proteinuria in the **nephrotic syndrome,** without uremia, of the idiopathic type or that due to lupus erythematosus
Gastrointestinal diseases, including ulcerative colitis and regional enteritis
Tuberculous meningitis with subarachnoid block or impending block (with appropriate antituberculous chemotherapy)
Trichinosis associated with neurological or myocardial involvement

ORAL DOSAGE

Adult: 20–240 mg/day or 10–120 ml (2–24 tsp)/day to start, followed by gradual reductions in dosage to lowest level possible consistent with maintaining an adequate clinical response; dosage must be individualized on the basis of the specific disease being treated, its severity, and clinical response

PARENTERAL DOSAGE

Adult: 15–240 mg/day IM to start, followed by gradual reductions in dosage to lowest level possible consistent with maintaining an adequate clinical response; in emergencies or when adequate preparation cannot be accomplished by the IM route, 100–500 mg IV, injected over a period of 30 s or more and repeated at intervals of 1, 3, 6, or 10 h, as determined by patient's response and clinical condition; dosage must be individualized on the basis of the specific disease being treated, its severity, and clinical response; larger than usual doses may be justified in certain overwhelming, acute, life-threatening situations

ADMINISTRATION/DOSAGE ADJUSTMENTS

Severe shock	Suggested regimens include 500 mg IV q4–6h; 1–2 g IV q2–6h; 1 g IV to start, followed by 50 mg/kg IV q24h; 50 mg/kg IV to start, repeated in 4 h, if necessary, or q24h. Therapy is initiated by IV administration of Solu-Cortef over a period of one to several minutes and should be continued only until patient's condition stabilizes (usually not beyond 48–72 h). Prophylactic antacid therapy may be indicated to prevent peptic ulceration.
Acute exacerbations of multiple sclerosis	Administer 800 mg/day PO or IM for 1 wk, followed by 320 mg every other day for 1 mo
Intra-articular administration in rheumatoid arthritis, synovitis of osteoarthritis, posttraumatic osteoarthritis, and acute gouty arthritis	Dose of suspension depends on joint size, and interval between doses on duration of relief obtained. For the knee, inject 25 mg to start and repeat when symptoms return (every 1–4 wk or longer); subsequent doses may be increased to 37.5 or 50 mg, if needed. For smaller joints, 10–15 mg may suffice. Injections must be made into the synovial space, where the synovial cavity is most superficial and most free of large vessels and nerves.
Acute and subacute bursitis, epicondylitis, acute nonspecific tenosynovitis	Inject 25–50 mg of the suspension directly into affected site; if needed, dose may be repeated in 3–5 days

Table continued on following page

CORTEF continued

ADMINISTRATION/DOSAGE ADJUSTMENTS continued

Cystic tumor of an aponeurosis or tendon (ganglion)	Inject 10.0–12.5 mg of the suspension directly into the ganglion cyst

CONTRAINDICATIONS

Systemic fungal infections	Injection into previously infected or unstable joints

WARNINGS/PRECAUTIONS

Patients subjected to unusual stress	Require increased dosage of rapidly acting corticosteroids before, during, and after emotionally or physically stressful situations
Infection	Clinical signs may be masked, new infections may appear, resistance may be decreased, and infections may be difficult to localize
Ocular damage	Prolonged use may produce posterior subcapsular cataracts and glaucoma, with possible damage to optic nerves, and may enhance development of secondary fungal or viral ocular infections
Dietary salt restriction and potassium supplementation	May be necessary to combat blood pressure elevation, salt and water retention, and increased potassium excretion with average and high-dose therapy
Immunization procedures	Especially against smallpox, should not be undertaken because of possible neurological complications and lack of antibody response
Active tuberculosis	Restrict use to fulminating or disseminated cases, as an adjunct to appropriate antituberculous therapy
Latent tuberculosis or tuberculin reactivity	Observe patient closely, since reactivation of the disease may occur; during prolonged therapy, employ antituberculous chemoprophylactic measures
Secondary adrenocortical insufficiency	May be minimized by gradual dosage reduction; since insufficiency may persist for months, reinstitute corticosteroid therapy in any stressful situation during this period, and administer salt and/or a mineralocorticoid concurrently to correct impaired mineralocorticoid secretion
Hypothyroidism, hepatic cirrhosis	May enhance effects of hydrocortisone
Corneal perforation	May occur in patients with ocular herpes simplex; use with caution
Special-risk patients	Use with caution in patients with nonspecific ulcerative colitis if impending perforation, abscess, or other pyogenic infection is likely, as well as in patients with diverticulitis, fresh intestinal anastomoses, active or latent peptic ulcer, renal insufficiency, hypertension, osteoporosis, or myasthenia gravis
Psychic derangements	May appear, ranging from euphoria, insomnia, mood swings, personality changes, and severe depression to frank psychotic manifestations; existing emotional instability or psychotic tendencies may be aggravated
Concomitant use with aspirin	Use with caution in patients with hypoprothrombinemia
Prolonged therapy	Routine laboratory studies (eg, urinalysis, 2-h postprandial blood sugar, blood pressure, body weight, chest film) should be made at regular intervals; in addition, an upper GI series is suggested in patients with an ulcer history or significant dyspepsia. Withdraw the drug gradually, rather than abruptly, when discontinuing long-term therapy.
Hypernatremia	May occur when massive doses of hydrocortisone must be continued beyond 48–72 h (eg, in cases of severe shock); under these circumstances, consider replacing the parenteral form with a corticosteroid that causes little or no sodium retention, such as methylprednisolone sodium succinate
Septic arthritis	May occur with intra-articular injection and require appropriate antimicrobial therapy; observe patient for suggestive symptoms (eg, increased pain, local swelling, further restrictions of joint mobility, fever, malaise) and examine joint fluid microscopically
Anaphylactoid reactions	Have occurred following parenteral corticosteroid administration; take appropriate precautionary measures before injecting hydrocortisone, especially in patients with a history of drug allergy

Table continued on following page

CORTEF continued

ADVERSE REACTIONS	
Fluid and electrolyte disturbances	Sodium retention, fluid retention, congestive heart failure in susceptible patients, loss of potassium, hypokalemic alkalosis, hypertension
Musculoskeletal	Muscle weakness, steroid myopathy, loss of muscle mass, osteoporosis, vertebral compression fractures, aseptic necrosis of femoral and humeral heads, pathological fracture of long bones
Gastrointestinal	Peptic ulcer with possible perforation and hemorrhage, pancreatitis, abdominal distention, ulcerative esophagitis
Dermatological	Impaired wound healing, thin fragile skin, petechiae and ecchymoses, facial erythema, increased sweating, suppressed reaction to skin tests
Neurological	Convulsions, increased intracranial pressure with papilledema (pseudotumor cerebri), vertigo, headache
Endocrinological	Menstrual irregularities, Cushingoid state, growth suppression in children, secondary adrenocortical and pituitary unresponsiveness, decreased carbohydrate tolerance, latent diabetes mellitus, increased insulin or oral hypoglycemic requirements
Ophthalmic	Posterior subcapsular cataracts, increased intraocular pressure, glaucoma, exophthalmos
Metabolic	Negative nitrogen balance
Additional reactions to parenteral therapy only	Hyperpigmentation or hypopigmentation, subcutaneous and cutaneous atrophy, sterile abscess, postinjection flare (following intra-articular use), Charcot-like arthropathy, blindness (rare) associated with intralesional therapy around the face and head, anaphylactoid reactions (eg, bronchospasm)

OVERDOSAGE	
Signs and symptoms	CNS changes, GI bleeding, hyperglycemia, hypertension, edema
Treatment	Discontinue medication; institute supportive measures, as required

DRUG INTERACTIONS	
Insulin, oral hypoglycemics	⇩ Hypoglycemic effect
Phenytoin, phenobarbital, ephedrine, rifampin	⇧ Metabolic clearance of hydrocortisone ⇩ Steroid blood level and physiological activity
Oral anticoagulants	⇧ or ⇩ Prothrombin time
Potassium-depleting diuretics	⇧ Risk of hypokalemia
Cardiac glycosides	⇧ Risk of arrhythmias or digitalis toxicity secondary to hypokalemia
Skin-test antigens	⇩ Reactivity
Immunizations	⇩ Antibody response

ALTERED LABORATORY VALUES	
Blood/serum values	⇧ Glucose ⇧ Cholesterol ⇧ Sodium ⇩ Potassium ⇩ Calcium ⇩ PBI ⇩ Thyroxine (T_4) ⇩ ^{131}I thyroid uptake ⇩ Uric acid
Urinary values	⇧ Glucose ⇧ Potassium ⇧ Calcium ⇧ Uric acid ⇩ 17-Hydroxycorticosteroids (17-OHCS) ⇩ 17-Ketosteroids

Use in children

Growth and development should be carefully observed in infants and children on prolonged therapy; general guidelines not established for dosage recommendations

Use in pregnancy or nursing mothers

Safe use has not been established during pregnancy or for nursing mothers. Infants born of mothers who have received substantial doses of corticosteroids during pregnancy should be carefully observed for signs of hypoadrenalism.

Note: Hydrocortisone also marketed as **HYDROCORTONE** (Merck, Sharp & Dohme); and hydrocortisone sodium succinate also marketed **A-HYDROCORT** (Abbott).

CORTISONE ACETATE various manufacturers

Tabs: 5, 10, 25 mg **Vials:** 25 mg/ml (10, 20 ml), 50 mg/ml (10 ml)

INDICATIONS

Endocrine disorders, including primary or secondary adrenocortical insufficiency, congenital adrenal hyperplasia, nonsuppurative thyroiditis, hypercalcemia associated with cancer, acute adrenocortical insufficiency (IM only), and preoperatively and in the event of serious trauma or illness in patients with known adrenal insufficiency or when adrenocortical reserve is doubtful (IM only)
Rheumatic disorders, including psoriatic arthritis, rheumatoid arthritis, juvenile rheumatoid arthritis, ankylosing spondylitis, acute and subacute bursitis, acute nonspecific tenosynovitis, acute gouty arthritis, posttraumatic osteoarthritis, synovitis of osteoarthritis, and epicondylitis (adjunctive, short-term therapy)
Collagen diseases, including systemic lupus erythematosus, acute rheumatic carditis, and systemic dermatomyositis (polymyositis) (IM only)
Dermatological diseases, including pemphigus, bullous dermatitis herpetiformis, severe erythema multiforme (Stevens-Johnson syndrome), exfoliative dermatitis, mycosis fungoides, severe psoriasis, and severe seborrheic dermatitis
Severe or incapacitating **allergic conditions** intractable to adequate trials of conventional treatment, including seasonal or perennial allergic rhinitis, bronchial asthma, contact dermatitis, atopic dermatitis, serum sickness, drug hypersensitivity reactions, urticarial transfusion reactions (IM only) and acute noninfectious laryngeal edema (IM only)
Ophthalmic diseases, including allergic conjunctivitis, keratitis, allergic corneal marginal ulcers, herpes zoster ophthalmicus, iritis and iridocyclitis, chorioretinitis, anterior segment inflammation, diffuse posterior uveitis and choroiditis, optic neuritis, and sympathetic ophthalmia
Respiratory diseases, including symptomatic sarcoidosis, Loeffler's syndrome not manageable by other means, berylliosis, fulminating or disseminated pulmonary tuberculosis (with appropriate antituberculous chemotherapy), aspiration pneumonitis
Hematological disorders, including idiopathic thrombocytopenic purpura (oral only), secondary thrombocytopenia in adults, acquired (autoimmune) hemolytic anemia, erythroblastopenia (RBC anemia), and congenital (erythroid) hypoplastic anemia
Palliative management of **neoplastic diseases,** including leukemias and lymphomas in adults and acute leukemia of childhood
To induce diuresis or remission of proteinuria in the **nephrotic syndrome,** without uremia, of the idiopathic type or that due to lupus erythematosus
Gastrointestinal diseases, including ulcerative colitis and regional enteritis
Tuberculous meningitis with subarachnoid block or impending block (with appropriate antituberculous chemotherapy)
Trichinosis associated with neurological or myocardial involvement

ORAL DOSAGE

Adult: 25–300 mg/day to start, followed by gradual reductions in dosage to lowest level possible consistent with maintaining an adequate clinical response; dosage must be individualized on the basis of the specific disease being treated, its severity, and clinical response

PARENTERAL DOSAGE

Adult: 20–300 mg/day IM to start, followed by gradual reductions in dosage to lowest level possible consistent with maintaining an adequate clinical response; dosage must be individualized on the basis of the specific disease being treated, its severity, and clinical response; larger than usual doses may be justified in certain overwhelming, acute, life-threatening situations

CONTRAINDICATIONS

Systemic fungal infections

WARNINGS/PRECAUTIONS

Patients subjected to unusual stress	Require increased dosage of rapidly acting corticosteroids before, during, and after emotionally or physically stressful situations
Infection	Clinical signs may be masked, new infections may appear, resistance may be decreased, and infections may be difficult to localize
Ocular damage	Prolonged use may produce posterior subcapsular cataracts and glaucoma, with possible damage to optic nerves, and may enhance development of secondary infections
Dietary salt restriction and potassium supplementation	May be necessary to combat the blood pressure elevation, salt and water retention, and increased potassium excretion with average and high-dose therapy
Immunization procedures	Especially against smallpox, should not be undertaken because of possible neurological complications and lack of antibody response
Active tuberculosis	Restrict use to fulminating or disseminated cases, as an adjunct to appropriate antituberculous therapy
Latent tuberculosis or tuberculin reactivity	Observe patient closely, since reactivation of the disease may occur; during prolonged therapy, employ antituberculous chemoprophylactic measures
Secondary adrenocortical insufficiency	May be minimized by gradual dosage reduction; since insufficiency may persist for months, reinstitute corticosteroid therapy in any stressful situation during this period, and administer salt and/or a mineralocorticoid concurrently
Hypothyroidism, hepatic cirrhosis	May enhance effects of cortisone acetate
Corneal perforation	May occur in patients with ocular herpes simplex; use with caution
Prolonged therapy	Routine laboratory studies (eg, urinalysis, 2-h postprandial blood sugar, blood pressure, body weight, chest film) should be made at regular intervals; in addition, an upper GI series is suggested in patients with an ulcer history or significant dyspepsia. Withdraw the drug gradually, rather than abruptly

Table continued on following page

CORTISONE ACETATE continued

WARNINGS/PRECAUTIONS continued

Special-risk patients	Use with caution in patients with nonspecific ulcerative colitis if impending perforation, abscess, or other pyogenic infection is likely, as well as in patients with diverticulitis, fresh intestinal anastomoses, active or latent peptic ulcer, renal insufficiency, hypertension, osteoporosis, or myasthenia gravis
Psychic derangements	May appear, ranging from euphoria, insomnia, mood swings, personality changes, and severe depression to frank psychotic manifestations; existing emotional instability or psychotic tendencies may be aggravated
Concomitant use with aspirin	Use with caution in patients with hypoprothrombinemia during therapy
Anaphylactoid reactions	Have occurred following parenteral corticosteroid administration; take appropriate precautionary measures before injecting cortisone acetate, especially in patients with a history of drug allergy

ADVERSE REACTIONS

Fluid and electrolyte disturbances	Sodium retention, fluid retention, congestive heart failure in susceptible patients, loss of potassium, hypokalemic alkalosis, hypertension
Musculoskeletal	Muscle weakness, steroid myopathy, loss of muscle mass, osteoporosis, vertebral compression fractures, aseptic necrosis of femoral and humeral heads, pathological fracture of long bones
Gastrointestinal	Peptic ulcer with possible perforation and hemorrhage, pancreatitis, abdominal distention, ulcerative esophagitis
Dermatological	Impaired wound healing, thin fragile skin, petechiae and ecchymoses, facial erythema, increased sweating, suppressed reaction to skin tests
Neurological	Convulsions, increased intracranial pressure with papilledema (pseudotumor cerebri), vertigo, headache
Endocrinological	Menstrual irregularities, Cushingoid state, growth suppression in children, secondary adrenocortical and pituitary unresponsiveness, decreased carbohydrate tolerance, latent diabetes mellitus, increased insulin or oral hypoglycemic requirements
Ophthalmic	Posterior subcapsular cataracts, increased intraocular pressure, glaucoma, exophthalmos
Metabolic	Negative nitrogen balance
Additional reactions to parenteral therapy only	Hyperpigmentation or hypopigmentation, subcutaneous and cutaneous atrophy, sterile abscess, postinjection flare (following intra-articular use), Charcot-like arthropathy, blindness (rare) associated with intralesional therapy around the face and head

OVERDOSAGE

Signs and symptoms	CNS changes, GI bleeding, hyperglycemia, hypertension, edema
Treatment	Discontinue medication; institute supportive measures, as required

DRUG INTERACTIONS

Insulin, oral hypoglycemics	⇩ Hypoglycemic effect
Phenytoin, phenobarbital, ephedrine, rifampin	⇧ Metabolic clearance of cortisone ⇩ Steroid blood level and physiological activity
Oral anticoagulants	⇧ or ⇩ Prothrombin time
Potassium-depleting diuretics	⇧ Risk of hypokalemia
Cardiac glycosides	⇧ Risk of arrhythmias or digitalis toxicity secondary to hypokalemia
Skin-test antigens	⇩ Reactivity
Immunizations	⇩ Antibody response

ALTERED LABORATORY VALUES

Blood/serum values	⇧ Glucose ⇧ Cholesterol ⇧ Sodium ⇩ Potassium ⇩ Calcium ⇩ PBI ⇩ Thyroxine (T_4) ⇩ ^{131}I thyroid uptake ⇩ Uric acid
Urinary values	⇧ Glucose ⇧ Potassium ⇧ Calcium ⇧ Uric acid ⇩ 17-Hydroxycorticosteroids (17-OHCS) ⇩ 17-Ketosteroids

Use in children

Growth and development should be carefully observed in infants and children on prolonged therapy;

Use in pregnancy or nursing mothers

Safe use has not been established during pregnancy or for nursing mothers. Infants born of mothers who received substantial doses of corticosteroids during pregnancy should be carefully observed for signs of hypoadrenalism.

DECADRON (Dexamethasone) Merck Sharp & Dohme

Tabs: 0.25, 0.5, 0.75, 1.5, 4.0 mg **Elixir:** 0.5 mg/5 ml

DECADRON PHOSPHATE (Dexamethasone sodium phosphate) Merck Sharp & Dohme

Syringe: 4 mg/ml (1 ml) **Vials:** 4 mg/ml (1, 5, 25 ml); 24 mg/ml (5, 10 ml) for IV use only

INDICATIONS

Endocrine disorders, including primary or secondary adrenocortical insufficiency, congenital adrenal hyperplasia, nonsuppurative thyroiditis, and hypercalcemia associated with cancer
Rheumatic disorders, including psoriatic arthritis, rheumatoid arthritis, juvenile rheumatoid arthritis, ankylosing spondylitis, acute and subacute bursitis, acute nonspecific tenosynovitis, acute gouty arthritis, posttraumatic osteoarthritis, synovitis of osteoarthritis, and epicondylitis (adjunctive, short-term therapy)
Collagen diseases, including systemic lupus erythematosus and acute rheumatic carditis
Dermatological diseases, including pemphigus, bullous dermatitis herpetiformis, severe erythema multiforme (Stevens-Johnson syndrome), exfoliative dermatitis, mycosis fungoides, severe psoriasis, and severe seborrheic dermatitis
Severe or incapacitating **allergic conditions** intractable to adequate trials of conventional treatment, including seasonal or perennial allergic rhinitis, bronchial asthma, contact dermatitis, atopic dermatitis, serum sickness, drug hypersensitivity reactions, urticarial transfusion reactions (IM, IV only), and acute noninfectious laryngeal edema (IM, IV only)
Ophthalmic diseases, including allergic conjunctivitis, keratitis, allergic corneal marginal ulcers, herpes zoster ophthalmicus, iritis and iridocyclitis, chorioretinitis, anterior segment inflammation, diffuse posterior uveitis and choroiditis, optic neuritis, and sympathetic ophthalmia
Respiratory diseases, including symptomatic sarcoidosis, Loeffler's syndrome not manageable by other means, berylliosis, fulminating or disseminated pulmonary tuberculosis (with appropriate antituberculous chemotherapy), and aspiration pneumonitis
Hematological disorders, including idiopathic thrombocytopenic purpura (oral, IV only) and secondary thrombocytopenia in adults, acquired (autoimmune) hemolytic anemia, erythroblastopenia (RBC anemia), and congenital (erythroid) hypoplastic anemia
Palliative management of **neoplastic diseases,** including leukemias and lymphomas in adults and acute leukemia of childhood
To induce a diuresis or remission of proteinuria in the **nephrotic syndrome,** without uremia, of the idiopathic type or that due to lupus erythematosus
Gastrointestinal diseases, including ulcerative colitis and regional enteritis
Tuberculous meningitis with subarachnoid block or impending block (with appropriate antituberculous chemotherapy)
Trichinosis associated with neurological or myocardial involvement

ORAL DOSAGE

Adult: 0.75–9 mg/day to start, followed by gradual reductions in dosage to lowest level possible consistent with maintaining an adequate clinical response; dosage must be individualized on the basis of the specific disease being treated, its severity, and clinical response; smaller doses than these may be sufficient in less severe diseases, while doses higher than 9 mg/day may be required in more severe diseases

PARENTERAL DOSAGE

Adult: 0.5–9 mg/day IM or IV to start, followed by gradual reductions in dosage to lowest level possible consistent with maintaining an adequate clinical response; dosage must be individualized on the basis of the specific diseases being treated, its severity, and clinical response; smaller doses than these may be sufficient in less severe diseases, while doses higher than 9 mg/day may be required in more severe diseases

DECADRON-LA Suspension (Dexamethasone acetate) Merck Sharp & Dohme

Vials: 8 mg/ml (1, 5 ml)

INDICATIONS

Same as Decadron Phosphate, except for adrenocortical insufficiency, pulmonary tuberculosis, and idiopathic thrombocytopenic purpura in adults

PARENTERAL DOSAGE

Adult: 8–16 mg IM, repeated at 1- to 3-wk intervals, if needed; dosage must be individualized on the basis of the specific disease being treated, its severity, and clinical response

ADMINISTRATION/DOSAGE ADJUSTMENTS

Unresponsive shock	Suggested regimens include 40 mg IV q2–6h; 1–6 mg/kg as a single IV injection; and 20 mg IV to start, followed by 3 mg/kg/24 h by continuous IV infusion. Treatment should be continued only until patient's condition stabilizes (usually not beyond 48–72 h). Prophylactic antacid therapy may be indicated to prevent peptic ulceration.
Cerebral edema associated with brain tumors, craniotomy, or head injury	Administer 10 mg Decadron Phosphate IV to start, followed by 4 mg IM q6h until symptoms subside; for palliative management, give 2 mg bid or tid, orally or parenterally
Intra-articular, soft-tissue, and intralesional administration (keloids, lichen planus lesions, psoriatic plaques, ganglia)	Employ only when the affected joints or areas are limited to one or two sites as follows: large joints (eg, knee), 2–4 mg; small joints (eg, interphalangeal, temporomandibular), 0.8–1.0 mg; bursal, 2–3 mg; tendon sheaths, 0.4–1.0 mg; soft-tissue infiltration, 2–6 mg; and ganglia, 1–2 mg. The frequency ranges from once every 3–5 days to once every week for Decadron Phosphate and 1–3 wk for Decadron-LA Suspension.
Dexamethasone suppression tests for Cushing's syndrome	Give 1 mg orally at 11:00 PM. Draw blood for plasma cortisol determination at 8:00 AM on the following morning. For greater accuracy, give 0.5 mg orally q6h for 48 h; collect a 24-h urine specimen for determination of 17-hydroxycorticosteroid excretion. To distinguish Cushing's disease from other causes of hypercortisolism, give 2 mg orally q6h for 48 h; collect a 24-h urine specimen for determination of 17-hydroxycorticosteroid excretion.

Table continued on following page

DECADRON continued

ADMINISTRATION/DOSAGE ADJUSTMENTS continued

Acute, self-limiting allergic disorders or acute exacerbations of chronic allergic disorders	Combine parenteral and oral therapy as follows: first day, 4–8 mg Decadron Phosphate IM; second and third days, 3 mg in two divided oral doses; fourth day, 1.5 mg in two divided oral doses; fifth and sixth days, 0.75 mg in a single oral dose; seventh day, no treatment; eighth day, follow up

CONTRAINDICATIONS

Sensitivity to dexamethasone or any other component ●

Injection into infected or unstable joints ●

Systemic fungal infections[1] ●

WARNINGS/PRECAUTIONS

Patients subjected to unusual stress	Require increased dosage of rapidly acting corticosteroids before, during, and after emotionally or physically stressful situations
Infection	Clinical signs may be masked, new infections may appear, resistance may be decreased, and infections may be difficult to localize; false-negative results may be obtained with nitroblue-tetrazolium test for bacterial infection
Latent amebiasis	May be activated; before instituting therapy, rule out latent or active amebiasis in any patient with unexplained diarrhea or who has spent time in the tropics
Ocular damage	Prolonged use may produce posterior subcapsular cataracts and glaucoma with possible damage to optic nerves, and may enhance development of secondary fungal or viral ocular infections
Dietary salt restriction and potassium supplementation	May be necessary to combat blood-pressure elevation, salt and water retention, and increased potassium excretion with average- and high-dose therapy
Immunization procedures	Especially against smallpox, should not be undertaken because of possible neurological complications and lack of antibody response, unless replacement therapy is being given for adrenocortical insufficiency
Active tuberculosis	Restrict use to fulminating or disseminated cases, as an adjunct to appropriate antituberculous therapy
Latent tuberculosis or tuberculin reactivity	Observe patient closely, since reactivation of the disease may occur; during prolonged therapy, employ antituberculous chemoprophylactic measures
Secondary adrenocortical insufficiency	May be minimized by gradual dosage reduction; since insufficiency may persist for months, reinstitute corticosteroid therapy in any stressful situation during this period, and administer salt and/or a mineralocorticoid concurrently to correct impaired mineralocorticoid secretion
Withdrawal symptoms	Including fever, myalgia, arthralgia, and malaise, may occur when drug is withdrawn following prolonged therapy, even in the absence of adrenal insufficiency
Hypothyroidism, hepatic cirrhosis	May enhance effects of dexamethasone
Corneal perforation	May occur in patients with ocular herpes simplex; use with caution
Special-risk patients	Use with caution in patients with nonspecific ulcerative colitis if impending perforation, abscess, or other pyogenic infection is likely, as well as in patients with diverticulitis, fresh intestinal anastomoses, active or latent peptic ulcer, renal insufficiency, hypertension, osteoporosis, or myasthenia gravis
Peptic ulcer, with possible perforation and hemorrhage	May occur, especially with large doses; risk may be minimized by administering with meals and taking antacids between meals
Psychic derangements	May appear, ranging from euphoria, insomnia, mood swings, personality changes, and severe depression to frank psychotic manifestations; existing emotional instability or psychotic tendencies may be aggravated
Concomitant use with aspirin	Use with caution in patients with hypoprothrombinemia during therapy
Concomitant use with oral anticoagulants	Check prothrombin time frequently; anticoagulant effect may be increased or decreased
Concomitant use with potassium-depleting diuretics	Monitor serum potassium level periodically; risk of hypokalemia is increased
Suppression tests	May be altered by phenytoin, phenobarbital, ephedrine, and rifampin; interpret with caution
Fertility	Motility and number of spermatozoa may be increased or decreased
Septic arthritis	May occur with intra-articular injection and require appropriate antimicrobial therapy; observe patient for suggestive symptoms (eg, increased pain, local swelling, further restrictions of joint mobility, fever, malaise) and examine joint fluid microscopically
Frequent intra-articular injection	May damage joint tissue
Overuse of joints	Caution patients who experience symptomatic relief against overusing joints as long as inflammatory process remains active

[1]Unless needed to control drug reactions due to amphotericin B

Table continued on following page

WARNINGS/PRECAUTIONS continued	
Anaphylactoid reactions	Have occurred following parenteral corticosteroid administration; take appropriate precautionary measures before injecting dexamethasone, especially in patients with a history of drug allergy

ADVERSE REACTIONS	
Fluid and electrolyte disturbances	Sodium retention, fluid retention, congestive heart failure in susceptible patients, loss of potassium, hypokalemic alkalosis, hypertension
Musculoskeletal	Muscle weakness, steroid myopathy, loss of muscle mass, osteoporosis, vertebral compression fractures, aseptic necrosis of femoral and humeral heads, pathological fracture of long bones, tendon rupture
Gastrointestinal	Peptic ulcer with possible perforation and hemorrhage, pancreatitis, abdominal distention, ulcerative esophagitis, increased appetite, nausea
Dermatological	Impaired wound healing, thin fragile skin, petechiae and ecchymoses, facial erythema, increased sweating, suppressed reactions to skin tests, allergic dermatitis, urticaria, angioneurotic edema
Neurological	Convulsions, increased intracranial pressure with papilledema (pseudotumor cerebri), vertigo, headache
Endocrinological	Menstrual irregularities, Cushingoid state, growth suppression in children, secondary adrenocortical and pituitary unresponsiveness, decreased carbohydrate tolerance, latent diabetes mellitus, increased insulin or oral hypoglycemic requirements
Ophthalmic	Posterior subcapsular cataracts, increased intraocular pressure, glaucoma, exophthalmos
Metabolic	Negative nitrogen balance, weight gain
Other	Anaphylactoid or hypersensitivity reactions, thromboembolism, malaise
Additional reactions to parenteral therapy only	Hyperpigmentation or hypopigmentation; subcutaneous and cutaneous atrophy; sterile abscess; postinjection flare (following intra-articular use); Charcot-like arthropathy; blindness associated with intralesional therapy around the face and head (rare); burning or tingling, especially in perineal area (with IV use); scarring; induration; inflammation; paresthesia; delayed pain or soreness; muscle twitching, ataxia, hiccoughs, and nystagmus (following use of suspension)

OVERDOSAGE	
Signs and symptoms	CNS changes, GI bleeding, hyperglycemia, hypertension, edema
Treatment	Discontinue medication; institute supportive measures, as required

DRUG INTERACTIONS	
Insulin, oral hypoglycemics	⇩ Hypoglycemic effect
Phenytoin, phenobarbital, ephedrine, rifampin	⇧ Metabolic clearance of dexamethasone ⇩ Steroid blood level and physiological activity
Oral anticoagulants	⇧ or ⇩ Prothrombin time
Potassium-depleting diuretics	⇧ Risk of hypokalemia
Cardiac glycosides	⇧ Risk of arrhythmias or digitalis toxicity secondary to hypokalemia
Skin-test antigens	⇩ Reactivity
Immunizations	⇩ Antibody response

ALTERED LABORATORY VALUES	
Blood/serum values	⇧ Glucose ⇧ Cholesterol ⇧ Sodium ⇩ Potassium ⇩ Calcium ⇩ PBI ⇩ Thyroxine (T_4) ⇩ ^{131}I thyroid uptake ⇩ Uric acid
Urinary values	⇧ Glucose ⇧ Potassium ⇧ Calcium ⇧ Uric acid ⇩ 17-Hydroxycorticosteroids (17-OHCS) ⇩ 17-Ketosteroids

Use in children

Growth and development should be carefully observed in infants and children on prolonged therapy; general guidelines not established for dosage recommendations Decadron and Decadron Phosphate. Dosage of Decadron-LA Suspension has not been established in children under 12 yr of age.

Use in pregnancy or nursing mothers

Safe use has not been established during pregnancy. Infants born of mothers who have received substantial doses of corticosteroids during pregnancy should be carefully observed for signs of hypoadrenalism. Corticosteroids appear in breast milk and may suppress growth, interfere with endogenous corticosteroid production, or cause other untoward effects. Patient should stop nursing if drug is prescribed.

DELTASONE (Prednisone) Upjohn

Tabs: 2.5, 5, 10, 20, 50 mg

INDICATIONS	ORAL DOSAGE
Endocrine disorders, including primary or secondary adrenocortical insufficiency, congenital adrenal hyperplasia, nonsuppurative thyroiditis, and hypercalcemia associated with cancer **Rheumatic disorders,** including psoriatic arthritis, rheumatoid arthritis, juvenile rheumatoid arthritis, ankylosing spondylitis, acute and subacute bursitis, acute nonspecific tenosynovitis, acute gouty arthritis, posttraumatic osteoarthritis, synovitis of osteoarthritis, and epicondylitis (adjunctive, short-term therapy) **Collagen diseases,** including systemic lupus erythematosus, acute rheumatic carditis and systemic dermatomyositis (polymyositis) **Dermatological diseases,** including pemphigus, bullous dermatitis herpetiformis, severe erythema multiforme (Stevens-Johnson syndrome), exfoliative dermatitis, mycosis fungoides, severe psoriasis, and severe seborrheic dermatitis Severe or incapacitating **allergic conditions** intractable to adequate trials of conventional treatment, including seasonal or perennial allergic rhinitis, bronchial asthma, contact dermatitis, atopic dermatitis, serum sickness, and drug hypersensitivity reactions **Ophthalmic diseases,** including allergic conjunctivitis, keratitis, allergic corneal marginal ulcers, herpes zoster ophthalmicus, iritis and iridocyclitis, chorioretinitis, anterior segment inflammation, diffuse posterior uveitis and choroiditis, optic neuritis, and sympathetic ophthalmia **Respiratory diseases,** including symptomatic sarcoidosis, Loeffler's syndrome not manageable by other means, berylliosis, fulminating or disseminated pulmonary tuberculosis (with appropriate antituberculous chemotherapy), and aspiration pneumonitis **Hematological disorders,** including idiopathic thrombocytopenic purpura and secondary thrombocytopenic purpura in adults, acquired (autoimmune) hemolytic anemia, erythroblastopenia (RBC anemia), and congenital (erythroid) hypoplastic anemia Palliative management of **neoplastic diseases,** including leukemias and lymphomas in adults and acute leukemia of childhood To induce a diuresis or remission of proteinuria in the **nephrotic syndrome,** without uremia, of the idiopathic type or that due to lupus erythematosus **Gastrointestinal disease,** including ulcerative colitis and regional enteritis **Tuberculous meningitis** with subarachnoid block or impending block (with appropriate antituberculous chemotherapy) **Trichinosis** associated with neurological or myocardial involvement	**Adult:** 5–60 mg/day to start, followed by gradual reductions in dosage to lowest level possible consistent with maintaining an adequate clinical response; dosage must be individualized on the basis of the specific disease being treated, its severity, and clinical response
Acute exacerbations of **multiple sclerosis**	**Adult:** 200 mg/day for 1 wk, followed by 80 mg every other day for 1 mo

ADMINISTRATION/DOSAGE ADJUSTMENTS

Alternate-day regimen	For patients requiring long-term steroid therapy, twice the usual daily dose may be given every other morning. Continue the initial suppressive dose level until a satisfactory clinical response is obtained (usually 4–10 days for many allergic and collagen diseases). Then change to alternate-day therapy and gradually reduce the dose given every other day, or first reduce the daily dose to the lowest effective level as quickly as possible and then change over to an alternate-day schedule. If an acute flare-up of the disease occurs, return to a full suppressive daily divided dosage regimen for control. Reinstate the alternate-day regimen when control is re-established. If difficulty is encountered in switching patients who have been on a daily regimen for long periods to alternate-day therapy, initially tripling or even quadrupling the daily maintenance dose and giving it every other day may be helpful.
Drug withdrawal	Withdraw drug gradually, rather than abruptly, after long-term therapy

CONTRAINDICATIONS

Systemic fungal infections

WARNINGS/PRECAUTIONS

Patients subjected to unusual stress	Require increased dosage of rapidly acting corticosteroids before, during, and after emotionally or physically stressful situations
Infection	Clinical signs may be masked, new infections may appear, resistance may be decreased, and infections may be difficult to localize
Ocular damage	Prolonged use may produce posterior subcapsular cataracts and glaucoma, with possible damage to optic nerves, and may enhance development of secondary fungal or viral ocular infections

Table continued on following page

WARNINGS/PRECAUTIONS continued	
Dietary salt restriction and potassium supplementation	May be necessary to combat blood-pressure elevation, salt and water retention, and increased potassium excretion with average- and high-dose therapy
Immunization procedures	Especially against smallpox, should not be undertaken because of possible neurological complications and lack of antibody response, unless replacement therapy is being given for adrenocortical insufficiency
Active tuberculosis	Restrict use to fulminating or disseminated cases, as an adjunct to appropriate antituberculous therapy
Latent tuberculosis or tuberculin reactivity	Observe patient closely, since reactivation of the disease may occur; during prolonged therapy, employ antituberculous chemoprophylactic measures
Secondary adrenocortical insufficiency	May be minimized by gradual dosage reduction; since insufficiency may persist for months, reinstitute corticosteroid therapy in any stressful situation during this period, and administer salt and/or a mineralocorticoid concurrently to correct impaired mineralocorticoid secretion
Hypothyroidism, hepatic cirrhosis	May enchance effects of prednisone
Corneal perforation	May occur in patients with ocular herpes simplex; use with caution
Special-risk patients	Use with caution in patients with nonspecific ulcerative colitis if impending perforation, abscess, or other pyogenic infection is likely, as well as in patients with diverticulitis, fresh intestinal anastomoses, active or latent peptic ulcer, renal insufficiency, hypertension, osteoporosis, or myasthenia gravis
Psychic derangements	May appear, ranging from euphoria, insomnia, mood swings, personality changes, and severe depression to frank psychotic manifestations; existing emotional instability or psychotic tendencies may be aggravated
Concomitant use with aspirin	Use with caution in patients with hypoprothrombinemia during therapy
ADVERSE REACTIONS	
Fluid and electrolyte disturbances	Sodium retention, fluid retention, congestive heart failure in susceptible patients, loss of potassium, hypokalemic alkalosis, hypertension
Musculoskeletal	Muscle weakness, steroid myopathy, loss of muscle mass, osteoporosis, vertebral compression fractures, aseptic necrosis of femoral and humeral heads, pathological fracture of long bones
Gastrointestinal	Peptic ulcer with possible perforation and hemorrhage, pancreatitis, abdominal distention, ulcerative esophagitis
Dermatological	Impaired wound healing, thin fragile skin, petechiae and ecchymoses, facial erythema, increased sweating, suppressed reaction to skin tests
Neurological	Convulsions, increased intracranial pressure with papilledema (pseudotumor cerebri), vertigo, headache
Endocrinological	Menstrual irregularities, Cushingoid state, growth suppression in children, secondary adrenocortical and pituitary unresponsiveness, decreased carbohydrate tolerance, latent diabetes mellitus, increased insulin or oral hypoglycemic requirements
Ophthalmic	Posterior subcapsular cataracts, increased intraocular pressure, glaucoma, exophthalmos
Metabolic	Negative nitrogen balance
OVERDOSAGE	
Signs and symptoms	CNS changes, GI bleeding, hyperglycemia, hypertension, edema
Treatment	Discontinue medication; institute supportive measures, as required
DRUG INTERACTIONS	
Insulin, oral hypoglycemics	⇩ Hypoglycemic effect
Phenytoin, phenobarbital, ephedrine, rifampin	⇧ Metabolic clearance of prednisolone ⇩ Steroid blood level and physiological activity
Oral anticoagulants	⇧ or ⇩ Prothrombin time
Potassium-depleting diuretics	⇧ Risk of hypokalemia
Cardiac glycosides	⇧ Risk of arrhythmias or digitalis toxicity secondary to hypokalemia
Skin-test antigens	⇩ Reactivity
Immunizations	⇩ Antibody response
Tetracycline	⇩ Absorption of tetracycline

Table continued on following page

ALTERED LABORATORY VALUES

Blood/serum values	⇧ Glucose ⇧ Cholesterol ⇧ Sodium ⇩ Potassium ⇩ Calcium ⇩ PBI ⇩ Thyroxine (T_4) ⇩ ^{131}I thyroid uptake ⇩ Uric acid
Urinary values	⇧ Glucose ⇧ Potassium ⇧ Calcium ⇧ Uric acid ⇩ 17-Hydroxycorticosteroids (17-OHCS) ⇩ 17-Ketosteroids

Use in children

Growth and development should be carefully observed in infants and children on prolonged therapy; general guidelines not established for dosage recommendations

Use in pregnancy or nursing mothers

Safe use has not been established during pregnancy or for nursing mothers. Infants born of mothers who have received substantial doses of corticosteroids during pregnancy should be carefully observed for signs of hypoadrenalism.

Note: Prednisone also marketed as **METICORTEN** (Schering) and **ORASONE** (Rowell).

MEDROL (Methylprednisolone) Upjohn

Tabs: 2, 4, 8, 16, 24, 32 mg

DEPO-MEDROL (Methylprednisolone acetate suspension) Upjohn

Syringe: 80 mg/ml (1 ml) **Vials:** 20 mg/ml (5 ml), 40 mg/ml (1, 5, 10 ml), 80 mg/ml (1, 5 ml)

INDICATIONS

Endocrine disorders, including primary or secondary adrenocortical insufficiency, congenital adrenal hyperplasia, nonsuppurative thyroiditis, hypercalcemia associated with cancer, acute adrenocortical insufficiency (IM only), and preoperatively and in the event of serious trauma or illness in patients with known adrenal insufficiency or when adrenocortical reserve is doubtful (IM only)
Rheumatic disorders, including psoriatic arthritis, rheumatoid arthritis, juvenile rheumatoid arthritis, ankylosing spondylitis, acute and subacute bursitis, acute non-specific tenosynovitis, acute gouty arthritis, posttraumatic osteoarthritis (adjunctive, short-term therapy)
Collagen diseases, including systemic lupus erythematosus, acute rheumatic carditis, and systemic dermatomyositis (polymyositis)
Dermatological diseases, including pemphigus, bullous dermatitis herpetiformis, severe erythema multiforme (Stevens-Johnson syndrome), exfoliative dermatitis, mycosis fungoides, severe psoriasis, and severe seborrheic dermatitis
Severe or incapacitating **allergic conditions** intractable to adequate trials of conventional treatment, including seasonal or perennial allergic rhinitis, bronchial asthma, contact dermatitis, atopic dermatitis, serum sickness, drug hypersensitivity reactions, urticarial transfusion reactions (IM only), and acute noninfectious laryngeal edema (IM only)
Ophthalmic diseases, including allergic conjunctivitis , keratitis, allergic corneal marginal ulcers, herpes zoster ophthalmicus, iritis and iridocyclitis, chorioretinitis, anterior segment inflammation, diffuse posterior uveitis and choroiditis, optic neuritis, and sympathetic ophthalmia
Respiratory diseases, including symptomatic sarcoidosis, Loeffler's syndrome not manageable by other means, berylliosis, fulminating or disseminated pulmonary tuberculosis (with appropriate antituberculous chemotherapy), and aspiration pneumonitis
Hematological disorders, including idiopathic thrombocytopenic purpura (oral only), secondary thrombocytopenia in adults, acquired (autoimmune) hemolytic anemia, erythroblastopenia (RBC anemia), and congenital (erythroid) hypoplastic anemia
Palliative management of **neoplastic diseases,** including leukemias and lymphomas in adults and acute leukemia of childhood
To induce diuresis or remission of proteinuria in the **nephrotic syndrome,** without uremia, of the idiopathic type or that due to lupus erythematosus
Gastrointestinal diseases, including ulcerative colitis and regional enteritis
Tuberculosis meningitis with subarachnoid block or impending block (with appropriate antituberculous chemotherapy)
Trichinosis associated with neurological or myocardial involvement

ORAL DOSAGE

Adult: 4–48 mg/day to start, followed by gradual reductions in dosage to lowest level possible consistent with maintaining an adequate clinical response; dosage must be individualized on the basis of the specific disease being treated, its severity, and clinical response

PARENTERAL DOSAGE

Adult: 4–48 mg, given in a single IM injection q24h, or, for prolonged effect, 7 times the daily oral dose, given in a single IM injection once a week; dosage must be individualized on the basis of disease severity and clinical response

SOLU-MEDROL (Methylprednisolone sodium succinate) Upjohn

Vials: 40 mg (1 ml), 125 mg (2 ml), 500 mg (8 ml), 1 g (16 ml)

INDICATIONS

Acute adrenocortical insuffiency
Acute rheumatic fever[1]
Systemic lupus erythematosus
Dermatological diseases, including pemphigus, severe erythema multiforme (Stevens-Johnson syndrome), exfoliative dermatitis, and generalized neurodermatitis[1]
Severe or incapacitating **allergic conditions** intractable to adequate trials of conventional treatment, including bronchial asthma, contact dermatitis, serum sickness, drug hypersensitivity reactions, angioedema,[2] urticaria,[2] and as an adjunct to epinephrine in anaphylaxis[2]
Ulcerative colitis
Overwhelming infections with severe toxicity (adjunctive therapy)[1]
Esophageal burns from ingestion of caustic[1]

PARENTERAL DOSAGE

Adult: 10–40 mg IV to start, repeated IV or IM at intervals dictated by patient's response and clinical condition; reduce dosage or discontinue gradually when administered for more than a few days

[1]Possibly effective
[2]Probably effective

Table continued on following page

ADMINISTRATION/DOSAGE ADJUSTMENTS

Alternate-day regimen	For patients requiring long-term steroid therapy, twice the usual daily oral dose may be given every other morning. Continue the initial suppressive dose level until a satisfactory clinical response is obtained (usually 4–10 days for many allergic and collagen diseases). Then change to alternate-day therapy and gradually reduce the dose given every other day, or first reduce the daily dose to the lowest effective level as quickly as possible and then change over to an alternate-day schedule. If an acute flare-up of the disease occurs, return to full suppressive daily divided dosage regimen for control. Reinstate the alternate-day regimen when control is reestablished. If difficulty is encountered in switching patients who have been on a daily regimen for long periods to alternate-day therapy, initially tripling or even quadrupling the daily maintenance dose and giving it every other day may be helpful.
Adrenogenital syndrome	As an alternative to daily oral therapy, a single 40-mg dose of the suspension injected once every 2 wk may be adequate for control
Systemic treatment of dermatological lesions	When oral therapy is not feasible, 40–120 mg of the suspension may be given in a single IM injection at weekly intervals for 1–4 wk. Relief of acute severe dermatitis due to poison ivy may result within 8–12 h following a single 80- to 120-mg IM dose. For chronic contact dermatitis, repeated IM injections at 5- to 10-day intervals may be required. For seborrheic dermatitis, a single weekly injection of 80 mg may be adequate.
Intralesional administration (keloids, lichen planus lesions, psoriatic plaques, etc)	Inject 20–60 mg of the suspension directly into the lesion. Large lesions may require repeated local injections of 20–40 mg; usually 1–4 injections are needed. Intervals between injections vary with the type of lesion being treated and the duration of improvement produced by the initial injection.
Allergic conditions	When oral therapy is not feasible in patients with bronchial asthma or allergic rhinitis (hay fever), the suspension may be given in a single IM injection of 80–120 mg. Relief of asthmatic symptoms may result within 6–48 h and persist for several days to 2 wk; relief of coryzal symptoms may be obtained within 6 h and persist for several days to 3 wk.
Intra-articular administration in rheumatoid arthritis and osteoarthritis	Dose of suspension is dependent on severity of condition and size of joint, as follows: large (eg, knee, ankle, shoulder), 20–80 mg; medium (eg, elbow, wrist), 10–40 mg; small (eg, metacarpophalangeal, interphalangeal, sternoclavicular, acromioclavicular), 4–10 mg. Injections may be repeated at intervals of 1–5 wk, depending on degree of relief obtained from the initial injection.
Bursitis, ganglia, tendinitis, tenosynovitis, epicondylitis	Dose of suspension varies with condition being treated, ranging from 4 to 30 mg per injection; repeated injections may be required in recurrent or chronic conditions. In treating such conditions as tendinitis and tenosynovitis, care should be taken to inject the suspension into the affected tendon sheath, rather than the tendon itself. In treating epicondylitis, the suspension should be infiltrated into the area of greatest tenderness. For ganglia, inject the suspension directly in the ganglion cyst.
Acute exacerbations of multiple sclerosis	Administer 160 mg/day PO or IM for 1 wk, followed by 64 mg PO or IM every other day for 1 mo
Ulcerative colitis	To tide the patient over a critical period, Solu-Medrol may be given in doses of 20–40 mg as a retention enema or by continuous drip 3–7 times/wk for periods of 2 wk or more[2]; many patients can be controlled with 40 mg administered in 1–10 fl oz of water, depending on the degree of involvement of the affected colonic mucosa
Severe shock	As an adjunct to standard methods of combating hemorrhagic, traumatic, surgical, or septic shock, concomitant IV use of large doses of Solu-Medrol may help restore hemodynamic function and improve survival.[1] Suggested regimens include 100 mg q2–6h or 250 mg q4–6h; 200 mg to start, followed by 100 mg q4–6h; 15 mg/kg q24h; and 30 mg/kg, repeated in 4 h, if needed. Therapy is initiated by IV administration over a period of one to several minutes and should be continued only until patient's condition stabilizes (usually not beyond 48–72 h). Prophylactic antacid therapy may be indicated to prevent peptic ulceration.
Overwhelming infections	As an adjunct to intensive antibiotic therapy, intensive treatment with Solu-Medrol may permit survival until the antibiotic has had time to take effect.[1] Treatment with the indicated antibiotic must be started before hormonal therapy is started. The corticosteroid must be administered for the briefest period necessary for adequate clinical response and must be stopped at least 3 days before the antibiotic therapy is discontinued. In surgical infections, clinical improvement resulting from hormonal therapy must not deter definitive surgical treatment, which should be scheduled as soon as the patient's condition permits.
Esophageal burns due to ingestion of caustic	As an adjunct to supportive fluid management and antibiotic therapy, concomitant corticosteroid therapy may lower the incidence of stricture formation and decrease morbidity.[1] Treatment with Solu-Medrol should be initiated within 48 h of the time the burn is sustained. Patients with esophageal damage, as demonstrated by esophagoscopy, may be continued on Depo-Medrol or, if tolerated, oral Medrol and, where required, antibiotics and bougienage.

Table continued on following page

ADMINISTRATION/DOSAGE ADJUSTMENTS continued

Croup	As an adjunct to other accepted therapeutic measures, IM administration of Solu-Medrol may be of value in the treatment of moderately severe and severe croup (acute laryngotracheobronchitis).[1] The recommended dose for infants and children is 40 mg IM, administered as early in the attack as possible. There is no evidence that such treatment decreases the incidence of tracheostomy or affects the acute epiglottic form of croup caused by *Hemophilus influenzae*. Transient bradycardia has been reported occasionally.
Preparation of parenteral solutions	Because of possible physical incompatibilities, Depo-Medrol should not be mixed or diluted with other solutions. Only the accompanying diluent should be used to prepare solutions of Solu-Medrol for IM or IV injection (consult manufacturer's labeling for directions). If desired, the prepared solution may be further diluted with Sterile Water for Injection or other suitable diluent or added to 5% dextrose-in-water, isotonic saline solution, or 5% dextrose in isotonic saline solution for IV infusion.

CONTRAINDICATIONS

Systemic fungal infections ●	Injection into unstable or previously infected joints ●

WARNINGS/PRECAUTIONS

Patients subjected to unusual stress	Require increased dosage of rapidly acting corticosteroids before, during, and after emotionally or physically stressful situations
Infection	Clinical signs may be masked, new infections may appear, resistance may be decreased, and infections may be difficult to localize
Ocular damage	Prolonged use may produce posterior subcapsular cataracts and glaucoma, with possible damage to optic nerves, and may enhance development of secondary fungal or viral ocular infections
Dietary salt restriction and potassium supplementation	May be necessary to combat blood pressure elevation, salt and water retention, and increased potassium excretion with average- and high-dose therapy
Immunization procedures	Especially against smallpox, should not be undertaken because of possible neurological complications and lack of antibody response
Active tuberculosis	Restrict use to fulminating or disseminated cases, as an adjunct to appropriate anti-tuberculous therapy
Latent tuberculosis or tuberculin reactivity	Observe patient closely, since reactivation of the disease may occur; during prolonged therapy, employ antituberculous chemoprophylactic measures
Secondary adrenocortical insufficiency	May be minimized by gradual dosage reduction; since insufficiency may persist for months, reinstitute corticosteroid therapy in any stressful situation during this period, and administer salt and/or a mineralocorticoid concurrently to correct impaired mineralocorticoid secretion
Hypothyroidism, hepatic cirrhosis	May enhance effects of methylprednisolone
Corneal perforation	May occur in patients with ocular herpes simplex; use with caution
Special-risk patients	Use with caution in patients with nonspecific ulcerative colitis if impending perforation, abscess, or other pyogenic infection is likely, as well as in patients with diverticulitis, fresh intestinal anastomoses, active or latent peptic ulcer, renal insufficiency, hypertension, osteoporosis, or myasthenia gravis
Psychic derangements	May appear, ranging from euphoria, insomnia, mood swings, personality changes, and severe depression to frank psychotic manifestations; existing emotional instability or psychotic tendencies may be aggravated
Concomitant use with aspirin	Use with caution in patients with hypoprothrombinemia
Cardiac arrhythmias and/or circulatory collapse	Have been reported primarily in renal-transplant recipients following rapid administration of large (>0.5 g) IV doses
Prolonged therapy	Routine laboratory studies (eg, urinalysis, 2-h postprandial blood sugar, blood pressure, body weight, chest film) should be made at regular intervals; in addition, an upper GI series is suggested in patients with an ulcer history or significant dyspepsia. When therapy has been continued for more than a few days, dosage must be reduced gradually.
Dermal and subdermal atrophy	May be minimized by not exceeding recommended doses; administer multiple small injections into lesion area whenever possible. Avoid injection into the deltoid muscle because of a high incidence of subcutaneous atrophy.
Suppression tests	May be altered by phenytoin, phenobarbital, ephedrine, and rifampin; interpret with caution
Septic arthritis	May occur with intra-articular injection and require appropriate antimicrobial therapy; observe patient for suggestive symptoms (eg, increased pain, local swelling, further restrictions of joint mobility, fever, malaise) and examine joint fluid microscopically

Table continued on following page

MEDROL continued

WARNINGS/PRECAUTIONS continued

Frequent intra-articular administration	May result in joint instability; in selected cases, follow-up x-ray examination to detect deterioration may be advisable
Overuse of joints	Caution patients who experience symptomatic relief against overusing joints as long as inflammatory process remains active
Tartrazine sensitivity	Presence of FD&C Yellow No. 5 (tartrazine) in 24-mg tablets may cause allergic-type reactions, including bronchial asthma, in susceptible individuals
Anaphylactoid reactions	Have occurred following parenteral corticosteroid administration; take appropriate precautionary measures before injecting methylprednisolone, especially in patients with a history of drug allergy

ADVERSE REACTIONS

Fluid and electrolyte disturbances	Sodium retention, fluid retention, congestive heart failure in susceptible patients, loss of potassium, hypokalemic alkalosis, hypertension
Musculoskeletal	Muscle weakness, steroid myopathy, loss of muscle mass, osteoporosis, vertebral compression fractures, aseptic necrosis of femoral and humeral heads, pathological fracture of long bones
Gastrointestinal	Peptic ulcer with possible perforation and hemorrhage, pancreatitis, abdominal distention, ulcerative esophagitis
Dermatological	Impaired wound healing, thin fragile skin, petechiae and ecchymoses, facial erythema, increased sweating, suppressed reaction to skin tests
Neurological	Convulsions, increased intracranial pressure with papilledema (pseudotumor cerebri), vertigo, headache
Endocrinological	Menstrual irregularities, Cushingoid state, growth suppression in children, secondary adrenocortical and pituitary unresponsiveness, decreased carbohydrate tolerance, latent diabetes mellitus, increased insulin or oral hypoglycemic requirements
Ophthalmic	Posterior subcapsular cataracts, increased intraocular pressure, glaucoma, exophthalmos
Metabolic	Negative nitrogen balance
Additional reactions to parenteral therapy only	Hyperpigmentation or hypopigmentation, subcutaneous and cutaneous atrophy, sterile abscess, postinjection flare (following intra-articular use), Charcot-like arthropathy, severe arthralgia, blindness (rare) associated with intralesional therapy around the face and head; arachnoiditis (following intrathecal administration)

OVERDOSAGE

Signs and symptoms	CNS changes, GI bleeding, hyperglycemia, hypertension, edema
Treatment	Discontinue medication; institute supportive measures, as required

DRUG INTERACTIONS

Insulin, oral hypoglycemics	⇩ Hypoglycemic effect
Phenytoin, phenobarbital, ephedrine, rifampin	⇧ Metabolic clearance of methylprednisolone ⇩ Steroid blood level and physiological activity
Oral anticoagulants	⇧ or ⇩ Prothrombin time
Potassium-depleting diuretics	⇧ Risk of hypokalemia
Cardiac glycosides	⇧ Risk of arrhythmias or digitalis toxicity secondary to hypokalemia
Skin-test antigens	⇩ Reactivity
Immunizations	⇩ Antibody response

ALTERED LABORATORY VALUES

Blood/serum values	⇧ Glucose ⇧ Cholesterol ⇧ Sodium ⇩ Potassium ⇩ Calcium ⇩ PBI ⇩ Thyroxine (T_4) ⇩ ^{131}I thyroid uptake ⇩ Uric acid
Urinary values	⇧ Glucose ⇧ Potassium ⇧ Calcium ⇧ Uric acid ⇩ 17-Hydroxycorticosteroids (17-OHCS) ⇩ 17-Ketosteroids

Use in children

Growth and development should be carefully observed in infants and children on prolonged therapy; general guidelines not established for dosage recommendations

Use in pregnancy or nursing mothers

Safe use has not been established during pregnancy or for nursing mothers. Infants born of mothers who received substantial doses of corticosteroids during pregnancy should be carefully observed for signs of hypoadrenalism.

PREDNISOLONE ACETATE various manufacturers

Vials: 25 mg/ml (5, 10, 30 ml), 50 mg/ml (10, 30 ml), 100 mg/ml (10 ml)

PREDNISOLONE SODIUM PHOSPHATE various manufacturers

Vials: 22 mg (equivalent to 20 mg prednisolone phosphate)/ml (2, 5, 10 ml)

INDICATIONS	PARENTERAL DOSAGE
Endocrine disorders, including primary or secondary adrenocortical insufficiency, congenital adrenal hyperplasia, nonsuppurative thyroiditis, hypercalcemia associated with cancer, acute adrenocortical insufficiency, and preoperatively and in the event of serious trauma or illness in patients with known adrenal insufficiency or when adrenocortical reserve is doubtful **Rheumatic disorders,** including psoriatic arthritis, rheumatoid arthritis, juvenile rheumatoid arthritis, ankylosing spondylitis, acute and subacute bursitis, acute nonspecific tenosynovitis, acute gouty arthritis, posttraumatic osteoarthritis, synovitis of osteoarthritis, and epicondylitis (adjunctive, short-term therapy) **Collagen diseases,** including systemic lupus erythematosus, acute rheumatic carditis, and systemic dermatomyositis (polymyositis) **Dermatological diseases,** including pemphigus, bullous dermatitis herpetiformis, severe erythema multiforme (Stevens-Johnson syndrome), exfoliative dermatitis, mycosis fungoides, severe psoriasis, and severe seborrheic dermatitis Severe or incapacitating **allergic conditions** intractable to adequate trials of conventional treatment, including seasonal or perennial allergic rhinitis, bronchial asthma, contact dermatitis, atopic dermatitis, serum sickness, drug hypersensitivity reactions, urticarial transfusion reactions, and acute noninfectious laryngeal edema **Ophthalmic diseases,** including allergic conjunctivitis, keratitis, allergic corneal marginal ulcers, herpes zoster ophthalmicus, iritis and iridocyclitis, chorioretinitis, anterior segment inflammation, diffuse posterior uveitis and choroiditis, optic neuritis, and sympathetic ophthalmia **Respiratory diseases,** including symptomatic sarcoidosis, Loeffler's syndrome not manageable by other means, berylliosis, fulminating or disseminated pulmonary tuberculosis (with appropriate antituberculous chemotherapy), and aspiration pneumonitis **Hematological disorders,** including idiopathic thrombocytopenic purpura (IV only) and secondary thrombocytopenia in adults, acquired (autoimmune) hemolytic anemia, erythroblastopenia (RBC anemia), and congenital (erythroid) hypoplastic anemia Palliative management of **neoplastic diseases,** including leukemias and lymphomas in adults and acute leukemia of childhood To induce diuresis or remission of proteinuria in the **nephrotic syndrome,** without uremia, of the idiopathic type or that due to lupus erythematosus **Gastrointestinal diseases,** including ulcerative colitis and regional enteritis **Tuberculous meningitis** with subarachnoid block or impending block (with appropriate antituberculous chemotherapy) **Trichinosis** associated with neurological or myocardial involvement	**Adult:** 4–60 mg/day IM (prednisolone acetate, prednisolone sodium phosphate) or IV (prednisolone sodium phosphate only) to start, followed by gradual reductions in dosage to lowest level possible consistent with maintaining an adequate clinical response; dosage must be individualized on the basis of the specific disease being treated, its severity, and clinical response; larger than usual doses may be justified in certain overwhelming, acute, life-threatening situations
Acute exacerbations of **multiple sclerosis**	**Adult:** 200 mg/day IM for 1 wk, followed by 80 mg every other day or 4–8 mg of dexamethasone every other day for 1 mo

CONTRAINDICATIONS

Systemic fungal infections ●	Injection into unstable or previously infected joints ●

WARNINGS/PRECAUTIONS

Patients subjected to unusual stress	Require increased dosage of rapidly acting corticosteroids before, during, and after emotionally or physically stressful situations
Infection	Clinical signs may be masked, new infections may appear, resistance may be decreased, and infections may be difficult to localize
Ocular damage	Prolonged use may produce posterior subcapsular cataracts and glaucoma, with possible damage to optic nerves, and may enhance development of secondary fungal or viral ocular infections
Dietary salt restriction and potassium supplementation	May be necessary to combat blood pressure elevation, salt and water retention, and increased potassium excretion with average and high-dose therapy
Immunization procedures	Especially against smallpox, should not be undertaken because of possible neurological complications and lack of antibody response
Active tuberculosis	Restrict use to fulminating or disseminated cases, as an adjunct to appropriate antituberculous therapy
Latent tuberculosis or tuberculin reactivity	Observe patient closely, since reactivation of the disease may occur; during prolonged therapy, employ antituberculous chemoprophylactic measures

Table continued on following page

PREDNISOLONE continued

WARNINGS/PRECAUTIONS continued	
Secondary adrenocortical insufficiency	May be minimized by gradual dosage reduction; since insufficiency may persist for months, reinstitute corticosteroid therapy in any stressful situation during this period, and administer salt and/or a mineralocorticoid concurrently to correct impaired mineralocorticoid secretion
Hypothyroidism, hepatic cirrhosis	May enhance effects of prednisolone
Corneal perforation	May occur in patients with ocular herpes simplex; use with caution
Special-risk patients	Use with caution in patients with nonspecific ulcerative colitis if impending perforation, abscess, or other pyogenic infection is likely, as well as in patients with diverticulitis, fresh intestinal anastomoses, active or latent peptic ulcer, renal insufficiency, hypertension, osteoporosis, or myasthenia gravis
Psychic derangements	May appear, ranging from euphoria, insomnia, mood swings, personality changes, and severe depression to frank psychotic manifestations; existing emotional instability or psychotic tendencies may be aggravated
Concomitant use with aspirin	Use with caution in patients with hypoprothrombinemia
Prolonged therapy	Routine laboratory studies (eg, urinalysis, 2-h postprandial blood sugar, blood pressure, body weight, chest film) should be made at regular intervals; in addition, an upper GI series is suggested in patients with an ulcer history or significant dyspepsia. Withdraw the drug gradually, rather than abruptly, when discontinuing long-term therapy.
Septic arthritis	May occur with intra-articular injection and require appropriate antimicrobial therapy; observe patient for suggestive symptoms (eg, increased pain, local swelling, further restrictions of joint mobility, fever, malaise) and examine joint fluid microscopically
Anaphylactoid reactions	Have occurred following parenteral corticosteroid administration; take appropriate precautionary measures before injecting dexamethasone, especially in patients with a history of drug allergy

ADVERSE REACTIONS	
Fluid and electrolyte disturbances	Sodium retention, fluid retention, congestive heart failure in susceptible patients, loss of potassium, hypokalemic alkalosis, hypertension, hypotensive or shock-like reactions
Musculoskeletal	Muscle weakness, steroid myopathy, loss of muscle mass, osteoporosis, vertebral compression fractures, aseptic necrosis of femoral and humeral heads, pathological fracture of long bones
Gastrointestinal	Peptic ulcer with possible perforation and hemorrhage, pancreatitis, abdominal distention, ulcerative esophagitis
Dermatological	Impaired wound healing, thin fragile skin, petechiae and ecchymoses, facial erythema, increased sweating, suppressed reaction to skin tests
Neurological	Convulsions, increased intracranial pressure with papilledema (pseudotumor cerebri), vertigo, headache
Endocrinological	Menstrual irregularities, Cushingoid state, growth suppression in children, secondary adrenocortical and pituitary unresponsiveness, decreased carbohydrate tolerance, latent diabetes mellitus, increased insulin or oral hypoglycemic requirements
Ophthalmic	Posterior subcapsular cataracts, increased intraocular pressure, glaucoma, exophthalmos
Metabolic	Negative nitrogen balance
Other	Anaphylactoid or hypersensitivity reactions
Additional reactions to parenteral therapy only	Hyperpigmentation or hypopigmentation, subcutaneous and cutaneous atrophy, sterile abscess, postinjection flare (following intra-articular use), Charcot-like arthropathy, blindness (rare) associated with intralesional therapy around the face and head

Table continued on following page

OVERDOSAGE

Signs and symptoms	CNS changes, GI bleeding, hyperglycemia, hypertension, edema
Treatment	Discontinue medication; institute supportive measures, as required

DRUG INTERACTIONS

Insulin, oral hypoglycemics	⇩ Hypoglycemic effect
Phenytoin, phenobarbital, ephedrine, rifampin	⇧ Metabolic clearance of prednisolone ⇩ Steroid blood level and physiological activity
Oral anticoagulants	⇧ or ⇩ Prothrombin time
Potassium-depleting diuretics	⇧ Risk of hypokalemia
Cardiac glycosides	⇧ Risk of arrhythmias or digitalis toxicity secondary to hypokalemia
Skin-test antigens	⇩ Reactivity
Immunizations	⇩ Antibody response

ALTERED LABORATORY VALUES

Blood/serum values	⇧ Glucose ⇧ Cholesterol ⇧ Sodium ⇩ Potassium ⇩ Calcium ⇩ PBI ⇩ Thyroxine (T_4) ⇩ ^{131}I thyroid uptake ⇩ Uric acid
Urinary values	⇧ Glucose ⇧ Potassium ⇧ Calcium ⇧ Uric acid ⇩ 17-Hydroxycorticosteroids (17-OHCS) ⇩ 17-Ketosteroids

Use in children

Growth and development should be carefully observed in infants and children on prolonged therapy; general guidelines not established for dosage recommendations

Use in pregnancy or nursing mothers

Safe use has not been established during pregnancy or for nursing mothers. Infants born of mothers who received substantial doses of corticosteroids during pregnancy should be carefully observed for signs of hypoadrenalism.

Skin Disorders

Acne

Acne vulgaris, the medical term for common acne, is a chronic disease that many people regard as a nuisance afflicting mostly teenagers. In many instances, it is a relatively mild, passing problem encountered during puberty and young adulthood. But for others, acne can be cruel and disfiguring, not only physically but psychologically, triggering emotional problems, such as embarrassment and low self-esteem, that may last a lifetime. Furthermore, acne can occur at any age. Some women (and men who use cosmetics), for instance, suffer from a low-grade condition called acne cosmetica, due to overuse of cosmetics containing such substances as vegetable oils, lanolin, and fatty acid; many men and women have recurrent acne as a result of irritation from clothing or athletic equipment; some women have a flare-up of acne during their menstrual periods. But the fact is that acne does occur most commonly in adolescence.

CAUSES OF ACNE

Acne originates in the sebaceous glands, which are located in the dermis, the layer of skin beneath the surface or epidermis. Most sebaceous glands are on the face, back, and chest, which is why acne occurs most often in those areas. The sebaceous gland is connected to the skin surface by a duct known as the sebaceous follicle—or pore—which also contains a hair follicle. The gland produces an oily, waxy substance, called sebum, that plays an essential role in the regenerative cycle of the follicle. In the normal process of regeneration, the old cells are shed from the lining just as they are shed from the surface of the skin. The sebum brings the dead cells to the surface.

Acne is triggered by an overproduction of sebum, which is attributed to increased hormone production, such as occurs during puberty. The dead cells become so sticky with sebum that they remain fixed to the walls of the follicle. Consequently, the duct narrows and the sebum backs up and becomes impacted, forming a comedo (pimple).

Basically, there are two types of comedones. When the opening of the follicle remains intact and all that is seen is a whitish or skin-colored pimple, it is a closed comedo or whitehead. If the follicle is open, it is an open comedo or blackhead. The reason it is black is not because of dirt, as is commonly assumed, but rather because of a chemical reaction when the comedo is exposed to the air.

Complications

Acne can be noninflammatory or inflammatory. The latter entails a far greater likelihood of permanent scarring. Inflammatory acne usually begins in closed comedones. Within a closed comedo, *Propionibacterium acnes* microorganisms may feed upon the sebum, converting it to fatty acids, which irritate the follicle walls. These bacteria may also release enzymes that rupture the walls of the follicle, permitting the sebum and the debris and microorganisms it contains to ooze through the tissues. The resulting inflammatory lesions are classified as pustules (near the skin surface), papules (somewhat deeper in the follicle), or abscesses (deep within the follicle).

FACTS AND FALLACIES ABOUT ACNE

There are a number of myths and half-truths about the causes, prevention, and treatment of acne. Many of these have been handed down for generations and perhaps centuries, and they tend to place the burden of acne on the sufferer, attributing it to bad habits or, worse, a lack of willpower. This, of course, increases the emotional ramifications of the disease, especially if the person is a self-conscious adolescent. The facts are these:

- *Diet* Although it is commonly assumed that people bring acne on themselves, or exacerbate it, by eating such things as chocolate, ice cream, pizzas, and greasy foods, there is no scientific evidence to support this.
- *Sex* It is also widely believed that masturbation can cause acne, and that an active heterosexual life can prevent it or clear it up. Neither is true.
- *Cleanliness* Failure to keep the skin clean is often blamed for acne, but since the process starts deep in the follicle, this is not true. However, gentle washing of the face is important in management because it helps remove excess sebum and may help keep the pores open. It also causes some drying of the skin, which may be beneficial. Some physicians recommend using ordinary soap, while others recommend medicated soaps and lotions. It is also important to keep the skin as free as possible of such things as greasy suntan lotions, oil-based cosmetics, and the grease from hair tonics.
- *Picking or squeezing pimples* This approach, as common wisdom has it, only worsens the condition.
- *Stress* Though not a direct cause of acne, stress can possibly aggravate it by affecting hormonal levels.
- *Sunlight and sunlamps* A moderate amount of exposure to sunlight might be beneficial, but some authorities discount the possible benefits of using an

ultraviolet sunlamp. (Elderly, fair-skinned people sometimes develop a form of acne as a result of too much exposure to sun over the years. It is called Favre–Racouchot syndrome, or "solar comedones.")

DRUG TREATMENT

Persons with just a few noninflammatory pimples should use their own judgment, perhaps based on their level of anxiety, in deciding whether to see a physician or attempt to manage the problem with the help of nonprescription topical drugs. If acne shows any sign of inflammation, however, a physician should be consulted.

Nonprescription Drugs

There are many soaps, gels, lotions, and creams for the treatment of minor acne. A major group of these drugs is the exfoliants, which work by irritating the skin and causing it to dry out and peel. A second group contains abrasive ingredients, such as aluminum oxide or pumice, and act on the skin much as sandpaper would. These products should be used with caution, since research has shown they may worsen the problem. A third group contains benzoyl peroxide, an oxidizing agent that has an antibacterial effect on the microorganisms in the follicles and also causes irritation and peeling of the skin. Many nonprescription products contain benzoyl peroxide, although some forms require a prescription.

Exfoliants The mildest of these drugs, and the ones that are often recommended first in treating noninflammatory acne, are those containing sulfur, resorcinol, or salicylic acid. Sometimes they are used in combination with each other or with other ingredients. Acnomel, for example—in either cream or cake form—is made up of sulfur, resorcinol, and alcohol; Liquimat lotion contains sulfur and alcohol; and Therapads, a wipe, contains salicylic acid and alcohol. Some of these products, such as Liquimat and Acne-Aid, also contain coloring agents that help mask the acne.

Prolonged use of some of these products has been found to cause dermatitis in susceptible persons. Consequently, people with fair, sensitive skin should be particularly careful, beginning treatment with the lowest available strengths to prevent or minimize irritation.

Benzoyl peroxide Although benzoyl peroxide products are considered among the most effective nonprescription drugs in the treatment of acne, they should be used with caution since they can be highly irritating. Solutions containing this ingredient should be kept away from the eyes, eyelids, and lips. Benzoyl peroxide is an oxidizing agent that may bleach fabrics, so one should avoid spilling it on clothes.

When it is first applied to the skin, benzoyl peroxide produces a mild stinging or burning sensation. If this is excessive or lasts for more than a few minutes, the preparation should be washed off, and not applied again until the next day. Some persons with sensitive skin may find it best to leave the benzoyl peroxide

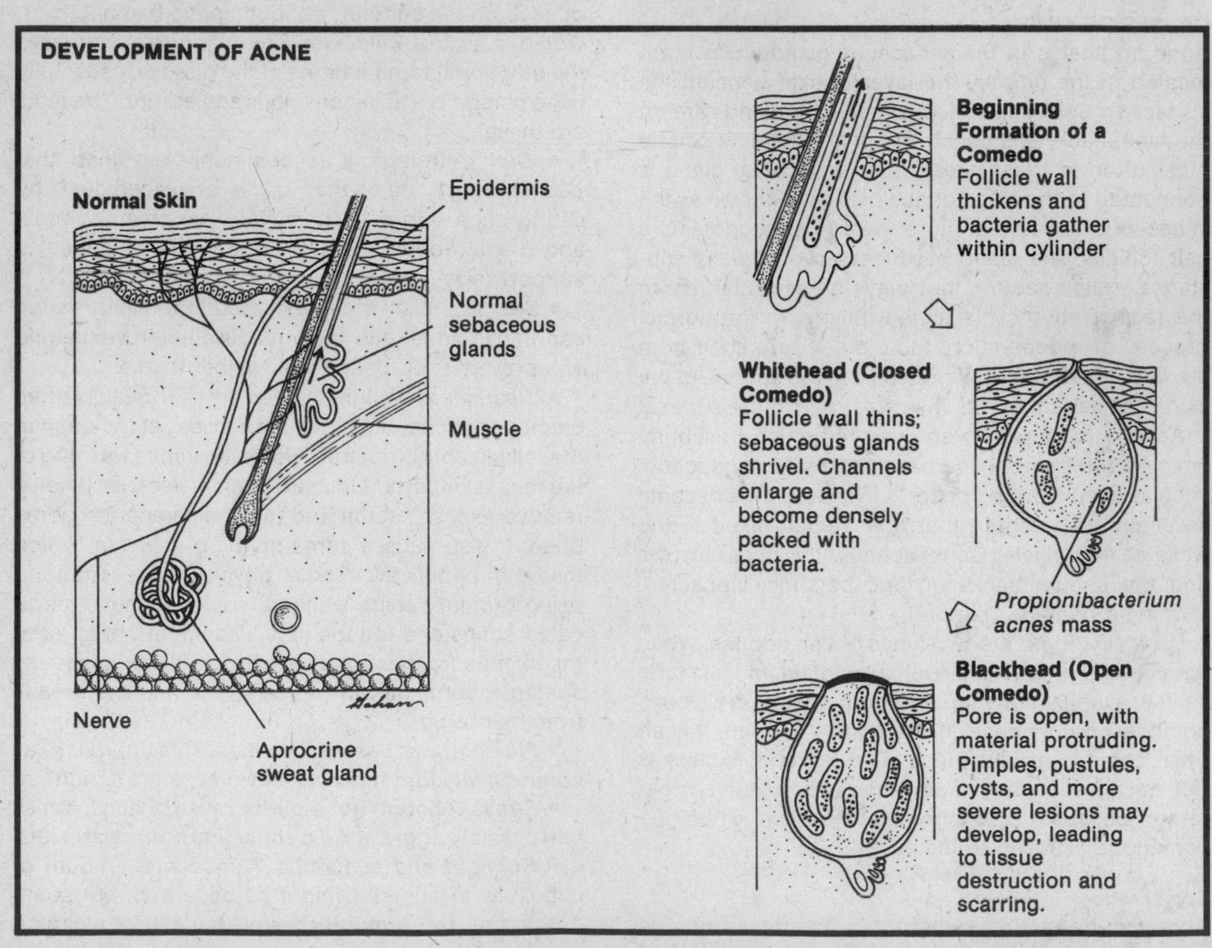

solutions on the skin for only two or three hours during the first few weeks of therapy and then, as the skin becomes less sensitive, increase the time. The water-base gels are not as irritating as the alcohol-base gels or the sulfur-benzoyl peroxide formulations. It may also be wise to start with the milder (2.5 or 5 percent) solutions, and, if necessary, gradually work up to the 10 percent strengths. The product labels or names (e.g., Oxy-5 or Oxy-10) indicate the concentration of benzoyl peroxide.

Miscellaneous cleansers and scrubs Antiseptic skin cleansers, such as Betadine, are sometimes used adjunctively in managing acne. Although no prescription is required, it is best to ask the advice of a physician. Soaps such as Neutrogena can also be helpful. Cleansers, such as Epi-Clear Scrub Cleanser, often come in fine, medium, or coarse concentrations of aluminum oxide or other abrasives.

Prescription Drugs

There are two major classifications of prescription acne preparations: antibiotics, both systemic (taken internally through oral or injected medication) and topical (applied to the skin), and vitamin A derivatives.

Antibiotics Although acne is not an infectious disease—indeed, the body's normal bacteria are usually the ones involved in rupturing the sebaceous follicle wall—antibiotics can nonetheless play an important role in controlling acne by suppressing the activity of the bacteria and combating secondary infection. Generally antibiotics are prescribed in conjunction with other acne medications, usually either tretinoin or benzoyl peroxide.

The oral antibiotics that have proved most effective in treating acne are the tetracyclines, such as Achromycin V and Sumycin; the tetracycline derivative, Minocin; the erythromycins, and clindamycin. The most common side effects are irritation of the gastrointestinal tract and the anogenital region. (See the section on *Bacterial Infections*, pages 339–443 for specific information on these drugs.)

Some newly developed topical antibiotic creams and lotions, containing derivatives of erythromycin, tetracycline, and clindamycin, also have proved effective in treating acne and have an added advantage of minimal or no systemic side effects. A 2% erythromycin and clindamycin lotion, often used in combination with tretinoin, is one of the more effective topical antibiotics for the treatment of acne.

Vitamin A Although vitamin A is essential to the normal functioning of skin cells, massive doses that would be required to treat acne would be in the toxic range. Instead, vitamin A acid, or tretinoin, is prescribed, often to prevent new comedones from forming. It works mainly by facilitating the flow of dead cells from the pores. Tretinoin is available as a topical medication (Retin-A) in gel, cream, or liquid form. Since tretinoin is also an irritant, it often makes the skin look worse before improvement becomes evident. Indeed, it may take from four to six weeks to work.

Because tretinoin *is* a strong irritant, it is important that patients using it do not irritate their skin in other ways. The skin should be washed with a mild soap, such as Neutrogena, and persons using it should avoid prolonged exposure to sun. It also should not be applied at the same time as benzoyl peroxide—if both these medications are used, one should be applied in the morning and the other at night.

Other Miscellaneous Treatments

In some cases of intractable acne, the physician may inject corticosteroids directly into the lesion. Although this has often been quite successful, the many side effects associated with steroids prohibit this approach except in severe and intractable cases. Other approaches include certain types of surgery, such as the abrading of scars.

IN CONCLUSION

The following charts cover the major prescription and nonprescription drugs used to treat acne. Other medications for severe acne may be found in the sections on *Bacterial Infections* (pages 339–443) and *Corticosteroids* (pages 1038–1066).

A/T/S (Erythromycin) **Hoechst-Roussel**

Sol: 20 mg/ml (60 ml)

INDICATIONS	**TOPICAL DOSAGE**
Acne vulgaris	**Adult:** moisten a pad with solution and rub over affected areas bid after thorough washing with soap and warm water

CONTRAINDICATIONS

Hypersensitivity to any component

WARNINGS/PRECAUTIONS

Contact with eyes, nose, mouth, or mucous membranes	Should be avoided
Concomitant topical acne therapy	Use with caution, since a cumulative irritant effect may occur, especially if peeling, desquamating, or abrasive agents are used
Proliferation of nonsusceptible organisms	May occur; discontinue use and institute appropriate therapy

ADVERSE REACTIONS

Local	Dry or scaly skin, pruritus, eye irritation, burning sensation

Use in children	**Use in pregnancy or nursing mothers**
General guidelines not established	Safe use not established during pregnancy or in nursing mothers

BENZAC (Benzoyl peroxide) **Owen**

Gel: 5% (60 g), 10% (60 g)

BENZAC W (Benzoyl peroxide) **Owen**

Gel (water base): 5%, 10% (60 g)

INDICATIONS	**TOPICAL DOSAGE**
Acne vulgaris (adjunctive therapy)	**Adult:** apply qd or bid after washing with a mild cleanser and water

ADMINISTRATION/DOSAGE ADJUSTMENTS

Degree of drying and peeling	Modify by adjusting dosage

CONTRAINDICATIONS

Hypersensitivity to any component

WARNINGS/PRECAUTIONS

For external use only	Avoid contact with eyes, eyelids, and other mucous membranes
Bleaching	May occur; avoid contact with hair and colored fabrics

ADVERSE REACTIONS

Local	Itching, redness, burning, swelling, dryness

Use in children	**Use in pregnancy or nursing mothers**
General guidelines not established	General guidelines not established

Note: Other prescription acne medications containing benzoyl peroxide include **5-BENZAGEL** and **10-BENZAGELd1 (Dermik); DESQUAM-X 5**, **DESQUAM-X 10**, and **DESQUAM-X WASH** (Westwood); **PERSA-GEL** (Owen); and **PAN OXYL** and **PANOXYL AQ** (Stiefel). Nonprescription benzoyl peroxide medications are listed in the chart Nonprescription Acne Medications.

CLEOCIN T (Clindamycin phosphate) Upjohn

Sol: equivalent to 10 mg clindamycin/ml (30, 60 ml)

INDICATIONS	TOPICAL DOSAGE
Acne vulgaris[1]	**Adult:** apply a thin film to affected areas bid

CONTRAINDICATIONS

Hypersensitivity to clindamycin or lincomycin●	History of regional enteritis or ulcerative colitis●	History of antibiotic-associated colitis●

WARNINGS/PRECAUTIONS

Severe colitis (possibly fatal)	Has occurred with both orally and parenterally administered clindamycin
Diarrhea	May occur; if significant, discontinue use. If severe, consider performing a large bowel endoscopic examination, which may reveal pseudomembranous colitis
Drug-induced colitis (including pseudomembranous colitis)	Has been reported with use of topical and systemic clindamycin; symptoms can occur within a few days, weeks, or months after start of clindamycin therapy, or up to several weeks after cessation of therapy, and usually consist of severe persistent diarrhea, severe abdominal cramps, and possibly, the passage of blood and mucus; discontinue use. Manage promptly with fluid, electrolyte, and protein supplementation, as indicated. Cholestyramine and colestipol resins have been shown to bind the toxin in vitro. Systemic corticoids and corticoid retention enemas may be helpful. For pseudomembranous colitis produced by *Clostridium difficile,* administer vancomycin, 500 mg orally q6h for 7–10 days. Do *not* use antiperistaltic agents, such as opiates and diphenoxylate with atropine.
Contact with eyes, abraded skin, or mucous membranes	Will cause burning and irritation, due to alcohol base; bathe with large amounts of cool tap water
Atopic patients	Use with caution
Unpleasant taste	Advise patients to exercise caution when applying clindamycin around the mouth
Concomitant use of other acne preparations (eg, benzoyl peroxide, retinoic acid)	Has been reported in uncontrolled studies

ADVERSE REACTIONS

Gastrointestinal	Diarrhea, bloody diarrhea, colitis, abdominal pain
Local	Contact dermatitis, dryness, oiliness, sensitization, irritation
Genitourinary	Urinary frequency, vaginitis
Central nervous system	Headache, fatigue
Other	Sore throat, stinging of the eyes, facial swelling, pain, Gram-negative folliculitis

DRUG INTERACTIONS

Neuromuscular blocking agents	⇧ Neuromuscular blockade
Chloramphenicol, erythromycin	⇩ Clindamycin effects

ALTERED LABORATORY VALUES

No clinically significant alterations in blood/serum or urinary values occur at therapeutic dosages

Use in children	Use in pregnancy or nursing mothers
General guidelines not established	Use during pregnancy only if clearly needed. Safe use not established in nursing mothers; as a general rule, nursing should not be undertaken while patient is receiving the drug

[1] In view of the potential for diarrhea, bloody diarrhea, and pseudomembranous colitis, the physician should consider whether other agents are more appropriate

RETIN-A (Tretinoin) Ortho

Cream: 0.05% (20, 45 g), 0.1% (20 g) **Gel:** 0.025%, 0.01% (15, 45 g) **Liq:** 0.05% (28 ml) **Swab:** saturated with 0.05% liquid

INDICATIONS	TOPICAL DOSAGE
Acne vulgaris, primarily grades I, II, and III, in which comedones, papules, and pustules predominate	**Adult:** apply to affected area qd at bedtime, for 2–3 wk or longer until a satisfactory response is obtained; for maintenance, apply less often or switch to other dosage forms

ADMINISTRATION/DOSAGE ADJUSTMENTS

Application of liquid	Apply with fingertip, gauze pad, or cotton swab. Do not oversaturate gauze or cotton to the extent that the medication would run into unaffected areas
Application of swab	One swab supplies enough medication to treat the entire face. If other sites are treated, such as the back, use additional swabs.
"Pilling" of gel	May occur with excessive application
Alterations of vehicle, drug concentration, or dose frequency	Should be closely monitored by careful observation of therapeutic response and skin tolerance
Use of cosmetics	Is permissible, but the areas to be treated should be cleansed thoroughly before applying the medication

CONTRAINDICATIONS

Hypersensitivity to any component

WARNINGS/PRECAUTIONS

Exposure to sun	Recent studies in hairless albino mice suggest that tretinoin may accelerate the tumorigenic potential of ultraviolet radiation; caution patients to avoid or minimize exposure to sun, especially if they are inherently sensitive to sunlight. If exposure is unavoidable, sunscreen products and protective clothing should be used. Patients with sunburn should not use tretinoin until fully recovered.
Weather extremes (wind or cold)	May cause irritation
For external use only	Avoid contact with eyes, mouth, angles of the nose, and mucous membranes
Severe local erythema and peeling	May occur at application site; use medication less often, discontinue use temporarily, or discontinue altogether, as warranted
Eczematous skin	Severe irritation may occur; use with extreme caution
Hypersensitivity reactions	Skin may become excessively red, edematous, blistered, or crusted; discontinue use temporarily, or adjust dosage to tolerable level. True contact allergy rarely occurs.
Unwarranted uses	Not effective in most cases of severe pustular and deep cystic nodular acne
Transitory warmth or slight stinging	May occur on application
Exacerbation of inflammatory lesions	May occur during early weeks of therapy due to action of medication on deep, previously unseen lesions; this should *not* be considered a reason to discontinue therapy
Excessive application	Will not improve results of therapy and may cause marked redness, peeling, or discomfort
Concomitant use of topical medications	May interact with tretinoin; use with caution, especially if medications contain peeling agents, such as sulfur, resorcinol, benzoyl peroxide, or salicylic acid. Before using tretinoin, the patient should allow the skin to "rest" until effect of peeling agent subsides.
Concomitant use of other topical products	May interact with tretinoin; use the following with caution: medicated or abrasive soaps and cleansers, soaps and cosmetics that have a strong drying effect, and products with high concentrations of alcohol, astringents, spices, or lime

ADVERSE REACTIONS[1]

Sensitivity	Excessively red, edematous, blistered, and/or crusted skin; temporary hypo- or hyperpigmentation; contact allergy (rare)
Local	Irritation, severe erythema, peeling, sensation of warmth, slight stinging

Use in children	**Use in pregnancy or nursing mothers**
General guidelines not established	General guidelines not established

[1]To date, all adverse reactions have been reversible upon discontinuation of therapy

TOPICYCLINE (Tetracycline hydrochloride) Procter & Gamble

Sol: 2.2 mg/ml after reconstitution (70 ml)

INDICATIONS	TOPICAL DOSAGE
Acne vulgaris	**Adult:** apply generously to affected areas bid, in AM and PM

ADMINISTRATION/DOSAGE ADJUSTMENTS

Application	Apply by tilting the bottle and rubbing the applicator top over the skin while gently applying pressure; control the rate of flow by increasing or decreasing pressure against the skin
Use of cosmetics	Is permissible

CONTRAINDICATIONS

Hypersensitivity to any component

WARNINGS/PRECAUTIONS

Liver damage in patients with renal impairment	Highly unlikely to occur; nonetheless, consider the warnings associated with the use of orally administered tetracycline before prescribing this topical tetracycline to patients with renal impairment
For external use only	Avoid contact with eyes, nose, and mouth
Superficial yellowing of skin	May occur at application site, particularly in fair-skinned patients; eliminate by washing

ADVERSE REACTIONS Frequent reactions are italicized

Local	*Transient stinging or burning upon application,* superficial yellowing of skin, fluorescence of treated areas under ultraviolet light, severe dermatitis (rare)

Use in children

General guidelines not established

Use in pregnancy or nursing mothers

General guidelines not established

NONPRESCRIPTION ACNE MEDICATIONS

Product (Manufacturer)	Ingredients	Actions
Acnaveen (Cooper) Bar **Dosage** Lather and massage into wet skin and rinse thoroughly 3 times/day	2% Sulfur	Peeling agent with irritant effect; reduces tendency to form comedones
	2% Salicylic acid	Peeling agent with irritant effect; reduces tendency to form comedones
	50% Colloidal oatmeal	Abrasive agent
Acne-Aid (Stiefel) Cream **Dosage** Apply to affected areas and rub in gently 2–3 times/day	2.5% Sulfur	Peeling agent with irritant effect; reduces tendency to form comedones
	1.25% Resorcinol	Peeling agent with irritant effect; reduces tendency to form comedones
	0.375% Chloroxynol	Antiseptic agent
Acne-Aid (Stiefel) Cream **Dosage** Apply to affected areas and rub in gently 2–3 times/day	10% Sulfur	Peeling agent with irritant effect; reduces tendency to form comedones
	10% Alcohol	Astringent
Acnomel (Smith Kline & French) Liquid **Dosage** Wash with cleanser and rinse thoroughly, 2–3 times/day	8% Sulfur	Peeling agent with irritant effect; reduces tendency to form comedones
	2% Resorcinol	Peeling agent with irritant effect; reduces tendency to form comedones
Betadine Skin Cleanser (Purdue-Frederick) Liquid **Dosage** Lather and massage into wet skin and rinse thoroughly, 2–3 times/day	7.5% Povidone-iodine	Anti-infective agent
	Detergents	Cleansing agent
Brasivol (Steifel) Liquid **Dosage** Lather and massage into wet skin and rinse thoroughly, 2–3 times/day	Aluminum oxide	Astringent
	Neutral soap	Cleansing agent
	Detergents	Cleansing agent
Clearasil Antibacterial Acne Lotion (Vicks) Lotion **Dosage** Rub gently into affected areas up to 2 times/day; if discomfort occurs, reduce number of applications	5% Benzoyl peroxide	Peeling agent with irritant effect; reduces tendency to form comedones

Table continued on following page

Product (Manufacturer)	Ingredients	Actions
Clearasil Medicated Cleanser (Vicks) Liquid **Dosage** Saturate cotton ball with cleanser and apply to skin without rinsing, several times/day	0.25% Salicylic acid	Peeling agent with irritant effect; reduces tendency to form comedones
	43% Alcohol	Astringent
	0.1% Allantoin	Healing agent
Cuticura (Purex) Ointment **Dosage** Massage ointment gently into clean, dry skin as needed	Precipated sulfur	Peeling agent with irritant effect; reduces tendency to form comedones
	8-Hydroquinoline	Antiseptic
	Mineral oil	Emollient
	Mineral wax	Hardener for ointment base
	Isopropyl palmitate	Hardener for ointment base
	Synthetic beeswax	Hardener for ointment base
	Phenol	Antimicrobial agent
	Pine oil	Emollient
	Rose geranium oil	Emollient
Cuticura Acne Cream (Purex) Cream **Dosage** Rub gently into affected areas 2–3 times/daily	5% Benzoyl peroxide	Peeling agent with irritant effect; reduces tendency to form comedones
	Alcohol	Astringent
Dry and Clear Acne Cream (Whitehall) Cream **Dosage** Rub gently into affected areas up to 3 times/day; if discomfort occurs, reduce number of applications	2% Sulfur	Peeling agent with irritant effect; reduces tendency to form comedones
	Salicylic acid	Peeling agent with irritant effect; reduces tendency to form comedones
	10% Benzoyl peroxide	Peeling agent with irritant effect; reduces tendency to form comedones
	Benzethonium chloride	Antibacterial agent
EPI-CLEAR (Squibb) Lotion **Dosage** Rub gently into affected areas several times/day; if discomfort occurs, reduce number of applications	10% Sulfur	Peeling agent with irritant effect; reduces tendency to form comedones
	10% Benzoyl peroxide	Peeling agent with irritant effect; reduces tendency to form comedones

Table continued on following page

Product (Manufacturer)	Ingredients	Actions
EPI-CLEAR Scrub Cleanser (Squibb) **Dosage** Lather and massage into wet skin for 2 to 3 min and rinse thoroughly with warm and then cool water, 2–3 times/day	65% Coarse aluminum oxide	Astringent and abrasive agent
	52% Medium aluminum oxide	Astringent and abrasive agent
	38% Fine aluminum oxide	Astringent and abrasive agent
Fostex (Westwood) Cream **Dosage** Rub gently into affected areas several times/day; if discomfort occurs, reduce number of applications	2% Sulfur	Peeling agent with irritant effect; reduces tendency to form comedones
	2% Salicylic acid	Peeling agent with irritant effect; reduces tendency to form comedones
Fostex (Westwood) Liquid **Dosage** Lather and massage into wet skin and rinse thoroughly, 2–3 times/day	2% Sulfur	Peeling agent with irritant effect; reduces tendency to form comedones
	2% Salicylic acid	Peeling agent with irritant effect; reduces tendency to form comedones
Fostex (Westwood) Soap **Dosage** Lather and massage into skin and rinse thoroughly with water, several times/day	2% Sulfur	Peeling agent with irritant effect; reduces tendency to form comedones
	2% Salicylic acid	Peeling agent with irritant effect; reduces tendency to form comedones
Fostril (Westwood) Lotion **Dosage** Apply a thin film to affected areas, 1–2 times/day	2% Sulfur	Peeling agent with irritant effect; reduces tendency to form comedones
	Laureth-4	Solvent
	Zinc oxide	Skin protective and masking agent
	Talc	Skin protective
Ionax Foam (Owen) Aerosol foam **Dosage** Massage small amount of foam into affected area and rinse well, 1–2 times/day	0.2% Benzalkonium chloride	Antiseptic agent
	Polyoxyethylene ethers	Cleansing agents
	Soapless surfactant	Cleansing agent
Klaron (Dermik) Lotion **Dosage** Massage small amount of lotion into affected area once or twice daily	5% Colloidal sulfur	Peeling agent with irritant effect; reduces tendency to form comedones
	2% Salicylic acid	Peeling agent with irritant effect; reduces tendency to form comedones
	13.1% Alcohol	Astringent

Table continued on following page

NONPRESCRIPTION ACNE MEDICATIONS

Product (Manufacturer)	Ingredients	Actions
Komex (Barnes-Hind) Liquid **Dosage** Massage cleanser into wet affected area for about 1 min., rinse thoroughly, and dry, 1–2 times/day	Sodium tetrahydrate decahydrate granules	Abrasive and cleansing agents
Liquimat (Texas Pharmacal) Lotion **Dosage** Massage into affected areas several times/day	5% Sulfur	Peeling agent with irritant effect; reduces tendency to form comedones
	22% Alcohol	Astringent
	Tinted bases	Masking agents
Lotio Alsulfa (Doak) Lotion **Dosage** Massage into affected areas several times/day	5% Colloidal sulfur	Peeling agent with irritant effect; reduces tendency to form comedones
	95% Colloidal clays	Data to come
Microsyn (Syntex) Lotion **Dosage** Massage into affected areas several times/day	2% Resorcinol	Peeling agent with irritant effect; reduces tendency to form comedones
	2% Salicylic acid	Peeling agent with irritant effect; reduces tendency to form comedones
	8% Sodium thiosulfate	Disinfectant
	Colloidal alumina	Absorbing agent and skin protective
	Menthol	Anti-irritant
Oxy-5 (Norcliff Thayer) Lotion **Dosage** Smooth lotion onto existing pimples and acne-prone areas several times/day	5% Benzoyl peroxide	Peeling agent with irritant effect; reduces tendency to form comedones
Oxy-10 (Norcliff Thayer) Lotion **Dosage** Smooth lotion onto existing pimples and acne-prone areas several times/day	10% Benzoyl peroxide	Peeling agent with irritant effect; reduces tendency to form comedones
Pernox Lotion (Westwood) Lotion **Dosage** Lather and massage lotion into wet skin for about 1 min. and rinse thoroughly, 1–2 times/day	2% Sulfur	Peeling agent with irritant effect; reduces tendency to form comedones
	1.5% Salicylic acid	Peeling agent with irritant effect; reduces tendency to form comedones
	Sufactants	Cleansing agents
	Polyethylene granules	Abrasive agents

Table continued on following page

Product (Manufacturer)	Ingredients	Actions
pHisoAc (Winthrop) Cream **Dosage** Massage cream into affected areas several times/day	6% Colloidal sulfur	Peeling agent with irritant effect; reduces tendency to form comedones
	1.5% Resorcinol	Peeling agent with irritant effect; reduces tendency to form comedones
	10% Alcohol	Astringent
pHisoderm (Winthrop) Cleanser **Dosage** Lather and massage into face for about one min. and rinse thoroughly, as needed	Entsufon sodium	Cleansing agent
	Petrolatum	Emollient
	Lanolin	Emollient
Stri-Dex Medicated Pads (Lehn & Fink) Medicated Pads **Dosage** Wash and dry face and wipe pad over entire face AM and PM	0.5% Salicylic acid	Peeling agent with irritant effect; reduces tendency to form comedones
	Sulfonated alkylbenzenes	Anti-infectives
	Citric acid	Acidifying agent
	Alcohol	Astringent
Therapads (Parke-Davis) Pads **Dosage** Wipe pad over affected areas several times/day	1.5% Salicylic acid	Peeling agent with irritant effect; reduces tendency to form comedones
	50% Alcohol	Astringent

Dermatitis and Psoriasis

The skin is a complex organ that performs a variety of essential functions in addition to acting as a protective cover for the body. These roles include temperature regulation, sensory and nerve functions, and chemical exchange as well as immunological processes.

Since the skin covers such a large area, is exposed to so many potential irritants and harmful substances, and performs a variety of functions, it is not surprising that it is afflicted by a large number of disorders. In addition, many systemic diseases, ranging from infectious disorders to chronic diseases and nutritional deficiencies, may have dermatological manifestations. In this section, the various types of inflammatory skin disorders (dermatitis) and psoriasis will be discussed. Skin disorders caused by fungi (e.g., athlete's foot or ringworm) are discussed in the section on *Fungal Infections* (pages 444–468).

DERMATITIS

Dermatitis, also referred to as eczema, is characterized by inflammation and itching, which may be intense. In the early stages, there is usually swelling due to edema (retention of fluids) and erythema (raised red rash). Typically, small, often oozing blisters known as vesicles will form, progressing to crusting and scaling. If the problem becomes chronic, the skin will thicken, and the pigmentation may become darker, or in some cases lighter, than unaffected skin. In time, the oozing vesicles usually give way to thickened, dry lesions that are hyperpigmented (darker than normal).

Atopic Dermatitis

Intense itching is a major characteristic of atopic dermatitis. As the term "atopic" signifies, this chronic type of dermatitis tends to run in families—about 70 percent of all persons with atopic dermatitis have a family history of the disorder. It is frequently seen in persons with asthma or rhinitis (inflammation of the nose). It characteristically begins in early childhood (see *Infant Skin Disorders*, page 1114), subsiding at about age four, only to recur during adolescence or young adulthood. By age fifty, most persons seem to have "outlived" the disorder.

The dermatitis is generally worse in the winter, but flare-ups are unpredictable. The areas most commonly affected are the face, neck, scalp, upper back, and body folds or creases, such as the bends of the elbows or knees. The disorder itself is not harmful to general health, but the intense itching often results in uncontrolled scratching and infection. In addition, persons with atopic dermatitis appear to be more susceptible to viral infections, particularly herpes simplex virus. Chronic eczema

TYPICAL SITES OF CONTACT DERMATITIS

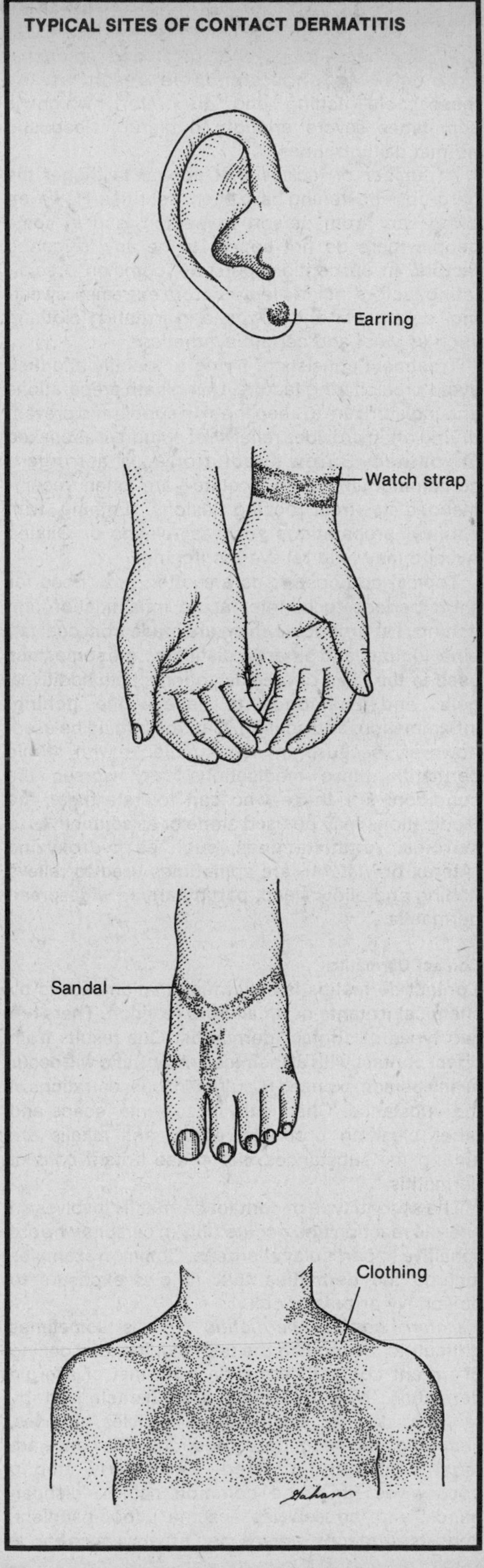

may also lead to psychological and emotional problems—an understandable result of the inescapable itching and discomfort, which is sometimes severe enough to disrupt sleep and normal daily routines.

A number of factors that appear to trigger the flare-ups and itching have been identified. However, these vary from person to person, and in some people there do not appear to be any triggering factors. In susceptible persons, common precipitating factors include temperature extremes, sweating, detergents and soaps, and irritating clothing such as wool and certain synthetics.

Treatment consists of trying to identify and then avoid precipitating factors. Using bath preparations and moisturizers to keep the skin supple and prevent drying often provides relief. Wet compresses soaked in diluted Burow's solution—an astringent containing aluminum acetate—are often recommended to treat oozing lesions. Bathing with oatmeal preparations such as Aveeno or Oilated Aveeno may help relieve the itching.

Topical corticosteroids are often prescribed for short periods to counter acute inflammation and itching. Tar products, which are made from coal tar, pine, juniper, and other tar distillates, are sometimes used in the form of creams, lotions, bath additives, gels, and shampoos to relieve the itching, inflammation, and scaling. Caution should be used, however, because in some patients with atopic dermatitis these medications may worsen the condition. For those who can tolerate them, the medications may be used alone or as adjunctives to steroids. Antihistamines, such as hydroxyzine (Atarax or Vistaril), are sometimes used to relieve itching and allow sleep, particularly in widespread dermatitis.

Contact Dermatitis

Contact dermatitis is skin inflammation caused by chemical irritants or an allergic reaction. There are two types of contact dermatitis. One results from direct contact with a chemical irritant, and will occur in any person exposed to sufficient concentrations of the substance. Chemicals in solvents, soaps and other cleaning products, acids, and alkalis are among the substances that cause irritant contact dermatitis.

The second type of contact dermatitis involves an allergic reaction and occurs only in persons who are sensitive to particular allergens. Common examples include the dermatitis that follows exposure to poison ivy or poison oak.

Irritant contact dermatitis It is sometimes difficult to distinguish the rash, itching, and oozing of irritant contact dermatitis from that of allergic dermatitis. Mild irritations are characterized by redness, itching, small oozing vesicles, dryness, chapping, and secondary infections. The hands are most commonly affected, particularly among housewives (thus the common names "dishpan hands" and "housewives' eczema"), food handlers, dentists, surgeons, nurses, and others whose hands are frequently exposed to irritants in soaps, detergents, and solvents. In more severe cases, drying and stiffening of the skin, with formation of fissures, may be seen. Exposure to harsh chemicals such as lye and strong solvents may result in blistering, ulcers, and erosion of the skin.

Allergic contact dermatitis Sensitivity to a particular allergen may take anywhere from a few days to years to develop. For example, a person may use a cosmetic or soap for years before developing an allergic reaction to it. In other instances, only a few exposures may be required, particularly if the allergen is a strong one such as poison ivy. In some instances, exposure to the sun heightens the allergic response—a phenomenon called photoallergic contact dermatitis.

Symptoms range from redness at the point of contact to severe swelling (edema) with blisters, generally accompanied by itching. In some instances, the dermatitis may spread from the initial point of exposure, or the allergen may be carried by the hands to other parts of the body.

Although almost any substance may provoke an allergic response in a hypersensitive individual, most allergic contact dermatitis can be attributed to six groups of substances.

- *Plants* More than 60 different plants commonly cause allergic contact dermatitis, with the most frequent being those in the *Toxicodendron* genus. These include poison ivy, poison oak, and poison sumac, which were formerly assigned to the *Rhus* genus. These plants are found in many places and commonly cause contact dermatitis even in persons with no other allergies.
- *Paraphenylenediamine (PPD)* PPD is a chemical used in dyes for hair, furs, and leathers. Persons sensitive to PPD may also react to similarly structured chemicals, such as procaine, benzocaine, and sulfonamide, as well as to topical forms of some antibiotics, such as streptomycin, chloramphenicol, and neomycin.
- *Nickel* Many metal objects that are worn close to the skin, such as watches, earrings, brassiere clips, zippers, and suspender clips, contain nickel. Allergic dermatitis in persons sensitive to nickel is usually easy to track down because it most often occurs at the point of contact, such as under or around a wristwatch.
- *Rubber compounds* Natural rubber rarely causes an allergic reaction, but antioxidants, accelerators, and peptizers used in synthetic rubber are common causes of dermatitis.
- *Chromates* This group of chemicals is used in many paints, varnishes, leather and fur dyes, and in electroplating solutions.
- *Formaldehyde and other chemical preservatives* Some chemical perservatives are used in the manufacture of permanent-press clothes; others are common ingredients in cosmetics, creams, perfumes, lanolin, and sunscreens.

Although the rash and symptoms of allergic contact dermatitis may resemble those of irritant dermatitis, the pattern of the skin lesions often

COMMON SOURCES OF PLANT DERMATITIS

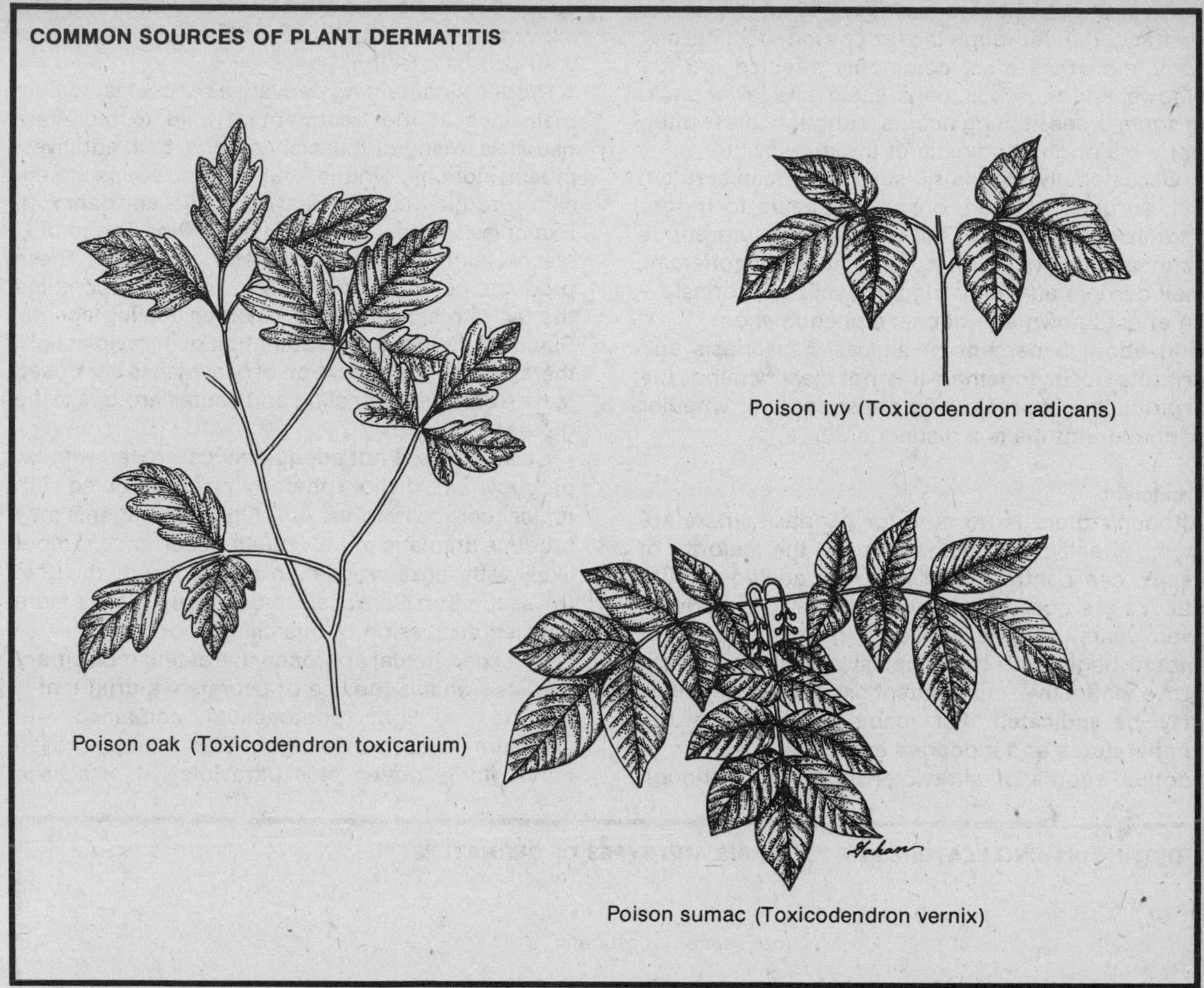

Poison oak (Toxicodendron toxicarium)

Poison ivy (Toxicodendron radicans)

Poison sumac (Toxicodendron vernix)

provides distinguishing clues. In many instances, the dermatitis will have distinct outlines that coincide with jewelry, items of clothing, or other objects.

In all instances of contact dermatitis, careful investigation of the total environment and activities is important in determining the cause of the irritation or allergic reaction. Avoiding the offending substances is the most effective treatment. Very often, the offending objects are job-related and impossible to avoid. When one's occupation necessitates daily contact with an irritating or sensitizing substance, it is advisable to wear gloves or other protective clothing to act as barriers against the substance(s). Creams and other chemical barriers *are not* effective protectants.

The rashes and lesions of most contact dermatitis will resolve with time and removal of the allergen. Washing thoroughly as soon as possible after exposure to an offending substance, such as poison ivy, may help lessen the reaction. Cold compresses soaked in a mild Burow's solution may help relieve the oozing and discomfort. Calamine or other soothing lotions also may relieve the itching. Severe cases with a good deal of edema and inflammation may be treated with topical corticosteroids. Chronic irritant dermatitis, particularly of the hands, also may be treated with corticosteroids. In severe cases, a sheet of plastic may be wrapped over a steroid cream or ointment to increase absorption and efficacy. However, this treatment, which is called an occlusive wrap, should be used only under a physician's supervision. Coal tar or similar products (e.g., Zetar, Doak, Estar, and others) are available as ointments, shampoos, lotions, creams, bath oils, and emulsions, and may be used to relieve itching and oozing.

PSORIASIS

Psoriasis, a chronic skin disease afflicting about 1 percent of all Americans, is characterized by patches of thick, scaling skin due to an overgrowth of epidermal cells. The cause is unknown, although a family history of psoriasis has been noted in up to 30 percent of all cases. Environment, climate, occupation, stress, and allergy all may be aggravating factors. The disease is characterized by unpredictable flare-ups and subsequent remissions, which may last for years.

Typically, psoriasis begins in young adulthood, although onset has been noted at all ages. Psoriatic eruptions may start as small red spots with white or silver scaling. Small areas may merge into larger ones or form bright red plaques covered by scales that resemble mica (micaceous) or oyster shells (ostraceous). Although the lesions may occur at any spot, the areas most commonly affected are the elbows, knees, hands, nails, scalp, and lower back. In some cases, itching occurs, although this is often not a major characteristic of the disease.

Occasionally, an injury, such as a deep scratch, cut, surgical incision, or burn, appears to trigger psoriasis at the site of the trauma. Pressure points such as those occurring on the hands of golfers or mail carriers also may trigger localized psoriasis—an effect known as Koebner's phenomenon.

In about 5 percent of all cases, psoriasis and arthritis occur together. It is not clear whether the arthritis is a characteristic of psoriasis, or whether psoriatic arthritis is a distinct entity.

Treatment

Although there is no cure for psoriasis, there are many effective treatments that, in the majority of cases, can control the disease. In addition, acute attacks are occasionally followed by long periods, even years, of quiescence. In general, treatment should begin with the simplest measures; if these prove ineffective, more potent or complex regimens may be indicated. For many individuals, warm temperatures and moderate exposure to the sun or another source of ultraviolet light help, although sunburn can worsen the condition. Unfortunately, many people are reluctant or embarrassed to expose their psoriatic lesions.

Products containing derivatives of coal tar remain mainstays in the treatment of mild to moderate psoriasis. Many of these shampoos, bath additives, creams, lotions, ointments, gels, and soaps are the same products used to treat dermatitis and dandruff. Examples include Tegrin, Packer's Pine Tar, Ionil T, Mazon, Alma Tar, Estar, Balnetar, and Zetar. These products contain various tars, and some combine the tar with salicylic acid or other peeling agents. Since the 1920's, the combination of ultraviolet light therapy and the application of coal tar has been used to help control the scaling and acute flare-ups of the disease.

Cases that are not adequately controlled with tar products and/or light therapy may be treated with topical corticosteroids. Although these agents may produce dramatic initial results, recurrence is more likely with these drugs than with tar products. (See the section on *Corticosteroids,* page xx, for a more detailed discussion of this class of drugs.)

An experimental approach to treating recalcitrant psoriasis entails the use of psoralen, a drug that is activated by light (photoactive), combined with exposure to ultraviolet light. This therapy, called PUVA (for psoralen plus ultraviolet A), has been

DISTINGUISHING FEATURES OF PSORIASIS AND TYPES OF DERMATITIS

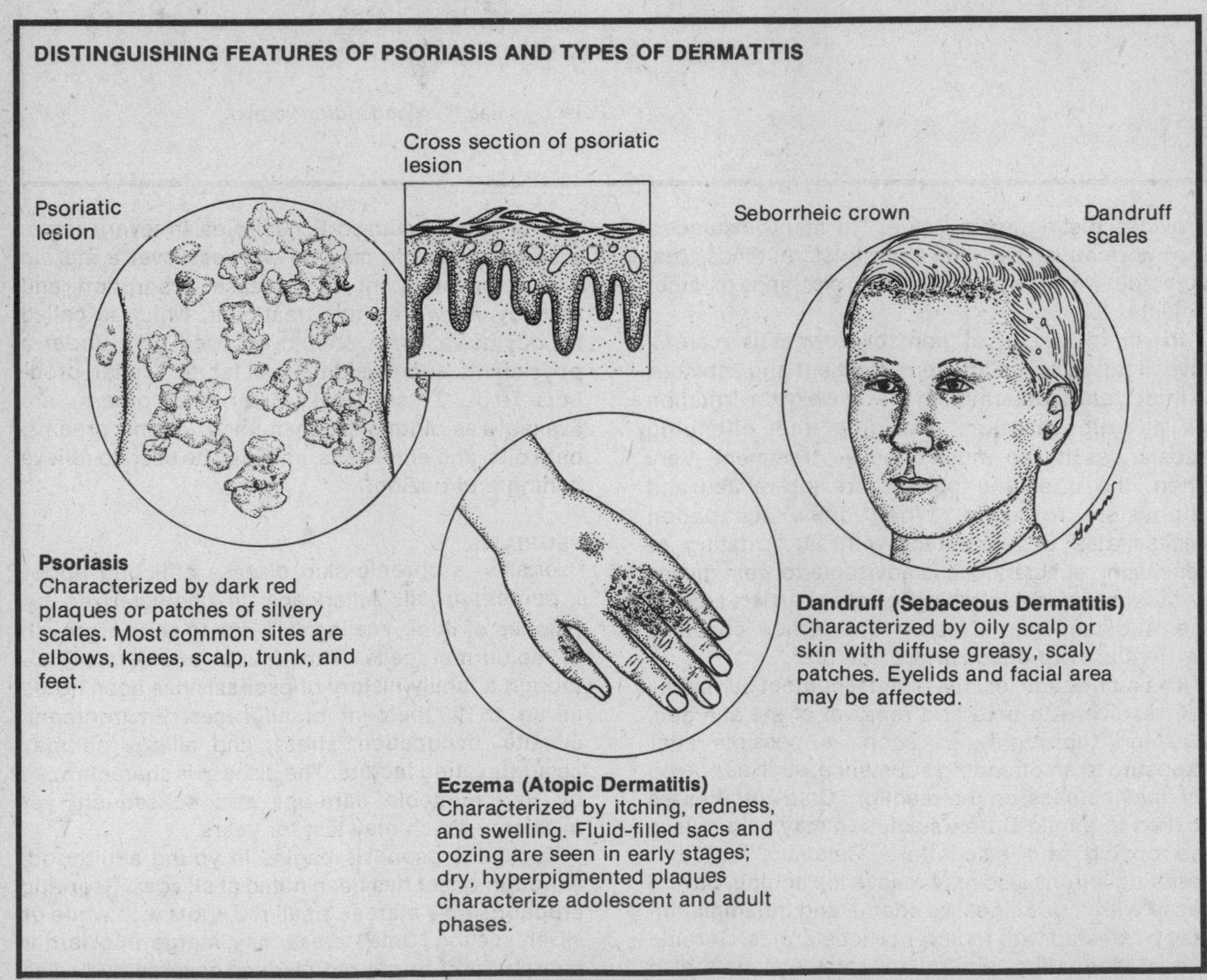

Psoriasis
Characterized by dark red plaques or patches of silvery scales. Most common sites are elbows, knees, scalp, trunk, and feet.

Eczema (Atopic Dermatitis)
Characterized by itching, redness, and swelling. Fluid-filled sacs and oozing are seen in early stages; dry, hyperpigmented plaques characterize adolescent and adult phases.

Dandruff (Sebaceous Dermatitis)
Characterized by oily scalp or skin with diffuse greasy, scaly patches. Eyelids and facial area may be affected.

used in research settings with reports of good results, but its long-term efficacy and possible adverse effects are unknown.

DANDRUFF

Dandruff is a noninflammatory scalp condition characterized by increased scaling of dry, white flakes as a result of a mild increase in the formation and shedding of epidermal cells. The cause of dandruff is unknown; at one time, it was believed that a microorganism might be involved, but this is not the case. Nor is the dandruff caused by increased production of sebum.

Most cases of dandruff can be effectively controlled with medicated shampoos—in many instances, the same products recommended for persons with dermatitis or psoriasis. Many of these products are available without prescription and contain a variety of active ingredients. They include selenium sulfide (Selsun Blue), zinc pyrithione (Head & Shoulders, Anti-Dandruff Brylcreem) coal tar (Zetar), and salicylic acid and sulfur (Sebulex). Selenium sulfide and zinc pyrithione slow cell turnover, while salicylic acid and sulfur act as peeling (keratolytic) agents, which loosen and promote shedding of the epidermal cells.

DRY SKIN

Although dry skin is unrelated to eczema, psoriasis, or dandruff, it sometimes accompanies these disorders. In many persons, dry skin is a seasonal reaction that is aggravated in the winter or when the humidity is low. Itchiness is a major symptom, although there also may be roughness, flaking, and formation of fissures.

Drying of the skin is usually accelerated with age, overexposure to the sun and wind, and low humidity. The primary treatment is prevention of further loss of moisture from the skin. Bath oils, moisturizers, creams, lotions, and emollients are often beneficial. Many of these are sold as cosmetic products, others as skin care medications. Common ingredients include mineral oil, lanolin, and other oils; water; petrolatum; vitamins A and D; glycerin; and other ingredients to promote retention of water in the skin (humectants). Selection of a product depends largely upon personal preference and whether or not it produces the desired results.

IN CONCLUSION

Common skin disorders such as dermatitis, psoriasis, and dandruff are more demoralizing and annoying than they are serious threats to health. They should not be dismissed as trivial, however, because of the discomfort, self-consciousness, and psychological damage they often produce. In addition, they may increase susceptibility to skin infections, especially in infants and others who may scratch and irritate the lesions in seeking relief.

A wide variety of drugs are available that, in most instances, can control these conditions. In general, therapy should begin with the milder nonprescription products, with the more potent corticosteroids and other such agents reserved for refractory cases or acute flare-ups. The following charts cover the more common nonprescription products used to treat dermatitis, psoriasis, dandruff, dry skin, poison ivy, and insect stings and bites, as well as topical corticosteroids and other prescription medications. It should be noted that in many instances these drugs are used to treat more than one skin disorder. Antihistamines, which may be prescribed to control itching, are in the section on *Allergic Disorders*, (pages 916–938).

CORDRAN (Flurandrenolide) **Dista**

Lotion: 0.05% (15, 60 ml) **Ointment:** 0.025% (30, 60, 225 g), 0.05% (15, 30, 60, 225 g)

CORDRAN-SP (Flurandrenolide) **Dista**

Cream: 0.025% (30, 60, 225 g), 0.05% (15, 30, 60, 225 g)

INDICATIONS	TOPICAL DOSAGE
Inflammatory manifestations of corticosteroid-responsive dermatoses	**Adult:** For moist lesions, gently rub a small amount of the cream or lotion into affected area bid or tid; for dry, scaly lesions, apply a thin film of ointment to affected area bid or tid

ADMINISTRATION/DOSAGE ADJUSTMENTS

Occlusive dressing technique	Remove superficial scales as much as possible by brushing, picking, or rubbing (soaking in a bath will help soften scales and permit easier removal). Rub cream, ointment, or lotion thoroughly into affected area and cover with plastic film. Additional moisture may be provided by placing a slightly dampened cloth or gauze over the lesion before applying film. Seal the edges with tape or a gauze wrapping. Dressing may be changed daily or left in place for 3–4 days in more resistant cases. To prevent relapse, continue treatment for at least a few days after lesions clear.

CONTRAINDICATIONS

Hypersensitivity to flurandrenolide or other components ●	Ophthalmic use ●

WARNINGS/PRECAUTIONS

Irritation	Discontinue use and institute appropriate therapy
Infection	Institute appropriate antifungal or antibacterial therapy; if infection persists, discontinue steroid therapy until a favorable response is achieved
Systemic absorption	Increases with extensive treatment or occlusive dressing technique; use with caution, especially in infants and children
Miliaria, folliculitis	May occur with use of occlusive dressing; treatment may be continued by inunction
Sensitivity	May develop to occlusive dressing material; substitute different material for dressing
Thermal regulation	May be impaired, especially with occlusive dressings and extensive treatment; discontinue use of occlusive dressing if temperature rises

ADVERSE REACTIONS[1]

Dermatological	Acneform eruptions, allergic contact dermatitis, burning, dryness, folliculitis, hypertrichosis, hypopigmentation, irritation, itching, perioral dermatitis, maceration, miliaria, secondary infection, skin atrophy, striae

Use in children

General guidelines not established

Use in pregnancy or nursing mothers

Safe use not established during pregnancy; use in large amounts, for prolonged periods, or over extensive areas is not recommended. General guidelines not established for use in nursing mothers.

[1]Includes reactions common to topical corticosteroids in general

CORDRAN-N (Flurandrenolide and neomycin sulfate) **Dista**

Cream: 0.5 mg flurandrenolide (0.05%) and 5 mg neomycin sulfate per gram (15, 30, 60 g) **Ointment:** 0.5 mg flurandrenolide (0.05%) and 5 mg neomycin sulfate per gram (15, 30, 60 g)

INDICATIONS	TOPICAL DOSAGE
Inflammatory manifestations of corticosteroid-responsive dermatoses complicated by bacterial infection[1]	**Adult:** Apply a small amount of cream or thin film of ointment to affected area bid or tid; cream should be rubbed gently into lesion

ADMINISTRATION/DOSAGE ADJUSTMENTS

Selection of appropriate formulation	For moist lesions, use the cream; for dry, scaly lesions, use the ointment

CONTRAINDICATIONS

Hypersensitivity to any of the components ●	Ophthalmic use ●

WARNINGS/PRECAUTIONS

Irritation	Discontinue use and institute appropriate therapy
Fungal or yeast infections	Institute additional appropriate antifungal therapy and observe patient frequently
Superinfection	Prolonged use may result in overgrowth of nonsusceptible organisms requiring appropriate therapy
Systemic absorption	Increases with extensive treatment or occlusive dressing technique; use with caution, especially in infants and children
Nephrotoxicity, ototoxicity	Avoid prolonged use or use of large amounts in the presence of extensive burns, trophic ulceration, and other conditions in which absorption of neomycin is possible
Neomycin sensitivity	Current literature indicates an increase in the prevalence of persons allergic to neomycin

ADVERSE REACTIONS[2]

Dermatological	Acneform eruptions, allergic contact dermatitis, burning, dryness, folliculitis, hypertrichosis, hypopigmentation, irritation, itching, perioral dermatitis, maceration, miliaria, secondary infection, atrophy, striae
Other	Ototoxicity, nephrotoxicity

Use in children

General guidelines not established

Use in pregnancy or nursing mothers

Safe use not established during pregnancy; use in large amounts, for prolonged periods, or over extensive areas is not recommended. General guidelines not established for use in nursing mothers.

[1]Possibly effective
[2]Includes reactions common to topical corticosteroids in general

CORTISPORIN Cream (Polymyxin B sulfate, neomycin sulfate, gramicidin, and hydrocortisone acetate) Burroughs Wellcome

Cream: 10,000 units polymyxin B sulfate, 5 mg neomycin sulfate, 0.25 mg gramicidin, and 5 mg hydrocortisone acetate (0.5%) per gram (7.5 g)

INDICATIONS

Topical bacterial infections caused by susceptible organisms in conditions requiring the anti-inflammatory and/or antiallergic action of a corticosteroid[1]

Atopic, contact, stasis, and infectious eczematoid dermatitis; neurodermatitis, eczema, and anogenital pruritus[1]

As an adjunct to systemic antibiotic therapy in certain **pyodermas,** such as impetigo[1]

TOPICAL DOSAGE

Adult: Apply a small amount of cream to affected area bid, tid, or qid, as needed; if conditions permit, cream should be gently rubbed into affected area

ADMINISTRATION/DOSAGE ADJUSTMENTS

Withdrawal of chronic therapy — Decrease frequency of application until cream is applied as infrequently as once a week; then discontinue treatment

CONTRAINDICATIONS

Ophthalmic use ●

Use in the external ear canal if the eardrum is perforated ●

Fungal or viral skin lesions, including herpes simplex, vaccinia, and varicella ●

Tuberculosis ●

Hypersensitivity to any of the components ●

WARNINGS/PRECAUTIONS

Nephrotoxicity and ototoxicity — Use with caution in the presence of extensive burns, trophic ulceration, or other extensive conditions in which systemic absorption of neomycin is possible; limit use to one application/day in burns covering >20% of body surface, especially in patients with renal impairment or those receiving other aminoglycoside antibiotics concurrently

Neomycin sensitization — May occur with prolonged use; discontinue medication if low-grade reddening with swelling, dry scaling, and itching occurs or lesion fails to heal

Superinfection — Overgrowth of nonsusceptible organisms, including fungi, may occur with prolonged use; institute appropriate anti-infective therapy.

Systemic corticosteroid therapy — May be required for generalized dermatological conditions

Spread of infection — May be encouraged by use of steroids on infected areas; discontinue treatment and institute appropriate antibacterial therapy

ADVERSE REACTIONS

Dermatological — Striae, cutaneous sensitization

Other — Ototoxicity, nephrotoxicity

Use in children

General guidelines not established

Use in pregnancy or nursing mothers

Safe use not established during pregnancy; use in large amounts, for prolonged periods, or over extensive areas is not recommended. General guidelines not established for use in nursing mothers.

[1]Possibly effective

CORTISPORIN Ointment (Polymyxin B sulfate, bacitracin zinc, neomycin sulfate, and hydrocortisone acetate) **Burroughs Wellcome**

Ointment: 5,000 units polymyxin B sulfate, 400 units bacitracin zinc, 5 mg neomycin sulfate, and 10 mg hydrocortisone acetate (1%) per gram (14.2 g)

INDICATIONS	TOPICAL DOSAGE
Topical bacterial infections caused by susceptible organisms in conditions requiring the anti-inflammatory and/or antiallergic action of a corticosteroid[1]	**Adult:** Apply a thin film of ointment to affected area bid, tid, or qid
Atopic, contact, stasis, and infectious eczematoid dermatitis, neurodermatitis, eczema, and anogenital pruritus[1]	
As an adjunct to systemic antibiotic therapy in certain **pyodermas,** such as impetigo[1]	

ADMINISTRATION/DOSAGE ADJUSTMENTS

Withdrawal of chronic therapy	Decrease frequency of application, until ointment is applied as infrequently as once a week; then discontinue treatment

CONTRAINDICATIONS

Use in the external ear canal if the eardrum is perforated ●	Hypersensitivity to any of the components ●	Ophthalmic use ●

WARNINGS/PRECAUTIONS

Nephrotoxicity and ototoxicity	Use with caution in the presence of extreme burns, trophic ulceration, or other extensive conditions in which systemic absorption of neomycin is possible; limit use to one application/day in burns covering >20% of body surface, especially in patients with renal impairment or receiving other aminoglycoside antibiotics concurrently
Neomycin sensitization	May occur with prolonged use; discontinue medication if low-grade reddening with swelling, dry scaling, and itching occurs or lesion fails to heal
Superinfection	Overgrowth of nonsusceptible organisms, including fungi, may occur with prolonged use; institute appropriate anti-infective therapy
Systemic corticosteroid therapy	May be required for generalized dermatological conditions
Spread of infection	May be encouraged by use of steroids on infected areas; discontinue treatment and institute appropriate antibacterial therapy

ADVERSE REACTIONS

Dermatological	Striae, cutaneous sensitization
Other	Ototoxicity, nephrotoxicity

Use in children

General guidelines not established

Use in pregnancy or nursing mothers

Safe use not established during pregnancy; use in large amounts, for prolonged periods, or over extensive areas is not recommended. General guidelines not established for use in nursing mothers.

[1]Possibly effective

CYCLOCORT (Amcinonide) Lederle

Cream: 0.1% (15, 60 g)

INDICATIONS	TOPICAL DOSAGE
Inflammatory manifestations of corticosteroid-responsive dermatoses	**Adult:** apply a light film to affected area bid or tid; cream should be rubbed in gently and thoroughly until it disappears

CONTRAINDICATIONS

Hypersensitivity to amcinonide or other components ●	Ophthalmic use ●

WARNINGS/PRECAUTIONS

Irritation	Discontinue use and institute appropriate therapy
Infection	Institute appropriate antifungal or antibacterial therapy; if infection persists, discontinue steroid therapy until infection is controlled
Systemic absorption	Increases with extensive treatment or occlusive dressing technique; use with caution, especially in infants and children

ADVERSE REACTIONS[1]

Dermatological	Burning, itching, irritation, dryness, folliculitis, hypertrichosis, acneform eruptions, hypopigmentation, perioral dermatitis, allergic contact dermatitis, maceration, secondary infection, skin atrophy, striae, miliaria

Use in children

General guidelines not established

Use in pregnancy or lactating mothers

Safe use not established during pregnancy; use in large amounts, for prolonged periods, or over extensive areas is not recommended. General guidelines not established for use in nursing mothers.

[1]Includes reactions common to topical corticosteroids in general

DECADERM (Dexamethasone) Merck Sharp & Dohme

Gel: 0.1% (15, 30 g)

INDICATIONS	TOPICAL DOSAGE
Inflammatory manifestations of corticosteroid-responsive dermatoses	**Adult:** Apply to affected areas tid or qid

CONTRAINDICATIONS

Hypersensitivity to dexamethasone or other components ●

Tuberculosis of the skin ●

Vaccinia or varicella ●

Herpes simplex infections ●

Fungal infections ●

Ophthalmic use ●

WARNINGS/PRECAUTIONS

Irritation	Discontinue use and institute appropriate therapy
Infection	Institute appropriate antifungal or antibacterial therapy; if infection persists, discontinue steroid therapy until a favorable response is achieved. If occlusive dressing technique is used, inspect lesions when changing dressing and discontinue technique if infection develops.
Systemic absorption	Increases with extensive treatment or occlusive dressing technique; use with caution, especially in infants and children
Thermal regulation	May be impaired, especially with occlusive dressing and extensive treatment; discontinue use of occlusive dressing if temperature rises
Steroid glaucoma	May result from prolonged ocular exposure; drug may enter eyes if applied to eyelids or skin near eyes
Weeping or exudative lesions	Do not use occlusive dressings

ADVERSE REACTIONS[1]

Dermatological	Burning, itching, irritation, dryness, folliculitis, hypertrichosis, acneform eruptions, hypopigmentation, perioral dermatitis, allergic contact dermatitis, maceration, secondary infection, skin atrophy, striae, miliaria

Use in children

General guidelines not established

Use in pregnancy or nursing mothers

Safe use not established during pregnancy; use in large amounts, for prolonged periods, or over extensive areas is not recommended. General guidelines not established for use in nursing mothers.

[1]Includes reactions common to topical corticosteroids in general

DIPROSONE (Betamethasone dipropionate) Schering

Cream: 0.05% (15, 45 g) **Lotion:** 0.05% (20, 60 ml) **Ointment:** 0.05% (15, 45 g) **Spray:** 0.1% (85 g)

INDICATIONS	TOPICAL DOSAGE
Inflammatory manifestations of corticosteroid-responsive dermatoses	**Adult:** Apply a thin film of the cream or ointment or a few drops of the lotion to affected areas bid (in AM and PM); lotion should be massaged gently into the lesion until the preparation disappears

ADMINISTRATION/DOSAGE ADJUSTMENTS

Spray (acute contact dermatitis)	Direct spray onto affected area from a distance of not less than 6 in, and apply for only 3 s tid; do not apply under occlusive dressings

CONTRAINDICATIONS

Hypersensitivity to betamethasone or other components ●	Ophthalmic use ●

WARNINGS/PRECAUTIONS

Irritation	Discontinue use and institute appropriate therapy
Infection	Institute appropriate antifungal or antibacterial therapy; if infection persists, discontinue steroid therapy until a favorable response is achieved
Systemic absorption	Increases with extensive treatment or occlusive dressing technique; use with caution, especially in infants and children

ADVERSE REACTIONS[1]

Dermatological	Burning, itching, irritation, dryness, folliculitis, hypertrichosis, acneform eruptions, hypopigmentation, perioral dermatitis, allergic contact dermatitis, maceration, secondary infection, skin atrophy, striae, miliaria

Use in children

General guidelines not established

Use in pregnancy or nursing mothers

Safe use not established during pregnancy; use in large amounts or for prolonged periods is not recommended. General guidelines not established for use in nursing mothers.

Note: Betamethasone valerate marketed as **VALISONE** (Schering).

[1] Includes reactions common to topical corticosteroids in general

FLORONE (Diflorasone diacetate) Upjohn

Cream, ointment: 0.05% (15, 30, 60 g)

INDICATIONS	TOPICAL DOSAGE
Inflammatory manifestations of corticosteroid-responsive dermatoses (adjunctive therapy)	**Adult:** Apply a small amount of cream and massage gently into affected area bid to qid, or apply a thin film of ointment to area qd to tid, without massage

CONTRAINDICATIONS

Hypersensitivity to diflorasone or other components ●	Vaccinia or varicella ●	Ophthalmic use ●

WARNINGS/PRECAUTIONS

Irritation	Discontinue use and institute appropriate therapy
Infection	Institute appropriate antifungal or antibacterial therapy; if infection persists, discontinue steroid therapy until a favorable response is achieved
Systemic absorption	Increases with extensive treatment or occlusive dressing technique; use with caution, especially in infants and children. If lesions are extensive, a sequential approach, occluding one portion of the body at a time, may be preferable.
Thermal regulation	May be impaired, especially with occlusive dressing and extensive treatment; discontinue use of occlusive dressing if temperature rises
Steroid withdrawal symptoms	May develop when drug is withdrawn after prolonged therapy, especially with occlusive dressings

ADVERSE REACTIONS[1]

Dermatological	Burning, itching, irritation, dryness, folliculitis, hypertrichosis, acneform eruptions, hypopigmentation, maceration, secondary infection, skin atrophy, striae, miliaria

Use in children	Use in pregnancy or nursing mothers
General guidelines not established	Safe use not established during pregnancy; use in large amounts, for prolonged periods, or over extensive areas is not recommended. General guidelines not established for use in nursing mothers.

[1] Includes reactions common to topical corticosteroids in general

HALOG (Halcinonide) Squibb

Cream: 0.025% (15, 60, 240 g), 0.1% (15, 30, 60, 240 g) **Ointment:** 0.025% (15, 60, 240 g), 0.1% (15, 30, 60, 240 g)
Sol: 0.1% (20, 60 ml)

INDICATIONS	TOPICAL DOSAGE
Inflammatory manifestations of corticosteroid-responsive dermatoses	**Adult:** Apply cream, solution, or thin film of ointment to affected area bid to tid; cream should be rubbed in gently after application

ADMINISTRATION/DOSAGE ADJUSTMENTS

Occlusive dressing technique	Apply solution or a thin film of ointment to the lesion and cover with plastic film. Alternatively, gently rub a small amount of cream into the lesion until the preparation disappears; reapply the cream, leaving a thin coating on the lesion, and cover with plastic film. Frequency of dressing changes should be determined on an individual basis; reapply medication with each change. If occlusive dressing is used only at night (12-h occlusion), additional medication should be applied, without occlusion, during the day.

CONTRAINDICATIONS

Hypersensitivity to halcinonide or other components ●	Ophthalmic use ●

WARNINGS/PRECAUTIONS

Irritation	Discontinue use and institute appropriate therapy
Infection	Institute appropriate antifungal or antibacterial therapy; if infection persists, discontinue steroid therapy until a favorable response is achieved
Systemic absorption	Increases with extensive treatment or occlusive dressing technique; use with caution, especially in infants and children. If lesions are extensive, a sequential approach, occluding one portion of the body at a time, may be preferable.
Thermal regulation	May be impaired, especially with occlusive dressings and extensive treatment; discontinue use if temperature elevation occurs
Steroid withdrawal symptoms	May develop when drug is withdrawn after prolonged therapy, especially with occlusive dressings

ADVERSE REACTIONS[1]

Dermatological	Burning, itching, irritation, dryness, folliculitis, hypertrichosis, acneform eruptions, hypopigmentation, perioral dermatitis, allergic contact dermatitis, maceration, secondary infection, skin atrophy, striae, miliaria

Use in children

General guidelines not established

Use in pregnancy or nursing mothers

Safe use not established during pregnancy; use in large amounts, for prolonged periods, or over extensive areas is not recommended. General guidelines not established for use in nursing mothers.

[1]Includes reactions common to topical corticosteroids in general

HYTONE (Hydrocortisone) **Dermik**

Cream: 0.5, 1.0% (30, 120 g), 2.5% (30 g)

INDICATIONS	TOPICAL DOSAGE
Inflammatory manifestations of corticosteroid-responsive dermatoses	**Adult:** Apply to affected areas tid or qid

CONTRAINDICATIONS

Hypersensitivity to hydrocortisone or other components ●	Ophthalmic use ●

WARNINGS/PRECAUTIONS

Irritation	Discontinue use and institute appropriate therapy
Infection	Institute appropriate antifungal or antibacterial therapy; if infection persists, discontinue steroid therapy until a favorable response is achieved
Systemic absorption	Increases with extensive treatment or occlusive dressing technique; use with caution, especially in infants and children

ADVERSE REACTIONS[1]

Dermatological	Burning, itching, irritation, dryness, folliculitis, hypertrichosis, acneform eruptions, hypopigmentation, perioral dermatitis, allergic contact dermatitis, maceration, secondary infection, skin atrophy, striae, miliaria

Use in children	Use in pregnancy or nursing mothers
General guidelines not established	Safe use not established during pregnancy; use in large amounts, for prolonged periods, or over extensive areas is not recommended. General guidelines not established for use in nursing mothers.

Note: Hydrocortisone or cortisol also marketed as **ALPHADERM** (Norwich-Eaton); **CETACORT** (Parke-Davis); **CORT-DOME** (Dome); **CORTEF** (Upjohn); **CORTRIL** (Pfipharmecs); and various other brands.

[1]Includes reactions common to topical corticosteroids in general

KENALOG (Triamcinolone acetonide) Squibb

Cream: 0.025% (15, 80, 240, 2,380 g), 0.1% (15, 60, 80, 240, 2,380 g), 0.5% (20, 240 g) **Ointment:** 0.025% (15, 80, 240 g), 0.1% (15, 60, 80, 240 g), 0.5% (20, 240 g) **Lotion:** 0.025% (60 ml), 0.1% (15, 60 ml) **Spray:** 0.2% following 2-s spray (23, 63 g)

KENALOG-H (Triamcinolone acetonide) Squibb

Cream: 0.1% (15, 60 g)

INDICATIONS	TOPICAL DOSAGE
Inflammatory manifestations of corticosteroid-responsive dermatoses (adjunctive therapy)	**Adult:** Apply cream, lotion, or thin film of ointment to affected areas bid to qid (if 0.025% strength is used) or bid to tid (if 0.1% or 0.5% strength is used); cream and lotion should be rubbed in gently after application

ADMINISTRATION/DOSAGE ADJUSTMENTS

Spray application	Follow directions on aerosol can; preparation may be applied to any part of the body, but if applied to face, care should be taken to avoid contact with eyes or inhalation of spray. Area may also be covered with occlusive dressing (see below). Three or four applications daily are generally adequate.
Occlusive dressing technique	Apply a thin film of ointment to affected area or gently massage a small amount of cream or lotion into affected area until preparation disappears. Reapply, leaving a thin coating, and cover with plastic film. Additional moisture may be provided by covering lesion with a damp cotton cloth or by briefly soaking affected area in water before applying film. Frequency of dressing changes should be determined on an individual basis; reapply medication with each change.

CONTRAINDICATIONS

Hypersensitivity to triamcinolone or other components ●	Ophthalmic use ●

WARNINGS/PRECAUTIONS

Irritation	Discontinue use and institute appropriate therapy
Infection	Institute appropriate antifungal or antibacterial therapy; if infection persists, discontinue steroid therapy until a favorable response is achieved
Systemic absorption	Increases with extensive treatment or occlusive dressing technique; use with caution, especially in infants and children. If lesions are extensive, a sequential approach, occluding one portion of the body at a time, may be preferable.
Thermal regulation	May be impaired, especially with occlusive dressing and extensive treatment; **discontinue use of occlusive dressing if temperature elevation occurs**
Steroid withdrawal symptoms	May develop when drug is withdrawn after prolonged therapy, especially with occlusive dressings

ADVERSE REACTIONS[1]

Dermatological	Burning, itching, irritation, dryness, folliculitis, hypertrichosis, acneform eruptions, hypopigmentation, perioral dermatitis, allergic contact dermatitis, maceration, secondary infection, skin atrophy, striae, miliaria

Use in children	Use in pregnancy or nursing mothers
General guidelines not established	Safe use not established during pregnancy; use in large amounts, for prolonged periods, or over extensive areas is not recommended. General guidelines not established for use in nursing mothers.

NOTE: Triamcinolone acetonide also marketed as **ARISTOCORT** (Lederle).

[1]Includes reactions common to topical corticosteroids in general

LIDEX (Fluocinonide) **Syntex**

Cream, ointment: 0.05% (15, 30, 60 g)

LIDEX-E (Fluocinonide) **Syntex**

Cream: 0.05% (15, 30, 60 g)

INDICATIONS	TOPICAL DOSAGE
Inflammatory manifestations of corticosteroid-responsive dermatoses	**Adult:** Apply small amount and massage gently into affected areas tid or qid

CONTRAINDICATIONS

Hypersensitivity to fluocinonide or other components ●	Ophthalmic use ●

WARNINGS/PRECAUTIONS

Irritation	Discontinue use and institute appropriate therapy
Infection	Institute appropriate antifungal or antibacterial therapy; if infection persists, discontinue steroid therapy until a favorable response is achieved
Systemic absorption	Increases with extensive treatment or occlusive dressing technique; use with caution, especially in infants and children

ADVERSE REACTIONS[1]

Dermatological	Burning, itching, irritation, dryness, folliculitis, hypertrichosis, acneform eruptions, hypopigmentation, perioral dermatitis, allergic contact dermatitis, maceration, secondary infection, skin atrophy, striae, miliaria

Use in children

General guidelines not established

Use in pregnancy or nursing mothers

Safe use not established during pregnancy; use in large amounts, for prolonged periods, or over extensive areas is not recommended. General guidelines not established for use in nursing mothers.

NOTE: Fluocinonide also marketed as **TOPSYN** (Syntex).

[1] Includes reactions common to topical corticosteroids in general

MYCOLOG (Nystatin, neomycin sulfate, gramicidin, and triamcinolone acetonide) Squibb

Cream, ointment: 100,000 units nystatin, neomycin sulfate equivalent to 2.5 mg neomycin base, 0.25 mg gramicidin, and 1 mg triamcinolone acetonide (1%) per gram (15, 30, 60, 120 g)

INDICATIONS	TOPICAL DOSAGE
Cutaneous candidiasis[1] **Superficial bacterial infections**[1] **Atopic, eczematoid, stasis, nummular, contact, or seborrheic dermatitis, neurodermatitis, and dermatitis venenata complicated by candidal and/or bacterial infection**[1] **Infantile eczema**[1] **Lichen simplex chronicus**[1]	**Adult:** Apply cream or a thin film of ointment to affected area bid or tid; cream should be gently rubbed in until it disappears
Pruritus ani and pruritus vulvae[1]	**Adult:** Apply cream to affected area bid or tid; cream should be gently rubbed in until it disappears

ADMINISTRATION/DOSAGE ADJUSTMENTS

Occlusive dressing technique	Gently rub a small amount of cream into the affected area until the preparation disappears; reapply the cream, leaving a thin coat on the lesion, and cover with plastic film. Alternatively, apply a thin coat of ointment over the affected area and cover with plastic film. Additional moisture may be provided by covering the lesion with a dampened, clean cotton cloth before applying the film or by briefly soaking the affected area in water. Frequency of dressing changes should be determined on an individual basis; reapply medication with each change

CONTRAINDICATIONS

Viral skin diseases ●	Hypersensitivity to any of the components ●	Use in the external ear canal if eardrum is perforated ●
Fungal skin lesions (except candidiasis) ●	Ophthalmic use ●	
Markedly impaired circulation ●		

WARNINGS/PRECAUTIONS

Nephrotoxicity and ototoxicity	Avoid prolonged use or use of large amounts in the presence of extensive burns, trophic ulceration, or other conditions in which systemic absorption of neomycin is possible
Superinfection	Overgrowth of nonsusceptible organisms, including fungi other than *Candida*, may occur with prolonged use; institute appropriate concomitant anti-infective therapy. If infection persists, discontinue topical steroid therapy until a favorable response is achieved.
Irritation	Discontinue use and institute appropriate therapy
Systemic absorption	Increases with extensive treatment or occlusive dressing technique; use with caution
Neomycin sensitivity	Current literature indicates an increase in the prevalence of persons allergic to neomycin

ADVERSE REACTIONS[2]

Dermatological	Burning sensations, itching, irritation, dryness, folliculitis, secondary infection, skin atrophy, striae, miliaria, hypertrichosis, acneform eruptions, maceration, hypopigmentation, contact sensitivity to dressing material or adhesive
Other	Ototoxicity, nephrotoxicity

Use in children

General guidelines not established

Use in pregnancy or nursing mothers

Safe use not established during pregnancy; use in large amounts, for prolonged periods, or over extensive areas is not recommended. General guidelines not established for use in nursing mothers.

[1]Possibly effective
[2]Includes reactions common to topical corticosteroids in general

NEO-SYNALAR (Neomycin sulfate and fluocinolone acetonide) Syntex

Cream: 5 mg neomycin sulfate (0.5%) and 0.25 mg fluocinolone acetonide (0.025%) per gram (15, 30, 60 g)

INDICATIONS	TOPICAL DOSAGE
Acute or chronic dermatoses, including atopic dermatitis, neurodermatitis, contact dermatitis, seborrheic dermatitis, eczematous dermatitis, pruritus ani, lichen simplex chronicus, postanal surgical infections, nummular eczema, stasis dermatitis, intertrigo, exfoliative dermatitis, and intertriginous psoriasis complicated by bacterial infections caused by neomycin-susceptible organisms (adjunctive therapy)[1]	**Adult:** Apply a small amount lightly to affected area bid or tid, as needed; the cream should be rubbed in gently and thoroughly until it disappears

CONTRAINDICATIONS

Hypersensitivity to any of the components ●	Ophthalmic use ●

WARNINGS/PRECAUTIONS

Irritation	Discontinue use and institute appropriate therapy
Persistent or severe local infection or systemic infection	Institute appropriate systemic antibacterial therapy based on susceptibility testing
Superinfection	Prolonged use may result in overgrowth of nonsusceptible organisms requiring appropriate therapy
Systemic absorption	Increases with extensive treatment or occlusive dressing technique; use with caution, especially in infants and children
Nephrotoxicity, ototoxicity	Avoid prolonged use or use of large amounts in the presence of extensive burns, trophic ulceration, and other conditions in which absorption of neomycin is possible
Neomycin sensitivity	Current literature indicates an increase in the prevalence of persons allergic to neomycin

ADVERSE REACTIONS[2]

Dermatological	Burning, itching, irritation, dryness, folliculitis, hypertrichosis, acneform eruptions, hypopigmentation, perioral dermatitis, allergic contact dermatitis, maceration, secondary infection, atrophy, striae, miliaria
Other	Ototoxicity, nephrotoxicity

Use in children

General guidelines not established

Use in pregnancy or nursing mothers

Safe use not established during pregnancy; use in large amounts, for prolonged periods, or over extensive areas is not recommended. General guidelines not established for use in nursing mothers.

[1]Possibly effective
[2]Includes reactions common to topical corticosteroids in general

SYNALAR (Fluocinolone acetonide) Syntex

Cream: 0.025% (15, 30, 60, 120, 425 g), 0.01% (15, 45, 60 g) **Ointment:** 0.025% (15, 30, 60, 425 g) **Sol:** 0.01% (20, 60 ml)

SYNALAR-HP (Fluocinolone acetonide) Syntex

Cream: 0.2% (12 g)

INDICATIONS	TOPICAL DOSAGE
Inflammatory manifestations of corticosteroid-responsive dermatoses	**Adult:** Apply a sparing amount, sufficient to cover affected area, tid to qid; preparation should be spread evenly over the surface and rubbed in gently until it disappears

ADMINISTRATION/DOSAGE ADJUSTMENTS

Hirsute sites	Hair should be parted to allow direct contact with lesion
Occlusive dressing technique	Apply preparation directly to affected area, leaving a visible thin coat on the surface qd or bid; cover completely with plastic film
Maximum dosage	Up to 2 g of the 0.2% cream may be applied daily; use of this preparation for prolonged periods is not recommended

CONTRAINDICATIONS

Hypersensitivity to fluocinolone or other components ●	Ophthalmic use ●

WARNINGS/PRECAUTIONS

Irritation	Discontinue use and institute appropriate therapy
Infection	Institute appropriate antifungal or antibacterial therapy; if infection persists, discontinue steroid therapy until a favorable response is achieved
Systemic absorption	Increases with extensive treatment or occlusive dressing technique; use with caution, especially in infants and children

ADVERSE REACTIONS[1]

Dermatological	Burning, itching, irritation, dryness, folliculitis, hypertrichosis, acneform eruptions, hypopigmentation, perioral dermatitis, allergic contact dermatitis, maceration, secondary infection, skin atrophy, striae, miliaria

Use in children

General guidelines not established; Synalar-HP is contraindicated in infants under 2 yr of age

Use in pregnancy or nursing mothers

Safe use not established during pregnancy; use in large amounts, for prolonged periods, or over extensive areas is not recommended. General guidelines not established for use in nursing mothers.

NOTE: Fluocinolone acetonide also marketed as **SYNEMOL** (Syntex).

[1]Includes reactions common to topical corticosteroids in general

TOPICORT (Desoximetasone) Hoechst-Roussel

Cream: 0.25% (5, 15, 60 g)

INDICATIONS	TOPICAL DOSAGE
Inflammatory manifestations of corticosteroid-responsive dermatoses	**Adult:** Massage a thin film of cream gently into affected area bid

CONTRAINDICATIONS

Hypersensitivity to desoximetasone or other components ●

Ophthalmic use ●

WARNINGS/PRECAUTIONS

Irritation	Discontinue use and institute appropriate therapy
Infection	Institute appropriate antifungal or antibacterial therapy; if infection persists, discontinue steroid therapy until a favorable response is achieved
Systemic absorption	Increases with extensive treatment or occlusive dressing technique; use with caution, especially in infants and children

ADVERSE REACTIONS[1]

Dermatological	Burning, itching, irritation, dryness, folliculitis, hypertrichosis, acneform eruptions, hypopigmentation, perioral dermatitis, allergic contact dermatitis, maceration, secondary infection, skin atrophy, striae, miliaria

Use in children

General guidelines not established

Use in pregnancy or nursing mothers

Safe use not established during pregnancy; use in large amounts, for prolonged periods, or over extensive areas is not recommended. General guidelines not established for use in nursing mothers.

TRIDESILON (Desonide) Dome

Cream: 0.05% (5, 15, 60, 2,270 g) **Ointment:** 0.05% (15, 60 g)

INDICATIONS	TOPICAL DOSAGE
Inflammatory manifestations of corticosteroid-responsive dermatoses	**Adult:** Apply a thin film to affected areas bid or tid and massage lightly

CONTRAINDICATIONS

Hypersensitivity to desonide or other components ●

Ophthalmic use ●

WARNINGS/PRECAUTIONS

Irritation	Discontinue use and institute appropriate therapy
Infection	Institute appropriate antifungal or antibacterial therapy; if infection persists, discontinue steroid therapy until a favorable response is achieved
Systemic absorption	May increase with extensive treatment or occlusive dressing technique; use with caution, especially in infants and children

ADVERSE REACTIONS[1]

Dermatological	Burning, itching, irritation, dryness, folliculitis, hypertrichosis, acneform eruptions, hypopigmentation, perioral dermatitis, allergic contact dermatitis, maceration, secondary infection, skin atrophy, striae, miliaria

Use in children

General guidelines not established

Use in pregnancy or nursing mothers

Safe use not established during pregnancy; use in large amounts, for prolonged periods, or over extensive areas is not recommended. General guidelines not established for use in nursing mothers.

[1]Includes reactions common to topical corticosteroids in general

VIOFORM-HYDROCORTISONE (iodochlorhydroxyquin and hydrocortisone) Ciba

Cream: 3% iodochlorhydroxyquin and 1% hydrocortisone (5, 20 g); 3% iodochlorhydroxyquin and 0.5% hydrocortisone (14.2, 28.4 g)
Ointment: 3% iodochlorhydroxyquin and 1% hydrocortisone (20 g); 3% iodochlorhydroxyquin and 0.5% hydrocortisone (28.4 g)
Lotion: 3% iodochlorhydroxyquin and 1% hydrocortisone (15 ml)

INDICATIONS

Acute and chronic dermatoses, including contact or atopic dermatitis, impetiginized eczema, nummular eczema, infantile eczema, endogenous chronic infectious dermatitis, stasis dermatitis, pyoderma, nuchal eczema and chronic eczematoid otitis externa, acne urticata, localized or disseminated neurodermatitis, lichen simplex chronicus, anogenital pruritus (vulvae, scroti, ani), folliculitis, bacterial dermatoses, mycotic dermatoses such as tinea (capitis, cruris, corporis, pedis), moniliasis, and intertrigo[1]

TOPICAL DOSAGE

Adult: apply a thin film of cream, ointment, or lotion to affected areas tid or qid

ADMINISTRATION/DOSAGE ADJUSTMENTS

Selection of appropriate formulation — For moist, weeping lesions, use the cream; for application behind the ears and in intertriginous areas of the body, use the lotion; for dry lesions accompanied by thickening and scaling of the skin, use the ointment; for lesions involving extensive body areas or less severe dermatoses, use the mild cream or mild ointment

CONTRAINDICATIONS

Ophthalmic use ●

Most viral skin lesions, including herpes simplex, vaccinia, and varicella ●

Tuberculosis of the skin ●

Hypersensitivity to any of the components or related compounds ●

WARNINGS/PRECAUTIONS

Irritation	May occur; discontinue medication
Staining of skin	May occur
Superinfection	May result in overgrowth of nonsusceptible organisms, requiring appropriate anti-infective therapy
Systemic infections	Use appropriate systemic antibiotics
Systemic absorption	Increases with extensive treatment, prolonged therapy, or occlusive dressing technique; use with caution, especially in infants and children
Thyroid-function tests	Wait at least 1 mo between discontinuation of therapy and performance of such tests

ADVERSE REACTIONS[2]

Dermatological — Rash, hypersensitivity, burning, itching, irritation, dryness, folliculitis, hypertrichosis, acneform eruptions, hypopigmentation, perioral dermatitis, allergic contact dermatitis, maceration, secondary infection, skin atrophy, striae, miliaria

ALTERED LABORATORY VALUES

Urinary values — ⇧ Phenylketones (with ferric chloride test)

No clinically significant alterations in blood/serum values occur at therapeutic dosages

Use in children

General guidelines not established

Use in pregnancy or nursing mothers

Safe use not established during pregnancy; use in large amounts, for prolonged periods, or over extensive areas is not recommended. General guidelines not established for use in nursing mothers.

[1]Possibly effective
[2]Includes reactions common to topical corticosteroids in general

Product (Manufacturer)	Ingredients	Actions
Americaine (Arnar-Stone) **Dosage** Spray liberally on affected area	10% Benzocaine	Local anesthetic
	0.1% Benzethonium chloride	Antiseptic
	Alcohol	Antiseptic and astringent
Caladryl (Parke-Davis) Cream **Dosage** Apply to affected areas 3–4 times daily	1% Diphenhydramine hydrochloride	Antihistamine
	0.1% Camphor	Anesthetic, antipruritic, and antiseptic
	Calamine	Astringent
Caladryl (Parke-Davis) Lotion **Dosage** Apply to affected areas 3–4 times daily	1% Diphenhydramine hydrochloride	Antihistamine
	0.1% Camphor	Anesthetic, antipruritic, and antiseptic
	Calamine	Astringent, antiseptic, and skin protectant
	2% Alcohol	Antiseptic and astringent
Calamatum (Blair) **Dosage** Spread thin film over affected area 3–4 times daily. Wash off once daily with warm water.	3% Benzocaine	Local anesthetic
	Camphor	Anesthetic, antipruritic, and antiseptic
	Phenol	Anesthetic, antipruritic, and antiseptic
	Zinc oxide	Astringent, antiseptic, and skin protectant
Calamox (Mallard) **Dosage** Apply to affected area 3 or 4 times daily	0.5% Camphor	Anesthetic, antipruritic, and antiseptic
	0.5% Phenol	Anesthetic, antipruritic, and antiseptic
Cortaid (Upjohn) Cream **Dosage** Apply to affected areas no more than 3–4 times daily. Do not use for children under 2 except under supervision of physician.	0.5% Hydrocortisone acetate	Anti-inflammatory agent
	Water-washable base	
Dalicote (Dalin) Lotion **Dosage** Apply to affected areas as needed	0.25% Diperodon hydrochloride	Mild anesthetic agent
	Pyrilamine maleate	Antihistamine and antirash agent
	Camphor	Anesthetic, antipruritic, and antiseptic
	Zinc oxide	Astringent
	Dimethyl polysiloxane	Skin protectant
	Silicone	Skin protectant
	Greaseless base	

Table continued on following page

NONPRESCRIPTION ALLERGIC CONTACT DERMATITIS (POISON IVY) MEDICATIONS

Product (Manufacturer)	Ingredients	Actions
Didelamine (Commerce) **Dosage** Apply to affected area 3 to 4 times daily or as directed by physician	Tripelennamine hydrochloride	Antihistamine
	Methapyrilene hydrochloride	Antihistamine
	Menthol	Antipruritic, anesthetic, and antiseptic
	Benzalkonium chloride	Antiseptic
Hist-A-Balm Medicated Lotion (Columbia Medical) **Dosage** Apply to affected area 3 to 4 times daily or as directed by physician	0.25% Diperodon hydrochloride	Anesthetic
	0.75% Phenyltoloxamine dihydrogen citrate	Antihistamine
	Menthol	Antipruritic, anesthetic, and antiseptic
	0.1% Benzalkonium chloride	Antiseptic
Hista-Calma Lotion (Rexall) **Dosage** Apply to affected area 3 to 4 times daily	1% Benzocaine	Anesthetic
	1% Phenyltoloxamine dihydrogen citrate	Antihistamine
	Calamine	Astringent, antiseptic, and skin protectant
Ivarest (Carbisulphoil-Blistex) **Dosage** Apply to affected area immediately after exposure. Repeat 3 to 4 times daily.	1% Benzocaine	Local anesthetic
	1.5% Pyrilamine maleate	Antihistamine
	0.7% Menthol	Antipruritic, anesthetic, and antiseptic
	0.3% Camphor	Anesthetic, antipruritic, and antiseptic
	10% Calamine	Astringent, antiseptic, and skin protectant
	4% Zirconium oxide	Astringent
Ivy Dry Cream (Ivy) **Dosage** Apply to affected area as needed to relieve itching or as directed by physician	Benzocaine	Local anesthetic
	Menthol	Antipruritic, anesthetic, and antiseptic
	Camphor	Anesthetic, antipruritic, and antiseptic
	8% Tannic acid	Astringent
	Methylparaben	Antifungal agent (preservative)
	Propylparaben	Antifungal agent (preservative)
	7.5% Isopropyl alcohol	Antiseptic
Ivy Dry Liquid (Ivy) **Dosage** Bathe skin, rinse dry, and apply to affected area. Repeat applications as needed.	Tannic acid	Anesthetic
	12.5% Isopropyl alcohol	Antiseptic

Table continued on following page

NONPRESCRIPTION ALLERGIC CONTACT DERMATITIS (POISON IVY) MEDICATIONS

Product (Manufacturer)	Ingredients	Actions
Ivy Surpa Dry (Ivy) **Dosage** Apply to affected area as needed to relieve itching or as directed by physician	Benzocaine	Anesthetic
	Menthol	Antipruritic, anesthetic, and antiseptic
	Camphor	Anesthetic, antipruritic, and antiseptic
	Tannic acid	Astringent
	35% Isopropyl alcohol	Antiseptic
	Methylparaben	Antifungal agent (preservative)
	Propylparaben	Antifungal agent (preservative)
Nupercainal Cream (Ciba) **Dosage** Apply liberally to affected area and rub in gently	0.5% Dibucaine	Anesthetic
	0.37% Acetone sodium bisulfite	Antioxidant
Nupercainal Ointment (Ciba) **Dosage** Apply to affected area gently. If needed, cover with a light dressing for protection.	1% Dibucaine	Anesthetic
	0.5% Acetone sodium bisulfite	Antioxidant
Poison Ivy Cream (McKesson) **Dosage** Apply to affected area as needed to relieve itching or as directed by physician	2.5% Benzocaine	Local anesthetic
	Pyrilamine maleate	Antihistamine
	Povidone	Antiseptic
	4% Zirconium oxide (as carbonated hydrous zirconia)	Astringent
Poison Ivy Spray (McKesson) **Dosage** Apply to affected area as needed to relieve itching or as directed by physician	0.5% Benzocaine	Local anesthetic
	Menthol	Antipruritic, anesthetic, and antiseptic
	Camphor	Anesthetic, antipruritic, and antiseptic
	2% Calamine	Astringent, antiseptic, and skin protectant
	1% Zinc oxide	Astringent, antiseptic, and skin protectant
	9.44% Isopropyl alcohol	Antiseptic
Pontocaine (Breon) **Dosage** Apply liberally, with gentle rubbing, to affected area; or, if preferred, spread lightly on gauze or cotton before topical application	Tetracaine hydrochloride (ointment, 0.5%; cream, 1%)	Anesthetic
	0.5% Menthol (ointment)	Antipruritic, anesthetic, and antiseptic
	Methylparaben (cream)	Antifungal agent (preservative)
	Sodium bisulfite (cream)	Antioxidant
	White petrolatum (ointment)	Emollient and lubricant
	White wax (ointment)	Ointment base hardener

Table continued on following page

NONPRESCRIPTION ALLERGIC CONTACT DERMATITIS (POISON IVY) MEDICATIONS

Product (Manufacturer)	Ingredients	Actions
Pyrabenzamine (Ciba) Cream **Dosage** Apply to affected areas as needed	2% Tripeiennamine	Antihistamine and antirash agent
	Water-washable base	
Pyribenzamine (Ciba) Ointment **Dosage** Apply to affected areas as needed	2% Tripelennamine	Antihistamine and antirash agent
	Petrolatum	Base
Rhuli Cream (Lederle) **Dosage** Apply to affected area 2 to 3 times daily and at bedtime, or as needed	1% Benzocaine	Anesthetic
	0.7% Menthol	Antipruritic, anesthetic, and antiseptic
	0.3% Camphor	Anesthetic, antipruritic, and antiseptic
	1% Zirconium oxide	Astringent
	8.8% Isopropyl alcohol	Antiseptic
Rhuligel (Lederle) **Dosage** Apply to affected area 2 to 3 times daily or as directed by physician	0.3% Menthol	Antipruritic, anesthetic, and antiseptic
	0.3% Camphor	Anesthetic, antipruritic, and antiseptic
	2% Benzyl alcohol	Antiseptic and antipruritic
	31% Alcohol	Antiseptic
Rhulihist (Lederle) **Dosage** Smooth on affected area by hand or with cotton 2 to 3 times daily and at bedtime, or as needed	1.153% Benzocaine	Anesthetic
	0.253% Camphor	Anesthetic, antipruritic, and antiseptic
	0.025% Menthol	Antipruritic, anesthetic, and antiseptic
	0.674% Benzyl alcohol	Antiseptic and antipruritic
	4.710% Calamine	Astringent, antiseptic, and skin protectant
	28.76% Alcohol	Antiseptic
Rhuli Spray (Lederle) **Dosage** Apply to affected area 3 to 4 times daily and at bedtime, or as needed	0.98% Benzocaine	Local anesthetic
	0.098% Camphor	Anesthetic, antipruritic, and antiseptic
	0.009% Menthol	Antipruritic, anesthetic, and antiseptic
	1% Zirconium oxide	Astringent
	0.98% Calamine	Astringent, antiseptic, and skin protectant
	9.5% Isopropyl alcohol	Antiseptic
Surfadil (Lilly) **Dosage** Apply 3 to 4 times daily or as directed by physician	0.5% Cyclomethycaine	Anesthetic
	2% Methapyrilene hydrochloride	Antihistamine
	5% Titanium dioxide (lotion)	Skin protectant
Tronothane Hydrochloride (Abbott) **Dosage** Apply locally 3 to 4 times daily or as directed by physician	1% Pramoxine hydrochloride	Anesthetic

Table continued on following page

NONPRESCRIPTION ALLERGIC CONTACT DERMATITIS (POISON IVY) MEDICATIONS

Product (Manufacturer)	Ingredients	Actions
Ziradryl (Parke-Davis) **Dosage** Cleanse affected area and apply generously 3 to 4 times daily	2% Diphenhydramine hydrochloride	Antihistamine
	0.1% Camphor	Anesthetic, antipruritic, and antiseptic
	2% Zinc oxide	Astringent, antiseptic, and skin protectant
	2% Alcohol	Antiseptic

NONPRESCRIPTION TAR-BASED ECZEMA MEDICATIONS

Product (Manufacturer)	Ingredients	Actions
Alma Tar (Schieffelin) Shampoo **Dosage** Add to bath water and soak affected areas	35% Juniper tar	Emollient that softens scaly skin and reduces itching and peeling
Alma Tar (Schieffelin) Liquid **Dosage** Lather into scalp, rinse, and repeat. Use as needed.	4% Juniper tar	Emollient that softens scaly skin and reduces itching and peeling
	Polyoxyethylene ether	Surfactant
	Edetate sodium	Binding agent
	Sulfonated castor oil	Emollient
	Coconut oil	Emollient
	Triethanolamine	Buffer
Alphosyl (Reed & Carnrick) Lotion **Dosage** Apply to affected areas as needed	2% Allantoin	Moisturizing agent and skin softener
	5% Coal tar extract	Emollient that softens scaly skin and reduces itching and peeling
	Hydrophilic base	
Alphosyl (Reed & Carnrick) Cream **Dosage** Apply to affected areas as needed	2% Allantoin	Moisturizing agent and skin softener
	5% Coal tar extract	Emollient that softens scaly skin and reduces itching and peeling
	Hydrophilic base	
Balnetar (Westwood) Liquid **Dosage** Add to bath water and soak	Equivalent to 5% coal tar	Emollient that softens scaly skin and reduces itching and peeling
	Mineral oil	Emollient
	Lanolin oil	Emollient
Denorex (Whitehall) Shampoo **Dosage** Lather into scalp, rinse, and repeat. Use every other day for first 10 days and 2–3 times/week thereafter.	Coal tar solution	Emollient that softens scaly skin and reduces itching and peeling
	Menthol	Prevents skin irritation
	7.5% Alcohol	Astringent

Table continued on following page

Product (Manufacturer)	Ingredients	Actions
Estar (Westwood) Gel **Dosage** Apply gel to affected areas and then wipe off excess after 5 min. Use each AM. and PM.	Equivalent to 5% coal tar	Emollient that softens scaly skin and reduces itching and peeling
	Hydroalcoholic gel	Suspending agent
Ionil T (Owen) Liquid **Dosage** Lather into scalp, rinse, and repeat. Use as needed.	2% Salicylic acid	Moisturizing agent and skin softener
	Equivalent to 5% coal tar	Emollient that softens scaly skin and reduces itching and peeling
	Polyoxyethylene ethers	Liquid base
	0.2% Benzalkonium chloride	Antiseptic
	12% Alcohol	Astringent
Mazon Cream (Norcliff Thayer) Cream **Dosage** Apply to affected areas as needed	1% Salicylic acid	Moisturizing agent and skin softener
	1% Resorcinol	Moisturizing agent and skin softener
	0.18% Coal tar	Emollient that softens scaly skin and reduces itching and peeling
	0.5% Benzoic acid	Antifungal agent
Mazon Shampoo (Norcliff Thayer) Liquid **Dosage** Lather into scalp, rinse, and repeat. Use as needed.	1% Sulfur	Moisturizing agent and skin softener
	0.5% Salicylic acid	Moisturizing agent and skin softener
	0.5% Coal tar	Emollient that softens scaly skin and reduces itching and peeling
Packer's Pine Tar Shampoo (Cooper) Liquid **Dosage** Lather into scalp, rinse, and repeat. Use as needed.	0.82% Pine tar	Emollient that softens scaly skin and reduces itching and peeling
	2.175% Isopropyl alcohol	Astringent
Packer's Pine Tar (Cooper) Bar **Dosage** Lather into affected areas and rinse. Use as needed.	6% Pine tar	Emollient that softens scaly skin and reduces itching and peeling
	93% Soap chips	Vehicle and cleansing agent
Pragmatar (Smith Kline & French) Cream **Dosage** Apply small amounts to affected areas. Use no more than once a day.	3% Salicylic acid	Moisturizing agent and skin softener
	3% Colloidal sulfur	Moisturizing agent and skin softener
	4% Cetyl alcohol–Coal tar	Emollient that softens scaly skin and reduces itching and peeling
	Emulsion base	

Table continued on following page

NONPRESCRIPTION TAR-BASED ECZEMA MEDICATIONS

Product (Manufacturer)	Ingredients	Actions
Tegrin (Block) Cream, Lotion **Dosage** Apply to affected areas 2-4 times/day	0.02% Allantoin	Moisturizing agent and skin softener
	5% Coal tar extract	Emollient that softens scaly skin and reduces itching and peeling
Tegrin (Block) Shampoo **Dosage** Lather into scalp, rinse, and repeat 2-4 times/week	0.02% Allantoin	Moisturizing agent and skin softener
	5% Coal tar extract	Emollient that softens scaly skin and reduces itching and peeling
Vaseline Pure Petroleum Jelly (Chesebrough-Pond's) Gel **Dosage** Apply to affected areas as needed	100% Petrolatum	Emollient

NONPRESCRIPTION DANDRUFF SHAMPOOS

Product (Manufacturer)	Ingredients	Actions
Anti-Dandruff Brylcreem (Beecham) Cream **Dosage** Apply shampoo, lather, rinse, and repeat. Use as needed.	0.1% Zinc pyrithione	Relieves scalp flaking, itching, and scaling
	Mineral oil	Emollient
	Propylene glycol	Solvent
	Paraffin wax	Lotion base
	Water	
	Excipients	Cosmetic and suspending agents
Breck One (Breck) Cream **Dosage** Massage small amount into affected areas no more than 3-4 times daily	1% Zinc pyrithione	Relieves scalp flaking, itching, and scaling
	15.6% Anionic surfactants	Cleansing agents and cream base
Breck One (Breck) Lotion **Dosage** Massage small amount into affected areas no more than 3-4 times daily	1% Zinc pyrithione	Relieves scalp flaking, itching, and scaling
	15.6% Anionic surfactants	Cleansing agents and lotion base
Breck One (Breck) Shampoo **Dosage** Apply shampoo, lather, rinse, and repeat. Use as needed.	1% Zinc pyrithione	Relieves scalp flaking, itching, and scaling
	15.6% Anionic surfactants	Cleansing agents and shampoo base
Cuticura Anti-Dandruff Shampoo (Purex) Shampoo **Dosage** Apply shampoo, lather, rinse, and repeat. Use as needed.	2% Sulfur	Relieves scalp flaking, itching, and scaling
	2% Salicylic acid	Relieves scalp flaking, itching, and scaling
	Protein	Conditioner
	Surfactants	Cleansing agents and lotion base

Table continued on following page

Product (Manufacturer)	Ingredients	Actions
Head & Shoulders Cream (Procter & Gamble) Shampoo **Dosage** Apply shampoo, lather, rinse, and repeat. Use as needed.	2% Zinc pyrithione	Relieves scalp flaking, itching, and scaling
	Anionic detergent	Cleansing agents
Head & Shoulders Lotion (Procter & Gamble) Shampoo **Dosage** Apply shampoo, lather, rinse, and repeat. Use as needed.	2% Zinc pyrithione	Relieves scalp flaking, itching, and scaling
	Lauryl sulfate	Wetting agent
	Cocamide	Sudsing agent
	Ethanolamine	Buffer
	Triethanolamine	Buffer
	Magnesium aluminum silicate	Absorbing agent
	Hydroxypropyl methylcellulose	Thickening agent
Klaron (Dermik) Lotion **Dosage** Massage small amount into affected areas no more than 3–4 times daily	5% Colloidal sulfur	Relieves scalp flaking, itching, and scaling
	2% Salicylic acid	Relieves scalp flaking, itching, and scaling
	13.1% Alcohol	Solvent and astringent
	Greaseless, hydroalcoholic vehicle	
Meted (Texas Pharmacal) Shampoo **Dosage** Apply shampoo, lather, rinse, and repeat. Use as needed.	3% Sulfur	Relieves scalp flaking, itching, and scaling
	2% Salicylic acid	Relieves scalp flaking, itching, and scaling
	Highly concentrated detergents	
Pernox (Westwood) Shampoo **Dosage** Apply shampoo, lather, rinse, and repeat. Use as needed.	Sodium laureth sulfate	Detergent
	Lauramide DEA	Thickening agent and foam stabilizer
	Quarternium 22	Conditioner
	Lanate 25	Conditioner
	Sodium chloride	Relieves itching and scaling
	Lactic acid	Acidifying agent
pHisoDan (Winthrop) Shampoo **Dosage** Apply shampoo, lather, rinse, and repeat. Use as needed.	5% Precipitated sulfur	Relieves scalp flaking, itching, and scaling
	0.5% Sodium salicylate	Relieves scalp flaking, itching, and scaling
	Entsufon sodium	Cleansing agent
	Lanolin	Shampoo base
	Cholesterols	Emulsifying agent
	Petrolatum	Shampoo base

Table continued on following page

Product (Manufacturer)	Ingredients	Actions
Rezamid Tinted (Dermik) Shampoo **Dosage** Apply shampoo, lather, rinse, and repeat. Use as needed.	2% Microsize sulfur	Relieves scalp flaking, itching, and scaling
	2% Salicylic acid	Relieves scalp flaking, itching, and scaling
Rezamid Tinted (Dermik) Lotion **Dosage** Massage small amount into affected areas no more than 3–4 times daily	5% Microsize sulfur	Relieves scalp flaking, itching, and scaling
	2% Resorcinol	Relieves scalp flaking, itching, and scaling
	0.5% Parachlorometaxylenol	Antiseptic agent
	28.5% Alcohol	Solvent and astringent
Rinse Away (Alberto Culver) Lotion **Dosage** Massage small amount into affected areas no more than 3–4 times daily	0.05% Benzalkonium chloride	Antiseptic agent
	0.05% Laurylisoquinolium bromide	Antiseptic agent
Sebucare (Westwood) Lotion **Dosage** Massage small amount into affected areas no more than 3–4 times daily	1.8% Salicylic acid	Relieves scalp flaking, itching, and scaling
	Laureth-4	Emulsifier and surfactant
	Alcohol	Solvent and astringent
	Water	Solvent
	Butyl ether	Emollient
	Dihydroabietyl alcohol	Conditioner
Sebulex (Westwood) Shampoo **Dosage** Apply shampoo, lather, rinse, and repeat. Use as needed.	2% Sulfur	Relieves scalp flaking, itching, and scaling
	2% Salicylic acid	Relieves scalp flaking, itching, and scaling
	Surfactants	
Sebutone (Westwood) Shampoo **Dosage** Apply shampoo, lather, rinse, and repeat. Use as needed.	2% Sulfur	Relieves scalp flaking, itching, and scaling
	2% Salicylic acid	Relieves scalp flaking, itching, and scaling
	0.5% Tar	Relieves scalp flaking, itching, and scaling
	Surfactants	
	Cleansing agents	
	Wetting agents	
Sulfur-8 Hair and Scalp Conditioner (Plough) Ointment **Dosage** Massage small amount into affected areas no more than 3–4 times daily	2% Sulfur	Relieves scalp flaking, itching, and scaling
	Menthol	Prevents skin irritation
	Triclosan	Antiseptic agent

Table continued on following page

Product (Manufacturer)	Ingredients	Actions
Acid Mantle (Dorsey) Cream **Dosage** Apply to affected areas as needed	Glycerin	Moisturizing agent and skin softener
	Aluminum acetate	Astringent and antiseptic
	Water	Solvent
	Cetearyl alcohol	Solvent
	Sodium lauryl sulfate	Wetting agent
	Petrolatum	Emollient
	Synthetic beeswax	Hardening agent
	Mineral oil	Emollient
	Methylparaben	Preservative
Alpha Keri (Westwood) Liquid **Dosage** Add to bathtub of water and soak affected areas for 10–20 minutes	Mineral oil	Emollient
	Lanolin oil	Emollient and liquid base
	Polyethylene glycol-4-dilaurate	Liquid base
	Benzophenone-3	Perfume fixative
	Fragrance	
Extra Strength Vaseline Intensive Care (Chesebrough-Pond's) Lotion **Dosage** Apply to affected areas as needed	Glycerin	Moisturizing agent and skin softener
	White petrolatum	Lotion base
	Zinc oxide	Skin protectant
Jergens Direct Aid (Jergens) Lotion **Dosage** Apply to affected areas as needed	Allantoin	Moisturizing agent and skin softener
	Deionized water	Lotion base
	Sorbitol	Moisturizer
	Stearic acid	Lotion base
	Glyceryl dilaurate	Lotion base
	Glyceryl stearate	Lotion base
	Lard glyceride	Lotion base
	Stearamide	Skin protectant
	Hydrogenated vegetable oil	Emollient
	Isopropyl palmitate	Thickening agent
	Polyethylene glycol	Lotion base
	100 stearate	Lotion base
	Dimethicone	Skin protectant
	Petrolatum	Emollient
	Sodium carbomer 941	Buffer
	Fragrance	

Table continued on following page

Product (Manufacturer)	Ingredients	Actions
Jergens Direct Aid (cont)	Propylparaben	Antifungal agent and preservative
	Methylparaben	Preservative
	Simethicone	Skin protectant
	Cetearyl alcohol	Solvent
Jergens Hand Cream (Jergens) Cream **Dosage** Apply to affected areas as needed	Allantoin	Moisturizing agent and skin softener
	Salicylic acid	Moisturizing agent and skin softener
	Glycerin	Moisturizing agent and skin softener
	Deionized water	Cream base
	Stearic acid	Cream base
	Alcohol	Antiseptic
	Potassium stearate	Thickening agent and cream base
	Propylene glycol dipelargonate	Cream base
	Fragrance	
	Lanolin oil	Emollient and cream base
	Potassium carbomer 941	Buffer
	Methylparaben	Preservative
	Polysorbate 81	Cream base
	Simethicone	Skin protectant
	Cellulose gum	Thickening agent
	Propylparaben	Antifungal agent and preservative
	Other unspecified ingredients	
Keri Cream (Westwood) Cream **Dosage** Apply to affected areas as needed	Water	Cream base
	Mineral oil	Emollient
	Talc	Skin protectant
	Sorbitol	Moisturizer
	Lanolin alcohol	Emollient and antiseptic
	Magnesium stearate	Cream base
	Glycerol oleate	Emollient
	Methylparaben	Preservative
	Propylparaben	Antifungal agent and preservative
	Fragrance	

Table continued on following page

Product (Manufacturer)	Ingredients	Actions
Lowila Cake (Westwood) Bar **Dosage** Lather into affected areas as needed	Urea	Moisturizing agent and skin softener
	Lactic acid	Moisturizing agent and skin softener
	Dextrin	Thickening agent
	Sodium lauryl sulfoacetate	Cleansing agent
	Boric acid	Antiseptic
	Sorbitol	Moisturizer
	Mineral oil	Emollient
	Polyethylene glycol 14-M	Bar base
	Cellulose gum	Thickening agent
	Dioctyl sodium sulfosuccinate	Wetting agent
Lubriderm (Texas Pharmacal) Cream **Dosage** Apply to affected areas as needed	Glycerin	Moisturizing agent and skin softener
	Lanolin derivatives	Emollients and cream base
	Cetyl alcohol	Emulsifying agent
	Petrolatum blend	Emollient
Sardo (Plough) Liquid **Dosage** Add to bathtub of water and soak affected areas	Mineral oil	Emollient
	Isopropyl myristate	Controls thickness of liquid
	Isopropyl palmitate	Thickening agent
Wibi (Owen) Lotion **Dosage** Apply to affected areas as needed	Emulsifying wax	Emulsifying and thickening agent
	Polyglycols	Lotion bases
	Alcohol	Astringent
	Menthol	Prevents skin irritation
	Glycerol	Emollient
Woodbury for Extra Dry Skin (Jergens) Lotion **Dosage** Apply to affected areas as needed	Allantoin	Moisturizing agent and skin softener
	Glycerin	Moisturizing agent and skin softener
	Deionized water	Lotion base
	Alcohol	Astringent
	Mineral oil	Emollient
	Triethanolamine stearate	Buffer
	Stearyl alcohol	Emulsifying agent
	Lanolin	Emollient and lotion base
	Hydrogenated vegetable oil	Emollient

Table continued on following page

NONPRESCRIPTION DRY SKIN PREPARATIONS

Product (Manufacturer)	Ingredients	Actions
Woodbury for Extra Dry Skin (cont)	Cetyl alcohol	Emulsifying agent
	Sodium carbomer 941	Buffer
	Methylparaben	Preservative
	Propylparaben	Antifungal agent and preservative
	Fragrance	

NONPRESCRIPTION BEE STINGS AND INSECT BITE MEDICATIONS

Product (Manufacturer)	Ingredients	Actions
Dermoplast (Ayerst) Spray **Dosage** Spray affected area 2–3 times daily or as directed by physician	Polyethylene glycol 400 monolaurate	Solvent and dispersing agent
	20% Benzocaine	Anesthetic
	2% Methylparaben	Antifungal agent (preservative)
	0.5% Menthol	Antipruritic, anesthetic, and antiseptic
	Polysorbate 80	Emulsifying, dispersing, and solubilizing agent
Dermtex Anti-Itch Lotion (Pfeiffer) Lotion **Dosage** Use as needed for relief	3% Benzocaine	Anesthetic
	1:750 Benzalkonium chloride	Antiseptic
	90% Alcohol	Antiseptic
Nupercainal Cream (Ciba) **Dosage** Apply liberally to affected area and rub in gently	0.5% Dibucaine	Anesthetic
	0.37% Acetone sodium bisulfate	Antioxidant
	Water-washable base	
Pyribenzamine (Ciba) Cream, Ointment **Dosage** Apply gently to affected area 3–4 times daily or as directed by physician	2% Tripelennamine	Antihistamine
	Water-washable base (cream)	
	Petrolatum base (ointment)	
Surfadil (Lilly) Lotion **Dosage** Apply 3–4 times daily or as directed by physician	2% Methapyrilene hydrochloride	Antihistamine
	0.5% Cyclomethycaine	Anesthetic
	5% Titanium dioxide (lotion)	Skin protectant
Tucks and Tucks Alongs (Parke-Davis) Pads **Dosage** Apply to affected areas for 15–30 min, as needed	50% Witch hazel	Astringent
	10% Glycerin	Emollient and vehicle
	0.1% Methylparaben	Antifungal agent (preservative)
	0.003% Benzalkonium chloride	Antiseptic

Infant Skin Problems

Despite what poets have written, a baby's skin is not necessarily synonymous with softness. An infant can suffer from a variety of skin diseases and conditions, ranging from cradle cap on the head to diaper rash on the buttocks. Some of these syndromes are innocent or temporary; others are physiological and episodic. However, aside from the skin conditions resulting from viral or genetic causes, scaly, irritated, and inflamed skin on a baby is usually amenable to time, topical treatment, or both. In severe cases, a skin problem may indicate an underlying disorder.

Neonatal skin is distinct from that of older children and adults. The skin cells of infants are more uniform in size than those of children and adults. Production of melanin (dark pigment) is low in the newborn, and thus the coloring of an infant is lighter than that of an older child. Sensitivity to sunlight is therefore more intense. In addition, the epidermis in the newborn is less adherent to the dermis, and there is a greater tendency for babies to blister, both from exposure to the sun and from rubbing or friction. Lubrication of the baby's skin with oil or lotion decreases friction, and may help prevent blistering.

TYPES OF INFANT SKIN DISORDERS

Seborrheic dermatitis—recurring skin inflammation characterized by scaling, crusting, and itching—or atopic dermatitis—eczema and other inflammatory skin disorders characterized by intense itching—are the most common skin disorders seen in early infancy.

Seborrheic dermatitis usually begins in the first few weeks of life as dry, scaly lesions that may or may not be greasy. These lesions, which occur most frequently on the scalp, face, and in body folds or creases, may be salmon or yellowish, with the color more evident on the periphery than in the center, which may be clear. There is no oozing or weeping, and itching (pruritus) may be present.

Atopic dermatitis is seldom seen in the first two months of life. Its lesions are often very red, particularly in the center. A family history of allergy is a strong predisposing factor. Edema (swelling due to retention of fluid) and oozing are common characteristics, as are vesicles (blisters) in the acute phases. Itching is severe and paroxysmal (recurrent).

This section will review the most common skin problems found in infancy and their treatment.

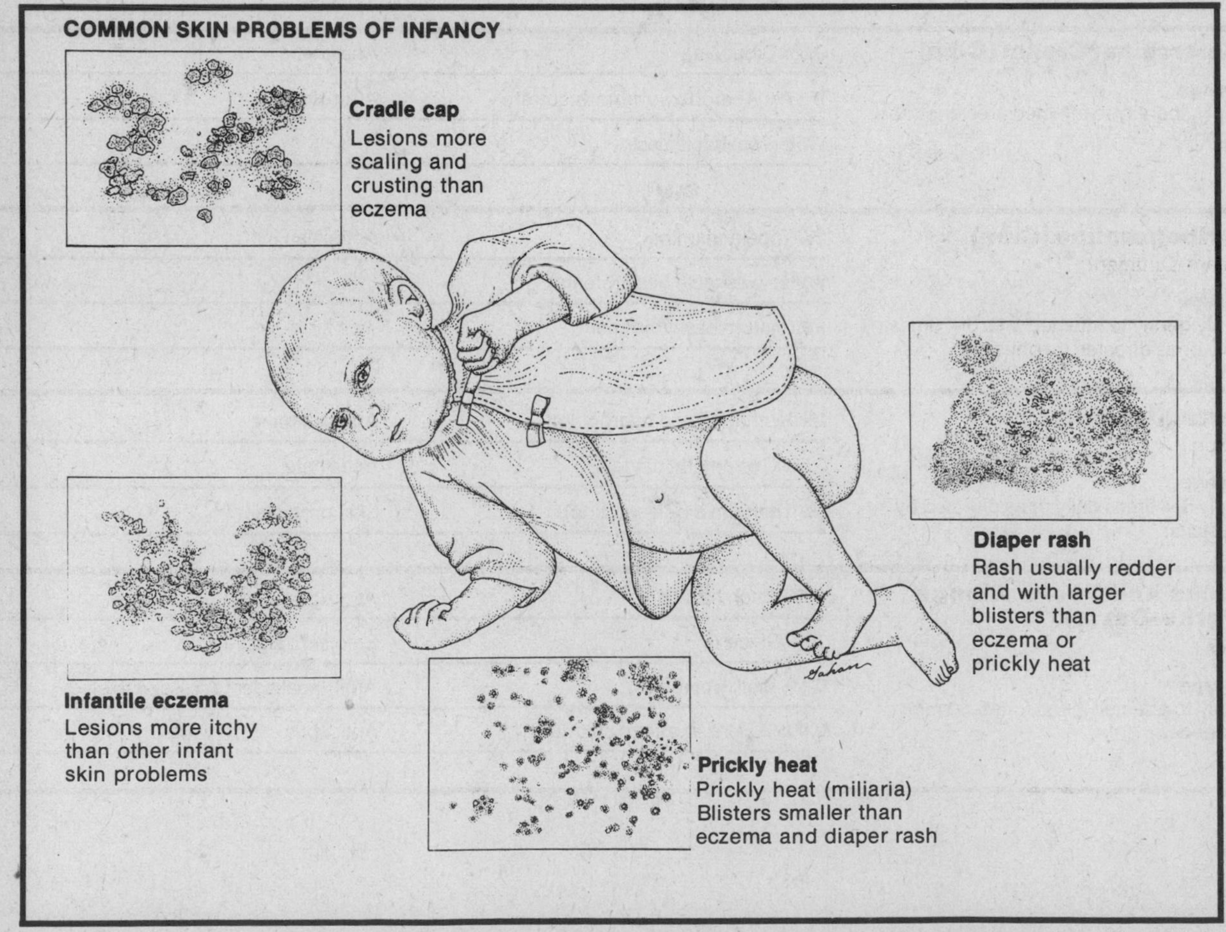

Diaper Rash

Almost all babies at one time or another suffer from diaper rash, which is an inflammation of the skin in the diaper area. Wetness and irritation from chafing, chemical irritants, sweat, and bacteria are among the common causes of diaper rash. Ammonia and other substances produced by urine are particularly irritating to a baby's skin. Since the normal infant urinates up to twenty times a day, it is hard to avoid exposure to the irritants found in urine. Keeping the baby dry and even free of diaper cover for short periods during the day helps to keep the rash and discomfort at a minimum. In babies who are particularly susceptible to diaper rash, cloth diapers may be preferable to the plastic-covered kind. In any case, frequent changing, careful cleansing and rinsing of the diaper area, and the use of drying powders and protective and soothing ointments will usually minimize the problem. A persistent diaper rash after six months of age may be a form of seborrheic or atopic dermatitis. The rash may intensify if it spreads, and, in severe cases, a steroid cream may be called for.

A more extreme rash on the buttocks can be caused by perianal irritation resulting from diarrhea. Frequent changing and extreme cleanliness are essential to control this, as is keeping the perianal area free of irritation. Control of the diarrhea and use of a soothing topical cream in the perianal area will usually suffice to control the problem.

If diaper rash is untreated or uncontrolled, an infection caused by bacteria or fungi may result. The warm, wet, alkaline environment of the diaper is especially conducive to the growth of certain fungi, particularly *Candida albicans,* a microorganism ordinarily found in the colon.

Bacterial infections caused by *Staphylococcus* or, less frequently, *Streptococcus* are other common complications of diaper rash, particularly if the skin is cut or broken.

Prickly Heat

Prickly heat is often confused with diaper rash, but it has several distinguishing characteristics. Prickly heat is caused by an obstruction of the sweat glands, which results in rupturing of the sweat ducts. It appears as clusters of tiny pink blisters or pimples surrounded by pink blotches. When the blisters dry up, the skin may take on a tan appearance. It occurs most often in the summer, but may also be seen during a high fever or when the baby is too warmly dressed. Keeping the baby cool with removal of clothing helps prevent prickly heat, especially during hot weather. Powders and lotions can help keep the baby cool and dry, and bathing the baby in a solution of a teaspoonful of bicarbonate of soda per cup of water also provides cooling relief from burning and/or itching.

Eczema

Eczema is the common term for atopic dermatitis. It can range from mild forms of red, rough skin to patches of extremely itchy, scaly, crusted skin. It most commonly appears in the folds of the body, such as in the crook of the elbow, behind the knee, or on the neck. Eczema can be particularly affected by changes in the climate and may appear in either very cold or very hot weather. Topical agents, such as astringents to reduce the oozing, cooling agents to relieve the itching, and certain ointments to protect and sooth the skin, are often sufficient. (See section on *Dermatitis and Psoriasis,* page 1079).

Cradle Cap

Cradle cap, a mild disorder that starts on the infant's head in the early weeks of life, is characterized by scaling or crusting. It responds well to washing with mild soap and water. Cradle cap causes little or no discomfort to the infant and with frequent washing, usually disappears within a few months.

Miscellaneous Skin Disorders

There are more serious skin diseases in the newborn and infant, but in most cases they are distinguished by more severe and persistent symptoms that require a physician's attention. These include bullous impetigo, a skin disease characterized by tiny blisters and caused by a staphylococcal microorganism. The diaper region is most frequently involved, with the blisters spreading to contiguous areas. Compresses of sterile water, normal saline solution, or 0.1 percent silver nitrate solution applied every four hours help dry the blisters. An antibiotic, given either topically or systemically, may also be prescribed.

A number of diseases, particularly infectious diseases associated with childhood (such as chicken pox, measles, and scarlet fever), manifest themselves as various types of skin rashes. Any persistent rash, or any rash accompanied by other symptoms, such as fever, vomiting, or sore throat, should be seen by a physician.

TREATMENT OF INFANT SKIN PROBLEMS

Most infant skin problems such as diaper rash and prickly heat can be treated with hygienic measures, such as frequent changing, cleanliness, and avoidance of irritants, overheating, or chafing. In addition, there are a variety of nonprescription baby powders, lotions, and ointments that can provide relief from symptoms and help prevent their recurrence. In general, these products are designed to keep the skin dry and prevent chafing (powders); provide a protective barrier (ointments and creams); and provide antiseptic protection against bacteria and fungi.

Ointments, Creams, and Lotions

Zinc oxide and petrolatum are the major protective ingredients in several infant ointments and creams. Zinc oxide, in addition to protecting the skin, has a mild antiseptic action. Petrolatum is easier to remove from skin and diapers than zinc oxide, and many products, such as Desitin Ointment, contain both. Lanolin, vitamins A and D, cod liver oil, and various other oils are among the ingredients in many ointments, creams, and lotions available to treat or prevent diaper rash and prickly heat. In selecting a particular product, one should note the various ingredients and match the action of these ingredients with the baby's needs.

Powders

Talc, corn starch, and zinc stearate are the major ingredients in baby powders. Their principal benefits are to keep the area dry and to help prevent chafing and rubbing. Some also have a mildly antiseptic effect.

Caution should be used in making sure the baby does not inhale the powder, since there have been reports of fatal chemical pneumonia suffered by infants who inhaled large amounts of baby powder.

Antiseptic Washes and Ointments

Ordinary mild soap is sufficient as a cleansing agent for most infant needs. Some antiseptic washes, such as hexachlorophene, that were once routinely used for babies are no longer recommended for the very young because of their possible toxic effects. Boric acid, another product commonly used in infants' products in the past because of its antibacterial and antifungal actions, is no longer recommended by the American Academy of Pediatrics Committee on Drugs because of possible toxicity.

However, a number of ointments, powders, lotions, and washes remain that do have mild antiseptic effects. Ingredients that have specific antiseptic actions include methylbenzethonium chloride, 8-hydroxyquinoline sulfate, bacitracin, polymyxin B sulfate, benzalkonium chloride, and calcium undecylenate.

IN CONCLUSION

In selecting a particular infant skin product, one should note the various ingredients and match their intended action with the problem to be treated. For example, an astringent agent may be useful in treating eczema or prickly heat, but may not be needed for controlling diaper rash. The following table lists the more common infant skin products, the major ingredients in these products, and their actions.

One should also remember that some babies' skins are more sensitive than those of others . Many will react to certain ingredients in a particular lotion or cream, but will be able to tolerate a different combination in some other product(s). A rash or irritation that appears related to a specific soap or skin preparation should be interpreted as a signal to switch products and to avoid the offending ingredients, at least until the baby is older and his or her skin is less sensitive.

The following charts cover the most commonly used nonprescription infant skin products, such as creams, lotions, powders, and washes. Other products that may be prescribed for more serious skin problems may be found in the sections on *Bacterial Infections* (page 339), *Fungal Infections* (page 444), and *Dermatitis and Psoriasis* (page 1079).

Product (Manufacturer)	Ingredients	Actions
A and D Ointment (Shering) Ointment **Dosage** Smooth small amount into affected areas as needed	Petrolatum	Emollient, ointment base and skin protective
	Anhydrous lanolin	Ointment base and skin protective
	Vitamins A and D	Promotes healing
Ammens Medicated Powder (Bristol-Myers) Powder **Dosage** Apply liberally to skin after bath or diaper change	45.06% Talc	Skin protective
	41% Starch	Skin protective
	9.1% Zinc oxide	Skin protective
	4.55% Boric acid	Antimicrobial agent
	.1% 8-Hydroxyquinoline	Antimicrobial agent
	.05% 8-Hydroxyquinoline sulfate	Antimicrobial agent
	.14% Aromatic oils	Fragrance
Aveeno Bar (Cooper) Cleanser **Dosage** Lather and massage gently into affected areas as needed	50% Colloidal oatmeal	Skin protective
	Mild sudsing agent	Cleanser
	Lanolin	Emollient and skin protective
Aveeno Colloidal Oatmeal (Cooper) Powder **Dosage** Apply liberally to skin after bath or diaper change	Oatmeal derivatives	Skin protective
Aveeno Lotion (Cooper) Lotion **Dosage** Smooth into affected areas as needed	10% Colloidal oatmeal	Skin protective
	Nonionic surfactants	Cleansers
	Emollients	
Aveeno Oilated (Cooper) Liquid **Dosage** Smooth into affected areas as needed	43% Colloidal oatmeal	Skin protective
	Lanolin fraction	Emollient
	Liquid petrolatum	Emollient and skin protective
Baby Magic Lotion (Mennen) Lotion **Dosage** Smooth into affected areas as needed	Benzalkonium chloride	Antimicrobial agent
	Lanolin	Emollient and skin protective
	Refined sterols	Emollient
Borofax (Burroughs Wellcome) Ointment **Dosage** Smooth small amount into affected areas as needed	5% Boric acid	Antimicrobial agent
	Lanolin	Emollient and skin protective

Table continued on following page

Product (Manufacturer)	Ingredients	Actions
Caldesene Medicated Powder (Pharmacraft) Powder **Dosage** Apply liberally to affected area 3–4 times/day	Talc	Skin protective
	10% Calcium undecylenate	Anti-fungal agent
Desitin Ointment (Leeming) Ointment **Dosage** Smooth into affected areas as needed	Zinc oxide	Skin protective
	Talc	Skin protective
	Cod liver oil	Emollient
	Petrolatum	Ointment base, emollient and skin protective
	Lanolin	Emollient
	Vitamins A and D	Promotes healing
Diaperene Baby Powder (Glenbrook) Powder **Dosage** Apply liberally to affected areas as needed	Magnesium carbonate	Skin protective
	Corn starch	Drying agent; absorbent
	Methylbenzethonium chloride, 1:1800	Antimicrobial agent
Diaperene Ointment (Glenbrook) Ointment **Dosage** Smooth into affected areas as needed	Methylbenzethonium chloride, 1:1000	Antimicrobial agent
	Petrolatum	Ointment base and emollient
	Glycerin	Skin protective
Diaperene Peri-Anal Creme (Glenbrook) Cream **Dosage** Smooth small amount into perianal area after cleansing and drying as needed	Methylbenzethonium chloride, 1:1000	Antimicrobial agent
	Cod liver oil	Emollient
	Water-repellent base	
Johnson & Johnson Medicated Powder (Johnson & Johnson) Powder **Dosage** Apply liberally to affected areas as needed	Zinc oxide	Skin protective
	Talc	Skin protective
	Menthol	Anti-rash agent
	Fragrance	Aesthetic
Johnson's Baby Cream (Johnson & Johnson) Cream **Dosage** Smooth into affected areas as needed	Mineral oil water	Emollient and ointment base
	Paraffin	Ointment base and skin protective
	Sodium borate	Buffer
	Lanolin	Ointment base and skin protective
	White beeswax	Hardening agent
	Ceresin	Hardening agent
	Glyceryl stearate	Ointment base and skin protective

Table continued on following page

Product	Ingredients	Actions
Johnson's Baby Powder (Johnson & Johnson) Powder **Dosage** Apply liberally to affected areas as needed	Talc	Skin protective
	Fragrance	Aesthetic
Methakote Pediatric Cream (Syntex) Cream **Dosage** Smooth small amount into affected areas as needed	Talc	Skin protective
	Benzethonium chloride	Antimicrobial agent
	Protein hydrolysate	Replenishes skin proteins
Panthoderm (USV) Lotion **Dosage** Smooth into affected areas as needed	2% Dexpanthenol	Relieves itching
	Water-miscible base	
Zincofax Cream (Burroughs Wellcome) Cream **Dosage** Smooth into affected areas as needed	15% Zinc oxide	Skin protective
	Petrolatum	Cream base, emollient and skin protective
	Lanolin	Emollient and skin protective

Sunburn

The sun is both friend and foe to mankind—its warmth and light make life on this planet possible, but prolonged exposure to its ultraviolet rays can be very detrimental to the human skin. Even a brief stint in the sun can result in painful sunburn under certain circumstances. And although a deep, year-round tan has become a symbol of youth, healthfulness, and success in our society, the amount of sun exposure required to keep and maintain such a tan results in premature aging and an increased risk of skin cancer. In addition, some persons are extremely sensitive to the sun and can tolerate very little exposure to it. A number of drugs and other substances also may lower tolerance to the sun.

DERMATOLOGIC EFFECTS OF THE SUN

A suntan may look healthy, but in actuality, it is nature's way of trying to minimize the damage from overexposure to the sun. When exposed to the ultraviolet rays of the sun (and other light sources), the skin is stimulated to produce more melanin—the pigmenting substance that darkens the skin. The outer layer of the skin thickens and becomes tougher or more leathery. While this process reduces the danger of sunburn, it also accelerates the aging of the skin by causing it to lose its elasticity and become dry and wrinkled. The adverse effects are not immediately apparent, but the damage is cumulative. By ages twenty-five to thirty-three, moderate to severe skin damage is present in about a third of all Americans. By age forty, chronically sun-exposed skin is comparable to what one would expect in someone fifty or older. The damage is more severe in persons who are light-haired with fair skin—for example, persons of Northern European extraction. Geography and season are also important—solar rays during the summer, when the tilt of the earth makes the sun's rays more direct, are more harmful than at other times of the year, and exposure to the sun at high altitudes or at the lower geographic latitudes (e.g., Florida, the American Southwest, and Southern California) also is more detrimental.

Photosensitizing Substances

A number of drugs and other substances increase photosensitivity, meaning less exposure will cause a sunburn. Medications that increase sun sensitivity include anticonvulsants; antihistamines; anticancer drugs; psychotropic drugs such as barbiturates, the phenothiazines (e.g., Thorazine and other chlorpromazines, Compazine, Stelazine, and others); certain antibiotics, such as demeclocycline, (e.g. Declomycin), erythromycin, and more rarely, tetracycline; quinidine; quinine; salicylates; sex hormones (including those in oral contraceptives); oral diabetes agents; sulfa drugs; and thiazide diuretics. Ingredients often used in cosmetics, perfumes, soaps, antiseptics, and topical medications, such as phenols, coal tars, wood tars, and oil of bergamot, also increase photosensitivity as does furocoumarin, a substance found in parsley, celery, carrots, and limes.

Sunscreens

A number of products effectively screen or block the sun's damaging rays. These may act either by chemically absorbing the ultraviolet rays or by forming a physical barrier to ultraviolet radiation. The major chemical absorbant is paraamino-benzoic acid (PABA) or one of its derivatives. Opaque compounds that block ultraviolet rays—in order of decreasing blocking actions—are zinc oxide, titanium dioxide, bentonite powders, and benzophenone.

Sunscreen manufacturers generally affix an SPF (sun protection factor) number to their products, which indicates the expected degree of protection and the concentration of sunscreening ingredients. Thus, PreSun 15 means that the product affords about fifteen times one's natural protection, and Coppertone 8 offers eight times one's natural protection. The greatest protection is afforded by products that contain at least one chemical and one blocking ingredient. Examples include Ban de Soleil Ultra Sun Block Cream, Super Shade, Total Eclipse Sunscreen, or PreSun 15, all which contain PABA derivatives and benzophenone. Products in this category are recommended for persons who burn easily and do not tan.

The most commonly used sunscreens allow some tanning while protecting against the most damaging rays. These generally contain PABA and its esters (compounds formed when PABA is combined with alcohol), cinnamates, benzophenones, and homomenthyl salicylate. The amount of PABA is important in determining the degree of sun protection; the most effective preparation is 5 percent PABA in 50 to 70 percent alcohol (Pabagel, PreSun, SunGer Sun Block). PABA, however, is likely to stain fabrics. Sunscreens containing PABA esters (Block Out, Pabafilm, Golden Tan, Sea & Ski Lotion, Uval Lotion) are less effective but do not stain as much. PABA also may irritate the skin or interact with photosensitizing substances such as thiazide diuretics or sulfonylureas (oral diabetes drugs) to permit sunburn. Cinnamates and benzophenones are effective against a relatively wide spectrum of ultraviolet rays and do permit slow tanning.

Homosalate preparations allow more ultraviolet rays to reach the skin, but when combined with oxybenzone (Coppertone Nosekote, Coppertone Shade Lotion), can give adequate protection. Salicylate preparations moisturize the skin but offer little protection from ultraviolet rays. In general, suntan lotions and oils do not contain screening agents; therefore, these products lubricate the skin but do not prevent sun damage or retard aging.

Sunscreens should be applied an hour or two

before exposure to the sun and should be reapplied after swimming or perspiring.

SUNBURN

A sunburn is just that—a burn caused by exposure to the sun. Reactions are similar to first-degree burns, with redness and tenderness beginning one to twenty-four hours after exposure. Blisters may form on both exposed or unexposed skin. If the sunburned area is large, malaise, nausea and vomiting, and chills and fever also may occur. Unless the person is particularly sensitive to the sun or the burn is very extensive, sunburn is usually benign and self-limiting. The pain is best alleviated with cold water or cool wet cloths or towels applied to the burned area. Soaking in a cool bath for thirty minutes several times a day is also helpful.

Preparations with local anesthetics may provide some relief, but they may be harmful under certain circumstances because burned skin is more likely to absorb the chemicals in these products, increasing the risk of systemic toxicity. Various creams, solutions, or sprays may relieve the burn by cooling the skin, but again, chemicals in these medications may be absorbed or may irritate the already sensitive skin. Ointments may be difficult to remove. Some sunburn products also contain antibiotics or other anti-infective agents—these are unnecesary unless there is a secondary infection, such as in cases of blistering and peeling. Very severe sunburn may be treated with systemic corticosteroids, given in a diminishing dosage over a week.

IN CONCLUSION

Although it is well known that the sun is harmful to the skin, it is impossible to avoid all exposure to it. The use of effective sunscreens before sunbathing or outdoor activity, especially when the risk of burning is increased (during the summer, in areas of high altitude or the lower geographic latitudes), will help minimize the adverse effects. Persons who are particularly sensitive to the sun or who are taking drugs that increase photosensitivity must exercise extra caution to avoid burning. The risk of sunburn also increases when the ultraviolet rays are reflected—on the water or a sandy beach, for example.

The following charts list the various nonprescription sunscreens and their major ingredients, as well as the rating of the sun protective factor (SPF) for those products. The section on sunburn products lists the most commonly used topical agents to relieve minor sunburn pain.

NONPRESCRIPTION SUNSCREENS

Product (Manufacturer)	Ingredients	Actions
Block Out (Sea & Ski) Lotion (10)* **Dosage** Apply evenly to exposed skin; reapply after swimming or exercise.	8% Octyldimethylaminobenzoic acid	Protects skin by absorbing damaging solar radiation
	70% Alcohol	Astringent
	Moisturizer	
	Fragrance	Aesthetic
Coppertone LipKote (Plough) **Dosage** Apply evenly over lips; reapply after swimming or exercise.	Homosulate	Protects skin by absorbing damaging solar radiation
Coppertone Nosekote (Plough) Balm **Dosage** Apply liberally and evenly over exposed part of nose; reapply after swimming or exercise.	7% Homosalate	Protects skin by absorbing damaging solar radiation
	Oxybenzone	Protects skin by absorbing damaging solar radiation
Coppertone Shade Lotion (Plough) Lotion (2, 4, 6)* **Dosage** Apply evenly to exposed areas; reapply after swimming or exercise.	8% Homosalate	Protects skin by absorbing damaging solar radiation
	3% Oxybenzone	Protects skin by absorbing damaging solar radiation
Golden Tan Lotion (Sea & Ski) Lotion (2)* **Dosage** Apply evenly to exposed areas; reapply after swimming or exercise.	1.7% Octyldimethylaminobenzoic acid	Protects skin by absorbing damaging solar radiation
	Cocoa butter	Emollient
	Mineral oil	Lotion base and emollient
	Lanolin	Lotion base and emollient
	Alcohol	Astringent
Pabafilm (Owen) Liquid (10)* **Dosage** Coat exposed skin evenly and let dry into film; reapply after swimming or exercise.	2.5% Isoasmyl N, *N*-dimethyl-aminobenzoate	Protects skin by absorbing damaging solar radiation
	70% Alcohol	Astringent
Q.T. Quick Tanning Lotion (Plough) Lotion (2)* **Dosage** Apply evenly to desired tanning areas at least 1 h before bathing; reapply after swimming or exercise.	8% Homosalate	Protects skin by absorbing damaging solar radiation
	Dihydroxyacetone	Artificial tanning agent
Sea & Ski Lotion (Sea & Ski) Lotion (8)* **Dosage** Apply evenly to exposed areas; reapply after swimming or exercise.	2.5% Octyldimethylaminobenzoic acid	Protects skin by absorbing damaging solar radiation
	Glycerin	Emollient
	Mineral oil	Emollient and lotion base
	Lanolin	Emollient and lotion base
	Sesame oil	Emollient and lotion base

Table continued on following page

Product (Manufacturer)	Ingredients	Actions
SunGer Extra Protection (Plough) Lotion (6)* **Dosage** Apply evenly to exposed areas; reapply after swimming or exercise.	Homosalate	Protects skin by absorbing damaging solar radiation
	Oxybenzone	Protects skin by absorbing damaging solar radiation
SunGer Sun Block (Plough) Lotion (15)* **Dosage** Apply evenly to exposed areas; reapply after swimming or exercise.	Padimate	Protects skin by absorbing damaging solar radiation
	Oxybenzone	Protects skin by absorbing damaging solar radiation
SunGer Sun and Weather Protection Stick (Plough) Stick (4)* **Dosage** Rub evenly over exposed areas; reapply after swimming or exercise.	Homosalate	Protects skin by absorbing damaging solar radiation
Tropic Sun Oil (Sea & Ski) Liquid (20)* **Dosage** Apply evenly to exposed areas; reapply after swimming or exercise.	1.1% Padimate	Protects skin by absorbing damaging solar radiation
	Cocoa butter	Emollient
	Cocoanut oil	Emollient
	Almond oil	Emollient
	Mineral oil	Emollient
	Lanolin	Emollient
Tropic Sun Butter (Sea & Ski) Lotion **Dosage** Apply evenly to exposed areas; reapply after swimming or exercise.	Cocoa butter	Emollient
	Cocoanut oil	Emollient
	Almond oil	Emollient
	Mineral oil	Emollient
	Lanolin	Emollient

*Sun protection factor

Product (Manufacturer)	Ingredients	Actions
Americaine (Arnar-Stone) Aerosol **Dosage** Spray affected areas as needed.	20% Benzocaine	Mild anesthetic agent that relieves minor pain, burning, and itching
Americaine (Arnar-Stone) Ointment **Dosage** Apply to affected areas as needed.	20% Benzocaine	Mild anesthetic agent that relieves minor pain, burning, and itching
	0.1% Benzethenonium chloride	Antimicrobial agent
	Polyethylene glycols	Ointment base
Betadine (Purdue-Frederick) Aerosol **Dosage** Spray affected areas as needed.	5% Povidone-Iodine	Antimicrobial agent
	Aqueous base	
Betadine (Purdue-Frederick) Ointment **Dosage** Apply to affected areas as needed.	10% Povidone-Iodine	Antimicrobial agent
	Water-miscible base	
Dermoplast (Ayerst) Aerosol **Dosage** Spray affected areas as needed.	20% Benzocaine	Mild anesthetic agent that relieves minor pain, burning, and itching
	0.5% Methol	Mild anesthetic agent that relieves minor pain, burning, and itching
	Methylparaben	Preservative
	Polyethylene glycol 400 monolaurate	Aerosol base
	Polysorbate 85	Cleansing agent
Medicone Dressing Cream (Medicone) Cream **Dosage** Apply to affected areas as needed.	5 mg/g Benzocaine	Mild anesthetic agent that relieves minor pain, burning, and itching
	0.5 mf/g 8-Hydroxyquinoline sulfate	Antimicrobial agent
	125 mg/g Cod liver oil	Healing agent
	125 mg/g Zinc oxide	Skin protective
	1.8 mg/g Menthol	Mild anesthetic agent that relieves minor pain, burning, and itching
	Petrolatum	Cream base
	Lanolin	Cream base
	Paraffin	Cream base
	Talc	Skin protective
	Perfume	Aesthetic
Medi-Quick (Lehn & Fink) Aerosol **Dosage** Spray affected areas as needed.	2.5% Lidocaine	Mild anesthetic agent that relieves minor pain, burning, and itching
	Benzalkonium chloride	Antimicrobial agent
	12% Isopropyl alcohol	Solvent and antiseptic

Table continued on following page

NONPRESCRIPTION SUNBURN MEDICATIONS

Product (Manufacturer)	Ingredients	Actions
Medi-Quick (Lehn & Fink) Pump Spray **Dosage** Spray affected areas as needed.	2.5% Lidocaine	Mild anesthetic agent that relieves minor pain, burning, and itching
	Benzalkonium chloride	Antimicrobial agent
	79% Isopropyl alcohol	Solvent and antiseptic
Nupercainal Cream (CIBA) Cream **Dosage** Apply to affected areas as needed.	0.5% Dibucaine	Mild anesthetic agent that relieves minor pain, burning, and itching
	0.37% Acetone sodium bisulfite	Cream base and solvent
	Water-washable base	
Nupercainal Ointment (CIBA) Ointment **Dosage** Apply to affected areas as needed.	1% Dibucaine	Mild anesthetic agent that relieves minor pain, burning, and itching
	0.5% Acetone sodium bisulfite	Ointment base and solvent
Panthoderm (USV) Cream **Dosage** Apply to affected areas as needed.	2% Dexpanthenol	Relieves itching
	Water-miscible base	
Panthoderm (USV) Lotion **Dosage** Apply to affected areas as needed.	2% Dexpanthenol	Relieves itching
	Water-miscible base	
Pyribenzamine (CIBA) Cream **Dosage** Apply to affected areas as needed.	2% Tripelennamine	Relieves itching
	Water-washable base	
Pyribenzamine (CIBA) Ointment **Dosage** Apply to affected areas as needed.	2% Tripelennamine	Relieves itching and swelling
	Petrolatum	Ointment base
Solarcaine Spray (Plough) Aerosol Spray **Dosage** Spray affected areas as needed.	9.4% (Benzocaine)	Mild anesthetic agent that relieves minor pain, burning and itching
	Triclosan	Antimicrobial agent
Solarcaine Spray (Plough) Pump Spray **Dosage** Spray affected areas as needed.	2% Benzocaine	Mild anesthetic agent that relieves minor pain, burning and itching
	Triclosan	Antimicrobial agent
	31% Isopropyl alcohol	Antiseptic and solvent

Table continued on following page

Product (Manufacturer)	Ingredients	Actions
Unguentine (Norwich) Ointment **Dosage** Apply to affected areas as needed.	Parahydracin	Antimicrobial agent
	1% Phenol	Antimicrobial agent
	Aluminum hydroxide	Emulsifier
	Zinc carbonate	Astringent and antiseptic
	Zinc acetate	Astringent and antiseptic
	Zinc oxide	Astringent and skin protective
	Eucalyptus oil	Emollient
	Thyme oil	Emollient
	Menthol	Mild anesthetic agent that relieves minor pain, burning and itching
Unguentine (Norwich) Aerosol **Dosage** Spray on affected areas as needed.	Benzocaine	Mild anesthetic agent that relieves minor pain, burning and itching
	Benzalkonium chloride	Antimicrobial agent
	Chloroxylenol	Antimicrobial agent
	1% Phenol	Antimicrobial agent
	Aluminum hydroxide	Emulsifier
	Zinc carbonate	Astringent and antiseptic
	Zinc acetate	Astringent and antiseptic
	Zinc oxide	Astringent and skin protective
	Eucalyptus oil	Emollient
	Thyme oil	Emollient
	Menthol	Mild anesthetic agent that relieves minor pain, burning and itching
	7% Alcohol	Astringent
Xylocaine (Astra) Ointment **Dosage** Apply to affected areas as needed.	2.5% Lidocaine	Mild anesthetic agent that relieves minor pain, burning and itching
	Polyethylene glycols	Ointment base
	Propylene glycol	Solvent

Table continued on following page

Miscellaneous and Recently Introduced Drugs

℞

DRUGS TO TREAT ALCOHOLISM

ANTABUSE (Disulfiram) **Ayerst**

Tabs: 250, 500 mg

INDICATIONS	ORAL DOSAGE
Alcoholism, as an adjunct to supportive and psychotherapeutic treatment in patients who want to remain in a state of enforced sobriety	**Adult:** up to 500 mg qd for 1–2 wk, followed by 125–500 mg/day for maintenance; average maintenance dosage: 250 mg/day

ADMINISTRATION/DOSAGE ADJUSTMENTS

Initiation of therapy	Requires that patient has abstained from alcohol at least 12 h beforehand
Duration of therapy	Maintenance therapy is required until the patient is fully recovered socially and a basis for permanent self-control is established
Trial with alcohol	If test reaction is deemed necessary, give 15 ml (½ oz) of 100-proof whiskey or equivalent after the first 1–2 wk of therapy with 500 mg/day; repeat test dose of alcoholic beverage once only. Once reaction develops, no more alcohol should be consumed. Do not test reaction in patients over 50 yr of age.

CONTRAINDICATIONS

Recent or concomitant use of metronidazole, paraldehyde, alcohol, or alcohol-containing preparations ●	Severe myocardial disease ●	Coronary occlusion ●
Psychoses ●	Hypersensitivity to disulfiram or other thiuram derivatives ●	Alcohol intoxication ●

WARNINGS/PRECAUTIONS

Disulfiram-alcohol reaction	Caution patients that this will occur with even small amounts of alcohol, up to 14 days after ingesting disulfiram, and may produce flushing, throbbing in head and neck, throbbing headache, respiratory difficulty, nausea, copious vomiting, sweating, thirst, chest pain, palpitation, dyspnea, hyperventilation, tachycardia, hypotension, syncope, marked uneasiness, weakness, vertigo, blurred vision, and confusion; in severe reactions, there may be respiratory depression, cardiovascular collapse, arrythmias, myocardial infarction, acute congestive heart failure, unconsciousness, convulsions, and death. For severe reactions, restore blood pressure and treat shock. Administer oxygen, carbogen (95% oxygen and 5% carbon dioxide), massive IV doses (1 g) of vitamin C, and ephedrine sulfate. Antihistamines have been used intravenously. Hypokalemia has been reported; monitor potassium levels, particularly in digitalized patients.
Alcohol-containing substances	Warn patients taking disulfiram to avoid alcohol in disguised forms, eg, in sauces, vinegars, cough mixtures, aftershave lotions, and back rubs
Alcohol intoxication	Do not administer to intoxicated patient or without patient's full knowledge; inform relatives accordingly
Concomitant use of phenytoin or its congeners	May lead to phenytoin intoxication; use disulfiram with caution. Obtain serum levels of phenytoin.
Concomitant use of oral anticoagulants	Requires prothrombin-time determinations (see DRUG INTERACTIONS)
Concomitant use of isoniazid	May produce unsteady gait or marked changes in mental status; discontinue disulfiram if such signs appear
Concomitant ingestion of nitrites	Has been reported to cause tumors in rats; significance of this finding in humans is not known
Special-risk patients	Use with caution in patients with diabetes mellitus, hypothyroidism, epilepsy, cerebral damage, chronic and acute nephritis, hepatic cirrhosis or insufficiency, coronary-artery disease, or hypertension
Patients with rubber contact dermatitis	Should be evaluated for hypersensitivity to thiuram derivatives before receiving disulfiram (see CONTRAINDICATIONS)

Table continued on following page

15

ANTABUSE continued

WARNINGS/PRECAUTIONS continued

Patient identification card	Should be carried by the patient, stating that patient is receiving disulfiram, and describing symptoms most likely to occur as a result of the disulfiram-alcohol reaction; the card should also indicate the physician or institution to be contacted in an emergency. (Cards may be obtained from the manufacturer upon request.)
Concomitant use of barbiturates	Possibility of initiating a new abuse should be considered
Hepatic dysfunction	May occur; perform baseline and follow-up transaminase tests every 10–14 days, as well as a complete blood count and a sequential multiple analysis-12 (SMA-12) test every 6 mo
Exposure to ethylene dibromide or its vapors	Has resulted in a higher incidence of tumors and mortality in disulfiram-treated rats; although correlation of this finding to humans has not been demonstrated, caution patients against exposure to this substance
Metallic or garlicky aftertaste	May occur during first 2 wk of therapy (see ADVERSE REACTIONS)

ADVERSE REACTIONS

Central nervous system	Optic neuritis, peripheral neuritis, polyneuritis, transient mild drowsiness, fatigability, headache, psychotic reactions[1]
Dermatological	Skin eruptions, acneform eruptions, allergic dermatitis
Genitourinary	Impotence
Gastrointestinal	Metallic or garlicky aftertaste
Other	Cholestatic hepatitis (1 case; causal relationship not established)

OVERDOSAGE

Signs and symptoms	See ADVERSE REACTIONS
Treatment	Treat symptomatically

DRUG INTERACTIONS

Oral anticoagulants	⇧ Anticoagulant effect
Isoniazid	Unsteady gait, mental changes, psychosis
Metronidazole	Psychosis
Paraldehyde	⇧ Adverse reactions
Phenytoin and its congeners	⇧ Serum phenytoin level

ALTERED LABORATORY VALUES

Blood/serum values	⇧ Cholesterol
Urinary values	⇩ VMA

Use in children

General guidelines not established

Use in pregnancy or nursing mothers

Safe use not established during pregnancy; general guidelines not established for use in nursing mothers

[1]In most cases attributable to high doses, concomitant use of metronidazole or isoniazid, or unmasking of underlying psychoses

CALCIPARINE (Heparin calcium) Choay

Amps: 12,500 units (0.5 ml), 20,000 units (0.8 ml) **Syringe:** 5,000 units (0.2 ml)

INDICATIONS	PARENTERAL DOSAGE
Venous thrombosis **Atrial fibrillation with embolism** **Pulmonary embolism** Acute and chronic **consumption coagulopathies** (disseminated intravascular coagulation) Prevention of **cerebral thrombosis** in evolving stroke **Coronary occlusion with acute myocardial infarction** (adjunctive therapy) **Peripheral arterial embolism** (adjunctive therapy)	**Adult:** 5,000 units (undiluted) IV followed by 10,000–20,000 units of concentrated solution SC (deeply) to start, followed by 8,000–10,000 units of concentrated solution SC (deeply) q8h or 15,000–20,000 units q12h; for intermittent IV injection, 10,000 units (undiluted or in 50–100 ml of isotonic NaCl) IV to start, followed by 5,000–10,000 units (undiluted or in 50–100 ml of isotonic NaCl) IV q4–6h; for continuous IV infusion, 5,000 units (undiluted) IV to start, followed by 20,000–40,000 units (in 1 liter of isotonic NaCl)/24 h
Prevention of postoperative deep venous thrombosis and pulmonary embolism	**Adult:** 5,000 units (undiluted) by deep SC injection 2 h before surgery, followed by 5,000 units q8–12h for 7 days or until patient is fully ambulatory, whichever is longer
Prevention of clotting in arterial and heart surgery	**Adult:** not less than 150 units/kg to start; for procedures lasting <60 min, 300 units/kg; for procedures lasting >60 min, 400 units/kg

ADMINISTRATION/DOSAGE ADJUSTMENTS

As an anticoagulant in extracorporeal dialysis	Follow equipment manufacturer's operating directions carefully
As an anticoagulant in blood transfusions	Add 400–600 units to each 100 ml of whole blood; usually, 7,500 units of heparin is first added to 100 ml of Sterile Sodium Chloride Injection, and then 6–8 ml of this solution is added to 100 ml of whole blood. WBC counts should be performed within 2 h of adding heparin. Heparinized blood should not be used for isoagglutinin, complement, or erythrocyte fragility tests or for platelet counts.
As an anticoagulant in blood samples for laboratory purposes	Add 70–150 units to 10–20 ml of whole blood (see comments above)
Selection of patients for low-dose prophylaxis of postoperative thromboembolism	Reserve for patients over 40 yr of age undergoing major surgery. Exclude patients with bleeding disorders, those having neurosurgery, spinal anesthesia, eye surgery, or potentially sanguinous operations, as well as patients receiving oral anticoagulants or drugs that interfere with platelet aggregation (see WARNINGS/PRECAUTIONS and DRUG INTERACTIONS).
Blood coagulation tests	Regulate dosage by frequent testing. During 1st day of treatment, determine clotting time just prior to each injection. Dosage is considered adequate when clotting time is 2½–3 times the control value. When using continuous IV infusion, perform coagulation tests q4h during early stages of therapy. When using intermittent IV or SC injections, perform coagulation tests before each injection during the early stages of therapy and daily thereafter. In patients with normal coagulation parameters, there is usually no need for daily monitoring of *low-dose* heparin therapy.
Concomitant use of coumarin anticoagulants	Since heparin may prolong the one-stage prothrombin time, wait at least 5 h after the last IV dose or 24 h after the last SC dose before drawing blood, in order to obtain valid prothrombin times

CONTRAINDICATIONS

When suitable blood coagulation tests cannot be performed at required intervals ●	Hypersensitivity to heparin ●	Uncontrollable bleeding ●

Table continued on following page

CALCIPARINE continued

WARNINGS/PRECAUTIONS	
Increased risk of bleeding and hemorrhage	Use with caution in patients with subacute bacterial endocarditis, arterial sclerosis, increased capillary permeability, hemophilia, some purpuras, thrombocytopenia, or inaccessible ulcerative lesions of the GI tract; during continuous tube drainage of the stomach or small intestine; and during and immediately after a spinal tap, spinal anesthesia, or major surgery (especially involving the brain, spinal cord, or eye)
Unduly prolonged coagulation tests or hemorrhage	Discontinue anticoagulation therapy promptly (see OVERDOSAGE); significant GI- or urinary-tract bleeding may indicate the presence of an underlying occult lesion
Antiplatelet therapy	Bleeding may occur with concomitant use of drugs, such as acetylsalicylic acid, that interfere with platelet-aggregation reactions (see DRUG INTERACTIONS); use with caution in patients receiving heparin
Febrile state	Increased doses of heparin may be required
Special-risk patients	Use with caution in patients with mild hepatic or renal disease, hypertension, or indwelling catheters, as well as during menstruation and in women over 60 yr of age
Hypersensitive patients	If feasible, administer a trial dose of 1,000 units before giving a therapeutic dose to a patient with a history of allergy
Acute adrenal hemorrhage or insufficiency	Discontinue anticoagulant therapy; measure plasma cortisol levels immediately and promptly institute vigorous IV corticosteroid therapy. Do not delay treatment for laboratory confirmation of diagnosis, as death may result.
Vasospastic reactions	May develop 6–10 days after initiating therapy, causing pain, ischemia, and cyanosis in the affected limb which may last 4–6 h. After repeated injection, the reaction may become generalized, with cyanosis, tachypnea, a feeling of oppression, and headache. Chest pain, increased blood pressure, arthralgias, and/or headache may also occur in the absence of definite peripheral vasospasm. Protamine has no effect on the reaction.
ACD-converted blood	Blood collected in heparin calcium and later converted to ACD blood may alter the coagulation system of the recipient, especially if ACD-converted blood is given in multiple transfusions; use with caution
ADVERSE REACTIONS	
Hematological	Bleeding, overly prolonged bleeding time, hemorrhage, acute reversible thrombocytopenia (with IV use), vasospasm
Hypersensitivity	Chills, fever, urticaria, asthma, rhinitis, lacrimation, anaphylactoid reactions, anaphylactic shock (following IV injection; rare)
Metabolic	Osteoporosis (with long-term, high-dose therapy), rebound hyperlipemia upon discontinuation of heparin therapy
Genitourinary	Suppression of renal function (with long-term, high-dose therapy), priapism
Other	Local irritation, mild pain, or hematoma at injection site (frequently with IM injection, less often with deep SC administration), histamine-like reactions at injection site, suppression of aldosterone secretion, delayed transient alopecia
OVERDOSAGE	
Signs and symptoms	See ADVERSE REACTIONS
Treatment	Administer 1.0–1.5 mg of 1% protamine sulfate by slow infusion for every 100 units of heparin to be neutralized (30 min after a dose of heparin, ~0.5 mg of protamine is usually sufficient to neutralize 100 units of heparin). No more than 50 mg should be given very slowly in any 10-min period. Blood or plasma transfusions may be necessary; such transfusions dilute but do not neutralize heparin.
DRUG INTERACTIONS	
Acetylsalicylic acid (aspirin), coumarin anticoagulants, dextran, dipyramidole, hydroxychloroquine, ibuprofen, indomethacin, oxyphenbutazone, phenylbutazone, streptokinase, sulfinpyrazone, urokinase	⇧ Risk of bleeding and hemorrhage

Table continued on following page

DRUG INTERACTIONS continued

Corticotropin, ethacrynic acid, glucocorticoids, mefenamic acid, nonsteroidal anti-inflammatory agents	⇧ Risk of GI bleeding and hemorrhage
Antihistamines, digitalis, nicotine, tetracyclines	⇩ Anticoagulant effect

ALTERED LABORATORY VALUES

Blood/serum values	⇧ Whole-blood clotting time ⇧ Activated partial thromboplastin time ⇧ Prothrombin time ⇧ Thyroxine (T_4) ⇧ Triiodothyronine (T_3) uptake False-positive BSP tests ⇩ Cholesterol (with doses of 15,000–20,000 units)

No clinically significant alterations in urinary values occur at therapeutic dosages

Use in children

General guidelines not established

Use in pregnancy or nursing mothers

Increases the risk of maternal hemorrhage; use with caution during pregnancy, especially during the last trimester and immediately postpartum. Heparin calcium does not cross the placental barrier. It is not excreted in human breast milk.

DITROPAN (Oxybutynin chloride) **Marion**

Tabs: 5 mg

INDICATIONS	ORAL DOSAGE
Symptomatic relief associated with voiding in patients with uninhibited neurogenic and reflex neurogenic bladder	**Adult:** 5 mg bid or tid, up to qid **Child (5–12 yr):** 5 mg bid, up to tid

CONTRAINDICATIONS

Glaucoma ●

Intestinal atony in elderly or debilitated patients ●

Unstable cardiovascular status in acute hemorrhage ●

Partial or complete GI-tract obstruction ●

Megacolon ●

Severe colitis ●

Myasthenia gravis ●

Paralytic ileus ●

Toxic megacolon complicating ulcerative colitis ●

Obstructive uropathy ●

WARNINGS/PRECAUTIONS

Drowsiness, blurred vision	Performance of potentially hazardous activities may be impaired; caution patients accordingly
Ulcerative colitis	Large doses may suppress intestinal motility and lead to paralytic ileus or precipitate or aggravate toxic megacolon
Special-risk patients	Use with caution in the elderly and in those with autonomic neuropathy, hepatic or renal disease, hyperthyroidism, coronary heart disease, congestive heart failure, cardiac arrhythmias, hypertension, tachycardia, prostatic hypertrophy, or hiatal hernia associated with reflux esophagitis
Fever and heat stroke	May occur in high environmental temperatures as a result of anaphoresis
Incomplete intestinal obstruction	May be manifested by diarrhea, especially in ileostomy or colostomy patients; therapy may be harmful under these circumstances

ADVERSE REACTIONS

Gastrointestinal	Dry mouth, nausea, vomiting, constipation, bloating
Genitourinary	Urinary hesitancy and retention, impotence
Dermatological	Decreased sweating
Ophthalmic	Blurred vision, pupillary dilatation, increased ocular tension, cycloplegia
Cardiovascular	Tachycardia, palpitations
Central nervous system	Drowsiness, weakness, dizziness, insomnia
Endocrinological	Suppression of lactation
Allergic	Urticaria and other dermatoses

OVERDOSAGE

Signs and symptoms	Intensification of usual side effects, CNS disturbances (restlessness, excitement, psychotic behavior), circulatory changes (flushing, decrease in blood pressure, circulatory failure), respiratory failure, curare-like effects (neuromuscular blockade, leading to muscle weakness and possible paralysis), coma
Treatment	Immediately empty stomach by gastric lavage; inject physostigmine, 0.5–2.0 mg IV, up to 5 mg as needed. Treat fever symptomatically (ice, alcohol). Manage excessive excitement with 2% sodium thiopental IV (slowly) or 100–200 ml of 2% chloral hydrate via rectal infusion. For paralysis of respiratory muscles, institute artificial respiration.

DRUG INTERACTIONS

Digoxin	⇧ Serum digoxin level
Belladonna alkaloids, anticholinergic agents, phenothiazines, tricyclic antidepressants, quinidine, antihistamines, procainamide	⇧ Cholinergic blockade

Table continued on following page

DITROPAN continued

ALTERED LABORATORY VALUES

No clinically significant alterations in blood/serum or urinary values occur at therapeutic dosages

Use in children	**Use in pregnancy or nursing mothers**
See INDICATIONS; safety and efficacy not established in children <5 yr of age	Safe use not established during pregnancy; general guidelines not established for use in nursing mothers

LUDIOMIL (Maprotiline hydrochloride) **Ciba**

Tabs: 25, 50 mg

INDICATIONS	ORAL DOSAGE
Depressive neurosis (dysthymic disorder) **Manic-depressive illness, depressed type** (major depressive disorder)	**Adult:** for outpatients with mild-to-moderate depression, 75 mg/day in a single daily dose or divided to start, followed by gradual increments in dosage up to 150 mg/day or (in some cases) 225 mg/day, as needed and tolerated; for more severely depressed hospitalized patients, 100–150 mg/day in a single daily dose or divided to start, followed by gradual increments in dosage up to 150–225 mg/day or (in some cases) 300 mg/day, as needed and tolerated

ADMINISTRATION/DOSAGE ADJUSTMENTS

Maintenance therapy	Reduce dosage to 75–150 mg/day; therapeutic response should guide subsequent dosage adjustments
Elderly patients	Use lower dosages for patients over 60 yr of age; give 50–75 mg/day to elderly patients who do not tolerate higher amounts

CONTRAINDICATIONS

Hypersensitivity	To maprotiline
Seizure disorders	Known or suspected
MAO inhibitor therapy	Wait at least 14 days after discontinuing MAO inhibitors before initiating maprotiline therapy; start with low doses and increase dosage gradually, with caution
Myocardial infarction	During acute phase

WARNINGS/PRECAUTIONS

Cardiovascular effects	Conduction defects, arrhythmias, myocardial infarction, stroke, and tachycardia may occur in patients with a history of myocardial infarction or when a history of or active cardiovascular disease is present; use with extreme caution
Potentially suicidal patients	Should not have access to large quantities of maprotiline; prescribe smallest amount feasible
Seizures	Have been reported in patients both with and without a past history of seizure disorders (causal relationship not established)
Hypomanic or manic episodes	May occur, especially in patients with manic-depressive illness, although incidence is rare
Elective surgery	Discontinue medication for as long as clinically feasible prior to surgery
Anticholinergic effect	Use with caution in patients with increased intraocular pressure, history of urinary retention, or history of narrow-angle glaucoma
Mental impairment, reflex-slowing	Performance of potentially hazardous activities may be impaired; caution patients accordingly and about the additive effects of alcohol and other CNS depressants
Fever and sore throat	May occur; discontinue therapy if leukocyte count and differential shows evidence of pathologic neutrophil depression
Electroconvulsive therapy (ECT)	Should be avoided because of lack of experience in this area
Potential for cardiovascular toxicity	Is enhanced in hyperthyroid patients and in those receiving thyroid medication; use with caution

ADVERSE REACTIONS[1]	Frequent reactions are italicized
Central nervous system and neuromuscular	*Drowsiness (16%), dizziness (8%), nervousness (6%), weakness/fatigue (4%), headache (4%), anxiety (3%), tremor (3%), insomnia (2%), agitation (2%);* rarely, numbness, tingling, motor hyperactivity, seizures, EEG alterations, tinnitus, confusional states (especially in the elderly), hallucinations, disorientation, delusions, restlessness, nightmares, hypomania, mania, exacerbation of psychosis, decrease in memory, feelings of unreality
Cardiovascular	Hypotension, hypertension, tachycardia, palpitation, arrhythmia, heart block, syncope
Anticholinergic	*Dry mouth (22%), constipation (6%), blurred vision (4%);* rarely, accommodation disturbances, mydriasis, urinary,retention, and delayed micturition
Allergic (rare)	Skin rash, petechiae, pruritus, photosensitization, edema, drug fever

[1]Although the following adverse reactions have not been reported with maprotiline, its pharmacological similarity to tricyclic antidepressants requires that each reaction be considered when administering this drug: bone marrow depression, including agranulocytosis, eosinophilia, purpura, and thrombocytopenia; myocardial infarction; stroke; peripheral neuropathy, sublingual adenitis; black tongue; stomatitis; paralytic ileus; gynecomastia in the male; breast enlargement and galactorrhea in the female; and testicular swelling.

Table continued on following page

ADVERSE REACTIONS continued

Gastrointestinal	*Nausea (2%)*; rarely, vomiting, epigastric distress, diarrhea, bitter taste, abdominal cramps, dysphagia, altered liver function, jaundice
Endocrinological (rare)	Increased or decreased libido, impotence, hypoglycemia
Other (rare)	Weight loss or gain, diaphoresis, flushing, urinary frequency, increased salivation, nasal congestion

OVERDOSAGE

Signs and symptoms	Based on limited clinical experience, signs and symptoms may include drowsiness, tachycardia, ataxia, vomiting, cyanosis, hypotension, shock, restlessness, agitation, hyperpyrexia, muscle rigidity, athetoid movements, mydriasis, cardiac arrhythmias, impaired cardiac condition, and, in severe cases, loss of consciousness and generalized convulsions; congestive heart failure, a manifestation of tricyclic antidepressant overdosage, may also occur.
Treatment	Empty stomach contents by emesis or gastric lavage; to help promote more rapid elimination of the drug, leave the tube in the stomach for irrigation and continual aspiration of stomach contents. To reduce the tendency to convulsions, darken the room, allowing only minimal external stimulation. IV administration of 1–3 mg of physostigmine has been reported to reverse the signs and symptoms of overdosage with tricyclic antidepressants; repeat doses at intervals of 30 to 60 min may be necessary. *Do not use barbiturates.* Paraldehyde may be used effectively in some children to counteract muscular hypertonus and convulsions with less likelihood of causing respiratory depression. Treat shock (circulatory collapse) with supportive measures, such as IV fluids, oxygen, and corticosteroids. Control hyperpyrexia by whatever means available, including ice packs. Employ rapid digitalization for congestive heart failure. Dialysis is of little value.

DRUG INTERACTIONS

Alcohol, sedative-hypnotics, and other CNS depressants	⇧ CNS depression
MAO inhibitors	Hyperpyrexia, excitability, severe convulsions, coma, death
Anticholinergic agents	Acute glaucoma, urinary retention, paralytic ileus
Guanethidine and similar agents	⇩ Antihypertensive effect
Sympathomimetic agents	Severe hypertension, hyperpyrexia
Thyroid preparations	⇧ Antidepressant effect and possible risk of arrhythmias

ALTERED LABORATORY VALUES

Blood/serum values	⇧ or ⇩ Glucose

No clinically significant alterations in urinary values occur at therapeutic dosages

Use in children

Safety and effectiveness not established in children under 18 yr of age

Use in pregnancy or nursing mothers

May be used during pregnancy only if clearly needed. It is not known whether maprotiline is excreted in breast milk; use with caution in nursing mothers.

SPECTROBID (Bacampicillin hydrochloride) Roerig

Tabs: 400 mg

INDICATIONS	ORAL DOSAGE
Upper respiratory tract infections caused by susceptible strains of streptococci, pneumococci, non-penicillinase-producing staphylococci, and *Haemophilus influenzae* **Urinary tract infections** caused by susceptible stains of *Escherichia coli, Proteus mirabilis,* and *Streptococcus faecalis* (enterococci) **Skin and skin-structure infections** caused by susceptible strains of streptococci and staphylococci	**Adult:** 400 mg q12h; for severe infections or those caused by less susceptible organisms, 800 mg q12h **Child (≥25 kg):** same as adult
Lower respiratory tract infections caused by susceptible strains of streptococci, pneumococci, non-penicillinase-producing staphylococci, and *Haemophilus influenzae*	**Adult:** 800 mg q12h **Child (≥25 kg):** same as adult
Acute uncomplicated **urogenital infections** caused by *Neisseria gonorrhoeae*	**Adult:** 1.6 g given simultaneously with 1 g probenecid

ADMINISTRATION/DOSAGE ADJUSTMENTS

Duration of treatment	Continue treatment for at least 48-72 h after patient has become asymptomatic or bacteria have been eradicated; hemolytic streptococcal infections should be treated for at least 10 days to prevent acute rheumatic fever and glomerulonephritis

CONTRAINDICATIONS

Hypersensitivity to penicillins	Concomitant use of disulfiram (see DRUG INTERACTIONS)

WARNINGS/PRECAUTIONS

Hypersensitivity	Serious and occasionally fatal anaphylactic reactions may occur, most likely in patients with a history of penicillin hypersensitivity and/or hypersensitivity to multiple allergens. Urticaria and other skin rashes may be controlled with anti-histamines and, if necessary, systemic corticosteroids. Drug should be discontinued unless the opinion of the physician dictates otherwise. Serious anaphylactoid reactions may necessitate emergency measures, such as immediate use of epinephrine, oxygen, IV corticosteroids, and airway management, including intubation; use with caution in patients who have experienced allergic reactions to cephalosporins.
Long-term therapy	Perform blood, renal, and hepatic studies periodically, particularly in premature infants, neonates, and patients with hepatic or renal impairment
Superinfection	Overgrowth of nonsusceptible organisms, including fungi, may occur
Venereal disease	If syphilis is suspected, perform dark-field examination before instituting therapy and perform serology testing monthly for at least 4 mo
Chronic urinary tract and intestinal infections	Require bacteriological and clinical appraisal during therapy, and possibly for several months afterward
Complications of gonorrheal urethritis, such as prostatitis and epididymitis	Prolonged and intensive therapy is recommended such as prostatitis and epididymltls
Patients with infectious mononucleosis	Ampicillin-class antibiotics should not be used in treatment; infectious mononucleosis is viral in origin, and a high percentage of patients who receive ampicillin develop skin rash

ADVERSE REACTIONS[1]

	Frequent reactions are italicized
Gastrointestinal	*Diarrhea (2%), epigastric upset (2%),* gastritis, stomatitis, nausea, vomiting, glossitis, black hairy tongue, enterocolitis, pseudomembranous colitis
Hypersensitivity	Rash, urticaria, erythema multiforme, exfoliative dermatitis, anaphylaxis (see WARNINGS/PRECAUTIONS)
Hematological	Anemia, thrombocytopenia, thrombocytopenic purpura, eosinophilia, leukopenia, agranulocytosis

[1]Includes reactions reported with ampicillin

Table continued on following page

SPECTROBID continued

OVERDOSAGE	
Signs and symptoms	See ADVERSE REACTIONS
Treatment	Discontinue medication; treat symptomatically

DRUG INTERACTIONS[2]	
Disulfiram	Risk of disulfiram-like reaction
Probenecid	⇧ Ampicillin blood level and/or toxicity

ALTERED LABORATORY VALUES	
Blood/serum values	⇧ SGOT ⇩ Estrogen (in pregnant women; transient)
Urinary values	⇧ Glucose (with Clinitest tablets)

Use in children

See INDICATIONS

Use in pregnancy or nursing mothers

May be used during pregnancy only if clearly needed. Ampicillin-class antibiotics are excreted in breast milk; use with caution in nursing mothers.

[2]Co-administration of allopurinol and ampicillin increases substantially the incidence of rashes in patients receiving both drugs as compared to patients receiving ampicillin alone. Whether this potentiation of ampicillin rashes is due to allopurinol or the hyperuricemia present is unknown. No data are available on the incidence of rash in patients treated concurrently with bacampicillin and allopurinol.

URISPAS (Flavoxate hydrochloride) Smith Kline & French

Tabs: 100 mg

INDICATIONS	ORAL DOSAGE
Symptomatic relief of **dysuria, urgency, nocturia, suprapubic pain, frequency,** and **incontinence** associated with cystitis, prostatitis, urethritis, and urethrocystitis/urethrotrigonitis	**Adult:** 100–200 mg tid or qid, followed by reduction in dosage as symptoms improve

CONTRAINDICATIONS

Pyloric or duodenal obstruction ●	Obstructive intestinal lesions or ileus ●	Obstructive uropathy of the lower urinary tract ●
GI hemorrhage ●	Achalasia ●	

WARNINGS/PRECAUTIONS

Suspected glaucoma	Use with caution
Drowsiness, blurred vision	Performance of potentially hazardous activities may be impaired; caution patients accordingly

ADVERSE REACTIONS

Gastrointestinal	Dry mouth, nausea, vomiting
Genitourinary	Dysuria
Hematological	Eosinophilia, leukopenia
Central nervous system	Headache, nervousness, vertigo, confusion (especially in the elderly), drowsiness, hyperpyrexia
Cardiovascular	Palpitations, tachycardia
Ophthalmic	Blurred vision, increased ocular tension, disturbance in eye accommodation
Dermatological	Urticaria, other dermatoses

OVERDOSAGE

Consult manufacturer

DRUG INTERACTIONS

Digoxin	⇧ Serum digoxin level
Belladonna alkaloids, anticholinergic agents, phenothiazines, tricyclic antidepressants, quinidine, antihistamines, procainamide	⇧ Cholinergic blockade

ALTERED LABORATORY VALUES

No clinically significant alterations in blood/serum or urinary values occur at therapeutic dosages

Use in children

Not recommended for use in children

Use in pregnancy or nursing mothers

Safe use not established during pregnancy; general guidelines not established for use in nursing mothers

YUTOPAR (Ritodrine hydrochloride) Merrell-National

Tabs: 10 mg **Amps:** 10 mg/ml (5 ml)

INDICATIONS	ORAL DOSAGE	PARENTERAL DOSAGE
Preterm labor	**Adult:** 10 mg 30 min before termination of IV therapy; for maintenance, 10 mg q2h for 24 h, followed by 10-20 mg q4-6h, up to 120 mg/day	**Adult:** 0.1 mg/min by IV drip, gradually increased by 0.05 mg/min until desired result is attained; usual dosage, 0.15-0.35 mg/min

ADMINISTRATION/DOSAGE ADJUSTMENTS

Preparation of infusion liquid	Dilute 150 mg ritodrine in 500 ml of 0.9% w/v sodium chloride, 5% w/v dextrose, 10% w/v dextran 40 in 0.9% w/v sodium chloride, 10% w/v invert sugar, Ringer's solution, or Hartmann's solution to a final concentration of 0.3 mg/ml
Control and dose titration	Adjust the rate of flow with a controlled infusion device; monitor rate of infusion and amount administered to avoid circulatory fluid overload. Frequently monitor maternal uterine contractions, heart rate, and blood pressure and fetal heart rate, and titrate dosage according to response.
Hypotension during administration	Maintain patient on her left side during infusion to minimize risk of hypotension, and pay careful attention to dehydration
Recurrence of unwanted preterm labor	Treat with repeated infusion of ritodrine
Duration of therapy	Continue infusion for at least 12 h after uterine contractions cease

CONTRAINDICATIONS

First 19 weeks of pregnancy ●

Intrauterine fetal death ●

Preexisting maternal medical conditions adversely affected by betamimetic drugs (eg, hypovolemia, cardiac arrhythmias associated with tachycardia or digitalis intoxication, uncontrolled hypertension, pheochromocytoma, bronchial asthma already treated with betamimetics and/or steroids) ●

Pulmonary hypotension ●

Antepartum hemorrhage demanding immediate delivery ●

Chorioamnionitis ●

Maternal hyperthyroidism ●

Hypersensitivity to any component ●

Eclampsia and severe preeclampsia ●

Maternal cardiac disease ●

Uncontrolled maternal diabetes mellitus (see WARNINGS/PRECAUTIONS) ●

WARNINGS/PRECAUTIONS

Pulmonary edema	May occur (rarely) and may be fatal (one case) in patients treated concomitantly with ritodrine and corticosteroids; discontinue use and treat edema by conventional means
Adverse cardiovascular effects	May occur, especially with IV use; closely monitor maternal pulse rate and blood pressure and fetal heart rate. Observe for maternal signs and symptoms of pulmonary edema. Occult cardiac disease may be unmasked.
Special-risk patients	Administer to patients with mild to moderate preeclampsia, hypertension, or diabetes only when potential benefits clearly outweigh risks
Premature rupture of membranes	Balance benefits of delaying delivery against risks of developing chorioamnionitis
Intrauterine growth retardation	Occurs in 9% of low-birth-weight infants; assess fetal maturity, particularly if in doubt. Continue or reinitiate ritodrine therapy accordingly.
Glucose and electrolyte levels	Should be monitored closely when treating diabetic patients or those receiving potassium-depleting diuretics
IV solution	Do not use if discolored or contains any precipitate or particulate matter

ADVERSE REACTIONS — Frequent reactions are italicized

With oral use

Cardiovascular	*Small increases in maternal heart rate (<50%), palpitation (10–15%), arrhythmia (1%)*
Central nervous system	*Tremor (10–15%), jitteriness (5–8%)*
Gastrointestinal	*Nausea (5–8%)*
Dermatological	*Rash (3–4%)*

With IV use

Cardiovascular	*Alterations in maternal heart rate and blood pressure and fetal heart rate (80–100%), palpitation (33%), chest pain or tightness (1–2%),* heart murmur
Central nervous system	*Tremor (10–15%), headache (10–15%), nervousness (5–6%), jitteriness (5–6%), restlessness (5–6%), emotional upsets or anxiety (5–6%), malaise (5–6%),* drowsiness, weakness
Gastrointestinal	*Nausea (10–15%), vomiting (10–15%),* epigastric distress, ileus, bloating, constipation, diarrhea
Respiratory	Dyspnea, hyperventilation
Dermatological	*Erythema (10–15%),* rash
Neonatal	Hypoglycemia, ileus, hypocalcemia, hypotension
Other	Anaphylactic shock, hemolytic icterus, glycosuria, lactic acidosis, sweating, chills

OVERDOSAGE

Signs and symptoms	Maternal and fetal tachycardia, palpitation, cardiac arrhythmia, hypotension, dyspnea, nervousness, tremor, nausea, vomiting
Treatment	For oral overdosage, empty stomach by emesis or gastric lavage, followed by activated charcoal. For IV overdose, discontinue use and administer an appropriate beta-adrenergic blocking agent. Dialysis may be helpful.

DRUG INTERACTIONS

Corticosteroids	⇧ Risk of pulmonary edema
Other sympathomimetics	⇧ Sympathomimetic effects
Beta-adrenergic blocking agents	⇩ Ritodrine effect
Anesthetics	⇧ Hypotensive effect

ALTERED LABORATORY VALUES

Blood/serum values	⇧ Glucose ⇩ Potassium
Urinary values	⇧ Glucose

Use in children

Not indicated

Use in pregnancy or nursing mothers

See INDICATIONS for use during pregnancy; not indicated for use in nursing mothers

Achieving Good Health

Facts and Fallacies

Americans are increasingly aware that each individual is responsible for his or her own good health. Physicians and other health care professionals can advise, diagnose, and treat, but it is up to each individual to follow through, to, in essence, "heal thyself." The major problem lies in who and what to believe. Americans are bombarded with health information; unfortunately, much of it is confusing, conflicting, or simply false. How does a person determine what is valid and what is nonsense? Sadly, there is no easy answer or simple formula, although in most instances, understanding the basic principles of medicine, such as those described in this book, and using judicious commonsense will point the way. In this chapter, some of the basics of sound preventive medicine will be reviewed, as well as examples of fads and fringe medicine that attract many followers but have little if any value in promoting or preserving good health.

PREVENTIVE MEDICINE

The concept that some diseases may be prevented or at least forestalled is a topic of growing interest and ongoing debate among both physicians and patients. American doctors are often accused of concentrating most of their attention on diagnosing and treating established diseases rather than preventing their occurrence. Many physicians counter by asserting that, with a few notable exceptions, there is little scientific proof that most chronic or disabling diseases can be prevented by currently available knowledge or techniques. The exceptions include diseases that can be prevented by immunization and those that are a direct result of cigarette smoking, alcohol or drug abuse, and certain nutritional deficiences.

Contrary to popular belief, there is no scientific proof that any specific dietary practice, exercise regimen, or other activity will unfailingly prevent heart disease, diabetes, strokes, arthritis, cancer, or any other chronic or degenerative disease. This does not mean, however, that life-style is unimportant or that preventive medicine is still beyond our reach. It is generally accepted that most degenerative diseases, the major causes of death in all Western or industrialized societies, are complex processes with multiple causes, many of which can be prevented by good hygiene, and others that are unknown, poorly understood, or beyond our control.

Cardiovascular disease is a good example. No one knows why one person will fall victim to a heart attack in the prime of life and others with a similar background will escape, but it is possible to identify risk factors that appear to increase vulnerability. By avoiding, altering, or minimizing these risk factors—controlling high blood pressure, not smoking, and lowering elevated cholesterol levels, among others—in population groups that are particularly susceptible—for example, middle-aged men—it should be possible to reduce the overall incidence of heart attacks and strokes. In fact, the ongoing Framingham Heart Study—one of the most extensive epidemiological studies undertaken in this country—has found that the probability of suffering a heart attack by age fifty-three is thirty times higher for a forty-five-year-old man who smokes, and has untreated high blood pressure and an elevated cholesterol level than for a man without these risk factors.[1]

Obviously, preventive medicine is not an exact science with clear-cut rules or formulas to follow. However, studies have found that adhering to a generally healthy life-style markedly affects the incidence of disease and longevity. For example, the Human Population Laboratory of Alameda County, California, studied the effects on health of seven simple life habits: (1) eating moderately, (2) eating meals at regular times, (3) eating breakfast, (4) not smoking cigarettes, (5) drinking little or no alcohol, (6) engaging in regular physical activity, and (7) sleeping seven to eight hours each night. The researchers found that persons who followed six or seven of these health practices enjoyed better health and could expect to live longer than those who practiced five or fewer. Specifically, the study found that the average health of persons seventy years old who followed all seven health habits was comparable to that of persons thirty-five to forty years old who followed fewer than three. A forty-five-year-old man who adhered to all seven health practices could expect to live eleven years longer than a man of the same age who followed only three or fewer.[2] It should be noted that none of these health practices requires extraordinary measures; instead, all are grounded in commonsense and moderation.

Even people who follow a healthy life-style and enjoy good health occasionally fall ill and require medical care. Treatment in the early stages of a disease often ensures a better outcome; therefore, even healthy people should be aware of the warning signs that are a signal to seek medical attention. These warning signs include:

- A sore that does not heal.
- Chronic indigestion.
- Unusual shortness of breath or chest pains, especially during or after exercise.
- Nagging cough, hoarseness, or difficulty in swallowing.
- Any unusual bleeding or discharge.
- A thickening or lump in the breast or elsewhere.
- An unexplained change in bowel or bladder habits.
- Obvious changes in a wart or mole.
- A fever that lasts more than a day or two or that is very high (more than 103° F).
- Any fainting, seizure, temporary paralysis, or altered state of consciousness.
- Persistent or unexplained pain.
- Unusual changes in sleep, weight, and other routine life patterns.

FINDING THE RIGHT MEDICAL CARE

The health-care delivery system is the third largest industry in the United States, accounting for a total expenditure of $200 billion a year. For many persons, however, the abundance of choices in health care is a mixed blessing; while the most advanced medical care in the world is available in this country, it is also possible to fall into the hands of incompetent or unscrupulous physicians or practitioners of fringe or alternative medicine. Very often, patients go from doctor to doctor, seeking out different specialists to diagnose and treat vague, poorly defined symptoms or provide relief where others have failed. Finding out whom to see or where to go for appropriate health care is, for many persons, a frustrating and expensive exercise.

Medicine, like many other facets of modern life, has changed greatly in recent decades. Improvements in curing or treating many diseases have resulted in increased expectations that, in some instances, still cannot be fulfilled. As a result, many Americans seek out an array of alternative practitioners who offer a variety of unorthodox approaches to health care.

UNORTHODOX MEDICINE

Unorthodox or alternative practitioners are often denounced by the medical establishment—physicians, nurses, pharmacists, and other recognized health professionals—as "faddists" or "quacks," although some, such as chiropractors, often call themselves doctors and offer treatments that border on accepted medicine. Whether or not these unorthodox practices have any merit, they often attract large numbers of followers—particularly among persons with chronic diseases for which there are no cures—and create considerable confusion among persons trying to assume a more educated approach to their own health care. The charlatan is often difficult to distinguish from the legitimate health professional, especially since many practice in gray areas, such as nutrition or psychiatry, in which even the most knowledgeable experts disagree.

HISTORIC PERSPECTIVE

It is important to understand that most of modern medicine has evolved only in this century. Until the late 1800s, much of medicine was still rooted in folk wisdom, the tradition of the early Greek and Roman physicians, the magic of the shaman or medicine man, some rather primitive surgical techniques, and an abiding belief that healing was an art rather than a science. Indeed, it took physicians centuries to learn that such practices as applying leeches, pouring boiling oil into wounds, or swallowing everything from pulverized emeralds and rubies in red wine to snake oil and concoctions of herbs was either absurd or harmful, and had little effect on whether the patient got better or worse.

Medicine today is increasingly dominated by science and technology. In recent decades, the introduction of antibiotics, effective psychotropic agents, and hosts of other drugs so numerous that only a fraction can be included in a volume of this size, has markedly changed that nature of medical practice. Other advances, such as kidney machines, organ transplants, and microsurgery, combined with improved nutrition, sanitation, and public health practices, give an ever-increasing number of people the opportunity to reach old age. But disease and suffering have not been eliminated, and it is unlikely that they ever will be. Therefore, it seems likely that people will continue to turn to unorthodox or fringe medicine for remedies beyond the power of conventional practices.

SOURCES OF CONFUSION

Medicine itself is in a state of constant change. What is accepted medical practice today may be considered outmoded, faddist, or absurd a decade from now; by the same token, what is looked upon as unproven fringe medicine may one day be accepted as standard treatment.

Doctors in one area or country often approach the same medical problem very differently, with equally effective results. Who is right and who is wrong? Where does one draw the lines between medical wisdom, doubt, malpractice, and outright quackery or fraud? Unfortunately, there is often no clear-cut answer, especially in dealing with subjective opinions and small effects. This is particularly true in the use of drugs. No one doubted that penicillin worked wonders. On the other hand, some drug investigations require years of controlled studies involving thousands of patients to determine long-term safety or true effectiveness. Other results are so subjective or conflicting—vitamin C in colds, for example — that definite proof probably will never be obtained on either side.

GUIDANCE FOR THE LAYMAN

As noted earlier, the major obstacle encountered by a layman attempting to become a more knowledgeable participant in his or her own health care is sorting out valid, useful information from useless or even harmful misinformation—a task further complicated by a lack of clear answers to many perplexing questions. Special interest groups quickly rally on all sides of virtually every issue, as witness the current controversies over the use of laetrile to treat cancer or the use of saccharin or nitrates in foods. While it is not possible to offer a foolproof checklist that will separate the legitimate health professional who can provide beneficial guidance or services from the faddist of little or no merit, there are certain claims or practices that should alert the consumer to the possibility of quackery. These include:

Nutrition therapists who offer vitamin, herbal or "natural" food cures In recent years we have seen a pronounced "back to nature" movement, spurred by health food stores, a proliferation of organic products, and a growing public suspicion of established medicine and the food and drug industries. Many people have the mistaken notion that so-called natural vitamins and foods are somehow metabolized differently from manufactured or processed ones. To be sure, many processed foods contain unnecessary, even potentially harmful additives and other substances, and the typical American diet could be improved. But blind adherence to unproved nutritional theories and consumption of large doses of "natural" vitamins and minerals also can be detrimental.

The growing popularity of herbal medicine warrants extra caution. Many people believe that herbs are safe alternatives to drugs, and turn to them on the basis of personal testimonials or outdated texts rooted in folk medicine. Many herbs, if taken in sufficient quantity, are poisonous, causing severe side effects and even death. While some herbs do have pharmacological properties similar to drugs, they are seldom as effective as a scientifically developed and tested drug; herbal products are not subjected to the same stringent quality control as drugs, and they generally are much more expensive. In addition, the use of herbs instead of the proper drugs often means that effective medical treatment is needlessly withheld or delayed, often with serious consequences. For example, drinking garlic juice to control blood pressure or treat an infection—to mention one current herbal fad—is of little if any medical benefit, especially when compared to the variety of safe, effective, and inexpensive drugs available for these medical conditions. In addition, deaths have been reported when pharmacological doses of garlic juice were administered to children.[3] Certain other herbal remedies may be even more dangerous. For example, teas brewed of foxglove contain digitoxin and other heart stimulants. This herbal drink may cause life-threatening overdoses in people with heart disease or patients already taking digitalis. Of course, many herbal and home treatments are harmless, and some may have marginal value. Still, one should always consult a physician or pharmacist before taking any herb treatment or home remedy that has pharmacological effects.

Diet "doctors" who promise painless weight loss without a need to lower food consumption or alter eating habits Millions of overweight Americans are constantly searching for that magic diet scheme that will melt away fat without exercise or reduced food intake. Sadly, there is no such diet. The only safe and effective way to lose large amounts of weight and then maintain one's ideal weight is to do so under the supervision of a physician or other recognized health professional who emphasizes the need to alter long-term eating behavior. Most crash or fad diets work initially, but unless eating habits are changed, the weight will be regained in a short time.

Schemes to restore youth, enhance sexual function, increase breast size or body build, and other such miracles The desire to be young, beautiful, and sexually attractive is as old as mankind; indeed, the search for eternal youth predates by centuries Ponce de Leon's quest for the magic fountain of youth. Nor have we grown any wiser through the centuries, as witness the billions of dollars spent each year on a mind-boggling array of creams, potions, and secret formulas promising to erase wrinkles, melt unsightly bulges, increase sexual performance, build muscles without exercise, or perform any number of other desired but generally impossible transformations. Most of these schemes and products are quite harmless and equally ineffective. They also tend to be expensive.

The use of the title "doctor" by persons without an M.D. or comparable degree Many faddist or fringe practitioners invoke a scientific or medical mystique by using the title doctor or listing strings of initials for unusual nonmedical degrees after their names. Common examples include Ms. D. for Doctor of Metaphysics, N.D. for Doctor of Naturopathy, or DHM for Doctor of Herbal Medicine. Some hold medical degrees but lack the advanced training and licenses required to practice medicine. Legitimate medical education and training can be verified by contacting a local medical society or looking up the doctor's name in any of several reference books available in public libraries. These references include *The Directory of Medical Specialists* and the *American Medical Association Directory*. These directories tell where and when a physician graduated from medical school and specify advanced training, area of specialty, and medical licensure.

Special caution should be exercised in consulting nonphysicians who offer cures or treatments for serious diseases such as cancer or arthritis that are unavailable elsewhere. Cancer quacks commonly claim their breakthroughs or cures have been withheld from the public by a conspiracy of the medical establishment and the government. Medical fraud and quackery are deplorable under any circumstance, but are particularly reprehensible when the targets are victims of cancer, arthritis, or other chronic, painful diseases. Unfortunately, conventional medicine often cannot cure or satisfactorily relieve these diseases, and in understandable desperation, the victim or family will grasp at anything that promises hope or relief. The unsuspecting victims may mistakenly believe they are receiving a legitimate experimental drug or therapy, but these are almost always administered in recognized medical settings, such as a teaching hospital or medical center, and are administered only by licensed medical practitioners. In contrast, the quack usually is not affiliated with an established medical facility, often does not have a medical degree, and will tell patients that he or she has been forced to operate in secret. In many instances, the patients must travel to Mexico or other countries to obtain the treatments because they have been proven harmful or ineffective and are barred in this country.

Undue emphasis on paying in advance, buying an entire course of treatments, equipment, or other expensive paraphernalia Gadgetry is a common characteristic of medical fraud, but it is often difficult for the unsuspecting patient to distinguish a legitimate medical device from a worthless gimmick. Claims that the practitioner's own invention is unavailable elsewhere or documentation of its efficacy by personal testimonials only rather than by unbiased scientific studies are warnings that medical fraud may be involved.

A mixture of medical with cultist theories and practices Again, this is an area rife with fraud, but one that is hard to control or eliminate because the promoters usually practice within the law. Some regimens require a rigid diet or life-style rooted in Eastern religious practices. The practices may be quite harmlesss, especially for healthy persons. But again, the regimens are of little or no medical value when applied to serious diseases, and can be quite harmful under certain circumstances. For example, a very restricted Zen macrobiotic diet can lead to serious malnutrition if followed by a pregnant woman or person debilitated by cancer or other wasting diseases.

THE PLACEBO EFFECT

If faddist or quack remedies are worthless, why do so many people insist they work? Very often, the answer lies in a little-understood phenomenon known as the placebo effect. "Placebo" is Latin for "I shall please" and refers to the beneficial effect patients experience after taking an inactive substance (such as a sugar pill) that the patient *thinks* will be therapeutic or beneficial. The placebo effect takes place for both useless and efficacious drugs, and occurs in about 30 percent of all patients, sometimes in even dire circumstances and for a surprisingly long time. In addition, verbal assurances also appear to have a placebo effect, especially against vague, often subjective disorders such as arthritis, pain syndromes, fatigue, insomnia, and cold. In many instances, simple assurance from a doctor or dentist that the pain will disappear or the condition improve helps make it happen.

Many diseases like arthritis have natural remissions and exacerbations of symptoms. If a remission of arthritis happens to coincide with the wearing of a copper bracelet or a session of bee-sting treatments, the natural tendency is to attribute the change to the therapy rather than to the natural course of the disease.

OTHER GRAY AREAS

An especially difficult and confusing area for consumers to judge involves practices that are beneficial under certain circumstances and fraud under others. Hypnosis, biofeedback, and various forms of psychiatric therapy are common examples of potentially useful techniques that are frequently misused. The setting in which the technique is offered can often help the patient decide. Hypnosis used for pain control by a dentist trained in the medical application of the technique is useful, especially for patients who cannot tolerate anesthetic. Similarly, biofeedback techniques taught at a recognized pain clinic or rehabilitation center may provide relief where conventional approaches have failed. But when the techniques are used outside a medical setting and are promoted by persons who are not medical professionals as miracle cures for serious diseases, investigate further before embarking on treatment.

A SPECIAL WARNING

Many of the fringe or alternative treatments discussed in this chapter are essentially harmless in and of themselves; their major harm lies in the fact that the patient may neglect or omit proper and potentially effective treatment while resorting to an expensive but worthless remedy. In some instances, however, the treatments themselves may be harmful, or even lethal. An example is the increasingly popular therapy advocated by some practitioners of "holistic" medicine that involves a regimen of vitamins, "natural foods," and periodic coffee enemas. At least two deaths—one of a forty-six-year-old woman with bronchopneumonia and the other of a thirty-seven-year-old woman with cancer—have been attributed to electrolyte imbalances as a result of coffee enemas every few hours.[4] In both instances, the women had refused conventional treatments that could have saved or prolonged their lives. Other examples of potentially dangerous unorthodox treatments include the use of DMSO (dimethyl sulfoxide) to treat arthritis and other painful conditions and thyroid hormone treatments to lose weight.

IN CONCLUSION

Fringe medicine, quackery, and alternative treatments have paralleled or reacted to the medical establishment for years. Within the last century, conventional medicine has proved its worth by bettering the lot of mankind. Today, most of the claims and absurdities of faddism and quackery can be dismissed through logic and scientific examination. But human nature, imagination, and frustration persist; therefore, it seems likely that fads, fringe medicine, and outright fraud will continue to flourish. Many of the practices are essentially harmless, and are of little or no value except to their promoters. Whenever straying from established medical practice and practitioners, the patient should be suspicious and wary. Any treatment or cure that seems almost too good to be true and yet is scorned or rejected by the medical community is likely to be just that—too good to be true.

---

1. Kannel, W.B. Some Lessons in Cardiovascular Epidemiology from Framingham, *American Journal of Cardiology*, 37:269-282, 1976.

2. Belloc, N.B., and Breslow, L. Relationships of Physical Health Status and Practices, *Preventive Medicine*, 1:409-421, 1972.

3. Spoerke, D.G. Herbal Medication: Use and Misuse, *Hospital Formulary*, 941-951, December, 1980.

4. Eisele, J.S., and Reay, D.T. Deaths Related to Coffee Enemas, *Journal of the American Medical Association*, 244 (14) 1608-1609, 1980.

Appendix

Glossary of common medical and drug-related terms

abscess • A pus-filled cavity that may occur almost anywhere in the body.

Absidia • A genus of fungi, some species of which cause disease in man and animals.

accommodation • Adjustment or adaptation; specifically, the ability of the eye to change its focus.

ACD • Acid, citrate, and dextrose; an anticoagulant solution used when collecting blood for transfusions.

acetone • A ketone (chemical formula CH_3COCH_3) that is normally found in the blood and urine. In diabetics, the level of acetone may be greatly increased.

acetonuria • Large amounts of acetone, an acidic substance, in the urine. Acetonuria frequently occurs in diabetics.

acetylation • Formation of compounds with the atomic group CH_3CO (acetyl), as in acetic acid.

acidosis • Abnormally high acidity of the blood, caused by faulty metabolism and elimination of acidic chemicals from the body.

acne urticaria • A form of acne with itching patches.

acne vulgaris • Simple, uncomplicated acne.

acrocyanosis • Mottled cyanosis (bluish coloration) of the hands and feet, caused by local constriction of the blood vessels, generally brought on by cold or strong emotion.

acroparesthesia • Numbness, tingling, "pins and needles" sensation, or pain in the extremities, caused by either restricted circulation or increased sensitivity of the nerves.

ACTH • Adrenocorticotrophic hormone; ACTH is secreted by the pituitary gland and influences the functioning of the adrenal and other glands.

actinic rash • Dermatitis caused by exposure to sunlight, x-rays, or other radiant energy.

Actinomyces • A genus of bacteria characterized by delicate branching filaments that tend to fragment.

actinomycosis • A fungal disease seen mostly in cattle and hogs that less commonly affects humans, characterized by chronic destructive abscesses that discharge; commonly known as "lumpy jaw."

activated charcoal • Charcoal that has been treated to increase its adsorptive power, frequently used as an antidote to absorb toxic substances.

acute • Of limited duration; having a rapid onset, distinct symptoms, and a short course; opposite of chronic.

Adams-Stokes syndrome • A syndrome usually caused by poor conduction of nerve impulses in the heart, characterized by slow or absent pulse, dizziness and fainting, alterations in breathing patterns, and convulsions.

Addison's disease • Insufficiency of the adrenal glands; symptoms include weakness, darkening of the skin, low blood pressure, and various gastrointestinal problems.

adenitis • Inflammation of a lymph node or gland.

adenoma • A tumor, usually benign, that forms a gland-like structure.

adenopathy • Any glandular disorder.

adenosine triphosphatase • An enzyme that breaks down adenosine triphosphate. Abbreviated ATPase.

adenosine triphosphate • A chemical that supplies energy to the cells for muscle activity and other cellular processes. Abbreviated ATP.

ADH • Antidiuretic hormone.

adjunctive • Supportive; a treatment that complements another form of therapy or helps to relieve secondary symptoms of a condition requiring therapy.

adnexa • Accessory parts or appendages of an organ.

adrenochrome • A red crystal produced by the oxidation of adrenaline; it is a strong stimulant but has no current therapeutic use.

adrenocorticotrophic hormone • The hormone that stimulates activity of the adrenal glands. Abbreviated ACTH.

adrenergic • Sympathetic nerves that liberate adrenaline and noradrenaline.

adventitious • Accidental; *or* coming from without; *or* pertaining to the outer coat of an organ or structure.

adynamic ileus • Bowel obstruction (ileus) caused by muscle weakness or paralysis (adynamia), usually accompanied by vomiting, fever, and severe pain.

aerophagia • Excessive swallowing of air.

aerotitis • An acute or chronic traumatic inflammation of the middle ear; often occurs on descent in an aircraft.

afebrile • Without fever.

African trypanosomiasis • African sleeping sickness.

agonist • A drug capable of combining with a cellular receptor to produce a specific response; *or* a muscle that contracts to make movement possible.

agranulocytosis • A decrease in the number of granulocytes—a type of white cell—in the blood.

akathisia • Restlessness and quivering; inability to remain sitting.

akinetic seizure • An epileptic attack characterized by lack of movement.

albumin • A simple protein that is one of the major components of animal tissue.

albuminuria • Presence of the protein albumin in the urine; proteinuria.

alimentary tract • The organs and general region involved in the ingestion and digestion of food.

alkaline phosphatase • A phosphatase—an enzyme that participates in several metabolic processes, including bone formation—that is active in alkaline media.

alkalosis • Excessive alkalinity of the blood, characterized by dizziness, jerky muscle movements, and other symptoms.

alkylating agents • Anticancer drugs that act by interfering with DNA function and disrupting cell division.

alopecia • Loss of hair.

alpha-hemolytic • Causing partial disintegration of red cells in a blood agar medium. The term is used to classify certain infectious bacteria; compare *beta-hemolytic.*

alveolar ventilation • The regular exchange of air in the alveoli, the tiny air sacs in the lungs.

alveolitis • Inflammation of a tooth socket, usually following removal of the tooth; also called dry socket.

amaurosis • Blindness due to a defect of the optic nerve.

amblyopia • Dim vision.

amebiasis • Parasitic infection caused by *Entamoeba histolytica* or other pathogenic amoebas.

amenorrhea • Absence or abnormal cessation of menses.

aminoglycoside • Any of a group of antibiotics derived from various species of *Streptomyces.*

amphetamine • A nervous system stimulant, similar in functions and structure to adrenaline.

amps • Ampuls.

ampul • A hermetically sealed glass container for holding sterile preparations, usually for injection.

ampullar • Pertaining to the mouth of a small canal or duct (ampulla).

amylase • A group of enzymes that are active in the metabolism of carbohydrates.

amyloidosis • A disease characterized by extracellular accumulation of amyloid (protein); the cause is unknown.

ANA • Antinuclear antibody.

anaerobic • Growing best in an oxygen-free environment.

analeptic • A drug that restores consciousness or stimulates increased activity of the central nervous system.

anaphylactoid • Resembling anaphylaxis.

anaphylaxis • A severe and sudden hypersensitivity reaction that may lead to sudden loss of consciousness, severe asthma, shock, and, if not reversed, death.

anastomosis • Interconnection, either surgical or natural, between blood vessels, nerves, or normally distinct hollow organs or spaces.

androgens • Hormones secreted by the testes and adrenal cortex that trigger the development of male secondary sex characteristics such as deepening of voice, muscular growth, and chest hair.

anetoderma • A skin rash characterized by small, discolored, inflamed spots; in later stages the spots may become wrinkled and depressed or raised.

aneurysm • A place in a blood vessel where the vascular wall has weakened, resulting in stretching and swelling of the vessel.

angiitis • Inflammation of a blood vessel or lymph node.

angina pectoris • Spasmodic pain in the chest and, sometimes, the arms, caused by an inadequate supply of blood and oxygen to the heart, usually brought on by exercise or emotion.

angioedema • A benign allergic disorder marked by the growth of local allergic wheals, accompanied by tissue swelling.

angioneurotic edema • A localized, temporary swelling under the skin; may occur in the face, neck, hands, feet, genitals, or, more rarely, elsewhere.

anhidrosis • Inability to sweat.

ankylosing spondylitis • Arthritis of the spine.

anogenital • Pertaining to the anus and the genital organs.

anorexia • Loss of appetite.

anovulation • Suspension or cessation of ovulation.

anovulatory infertility • Infertility due to a permanent or temporary failure to ovulate.

antagonist • A drug that specifically counteracts another drug; *or* a muscle that counteracts the action of another muscle.

antibody • A component of the immune system that attacks foreign protein, bacteria, or other substances, thereby killing them or neutralizing their effects.

anticholinergic • Blocking the actions of the parasympathetic nervous system; inhibiting slowing of heartbeat, dilation of blood vessels, and other parasympathetic functions.

anticoagulant drugs • Drugs that retard or prevent the formation of blood clots.

antidiuretic hormone • A hormone that stimuilates constriction of the smooth muscles of the blood vessels, thus raising blood pressure and countering the effects of diuretics, which tend to lower blood pressure. Also called vasopressin. Abbreviated ADH.

antiemetic • A drug that prevents or relieves nausea and vomiting.

antihistamine • A drug acting as a histamine antagonist; used to treat allergy symptoms.

antimuscarinic • Countering the effects of a muscarine, a parasympathomimetic, and similar drugs. Antimuscarinic drugs inhibit dilation of blood vessels, salivation and other secretions, gastrointestinal activity, and other responses triggered by the parasympathetic nervous system.

antinuclear antibody • An antibody that attacks components of a cell's nucleus, particularly DNA; its presence in the blood is a common indicator of certain arthritic disorders, such as systemic lupus erythematosus.

antiperistaltic • Impeding or arresting peristalsis, the movement of the intestines that propels food through the digestive tract.

antipyretic • An agent tending to reduce fever.

antithrombin • A substance that inhibits the effects of thrombin, preventing the blood from clotting.

antitussive • A cough reliever.

anuria • Inability to urinate or greatly reduced urination, caused either by kidney failure or by obstruction of the urinary tract.

aortic stenosis • Abnormal narrowing of the aorta, the large trunk artery leading from the heart.

aphakia • Absence of the lens of the eye.

aphonia • Inability to speak because of disease or injury to the vocal organs.

aplasia • Defective development of a tissue or organ.

aplastic anemia • Abnormally low levels of red blood cells and other blood elements, caused by failure of cell formation in the bone marrow.

apnea • Suspension or stopping of breathing, usually by inhibition of the breathing reflex.

arachnoiditis • Inflammation of the web-like membrane (arachnoid membrane) covering the brain and spinal cord.

arteriole • A very small artery.

arteriosclerosis • Thickening and hardening of the artery walls, usually associated with aging.

arteriosclerosis obliterans • Arteriosclerosis in which the blood vessel walls grow so thick that they obstruct the flow of blood. The lower legs are often affected, leading to difficulty in walking.

arteriospasm • A spasm in the smooth muscle of an artery.

arthralgia • Pain in a joint.

ASA • Acetylsalicylic acid (aspirin).

ascites • Excess fluid in the abdominal cavity.

aspect • The part or side that faces in a particular position; the particular appearance, as of a face.

aspergillosis • A fungal infection caused by *Aspergillus,* affecting mostly the lungs and bronchi.

Aspergillus niger • A disease-causing fungus with black spores, often present in the external opening of the auditory canal.

aspiration • Inhalation of a liquid; *or* removal of fluid by suction from a body cavity; *or,* when administering a hypodermic injection, periodically pulling back the plunger to draw some of the injected fluid back into the syringe.

aspiration pneumonitis • Inflammation of the lungs due to inhalation of a foreign body into the bronchi.

asterixis • Involuntary jerking movements, especially of the hands, often called "liver flap" because it is a sign of impending hepatic coma.

asthenia • Weakness.

astringent • A substance that shrinks or puckers tissues or mucous membranes and stops secretions or bleeding.

asystole • Cardiac standstill; absence of heart contractions.

ataxia • Lack of muscle control, resulting in jerking movements.

atelectasis • Airlessness, incomplete expansion, or collapse of the lungs.

atherosclerosis • Arteriosclerosis accompanied by deposits of fats, carbohydrates, and other substances along the inner arterial walls.

athetoid • Characterized by slow, writhing involuntary movements, usually of the upper and sometimes of the lower limbs.

atopic dermatitis • A red, extremely itchy rash; eczema.

atopy • Hereditary allergy such as hay fever, eczema, or asthma.

atropine • An extract of belladonna, or deadly nightshade, often used to control convulsions.

ATP • Adenosine triphosphate.

ATPase • Adenosine triphosphatase.

atrial fibrillation • Rapid, irregular, ineffective beating of the atrium, the upper chamber on either side of the heart that receives blood from the veins.

atrial flutter • Rapid, regular beats of the atrium (about 250–400 beats per min), usually accompanied by ventricular beats at half the atrial rate.

atrioventricular • Referring to the atria, the upper heart chambers that receive blood from the veins, and the ventricles, the lower pumping chambers of the heart.

attention deficit disorder • Hyperactivity, hyperkinesis or minimal brain dysfunction, especially in children.

audiogram • A chart showing acuity of hearing as measured by an audiometer.

aura • A sensation preceding an epileptic seizure; may include tingling in parts of the body, perception of sounds or flashes of light, and vertigo.

auricle • The outer ear.

autogenous • Self-generated; originating within the body.

autoimmunity • A condition in which the body develops antibodies against its own substances and cells.

autoimmune hemolytic anemia • Anemia caused when the body develops antibodies to its own red blood cells.

autonomic nervous system • The part of the nervous system controlling involuntary movement, such as the heartbeat, intestinal movement, and dilation and contraction of the blood vessels.

AV • Atrioventricular; referring to the upper and lower heart chambers.

AV block • Atrioventricular block; impairment of normal conduction of nerve impulses between heart chambers.

azoospermia • Absence of live sperm cells in the semen.

azotemia • An excess of nitrogen and nitrogen compounds in the blood.

Bacillus anthracis • A rod-shaped, aerobic, spore-forming bacterium that causes anthrax.

bacteremia • The presence of bacteria in the bloodstream.

bacteriostatic • Inhibiting the growth of bacteria.

Bacteroides • A genus of non-spore-forming, anaerobic, rod-shaped bacteria normally present in the digestive, respiratory, and genital tracts and frequently found in abscesses.

Bartonella bacilliformis • The causative agent of bartonellosis, an infection characterized by an acute feverish anemic stage followed by a nodular skin eruption.

basal ganglia • Masses of grey nerve cells at the cerebral base that are concerned with voluntary muscle movement.

basal metabolism • The minimal energy necessary to sustain breathing, blood circulation, and other vegetative body functions.

Basidiobolus • A genus of fungi of the class Phycomycetes.

bejel • Nonvenereal syphilis occurring in the Middle East.

Bell's palsy • Paralysis of one side of the face.

Benedict's solution • A preparation used in testing urine for glucose.

berylliosis • Pneumonia resulting from inhalation of beryllium, a metallic element.

beta-adrenergic receptor • A tissue site capable of selective activation and blockade by adrenergic (sympathomimetic) drugs, resulting in various physiological responses.

beta blocker • An agent that causes blockade of the site in nerve pathways where inhibitory responses occur.

beta cells • Insulin-producing cells, located in the islets of Langerhans of the pancreas.

beta-hemolytic • Causing complete disintegration of red cells around a colony on a blood agar medium, resulting in a clear zone around the colony. (Compare *alpha-hemolytic*.)

bid • *Bis in die,* twice a day.

biliary • Involving bile or the bile duct.

biliary cirrhosis • Progressive liver disease due to bile-duct obstruction.

biliary stasis • Stagnation of bile in the liver, usually due to blockage of the bile duct.

bilirubin • An orange-red pigment secreted by the liver in bile; excessive amounts of bilirubin in the blood account for the yellow coloring of jaundice. Bilirubin is also produced by the breakdown of red blood cells.

black tongue • Appearance of blackish, yellowish, brownish, or hairy patches on the tongue, usually due to a fungal infection.

blastomycosis • Infection caused by yeast-like fungi, especially *Blastomyces* species.

blepharospasm • Uncontrolled, spasmodic twitching, quivering, or winking of the eyelid.

bone-marrow depression • A condition in which the functions of the bone marrow (chiefly the manufacture of red blood cells) are reduced.

bradyarrhythmia • A disturbance in the heart's rhythm that causes the heart to beat abnormally slowly (less than 60 beats per minute).

bradycardia • Abnormal slowing of the heartbeat; usually, to fewer than 60 beats per minute.

bradykinesia • Extreme slowness in movement.

brawny edema • Thick, hard swellings.

breakthrough bleeding • Prolonged or excessive vaginal bleeding at irregular times in the menstrual cycle, usually seen in women using oral contraceptives.

bromhidrosis • Foul-smelling perspiration.

bronchiectasis • Permanent dilation of one or both bronchi, usually due to bronchial obstruction and infection.

bronchodilation • Dilation or enlargement of the bronchus or the bronchial tubes.

bronchodilator • A drug that causes an increase in the diameter of a bronchus or bronchial tube; used to treat asthma.

bronchogenic • Originating in the bronchial tubes.

bronchogram • X-ray film of the lungs after the introduction of a radiopaque substance.

bronchopneumonia • Inflammation of the walls of the smaller bronchial tubes, sometimes leading to inflammation of the alveolar ducts, cell death, and the formation of abscesses in the lungs.

bronchospasm • Narrowing of the bronchi due to sudden contractions of the bronchial smooth muscle; adjective, *bronchospastic*.

bronchospirometry • The determination of the functional capacity of a single lung or lung segment.

brucellosis • An infectious disease caused by bacteria of the genus *Brucella,* transmitted to man from cattle, hogs, and goats. Also called Malta or Mediterranean fever.

bruxism • Unconscious grinding of the teeth, or grinding of the teeth while asleep.

BSP • Sulfobromophthalein sodium; a substance used to test liver function.

buccal • Of the cheeks; when referring to a drug, a dosage form that is administered to the cheeks.

bullous dermatitis herpetiformis • A blistered or bubbled skin inflammation resembling herpes.

bullous impetigo • Impetigo characterized by large blisters within or beneath the skin, filled with lymphatic fluid.

BUN • Blood urea nitrogen.

bundle branch block • Delay or blockage of electrical impulses through a portion of the heart known as the bundle of His, resulting in irregular heartbeat.

Burkitt's lymphoma • A malignant lymphoma, usually found in Central Africa, involving the facial bone, ovaries, and abdominal lymph nodes.

bursitis • Inflammation of the synovial sacs in a joint.

C • Degrees Celsius.

cachexia • Severe weakness; emaciation.

calcaneal spur • A bony spur of the heel that often forms after an injury or chronic irritation.

calcification • Hardening of an organic substance caused by deposits of calcium.

calculus • A small solid deposit within the body, such as a kidney stone; plural, calculi.

Camplyobacter fetus • A species of bacteria found in the reproductive organs of animals and in the intestinal tract of animals and man.

Candida albicans • A yeast-like organism that under certain conditions may infect the mouth, vagina, gastrointestinal tract, or other areas of the body.

candidiasis • Infection by organisms of the genus *Candida,* usually *Candida albicans*.

canker sore • A small ulcer or inflammation in the mouth.

caps • Capsules.

carbohydrate • A class of organic compounds, composed of carbon, oxygen, and hydrogen, that includes sugars, starches, dextrins, and celluloses.

carbonic anhydrase • An enzyme present in red blood cells that catalyzes the union of water and carbon dioxide to form carbonic acid.

carcinoma • Any cancerous tumor or growth.

cardiac asthma • Difficult breathing due to heart disease.

cardiac decompensation • Failure or inability of the heart to respond adequately to increased demands upon the circulatory system.

cardiac reserve • The capacity of the heart to increase its output of blood and raise blood pressure to meet body requirements.

cardiogenic • Of cardiac (heart) origin.

cardiomyopathy • Disease of the myocardium (heart muscle).

cardiospasm • Dilatation of the esophagus, due to spasmodic constriction of the lower portion, which is called the cardiac sphincter.

cardioversion • The application of an electric shock to the heart to restore its normal rhythm.

carditis • Inflammation of the heart.

catatonia • Stupor associated with fixed positions, with occasional outbursts or panic attacks.

catecholamines • Compounds such as dopamine, norepinephrine and epinephrine, that have a sympathomimetic action.

cathartic • A drug that causes evacuation of the bowels.

catheter • A flexible hollow tube with numerous uses, including removing or inserting fluid into a body cavity, or examining an internal organ, such as the heart.

CBC • Complete blood count.

CCr • Creatinine clearance rate; measured in testing kidney function.

cellulitis • Inflammation of the connective tissues, especially subcutaneous tissue.

central nervous system • The brain and spinal cord.

centrencephalic epilepsy • A form of epilepsy in which the seizures arise in the interconnecting neurons between hemispheres of the brain, so that both sides of the brain are affected.

cephalosporin • Any of a group of broad-spectrum antibiotics derived from certain species of *Cephalosporium.*

cerebral thrombosis • The formation of a blood clot within the blood vessels of the cerebrum.

cerebrospinal fluid • The fluid surrounding the brain and the spinal cord. Abbreviated CSF.

cerebrum • The largest, upper section of the brain; the seat of the higher mental functions such as perception, thought, and voluntary activity.

ceruloplasmin • A blue, copper-containing component of blood plasma.

cervical erosion • The alteration of the outer surface of the cervix as a result of irritation by infection.

cervicitis • Inflammation of the cervix of the uterus.

cervix • A narrow or constricted portion of any organ; specifically, the cervix uteri, the opening of the uterus.

Chagas' disease • Infection with a South American form of *Trypanosoma,* a blood parasite that causes fever, swellings, and in some cases chronic heart disease.

chancroid • A highly infectious, nonsyphilitic venereal ulcer.

cheilosis • Drying, chapping, and cracking of the lips caused by a vitamin B_2 deficiency.

chelating agent • An organic molecule that is able to bond a metal atom so that the resulting compound is a ring-type structure.

chemoprophylactic • Any chemical or drug used to prevent a specific disease.

chemotherapy • The treatment of a disease with chemical agents.

Cheyne-Stokes respiration • Cyclical waxing and waning of respiration; alternating hyperpnea and apnea.

chilblains • Mild frostbite; redness or inflammation of the hands and feet from cold or dampness, sometimes becoming chapped, ulcerated, or itchy.

chlamydial • Caused by virus-like bacteria of the genus *Chlamydia.*

chloasma • Extensive, irregular brown patches on facial skin and elsewhere, also called the "mask" of pregnancy; occurs during pregnancy and with oral contraceptive use.

cholelithiasis • Stones in the gallbladder or bile ducts; gallstones.

cholestatic jaundice • Jaundice caused by stoppage of the normal flow of bile into the digestive system.

chorea • Involuntary jerking or twitching caused by spasms of muscles in the limbs or face; chorea is a principal characteristic of St. Vitus's dance in children and Huntington's disease.

choreiform movements • Involuntary, irregular writhing and twisting movements of the limbs and face, characteristic of Huntington's disease.

choriocarcinoma • A highly malignant cancer, usually arising in the uterus and rapidly spreading to the lungs, liver, brain, vagina, and other pelvic organs.

chorioretinitis • Inflammation of the retina and the choroid, the outer membrane covering most of the eyeball.

choroiditis • Inflammation of the choroid, the outer membrane covering most of the eyeball.

chromoblastomycosis • A pigmented fungus infection of the skin and subcutaneous tissues.

chrysiasis • A change in skin color caused by injection of gold salts or other gold preparations.

ciliary • Referring to the eyelashes and hairlike structures, particularly the muscles of the iris.

cinchonism • Poisoning by cinchona (dried bark, root, and stem of the *Cinhcona* species), quinine, or quinidine; characterized by ringing in the ears (tinnitus), deafness, headache, and shock.

circumoral • Around the mouth.

cisterna • Any closed body cavity or space that serves as a reservoir for body fluid.

Citrobacter • A genus of bacteria that utilize citrate as a sole source of carbon.

claudication • Limping; lameness.

climacteric • The glandular, metabolic, and psychological changes in women that precede and bring about menopause.

clonus • Rapid, successive muscular contractions and relaxations resulting in convulsive movements.

Clostridium difficile • A species of bacteria found in the feces of newborn infants.

cluster headaches • A migraine variant in which the attacks, lasting 15–30 min, usually occur in clusters. Cluster headaches are characterized by severe pain over the eye and forehead and are accompanied by fever, tearing, and runny nose.

CNS • Central nervous system.

coagulation • The congealing of blood into a clot.

coagulopathy • Any disease affecting blood clotting.

coal tar • A coal by-product used to treat skin diseases, such as psoriasis.

coccidioidomycosis • A fungal infection, commonly referred to as desert fever, usually caused by inhaling spores of *Coccidioides immitis,* endemic in southwestern United States and Mexico.

cochlea • The shell-like structure in the inner ear where sound impulses come in contact with the auditory nerve.

colitis • Inflammation of the colon.

collagen • The protein that forms the white fibers of the body: the cartilage, connective tissues, tendons, and bones.

colon • The large intestine, divided into three major sections, called ascending colon, transverse colon, and descending colon.

comedo • A pimple; plural, comedones.

compression fracture • A fracture in which a surface of a bone is driven toward another bony surface; commonly found in vertebral bodies.

conc • Concentrate.

congestive heart failure • Inability of the heart to maintain an adequate outflow of blood, resulting in congestion or stretching of certain veins and organs and inadequate supply of blood to other areas of the body.

conjunctiva • The membranes lining the inner eyelid and anterior portion of the eyeball.

conjunctival injection • Increased flow of blood in conjunctiva, causing distended blood vessels.

conjunctivitis • Inflammation of the conjunctiva; pinkeye.

contact dermatitis • Skin inflammation acquired by contact with a chemical irritant.

Coombs' test • A blood test to determine whether red blood cells are coated with antibodies; Coombs' tests are often performed on the cord blood of newborn infants of Rh-negative mothers.

cord blood • Blood drawn from the umbilical cord of a gestating fetus.

coronary occlusion • Blockage of the arteries that supply blood to the heart muscle.

cor pulmonale • Strain of the right side of the heart (the side that pumps blood to the lungs), resulting from lung disease or pulmonary hypertension.

corticoid • Having an action similar to that of a steroid hormone of the adrenal cortex.

corticosteroids • Steroid hormones produced by the adrenal cortex, used to treat many inflammatory diseases, as well as to suppress tumor growth.

cortisol • Hydrocortisone, an essential adrenal hormone and the most potent naturally occurring glucocorticoid.

Corynebacterium diptheria • The causative organism of diptheria.

Corynebacterium minutissimum • The causative organism of erythrasma, a contagious skin disease that attacks the armpits or groin.

coryza • Common cold or infection of the upper respiratory tract.

costovertebral • Pertaining to the junction of the ribs and vertebrae and the surrounding area.

cradle cap • An infant skin disease characterized by heavy, greasy crusts on the baby's skull.

craniotomy • A surgical opening of the skull made to relieve pressure, stop hemorrhage, or remove a tumor.

creatinine phosphokinase • An enzyme found in heart and skeletal muscles, used to diagnose heart attacks and certain muscle diseases.

creatinine clearance rate • The rate at which creatinine, a waste product of muscular activity, is excreted by the kidneys; used as a measure of overall kidney function. Abbreviated CCr.

croup • Disease characterized by suffocative and difficult breathing, laryngeal spasm, and sometimes by the formation of a membrane in the breathing passages.

cryptococcosis • A fungal or yeast infection that may affect the central nervous system, causing meningitis, and less commonly the lungs, bone, and skin. Caused by *Cryptococcus neoformans.*

cryptorchidism • Presence of an undescended testicle.

crystalluria • Crystals in the urine; moderate amounts of crystals are a normal condition.

CSF • Cerebrospinal fluid.

curare • An extract from a South American plant used in surgery to produce complete muscle relaxation.

curariform • Having an action like curare.

Cushing's syndrome • Excessive secretion of adrenal hormones, caused by a tumor of the adrenal gland; symptoms include hypertension, obesity (especially about the face), abnormal carbohydrate metabolism, and, in women, menstrual abnormalities and hirsutism.

Cushingoid • Resembling Cushing's syndrome.

cutaneous • Referring to the skin.

CVP • Cardiovascular pressure.

cyanosis • Bluish discoloration of the skin and mucous membranes due to the presence of large amounts of reduced hemoglobin (venous blood) in the capillaries.

cyclic disorder • A psychological disease, such as manic depression, in which the different states alternate in regular progression.

cycloplegia • Loss of ability of the eye to change focus or respond to changes in light intensity.

cylindruria • The presence of casts—tube-like bodies that taper to a slender tail—in the urine.

cyst • An abnormal sac containing gas, fluid, or semisolid material; a bladder.

cystine • A common amino acid, found in many proteins.

cystinuria • Presence of cystine in the urine due to the kidneys' inability to reabsorb certain amino acids.

cystitis • Inflammation of the urinary bladder.

cystoscopy • A procedure in which a tubular, lighted instrument is inserted via the urethra into the bladder, allowing the physician to examine it visually.

cytology • The life processes of a cell. *Also* the study of those processes.

cytotoxic • Having the ability to kill cells.

dacryocystitis • Inflammation of the tear-producing glands and their ducts.

dark-field examination • Microscopic examination using oblique, rather than the usual direct, lighting, so that transparent and submicroscopic particles appear illuminated against a dark background.

decubital ulcers • Bed sores.

deep-tendon reflex • An involuntary muscular contraction following impact on muscle, tendons, or bone.

degmacyte • A type of damaged red blood cell.

delirium tremens • Delirium due to alcohol poisoning, characterized by mental confusion, hallucinations, sweating, trembling, anxiety, and other symptoms.

deltoid muscle • The shoulder muscle, extending from the neck down the collar bone to the upper arm.

demulcent • A soothing agent.

dermatitis • Inflammation of the skin. Plural, dermatitides.

dermatitis venenata • Skin inflammation resulting from direct contact with a chemical or other substance. Also called contact dermatitis.

dermatographism • A condition in which the skin is extremely susceptible to irritation; tracing over the skin with a fingernail or instrument leaves red wheals.

dermatomyositis • An inflammatory disorder involving skin and muscles.

dermatophyte • A superficial skin fungus.

dermatosis • Any disease of the skin.

dermis • The layer of skin below the epidermis, containing nerves, blood vessels, sweat glands, hair follicles, and other structures.

dermoid cyst • A congenital cyst, usually on the ovary, that contains elements of nails, hair, and skin.

desmosterol • An intermediate step in the formation of cholesterol, normally not present in the blood in measurable amounts.

desquamating agent • An agent that causes scaly skin to peel off.

diabetes insipidus • A chronic disease characterized by excretion of large amounts of pale, dilute urine and excessive thirst; a metabolic disease originating in the hypothalamus rather than the pancreas (see *diabetes mellitus*).

diabetes mellitus • A chronic disease in which the pancreas secretes an insufficient amount of insulin, reducing the body's ability to metabolize glucose.

dialysis • Filtration of a liquid through a semipermeable membrane to remove large molecules and substances in colloidial suspension; specifically, artificial filtration of the blood to assist the kidneys in removing wastes or other unwanted substances.

diaphoresis • Increased sweating.

diastole • The phase in the heart's pumping rhythm in which the chambers expand and fill with blood.

differential count • A count of each variety of white blood cell, by percentage of the total sample.

digitalization • The introduction into the bloodstream of sufficient amounts of the drug digitalis to have a therapeutic effect on the heart.

dilutional hyponatremia • Low sodium (salt) concentrations in the blood.

diplopia • Double vision.

disc • A thin, round plate of cartilage at the junction oftwo bones; specifically, an invertebral disc.

discogram • An x-ray picture of the intervertebral disc space after a contrasting substance has been injected into it.

diuresis • Increased excretion of urine.

diuretic • A drug that stimulates diuresis.

div • In equally divided doses.

dl • Deciliters.

DNA • Deoxyribonucleic acid. Long, helical chains of molecules found in cell nuclei; the carriers of genetic information from one generation to the next.

dopamine • A substance closely related to adrenaline and noradrenaline that increases the heart's output and blood flow to the kidneys but does not constrict peripheral blood vessels.

Down's syndrome • A group of congenital defects characterized by mental retardation and distinct facial features, formerly called mongolism.

ductus arteriosus • A fetal blood vessel connecting the aorta with the pulmonary artery. The ductus arteriosus generally turns into connective tissue shortly after birth.

duodenal • Of the duodenum.

duodenum • The first 8 or 10 inches of the small intestine, descending from the stomach, containing the openings of the pancreatic duct and the common bile duct.

dysarthria • Any disorder of the tongue or speech muscle that impairs the ability to speak.

dyscrasia • Any abnormal state or disorder.

dysdiadochokinesis • Impairment of the power of smooth, rhythmic alternating movement, such as flexing and extending a limb. Often a sign of minor brain damage.

dysmenorrhea • Painful or difficult menstruation.

dyspareunia • Painful or difficult sexual intercourse.

dysphagia • Difficulty in swallowing.

dysphoria • An uneasy feeling; anxiety; discomfort.

dysplasia • Abnormal cell growth.

dyspnea • Difficulty in breathing.

dysrhythmia • Defective rhythm.

dystonia • Alteration or loss of normal muscle tone.

dysuria • Painful or difficult urination.

ecchymosis • An area where blood has infiltrated from the vessel into the surrounding tissue, causing discoloration of the skin.

eclampsia • A convulsive attack or seizure; particularly, a syndrome occurring in women after childbirth, characterized by convulsions and coma.

ECT • Electroconvulsive therapy.

ectopic • Occurring in the wrong place or at the wrong time.

ectopic pregnancy • A pregnancy in which the embryo is implanted outside the uterus, usually in a fallopian tube.

eczema • Atopic dermatitis; a red, itchy skin rash of unknown cause. Rashes may also be pustulant, scaly, swollen, and weeping.

eczematoid • Resembling eczema.

edema • Swelling of tissue due to excessive accumulation of fluid.

EEG • Electoencephalogram.

effusion • The escape of fluid into a body tissue or cavity.

eighth nerve • The eighth cranial nerve; the nerve that serves the ears and organs of balance.

elastosis • Degeneration of the elastic or connective tissue.

electrocardiogram • A graphic record of the heart's action obtained by monitoring its electric forces with an electrocardiograph. Abbreviated ECG or EKG.

electroconvulsive therapy • Shock therapy; inducing a convulsion by passing an electric current through the brain, as a treatment for mental diseases. Abbreviated ECT.

electroencephalogram • A graphic record of the brain's electrical impulses, as monitored by an electroencephalograph. Abbreviated EEG.

electrophoresis • The movement of particles in an electric field to either pole, anode or cathode.

embolism • Partial or complete blockage of a blood vessel, either by a clot (thromboembolism) or by some other substance.

embryotoxicity • A toxic or poisonous effect on the fetus during the early months of pregnancy.

emesis • Vomiting, especially that which is deliberately induced.

emphysema • A progressive lung disease characterized by loss of elasticity of the lung tissue, making it impossible to fully exhale.

empyema • The presence of pus in a cavity.

encephalitis • Inflammation of the brain.

encephalopathy • Any disease of the brain.

encopresis • Involuntary defecation.

endocarditis • Inflammation of the membrane lining the heart's interior.

endocervicitis • Inflammation of the mucous membrane of the uterine cervix.

endocrine • Secreting internally; referring to an internally secreting gland or the glandular system.

endogenous • Originating in or produced by the body.

endometriosis • The growth of endometrial cells (the type of cells present in the uterus lining, or endometrium) in abnormal places.

endometritis • Inflammation of the mucous membrane lining the uterus.

endometrium • The mucous membrane of the uterus.

endoscopy • The insertion of a lighted instrument into a body cavity for the purpose of visual examination.

endotracheal intubation • The insertion of a tube into the windpipe (trachea) to assist respiration.

Entamoeba histolytica • The causative agent of tropical or amebic dysentery.

enteric • Relating to the intestines.

enteritis • Inflammation of the intestinal tract.

Enterobacter • A genus of rod-shaped intestinal bacteria.

Enterobacter aerogenes • A species of bacteria found in the feces of man and other animals, sewage, soil, water, and dairy products.

enterocolitis • Inflammation of the intestines.

enteropathogenic • Causing intestinal disease.

Entomophthora • A genus of fungi, generally parasitic on insects.

enuresis • Involuntary urination in people old enough to be toilet trained; bed-wetting.

eosinophil • A type of white blood cell that is stained red by eosin, an acid dye.

eosinophilia • An abnormal increase in the concentration of eosinophils in the blood.

eosinophilic pneumonia • Inflammation of the lungs accompanied by an increase in eosinophils in the blood, usually associated with a parasitic infection of the lungs.

epicondylitis • Infection or inflammation of bone ends.

epidermis • The outer layer of skin.

Epidermophyton floccosum • A fungus, commonly the cause of tinea pedis (athlete's foot, Hong Kong toe), tinea cruris (jock itch), and other superficial skin infections.

epididymitis • Inflammation of the portion of the seminal duct lying behind the testis.

epigastrium • The region just above the stomach.

epileptiform • Resembling epilepsy.

epinephrine • A hormone secreted by the inner part of the adrenal gland that is the most potent stimulant of adrenergic alpha- and beta-receptors; it constricts blood vessels, thus raising blood pressure. Also called adrenaline.

epiphyseal closure • Hardening of the growth plate of a long bone (epiphysis), bringing further growth to a halt.

epiphysis • A growing part of a long bone that is separated from the main shaft by a cartilage plate (epiphyseal or growth plate) that closes or hardens when growth stops.

epistaxis • Nosebleed.

epithelium • The layer of cells that covers the internal and external surfaces of the body, including the linings of glands, vessels, and other small cavities.

ergot • A fungus that grows on rye plants. As a drug, it causes the arteries to constrict, raising blood pressure; it also causes contraction of the uterine muscle and is often used to stop uterine bleeding.

ergotism • A toxic reaction caused by ingestion of grain contaminated with ergot fungus; symptoms include vomiting, paresthesias, convulsions, and psychotic behavior.

eructation • Belching.

erysipelas • An acute contagious disease, caused by streptococcus and characterized by localized inflammation of the skin, with pain and fever.

erythema • Red patches or rash on the skin which may have a number of causes.

erythema multiforme • A red skin rash, usually on the body and limbs, that results from an allergy or as a reaction to drugs.

erythema nodosum • Erythema characterized by clumps of tender red nodules, usually on the legs, often associated with rheumatic fever or drug allergy.

erythrasma • A skin disease, bacterial in origin, characterized by reddish-brown patches in the armpits and groin.

erythroblastopenia • A primary deficiency in bone marrow seen in aplastic anemia.

erythrocyte • Red blood cell.

erythroid • Reddish.

erythropoiesis • The formation and development of red blood cells (erythrocytes).

Escherichia coli • A common intestinal bacterium. Abbreviated *E coli*.

esophagitis • Inflammation of the esophagus.

estriol • An estrogenic hormone found in the urine of the female.

estrogen • A female sex hormone manufactured by the ovaries; it stimulates the female reproductive cycle and the development of female secondary sex characteristics.

eunuchoidism • A condition in which the testes are present but fail to function.

eustachian tube • The auditory tube, extending from the middle ear to the pharynx.

euthyroid • Having a normally functioning thyroid gland.

exanthema • A general disease accompanied by skin eruptions, such as measles.

exchange transfusion • The replacement of most or all of the recipient's blood in small amounts at a time by blood from a donor.

exfoliative dermatitis • Extensive, abnormal peeling of the skin, including loss of hair.

exogenous • Originating or produced outside of an organism or one of its parts.

exophthalmos • Bulging of the eyeballs, usually as a result of an overactive thyroid, often accompanying goiter (exophthalmic goiter).

expectorant • An agent that increases bronchial secretion of mucus and facilitates its expulsion.

extracorporeal • Occurring outside of the body.

extrapyramidal • Of the extrapyramidal motor system; a general term denoting all nerves controlling movement.

extrasystole • A premature heartbeat; a beat outside the heart's normal rhythm.

extravasation • A discharge or escape (as of blood, lymph, or an injected drug) from a vessel into tissue.

F • Degrees Farenheit.

FBS • Fasting blood sugar level, measured to confirm a diagnosis of diabetes mellitus.

febrile • Pertaining to or characterized by fever.

fecal impaction • Blockage of the large intestine by difficult-to-move masses of solidified feces.

fecal vomiting • Vomiting of fecal matter, usually caused by intestinal obstruction.

fetal resorption • Absorption of the remains of a dead fetus in the uterus.

fibrillation • Uncoordinated, quivering muscle contractions. Usually a very rapid, unsynchronized, and unproductive heartbeat that may lead to death.

fibrin • The fibrous, insoluble protein that gives blood clots their semisolid consistency.

fibrinogen • A soluble protein that interacts with thrombin to form fibrin.

fibrinolytic • Able to dissolve fibrin.

fibrocystic • Pertaining to the development of cysts, especially in a gland, accompanied by an overgrowth of fibrous tissue.

fibrosis • An increase or proliferation of fibrous connective tissue.

filariasis • Infestation with filaria worms, threadlike parasites affecting connective, lymphatic, and other tissues in the adult stage and the blood in the embryonic stage.

flatus • Gas in the stomach or intestine.

fl oz • Fluid ounces.

focal seizure • An epileptic attack of a limited nature, usually without loss of consciousness, due to localized scarring, inflammation, or tumor of the brain.

follicular lymphoma • A malignant lymphoma in which the cancerous cell growth resembles the follicles of normal lymph nodes.

folliculitis • Inflammation of a group of follicles (small glands giving rise to secretions). Hair follicles are most frequently involved.

fontanel • The soft membranous space between the skull bones of the fetus and newborn.

formication • A feeling that insects are crawling on one's skin. The symptom is common in diseases of the spinal cord and peripheral nerves and may also be a hallucination associated with drug reactions or alcohol withdrawal.

Francisella tularensis • The causative organism of tularemia (rabbit fever), a disease seen frequently in wild animals, birds, and insects that may be transmitted to humans.

friability • The ease with which a thing is broken or crumbles.

FSH • Follicle-stimulating hormone.

funduscopy • Examination of the interior of the eye.

fungal meningitis • A fungal inflammation of the membranes lining the brain or spinal cord.

Fusobacterium fusiforme • A spindle- or cigar-shaped bacterium normally found in the mouth and associated with gum disease, lung abscesses, and other infections.

fusospirochetosis • An infection associated with fusobacteria and other microorganisms that thrive in oxygen-free environments (anaerobic bacteria). Most commonly found in gum and other mouth infections, lung abscesses, and vulvovaginitis.

g • Grams.

gal • Gallons.

galactorrhea • Excessive flow of milk.

ganglion • A group of nerve cells located outside the brain and spinal cord (central nervous system). There are many types of ganglia throughout the body.

ganglionic blocking agent • An anesthetic that works by inhibiting nerve impulses in the ganglia.

gastric lavage • Cleaning out the stomach by repeated infusions of water administered through a rubber tube, often used to treat poisoning or drug overdoses.

gastric ulcer • A stomach ulcer.

gastritis • Inflammation of the stomach.

gastrointestinal • Pertaining to the stomach and intestines, and, loosely, to the entire alimentary canal.

GI • Gastrointestinal.

giardiasis • An intestinal infection caused by parasitic protozoa of the genus *Giardia*, giving rise to diarrhea, often containing fatty substances (steatorrhea).

Gilles de la Tourette's syndrome • Progressively violent muscular jerks of the face and body, beginning in childhood, and subsequent development of spasmodic grunting or explosive noises, which are choked-off obscenities.

gingiva • The gums.

gingivitis • Inflammation of the gums.

gingivostomatitis • Inflammation of the gums and mucous membranes of the mouth.

globus hystericus • The choking sensation, or so-called lump in the throat, occurring in hysteria.

glomerulus • A small tuft of capillaries in the uriniferous tubules of the kidneys; the point where wastes are filtered out of the blood to become urine. Plural, glomeruli.

glomerulitis • Inflammation of the glomeruli.

glomerulonephritis • A kidney disease, usually affecting both kidneys, characterized by glomerulitis.

glossitis • Inflammation of the tongue.

glucocorticoid • One of the adrenal hormones that affects the metabolism of sugar (glucose).

glucose • A sugar (chemical formula $C_6H_{12}O_6$); the usual form in which carbohydrates are absorbed by the body for energy.

glutathione • A substance found in plant and animal tissues that is important in tissue oxidation.

gluteal • Referring to the buttocks; e.g., gluteal muscles are those located in the buttocks and upper thigh.

glycosuria • The presence of glucose in the urine.

goitrogen • Any substance that causes goiter.

gonad • A sex gland; in men, the testes, and in women, the ovaries.

gonadotropin • A gonad-stimulating hormone.

gout • A painful arthritic disease caused by a genetic metabolic defect, resulting in a buildup of uric acid. Acute gouty attacks result from accumulation of uric acid crystals, usually in a big toe, knee, earlobe, or finger joint.

gr • Grains.

gram-negative • A pink result of Gram's stain in a test to differentiate bacteria.

gram-positive • A purplish-black result of Gram's stain in a test to differentiate bacteria.

grand mal seizure • A generalized epileptic seizure; the most severe form of epilepsy.

granulocyte • A mature white blood cell that contains granules in its cytoplasm.

granulocytopenia • An abnormally low level of granulocytes in the blood.

granuloma inguinale • A chronic encapsulated ulcer or sore of the external genitalia. Often results in tissue destruction.

gray syndrome • A failure of the vasomotor response, which controls the expansion and constriction of blood vessels, as a result of a toxic reaction to the antibiotic drug chloramphenicol. Seen primarily in infants under the age of four months.

gynecomastia • Overdevelopment of the breasts in men.

h • Hours.

Haemophilus ducreyi • Species of bacteria that causes chancroid, a venereal disease characterized by ulceration and painful enlargement of the regional lymph nodes.

Haemophilus influenzae • Bacteria that cause a number of serious infections, especially in children, such as meningitis, bacteremia, pneumonia, otitis media, and sinusitis.

Haemophilus vaginalis • Bacteria that causes a type of vaginitis unrelated to candida or other vaginal yeast infections.

half-life • The time required for half of a given amount of a drug, once absorbed, to be metabolized or excreted from the body.

hallucinosis • The state of having hallucinations more or less persistently.

hallux rigidus • Stiffness or restricted movement of the big toe; often occurs in arthritis.

Hashimoto's disease • Enlargement of the thyroid gland with infiltration of lymph cells, resulting in destruction of thyroid tissue and eventual hypothyroidism.

HCG • Human chorionic gonadotropins; a hormone obtained from the placenta, used to treat undescended testes.

heart block • A cardiac condition in which transmission of nerve impulses from the atrium to the ventricle is slowed or stopped.

hebetude • Emotional dullness and disinterest.

Heinz body • Minute bodies found in the cytoplasm of red blood cells.

helminth • An intestinal worm or wormlike parasite.

heloma durum • A hard corn.

heloma molle • A soft corn.

hemangioma • A benign tumor made up of newly formed blood vessels.

hematemesis • Vomiting of blood.

hematocrit • The percentage volume of red cells in the blood, *or* the tube or procedure used to determine this percentage.

hematological • Pertaining to the blood.

hematoma • A swelling or mass of blood (usually clotted) within a tissue or body part, which is caused by a break in a blood vessel.

hematopoietic • Related to blood cell formation.

hematuria • Blood in the urine.

hemeralopia • A type of blindness that occurs in daylight, as opposed to night blindness.

hemicrania • Pain on one side of the head.

hemiparesis • A partial paralysis on one side of the body.

hemochromatosis • Excessive deposits of iron in the body; manifestations include cirrhosis of the liver, skin pigmentation, and cardiac failure.

hemoconcentration • A decrease in the volume of blood plasma relative to red blood cell count; increased red blood cell concentration.

hemodialysis • A process of filtering impurities from the blood.

hemoglobin • The pigment in red blood cells that absorbs oxygen from the lungs and carries it throughout the body.

hemogram • A detailed count of the blood elements, and an examination of their health; a record of such a count and examination.

hemolytic • Destructive to red blood cells, causing the release of hemoglobin.

hemolytic anemia • Anemia caused by destruction of red blood cells.

hemoperitoneum • The escape of blood into the abdominal and pelvic cavities (peritoneal cavity).

hemophilia • A hereditary disease in which the ability to form blood clots is reduced or absent.

hemoptysis • Spitting of blood from the lungs, bronchi, or trachea.

hemostasis • The stopping of circulation in a blood vessel or part of the body; the stopping of bleeding.

heparin • An acidic substance found in lung and liver tissue that interferes with blood clotting, often used to treat thrombosis and other clotting disorders.

hepatic • Relating to the liver.

hepatic coma • Profound unconsciousness precipitated by cirrhosis, hepatitis, or other liver disease.

hepatocellular • Pertaining to or affecting liver cells.

hepatomegaly • Enlargement of the liver.

hepatotoxic • Having a destructive or poisonous effect upon the liver.

herpes simplex • A group of diseases, often recurring, caused by herpes simplex virus, usually affecting the skin, mouth, eyes, or genital organs.

herpes zoster • A painful viral infection of nerves and nerve endings, commonly called shingles.

Herxheimer reaction • A type of hypoglycemia (low blood sugar) caused by blockage of pancreatic secretions.

5-HIAA • 5-hydroxyindoleacetic acid. A substance found in the cerebrospinal fluid and in small amounts in the urine. An increase in the urine concentration is a symptom of a liver disorder known as carcinoid syndrome.

hiatus hernia • A rupture (hernia) of the opening where the esophagus passes through the diaphragm, permitting a part of the stomach to protrude into the diaphragm.

hirsutism • Hairiness; the growth of an excessive amount of hair, or of hair in unusual places.

histamine • A chemical substance found in body tissue that, in small amounts, has diverse effects on muscles, gastric secretions, and capillaries. Excessive or sudden release of histamine, often in response to allergens, causes many of the symptoms of allergic reactions.

histaminic cephalalgia • A headache brought on by histamines; an allergic reaction.

histoplasmosis • An infectious disease caused by *Histoplasma capsulatum*, a fungus, that is often asymptomatic but may produce symptoms of pneumonia or tuberculosis.

Horner's syndrome • Contraction of the pupil, drooping of the upper eyelid, retraction of the eyeball in its orbit, diminished sweating, and flushing of the face, due to paralysis of the cervical sympathetic nerve trunk on one side.

human chorionic gonadotropins • A gonad-stimulating hormone produced by the placenta and derived from the urine of pregnant women, often used to treat undescended testes.

Huntington's chorea • A heredity progressive disease characterized by uncontrolled twitchings and movements and progressive degeneration of mental faculties, also called hereditary chorea.

hydatiform • Resembling a hydatid, a cyst formed by tapeworm larvae; these larvae may be passed from dogs to humans and are usually in the lungs or liver.

hydrate • Replace lost body fluids.

17-hydroxycorticosteroid • Formal name of hydrocortisone, an adrenal steroid that occurs naturally in the body or may be made synthetically. It is more potent than cortisone, and is used as an anti-inflammatory agent to treat a number of diseases.

hymenopteran • An order of insects with well-developed, membranous wings, including bees, wasps, ants, and certain flies.

hyperacusis • Abnormal sensitivity to sound.

hyperaldosteronism • Excessive secretion of aldosterone, an adrenal corticosteroid; symptoms include potassium loss, weakness, high blood pressure, and high blood concentrations of sodium.

hyperbilirubinemia • An excess of bilirubin (red bile pigment) in the blood.

hypercalcemia • An excess of calcium in the blood.

hypercapnea • An excess of carbon dioxide in the blood.

hypercholesterolemia • An excess of cholesterol in the blood, believed to be a precipitating factor in gallstones and atherosclerosis.

hyperesthesia • Excessive sensitivity to touch, pain, or other sensory stimuli.

hyperglycemia • A high level or excess of sugar in the blood.

hyperhidrosis • Excessive or profuse sweating.

hyperkalemia • An excess of potassium in the blood.

hyperlipidemia • An abnormally high concentration of fats (lipids) in the blood.

hypermenorrhea • An excessive menstrual flow.

hypermetabolism • Production of excessive body heat, often associated with an overactive thyroid.

hypermotility • Excessive or abnormally increased spontaneous motion (motility), particularly of the intestines.

hyperosmotic agent • An agent that draws off water to reduce cerebral swelling.

hyperplasia • An increased number of cells in a tissue or organ, excluding tumors.

hyperpnea • Rapid, deep breathing.

hyperpyrexia • Extremely high fever; also called hyperthermia.

hyperreflexia • A condition in which deep-tendon reflexes are exaggerated.

hypertension • High blood pressure.

hyperthermia • Unusually high body temperature or fever; also called hyperpyrexia.

hyperthyroidism • Excessive secretion of thyroid hormones.

hypertonia • Increased tension (tone) of the muscles or arteries.

hypertonic • Referring to a fluid having a greater osmotic pressure than another fluid, as in hypertonic saline, which has a greater osmotic pressure than normal body fluid. *Also,* of or related to hypertonia.

hypertonicity • Increased effective tension or osmotic pressure of body fluids.

hypertonus • Excess of muscular tension.

hypertrichosis • Excessive hair growth (as in bearded women).

hypertriglyceridemia • An elevated triglyceride concentration in the blood.

hypertrophic subaortic stenosis • A general, nontumorous overgrowth narrowing the left ventricle of the heart.

hypertrophy • Overgrowth; a general, nontumorous increase in bulk of a part or organ.

hyperuricemia • High levels of uric acid in the blood.

hyperventilation • Abnormally prolonged, rapid, deep breathing, often resulting in dizziness or, more rarely, fainting.

hypervolemia • Abnormally high blood volume.

hyphema • Blood in the forward chamber of the eye between the cornea and the lens.

hypoadrenalism • Abnormally lowered activity of the adrenal gland.

hypoalbuminemia • Abnormally low levels of albumin (protein) in the blood.

hypochloremic alkalosis • Alkaline intoxication induced by an excess of chloride ions in the blood.

hypocholesterolemia • An abnormally low level of serum cholesterol.

hypofibrinogenemia • A decrease in plasma fibrinogen, a protein essential in blood clotting process.

hypoglycemia • Abnormally low levels of glucose in the bloodstream.

hypogonadism • Diminished internal secretion of the testes or ovaries, with retardation of growth and sexual development.

hypokalemia • Abnormally low potassium ion concentration in the blood.

hypomania • A degree of elation, excitement, and activity higher than normal but less severe than that present in mania.

hyponatremia • Abnormally low sodium ion concentration in the blood.

hypophosphatemia • Abnormally low phosphate concentration in the blood.

hypopituitarism • A condition resulting from diminished secretion of pituitary hormones.

hypoplasia • Defective or incomplete development of an organ or part.

hypoplastic anemia • Anemia resulting from greatly depressed bone marrow function.

hypoprothrombinemia • Abnormally low prothrombin (blood clotting factor II) levels in the blood.

hypospadias • An anomaly in which the urethra (in males) opens on the underside of the penis or (in females) opens into the vagina.

hypostatic pneumonia • Pneumonia seen in patients who remain in one position for long periods of time; gravity causes blood to become congested in one part of the lung.

hyposthenuria • Consistent production of abnormally watery urine (low specific gravity).

hypotension • Low blood pressure.

hypothalamus • Lower part of the brain whose functions include release of hormones that activate the release of pituitary hormones and various autonomic functions, such as control of the appetite, body temperature, and gastric secretion.

hypothermia • Subnormal body temperature, or the artificial reduction of body temperature to below normal to slow physiological processes.

hypothyroidism • Inadequate secretion of thyroid hormones; manifestations of this condition vary with the patient's age and the degree of inadequacy.

hypotonia • Reduced tension or loss of muscular tonicity.

hypoventilation • A state of reduced inhalation, resulting in increased carbon dioxide tension.

hypovolemia • A reduced amount of blood in the body.

hypoxemia • Deficiency of oxygen.

hypoxia • A decreased amount of oxygen in organs and tissues.

hysterosalpinography • X-ray of the uterus and uterine tubes after injection of radiopaque material.

^{131}I • A radioactive isotope of iodine used to treat overactive thyroid; absorption of ^{131}I over a 24-hour period is also used as a test of thyroid function.

IA • Intra-arterial; within the arteries; refers to injections administered directly into an artery.

ichthyosis • A congenital skin disease, commonly called Fishkin's disease, characterized by dry, scaly skin.

icterus • Jaundice.

idiopathic • Of unknown cause.

idioventricular rhythm • An abnormal heart rhythm that originates in the ventricles.

ileitis • Inflammation of the ileum, the lower three fifths of the small intestine.

ileostomy • Creation of a surgical passage through the abdominal wall into the ileum (lower portion of the small intestine).

ileus • Bowel obstruction, accompanied often by colicky pain, vomiting, fever, and dehydration.

IM • Intramuscular.

impetigo • An inflammatory skin disease caused by streptococci or staphylococci and marked by large boil-like abscesses that rupture and develop yellow crusts.

induration • The process of becoming extremely firm or hard; a region of indurated tissue.

infarction • Cell death and tissue damage caused by an inadequate supply of blood to a local area.

inguinal • Relating to the groin.

inspissate • To thicken by evaporation.

insulin • A hormone, secreted by the beta cells in the islets of Langerhans of the pancreas, which helps to regulate the metabolism of fats and carbohydrates, particularly glucose.

insulin-dependent diabetes • A severe form of diabetes mellitus that often begins in childhood or adolescence and is characterized by lack of insulin. Also called juvenile-onset diabetes or growth-onset diabetes.

insulin-resistant diabetes • A form of diabetes mellitus, often seen in obese adults over 35, in which the beta cells continue to produce insulin, but the hormone is not fully utilized in glucose metabolism. Also called maturity-onset diabetes.

intercurrent • Arising as a second disease in an already ill individual.

interphalangeal • Between the fingers or toes, usually referring to the joints between the knucklebones.

interstitial fibrosis • The formation of fibrous tissue (a healing process, usually) to fill a hole in an organ or tissue.

interstitial myocarditis • Inflammation of the gaps and spaces in the heart muscle.

interstitial nephritis • Inflammation of the gaps and spaces in one or both kidneys.

intertriginous • Characterized by or related to intertrigo, dermatitis occuring within folds of skin or between contacting parts, such as the thighs and groin.

intertrigo • Skin blisters caused by friction or rubbing of adjacent parts.

intra-arterial • Into or within an artery.

intrabursal • Within the bursa, the small fluid-filled sacs that separate parts that move upon each other, such as the bones forming a joint.

intracranial • Within the skull, usually not including the mouth.

intradermal • Between layers of the skin.

intrahepatic cholestasis • An arrest in the flow of bile in the liver.

intrahepatic cholestatic jaundice • Jaundice resulting from arrested bile flow in the liver.

intralesional • Within a lesion, the change in tissue that occurs as a result of disease or injury. A drug that is administered intralesionally is one that is introduced directly into the diseased area.

intramuscular • Into or within a muscle.

intrasynovial • Within the synovial sac of a joint.

intratendinous • Within a tendon, the band of thick, fibrous tissue that forms the attachment between the muscle and bone.

intrathecal • Within a sheath.

intratracheal • Within the windpipe (trachea).

intrauterine device • A device inserted into the uterus to prevent implantation of the embryo in the uterine wall. Abbreviated IUD.

intravenous • Into or within a vein.

intraventricular • Within a ventricle of the brain or heart.

in utero • Within the uterus.

in vitro • A process or reaction carried out in a test tube or a culture dish.

in vivo • A process or reaction carried out in a living organism as opposed to a test tube.

involutional depression • A severe mental disorder occurring in late middle life, marked by depression, agitation, worry, bodily preoccupation, insomnia, and sometimes paranoid reactions.

iodism • Iodine poisoning.

IPPB • Intermittent positive pressure breathing. A technique that involves deep breathing and forced exhaling to improve lung function in persons with chronic pulmonary diseases or patients following surgery to prevent lung problems.

iridocyclitis • Inflammation of both the iris and the ciliary body of the eye.

iritis • Inflammation of the iris.

ischemia • Localized blood deficiency caused by constriction or obstruction of the blood vessels that supply the affected area.

ischemic ulcer • An ulcer in which cell regeneration is impeded by a loss of blood supply (ischemia).

islets of Langerhans • A group of cells that comprise the endocrine portion of the pancreas; they secrete insulin and other hormones.

isotonic saline • A salt solution that is compatible with body tissues and fluids.

IU • International units.

IV • Intravenous.

Jacksonian seizure • A localized seizure with spasms confined to one part or one group of muscles.

Jarisch-Herxheimer reaction • An acute reaction following the initial dose of a drug. Symptoms include fever, chills, malaise, headache, and aches.

juvenile rheumatoid arthritis • Arthritis occurring in children and, rarely, young adults; in addition to joint inflammation, it is characterized by fever, rash, conjunctivitis, anemia, and other complications. Also called Still's disease.

kaliuresis • Increased urinary excretion of potassium.

keloid • A new growth of scar tissue or tumor of the skin; these growths tend to recur after removal, and are sometimes tender or painful.

keratitis • Inflammation of the cornea.

keratolytic • Associated with shedding of the epidermis or the upper skin layer.

keratosis nigricans • An eruption of horny growths or warts, with hyperpigmentation.

kernicterus • Discoloration and degeneration of the brain and other nerve structures seen in newborns suffering from an excess of bilirubin.

ketoacidosis • Acidosis associated with an excess of ketone bodies in the blood; it may occur with diabetes mellitus, pregnancy, starvation, or other conditions.

ketone body • A ketone; an organic compound related to acetone, formed when the body metabolizes its own fat cells.

ketonuria • An increased level of ketone bodies in the urine.

ketosteroid • A steroid found in urine; urinary androgens.

ketotic • Associated with ketosis, acid intoxication seen sometimes in severe diabetes.

kg • Kilograms

Klebsiella pneumoniae • Gram-negative, rod-shaped bacterium causing a serious type of pneumonia as well as other diseases.

Koebner's phenomenon • The appearance of psoriatic skin lesions at sites of injury or pressure; may also refer to trauma-induced lesions of other skin diseases, such as dermatitis.

kraurosis vulvae • A degenerative condition of the vaginal entrance associated with postmenopausal lack of estrogen.

l • Liters.

labile • Unstable, unsteady; not fixed; in psychiatry, emotionally unstable.

labyrinthine artery • The artery that supplies the inner ear.

lacrimation • The secretion of tears, especially in excess.

lactate • To produce breast milk; *also* a salt of lactic acid.

lactate dehydrogenase • An enzyme that rises after death of heart tissue, and therefore is used to diagnose a heart attack.

lactation • The production of milk; the time beginning immediately after childbirth when milk forms in the breasts.

lactobaccillus • A species of intestinal bacteria that produce lactic acid and thereby aid in the digestion of milk.

laparoscope • An examining instrument inserted into the abdominal or pelvic (peritoneal) cavities.

laparoscopy • Examination of the abdominal or pelvic cavity with a laparoscope.

laparotomy • Incision into the abdominal wall, usually for surgery or introduction of a laparoscope.

laryngeal stridor • An abnormal narrowing of the larynx.

laryngospasm • Spasmodic closure of the larynx (voice box).

lassitude • Weakness, exhaustion.

lb • Pounds

LDH • Lactate dehydrogenase; an enzyme found in five different forms in the body. LDH-1 is found in the heart and an increased level of it often signifies a heart attack.

LE • Lupus erythematosus, more properly called systemic lupus erythematosus.

leiomyoma • A benign growth derived from smooth muscle. Plural, leiomyomata.

leishmaniasis • Infection by bacteria of the genus *Leishmania.*

Lennox-Gastaut syndrome • An epileptic disorder of childhood.

lenticular • Pertaining to the lens of the eye.

Leriche syndrome • Intermittent blockage of circulation to the lower back and extremities, causing leg cramps, muscular atrophy, pallor of the legs, and sometimes impotence.

lesion • Any alteration in tissue caused by disease.

lethargic encephalitis • Epidemic inflammation of the brain, probably of viral origin, marked by lethargy, paralysis of the eye muscles, excessive movement, and neurologic disability.

leukemia • A malignant disease characterized by the proliferation of abnormal leukocytes in the blood or bone marrow.

leukocyte • A white blood cell.

leukocytosis • An abnormally high white blood cell count, often observed in acute infections.

leukopenia • A lower-than-normal white blood cell count.

LH • Luteinizing hormone; the hormone that promotes release of progesterone and of the mature egg from the ovary.

libido • Conscious or unconscious sexual desire; creative energy.

lichenoid • Resembling lichen (as in eruptions on the skin); heightened skin markings.

ligament • A band or sheath of tough, fibrous tissue that connects two or more bones. (Compare *tendon.*)

lingual frenulum • The membrane extending from the mouth floor to the midline of the underside of the tongue.

lipase • A fat-splitting (lipolytic) enzyme.

lipid • A fat; fat-soluble.

lipodystrophy • Defective metabolism of fat.

lipoprotein • A complex or compound containing lipid and protein.

liq • Liquid.

Listeria monocytogenes • Gram-positive microorganism occurring primarily in lower animals but sometimes infecting man to produce an upper respiratory disease with inflammation of the mouth and throat, lymph nodes, and/or the membrane lining of the eye.

lithiasis • A predisposition to an excess of uric acid.

livedo reticularis • Semipermanent bluish mottling of the skin of the legs and hands, which worsens on exposure to cold.

loading dose • Initial dosage to achieve a therapeutic effect.

lobar pneumonia • Acute febrile disease marked by inflammation of one or more lobes of the lung.

Loeffler's syndrome • A condition chracterized by transient infiltrations of the lungs associated with an increase of the eosinophilic leukocytes in the blood; called also Loffler's eosinophilia.

lordosis • Forward curvature of the spine.

lumbago • Pain in the middle and lower back (a descriptive, not specific, term).

lumbosacral • Pertaining to the lower part of the spine, below the rib cage.

luteal phase • A portion of the menstrual cycle, from the formation of the corpus luteum to the onset of menstrual flow (usually fourteen days).

luteinizing hormone • A cell-stimulating hormone that prompts progesterone release and ovulation.

lymphadenopathy • A disease affecting the lymphatic system.

lymphoblast • An immature white blood cell of a type formed by the lymph nodes.

lymphoblastic leukemia • A form of leukemia in which the cancerous cells are primarily of the type commonly found in lymphatic tissue.

lymphocyte • A cystic mass containing lymph.

lymphocytosis • High white blood cell count (actual or relative) and increased lymphocyte production.

lymphogranuloma venereum • Tropical veneral disease caused by a virus.

lymphoma • Any neoplastic disease of the lymphoid tissue (including Hodgkin's disease).

lymphomonocytosis • Excess of lymphomonocytes—a type of large leukocytes—in the blood.

M • Molar; containing a gram molecule of solute in 1,000 milliliters of solution.

m • Meters.

maceration • Softening by the action of a liquid.

macrocytosis • The presence of macrocytes, or abnormally large red cells, in the blood.

macular • Spotted.

maculopapular rash • A spotty, elevated skin rash.

maculopathy • Any disease of the yellow spot in the center of the retina, which provides the most acute vision.

malabsorption syndrome • Loss of weight with large amounts of fat in the stool caused by lesions of the small intestine, lack of digestive enzymes, or surgery.

malaise • A feeling of illness and discomfort.

Malassezia furfur • A fungus that causes brownish-yellow, branny patches on the skin of the trunk.

mammogram • A breast x-ray.

manic depression • A type of mental disorder which alternates between phases of euphoria and phases of depression.

MAO • Monoamine oxidase, an enzyme that aids in the breakdown of serotonin and catecholamines in the brain.

MAO inhibitor • Monoamine oxidase inhibitor; a drug that blocks the actions of monoamine oxidase. MAO inhibitors are prescribed as antidepressants.

mastalgia • Pain in the breast.

mast cell • A connective tissue cell associated with formation and storage of histamine, heparin, and other pharmacologically active substances.

masticatory • Related to chewing.

mastodynia • Pain in the breast.

mastoid bone • A nipple-shaped part of the temporal bone.

mediastinal • In the space in the chest between the lungs.

megaloblastosis • Presence in the bloodstream or bone marrow of large, immature (nucleated) red blood cells of a characteristic type called megaloblasts, often caused by a vitamin B_{12} or folic acid deficiency.

meibomianitis • Inflammation of the sebaceous glands of the eyelids.

melanin • A dark brown pigment produced by the skin and other organs.

melanoma • A malignant tumor composed primarily of melanin-forming cells.

melasma • Abnormal darkening of the skin.

melena • Stools that are black and tarry from the presence of altered blood.

membranous • Pertaining to or resembling a membrane.

Meniere's syndrome • Excess fluid in the inner ear, causing ringing in the ears, dizziness and other balance problems, and in some instance deafness.

meningeal leukemia • A leukemia in which cancer cells infiltrate the membranes of the brain or spinal cord.

meningitis • Inflammation of the meninges—the membranes surrounding the brain and the spinal cord.

menorrhagia • Excessive menstrual flow on a regular basis.

menses • Menstrual bleeding.

mEq • Milliequivalent; one thousandth of an equivalent or specific weight measurement.

mesenteric • Relating to the mesentery, a fold in the viscera enveloping a portion of the intestines.

metabolic acidosis • Actual or relative depletion of the body's alkali reserve due to accumulation of strong acids or abnormal losses of fixed base from the body, as in diarrhea or renal disease.

metabolic alkalosis • Alkaline intoxication in the blood and body organs.

metabolite • Any product of metabolism.

metacarpophalangeal • Pertaining to or related to the bones of the hands and fingers.

metaphase • A stage of cell division (mitosis or meiosis).

metastasis • The spread of a disease from one part of the body or organ to another, discontiguous part.

methemoglobinemia • The presence of methemoglobin, a form of hemoglobin that cannot transport oxygen, in the blood, usually seen following poisoning with cyanide or other chemicals.

mg • Milligrams; one thousandth of a gram.

μg • Micrograms; one millionth of a gram.

microcephaly • Abnormally small head.

microhematuria • Blood in the urine that is detectable only by microscope.

micronodular • Characterized by minute nodules or grains.

Microsporum audouini • The fungus that causes ringworm, especially of the scalp.

Microsporum canis • A common cause of ringworm in dogs and cats, often transmitted to children.

Microsporum gypseum • A fungus resembling *M canis* but found in soil.

micturition • Urination.

migraineur • A person who suffers from migraine headaches.

miliaria • Prickly heat, or heat rash. Eruption occurring mainly in hot, wet climates, and characterized by tiny blisters and itching, in skin folds. Most commonly seen in babies.

min • Minutes or minims.

mineralocorticoid • An adrenal hormone that regulates salt and mineral metabolism and, indirectly, fluid balance.

minim • A unit of liquid measure equal to 1/60 fluidram, or about one drop.

miosis • The period of decline in a disease's progress when symptoms begin to diminish; *also* contraction of the pupil of the eye.

miotic • Pertaining to contraction of the pupil.

mitral insufficiency • A defect in the closure of the mitral valve allowing blood to flow backwards past the closed valve.

mitral valve • The valve between the left atrium and ventricle of the heart; also called bicuspid valve or left atrioventricular valve.

ml • Milliliters; one thousandth of a liter.

mm • Millimeters; one thousandth of a meter.

mo • Months.

moiety • One of two or more parts into which something is divided.

monilial vaginitis • A fungal infection of the vagina and possibly adjacent areas; also called vaginal candidiasis.

moniliasis • Infection by fungi of the order Monilia; candidiasis.

monocytosis • An increased number of monocytes (large leukocytes with a single nucleus) in circulating blood; also called mononucleosis.

mononucleosis • An increase in the number of circulating mononuclear cells (large white cells with a single nucleus) in the blood.

morbilliform • Resembling the skin rash of measles.

Moro reflex • The startle reflex in infants, consisting of extension of all extremities, followed by flexing, in response to changes of position and loud noises. The reflex normally disappears after six months.

motility • The power of spontaneous movement.

msec • Milliseconds; one thousandth of a second.

mu • Milliunits; one thousandth of a unit.

mucocutaneous • Pertaining to mucous membrane and skin.

mucolytic • Causing dissolution of mucus.

Mucor • A genus of molds frequently found on dead and decaying vegetable matter, especially bread.

mucosa • Mucous membranes.

mucous membrane • A membrane containing glands that secrete mucus, lining the body cavities and passages leading to the exterior of the body.

multinodular goiter • A goiter (enlarged thyroid gland) with several nodules.

multiple myeloma • A disease in which many small nodules of cancerous marrow cells form in the bones and occasionally elsewhere in the body.

multiple sclerosis • Formation of sharply defined lesions or hardening in various areas of the brain and spinal cord, leading to episodes of focal disorder of the optic nerves, brain, or spinal cord.

mural • Relating to the wall of any cavity, organ, or vessel.

mural thrombus • A blood clot on a cavity, organ, or vessel wall.

mutagenic • Capable of causing a genetic mutation.

myalgia • Muscular pain.

myasthenia • Muscular weakness.

myasthenia gravis • Chronic, progressive weakness of the voluntary muscles, especially those of the eyes and face.

Mycoplasma pneumoniae • The causative agent of primary atypical pneumonia in man, a relatively mild pneumonia marked by cough, fever, and pulmonary infiltration.

mycosis • Disease caused by any fungus.

mycosis fungoides • A progressive, often fatal proliferation of abnormal cancer-like cells in the inner layer of skin, that eventually develop ulcerating tumors. Unrelated to fungal infection.

mycotic • Relating to or caused by a fungus.

mydriasis • Dilation of the pupils.

mydriatic • Causing dilation of the pupil.

myeloblastic • Characterized by the presence of myeloblasts—the earliest stage in the formation of granulocytes, a type of white blood cell.

myelocytic • Characterized by the presence of myelocytes, an intermediate stage in the formation of granulocytes.

myelogram • An x-ray picture of the spinal column made after injection of a contrasting substance.

myelosuppression • Suppression or reduction of bone marrow activity.

myocardial infarction • Death of heart muscle resulting from an inadequate supply of blood to the heart, commonly called heart attack.

myocardium • The muscular tissue of the heart.

myocarditis • Inflammation of the heart muscle.

myoclonus • Shocklike spasms or twitching of one or a set of muscles, usually one-sided; but bilateral myoclonus affects both sides of the body.

myopathy • Any disease or abnormality of the muscular tissues.

myopia • Nearsightedness.

myxedema • A condition caused by deficiency of thyroid hormone, characterized by slowed movements, mental dullness, slow heartbeat, dry skin, lowered body temperature, and swelling of the face and limbs. May lead to myxedema coma, a life-threatening medical emergency.

narcolepsy • A recurrent, uncontrollable tendency to fall asleep at inappropriate times.

narcosis • Stupor or general anesthesia resulting from narcotic use.

narcotic antagonist • An agent that neutralizes (antagonizes) the action of a narcotic drug.

narrow-angle glaucoma • Buildup of fluid pressure inside the eye (glaucoma) caused by a blockage in the drainage canal.

nasal polyp • A bulging, visible tissue mass in or around the nose.

natriuretic • Increasing or causing excessive excretion of sodium in the urine.

necrolysis • Pathologic death and loosening of tissue.

necrosis • Cell death.

necrotizing vasculitis • Irreversible cell loss in the blood vessels.

Neisseria catarrhalis • A species of bacteria found in the mucous membranes of the human respiratory tract and sometimes causing disease.

Neisseria gonorrhoeae • A species of bacteria which causes gonorrhea and other infections in man.

Neisseria meningitidis • A bacterial species found in the nose and throat of man and causing epidemic meningitis.

neonate • A baby less than one month old.

neoplasia • Pathological formation of new tissue.

neoplasm • Growth of abnormal new cells; tumor formation and growth.

nephrocalcinosis • Calcium deposits in the kidneys.

nephrosis • Any degenerative, noninflammatory change in the kidney.

nephrotic syndrome • An inflammatory kidney disease characterized by edema, peculiar susceptibility to toxins and infections, and changes in the blood and urine.

nephrotoxicity • Poisonous effect on the cells of the kidney.

neuralgia • Sharp, strong, stabbing, usually brief pain along the path of a nerve.

neuroblastoma • A malignant tumor formed primarily of immature nerve cells.

neurodermatitis • Leathery, thickened patches of skin resulting from chronic itching and scratching associated with emotional tension.

neurogenic • Originating within or forming nervous tissue; *also*, stimulating nervous energy.

neuroleptic • Acting on the nervous system.

neuromuscular • Relating to nerves and muscles, or to the nerve supply of a muscle.

neuromuscular blockade • Inhibition of nerve impulse transmission at the junction between the nerve and the muscle, induced by a drug such as curare.

neuro-ocular • Pertaining to the nerves in the eye.

neurosis • An emotional or psychological disorder that is not severe enough to prevent the individual from functioning in society.

neurosyphilis • Infection of the brain, spinal cord, or both by *Treponema pallidum.*

neurotoxicity • Poisonous effect on the nerves.

neutropenia • An abnormally low level of white blood cells in circulating blood.

ng • Nanograms; one billionth of a gram.

nocardosis • Any condition resulting from infection with bacteria of the genus *Nocardia.*

nocturia • Frequent urination at night.

nodule • A small knob or swelling.

norepinephrine • A stimulant hormone; when produced synthetically it is used to maintain adequate blood pressure during surgery or in other situations in which blood pressure is dangerously low.

normochromic anemia • Any anemia in which the hemoglobin content of the red blood cells is within normal ranges.

normocytic anemia • Any anemia in which erythrocytes (red corpuscles) are normal in size.

nosocomial • A new illness, usually an infection, contracted in hospital.

nuchal • Relating to the back of the neck.

nulliparous • Never having borne a child.

nummular • Coin-shaped or resembling rolls of coins.

nystagmus • Abnormal oscillation or repetitive jerky movements of the eyeballs.

oat-cell lung cancer • A carcinoma in which the cancerous cells resemble oats.

obliterative bronchiolitis • Complete blockage of the small bronchial tubes.

obstipation • Absolute inability to move the bowels; complete constipation.

obtundation • Blunting or deadening of sensation, particularly pain or irritation.

occlusive dressing • Covering of a lesion or wound that seals it from contact with air or bacteria.

occult • Of unknown cause; hidden or concealed; or detectable only by microscope (as in occult blood in the stools).

oculogyric • Referring to the movements of the eyeball.

17-OHCS • 17-hydroxycorticosteroid. See *hydroxycorticosteroid.*

oleaginous • Oily or greasy.

oligospermia • An abnormally low number of sperm cells in the ejaculate.

oliguria • Scanty urination.

omphalocele • A hernia in the umbilical cord.

onycholysis • Loosening of a toe- or fingernail.

onychomycosis • Ringworm or fungus infection of the fingernails or toenails.

open-angle glaucoma • Glaucoma in which the buildup of fluid pressure in the eye is not caused by constriction of the drainage canal (angle); open-angle glaucoma is usually chronic and progressive, affects both eyes equally, and often causes loss of vision if untreated.

opioid • A synthetic compound not obtained from opium but having similar effects.

opisthotonos • A spasm of the muscles of the back causing such arching that only the head and the feet touch the bed, often seen in tetanus.

opportunistic fungi • Fungi that are harmless to a healthy individual, but capable of producing disease in a person already weakened by illness; infection by opprotunistic fungi is common in persons undergoing cancer chemotheraphy or with weakened immune defenses.

optic neuritis • Inflammation of the optic nerve.

oral contraceptive • A drug taken by mouth to prevent conception.

oral hypoglycemic agent • A chemical taken by mouth that lowers the levels of glucose in the blood.

organic brain syndrome • Any mental disorder associated with impaired function of the brain tissue. Frequently used to refer to senility.

ornithosis • Human illness resulting from disease of birds.

oropharyngeal • Pertaining to the mouth and pharynx.

orthostatic • Caused by standing upright.

osmolarity • The concentration of osmotically active particles in solution.

osmotic • Pertaining to osmosis, or the passage of water or other solvent through a membrane caused by unequal concentrations of the solution on the two sides of the membrane.

ossicles • Small bones or bonelets, particularly in the middle ear.

ossification • The changing of soft tissue into bone.

osteoarthritis • Chronic degeneration of cartilage and joints, usually occurring in hands and weight-bearing joints, particularly in older persons.

osteomalacia • A gradual softening and bending of the bones with more or less severe pain, most common in persons with kidney failure.

osteomyelitis • Inflammation of bone marrow.

osteoporosis • Degeneration or thinning of the bone tissue, resulting in decreased thickness, enlarged marrow, and structural weakness.

osteosarcoma • A sarcoma growing from the bone.

otalgia • Earache.

OTC • Over the counter; sold without a prescription.

otitis • Inflammation of the ear.

otitis externa • Inflammation of the outer ear.

otitis media • Inflammation of the middle ear.

otomycosis • An infection in the ear canal believed to be caused by bacteria with subsequent (secondary) fungal infection.

ototoxicity • A harmful effect on the ear, especially the nerves.

ovulate • To release an egg cell (ovum) from the ovary into the uterus.

oz • Ounces.

palilalia • The pathologic repetition of words or phrases.

palliative • A treatment or medicine that affords relief but does not cure.

palpitation • Rapid and forceful heartbeat that is perceived by the individual.

pancreas • A large compound gland, located at the back of the abdomen beneath the stomach, that secretes digestive enzymes and insulin.

pancreatectomy • Removal of part or all of the pancreas.

pancreatitis • Inflammation of the pancreas.

pancytopenia • Pronounced reduction of three types of blood cells—red and white cells and platelets.

panhypopituitarism • Generalized effects due to the absence or damage of the pituitary gland, such as dwarfism and regression of secondary sex characteristics.

pantothenic acid • One of the essential B-complex vitamins widely distributed in animal and plant tissue; human deficiency has not been documented.

Papanicolaou smear • The microscopic evaluation of a cell specimen from the patient's body for various clinical purposes; Pap test or smear.

papilla • A minute nipple-shaped eminence.

papillary edema • Accumulation of fluid in a nipple-like or cone-shaped projection.

papilledema • Accumulation of fluid in the optic disk, the area of the retina that adjoins the optic nerve.

papule • A small elevation in the skin, generally formed in deeper layers than pustules.

paracoccidioidomycosis • Fungal infection of skin and mucous membranes caused by the paracoccidioides microorganism (also *Blastomyces brasiliensis*), seen primarily in South America.

paralysis agitans • A degenerative form of Parkinson's disease, beginning in middle age and growing progressively worse (see *parkinsonism*).

paralytic ileus • A bowel obstruction resulting from bowel wall paralysis.

parapsoriasis varioliformis acuta • An acute skin eruption characterized by pustules that later form crusts and then scars.

parasympathetic nervous system • A part of the autonomic (involuntary) nervous system whose functions are roughly opposite to those of the sympathetic nervous system. Parasympathetic functions include stimulation of secretions, slowing of heartbeat, dilation of blood vessels, bronchoconstriction, and gastrointestinal stimulation. (Compare *sympathetic nervous system*.)

parasympathomimetic • A drug that imitates the actions of the parasympathetic nervous system.

parathyroid • Parathyroid gland; a gland embedded in the underside of the thyroid that is active in phosphorus and calcium metabolism.

parenchyma • The parts of an organ concerned with its main function.

parenchymatous • Pertaining to parenchyma.

parenteral • Administration of drugs, fluids, or food other than by mouth; specifically, by injection.

paresthesia • An abnormal spontaneous sensation, such as a burning, pricking, or numbness.

parkinsonism • A group of nervous diseases related to and including Parkinson's disease, characterized by shuffling gait, tremor of the limbs, mask-like facial expression, and muscular rigidity.

paronychias • Inflammation of the nail fold, from bacteria, fungi, or mold.

parotid gland • The salivary gland situated near the external ear.

parous • Having borne children.

paroxysmal • Recurring in sudden attacks or fits; increasing suddenly in severity.

parturition • The act of child-bearing.

patent • Open, as in a breathing passage or blood vessels.

pathogen • Any virus, bacteria, or other microorganism or substance (usually living) capable of causing disease.

PBI • Protein-bound iodine.

pectus excavatum • A hollow in the lower chest caused by displaced cartilage, sometimes referred to as funnel chest.

ped • Pediatric.

pediculosis • Infestation with body or head lice, causing intense itching and rash.

peliosis hepatitis • The presence of multiple microscopic pools of blood in the liver.

pellagra • A disease caused by deficiency of B vitamins, particularly niacin or tryptophan, manifested by dermatitis, tongue inflammation, neuritis, spinal cord changes, anemia, and mental confusion.

pelvic cellulitis • Inflammation of the pelvic connective tissue.

pemphigus • A potentially serious skin disease characterized by clusters of large flaccid blisters (bullae).

penicillinase • An enzyme which destroys penicillin.

peptic ulcer • An ulcer that is exposed to gastric secretions in the stomach.

Peptococcus • A genus of gram-positive anaerobic bacteria found in the upper respiratory, gastrointestinal, and genitourinary tracts as harmless parasites.

Peptostreptococcus • A genus of anaerobic streptococci occurring as harmless parasitic inhabitants of the intestinal tract.

percutaneous • Performed or administered through the skin, as an injection.

perianal • Around the anus.

periarteritis nodosa • An inflammatory disease of the external coats of the small and medium-sized arteries.

pericardial • Pertaining to the pericardium, the membranous sac surrounding the heart.

pericardiocentesis • Surgical puncture of the pericardium.

pericarditis • Inflammation of the pericardium.

periderm • The outer layer of skin cells in an unborn fetus and newborn baby; these cells are replaced by ordinary epidermal cells shortly after birth.

perioperative • Related to an operation.

perioral • Situated or occurring around the mouth.

periorbital • Situated around the eye socket.

peripheral edema • Accumulation of fluid in limbs and other external body parts.

peripheral neuropathy • Any disease in the peripheral nervous system.

peripheral thrombosis • Formation of a blood clot in the vessels of the extremities.

peritoneal dialysis • The filtering of impurities from the blood through the membrane lining the abdominal cavity.

perivascular • Surrounding a blood or lymph vessel.

perivascular granulomata • Granular tumors (neoplasms) in the areas surrounding blood or lymph vessels.

peroral • Performed through the mouth.

petechiae • Small spots of bleeding on the skin or on a mucous membrane.

petit mal seizure • A brief, recurrent epileptic seizure characterized by flickering of the eyelids, sudden transient loss of consciousness or suspended animation, a blank stare, and, in some persons, strange movements such as lip smacking or stereotyped hand movements; also called absence attacks.

petrolatum • Petroleum jelly.

Peyronie's disease • A disease in which plaques or strands of fibrous tissue cause penis deformity and painful erection.

pH • Hydrogen ion concentration; the standard method of measuring acidity or alkalinity of a liquid.

pharyngitis • Inflammation of the pharynx and its mucous membrane.

pheochromocytoma • A benign tumor of the parasympathetic nervous system, usually derived from adrenal medullary cells, that secretes substances (catecholamines) that cause high blood pressure, headache, blurred vision, disturbed heart rhythm, and other symptoms.

phospholipid • A fat or fat-soluble substance containing phosphorus.

photodermatitis • An abnormal condition of the skin produced largely by the effect of light.

photophobia • Fear of or abnormal sensitivity to light.

photosensitivity • The capacity to be activated or stimulated by light; *also* increased sensitivity to light.

photosensitization • The development of abnormally high reactivity of the skin to sunlight.

phototoxicity • Injury from overexposure to light, gamma rays, or x-rays; increased sensitivity to light.

phycomycosis • A fungal infection caused by Phycomycetes, usually affecting persons with an underlying disease, such as diabetes.

picrotoxin • A bitter crystalline stimulant and convulsive drug used intravenously as an antidote for barbiturate poisoning.

pigmentary retinopathy • A chronic progressive inflammation and atrophy of the retina leading to contraction of the field of vision.

pinta • A disease widespread in Mexico and Central America, caused by a spirochete and marked by an eruption of patches of varying color that finally become white.

plasmin • An enzyme that slowly dissolves blood clots.

Plasmodium falciparum • Species of microscopic blood parasites causing the most severe form of malaria in man.

platelet • A tiny disc of protoplasm circulating in the bloodstream; platelets are active in the clotting process.

pleura • The membrane covering the lung surface and a portion of the chest wall.

pleural effusion • The presence of excess liquid in the space surrounding the lungs.

pneumococcal infection • Disease caused by microorganism *Streptococcus pneumoniae,* the most common causative agent of acute inflammation of the lung.

Pneumocystis carinii • A species of microorganisms causing a highly contagious, epidemic form of lung inflammation, particularly in young children.

pneumonitis • Inflammation of the lungs.

PO • *per os,* by mouth.

polyarteritis • Simultaneous inflammation of numerous arteries.

polyarthralgia • Simultaneous pain in several joints.

polyarthropathy • Any disease affecting several joints at the same time.

polycystic disease • Hereditary kidney cysts that eventually lead to kidney failure.

polycythemia • An increased number of red blood cells.

polydactyly • Extra fingers or toes.

polydipsia • Excessive thirst.

polymyalgia rheumatica • Pain and stiffness in the muscles, occuring most commonly in older persons.

polymyositis • Simultaneous inflammation in numerous muscles.

polypeptide • A chain of amino acids, as in a protein.

polyphagia • Overeating; gluttony.

polyuria • Excessive urination, often as a symptom of diabetes mellitus.

porphyria • A congenital metabolic disorder that causes abnormalities in nerve and muscle tissue and, occasionally, psychiatric disturbances.

porphyria cutanea tarda • A heriditary disease characterized by skin sensitivity to light and chemical changes in the feces.

postencephalitic parkinsonism • A form of parkinsonism occurring as a sequel to lethargic encephalitis, marked by onset before age 40, lethargy, and slow but steady evolution of the classical symptom complex.

postpartum • Pertaining to, or occurring during, the period immediately following childbirth.

postural hypotension • A marked drop in blood pressure caused by a change in position.

precordial • Relating to the area of the chest immediately over the heart.

pre-eclampsia • A condition arising in the latter part of pregnancy, marked by the presence of albumin in the urine, fluid retention, hypertension, headache, and visual disturbances.

pregnanediol • A metabolite of progesterone that is present in the urine during the progestational phase of the menstrual cycle.

prepartum • Just before labor, delivery, or childbirth; also called antepartum.

prerenal azotemia • Increased nitrogen in the blood as a result of decreased blood flow to the kidney or a cause other than primary kidney disease.

pressor • Producing a rise in blood pressure.

pressor amine • A substance derived from ammonia (an amine) that increases blood pressure.

priapism • Persistent erection of the penis independent of sexual arousal.

proctitis • Inflammation of the anus or rectum.

progesterone • A hormone secreted by the ovary that plays an important part in the regulation of the menstrual cycle and in pregnancy.

progestin • Any hormone conducive to gestation.

progestogen • Any agent capable of producing biological effects similar to those of progesterone.

prolactin • A hormone that stimulates milk production and, during pregnancy, breast growth.

proptosis • Bulging of an organ; specifically, of the eyeball.

prostaglandins • A class of physiologically active compounds found in many body tissues that affect circulation, the nervous system, metabolism, female reproductive functions, and other body processes.

prostate • The organ that surrounds the inner end of the male urethra. The prostate secretes a milky fluid that is discharged with semen at ejaculation.

prostatism • A condition caused by chronic disorders of the prostate, especially obstruction of urination by prostatic enlargement.

protein-bound iodine • Iodine attached to protein; protein-bound iodine levels accurately reflect the amount of thyroid hormone in the bloodstream. Abbreviated PBI.

proteinuria • Presence of protein (albumin) in the urine.

Proteus • Genus of bacteria normally found in GI tract. May cause disease in infants. Genus includes *P. vulgaris, P. mirabilis, P. rettgeri, and P. morganii.*

prothrombin • A protein in the bloodstream that helps activate the clotting of blood.

prothrombin time • A test to measure the time required for blood to clot.

pruritus • Itching.

pruritus ani • Itching around the anus.

pruritus scroti • Itching of the scrotum.

pruritus vulvae • Itching of the vulva and, occasionally, adjacent areas.

pseudomembranous colitis • Inflammation of the colon marked by the presence of a false membrane.

Pseudomonas aeruginosa • Species of bacteria that causes suppurative infections in humans. Organism's pigments give pus characteristic blue-green color.

pseudoparkinsonism • Symptoms of Parkinson's disease without organic manifestations.

pseudotumor cerebri • A nontumorous condition producing symptoms of tumor in the brain.

psittacosis • Form of pneumonia and systemic infection caused by *Chlamydia* microorganism and generally acquired by humans from parrots, parakeets, and other pet birds.

psoriasis • A chronic, recurrent, silver-gray, and patchy skin inflammation.

psychogenesis • The appearance of physical symptoms without apparent organic causes; also known as hysterical symptoms, as in hysterical paralysis.

psychomotor • Referring to physical activity as mediated by the brain.

psychomotor seizure • An epileptic seizure characterized by an aura or sensation of sights, sounds, or odors, and performance of activities that are blocked from memory.

psychotropic • Drug or other substance that has an effect on the mind.

pt • Pints.

ptosis • Drooping or falling down; particularly a drooping of the upper eyelid as in myasthenia gravis.

pulmonary embolism • An embolism (blood clot) in the lungs.

pulmonary infiltration • The accumulation of foreign organisms or substances, such as excess fluids, in the lungs.

punctate • Dotted or filled with minute points.

purpura • A spontaneous, nontraumatic seeping of blood (hemorrhage) from capillaries into the skin, that may take the form of small red patches (petechiae), or large, sometimes oozing plaques (ecchymoses). Purpura should not be confused with bruising that results from injury or other trauma.

pustule • A small infection on the surface of the skin, containing pus; a pimple.

pyelitis • Inflammation of the pelvis (basin-shaped cavity) of the kidney.

pyelonephritis • A kidney disorder caused by bacterial or other infection of the kidney.

pyloric valve • The valve in the lower portion of the stomach that controls flow into the intestine.

pyoderma • Any skin lesion that produces pus.

pyogenic • Pus-forming; related to pus formation.

pyrosis • Heartburn caused by a backflow of gastric juices from the stomach into the esophagus.

pyuria • Pus in the urine.

q • *Quaque*, every, as in q4h, every 4 hours.

qd • *Quaque die*, every day.

qh • Every hour.

qid • *Quater in die*, four times a day.

qs • *Quantum sufficit*, as much as is needed.

radiation therapy • Treatment of a cancerous tumor by exposing it to x-rays or other ionizing radiation.

radiotherapy • Radiation therapy.

RAI • Radioactive iodine, used to treat overactive thyroid.

Raynaud's phenomenon • Pallor, redness, or blueness in the toes, brought on by cold or strong emotion; when chronic, Raynaud's disease.

RBC • Red blood cell *or* red blood count.

RDA • Recommended daily allowance.

red cell aplasia • Defective, retarded, or incomplete development of the red blood cells; or a cessation in their regeneration.

reflux • A backward flow or regurgitation, as of gastric acid from the stomach into the esophagus, or of urine from the bladder into the kidney.

Reiter's syndrome • A rheumatic condition characterized by urethritis, eye inflammation, and arthritis. The cause is unknown, but it is often associated with venereal disease, particularly gonorrhea.

REM • Rapid eye movement; the stage of sleep associated with rapid eye movement, dreaming, and a characteristic EEG pattern.

renal • Pertaining to the kidneys.

renal tubule • Parts of the kidney that extract urine from the circulation.

renin • An enzyme produced in the kidneys that is transformed by other body tissues into the polypeptide angiotensin, which raises blood pressure by constricting blood vessels.

respiratory alkalosis • Buildup of hydrogen in the blood resulting from accelerated pulmonary removal of carbon dioxide from the body, often as a result of panting or hyperventilation.

respiratory reserve • The difference between the amount of air breathed under normal resting conditions and maximum breathing capacity.

reticulocyte • Immature red blood cell.

reticulocytosis • An excess of immature normal red blood cells (reticulocytes), which occurs in some types of anemia and during blood regeneration, such as after a large wound.

reticulum • A fine network formed by cells, connective fibers between cells, or by structures within a cell.

retinopathy • Any of several degenerative diseases of the retina that do not cause inflammation.

retrocollis • Retraction that accompanies wry neck (torticollis).

retroperitoneal • At the back of the abdomen.

Reye's syndrome • Serious disease seen in children, characterized by severe vomiting, swelling of the brain and fatty infiltration of the liver; usually follows viral infection.

rhinitis • Inflammation of the nasal mucous membrane, particularly during a cold or allergic response.

rhinorrhea • Runny nose.

rhinovirus • A virus group that causes the common cold.

Rhizopus • A genus of fungi, found in the nose, ear, tongue, and lungs; they may act as allergens in common molds.

Rickettsiae • Genus of bacteria that causes Rocky Mountain spotted fever and other spotted fever diseases.

RNA • Ribonucleic acid; a chemical similar to DNA found in cell cytoplasm; it carries the genetic information encoded in the DNA and transforms it into specific cellular activities.

rouleau • A roll of red blood cells that are stacked one atop the other, similar to a roll of coins.

s • Seconds.

salicylate • An organic crystallized salt in aspirin and other analgesics, used to treat pain and fever.

Salmonella • Genus of gram-negative bacteria that causes disease in all warm-bodied animals.

Salmonella typhi • Bacteria that causes typhoid fever. Also called *S. typhosa.*

salpingitis • Inflammation of the uterine tube; *also*, inflammation of the auditory tube in the ear.

saluretic • A substance that facilitates excretion of salt by the kidneys.

sanguinous • Pertaining to the blood; involving much bleeding.

sarcoidosis • A disorder most commonly affecting the lungs, lymph nodes, spleen, liver, skin, eyes, and glands, characterized by abnormal cell shape in all affected areas.

sarcoma • A malignant tumor formed of cells of connective tissue.

SC • Subcutaneous.

scabies • An intensely itchy rash caused by infection with mites (*Sarcoptes scabiei*), which burrow under the skin to lay their eggs, causing the irritation.

scarlatiniform • Disease or symptoms resembling scarlet fever.

schistosomiasis • A parasitic disease caused by blood flukes (worms of the genus *Schistosoma*); depending on the species, symptoms may range from mild dysentery to liver and spleen enlargement and severe lung damage.

sciatica • Throbbing pain radiating down the back of the thigh, usually caused by pressure on the sciatic nerve.

sclera • The white of the eye; plural, sclerae.

scleral injection • Bloodshot eyes, caused by increased blood flow in the sclerae, resulting in distended blood vessels.

sclerosis • Chronic, inflammatory hardening of tissue; particularly, hardening of nerves through overgrowth of fibrous connective tissue and decay of nerve cells.

scoliosis • Lateral curvature of the spine.

scotomata • Blind spots in the visual field or areas of depressed vision; "seeing stars"; singular, scotoma.

scrotum • The sac holding the testes.

sebaceous glands • Glands in the skin that secrete sebum.

seborrheic dermatitis • Inflammation of the skin, characterized by dry or greasy scales, yellowish, crusty patches, and itching.

sebum • An oily substance secreted onto the surface of the skin, composed primarily of fats and dead cells.

semicircular canals • Three fluid-filled canals in the inner ear, each at right angles to the others; the organ for sensing balance.

sensorium • The hypothetical "seat of sensation"; in psychiatry, synonymous with consciousness; also used as a generic term for the intellectual functions.

sepsis • The presence of bacteria or other infecting organisms or their toxins.

septicemia • Severe bacterial infection that invades the blood stream.

serous • Pertaining to serum.

serum • The amber-colored or clear fluid in blood and body fluid.

serum sickness • A reaction to the administration of a foreign serum; symptoms usually appear in 8 to 12 days and include rash, swollen lymph nodes, joint pain, and fever.

sex hormones • Any of the substances usually secreted by the ovaries or testes that stimulate development of the secondary sexual characteristics.

SGOT • Serum glutamic oxaloacetic transaminase, an enzyme released by tissue injury. An elevated level of SGOT in the blood indicates heart attack, liver disease, or other disorder characterized by tissue damage.

SGPT • Serum glutamic pyruvic transaminase, an enzyme manufactured in the liver. An increased level in the blood indicates liver disease.

Shigella • Genus of gram-negative bacteria that cause dysentery. Subgroups include *S dysenteriae, S flexneri, S boydii*, and *S sonnei*.

sialadenitis • Inflammation of a salivary gland.

sialorrhea • Salivation or production of saliva.

sick sinus syndrome • Severe slowing of the heartbeat due to incomplete conduction of nerve impulses in the heart.

sigmoid • The sigmoid, or descending, colon; the last section of the large intestine, terminating at the rectum.

sigmoidoscopy • Use of special instruments to view the inner part of the colon.

sinusitis • Inflammation of the sinus cavities of the head.

sinus tachycardia • Heart rhythm of more than 100 beats per minute originating in the sinus node of the heart.

Sjogren's syndrome • A glandular syndrome often seen in menopausal women; symptoms include drying of mucous membranes, spots on the face, and swollen salivary glands.

sol • Solution.

somatic • Relating to the framework of the body, as in somatic pain.

spasticity • Increased tension of a muscle or muscles with exaggeration of deep reflexes and often with some loss of muscle control.

spermatogenesis • The formation and development of male sperm cells.

spermatozoon • A mature male reproductive cell produced in the testes.

spermicidal • Poisonous to sperm cells.

sphincter of Oddi • The smooth muscle at the point where the common bile duct and pancreatic duct open into the duodenum.

sphygmomanometer • An instrument used to measure blood pressure.

spider telangiectases • Dilation of the small blood vessels just beneath the skin, appearing as a weblike pattern, usually on the legs.

spina bifida occulta • A minor, usually asymptomatic, congenital spinal defect in which parts of the vertebrae are incompletely joined, usually discoverable only by x-ray.

spirochete • Any spiral-shaped microorganism of the Spirochaetales order.

splenomegaly • Enlargement of the spleen.

sporotrichosis • A chronic fungal infection, usually picked up from soil, causing inflamed lymph nodes and sometimes affecting bones and other organs.

sputum • Discharge from the throat, air passages, or mouth.

squamous-cell carcinoma • A carcinoma arising from the external body surfaces and membranes, characterized by flat, scale-like cells.

Staphylococcus albus • *Staphylococcus epidermidis*.

Staphylococcus aureus • Species of staphylococci responsible for a variety of human diseases, including abscesses, endocarditis, pneumonia, and septicemia. May also inhabit skin or mucuous membranes without causing disease.

Staphylococcus epidermidis • Species of staphylococci microorganisms that in rare instances may be associated with heart and brain infection.

stasis dermatitis • Chronic inflammation of the skin of the legs due to impeded circulation.

status asthmaticus • A prolonged and refractory asthma attack.

steatorrhea • Large amounts of fat in the stool.

stenosis • Narrowing, especially of an orifice or vessel.

steroid hormone • One of a number of hormones sharing a similar chemical structure, including sex hormones and adrenal cortical hormones.

Stevens-Johnson syndrome • A severe, occasionally fatal form of erythema multiforme, in which skin eruptions are complicated by systemic symptoms and inflammation of the mucous membranes of the mouth and eyes.

stomatitis • Inflammation of the mucous membrane and other soft tissues of the mouth.

strabismus • Cross-eyes; the eyes not focused parallel on the visual axis.

Strept coccus faecalis • A species of bacteria that normally inhabit the intestinal tract and that are causative organisms of endocarditis and genitourinary and wound infections.

Streptococcus pneumoniae • One of the causative organisms of pneumonia and other infectious diseases, such as meningitis, middle ear infection, and arthritis.

Streptococcus pyogenes • The causative organism of scarlet fever, infectious sore throat, and various pus-forming infections.

stria • A stripe or streak distinguished from surrounding tissue by color, texture, or elevation. Plural, striae.

stromal • Of the connective tissue.

strychnine • A bitter, poisonous alkaloid that acts as a stimulant to the central nervous system.

subarachnoid • Beneath the arachnoid membrane, the delicate covering of the brain and spinal cord.

subarachnoid block • A condition in which some mass prevents the normal flow of cerebrospinal fluid.

subclinical • Pertaining to a disease in which manifestations are so slight as to be unnoticeable or undemonstrable.

subconjunctival • Situated beneath the membranes lining the inner eyelid and anterior portion of the eyeball.

subcutaneous • Just beneath the skin.

sublingual • Beneath the tongue.

substernal • Beneath the breast bone.

sulfobromophthalein • A water-soluble chemical excreted by the liver; its presence in the blood is often used to test liver function. Abbreviated BSP.

sulfonamide • One of a class of antibiotic drugs derived from the chemical sulfanilamide; a sulfa drug.

sulfonylurea • One of a class of related compounds that lower blood sugar (glucose); an oral hypoglycemic.

superinfection • A second infection added onto one already present.

supp • Suppository.

suppository • A solid body intended for insertion into the rectum, vagina, or urethra. Most suppositories are made of fatty substances that are solid at room temperature but soften or melt inside the body, thus releasing medication.

suppurative • Characterized by pus formation.

supraorbital • Situated above the bony cavity containing the eye.

suprapubic • Above the pubic bones.

suprarenal gland • Tiny endocrine gland just above each kidney; also called adrenal gland.

supraventricular arrhythmia • Irregular heart rhythm originating above the ventricles, usually in the atria.

susp • Suspension.

sust rel • Sustained release.

sympathetic nervous system • The part of the autonomic (involuntary) nervous system that is stimulated by adrenaline; it decreases secretions, increases heart activity, and causes the blood vessels to constrict. (Compare *parasympathetic nervous system*.)

sympathetic ophthalmia • Inflammation of the iris and ciliary body of the eye that results from an injury or disease in the other eye; it may eventually lead to bilateral blindness.

sympathomimetic agent • A drug able to imitate the actions of the sympathetic nervous system.

syncope • Fainting; loss of consciousness due to a sudden drop in blood pressure.

syndactyly • Webbing or fusion of the fingers or toes.

synovia • A clear fluid secreted by joints, tendon sheaths, and bursas for lubrication. Also called synovial fluid.

synovitis • Inflammation of an area lubricated by synovial fluid, particularly a joint; usually synonymous with arthritis.

systemic lupus erythematosus • An inflammatory connective tissue disease with variable symptoms including fever, muscle and joint pain, anemia, skin changes or rash, and sun sensitivity; the kidneys, spleen, heart, and skin are often involved. Abbreviated SLE (formerly LE).

systole • The phase in the heart's pumping rhythm in which the lower chambers contract.

T_3 suppression test • A test for evidence of decreased thyroid function; T_3 is the symbol for triiodothyronine, one of the thyroid hormones.

tab • Tablet.

tachycardia • Excessively rapid heartbeat.

tachypnea • Rapid breathing.

tamponade • Decreased heart capacity caused by accumulation of fluid in the sac surrounding the heart and resultant increased pressure on the heart.

tardive dyskinesia • Uncontrolled movements of the face, lips, and tongue, and to a lesser degree jerking of the limbs and trunk, usually induced by long-term use of certain antipsychotic drugs.

tbsp • Tablespoons.

telangiectases • Localized dilation of small blood vessels. Singular, telangiectasis.

temporal arteritis • Inflammation of the temporal or cranial arteries, seen most often in the elderly.

temporal bone • One of the two irregular bones forming part of the lateral surfaces and base of the skull, and housing the hearing organs.

temporal lobe seizure • An epileptic seizure, characterized by loss of consciousness, amnesia, some limb movement, and sometimes hallucinations.

tendon • A tough, fibrous cord that connects a muscle to a bone or other structure. (Compare *ligament*.)

tenesmus • A painful, ineffectual straining to empty the bowel or bladder.

tenosynovitis • Inflammation of a tendon and its enveloping sheath.

teratogenic • Capable of causing birth defects.

teratomatous • Having the properties of a teratoma, a tumor of chaotically arranged cells of an origin foreign to the tissue where they are located.

tertiary syphilis • Late syphilis, including all the symptoms of the disease occurring after the fourth year of infection.

tetany • A nervous disorder in which even mild stimuli produce muscle spasms and cramps, associated with vitamin D and calcium deficiencies.

thalamus • A mass of grey matter at the base of the cerebrum that relays sensory stimuli to the cerebral cortex.

thrombin • An enzyme produced from prothrombin during the blood clotting process; it, in turn, converts to fibrin.

thromboangiitis obliterans • Inflammation of the entire wall and connective tissue surrounding medium-sized arteries and veins, to the extent that blood flow is largely or completely obstructed, commonly resulting in gangrene.

thrombocytopenia • An abnormally low level of platelets in the blood.

thrombocytopenic purpura • A serious systemic illness marked by hemorrhage into the skin, mucous membrane bleeding, anemia, and low platelet count.

thromboembolism • Partial or complete obstruction of blood flow in a vein or artery or in the heart, caused by a blood clot.

thrombophlebitis • Inflammation of a vein associated with a blood clot.

thromboplastin • One of a group of substances that hasten blood clotting by accelerating the conversion of prothrombin to thrombin.

thrombosis • The formation of a blood clot within the heart or blood vessels.

thrombotic • Relating to a blood clot or its formation.

thrombus • A blood clot formed within the blood vessels or heart.

thrush • Fungal mouth infection caused by *Candida albicans*.

thyroactive • Capable of increasing activity of the thyroid gland.

thyroid hyperplasia • A nontumorous overgrowth or enlargement of the thyroid gland.

thyroid storm • A medical emergency caused by extreme overproduction of thyroid hormone, leading to severe rapid heartbeat (tachycardia), muscle weakness, coma, and, if untreated, death; also called thyrotoxic crisis.

thyroiditis • Inflammation of the thyroid gland.

thyrotoxicosis • Surplus thyroid hormone production.

thyroxine • An iodine-containing hormone secreted by the thyroid gland.

tic douloureux • Neuralgia of the trigeminal nerve, which serves the lower jaw, upper jaw, and eyes. Also called trigeminal neuralgia.

tidal volume • The amount of air normally inhaled and exhaled in resting respiration.

tid • *ter in die*, three times a day.

tinea barbae • Ringworm of the beard.

tinea capitis • Ringworm of the scalp.

tinea corporis • Fungal infection of the smooth non-hairy skin surfaces.

tinea cruris • Jock itch; ringworm of the inner thighs, groin, and perineal region.

tinea manus • Fungal infection of the hand, caused by *Trichophyton purpureum*.

tinea pedis • Athlete's foot; ringworm of the foot, particularly the skin between the toes.

tinea unguium • Fungal infection of the nails.

tinea versicolor • A chronic fungal infection causing brownish-yellow patches on the skin of the trunk, caused by *Malassezia furfur*.

tinnitus • Ringing in the ears; or, sometimes, a hissing or roaring sound.

titer • The amount of one substance that is equivalent to a stated quantity of another substance.

titrate • To measure out the amount of one substance that will be equivalent in strength or chemical reactivity to another substance; specifically, to measure out the amount of a drug that will be sufficient to have a specific therapeutic effect.

tonic-clonic seizure • An epileptic seizure in which there is both a rigid (tonic) and a convulsive (clonic) stage.

tonsillopharyngeal • Pertaining to the tonsils and pharynx.

tophaceous • Sandy; gritty; pertaining to or resembling a tophus, a mineral deposit or concentration such as sodium urate deposits seen in gout.

topical • Local; in drug administration, applied to specific areas of the skin.

torticollis • Stiff neck caused by spasmodic contraction of the neck muscles on one side only, resulting in an abnormal position of the head.

torulosis • An infection that may involve the skin, lungs, or other parts, but has a predilection for the central nervous system; also called cryptococcosis.

toxemia • The presence of poisonous toxins and other substances in the blood.

toxic amblyopia • Chronic dimness of vision or loss of sight resulting from toxemia caused by kidney disease, diabetes, or other disorders, as well as by ingestion of poisonous substances such as lead or methyl alcohol.

toxic megacolon • Acute dilatation of the colon that may progress to rupture.

toxoid • A toxin deprived of some harmful properties but still capable of producing immunity on injection.

toxoplasmosis • A condition of enlarged glands and fever caused by *Toxoplasma*, protozoa that commonly occur in mammals and birds and may infect man, sometimes causing severe disorders in infants born of infected mothers.

tracheobronchitis • Inflammation of the trachea and bronchi.

tracheostomy • The surgical creation of an opening into the trachea through the neck to facilitate breathing or remove secretions.

trachoma • A contagious conjunctivitis of viral origin, marked by inflammatory tissue formation on the membrane.

transcortin • A protein in the blood that binds active hydrocortisone and other corticosteroids in order to transport them through the body.

transient ischemic attacks • Transient attacks of numbness, partial paralysis, difficulty of speech, or other symptoms, caused by ischemia of a localized area of the brain. Also called TIAs; they may signal an impending stroke.

trephining • Removal of a circular section of bone, usually from the skull.

Treponema pertenue • The organism that causes yaws.

trichinosis • Infection with trichina worms, acquired by eating inadequately cooked, infected meat (usually pork or meat contaminated by infected pork); mild cases may mimic intestinal flu, but severe infections may cause inflammation of the skin, muscles, lungs, heart muscle, and other organs, possibly leading to death.

trichomonad • Pertaining to or resembling the flagellates belonging to the genus *Trichomonas*.

Trichomonas vaginalis • The species of flagellate protozoa that has been implicated in vaginitis.

trichomoniasis • Infection caused by *Trichomonas* protozoa, usually of the vaginal or urethral areas.

Trichophyton • A genus of fungi that attack the hair, skin, and nails, causing athlete's foot and ringworm; species includes *T crateriform, T gallinae, T interdigitalis, T megnini, T mentagrophytes, T rubrum, T schoenleini, T sulphureum, T tonsurans,* and *T verrucosum.*

tricyclic antidepressants • Drugs with three-ring molecular structure used for the treatment of depression.

trifascicular • Involving all three parts (fascicles) of the heart's ventricular conduction system.

trigeminal neuralgia • A severe sharp pain along the course of a facial nerve; also called tic douloureaux.

trigeminy • A disturbance of cardiac rhythm in which heartbeats are grouped in threes.

triglyceride • A lipid (fat) that is a major component of both animal and vegetable fats.

trigonitis • Inflammation of the urinary bladder, localized in the mucous membrane at the trigonum, the triangular area at the base of the bladder.

triiodothyronine • An iodine-containing hormone secreted by the thyroid gland.

trismus • Spasm of the muscles of the jaw; lockjaw.

trophic • Pertaining to nutrition.

TSH • Thyroid-stimulating hormone.

tsp • Teaspoons.

tuberculin • A sterile extract prepared from the tubercle bacillus and injected to determine the presence of a tuberculosis infection.

tularemia • An acute, plague-like infectious disease transmitted to man by the bite of an infected insect or by direct contact with infected animals or animal products; also called tick fever or rabbit fever.

tumorigenic • Tumor-forming.

T-wave • The electrocardiographic deflection due to repolarization of the ventricles; it may be positive or negative.

tympanic membrane • The eardrum.

tyramine • A chemical produced by the breakdown of an amino acid; it appears in wine, cheese, and other fermented substances.

ulcer • A perforation or lesion on the skin or a mucous surface, caused by superficial tissue loss, usually with inflammation.

unctuous • Oily; greasy.

urate • A salt of uric acid.

uremia • A toxic condition associated with renal insufficiency and the retention in the blood of nitrogenous substances normally excreted by the kidney.

ureter • The tube conducting urine from the kidney to the bladder.

urethritis • Inflammation of the canal through which urine is discharged from the bladder.

urethrocystitis • Inflammation of the urethra and urinary bladder.

urethrotrigonitis • Inflammation of the urethra and triangular base of the bladder.

uric acid • An acid found in the blood and urine; a product of the metabolization of protein.

uricosuric • Promoting the excretion of uric acid in the urine.

urolithiasis • The formation of urinary stones.

uropathy • Any disease affecting the urinary tract.

urticaria • Hives; an eruption of itching wheals, usually of systemic origin, possibly due to hypersensitivity or allergy.

uveitis • Inflammation of the entire uveal tract of the eye, which includes the iris, ciliary body, and choroid.

vaccinia • A disease resembling smallpox that affects animals and man; also called cowpox.

vacuolization • Formation of vacuoles (clear spaces in cell protoplasm filled with fluid or air).

vaginal cuff • Band-like structure encircling the vagina.

vaginitis • Inflammation of the vagina.

vagolytic • Inhibiting the vagus nerve.

vagus nerve • The wanderer nerve, which has numerous branches and is composed of both sensory and motor fibers; it has wide distribution in the neck, chest, and abdomen, with major branches to the heart, lungs, stomach, and other organs.

vanillylmandelic acid • A product of the breakdown of adrenal hormones; its concentration in the urine is used to test for pheochromocytoma.

varicella • Chickenpox.

varicocele • Varicose enlargement of spermatic cord veins, a common cause of male infertility.

varicose • Characterizing blood vessels, particularly veins, that have become excessively tortuous and dilated, sometimes to the point where the valves no longer work, and blood flows in both directions.

varicose ulcer • An ulcer arising from dilated or varicose vein or veins.

vascular • Of the blood vessels; containing blood vessels.

vasculitis • Angiitis; inflammation of a blood or lymphatic vessel.

vasoconstrictor • A drug or enzyme that causes the smooth muscles of the blood vessels to contract, thus constricting the vessels and raising blood pressure.

vasodilator • A drug or enzyme that causes the blood vessels to dilate, usually by relaxing the vascular muscles.

vasomotor • Causing or involving dilation or constriction of the blood vessels.

vasomotor rhinitis • Congestion of the nasal mucous membrane without infection or allergy.

vasopressor • A substance that produces narrowing or constriction of the blood vessels, resulting in a rise in blood pressure. Synonym, vasoconstrictor.

vasospasm • The constriction of blood vessels.

vasovagal attack • Syncope; a paroxysmal condition marked by slowed pulse, falling blood pressure, and, sometimes, convulsions, probably due to sudden vagus nerve stimulation.

venipuncture • The puncture of a vein, as by a hypodermic needle.

venogram • An x-ray picture of the veins in a particular area of the body after a contrasting substance has been injected into them.

venous thrombosis • The formation of a blood clot in a vein.

ventricle • A small cavity, especially in the brain or heart; specifically, the lower chambers of the heart.

ventricular tachycardia • Rapid, paroxysmal heartbeat originating in the ventricles.

vertigo • Dizziness, giddiness; a sensation of irregular or whirling motion, often a result of overstimulation of the semicircular canals in the inner ear.

vesical sphincter • The circular muscle controlling the urinary bladder opening.

vesicle • A bladder; a small sac containing fluid.

vesiculobullous • Having both small and large water-filled blisters.

vestibular • Pertaining to those parts of the inner ear concerned with balance.

Vibrio comma • The causative agent of cholera, shaped like a comma in fresh culture.

Vincent's infection • A noncontagious infection of the oral mucous membranes, marked by ulceration and formation of a gray false membrane.

viridans • A group of streptococci that produce a zone of greenish discoloration about the colonies on a blood-agar medium.

visceral • Referring to the viscera, the organs in the cranial, chest, abdominal, or pelvic cavities.

vitreous • Glassy; resembling glass; transparent. *Also*, the vitreous humor, the viscous fluid filling the eyeball between the lens and the retina.

VMA • Vanillylmandelic acid; a by-product of the breakdown of adrenal catecholamines that is secreted in urine; VMA measurement is a test for pheochromocytoma.

vomitus • Vomited matter or the act of vomiting.

vulva • The external female genital organs.

vulvar • Relating to the vulva.

vulvovaginitis • Inflammation of the vulva and vagina, or of the vulvovaginal glands.

water intoxication • Cramps, dizziness, headache, vomiting, convulsions, and coma, resulting from ingestion of large quantities of water or from water retention.

WBC • White blood cell *or* white blood count.

wheal-and-flare reaction • An immunological response occurring within minutes of injection of an antigen into the skin; itching at the site of injection is followed by the appearance of a raised welt (wheal); often seen in bee stings and insect bites.

Wilms' tumor • A malignant tumor of the kidney, usually affecting infants and children.

Wilson's disease • A hereditary disorder of faulty copper metabolism, associated with degenerative changes in the liver and central nervous system.

wk • Weeks.

w/v • Weight per volume.

xanthine • A precursor of uric acid occurring in many organs and in urine, occasionally forming urinary calculi.

xanthine calculi • Hard, brown to red stones found (rarely) in the urinary bladder.

xanthoma • Cholesterol-filled nodules that appear under the skin, especially on the eyelids and around the tendons.

xanthopsia • Yellow vision that sometimes occurs with jaundice.

xerostomia • Dryness of the mouth caused by insufficient secretion of saliva.

yaws • An infectious tropical disease marked by fever, pain in the joints, and a characteristic skin lesion called a yaw.

Yersinia pestis • Causative organism of plague in man and rodents, transmitted by the rat flea.

yr • Years.

Drug Identification

On the following pages are photographs showing more than 1,000 pills and capsules in their actual color, size, and shape. To facilitate identification of an unknown drug, the medications are arranged by color, and within each color grouping by shade, thus making it easier to match the pill or capsule with the photograph.

In each grouping, the solid-color medications are pictured first, followed by two-color capsules and pills. Capsules are grouped according to the color of the overlapping shell. For example, if you have a red and blue capsule, the medication will be found in the red section, if that is the color of the larger end of the capsule that fits over the opening of the blue half. To find a multicolor layered pill, look for the manufacturer's code, name, or number—this is the side that will determine color placement.

Under each photograph, you will find the brand name of the drug, dosage strength, and manufacturer. You can then look up the brand name in the index to find the page on which the medication is described.

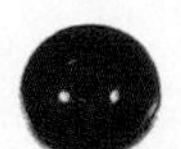
PLACIDYL 200 mg
Abbott

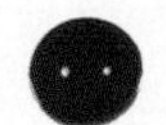
PLACIDYL 100 mg
Abbott

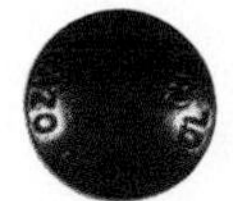
AZO GANTANOL
Roche

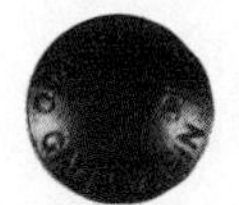
AZO GANTRISIN
Roche

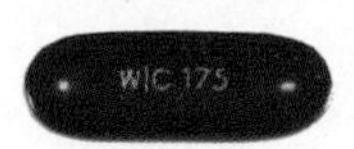

AZO-MANDELAMINE
Parke-Davis

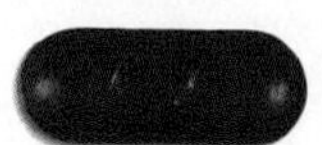
TriHEMIC 600
Lederle

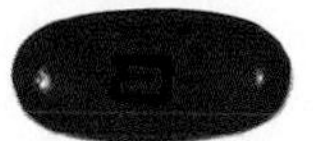
IBERET-FOLIC-500
Abbott

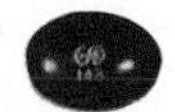
POLARAMINE 6 mg
Schering

DIETHYLSTILBESTROL 1 mg
Lilly

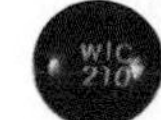

CHOLEDYL 100 mg
Parke-Davis

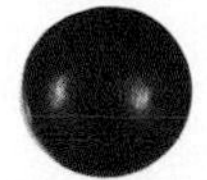
DISOPHROL CHRONOTAB
Schering

SUDAFED 30 mg
Burroughs Wellcome

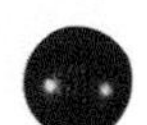
ETRAFON FORTE 4-25
Schering

DECLOMYCIN 300 mg
Lederle

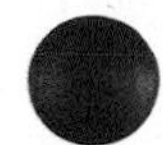
DECLOMYCIN 150 mg
Lederle

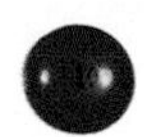
SERENTIL 10 mg
Boehringer-Ingelheim

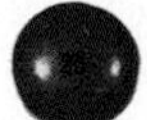
SERENTIL 25 mg
Boehringer-Ingelheim

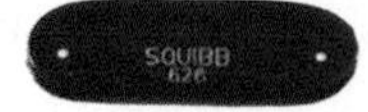

NOCTEC 500 mg
Squibb

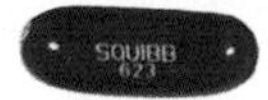

NOCTEC 250 mg
Squibb

MEPERGAN FORTIS
Wyeth

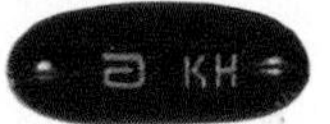

PLACIDYL 500 mg
Abbott

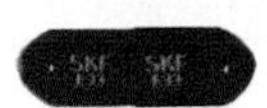

DIBENZYLINE 10 mg
Smith Kline & French

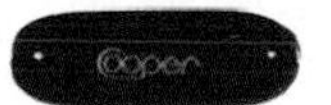

ELIXOPHYLLIN 200 mg
Cooper

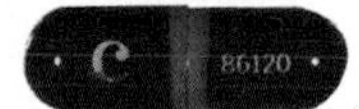

MIDRIN
Carnrick

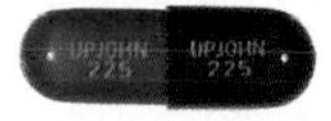

CLEOCIN 150 mg
Upjohn

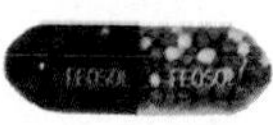

FEOSOL
Menley & James

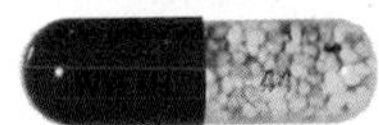
EQUANIL 400 mg
Wyeth

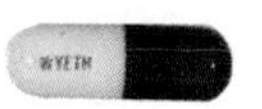

SERAX 30 mg
Wyeth

DURICEF 500 mg
Mead Johnson

SUDAFED 120 mg
Burroughs Wellcome

POLYCILLIN 500 mg
Bristol

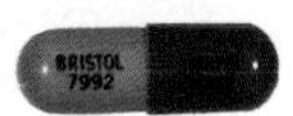

POLYCILLIN 250 mg
Bristol

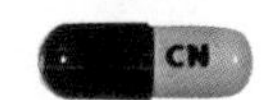

TRANXENE 7.5 mg
Abbott

SYNALGOS
Ives

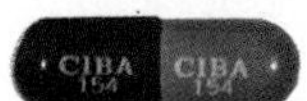

RIMACTANE 300 mg
Ciba

SINEQUAN 10 mg
Pfizer

POLYMOX 250 mg
Bristol

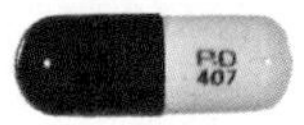

CYCLOPAR 250 mg
Parke-Davis

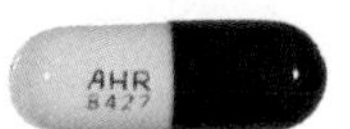

ROBITET 500 mg
Robins

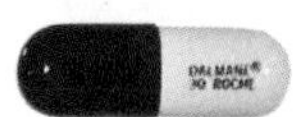
DALMANE 30 mg
Roche

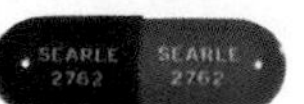

NORPACE 150 mg
Searle

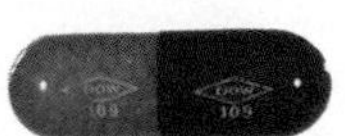
NOVAFED A
Dow

FIORINAL w/CODEINE
Sandoz

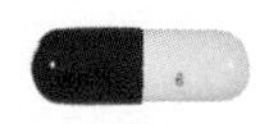
SERAX 15 mg
Wyeth

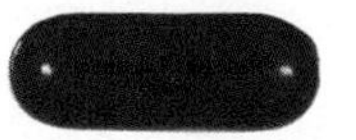
RONIACOL TIMESPAN
Roche

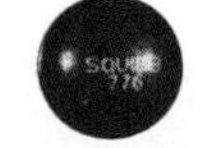
RAUDIXIN 100 mg
Squibb

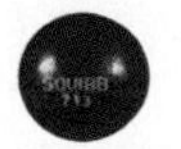
RAUDIXIN 50 mg
Squibb

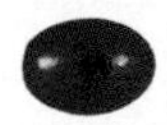
POLARAMINE 4 mg
Schering

RAUTRAX
Squibb

THIOSULFIL-A
Ayerst

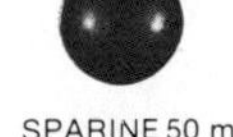
SPARINE 50 mg
Wyeth

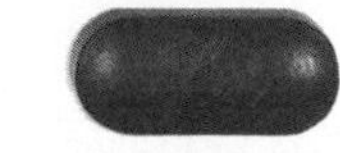
DARVOCET-N 100
Lilly

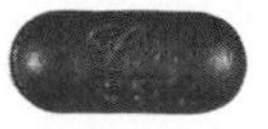
DARVOCET-N 50
Lilly

MEPERGAN FORTIS
Wyeth

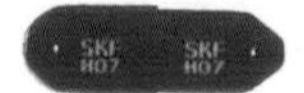

DYRENIUM 100 mg
Smith Kline & French

DYRENIUM 50 mg
Smith Kline & French

DYAZIDE
Smith Kline & French

TYLOX
McNeil

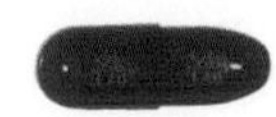

SECONAL 100 mg
Lilly

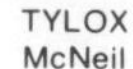

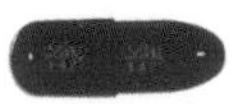

SECONAL 50 mg
Lilly

TUINAL 200 mg
Lilly

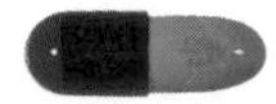

TUINAL 100 mg
Lilly

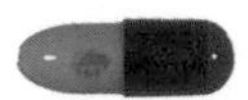

TUINAL 50 mg
Lilly

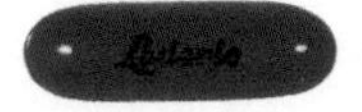

DECLOMYCIN 150 mg
Lederle

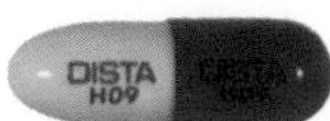

ILOSONE 250 mg
Dista

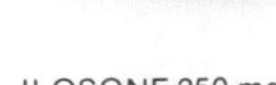

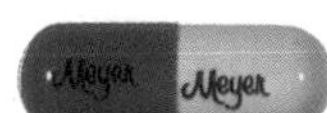

VICON-C
Meyer

TETREX 250 mg
Bristol

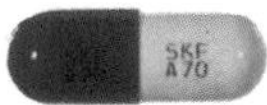

ANSPOR 250 mg
Smith Kline & French

BUTAZOLIDIN ALKA
Geigy

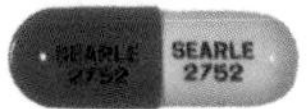

NORPACE 100 mg
Searle

DANTRIUM 50 mg
Norwich-Eaton

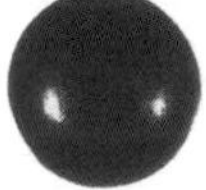

MILPREM 400
Wallace

FERO-FOLIC-500
Abbott

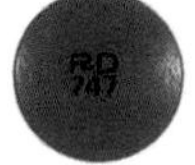

POVAN 50 mg
Parke-Davis

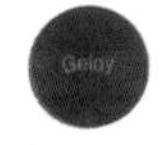

BUTAZOLIDIN 100 mg
Geigy

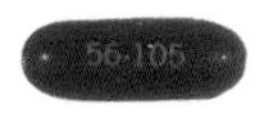

SYMMETREL 100 mg
Endo

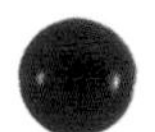

DIETHYLSTILBESTROL 0.5 mg (e-c)
Lilly

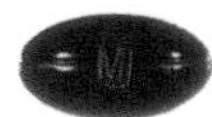

PERI-COLACE 30 mg
Mead Johnson

COLACE 100 mg
Mead Johnson

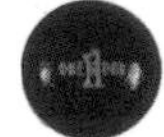

ONE-A—DAY VITAMINS
Miles

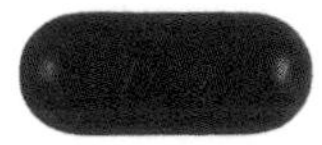

STRESSTABS 600 with IRON
Lederle

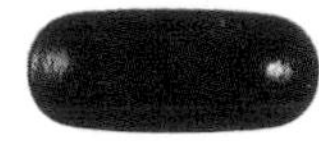

ONE-A-DAY VITAMINS PLUS MINERALS
Miles

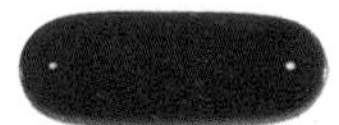

SURFAK 240 mg
Hoechst-Roussel

COLACE 50 mg
Mead Johnson

DEXATRIM EXTRA STRENGTH 275 mg
Thompson Medical

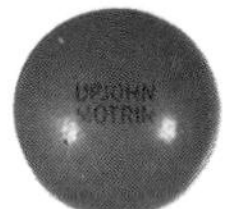

MOTRIN 400 mg
Upjohn

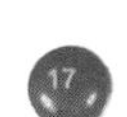

PERSANTINE 25 mg
Boehringer-Ingelheim

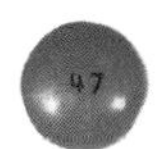

TARACTAN 50 mg
Roche

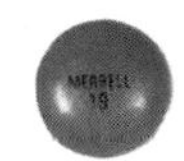

NORPRAMIN 75 mg
Merrell-National

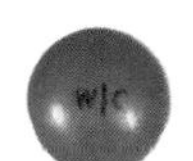

NARDIL 15 mg
Parke-Davis

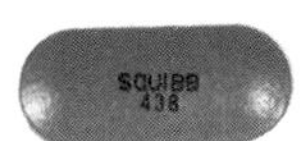

PRONESTYL 500 mg
Squibb

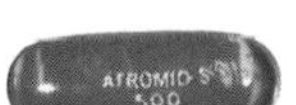

ATROMID-S 500 mg
Ayerst

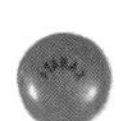

ATARAX 10 mg
Roerig

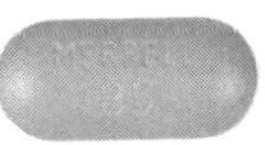

TRICLOS 750 mg
Merrell-National

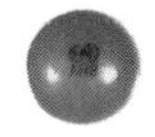

ETRAFON-A (4/10)
Schering

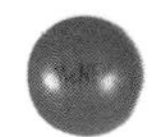

CLISTIN R-A 8 mg
McNeil

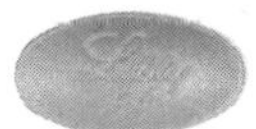

DARVON-N w/A.S.A.
Lilly

PRONESTYL 375 mg
Squibb

DEPAKENE 250 mg
Abbott

ATARAX 100 mg
Roerig

CRYSTODIGIN 0.05 mg
Lilly

STRESSTABS 600
Lederle

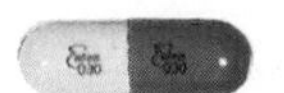

DANTRIUM 25 mg
Norwich-Eaton

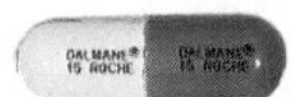

DALMANE 15 mg
Roche

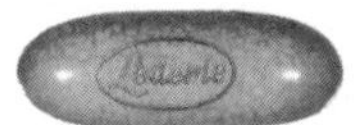

DIAMOX 500 mg
Lederle

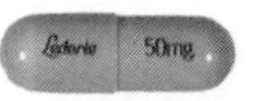

MINOCIN 50 mg
Lederle

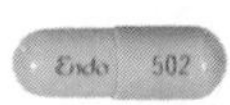

AZENE 6.5 mg
Endo

THORAZINE 300 mg
Smith Kline & French

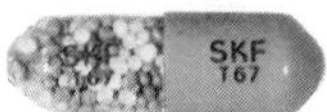

THORAZINE 200 mg
Smith Kline & French

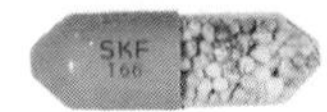

THORAZINE 150 mg
Smith Kline & French

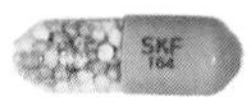

THORAZINE 75 mg
Smith Kline & French

THORAZINE 30 mg
Smith Kline & French

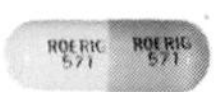

NAVANE 1 mg
Roerig

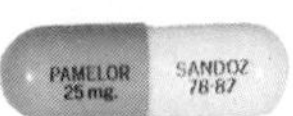

PAMELOR 25 mg
Sandoz

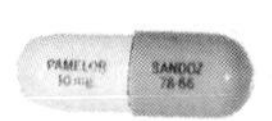

PAMELOR 10 mg
Sandoz

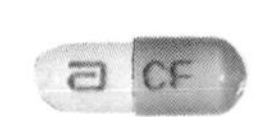

NEMBUTAL 50 mg
Abbott

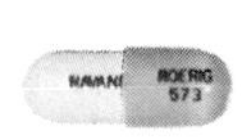

NAVANE 5 mg
Roerig

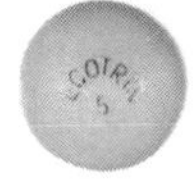

ECOTRIN
Menley & James

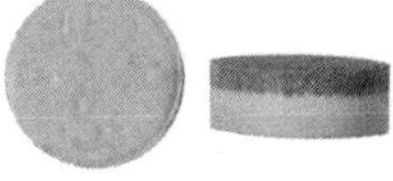

EQUAGESIC
Wyeth

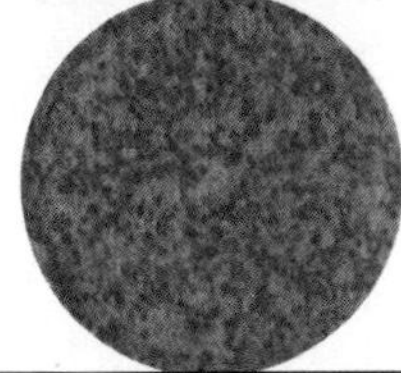

K-LYTE 25 mEq
Mead Johnson

ENDEP 10 mg
Roche

ENDEP 25 mg
Roche

ENDEP 50 mg
Roche

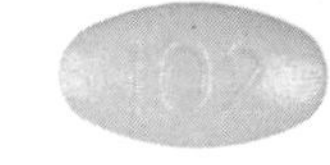

AZULFIDINE EN-TABS 500 mg
Pharmacia

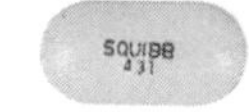

PRONESTYL 250 mg
Squibb

NALFON 600 mg
Dista

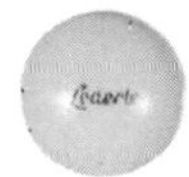

PATHIBAMATE 200 mg
Lederle

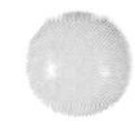

SPARINE 25 mg
Wyeth

ATARAX 50 mg
Roerig

AZULFIDINE 500 mg
Pharmacia

CLINORIL 200 mg
Merck Sharp & Dohme

CLINORIL 150 mg
Merck Sharp & Dohme

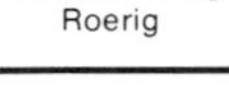

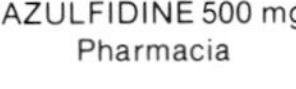

ISMELIN 10 mg
Ciba

PRO-BANTHINE w/PB
Searle

THYROLAR-3
Armour

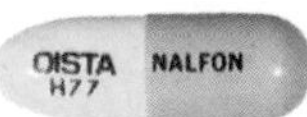

NALFON 300 mg
Dista

TERRAMYCIN 250 mg
Pfizer

IONAMIN 30 mg
Pennwalt

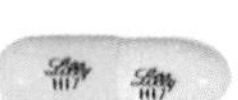

AVENTYL HCL 10 mg
Lilly

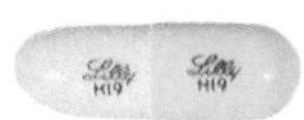

AVENTYL HCL 25 mg
Lilly

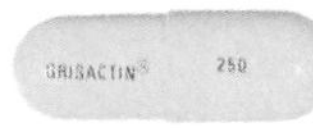

GRISACTIN 250 mg
Ayerst

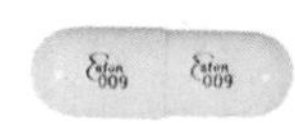

MACRODANTIN 100 mg
Norwich-Eaton

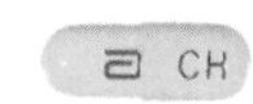

NEMBUTAL 100 mg
Abbott

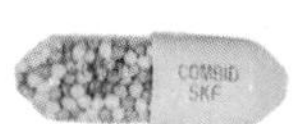

COMBID
Smith Kline & French

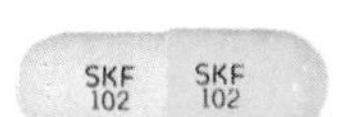

SK-AMPICILLIN 500 mg
Smith Kline & French

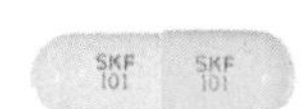

SK-AMPICILLIN 250 mg
Smith Kline & French

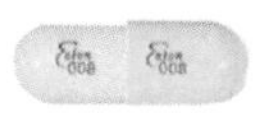

MACRODANTIN 50 mg
Norwich-Eaton

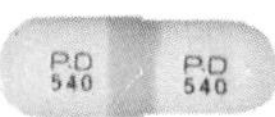

PONSTEL 250 mg
Parke-Davis

LAROTID 500 mg
Roche

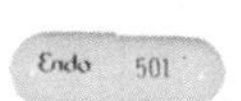

AZENE 3.25 mg
Endo

MENEST 0.3 mg
Beecham

VIVACTIL 10 mg
Merck Sharp & Dohme

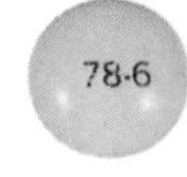

MELLARIL 150 mg
Sandoz

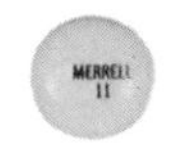

NORPRAMIN 25 mg
Merrell-National

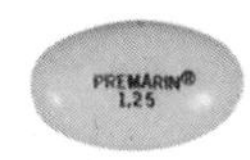

PREMARIN 1.25 mg
Ayerst

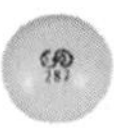

ETRAFON 2-10
Schering

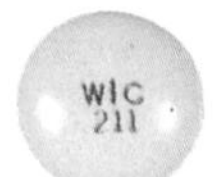

CHOLEDYL 200 mg
Parke-Davis

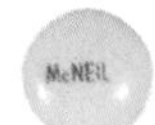

CLISTIN R-A 12 mg
McNeil

PROLIXIN 2.5 mg
Squibb

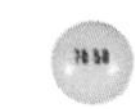

SANSERT 2 mg
Sandoz

REPOISE 5 mg
Robins

ENDEP 75 mg
Roche

COMPAZINE 25 mg
Smith Kline & French

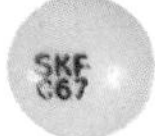

COMPAZINE 10 mg
Smith Kline & French

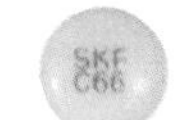

COMPAZINE 5 mg
Smith Kline & French

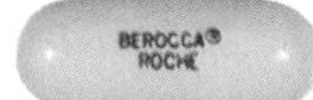

BEROCCA
Roche

ELAVIL 25 mg
Merck Sharp & Dohme

GEOCILLIN
Roerig

TRIAMINICIN
Dorsey

DRAMAMINE 50 mg
Searle

NORINYL 1 + 80 28-DAY
Syntex

TRIAMINIC
Dorsey

ISORDIL Sublingual 2.5 mg
Ives

SORBITRATE Chewable 10 mg
Stuart

TRIAVIL 4-25
Merck Sharp & Dohme

MELLARIL 100 mg
Sandoz

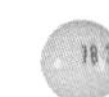

MELLARIL 10 mg
Sandoz

DYMELOR 500 mg
Lilly

FURADANTIN 100 mg
Norwich-Eaton

FURADANTIN 50 mg
Norwich-Eaton

ESIDRIX 50 mg
Ciba

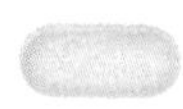

AMYTAL 30 mg
Lilly

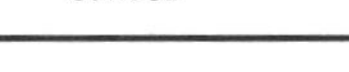

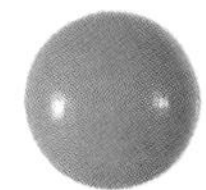

KAON
Warren-Teed

QUIBRON
Mead Johnson

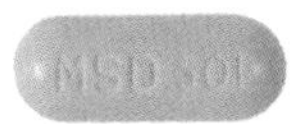

BENEMID 0.5 g
Merck Sharp & Dohme

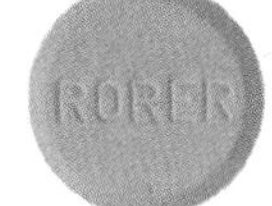

MAALOX PLUS
Rorer

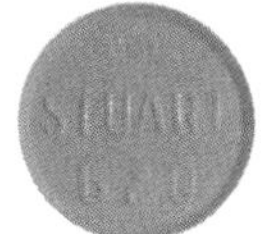

MYLANTA
Stuart

METHOTREXATE 2.5 mg
Lederle

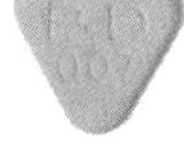

DILANTIN INFATABS 50 mg
Parke-Davis

ORTHO-NOVUM 1/50 □ 21
Ortho

ORTHO-NOVUM 1/50 □ 28
Ortho

NORINYL 1 + 80 21-DAY
Syntex

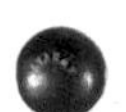

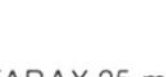

ATARAX 25 mg
Roerig

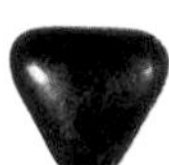

FEOSOL
Menley & James

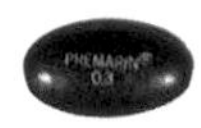

PREMARIN 0.3 mg
Ayerst

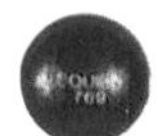

RAUZIDE
Squibb

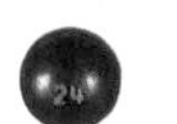

MENRIUM 5-4
Roche

PLACIDYL 750 mg
Abbott

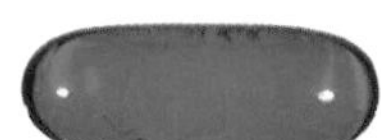

TACE 12 mg
Merrell-National

DRIXORAL
Schering

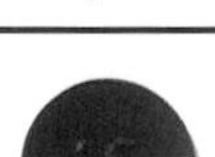

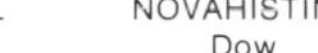

NOVAHISTINE
Dow

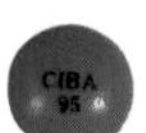

PBZ 25 mg
Geigy

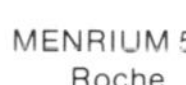

MENRIUM 5-2
Roche

WYGESIC
Wyeth

CAFERGOT P-B
Sandoz

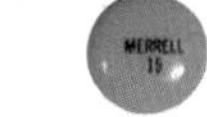

NORPRAMIN 50 mg
Merrell-National

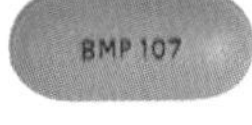

CONAR-A
Beecham

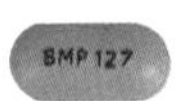

MENEST 1.25 mg
Beecham

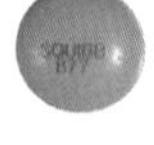

PROLIXIN 5 mg
Squibb

DONNATAL EXTENTABS
Robins

ALDOCLOR-250
Merck Sharp & Dohme

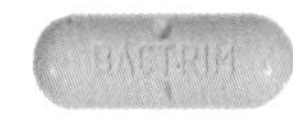

BACTRIM
Roche

HALDOL 5 mg
McNeil

NATURETIN 5 mg
Squibb

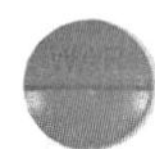

GITALIGIN 0.5 mg
Schering

ANDROID-10
Brown

HYDROPRES-25
Merck Sharp & Dohme

HYDROPRES-50
Merck Sharp & Dohme

PERITRATE 20 mg
Parke-Davis

ISORDIL Oral 20 mg
Ives

PARAFON FORTE
McNeil

SALUTENSIN
Bristol

ISORDIL TEMBIDS 40 mg
Ives

SYNTHROID 0.3 mg
Flint

GANTANOL 500 mg
Roche

HALOTESTIN 10 mg
Upjohn

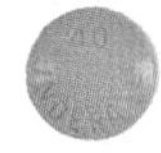

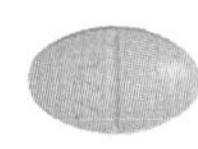

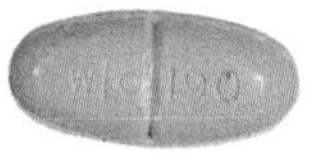
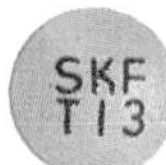

INDERAL 40 mg
Ayerst

SORBITRATE Chewable 5 mg
Stuart

SORBITRATE Oral 5 mg
Stuart

MOBAN 25 mg
Endo

UTIBID 750 mg
Parke-Davis

TAGAMET 300 mg
Smith Kline & French

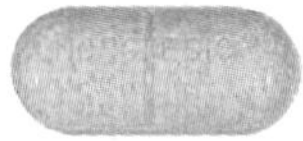
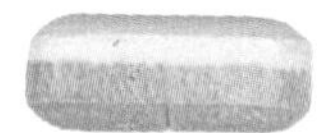
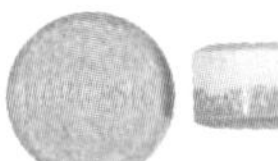
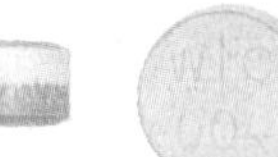
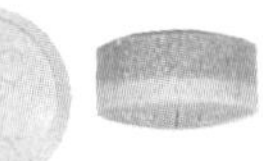

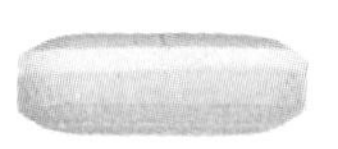

NORGESIC FORTE
Riker

NORGESIC
Riker

PERITRATE SA 80 mg
Parke-Davis

PHENERGAN COMPOUND
Wyeth

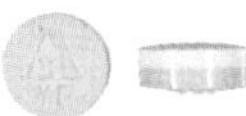

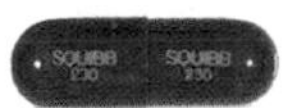
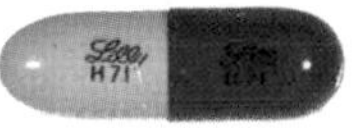
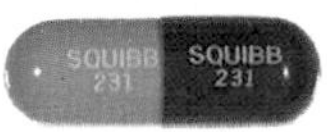

THYROLAR-2
Armour

ANTURANE 200 mg
Ciba

TRIMOX 250 mg
Squibb

KEFLEX 500 mg
Lilly

TRIMOX 500 mg
Squibb

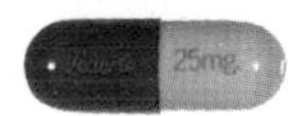
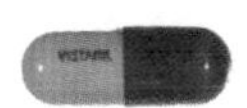
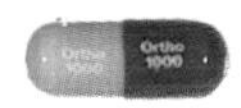
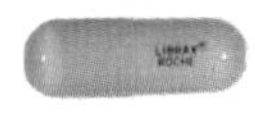
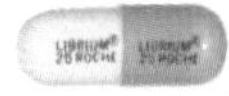

TACE 25 mg
Merrell-National

LOXITANE 25 mg
Lederle

VISTARIL 25 mg
Pfizer

IMODIUM 2 mg
Ortho

LIBRAX
Roche

LIBRIUM 25 mg
Roche

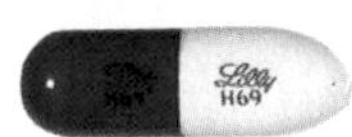
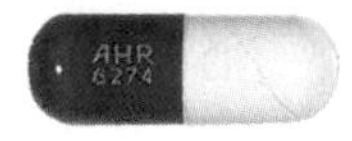
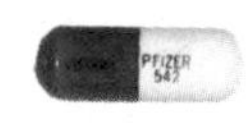
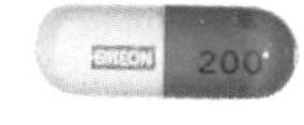
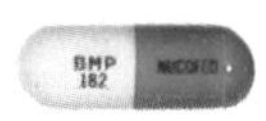
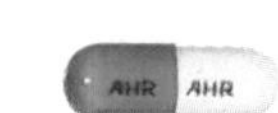

KEFLEX 250 mg
Lilly

PHENAPHEN w/CODEINE #4
Robins

VISTARIL 50 mg
Pfizer

BRONKODYL 200 mg
Breon

NUCOFED
Beecham

DONNATAL
Robins

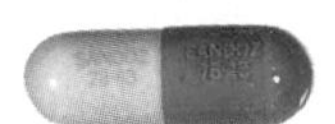
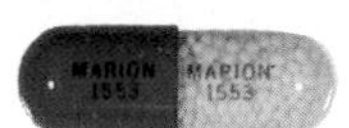
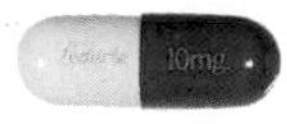
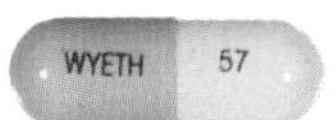
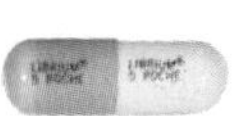

FIORINAL
Sandoz

NITRO-BID 9 mg
Marion

LOXITANE 10 mg
Lederle

UNIPEN 250 mg
Wyeth

LIBRIUM 5 mg
Roche

ADAPIN 25 mg
Pennwalt

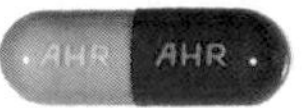
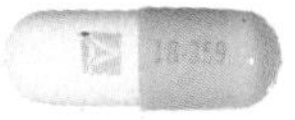
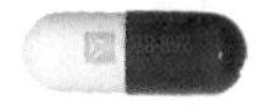
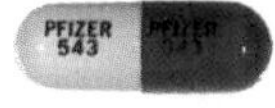
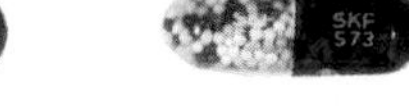
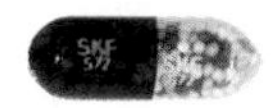

DIMACOL
Robins

ADAPIN 100 mg
Pennwalt

TUSSIONEX
Pennwalt

VISTARIL 100 mg
Pfizer

TELDRIN 12 mg
Menley & James

TELDRIN 8 mg
Menley & James

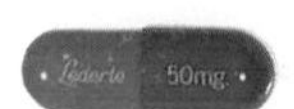
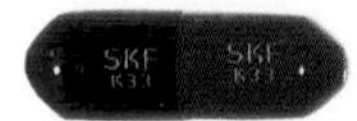
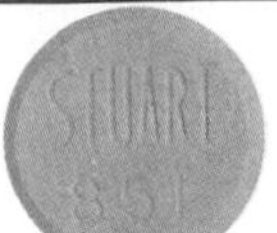

LOXITANE 50 mg
Lederle

FEOSOL PLUS
Menley & James

Z-BEC
Robins

MYLANTA-II
Stuart

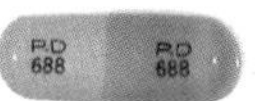
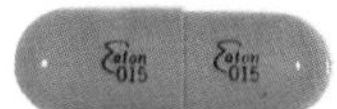

VECTRIN 100 mg
Parke-Davis

DOPAR Capsules
Norwich-Eaton

ALLBEE with C
Robins

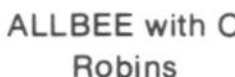

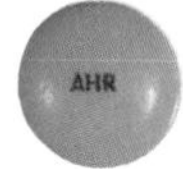

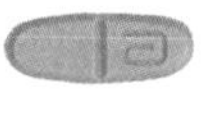
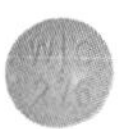

ESTRACE 2 mg
Mead Johnson

DIMETAPP EXTENTABS
Robins

BUTISOL SODIUM 30 mg
McNeil

DISALCID 500 mg
Riker

OGEN 2.5 mg
Abbott

VERSTRAN 10 mg
Parke-Davis

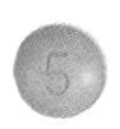
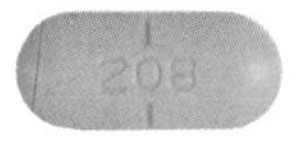

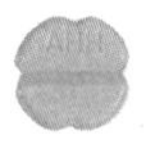

ZAROXOLYN 5 mg
Pennwalt

CORGARD 80 mg
Squibb

CORGARD 120 mg
Squibb

HYGROTON 50 mg
USV Laboratories

TENUATE 25 mg
Merrell-National

NAQUA 4 mg
Schering

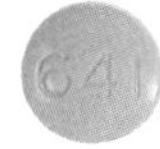

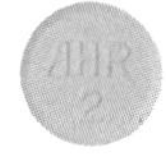

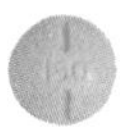

PROBANTHINE w/DARTAL
Searle

APRESOLINE 50 mg
Ciba

PBZ 50 mg
Geigy

ROBINUL-PH FORTE
Robins

ROBINUL PH
Robins

INDERAL 20 mg
Ayerst

SYNTHROID 0.15 mg
Flint

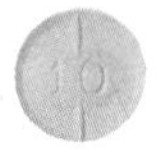

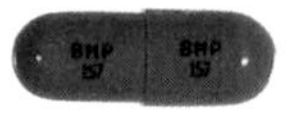

VALIUM 10 mg
Roche

RENESE-R
Pfizer

HALDOL 10 mg
McNeil

DECADRON 0.75 mg
Merck Sharp & Dohme

BENTYL 10 mg
Merrell-National

TIGAN 250 mg
Beecham

VELOSEF 500 mg
Squibb

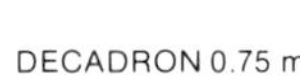
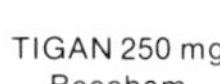

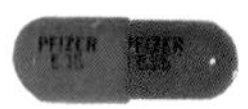
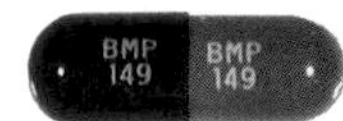
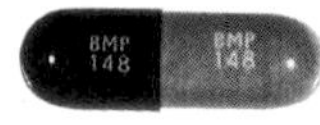
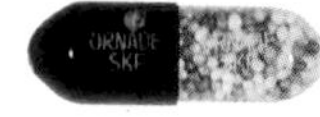
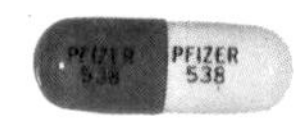
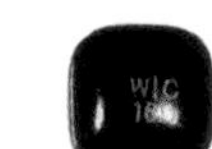

SINEQUAN 25 mg
Pfizer

AMOXIL 500 mg
Beecham

AMOXIL 250 mg
Beecham

ORNADE
Smith Kline & French

SINEQUAN 100 mg
Pfizer

DOLONIL
Parke-Davis

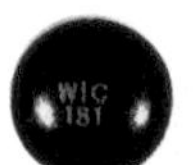
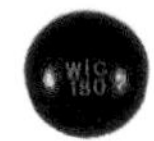
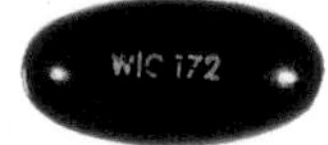
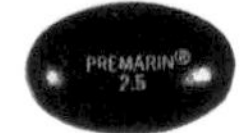
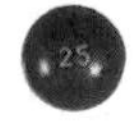

PYRIDIUM 200 mg
Parke-Davis

PYRIDIUM 100 mg
Parke-Davis

MANDELAMINE 1 g
Parke-Davis

PREMARIN 2.5 mg
Ayerst

MENRIUM 10-4
Roche

BUTISOL 15 mg
McNeil

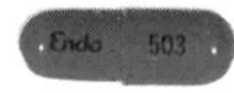
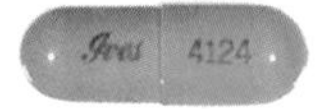
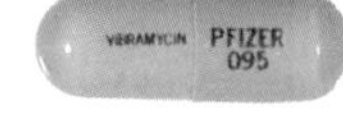
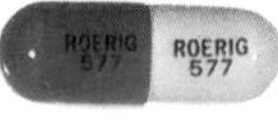

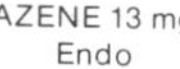
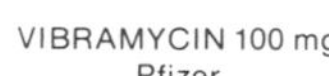

SINEQUAN 150 mg
Pfizer

AZENE 13 mg
Endo

CYCLOSPASMOL 200 mg
Ives

VIBRAMYCIN 100 mg
Pfizer

LINCOCIN 500 mg
Upjohn

NAVANE 20 mg
Roerig

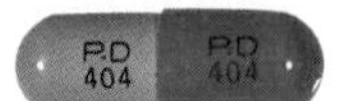

AMCILL 500 mg
Parke-Davis

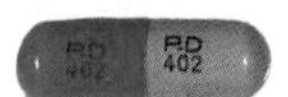

AMCILL 250 mg
Parke-Davis

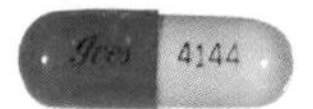

SYNALGOS-DC
Ives

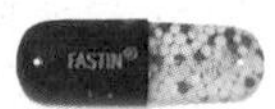

FASTIN
Beecham

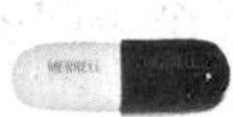
BENTYL w/PHENOBARBITAL 10 mg
Merrell-National

ORNEX
Menley & James

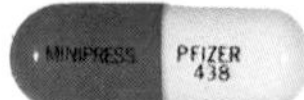

MINIPRESS 5 mg
Pfizer

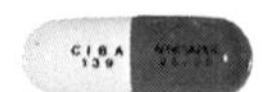
APRESAZIDE 25/25
Ciba

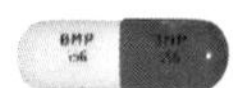
TIGAN 100 mg
Beecham

DYNAPEN 250 mg
Bristol

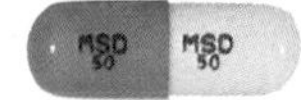

INDOCIN 50 mg
Merck Sharp & Dohme

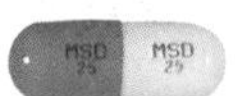

INDOCIN 25 mg
Merck Sharp & Dohme

ISORDIL Tembids 40 mg
Ives

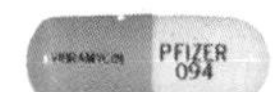

VIBRAMYCIN 50 mg
Pfizer

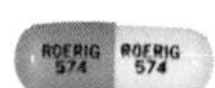

NAVANE 10 mg
Roerig

ACHROMYCIN V 500 mg
Lederle

ACHROMYCIN V 250 mg
Lederle

FIORINAL w/CODEINE #3
Sandoz

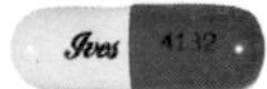

SURMONTIL 25 mg
Ives

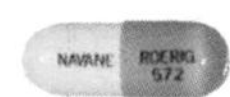

NAVANE 2 mg
Roerig

CYCLOSPASMOL 400 mg
Ives

MINOCIN 100 mg
Lederle

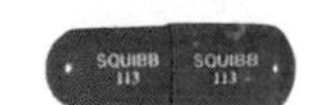

VELOSEF 250 mg
Squibb

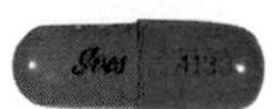

SURMONTIL 50 mg
Ives

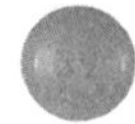
APRESOLINE 25 mg
Ciba

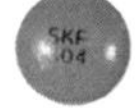

STELAZINE 2 mg
Smith Kline & French

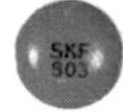

STELAZINE 1 mg
Smith Kline & French

TRANXENE SD 11.25 mg
Abbott

CORGARD 40 mg
Squibb

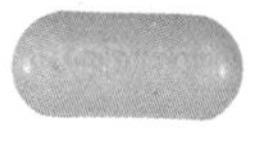
ELAVIL 150 mg
Merck Sharp & Dohme

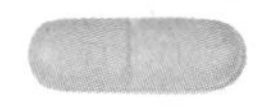
LOPRESSOR 100 mg
Geigy

BENTYL 20 mg
Merrell-National

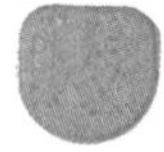
DIABINESE 250 mg
Pfizer

DIABINESE 100 mg
Pfizer

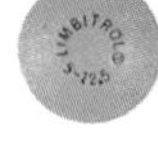

LIMBITROL 5-12.5
Roche

ISORDIL Oral 30 mg
Ives

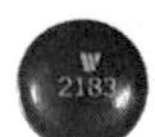

URISED
Webcon

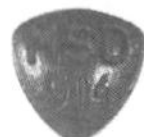
TRIAVIL 2-10
Merck Sharp & Dohme

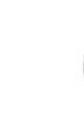

ELAVIL 10 mg
Merck Sharp & Dohme

COMBIPRES 0.2 mg
Boehringer-Ingelheim

SLO-PHYLLIN 250 mg capsules
Dooner

DITROPAN 5 mg
Marion

SINEQUAN 25 mg
Roerig

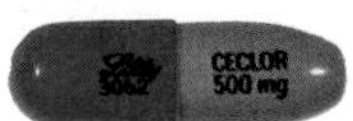

CECLOR 500 mg
Lilly

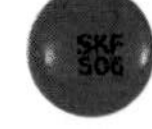

STELAZINE 5 mg
Smith Kline & French

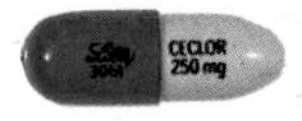

CECLOR 250 mg
Lilly

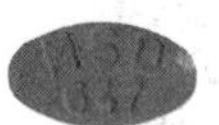

SINEMET 10/100
Merck Sharp & Dohme

COUMADIN 7.5 mg
Endo

SERPASIL-APRESOLINE #2
Ciba

DIDREX 25 mg
Upjohn

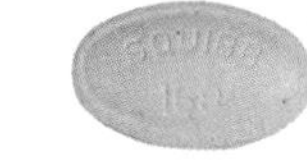

PENTIDS 500 mg
Squibb

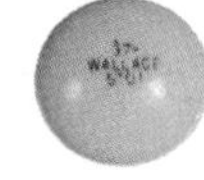
MILPATH 200 mg
Wallace

PERCODAN
Endo

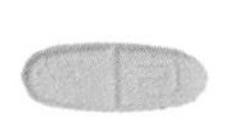      

OGEN 0.625 mg Abbott	MILPATH 400 mg Wallace	APRESOLINE 10 mg Ciba	INDERAL 80 mg Ayerst	VORANIL 50 mg USV Laboratories	CANTIL 25 mg Merrell-National	LANOXIN 0.125 mg Burroughs Wellcome

  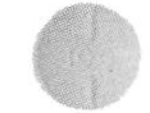  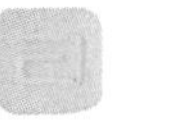 

METANDREN Linguets 10 mg Ciba	SYNTHROID 0.1 mg Flint	HYDROMOX R Lederle	ENDURONYL Abbott	CHOLOXIN 2 mg Flint	TEDRAL-25 Parke-Davis

 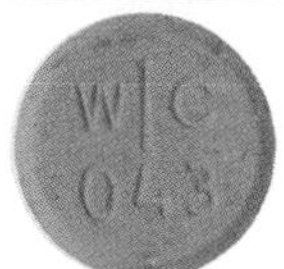   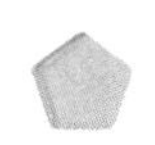 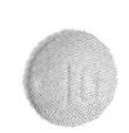

PATHIBAMATE-400 Lederle	GELUSIL-II Parke-Davis	HALOTESTIN 5 mg Upjohn	THIOSULFIL-A Forte Ayerst	DECADRON 0.5 mg Merck Sharp & Dohme	ZAROXOLYN 10 mg Pennwalt

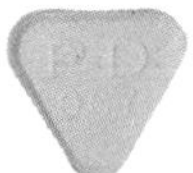 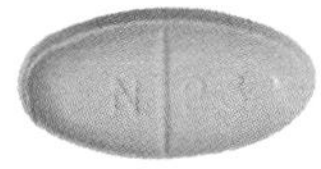 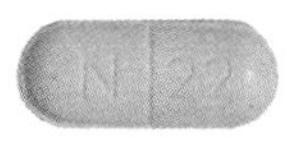 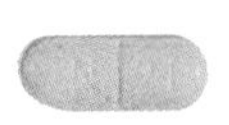  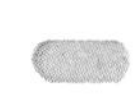

DILANTIN 50 mg Parke-Davis	NEGGRAM 1 g Winthrop	NEGGRAM 500 mg Winthrop	NEGGRAM 250 mg Winthrop	PLEGINE 35 mg Ayerst	ARISTOCORT 1 mg Lederle

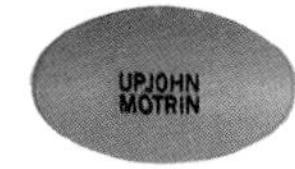 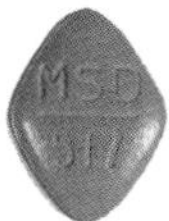 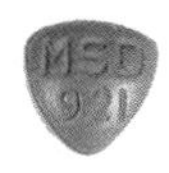 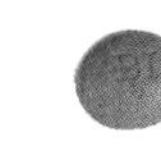 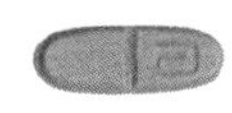

MOTRIN 600 mg Upjohn	TRIAVIL 4-50 Merck Sharp & Dohme	TRIAVIL 2-25 Merck Sharp & Dohme	CATAPRES 0.2 mg Boehringer-Ingelheim	OGEN 1.25 mg Abbott

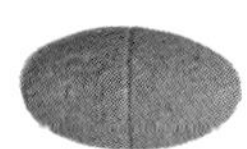 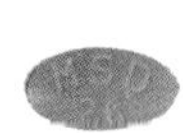 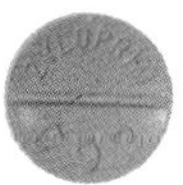 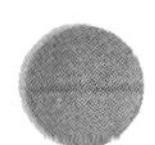  

KINESED Stuart	VIVACTIL 5 mg Merck Sharp & Dohme	ZYLOPRIM 300 mg Burroughs Wellcome	PHENERGAN 12.5 mg Wyeth	EVEX 0.625 mg Syntex	MARPLAN 10 mg Roche	DILAUDID 2 mg Knoll

 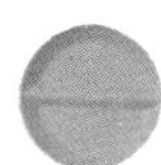 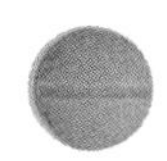 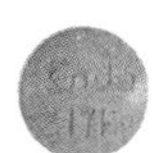  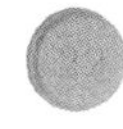

INDERAL 10 mg Ayerst	HEXADROL 1.5 mg Organon	ISORDIL w/PHENOBARBITAL 15 mg Ives	COUMADIN 2.5 mg Endo	ESTINYL 0.5 mg Schering	HYGROTON 25 mg USV Laboratories

  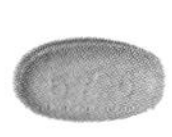 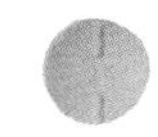  

ENDURON 2.5 mg Abbott	HydroDIURIL 50 mg Merck Sharp & Dohme	RONDEC T Ross	SYNTHROID 0.025 mg Flint	HydroDIURIL 25 mg Merck Sharp & Dohme	SOMA COMPOUND Wallace

  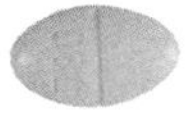  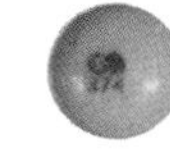 

HALDOL 1 mg McNeil	DARANIDE 50 mg Merck Sharp & Dohme	SORBITRATE Oral 10 mg Stuart	ISORDIL Chewable 10 mg Ives	CHLOR-TRIMETON 8 mg Schering	VALIUM 5 mg Roche

CHLOR-TRIMETON ALLERGY 4 mg
Schering

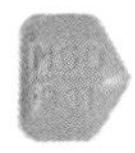
FLEXERIL 10 mg
Merck Sharp & Dohme

ZACTANE 75 mg
Wyeth

ANDROID-25
Brown

ALDACTONE 25 mg
Searle

NAQUIVAL
Schering

MIDICEL
Parke-Davis

ORETON 25 mg
Schering

ALDOMET 500 mg
Merck Sharp & Dohme

ALDOMET 250 mg
Merck Sharp & Dohme

ALDOMET 125 mg
Merck Sharp & Dohme

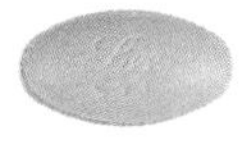
DARVON N 100 mg
Lilly

EXNA 50 mg
Robins

CLOMID 50 mg
Merrell-National

DILAUDID 4 mg
Knoll

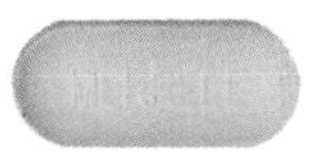
HIPREX 1 g
Merrell-National

NAPROSYN 250 mg
Syntex

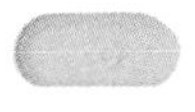
ARISTOCORT 8 mg
Lederle

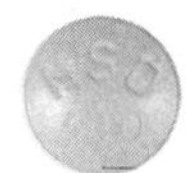
ELAVIL 75 mg
Merck Sharp & Dohme

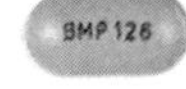

MENEST 0.625 mg
Beecham

PONDIMIN 20 mg
Robins

BUTISOL SODIUM 50 mg
McNeil

DEXEDRINE 5 mg
Smith Kline & French

ENDEP 100 mg
Roche

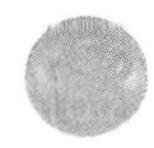
ELAVIL 50 mg
Merck Sharp & Dohme

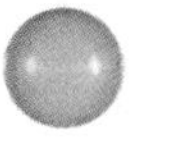
MELLARIL 25 mg
Sandoz

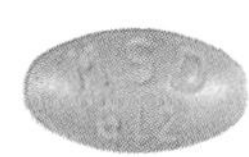
ALDOCLOR-150
Merck Sharp & Dohme

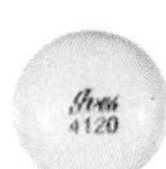

CYCLOSMASMOL 100 mg
Ives

E-MYCIN 250 mg
Upjohn

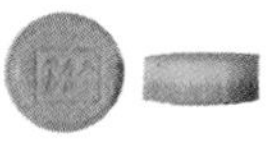
PHENERGAN-D
Wyeth

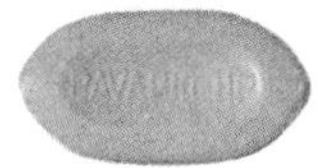
PAVABID HP 300 mg
Marion

APRESOLINE-ESIDRIX
Ciba

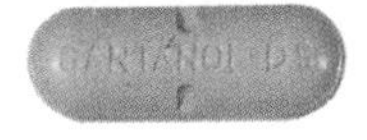
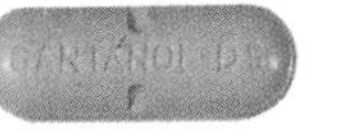

GANTANOL DS
Roche

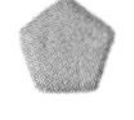
DECADRON 0.25 mg
Merck Sharp & Dohme

MEDROL 8 mg
Upjohn

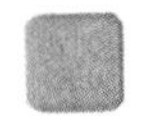
EUTHROID 0.5 gr
Parke-Davis

PROVERA 2.5 mg
Upjohn

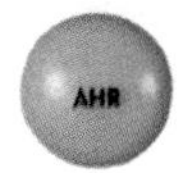

DIMETANE 12 mg
Robins

FORHISTAL 2.5 mg
Ciba

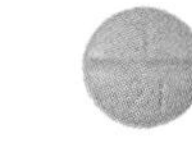
TALWIN 50 mg
Winthrop

VALPIN 50 mg
Endo

EMPRAZIL
Burroughs Wellcome

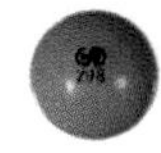
ESTINYL 0.02 mg
Schering

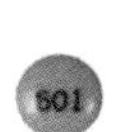

PRO-BANTHINE 15 mg
Searle

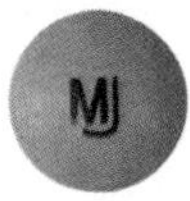

KLOTRIX
Mead Johnson

BAYER CHILDREN'S CHEWABLE ASPIRIN 81 mg (1¼ gr)
Glenbrook

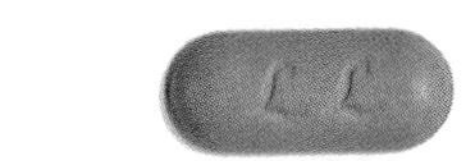
STRESSTABS 600 with ZINC
Lederle

VERMOX 100 mg
Janssen

OVCON-35
Mead Johnson

LACTINEX 250 mg
Hynson, Westcott & Dunning

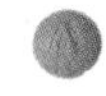
ARMOUR THYROID ¼ gr
Armour

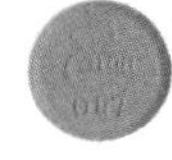
DUVOID 50 mg
Norwich Eaton

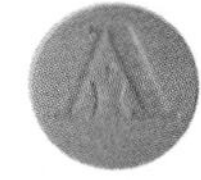
ARMOUR THYROID 5 gr
Armour

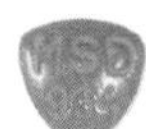
TRIAVIL 4-10
Merck Sharp & Dohme

LAROTID 250 mg
Roche

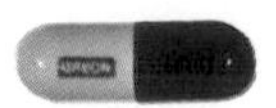
BRONKODYL 100 mg
Breon

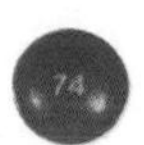
TOFRANIL 50 mg
Geigy

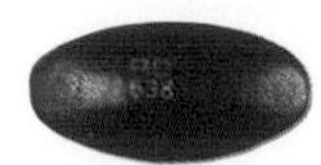
TABRON
Parke-Davis

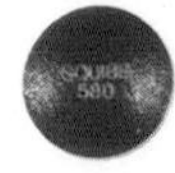
MYCOSTATIN
Squibb

TOFRANIL 25 mg
Geigy

TOFRANIL 10 mg
Geigy

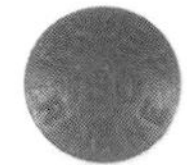

ENDEP 150 mg
Roche

E.E.S. 400 mg
Abbott

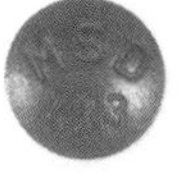
ALDORIL-15
Merck Sharp & Dohme

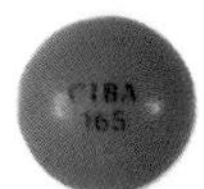
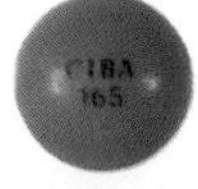
SLOW-K 600 mg
CIBA

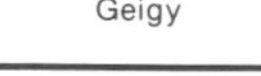
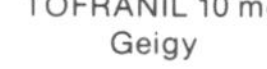
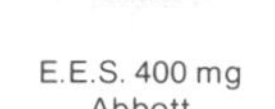
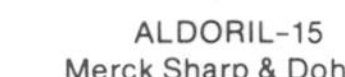

TOFRANIL-PM 150 mg
Geigy

TOFRANIL-PM 75 mg
Geigy

TOFRANIL-PM 125 mg
Geigy

TOFRANIL-PM 100 mg
Geigy

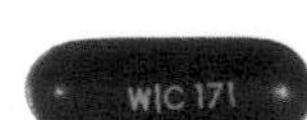

MANDELAMINE 0.5 g
Parke-Davis

THORAZINE 50 mg
Smith Kline & French

THORAZINE 25 mg
Smith Kline & French

THORAZINE 10 mg
Smith Kline & French

CHLOR-TRIMETON 12 mg
Schering

THORAZINE 200 mg
Smith Kline & French

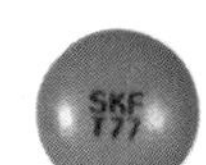
THORAZINE 100 mg
Smith Kline & French

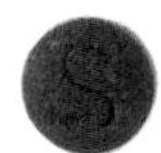
SENOKOT
Purdue Frederick

DOXIDAN
Hoechst-Roussel

EX-LAX
Ex-Lax

THERAGRAN
Squibb

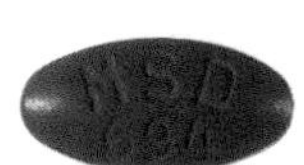
ALDORIL D30
Merck Sharp & Dohme

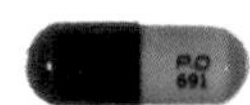
VECTRIN 50 mg
Parke-Davis

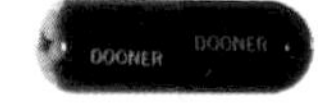
SLO-PHYLLIN 125 mg capsules
Dooner

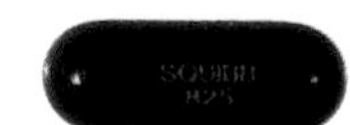
THERAGRAN-M
Squibb

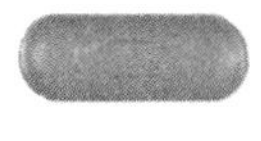
RYNATUSS
Wallace

TRANXENE-SD 22.5 mg
Abbott

CANTIL w/PHENOBARBITAL
Merrell-National

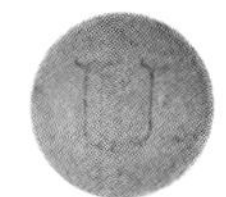
MAOLATE 400 mg
Upjohn

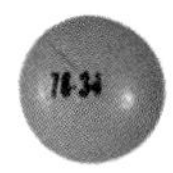
CAFERGOT
Sandoz

EUTHROID-1
Parke-Davis

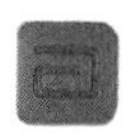
ENDURONYL FORTE
Abbott

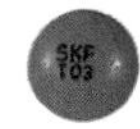
TEMARIL 2.5 mg
Smith Kline & French

EUTHROID 3
Parke-Davis

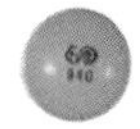
TRILAFON 4 mg
Schering

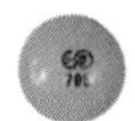
TRILAFON 2 mg
Schering

PROLOID 3 gr
Parke-Davis

PROLOID 2 gr
Parke-Davis

PROLOID 1.5 gr
Parke-Davis

PROLOID 1 gr
Parke-Davis

PROLOID 0.5 gr
Parke-Davis

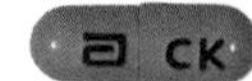
TRANXENE 15 mg
Abbott

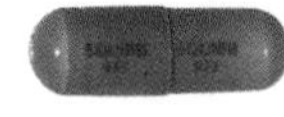
PRINCIPEN 250 mg
Squibb

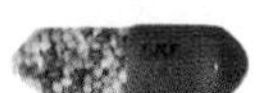

TEMARIL 5 mg
Smith Kline & French

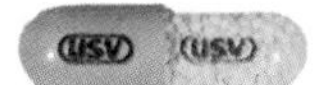

HISTASPAN-D
USV Laboratories

FIORINAL w/CODEINE #2 0.25 gr
Sandoz

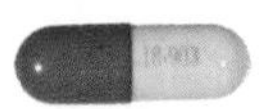

IONAMIN 15 mg
Pennwalt

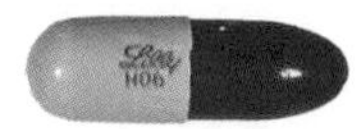

DARVON COMPOUND 65 mg
Lilly

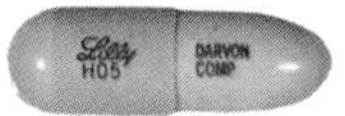

DARVON COMPOUND 32 mg
Lilly

COUMADIN 2 mg
Endo

TRILAFON 16 mg
Schering

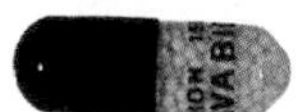

PAVABID 150 mg
Marion

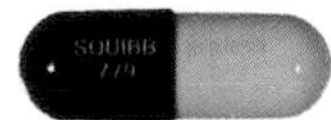

MYSTECLIN-F 250 mg
Squibb

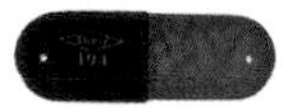

NOVAFED
Dow

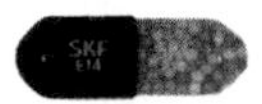

DEXEDRINE 15 mg
Smith Kline & French

DEXEDRINE 10 mg
Smith Kline & French

DEXEDRINE 5 mg
Smith Kline & French

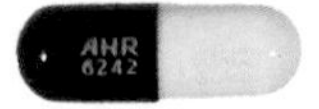

PHENAPHEN w/CODEINE #2
Robins

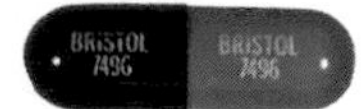

TEGOPEN 500 mg
Bristol

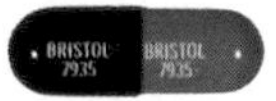

TEGOPEN 250 mg
Bristol

NITRO-BID 6.5 mg
Marion

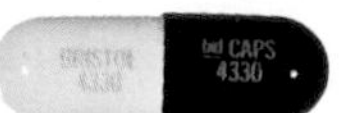

TETREX 500 mg
Bristol

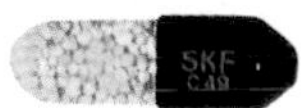

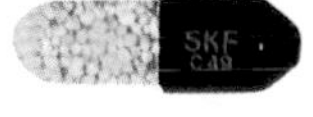

COMPAZINE 75 mg
Smith Kline & French

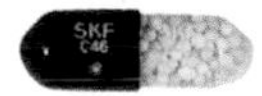

COMPAZINE 15 mg
Smith Kline & French

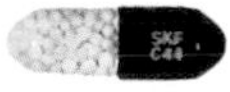

COMPAZINE 10 mg
Smith Kline & French

PHENAPHEN w/CODEINE #3
Robins

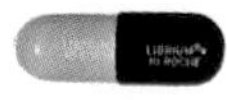

LIBRIUM 10 mg
Roche

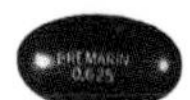

PREMARIN 0.625 mg
Ayerst

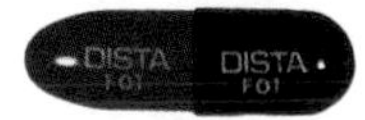

TRINSICON
Dista

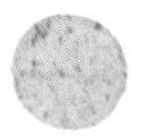

DISOPHROL
Schering

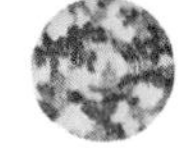

BELLERGAL-S
Dorsey

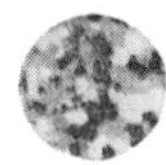

BELLADENAL-S
Sandoz

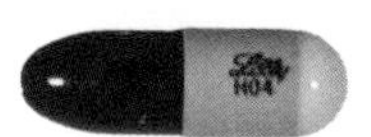

DARVON w/A.S.A.
Lilly

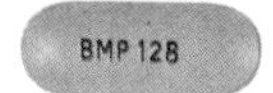

MENEST 2.5 mg
Beecham

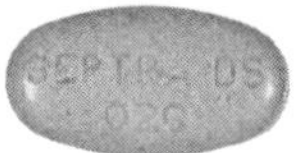

SEPTRA DS
Burroughs Wellcome

SEPTRA
Burroughs Wellcome

DARICON PB
Beecham

GRISACTIN 500 mg
Ayerst

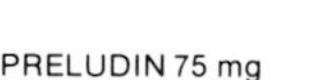

PRELUDIN 75 mg
Boehringer-Ingelheim

CLISTIN 4 mg
McNeil

BUTISOL 100 mg
McNeil

EVEX 1.25 mg
Syntex

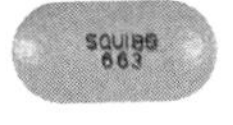

SUMYCIN 250 mg
Squibb

PERITRATE 40 mg
Parke-Davis

ILOSONE 250 mg
Dista

ILOSONE 125 mg
Dista

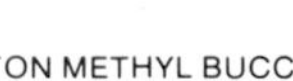

ORETON METHYL BUCCALS 10 mg
Schering

DILAUDID 3 mg
Knoll

CELESTONE 0.6 mg
Schering

NAQUA 2 mg
Schering

ARISTOCORT 2 mg
Lederle

SYNTHROID 0.2 mg
Flint

COUMADIN 5 mg
Endo

BONINE 25 mg
Pfizer

SER-AP-ES
Ciba

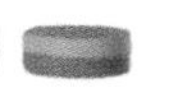
THYROLAR-½
Armour

RAUTRAX-N
Squibb

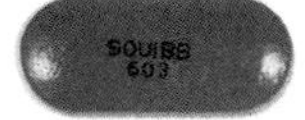
SUMYCIN 500 mg
Squibb

METHERGINE 0.2 mg
Sandoz

SINGLET
Dow

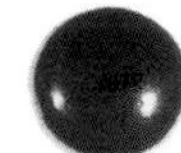
DIMETANE 8 mg
Robins

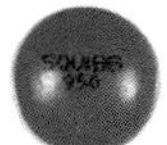
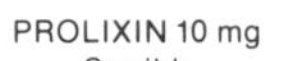
PROLIXIN 10 mg
Squibb

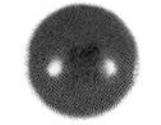
ETRAFON 2/25
Schering

TARACTAN 25 mg
Roche

TARACTAN 10 mg
Roche

POLARAMINE 2 mg
Schering

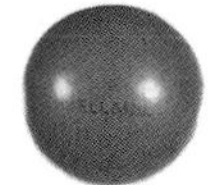
MELLARIL 200 mg
Sandoz

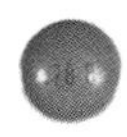
MELLARIL 15 mg
Sandoz

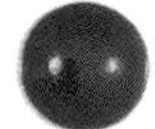
ESTINYL 0.05 mg
Schering

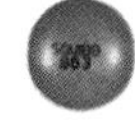
PROLIXIN 1 mg
Squibb

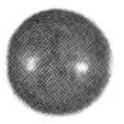
PATHILON 25 mg
Lederle

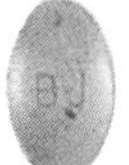
ORETON PROPIONATE BUCCALS 10 mg
Schering

COMBIPRES 0.1 mg
Boehringer-Ingelheim

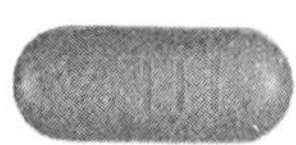
MAGAN
Warren-Teed

BUTIBEL
McNeil

TRIAMINIC JUVELETS
Dorsey

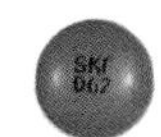
DARBID
Smith Kline & French

TUSSAGESIC
Dorsey

ENDURON 5 mg
Abbott

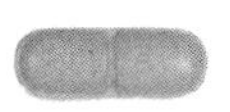
LOPRESSOR 50 mg
Geigy

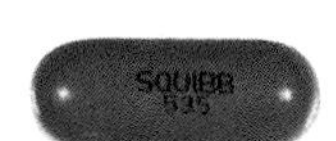
THERAGRAN HEMATINIC
Squibb

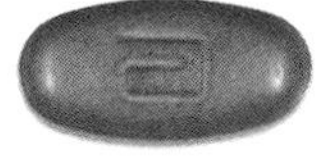
ERYTHROCIN 500 mg
Abbott

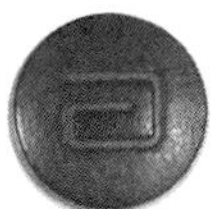
ERYTHROCIN 250 mg
Abbott

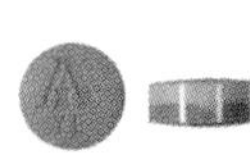
THYROLAR-1
Armour

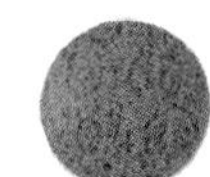
HYCOMINE COMPOUND
Endo

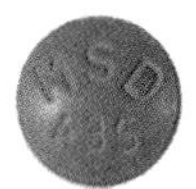
ELAVIL 100 mg
Merck Sharp & Dohme

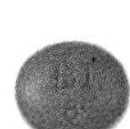
CATAPRES 0.1 mg
Boehringer-Ingelheim

DIDREX 50 mg
Upjohn

NORLUTATE 5 mg
Parke-Davis

PHENERGAN 50 mg
Wyeth

REGROTON
USV Laboratories

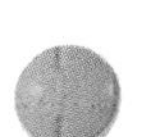
ESIDRIX 25 mg
Ciba

DECADRON 1.5 mg
Merck Sharp & Dohme

MEDROL 2 mg
Upjohn

DIUPRES-500
Merck Sharp & Dohme

DIUPRES-250
Merck Sharp & Dohme

ISORDIL Oral 5 mg
Ives

ROBINUL 1 mg
Robins

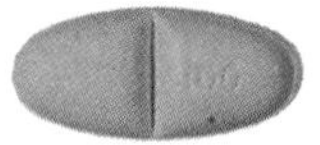
SINUBID
Parke-Davis

HALDOL 2 mg
McNeil

ISORDIL Sublingual 5 mg
Ives

SORBITRATE Sublingual 5 mg
Stuart

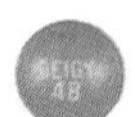
PBZ-SR 100 mg
Geigy

EUTHROID 2 gr
Parke-Davis

MOBAN 10 mg
Endo

ZAROXOLYN 2.5 mg
Pennwalt

METATENSIN 4 mg
Merrell-National

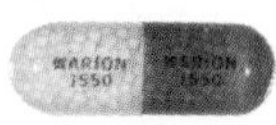
NITRO-BID 2.5 mg
Marion

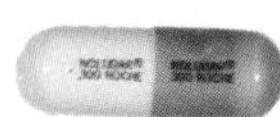
NOLUDAR 300 mg
Roche

POLYMOX 500 mg
Bristol

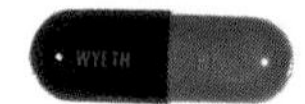

OMNIPEN 250 mg
Wyeth

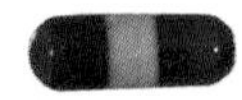
BENADRYL 50 mg
Parke-Davis

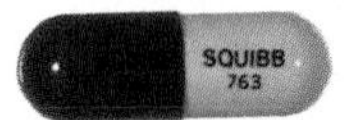

SUMYCIN 500 mg
Squibb

DIALOSE
Stuart

KAON-CL TABS
Warren-Teed

APRESAZIDE 50/50
Ciba

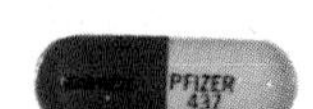

MINIPRESS 2 mg
Pfizer

BENADRYL 25 mg
Parke-Davis

SERAX 10 mg
Wyeth

SINEQUAN 50 mg
Roerig

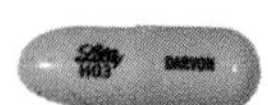

DARVON 65 mg
Lilly

ORGANIDIN 30 mg
Wallace

URECHOLINE 10 mg
Merck Sharp & Dohme

CRYSTODIGIN 0.1 mg
Lilly

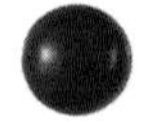
MODANE MILD 37.5 mg
Warren-Teed

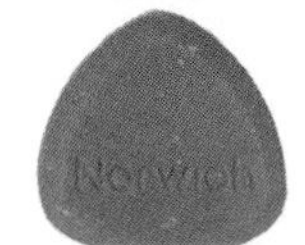

PEPTO-BISMOL 300 mg
Norwich-Eaton

EQUANIL 200 mg
Wyeth

PRELUDIN 25 mg
Boehringer-Ingleheim

CARDILATE 10 mg
Burroughs Wellcome

DECADRON 4 mg
Merck Sharp & Dohme

ROBAXISAL
Robins

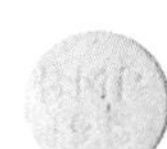
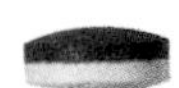
ENARAX 10
Beecham

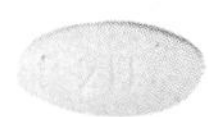

ANTIVERT 25 mg
Roerig

ANTIVERT 12.5 mg
Roerig

NALDECON
Bristol

DIUTENSEN-R
Wallace

DIUTENSEN
Wallace

PROLOID 0.25 gr
Parke-Davis

TAO 250 mg
Roerig

ELIXOPHYLLIN SR 125 mg
Cooper

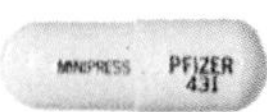

MINIPRESS 1 mg
Pfizer

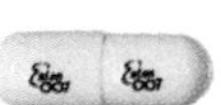
MACRODANTIN 25 mg
Norwich-Eaton

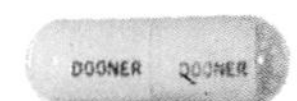

SLO-PHYLLIN GYROCAPS 60 mg
Dooner

ELIXOPHYLLIN SR 250 mg
Cooper

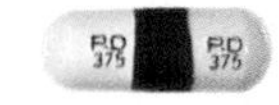

DILANTIN w/PHENOBARBITAL 0.25 gr
Parke-Davis

DILANTIN 100 mg
Parke-Davis

CARBRITAL
Parke-Davis

CHLOROMYCETIN 250 mg
Parke-Davis

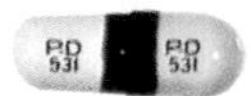

DILANTIN w/PHENOBARBITAL 0.5 gr
Parke-Davis

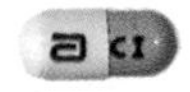
TRANXENE 3.75 mg
Abbott

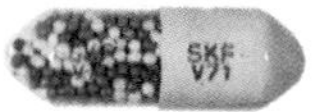

TUSS-ORNADE
Smith Kline & French

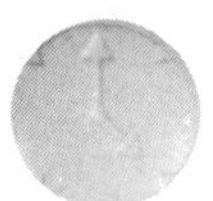

QUINAGLUTE DURA-TABS 324 mg
Cooper

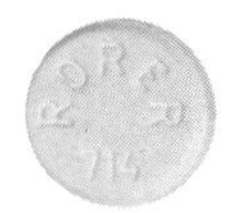

QUAALUDE 300 mg
Lemmon

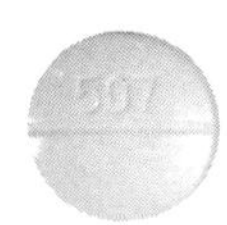

FULVICIN P/G 250 mg
Schering

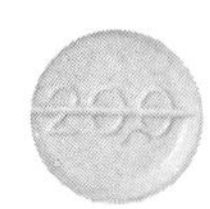

TOLECTIN 200 mg
McNeil

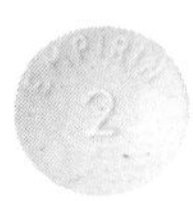

EMPIRIN w/CODEINE #2
Burroughs Wellcome

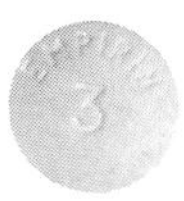

EMPIRIN w/CODEINE #3
Burroughs Wellcome

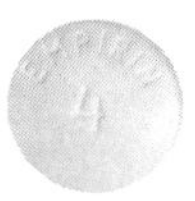

EMPIRIN w/CODEINE #4
Burroughs Wellcome

PERCOGESIC w/CODEINE
Endo

EMPRAZIL-C
Burroughs Wellcome

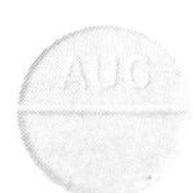

FULVICIN-U/F 500 mg
Schering

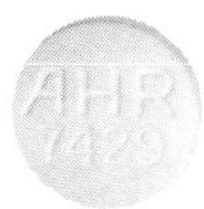

ROBAXIN 500 mg
Robins

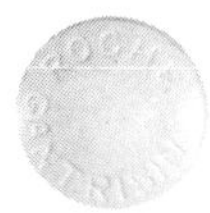

GANTRISIN
Roche

GRIFULVIN V 500 mg
McNeil

SOMA 350 mg
Wallace

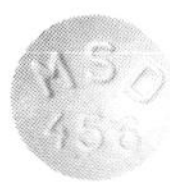

ALDORIL-25
Merck Sharp & Dohme

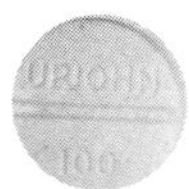

ORINASE 0.5 g
Upjohn

PERCOCET-5
Endo

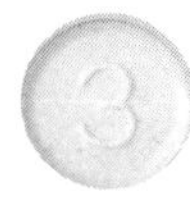

TYLENOL w/CODEINE #3
McNeil

MILTOWN 400 mg
Wallace

TYLENOL w/CODEINE #4
McNeil

FIORINAL
Sandoz

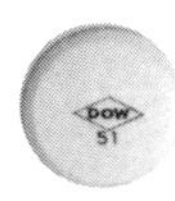

LORELCO 250 mg
Dow

NOLUDAR 200 mg
Roche

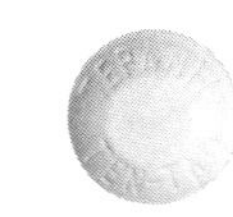

TEPANIL TEN-TAB 75 mg
Riker

PEN-VEE K 500 mg
Wyeth

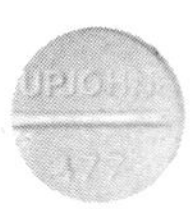

TOLINASE 500 mg
Upjohn

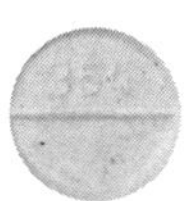

DORIDEN 0.5 g
USV Laboratories

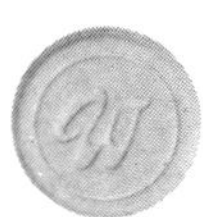

QUINAMM
Merrell-National

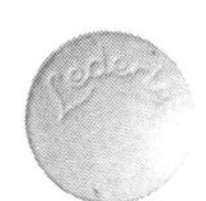

DIAMOX 250 mg
Lederle

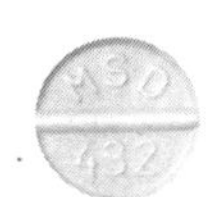

DIURIL 500 mg
Merck Sharp & Dohme

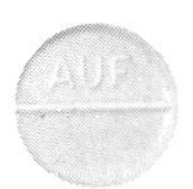

FULVICIN-U/F 250 mg
Schering

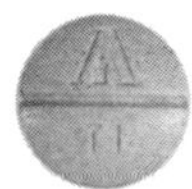

THYROID 5 gr
Armour

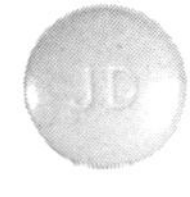

ORETON 10 mg
Schering

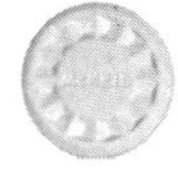

GRIFULVIN V 250 mg
McNeil

TYLENOL w/CODEINE #2
McNeil

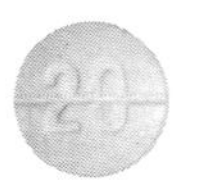

VASODILAN 20 mg
Mead Johnson

TOLINASE 250 mg
Upjohn

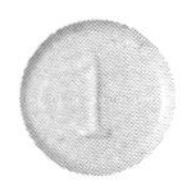

TYLENOL w/CODEINE #1
McNeil

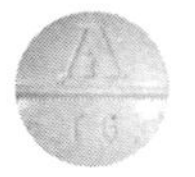

THYROID 3 gr
Armour

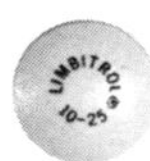

LIMBITROL 10-25
Roche

QUAALUDE 150 mg
Lemmon

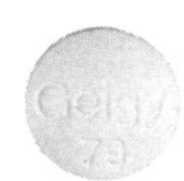

PRELUDIN 50 mg
Boehringer-Ingelheim

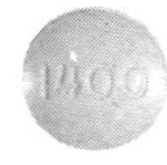

VENTAIRE 2 mg
Marion

ORINASE 250 mg
Upjohn

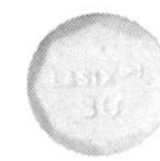

LASIX 80 mg
Hoechst-Roussel

DIURIL 250 mg
Merck Sharp & Dohme

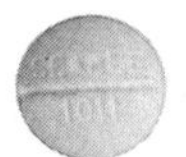
ALDACTAZIDE
Searle

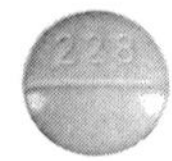
FULVICIN P/G 125 mg
Schering

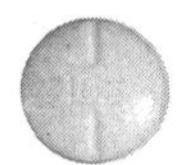
ISMELIN 25 mg
Ciba

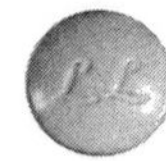
LEDERCILLIN VK 250 mg
Lederle

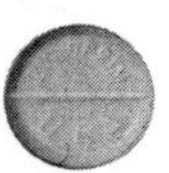
ZYLOPRIM 100 mg
Burroughs Wellcome

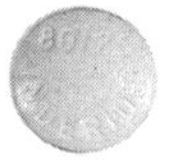
INDERIDE 80/25
Ayerst

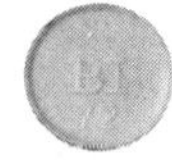
ALUPENT 20 mg
Boehringer-Ingelheim

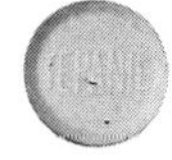
TEPANIL 25 mg
Riker

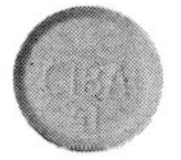

ANTURANE 100 mg
Ciba

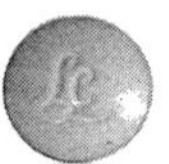
QUINIDINE SULFATE, U.S.P. 200 mg
Lederle

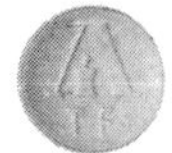
THYROID 2 gr
Armour

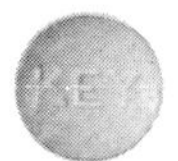

THEO-DUR 100 mg
Key

GYNOREST 5 mg
Mead Johnson

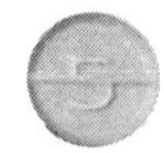

DUPHASTON 5 mg
Philips Roxane

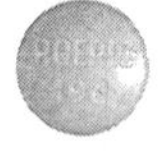
ENARAX 5
Beecham

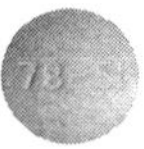
HYDERGINE Sublingual 0.5 mg
Sandoz

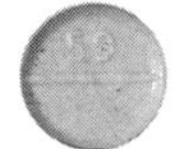
PEN-VEE K 250 mg
Wyeth

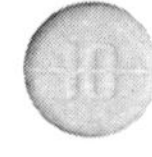

GYNOREST 10 mg
Mead Johnson

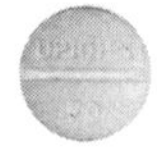
TOLINASE 100 mg
Upjohn

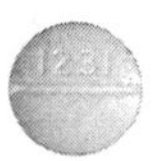
, AMINOPHYLLIN 100 mg
Searle

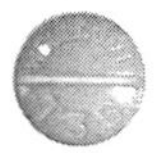
CARDILATE-P
Burroughs Wellcome

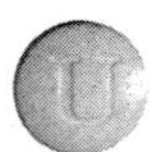

CORTEF 10 mg
Upjohn

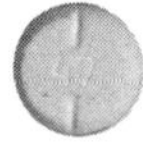
ESIMIL
Ciba

PRANTAL 100 mg
Schering

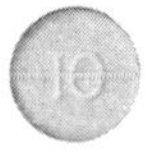

DUPHASTON 10 mg
Philips Roxane

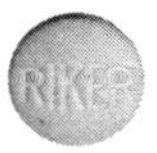

NORFLEX 100 mg
Riker

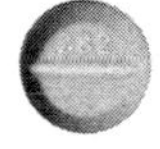
OPTIMINE 1 mg
Schering

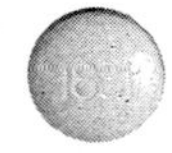
FLAGYL 250 mg
Searle

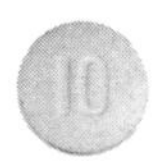

VASODILAN 10 mg
Mead Johnson

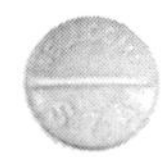
SUDAFED 60 mg
Burroughs Wellcome

COUMADIN 10 mg
Endo

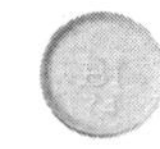
ALUPENT 10 mg
Boehringer-Ingelheim

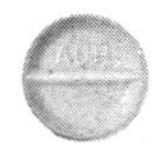
FULVICIN-U/F 125 mg
Schering

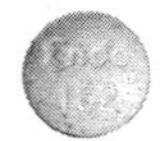
VALPIN 50-PB
Endo

BRETHINE 5 mg
Geigy

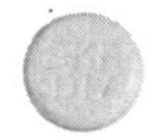
CYTOMEL 50 mcg
Smith Kline & French

VALIUM 2 mg
Roche

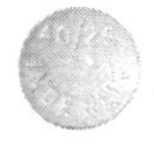
INDERIDE 40/25
Ayerst

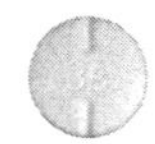
SERPASIL 0.25 mg
Ciba

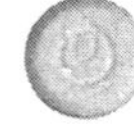
HEXADROL 0.75 mg
Organon

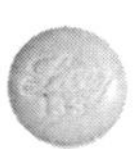
PHENOBARBITAL 100 mg
Lilly

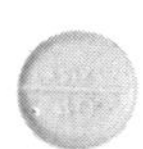
LASIX 40 mg
Hoechst-Roussel

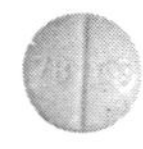
SANOREX 2 mg
Sandoz

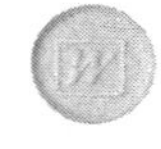
PHENERGAN 25 mg
Wyeth

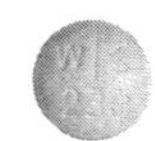
TEDRAL
Parke-Davis

SALURON 50 mg
Bristol

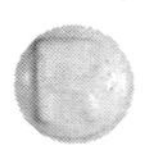
DONNATAL TABLETS
Robins

ARLIDIN 12 mg
USV Laboratories

HYDERGINE 1 mg
Sandoz

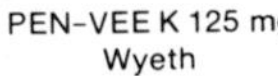
PEN-VEE K 125 mg
Wyeth

DEMEROL 100 mg
Winthrop

ISORDIL Oral 10 mg
Ives

SERPASIL 0.1 mg
Ciba

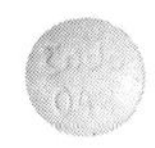

HYCODAN
Endo

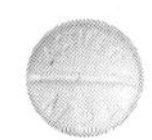

ACTIFED
Burroughs Wellcome

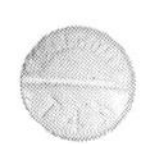

MAREZINE 50 mg
Burroughs Wellcome

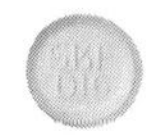

CYTOMEL 25 mcg
Smith Kline & French

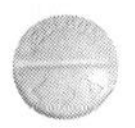

ACTIDIL 2.5 mg
Burroughs Wellcome

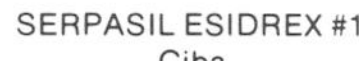

SERPASIL ESIDREX #1
Ciba

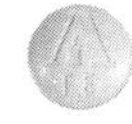

THYROID 1 gr
Armour

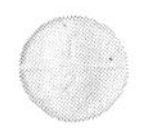

HALDOL 0.5 mg
McNeil

BENTYL w/PHENOBARBITAL 20 mg
Merrell-National

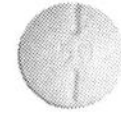

SYNTHROID 0.05 mg
Flint

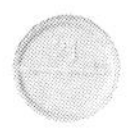

HYGROTON 100 mg
USV Laboratories

PROVERA 10 mg
Upjohn

LANOXIN 0.25
Burroughs Wellcome

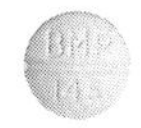

DARICON 10 mg
Beecham

TAVIST 2.68 mg
Dorsey

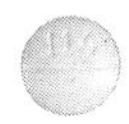

PURODIGIN 0.2 mg
Wyeth

PERIACTIN 4 mg
Merck Sharp & Dohme

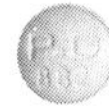

NORLUTIN 5 mg
Parke-Davis

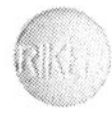

DIAFEN 2 mg
Riker

ERGOTRATE 0.2 mg
Lilly

DEMI-REGROTON
USV Laboratories

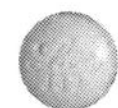

PHENOBARBITAL 30 mg
Lilly

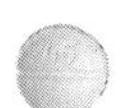

ARLIDIN 6 mg
USV Laboratories

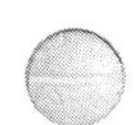

CARDILATE 5 mg
Burroughs Wellcome

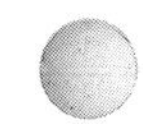

DEMEROL 50 mg
Winthrop

LOMOTIL 2.5 mg
Searle

CYTOMEL 5 mcg
Smith Kline & French

PHENOBARBITAL 15 mg
Lilly

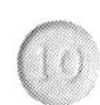

ISORDIL Sublingual 10 mg
Ives

CODEINE SULFATE 60 mg
Lilly

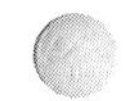

CODEINE SULFATE 30 mg
Lilly

CODEINE SULFATE 15 mg
Lilly

DIETHYLSTILBESTROL 0.1 mg
Lilly

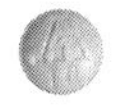

THYROID 0.5 gr
Armour

COLCHICINE 0.6 mg
Lilly

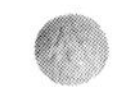

THYROID 0.25 gr
Armour

ATIVAN 0.5 mg
Wyeth

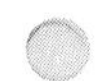

NITROGLYCERIN 0.6 mg
Lilly

NITROGLYCERIN 0.4 mg
Lilly

NITROGLYCERIN 0.3 mg
Lilly

NITROGLYCERIN 0.15 mg
Lilly

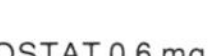

NITROSTAT 0.6 mg
Parke-Davis

NITROSTAT 0.4 mg
Parke-Davis

NITROSTAT 0.3 mg
Parke-Davis

NITROSTAT 0.15 mg
Parke-Davis

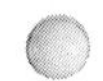

SORBITRATE Sublingual 2.5 mg
Stuart

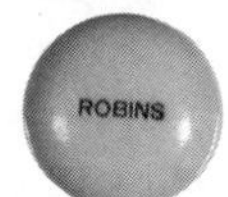

QUINIDEX EXTENTABS 300 mg
Robins

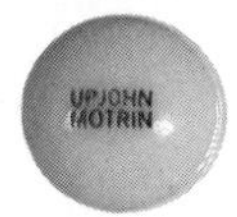

MOTRIN 300 mg
Upjohn

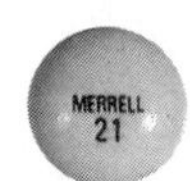

NORPRAMIN 150 mg
Merrell-National

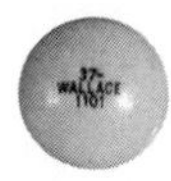
MILTOWN 200 mg
Wallace

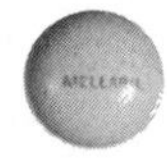
MELLARIL 50 mg
Sandoz

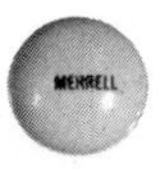

BENDECTIN
Merrell-National

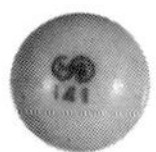
TRILAFON 8 mg
Schering

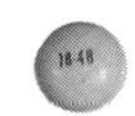
GYNERGEN
Sandoz

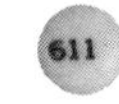

PRO-BANTHINE 7.5 mg
Searle

Gris-PEG 125 mg
Dorsey

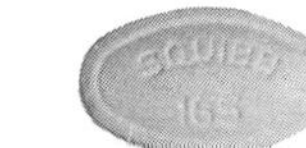
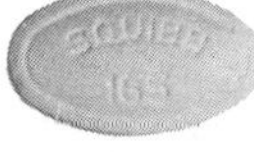
PENTIDS 250 mg
Squibb

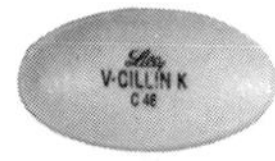
V-CILLIN K 500 mg
Lilly

AMINODUR 300 mg
Cooper

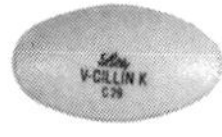
V-CILLIN K 250 mg
Lilly

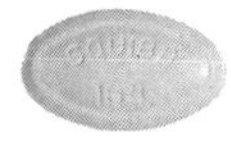
PENTIDS 125 mg
Squibb

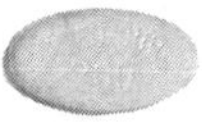
THEO-DUR 200 mg
Key

THIOSULFIL 0.25 g
Ayerst

BRETHINE 2.5 mg
Geigy

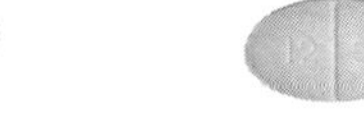
AMINOPHYLLIN 200 mg
Searle

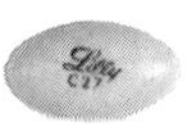
V-CILLIN K 125 mg
Lilly

HYDERGINE Sublingual 1 mg
Sandoz

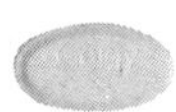
LIORESAL 10 mg
Geigy

MEDROL 16 mg
Upjohn

DIUCARDIN 50 mg
Ayerst

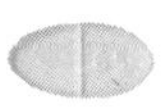
ATIVAN 2 mg
Wyeth

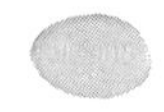
MEDROL 4 mg
Upjohn

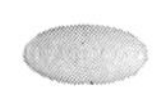
LASIX 20 mg
Hoechst-Roussel

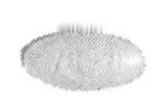
SANOREX 1 mg
Sandoz

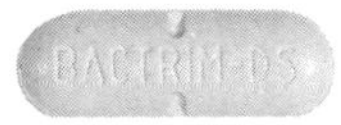

BACTRIM DS
Roche

UNIPEN 500 mg
Wyeth

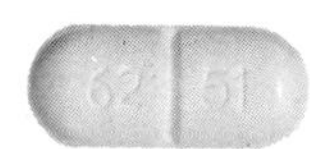

PHENAPHEN-650 w/CODEINE
Robins

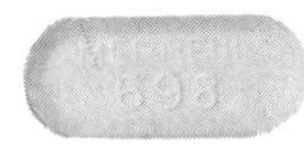
TENUATE DOSPAN
Merrell-National

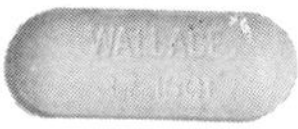
MILTOWN 600 mg
Wallace

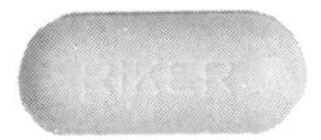

UREX 1 g
Riker

ROBAXIN 750 mg
Robins

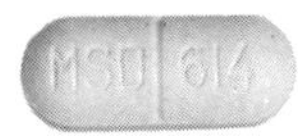

Col BENEMID
Merck Sharp & Dohme

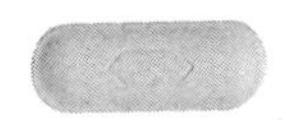
RYNATAN
Wallace

ANDROID-5
Brown

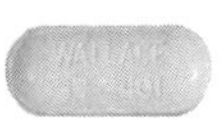
SOMA COMPOUND w/CODEINE
Wallace

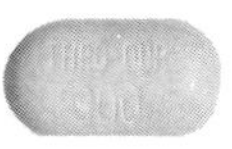
THEO-DUR 300 mg
Key

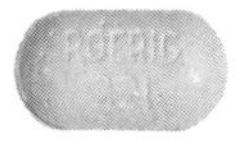
SUSTAIRE 300 mg
Roerig

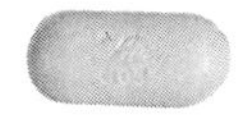
DYMELOR 250 mg
Lilly

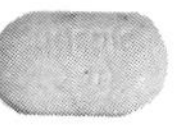
SUSTAIRE 100 mg
Roerig

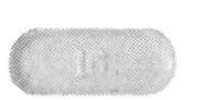
ARISTOCORT 16 mg
Lederle

ATIVAN 1 mg
Wyeth

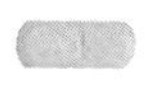
ARISTOCORT 4 mg
Lederle

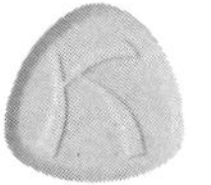
THEOPHYL-225
Knoll

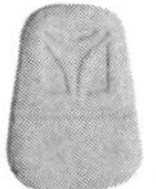
TUSSIONEX
Pennwalt

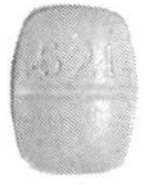
LUFYLLIN 200 mg
Wallace

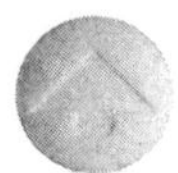
ANACIN
Whitehall

MAXIMUM STRENGTH ANACIN
Whitehall

URECHOLINE 5 mg
Merck Sharp & Dohme

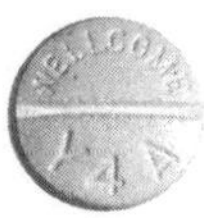
ANTEPAR 550 mg
Burroughs Wellcome

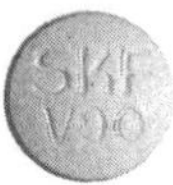

URISPAS 100 mg
Smith Kline & French

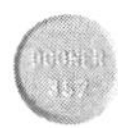
SLO-PHYLLIN 200 mg tablets
Dooner

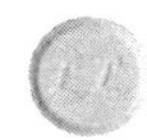
ARTANE 2 mg
Lederle

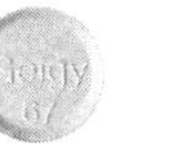
TEGRETOL 200 mg
Geigy

MARAX
Roerig

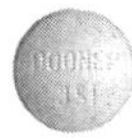
SLO-PHYLLIN 100 mg tablets
Dooner

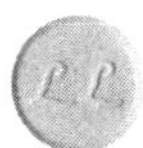
ARTANE 5 mg
Lederle

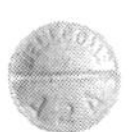
ALKERAN 2 mg
Burroughs Wellcome

LO/OVRAL
Wyeth

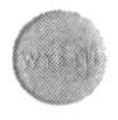
OVRAL
Wyeth

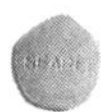
OVULEN
Searle

COGENTIN 2 mg
Merck Sharp & Dohme

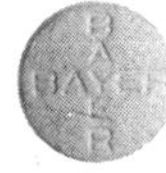
BAYER ASPIRIN 325 mg
Glenbrook

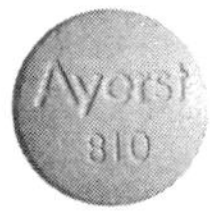

ANTABUSE 500 mg
Ayerst

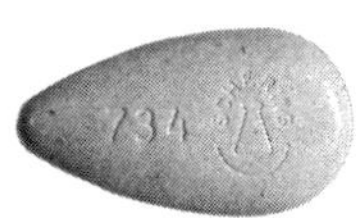

GYNE-LOTRIMIN 100 mg
Schering

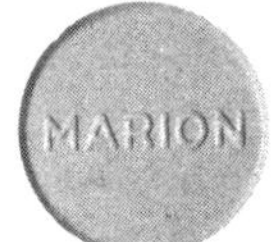

GAVISCON
Marion

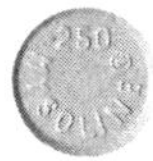
MYSOLINE 250 mg
Ayerst

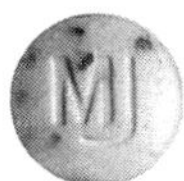

CYTOXAN 50 mg
Mead Johnson

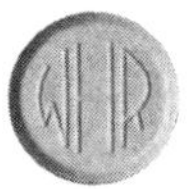

ASCRIPTIN
Rorer

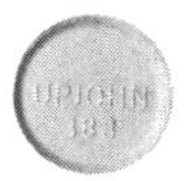
DELTASONE 50 mg
Upjohn

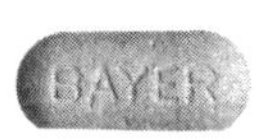

BAYER TIMED-RELEASE 650 mg
Glenbrook

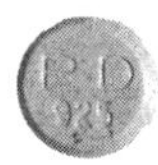
RENOQUID 250 mg
Parke-Davis

KANTREX 500 mg
Bristol

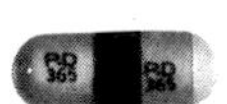
DILANTIN 30 mg
Parke-Davis

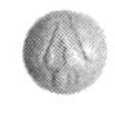
ARMOUR THYROID ½ gr
Armour

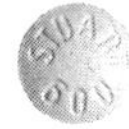
NOLVADEX 10 mg
Stuart

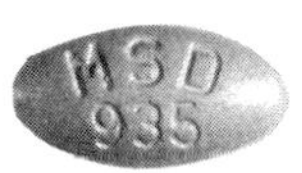

ALDORIL D50
Merck Sharp & Dohme

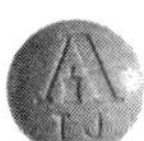
ARMOUR THYROID 1½ gr
Armour

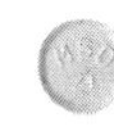
COGENTIN 0.5 mg
Merck Sharp & Dohme

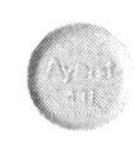
MYSOLINE 50 mg
Ayerst

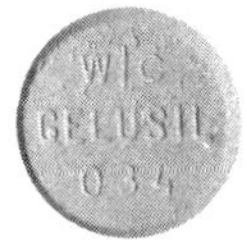

GELUSIL
Parke-Davis

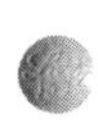
DIETHYLSTILBESTROL 0.1 mg (e-c)
Lilly

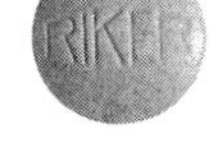

TITRALAC 0.42 g
Riker

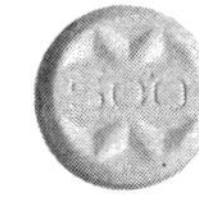

EXTRA-STRENGTH TYLENOL 500 mg
McNeil Consumer Products

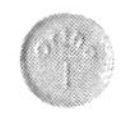
ORTHO-NOVUM 1/80 □ 21
Ortho

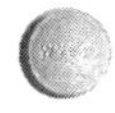
LO/OVRAL-28
Wyeth

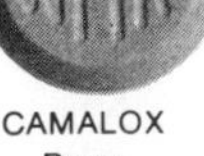

CAMALOX
Rorer

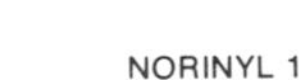
NORINYL 1 + 50 21-DAY
Syntex

DIETHYLSTILBESTROL 5 mg
Lilly

OVULEN-28
Searle

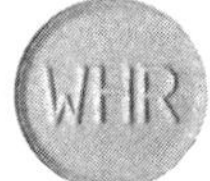

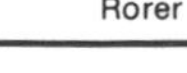
MAALOX No. 1
Rorer

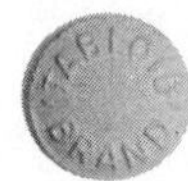

EMPIRIN ANALGESIC TABLETS 325 mg
Burroughs Wellcome

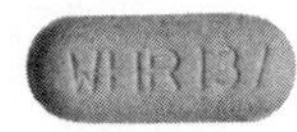

ASCRIPTIN A/D
Rorer

DEMULEN-28
Searle

MODICON
Ortho

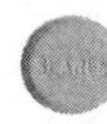

DEMULEN
Searle

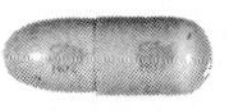

DARVON 32 mg
Lilly

PROSTAPHLIN 500 mg
Bristol

PROSTAPHLIN 250 mg
Bristol

SINEQUAN 75 mg
Roerig

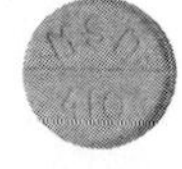

HydroDIURIL 100 mg
Merck Sharp & Dohme

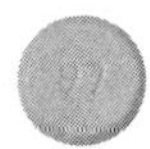

SERPASIL-ESIDRIX #2
Ciba

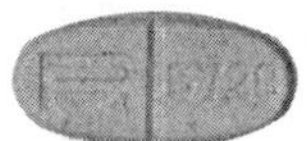

RONDEC C
Ross

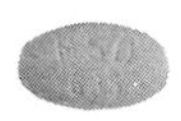

COGENTIN 1 mg
Merck Sharp & Dohme

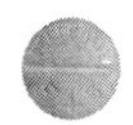

KEMADRIN 2 mg
Burroughs Wellcome

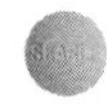

OVULEN-21
Searle

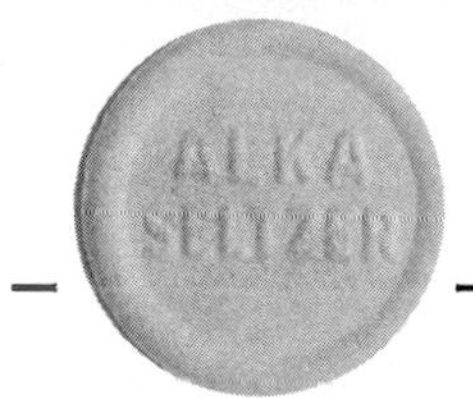

ALKA-SELTZER
Miles Laboratories

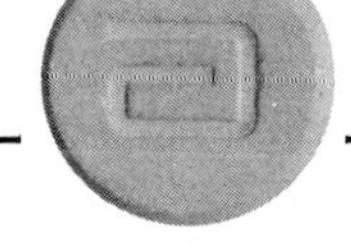

E.E.S. 200 mg
Abbott

Selected Bibliography

In preparing *The Physicians' Drug Manual,* hundreds of different medical texts, journals, and other sources were consulted. Space does not permit a complete listing of these sources, but following are the major references used.

General References - Drugs

Adverse Drug Reactions in the United States: An Analysis of the Scope of the Problem and Recommendations for Future Approaches. Washington, D.C.: Medicine in the Public Interest, Inc., 1974.

AMA Drug Evaluations (Fourth Edition). Chicago: American Medical Association, 1980.

Avery, Graeme S. (editor). *Drug Treatment: Principles and Practice of Clinical Pharmacology and Therapeutics* (Second Edition). New York: ADIS Press, 1980.

Avido, Domingo M. *Krantz and Carr's Pharmacologic Principles of Medical Practice* (Eighth Edition). Baltimore: Williams & Wilkins Company, 1972.

Cluff, Leighton E.; Caranasos, G.J.; and Stewart, R.B. (editors). *Clinical Problems with Drugs.* Philadelphia: W.B. Saunders Company, 1975.

Creasey, William A. *Drug Disposition in Humans.* New York: Oxford University Press, 1979.

DiCyan, Erwin, and Hessman, Lawrence. *Without Prescription.* New York: Simon and Schuster, 1973.

Gibaldi, Milo. *Biopharmaceutics and Clinical Pharmacokinetics.* Philadelphia: Lea and Febiger, 1977.

Gilman, Alfred Goodman; Goodman, Louis S.; and Gilman, Alfred (editors). *Goodman and Gilman's The Pharmacological Basis of Therapeutics* (Sixth Edition). New York: Macmillan Publishing Company, 1980.

Handbook of Nonprescription Drugs (Sixth Edition). Washington, D.C.: American Pharmaceutical Association, 1980.

Hansten, Philip C. *Drug Interactions* (Third Edition). Philadelphia: Lea and Febiger, 1979.

La Du, Bert N.; Mandel, H. George; and Way, Leong E. (editors). *Fundamentals of Drug Metabolism and Disposition.* Baltimore: Williams & Wilkins Company, 1971.

Lasagna, Louis (editor). *Controversies in Therapeutics.* Philadelphia: W.B. Saunders Company, 1980.

Levine, R.R. *Drug Actions and Reactions* (Second Edition). Boston: Little, Brown and Company, 1978.

Melmon, Kenneth L., and Morrelli, Howard F. (editors). *Clinical Pharmacology: Basic Principles in Therapeutics.* New York: Macmillan Publishing Company, 1972.

Miller, Russell R., and Greenblatt, David J. (editors). *Handbook of Drug Therapy.* New York: Elsevier, 1971.

Modell, Walter (editor). *Drugs of Choice 1980-81.* St. Louis: C.V. Mosby Company, 1980.

Talalay, Peter (editor). *Drugs in Our Society.* Baltimore: The Johns Hopkins University Press, 1964.

Internal Medicine

Beeson, Paul B., and McDermott, Walsh (editors). *Textbook of Medicine* (Fourteenth Edition). Philadelphia: W.B. Saunders Company, 1975.

Hurst, J. Willis (editor). *Heart* (Fourth Edition). New York: McGraw-Hill, 1978.

Krupp, Marcus A., and Chatton, Milton J. (editors). *Current Medical Diagnosis and Treatment 1979.* Los Altos, Calif.: Lange Medical Publications, 1979.

Krupp, Marcus A.; Sweet, Norman J.; Jawetz, Ernst; Biglieri, Edward G.; and Roe, Robert. *Physician's Handbook* (Nineteenth Edition). Los Altos, Calif.: Lange Medical Publications, 1979.

Thorn, G.W.; Adams, R.D.; Braunwald, Eugene; Isselbacher, Kurt J.; and Petersdorf, Robert G. (editors). *Harrison's Principles of Internal Medicine* (Eighth Edition). New York: McGraw-Hill, 1977.

Widmann, Frances K. *Clinical Interpretation of Laboratory Tests* (Eighth Edition). Philadelphia: F.A. Davis Company, 1979.

Young, D.S.; Postaner, L.C.; and Gibberman, Val. "Effects of Drugs on Clinical Laboratory Tests," *Clinical Chemistry 21.* Washington, D.C.: American Association of Clinical Chemists, 1975.

Miscellaneous

Arndt, Kenneth A. *Manual of Dermatologic Therapeutics with Essentials of Diagnosis* (Second Edition). Boston: Little, Brown and Company, 1978.

Bressler, Rubin. *Use of Psychopharmacologic Drugs in the Elderly.* St. Louis: C.V. Mosby Company, 1980.

Durand, John L., and Bressler, Rubin. "Clinical Pharmacology of the Steroidal Oral Contraceptives," *Advances in Internal Medicine, Vol. 24.* Chicago: Yearbook Medical Publishers, 1979.

Hollister, Leo E. *Clinical Pharmacology of Psychotherapeutic Drugs.* New York: Churchill Livingstone, 1978.

Houston, Merritt, H. *Textbook of Neurology* (Fifth Edition). Philadelphia: Lea and Febiger, 1973.

Newell, Frank W. *Ophthalmology: Principles and Concepts* (Fourth Edition). St. Louis: C.V. Mosby Company, 1978.

Shirkey, Harry C. *Pediatric Dosage Handbook* (Second Edition). Washington, D.C.: American Pharmaceutical Association, 1979.

Pediatric Drug Handbook. Philadelphia: W.B. Saunders Company, 1977.

Strauss, Maurice B., and Welt, Louis G. *Diseases of the Kidney* (Second Edition). Boston: Little, Brown and Company, 1971.

Williams, Robert H. (editor). *Textbook of Endocrinology* (Fifth Edition). Philadelphia: W.B. Saunders Company, 1974.

Directory of Major Pharmaceutical Manufacturers

The following list includes the addresses and telephone numbers of the major pharmaceutical manufacturers in the United States. Although every effort has been made to include all of the manufacturers whose products appear in *The Physicians' Drug Manual*, a complete listing of the hundreds of different producers of prescription and nonprescription drugs in the U.S. is beyond the scope of this book.

Abbott Laboratories
Abbott Park
P.O. Box 68
North Chicago, Ill. 60064
(312) 937-3899

Adria Laboratories Inc.
P.O. Box 16529
Columbus, Ohio 43216
(614) 764-8100

Alcon/bp
6201 South Freeway
P.O. Box 1959
Fort Worth, Tex. 76101
(817) 293-0450

Alleghany Pharmacal Corporation
535 Fifth Avenue
New York, N.Y. 10017
(212) 661-3640

Allergan Pharmaceuticals, Inc.
2525 Dupont Drive
Irvine, Calif. 92713
(714) 752-4500 Ext. 4586

Almay Hypoallergenic
Cosmetics & Toiletries
850 Third Avenue
New York, N.Y. 10022
(212) 888-1990

American Critical Care
McGaw Park, Ill.
(312) 473-3000

Ames Division
Miles Laboratories, Inc.
1127 Myrtle Street
P.O. Box 70
Elkhart, Ind. 46515
(219) 264-8901

Anabolic Laboratories, Inc.
17802 Gillette Avenue
Irvine, Calif. 92714
(714) 546-8901

Arco Pharmaceutical
105 Orville Drive
Bohemia, N.Y. 11716
(516) 567-9500

Armour Pharmaceutical Company
P.O. Box 1849
Scottsdale, Ariz. 85252
(602) 941-2924

Astra Pharmaceutical Products, Inc.
7 Neponset Street
Worcester, Mass. 01606
(617) 620-0600

Ayerst Laboratories
685 Third Avenue
New York, N.Y. 10017
(212) 986-1000 Ext. 555

Barnes-Hind Pharmaceuticals, Inc.
895 Kifer Road
Sunnyvale, Calif. 94086
(408) 736-5462

Beach Pharmaceuticals
5220 S. Manhattan Avenue
Tampa, Fla. 33611
(813) 839-6565

Becton Dickinson Consumer Products
365 W. Passaic Street
Rochelle Park, N.J. 07662
(201) 368-7324

Beecham Laboratories
501 Fifth Street
Bristol, Tenn. 37620
(615) 764-5141 Ext. 363

Berlex Laboratories
101 East Hanover Avenue
Cedar Knolls, N.J. 07927
(201) 540-8700

Bio-Dynamics Home
Healthcare Company, Inc.
6405 Castleway Court
Indianapolis, Ind. 46250
(317) 849-4110

Blair Laboratories
50 Washington Street
Norwalk, Conn. 06856
(203) 853-0123

Boehringer Ingelheim Ltd.
90 East Ridge
P.O. Box 368
Ridgefield, Conn. 06877
(203) 438-0311

Boots Pharmaceuticals, Inc.
6540 Line Avenue
Shreveport, La. 71106
(318) 869-3551

Breon Laboratories Inc.
90 Park Avenue
New York, N.Y. 10016
(212) 972-2631

Bristol-Myers Products
345 Park Avenue
New York, N.Y. 10022
(212) 644-4287

Brown Pharmaceutical Company, Inc.,The
2500 West Sixth Street
Los Angeles, Calif. 90057
(213) 389-1394

Burroughs Wellcome Company
3030 Cornwallis Road
Research Triangle Park, N.C. 27709
(919) 541-9090

Burton, Parsons & Company, Inc.
120 Westhampton Avenue
Washington, D.C. 20027
(301) 336-5700

Carnation Company
5045 Wilshire Blvd.
Los Angeles, Calif. 90036
(213) 932-6000

Carnrick Laboratories, Inc.
Cedar Knolls, N.J. 07927
(201) 267-2675

Carter Products
767 Fifth Avenue
New York, N.Y. 10022
(212) 758-4500

Chesebrough-Pond's, Inc.
33 Benedict Place
Greenwich, Conn. 06830
(203) 661-2000

CIBA Pharmaceutical Company
556 Morris Avenue
Summit , N.J. 07901
(201) 277-5000

Colgate-Palmolive Company
300 Park Avenue
New York, N.Y. 10022
(212) 751-1200

Comatic Laboratories, Inc.
P.O. Box 42300
Houston, Tex. 77042
(713) 783-2032

Combe Inc.
1101 Westchester Avenue
White Plains, N.Y. 10604
(914) 694-5454

Cooper Dermatology Division
Division of Cooper Laboratories, Inc.
305 Fairfield Avenue
Fairfield, N.J. 07006
(201) 575-3363

Creighton Products Corp.
605 Third Avenue
New York, N.Y. 10016
(212) 687-7575

Cutter Medical
Fourth & Parker Streets
Berkeley, Calif. 94710
(415) 420-4000

Dalin Pharmaceuticals, Inc.
1750 New Highway
Farmingdale, N.Y. 11735
(516) 454-9282

Daywell Laboratories, Corp.
78 Unquowa Place
Fairfield, Conn. 06430
(203) 255-3154

Dermik Laboratories, Inc.
500 Virginia Drive
Fort Washington, Pa. 10934
(215) 628-6429

Dewitt International Corporation
5 North Watson Road
Taylors, S.C. 29687
(803) 244-8521

Diagnostic Testing, Inc.
767 Fifth Avenue
New York, N.Y. 10022
(212) 758-4500

Dista Products Company
Division of Eli Lilly and Company
307 East McCarty Street
P.O. Box 618
Indianapolis, Ind. 46206
(317) 261-3714

Dome Division
Miles Laboratories, Inc.
400 Morgan Lane
West Haven, Conn. 06516
(203) 934-9221

Dooner Laboratories, Inc.
500 Virginia Drive
Fort Washington, Pa. 19034
(215) 628-6296

Dorsey Laboratories
Division of Sandoz, Inc.
P.O. Box 83288
Lincoln, Neb. 68501
(402) 464-6311

Dow Pharmaceuticals
P.O. Box 68511
Indianapolis, Ind. 46268
(317) 873-7338

Elkins-Sinn, Inc.
Sub. of A.H. Robins Co.
2 Esterbrook Lane
P.O. Box 5483
N.J. 08034
(609) 424-3700 Ext. 21

Endo Laboratories, Inc.
Sub. of Dupont Co.
1000 Stewart Avenue
Garden City, N.Y. 11530
(516) 832-2123

Ex-Lax Pharmaceutical Company, Inc.
605 Third Avenue
New York, N.Y. 10016
(212) 687-7575

Fisions Corporation
Pharmaceutical Division
Two Preston Court
Bedford, Mass. 01730
(617) 275-1000 Ext. 246

Fleet Co., Inc., C.B.
4615 Murray Place
Lynchburg, Va. 24506
(800) 446-0991

Fleming & Company
1600 Fenpark Drive
Fenton, Mo. 63026
(314) 343-8200

Flint Laboratories
Division of Travenol Laboratories, Inc.
Deerfield, Ill. 60015
(312) 480-5220

Fox Pharmacal, Inc.
1750 West McNab Road
Fort Lauderdale, Fla. 33310
(305) 971-4100

G & W Laboratories, Inc.
111 Coolidge Street
South Plainfield, N.J. 07080
(201) 753-2000

Garden Pharmaceuticals, Inc.
Farmingdale, N.Y. 11735
(516) 454-9282

GEIGY Pharmaceuticals, Inc.
Division of CIBA-GEIGY Corp.
Ardsley, N.Y. 10502
(201) 277-5000

Gerber Products Company
Fremont, Mich. 49412
(616) 928-2000

Glaxo Inc.
1900 West Commercial Blvd.
Fort Lauderdale, Fla. 33309
(305) 776-5300 (8 AM-4:30 PM)

Glenbrook Laboratories
Division of Sterling Drug Inc.
90 Park Avenue
New York, N.Y. 10016
(212) 972-4141

Goody's Manufacturing Corporation
436 Salt Street
Winston-Salem, N.C. 27108
(919) 723-1831

Health Care Industries, Inc.
4295 South Ohio Street
Michigan City, Ind. 46360
(219) 879-8227

Herbert Laboratories
Dermatology Division of Allergan
Pharmaceuticals, Inc.
2525 DuPont Drive
Irvine, Calif. 92713
(714) 752-4500

Hickam, Inc., Dow B.
P.O. Box 35413
Houston, Tex. 77035
(713) 723-0690

Hoechst-Roussel Pharmaceuticals Inc.
Routes 202-206 North
Sommerville, N.J. 08876
(201) 685-2611

Holland-Rantos Company, Inc.
P.O. Box 385
865 Centennial Avenue
Piscataway, N.J. 08854
(201) 885-5777

Hynson, Westcott & Dunning
Division of Becton Dickinson and Co.
Charles & Chase Streets
Baltimore, Md. 21201
(301) 837-0890

Ives Laboratories Inc.
685 Third Avenue
New York, N.Y. 10017
(212) 986-1000

Jamol Laboratoires Inc.
13 Ackerman Avenue
Emerson, N.J. 07630
(201) 262-6363

Janssen Pharmaceutica Inc.
501 George Street
New Brunswick, N.J. 08903
(201) 594-9591

Jayco Pharmaceuticals
890 Poplar Church Drive
Suite 305
Camp Hill, Pa. 17011
(717) 763-7687

Johnson & Johnson
501 George Street
New Brunswick, N.J. 08903
(201) 524-0400

Key Pharmaceuticals, Inc.
50 N.W. 176th Street
Miami, Fla. 33169
(800) 327-9054 (8 AM-6 PM)

Knoll Pharmaceutical Company
30 North Jefferson Road
Whippany, N.J. 07981
(201) 887-8300 Ext. 177, 130

Kremers-Urban Company
P.O. Box 2038
Milwaukee, Wis. 53201
(800) 558-5114 (7:30 AM-4 PM)

Lannett Company, Inc., The
9000 State Road
Philadelphia, Pa 19136
(215) 333-9000

Lederle Laboratories Division of American Cyanamid Co.
Wayne, N.J. 07470
(914) 735-5000 Ext. 3642, 43, 44

Leeming Division
Pfizer Inc.
100 Jefferson Road
Parsippany, N.J. 07054
(201) 887-2100

Lehn & Fink Products Company
Division of Sterling Drug Inc.
225 Summit Avenue
Montvale, N.J. 07645
(201) 391-8500

Lemmon Company
P.O. Box 30
Sellersville, Pa. 18960
(215) 723-5544

Lilly and Company, Eli
307 E. McCarty Street
P.O. Box 618
Indianapolis, Ind. 46225
(317) 261-3714

Loma Linda Foods
Riverside, California 92515
(714) 785-2415

Macsil, Inc.
1326 Frankford Avenue
Philadelphia, Pa. 19125
(215) 423-5566

Marion Laboratories, Inc.
10236 Bunker Ridge Road
Kansas City, Mo. 64137
(800) 821-2130

McNeil Consumer Products Company
Fort Washington, Pa. 19034
(215) 836-4500

McNeil Pharmaceutical
Spring House, Pa.
(215) 628-5000

Mead Johnson Pharmaceutical
Division Mead Johnson & Company
2404 W. Pennsylvania Street
Evansville, Ind. 47721
(812) 426-6003 (7:30 AM-4 PM)

Medicone Company
225 Varick Street
New York, N.Y. 10014
(212) 924-5166

Menley & James Laboratories
Professional Products Division
a SmithKline Company
P.O. Box 8082
Philadelphia, Pa. 19101
(215) 854-4969

Merck Sharp & Dohme
West Point, Pa. 19486
(215) 699-5848

Mericon Industries
420 S.W. Washington Street
Peoria, Ill. 61602
(309) 676-0744

Merrell-National Laboratories
Division of Richardson-Merrell Inc.
Cincinnati, Ohio 45215
(513) 948-9111

Merrick Medicine Company
501-503 South Eighth
P.O. Box 1489
Waco, Tex. 76706
(817) 753-3461

Miles Laboratories, Inc.
1127 Myrtle Street
Elkhart, Ind. 46514
(219) 264-8111

Milles Marton Company
Richmond, Va. 23230
(804) 257-2727

Nature's Bounty, Inc.
105 Orville Drive
Bohemia, N.Y. 11716
(516) 567-9500

Naturslim Corporation
P.O. Box 3609
Santa Rosa, Calif. 95402
(707) 528-7311

Neutrogena Corporation
5755 West 96th Street
P.O. Box 45036
Los Angeles, Calif. 90045
(213) 776-5223

Nion Corporation
11581 Federal Drive
El Monte, Calif. 91731
(213) 443-0126

Norcliff Thayer Inc.
One Scarsdale Road
Tuckahoe, N.Y. 10707
(914) 969-8383

Norwich-Eaton Pharmaceuticals
17 Eaton Avenue
Norwich, N.Y. 13815
(607) 335-2565

Nutrition Control Products
Division of Pharmex, Inc.
2113 Lincoln Street
Hollywood, Fla. 33022
(305) 923-2821

O'Connor Products Company
24400 Capitol
Redford, Mich. 48239
(800) 521-9522

O'Neal, Jones & Feldman Pharmaceuticals
2510 Metro Blvd.
Maryland Heights, Mo. 63043
(314) 569-3610

Organon Pharmaceuticals
375 Mount Pleasant Avenue
West Orange, N.J. 07052
(201) 325-4500

Ortho Pharmaceutical Corporation
Raritan, N.J. 08869
(201) 254-0400

Parke-Davis
Division of Warner-Lambert Company
201 Tabor Road
Morris Plains, N.J. 07950
(201) 540-2000

Pennwalt Pharmaceutical Division
Pennwalt Corporation
755 Jefferson Road
Rochester, N.Y. 14623
(716) 475-9000 Ext. 375

Pfipharmecs Division
Pfizer Inc.
235 East 42nd Street
New York, N.Y. 10017
(212) 573-2323

Pfizer Laboratories Division
Pfizer Inc.
235 East 42nd Street
New York, N.Y. 10017
(212) 573-2422

Pharmacia Laboratories
Division of Pharmacia Inc.
800 Continental Avenue
Piscataway, N.J. 08854
(800) 526-3575

Pharmacraft Consumer Products
Pharmaceutical Division
Pennwalt Corp.
755 Jefferson Road
Rochester, N.Y. 14623
(716) 475-9000 Ext. 375

Phillips Roxane Laboratories, Inc.
333 Oak Street
Columbus, Ohio 43216
(614) 228-5403 Ext. 229

Plough, Inc.
3030 Jackson Avenue
Memphis, Tenn. 38151
(901) 320-2660

Polythress & Company, Inc., Wm. P.
16 North 22nd Street
P.O. Box 26946
Richmond, Va. 23261
(804) 644-8591

Proctor & Gamble
P.O. Box 171
Cincinnati, Ohio 45201
(513) 977-5547

Purdue Frederick Company, The
50 Washington Street
Norwalk, Conn. 06856
(800) 243-5666 Ext. 222 (8:30 AM-5 PM)

Reed & Carnick
30 Bright Avenue
Kenilworth, N.J. 07033
(201) 272-6600

Requa Manufacturing Company, Inc.
1 Seneca Place
Greenwich, Conn. 06830
(203) 869-2445

Revlon
Etherea Division
767 Fifth Avenue
New York, N.Y. 10022
(212) 572-5000

Riker Laboratories, Inc.
Sub. of 3M Company
19901 Nordhoff Street
Northridge, Calif. 91324
(213) 341-1300 Ext. 421

Robins Company, A.H.
1407 Cummings Drive
Richmond, Va. 23220
(804) 257-2000

Roche Laboratories
Division of Hoffman-LaRoche Inc.
Nutley, N.J. 07110
(201) 235-2355

Roerig
A Division of Pfizer Pharmaceuticals
235 East 42nd Street
New York, N.Y. 10017
(212) 573-2187

Rorer, Inc., William H.
500 Virginia Drive
Fort Washington, Pa. 19034
(215) 628-6296

Ross Laboratories
Division of Abbott Laboratories
Columbus, Ohio 43216
(614) 227-3333

Rowell Laboratories
210 Main Street, W.
Baudette, Minn. 55623
(800) 346-5040

Rystan Company, Inc.
470 Mamaroneck Avenue
White Plains, N.Y. 10605
(914) 761-0044

SDA Pharmaceuticals, Inc.
919 Third Avenue
New York, N.Y. 10022
(212) 688-4420

S.S.S. Company
71 University Avenue, SW
Atlanta, Ga. 30315
(404) 521-0857

Sandoz Pharmaceuticals
Division of Sandoz, Inc.
Route 10
East Hanover, N.J. 07936
(201) 386-7764

Schering Corporation
Galloping Hill Road
Kenilworth, N.J. 07033
(201) 931-2908

Schmid Products Company
Division of Schmid Laboratories, Inc.
Route 46 West
Little Falls, N.J. 07424
(201) 256-5500

Scott Tussin Pharmacal Company, Inc.
50 Clemence Street
P.O. Box 8217
Cranston, R.I. 02920
(401) 942-8555

Searle Laboratories
Division of Searle Pharmaceuticals Inc.
Box 5110
Chicago, Ill. 60680
(312) 982-7963

Smith Kline & French Laboratories
Division of SmithKline Corp.
1500 Spring Garden Street
Philadelphia, Pa 19101
(215) 854-5231,5232

Squibb & Sons, Inc., E.R.
P.O. Box 4000
Princeton, N.J. 08540
(609) 921-4006 Ext. 4162

Stanback Company LTD
1500 South Main Street
Salisbury, N.C. 28144
(704) 633-9231

Steifel Laboratories, Inc.
2801 Ponce de Leon Blvd.
Coral Gables, Fla. 33134
(305) 443-3807 (8:30 AM-5 PM)

Stuart Pharmaceuticals
Division of ICU Americas Inc.
Wilmington, Del. 19897
(800) 441-7758

Sugarlo Company
3540 Atlantic Avenue
P.O. Box 1017
Atlantic City, N.J. 08404
(609) 348-3148

Syntex Laboratories, Inc.
3401 Hillview Avenue
Palo Alto, Calif. 94304
(415) 855-5545

Thompson Medical Company, Inc.
919 Third Avenue
New York, N.Y. 10022
(212) 688-4420

Tutag Pharmaceuticals, Inc.
2599 W. Midway Blvd.
Broomfield, Colo. 80020
(303) 466-8841 Ext. 350,310,368

USV Laboratories
Division USV Pharmaceutical Corp.
1 Scarsdale Road
Tuckahoe, N.Y. 10707
(914) 779-6300

Upjohn Company, The
7000 Portage Road
Kalamazoo, Mich. 49001
(616) 323-6615

Vicks Toiletry Products Division
Richardson-Merrell Inc.
10 Westport Road
Wilton, Conn. 06897
(914) 664-5000

Wallace Laboratories
Half Acre Road
Cranbury, N.J. 08512
(609) 655-6000

Walker, Corporation & Company, Inc.
20 East Hampton Place
Syracuse, N.Y. 13206
(315) 463-4511

Warner-Lambert Company
201 Tabor Road
Morris Plains, N.J. 07950
(201) 540-3204

Warren-Teed Laboratories
Division of Adria Laboratories Inc.
582 West Goodale Street
Columbus, Ohio 43215
(614) 764-8100

Webcon Pharmaceuticals
Division of Alcon Laboratories
(Puerto Rico), Inc.
P.O. Box 1629
Fort Worth, Tex. 76101
(817) 293-0450

Westwood Pharmaceuticals Inc.
468 Dewitt Street
Buffalo, N.Y. 14213
(716) 887-3400

Whitehall Laboratories
Division of American Home
Products Corp.
685 Third Avenue
New York, N.Y. 10017
(212) 878-5508

Williams Company, Inc. The J.B.
767 Fifth Avenue
New York, N.Y. 10022
(212) 752-5700

Winthrop Laboratories
90 Park Place
New York, N.Y. 10016
(212) 972-4095

Wyeth Laboratories
Division of American Home
Products Corp.
P.O. Box 8299
Philadelphia, Pa. 19101
(215) 688-4400

Index

IN